Obstetrics and Gynaecology

LEAD EDITORS

David M. Luesley MA MD FRCOG
Lawson Tait Professor of Gynaecological Oncology, Department of Reproductive and Child Health
University of Birmingham, Birmingham; and
Honorary Consultant Gynaecological Oncologist
Birmingham Women's Healthcare NHS Trust, Birmingham

Philip N. Baker DM BMedSci BM BS FRCOG
Professor of Maternal and Fetal Health and Director of the Maternal and Fetal Health Research Centre
St Mary's Hospital, University of Manchester, Manchester

SECTION EDITORS

Linda Cardozo MD FRCOG
Professor of Urogynaecology
King's College Hospital, London

James Drife MD FRCOG FRCPEd FRCSEd
Professor, Department of Obstetrics and Gynaecology
Leeds General Infirmary, Leeds

Lucy Kean DM MA MRCOG
Consultant Obstetrician (Subspecialist in Maternal and Fetal Medicine)
City Hospital, Nottingham

Mark D. Kilby MD MRCOG
Professor in Maternal and Fetal Medicine, Division of Reproduction and Child Health
Birmingham Women's Hospital, University of Birmingham, Birmingham

Henry C. Kitchener MD FRCOG FRCS(Glasgow)
Professor of Gynaecological Oncology and Head, Academic Unit of Obstetrics and Gynaecology
University of Manchester, Manchester

William L. Ledger MA DPhil(Oxon) MB ChB FRCOG
Head of Section of Reproductive and Developmental Medicine; and Professor of Obstetrics and Gynaecology
Royal Hallamshire Hospital, Sheffield

ALSO AVAILABLE

MCQs and Short Answer Questions for the MRCOG: An aid to revision and self-assessment,
edited by David M. Luesley and Philip N. Baker with additional contributions from Jeremy C. Brockelsby (0 340 80874 8)

Obstetrics and Gynaecology

An evidence-based text for MRCOG

Lead Editors

DAVID M. LUESLEY
and
PHILIP N. BAKER

Section Editors

Linda Cardozo
James Drife
Lucy Kean
Mark D. Kilby
Henry C. Kitchener
and
William L. Ledger

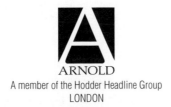

ARNOLD
A member of the Hodder Headline Group
LONDON

First published in Great Britain in 2004 by
Arnold, a member of the Hodder Headline Group,
338 Euston Road, London NW1 3BH

http://www.arnoldpublishers.com

Distributed in the United States of America by
Oxford University Press Inc.,
198 Madison Avenue, New York, NY10016
Oxford is a registered trademark of Oxford University Press

Whilst the advice and information in this book are believed to be true and
accurate at the date of going to press, neither the authors nor the publisher
can accept any legal responsibility or liability for any errors or omissions
that may be made. In particular (but without limiting the generality of the
preceding disclaimer) every effort has been made to check drug dosages;
however, it is still possible that errors have been missed. Furthermore,
dosage schedules are constantly being revised and new side-effects
recognized. For these reasons the reader is strongly urged to consult the
drug companies' printed instructions before administering any of the drugs
recommended in this book.

British Library Cataloguing-in-Publication Data
A catalogue record for this book is available from the British Library

Library of Congress Cataloging-in-Publication Data
A catalog record for this book is available from the Library of Congress

ISBN 0 340 80875 6
ISBN 0 340 80876 4 (International Students' Edition, restricted
                                territorial availability)

1 2 3 4 5 6 7 8 9 10

Commissioning Editor: Joanna Koster
Development Editor: Sarah Burrows
Project Editor: Wendy Rooke
Production Controller: Deborah Smith
Cover Design: Lee-May Lim

Typeset in 9.5/12 Rotis serif by Charon Tec Pvt. Ltd, Chennai, India
Printed and bound in India

What do you think about this book? Or any other Arnold title?
Please send your comments to feedback.arnold@hodder.co.uk

To my daughters, Alice and Megan (DL)
To my elder daughter, Charlotte (PB)

Contents

INTRAPARTUM

Section C   Late pregnancy/intrapartum events

POST-DELIVERY

PART THREE   GYNAECOLOGY   Senior section editor: David M. Luesley

Contributors

Philip N. Baker DM BMedSci BM BS FRCOG
Professor of Maternal and Fetal Health and Director of the
Maternal and Fetal Health Research Centre, St Mary's Hospital,
University of Manchester, Manchester

James Balmforth MB BS BSc MRCOG
Clinical Research Fellow, Department of Urogynaecology,
King's College Hospital, London

Sandie Bohin MB ChB DCH MRCP FRCPCH
Consultant Neonatal Paediatrician, Neonatal Unit, Royal
Infirmary, Leicester

Linda Cardozo MD FRCOG
Professor of Urogynaecology, King's College Hospital, London

Margaret E. Cruickshank MB ChB MD FRCOG
Senior Lecturer in Gynaecological Oncology, Department of
Obstetrics and Gynaecology, Aberdeen Maternity Hospital,
Aberdeen

Andrew Currie BM DCH FRCPCH FRCP(Ed)
Consultant Neonatologist, Leicester Royal Infirmary, University
Hospitals of Leicester NHS Trust, Leicester

James Drife MD FRCOG FRCPEd FRCSEd Hon FCOGSA
Professor, Department of Obstetrics and Gynaecology, General
Infirmary, Leeds

Ian J. Etherington MB ChB MD MRCOG
Consultant Obstetrician and Gynaecologist, City Hospital,
Birmingham

Diana Fothergill BSc (Med Sci) Hons MB ChB FRCOG
Consultant Obstetrician and Gynaecologist, The Jessop Wing,
Sheffield Teaching Hospitals NHS Trust, Sheffield

Harold Gee MD FRCOG
Consultant Obstetrician, Director of Postgraduate Education,
Medical Director, RCOG Examiner, Birmingham Women's
Hospital, Birmingham

Joanna C. Gillham BSc MB BS MRCOG
Clinical Research Fellow, Maternal and Fetal Health Research
Centre, Academic Unit of Obstetrics and Gynaecology and
Reproductive Health Care, St Mary's Hospital, Manchester

Barry W. Hancock MD FRCP FRCR
YCR Professor of Clinical Oncology and Director of Trophoblastic
Disease Centre, Weston Park Hospital, Sheffield

Richard Hayman BSc MB BS MRCOG DM
Consultant in Obstetrics and Gynaecology, Gloucester Royal
Hospital, Gloucester

Susan J. Houghton MB ChB MRCOG
Consultant Obstetrician and Gynaecologist, Good Hope Hospital,
Sutton Coldfield

Tracey A. Johnston MD MRCOG
Consultant in Fetal and Maternal Medicine, St. Mary's Hospital
for Women and Children, Manchester

Griff Jones BSc MB BS MRCOG FRCSC
Consultant Obstetrician and Gynaecologist, Winchester District
Memorial Hospital, Winchester, Ontario, Canada

Lucy Kean DM MA MRCOG
Consultant Obstetrician (Subspecialist in Maternal and Fetal
Medicine), City Hospital, Nottingham

Louise Kenny MB ChB DFFP MRCOG PhD
Clinical lecturer, Maternal and Fetal Health Research Centre,
St Mary's Hospital, Manchester

Mark D. Kilby MD MRCOG
Professor in Maternal and Fetal Medicine, Division of Reproduction
and Child Health, Birmingham Women's Hospital, Birmingham

Henry C. Kitchener MD FRCOG FRCS (Glasgow)
Professor of Gynaecological Oncology and Head, Academic Unit of
Obstetrics and Gynaecology, University of Manchester, Manchester

Justin C. Konje MD FWACS MRCOG
Senior Lecturer and Honorary Consultant Obstetrician and
Gynaecologist, University of Leicester and Leicester Royal
Infirmary, Leicester

Sailesh Kumar MB BS MMed(O&G) FRCS MRCOG FRANZCOG DPhil(Oxon)
Honorary Senior Lecturer and Consultant in Maternal and Fetal
Medicine, Centre for Fetal Care, Imperial College London, Queen
Charlotte's and Chelsea Hospital, London

Hany A.M.A. Lashen MD MRCOG MB BCh
Senior Lecturer and Honorary Consultant in Reproductive
Medicine, Sheffield Teaching Hospitals Trust, Sheffield

William L. Ledger MA DPhil(Oxon) MB ChB FRCOG
Head of Section of Reproductive and Developmental Medicine;
and Professor of Obstetrics and Gynaecology, Royal Hallamshire
Hospital, Sheffield

David M. Levy FRCA
Consultant Obstetric Anaesthetist, Anaesthetics Directorate,
Queen's Medical Centre, Nottingham

Murray Luckas BSc MD MRCOG
Consultant Obstetrician and Gynaecologist, Leighton Hospital,
Crewe

David M. Luesley MA MD FRCOG
Lawson Tait Professor of Gynaecological Oncology, Department
of Reproductive and Child Health, University of Birmingham; and
Honorary Consultant Gynaecological Oncologist, Birmingham
Women's Healthcare NHS Trust, Birmingham

Melanie C. Mann MB ChB MRCOG MFFP Dip GUM
Consultant in Contraception and Reproductive Health, South Worcestershire PCT, Arrowside Unit, Alexandra Hospital, Redditch

Pierre L. Martin-Hirsch MRCOG
Consultant Gynaecological Oncologist, Central Lancashire Teaching Hospitals, Preston

Lawrence J. Mascarenhas MD MD MRCOG MFFP MEd
Consultant Obstetrician and Gynaecologist, Emergency Gynaecology Unit, St Thomas' Hospital, London

Alec McEwan BA BM BCh MRCOG
Subspecialty Trainee in Fetomaternal Medicine, Queen's Medical Centre, Nottingham

Sheila McLean LLB MLitt PhD LLD(Abertay, Edin) FRSE FRCGP FRCP(Edin) FRSA
International Bar Association Professor of Law and Ethics in Medicine, University of Glasgow, Glasgow

Enda McVeigh MB BCh BAO MPhil MRCOG
Subspecialist in Reproductive Medicine and Surgery, University of Oxford, and Honorary Consultant Obstetrician and Gynaecologist, John Radcliffe Hospital, Oxford

Catherine Minto MB ChB
Gynaecology Research Fellow, Academic Department of Obstetrics and Gynaecology, University College London, London

Michele P. Mohajer BM BS FRCOG MD
Consultant in Feto-Maternal Medicine, Royal Shrewsbury Hospital NHS Trust, Shrewsbury

Catherine Nelson-Piercy MA FRCP
Consultant Obstetric Physician, Guy's and St Thomas' Hospitals, London

David Nunns MD MRCOG
Consultant Gynaecological Oncologist, Nottingham City Hospital, Nottingham

Michael E.L. Paterson MB ChB MD FRCOG FRCS(Ed)
Consultant Gynaecologist, Royal Hallamshire Hospital, Sheffield

Richard Porter MA MSc FRCOG
Consultant Obstetrician and Gynaecologist, Royal United Hospital, Bath

Charles Redman MB ChB FRCOG FRCS(Ed)
Consultant Gynaecologist, City General, North Staffordshire Hospital, Stoke-on-Trent

Fiona M. Reid MB ChB MRCOG
Clinical Research Fellow, The Warrell Unit, St Mary's Hospital, Manchester

Karina Reynolds MD FRCS MRCOG
Senior Lecturer in Gynaecological Oncology, Barts and The London, Queen Mary School of Medicine, London

Dudley Robinson MB BS MRCOG
Subspecialty Trainee in Urogynaecology, Department of Urogynaecology, King's College Hospital, London

Jane Rufford
Department of Urogynaecology, King's College Hospital, London

Andrew Shennan MB BS MD FRCOG
Professor of Obstetrics, Maternal and Fetal Research Unit, St Thomas' Hospital, London

Anthony R.B. Smith MD FRCOG
Consultant Gynaecologist, The Warrell Unit, St Mary's Hospital, Manchester

David Somerset BM DM MRCOG
Clinical Lecturer in Obstetrics and Gynaecology, Division of Reproductive Medicine and Child Health, Birmingham Women's Hospital, University of Birmingham, Birmingham

John A.D. Spencer MB BS BSc AKC FRCOG
Consultant Obstetrician and Gynaecologist, Northwick Park Hospital, Harrow, and Honorary Clinical Senior Lecturer, Imperial College Medical School, University of London

John Tidy MD FRCOG
Consultant Gynaecological Oncologist, The Jessop Wing, Sheffield

Jane Thomas MB ChB MSc and MRCOG
Director, National Collaborating Centre, Women's and Children's Health, and Honorary Consultant Obstetrician and Gynaecologist, Nuffield Department of Obstetrics and Gynaecology, Oxford

Peter J. Thompson MB BS MRCOG
Consultant Obstetrician, Birmingham Women's Hospital, Birmingham

Christine P. West MD FRCOG
Consultant Obstetrician and Gynaecologist, Simpson Centre for Reproductive Health, Royal Infirmary, Edinburgh

Preface

There are many demands made on modern medical practitioners. First, to provide high-quality patient-focused care that should be based upon the best evidence available. Next, to compare the care delivered with agreed standards with the objective of continuing to improve the process. There is also a duty to work towards filling the gaps in the evidence base through properly constructed and conducted research. Not least, there is a responsibility to disseminate new ideas and information through teaching and educational programmes.

This book recognizes the importance of a solid evidence-based foundation for obstetrical and gynaecological practice, and in certain instances moves away from traditional or 'enteric-based' practice. We have deviated somewhat from the established textbook model to accommodate the need to base each section, where applicable, on evidence and to include a critique of such evidence. To achieve this, we have developed a simple template to link MRCOG syllabus criteria with the evidence that underlies practice. It will be obvious to most readers that the strength of evidence varies widely and in some instances it can hardly be recognized at all. Our contributors have worked hard to provide both balance and breadth to the sections that they have addressed. Sections are broken down into separate chapters, but we feel that a sense of continuity has been imparted to a recognized area of obstetric or gynaecological care. Contributors were chosen because of their expertise, but also because they are currently involved in the shaping of care and therefore have a first-hand feel for the evidence. The members of the editorial team have worked closely with each other and the contributors to try to maintain the original template-format emphasis on evidence and its strength, with continued close reference to the MRCOG syllabus. We not only feel that the final product will help trainees come to appreciate and understand the core knowledge of their chosen discipline, but also hope it will fire their enthusiasm to seek more information and continue to strive for excellence in all aspects of their professional careers.

Textbooks do not make good doctors, but good doctors must practise from a sound basis of knowledge, and this text aims to provide in some measure the foundation of core knowledge required of a practising obstetrician and gynaecologist.

David M. Luesley and Philip N. Baker

Acknowledgements

We would like to acknowledge the help of Dr Jeremy Brockelsby in reviewing the manuscripts and assisting the editorial process.

Glossary

ABC	Airway, breathing and circulation
AC	Abdominal circumference
ACA	Anticardiolipin antibody
ACE	Angiotensin-converting enzyme
AChe	Acetylcholinesterase
ACTG	AIDS Clinical Trial Group
ACTH	Adrenocorticotrophic hormone
ACTION	Adjuvant Chemotherapy in Ovarian Neoplasm Trial
aCL	anticardiolipin
ACOG	American College of Obstetricians and Gynecologists
ACTH	Adrenocorticotrophic hormone
AED	Anti-epileptic drug
AEDF	Absent end-diastolic flow
AFE	Amniotic fluid embolism
AFI	Amniotic fluid index
AFLP	Acute fatty liver of pregnancy
aFP	Alpha-fetoprotein
AFS	American Fertility Society
AFV	Amniotic fluid volume
AGUM	Association for Genito Urinary Medicine
AIDS	Acquired immunodeficiency syndrome
AIS	Adenocarcinoma-in-situ
ALT	Alanine transaminase
AMH	Anti-Müllerian hormone
ANA	Antinuclear antibody
APA	Antiphospholipid antibody
APAS	Antiphospholipid antibody syndrome
APC	Activated protein C
APH	Antepartum haemorrhage
aPL	Antiphospholipid antibody
APS	Antiphospholipid syndrome
ARBD	Alcohol-related birth defect
ART	Antiretroviral therapy
ART	Assisted reproductive technology
ASA	American Society of Anesthesiologists
ASCUS	Atypical squamous cells of undetermined significance
ASD	Atrial septal defect
AST	Aspartamine transaminase
ASTEC	A Study in the Treatment of Endometrial Cancer
ATP	Adenosine triphosphate
AUM	Ambulatory urodynamic monitoring
AV	Atrioventricular
AVM	Arteriovenous malformation
AZT	Zidovudine
BCG	Bacille Calmette Guérin
BCPT	Breast Cancer Prevention Trial
BDA	British Diabetic Association
BD	Base deficit
BE	Base excess
BHIVA	British Human Immunodeficiency Virus Association
BMI	Body mass index
BP	Blood pressure
bpm	Beats per minute
BPP	Biophysical profile
BSID	Bayley Scales of Infant Development
BV	Bacterial vaginosis
bvm	Bag-valve-mask
CAH	Chronic active hepatitis
CAIS	Complete androgen insensitivity syndrome
CASA	Computer-assisted sperm analysis
CCAML	Congenital cystic malformation of the lung
CDC	Centers for Disease Control
CEA	Carcinoembryonic antigen
CEE	Conjugated equine (o)estrogens
CEMACH	Confidential Enquiries into Maternal and Child Health
CEMD	Confidential Enquiries into Maternal Deaths
CEPOD	Confidential Enquiries into Perioperative Deaths
CESDI	Confidential Enquiry into Stillbirths and Deaths in Infancy
cfu	Colony-forming units
CHD	Coronary heart disease
CHM	Complete hydatidiform mole
CI	Confidence interval
CIGN	Cervical intraepithelial glandular neoplasia
CIN	Cervical intraepithelial neoplasia
CIS	Carcinoma-in-situ
CISH	Confidential Inquiry into Suicides and Homicides [by People with Mental Illness]
CLASP	Collaborative Low-dose Aspirin Study in Pregnancy
ClaSS	Chlamydia Screening Study
CMV	Cytomegalovirus
CNS	Central nervous system
CNST	Clinical Negligence Scheme for Trusts
COC	Combined oral contraception
COCP	Combined oral contraceptive pill
COMET	Comparative Obstetric Mobile Epidural Trial
COS	Controlled ovarian stimulation
COX-2	Cyclooxygenase-2
CPAP	Continuous positive airway pressure
CPD	Cephalo-pelvic disproportion
CPR	Cardiopulmonary resuscitation
CPS	Crown Prosecution Service
CREST	Calcinosis, Raynaud's phenomenon, (o)esophageal involvement, sclerodactyly and telangiectasia [syndrome]
CRH	Corticotrophin-releasing hormone

CRL	Crown–rump length
CRP	C-reactive protein
CRS	Congenital rubella syndrome
CSE	Combined spinal–epidural
CSF	Cerebrospinal fluid
CT	Computerized tomography
CTG	Cardiotocography
CVA	Cerebrovascular accident
CVP	Central venous pressure
CVS	Chorionic villus sampling
CXR	Chest X-ray
D&C	Dilatation and curettage
DDAVP	Desmopressin acetate
DES	Diethylstilboestrol
DFA	Direct fluorescent antibody [test]
7-DHCO	7-Dehydrocholesterol
DHEA	Dehydroepiandrosterone
DHEAS	Dehydroepiandrosterone sulphate
DHT	Dihydrotestosterone
DI	Donor insemination
DIC	Disseminated intravascular coagulopathy
DO	Detrusor over-activity
DMPA	Depot medroxyprogesterone acetate
DMSO	Dimethyl sulphoxide
DSM-IV	*Diagnostic and Statistical Manual of Mental Disorders*, Fourth Edition
DSU	Day surgery unit
DUB	Dysfunctional uterine bleeding
DVP	Deepest vertical pool
DVT	Deep vein thrombosis
E3	(O)estriol
E3G	(O)estrone-3-glucuronide
EBV	Epstein–Barr virus
ECG	Electrocardiogram
ECMO	Extracorporeal membrane oxygenation
ECV	External cephalic version
EDD	Estimated date of delivery
EDF	End-diastolic flow
EE	Ethinyl(o)estradiol
EEG	Electroencephalogram
EFM	Electronic fetal monitoring
EIA	Enzyme immunoassay
ELISA	Enzyme-linked immunosorbant assay
EMG	Electromyography
ENA	Extractable nuclear antigen
EORTC	European Organisation for Research and Treatment of Cancer
ER	(O)estrogen receptor
ERCP	Evacuation of retained products of conception
ERT	(O)estrogen replacement therapy
ESR	Erythrocyte sedimentation rate
ET	Embryo transfer
FAS	Fetal alcohol syndrome
FBC	Full blood count
FBS	Fasting blood sugar
FDP	Fibrin degradation product

FDV	First desire to void
FEV_1	Forced expiratory volume in 1 second
fFN	Fetal fibronectin
FFP	Fresh frozen plasma
FGR	Fetal growth restriction
FH	Fetal heart
FHM	Fundal height measurement
FIGO	International Federation of Gynecology and Obstetrics
FISH	Fluorescence in-situ hybridization
FMC	Fetal movement counting
FME	Forensic medical examiner
FSE	Fetal scalp electrode
FSH	Follicle-stimulating hormone
FTA-ABS	Fluorescent-treponemal antibody–absorbed test
5FU	5-Fluorouracil
FVL	Factor V Leiden
GA	General anaesthesia
GABA	Gamma-aminobutyric acid
GABA-A	Gamma-aminobutyric acid type A receptor
GAG	Glycosaminoglycan
GAX	Gluteraldehyde cross-linked
GBS	Group B streptococcus
GDM	Gestational diabetes mellitus
GIFT	Gamete intrafallopian transfer
GIT	Gastrointestinal tract
GnRH	Gonadotrophin-releasing hormone
GP	General practitioner
G6PD	Glucose-6-phosphate dehydrogenase
GRIT	Growth Restriction Intervention Trial
GTD	Gestational trophoblastic disease
GTN	Glyceryl trinitrate
GUM	Genitourinary medicine
HAART	Highly active antiretroviral therapy
Hb	Haemoglobin
HbA1C	Glycosylated haemoglobin
HbcAg	Hepatitis A core antigen
HbeAg	Hepatitis A e antigen
HbsAg	Hepatitis A surface antigen
HBV	Hepatitis B virus
hCG	Human chorionic gonadotrophin
HCV	Hepatitis C virus
HDL	High-density lipoprotein
HDU	High dependency unit
HELLP	Haemolysis, increased liver enzymes and low platelets
HERS	Heart and Estrogen/Progestin Replacement Study
HFEA	Human Embryology and Fertilisation Authority
HHC	Hyperhomocysteinaemia
HIE	Hypoxaemic–ischaemic encephalopathy
HIT	Heparin-induced thrombocytopenia
HIV	Human immunodeficiency virus
HLA	Human leucocyte antigen

hMG	Human menopausal gonadotrophin	LMP	Last menstrual period
HNPCC	Hereditary non-polyposis colorectal cancer	LMWH	Low-molecular-weight heparin
HOCM	Hypertrophic obstructive cardiomyopathy	LNG-IUS	Levonorgestrel-releasing intrauterine system
hPL	Human placental lactogen	LSCS	Lower segment caesarean section
HPLC	High performance liquid chromatography	LSIL	Low-grade squamous intraepithelial lesion
HPV	Human papillomavirus	LUNA	Laparoscopic uterine nerve ablation
HRT	Hormone replacement therapy	MAP	Mean arterial pressure
HSIL	High-grade squamous intraepithelial lesion	MAR	Mixed antibody reaction [test]
HSV	Herpes simplex virus	MAS	Meconium aspiration syndrome
HUS	Haemolytic uraemic syndrome	MCA	Middle cerebral artery
HWY	Hundred woman-years	MCH	Mean corpuscular haemoglobin
HyCoSy	Hysterosalpingo contrast sonography	MCHC	Mean corpuscular haemoglobin concentration
IBD	Irritable bowel disease	MCV	Mean corpuscular volume
IBIS	International Breast Cancer Intervention Study	MDKD	Multicystic dysplastic kidney disease
ICP	Intracranial pressure	MDMA	3,4-Methylenedioxymethamphetamine
ICS	International Continence Society		('Ecstasy')
ICSI	Intracytoplasmic sperm injection	MFPR	Multi-fetal pregnancy reduction
ICU	Intensive care unit	MG	Myasthenia gravis
IDDM	Insulin-dependent diabetes mellitus	MHA-TP	Microhaemaglutination assay for *Treponema*
β-IFN	Beta-interferon		*pallidum*
IGF	Insulin-like growth factor	MI	Myocardial infarction
Ig	Immunoglobulin	MIN	Multicentric intraepithelial neoplasia
IH	Immune (fetal) hydrops	MIS	Müllerian inhibiting substance
ILCOR	International Liaison Committee on	MLS	Maternal Lifestyles Study
	Resuscitation	MMP	Matrix metalloproteinases
i.m.	Intramuscular	MMR	Maternal mortality rate
INR	International normalized ratio	MMR	Measles, mumps and rubella
IPPV	Intermittent positive pressure ventilation	MMT	Methadone maintenance treatment
IQ	Intelligence quotient	MOM	Multiple of the normal median
ISSHP	International Society for the Study of	MPA	Medroxyprogesterone acetate
	Hypertension in Pregnancy	MRC	Medical Research Council
ISSVD	International Society for the Study of Vulvar	MRI	Magnetic resonance imaging
	Diseases	MRKH	Mayer–Rokitansky–Kuster–Hauser [syndrome]
ITP	Idiopathic thrombocytopenic purpura	MS	Multiple sclerosis
IUCD	Intrauterine contraceptive device	MSAFP	Maternal serum alpha-fetoprotein
IUD	Intrauterine death	MSSVD	Medical Society for the Study of Venereal
IUFD	Intrauterine fetal death		Diseases
IUGR	Intrauterine growth restriction	MSU	Midstream urine
IUI	Intrauterine insemination	MTT	N-methylthiotetrazole
IUP	Intrauterine pregnancy	MUFR	Maximum urine flow rate
i.v.	Intravenous	MUP	Motor nerve unit potential
IVC	Inferior vena cava	NAAT	Nucleic acid amplification technique
IVF	In-vitro fertilization	NAS	Neonatal abstinence syndrome
IVF-ET	In-vitro fertilization and embryo transfer	NBAS	[Brazleton] Neonatal Behavioural Assessment
IVS	Intravaginal slingplasty		Scale
IVU	Intravenous urogram	NCRI	National Cancer Research Institute
JVP	Jugular venous pressure	NET	Norethisterone
KCl	Potassium chloride	NET-EN	Norethisterone (o)enanthate
KUB	Kidney, ureter, bladder	NHS	National Health Service
LA	Lupus anticoagulant	NICE	National Institute for Clinical Excellence
LAVH	Laparoscopically assisted vaginal hysterectomy	NIDDM	Non-insulin-dependent diabetes mellitus
LDH	Lactate dehydrogenase	NIH	Non-immune (fetal) hydrops
LDL	Low-density lipoprotein	NMG	Neonatal myasthenia gravis
LFT	Liver function test	NNH	Number needed to harm
LGA	Large for gestational age	NNT	Number needed to treat
LH	Luteinizing hormone	NSAID	Non-steroidal anti-inflammatory drug

NST	Non-stress test
NT	Nuchal translucency
NTD	Neural tube defect
OCP	Oral contraceptive pill
OGTT	Oral glucose tolerance test
OHSS	Ovarian hyperstimulation syndrome
OR	Odds ratio
PAIS	Partial androgen insensitivity syndrome
Pap	Papanicolaou [smear test]
PAPP-A	Pregnancy-associated plasma protein A
PAT	Pregnancy-associated thrombocytopenia
PBC	Primary biliary cirrhosis
PCA	Patient-controlled analgesia
PCO	Polycystic ovary
PCOS	Polycystic ovary syndrome
PCR	Polymerase chain reaction
PCRH	Placental corticotrophin-releasing hormone
PDL	Primary dysfunctional labour
PDS	Polydioxanone suture
PE	Pulmonary embolism
PEEP	Positive end-expiratory pressure
PEFR	Peak expiratory flow rate
PEP	Post-exposure prophylaxis
PET	Positron emission tomography
PGD	Pre-implantation genetic diagnosis
PGM	Prothrombin gene mutation
PID	Pelvic inflammatory disease
PIH	Pregnancy-induced hypertension
PIVKA	Prothrombin induced by vitamin K absence
PMB	Postmenopausal bleeding
PMDD	Premenstrual dysphoric disorder
PMR	Perinatal mortality rate
PMS	Premenstrual syndrome
PMSG	Pregnant mare serum gonadotrophin
PND	Postnatal depression
POD	Pouch of Douglas
POP	Progestogen-only pill
POP-Q	Pelvic Organ Prolapse Quantification
PPH	Postpartum haemorrhage
PPROM	Preterm premature rupture of membranes
PR	Progesterone receptor
PROM	Pre-labour rupture of membranes
PSN	Presacral neurectomy
PT	Prothrombin
PTSD	Post-traumatic stress disorder
PTU	Propylthiouracil
PUVA	Psoralen plus ultraviolet A
QoL	Quality of life
RA	Rheumatoid arthritis
RCOG	Royal College of Obstetricians and Gynaecologists
RCT	Randomized, controlled trial
RDS	Respiratory distress syndrome
rec. FSH	Recombinant follicle-stimulating hormone
REDF	Reversed end-diastolic flow
REM	Rapid eye movement
Rh	Rhesus
RMI	Risk of Malignancy Index
RPR	Rapid plasma regain [test]
RR	Relative risk
RTA	Road traffic accident
RT-PCR	Reverse transcriptase–polymerase chain reaction
SAFP	Serum alpha-fetoprotein
SANDS	Stillbirth and Neonatal Death Society
SCBU	Special care baby unit
SDV	Strong desire to void
sEMG	Surface electromyography
SERMS	Selective (o)estrogen receptor modulators
SGA	Small for gestational age
SGOT	Serum glutamic-oxaloacetic transaminase
SGPT	Serum glutamic pyruvic transaminase
SHBG	Sex hormone-binding globulin
SIDS	Sudden infant death syndrome
SLE	Systemic lupus erythematosus
SMR	Severe mental retardation
SOAP	Subjective, objective, assessment, plan [acronym for daily postoperative assessments]
SSRI	Selective serotonin reuptake inhibitor
STD	Sexually transmitted disease
STI	Sexually transmitted infection
STV	Short-term variability
SUZI	Subzonal sperm injection
SVT	Supraventricular tachycardia
T3	Triiodothyronine
T4	Thyroxine
TAH/BSO	Total abdominal hysterectomy and bilateral salpingo-oophorectomy
TB	Tuberculosis
TBG	Thyroid-binding globulin
TDF	Testes-determining factor
TED	Thromboembolic deterrent
TENS	Transcutaneous electrical nerve stimulation
THRIFT	Thromboembolic Risk Factors [Consensus Group]
TIBC	Total iron-binding capacity
TOMBOLA	Trial of the Management of Borderline and Low-grade Abnormalities
TOP	Termination of pregnancy
TORC	[infection] Toxoplasmosis, rubella and cytomegalovirus
TPHA	*Treponema pallidum* haemagglutination assay
TPI	*Treponema pallidum* immobilization [test]
TRAP	Twin reversed arterial perfusion
TRH	Thyrotropin-releasing hormone
TSH	Thyroid-stimulating hormone
TTN	Transient tachypnoea of the newborn
TTP	Thrombotic thrombocytopenic purpura
TTTS	Twin–twin transfusion syndrome
T_V	Tidal volume
TVS	Transvaginal ultrasound
TVT	Tension-free vaginal tape

UA	Umbilical artery	VCO_2	Carbon dioxide output
UADW	Umbilical artery Doppler waveform	VCU	Videocystourethrogram
UDCA	Ursodexycholic acid	VDRL	Venereal Disease Research Laboratory
U & E	Urea and electrolytes	V_E	Minute ventilation
uE3	Unconjugated (o)estriol	VF	Ventricular fibrillation
UK CTOCS	United Kingdom Collaborative Trial of Ovarian Cancer Screening	VIN	Vulval intraepithelial neoplasia
		VO_2	Oxygen uptake
UNFPA	United Nations Population Fund	VSD	Ventricular septal defect
UNICEF	United Nations Children's Fund	VT	Ventricular tachycardia
UPP	Urethral pressure profilometry	VTE	Venous thromboembolism
USI	Urodynamic stress incontinence	vWD	von Willebrand's disease
UTI	Urinary tract infection	vWF	von Willebrand factor
V_A	Alveolar ventilation	VZIG	Varicella zoster immunoglobulin
VACTERAL	Vertebral, anal, cardiovascular, tracheo-(o)esophageal, renal, radial and limb [malformations that can result from the prolonged use of steroids]	VZV	Varicella zoster virus
		WHI	Women's Health Initiative [Trial]
		WHO	World Health Organization
		ZD	Zona drilling
VaIN	Vaginal intraepithelial neoplasia	ZDV	Zidovudine
VBAC	Vaginal birth after caesarean section	ZIFT	Zygote intrafallopian transfer

Text Features

MRCOG standards

An MRCOG standards box appears at the start of every chapter listing the relevant standards and/or skills relating to the topic.

EVIDENCE-BASED MEDICINE

Red-outlined evidence-based medicine boxes are included to provide a rapid summary of the evidence relating to the interventions and treatments discussed in each chapter. Where evidence is limited, this is also stated.

KEY POINTS

Pink key points boxes are included where relevent in the chapters to summarize the main points in a section.

EVIDENCE SCORING

It is important to assess the quality and applicability of available evidence. The evidence considered in this book has been graded according to the structure below, in accord with the system used in the RCOG Green-top Guidelines. This represents a modification of standard evidence tables used by the Scottish Intercollegiate Guidelines Network (SIGN).

Classification of evidence levels

Ia   Evidence obtained from meta-analysis of randomized, controlled trials.

Ib   Evidence obtained from at least one randomized, controlled trial.

II   Evidence obtained from at least one well-designed controlled study without randomization, or from at least one other type of well-designed quasi-experimental study.

III   Evidence obtained from well-designed non-experimental descriptive studies, such as comparative studies, correlation studies and case studies.

IV   Evidence obtained from expert committee reports or opinions and/or clinical experience of respected authorities.

PART ONE

General

PART ONE

Evidence-based Medicine and Medical Informatics

Jane Thomas

INTRODUCTION

This chapter outlines what evidence-based medicine is and how to practise it and some key epidemiological and statistical concepts that will help you to understand the terms used within this book, in clinical research and in the MRCOG examination.

In order to keep up to date, doctors need to be able to evaluate research evidence critically and integrate it into their practice. Evidence-based medicine is the conscientious, explicit and judicious use of current best evidence in making decisions about health care. The 'best evidence' is patient-centred clinical research on the precision of diagnostic tests, the power of prognostic markers and the effectiveness and safety of therapeutic interventions. Individual clinical expertise is the proficiency and judgement that individual clinicians acquire through clinical experience and clinical practice. Evidence and expertise need to be incorporated into decision making whilst taking into account patient preferences, concerns and expectations.[1] The concept of evidence-based medicine fits into the model of lifelong learning and clinical accountability of clinical governance.

The volume of published medical research and the average time a doctor has available for reading mean that it is not possible for clinicians to read all the research literature published.[1] However, developments in information technology and the Internet have made practising evidence-based medicine technically feasible. The practice of evidence-based medicine comprises five steps:

1. defining a clinical question,
2. finding the best evidence,
3. appraising the evidence for its validity (closeness to the truth), impact (size of effect) and applicability (usefulness in clinical practice),
4. integrating the findings of the critical appraisal with clinical expertise and patient values,
5. reviewing (auditing) clinical practice and the efficiency of the above steps.

STEP 1. SETTING THE CLINICAL QUESTION

Generating an answerable clinical question that is precise and specific is the basis of evidence-based medicine. The development of a search strategy will flow from this. Focused clinical questions include four components – 'PICO':[1,2]

- P – the population: a description of the patients, such as their age, parity, clinical problem and the healthcare setting;
- I – the intervention(s) (or exposure): these are the main actions, such as treatment, diagnostic test or risk factor;
- C – the comparison group: for example placebo or alternative treatment;
- O – the outcome: for example the change in health expected as a result of the intervention.

The type of studies that will be sought is determined by the type of clinical question. For example, for a question about therapy, the highest level of evidence is based on randomized controlled trials (RCTs); for a question about aetiology, cohort or case control may be more appropriate. For observational studies, the intervention is often an exposure and additional factors (length of follow-up or time) may be included. This is sometimes a population, exposure, comparison, outcome and time (PECOT) question.[3]

An example of a vague clinical question is: 'Should we use antibiotic prophylaxis at caesarean section?'. This question could be focused in a number of ways.

- *Population.* Are you interested in all caesarean sections, or a specific subgroup such as emergency or repeat caesarean section?
- *Intervention*: antibiotic prophylaxis. Do you want to specify the antibiotic? Are you interested in the dose/duration of use?
- *Comparison.* Is this compared to no antibiotics or another intervention or another antibiotic – or a different dose or treatment schedule?
- *Outcomes.* What do you anticipate the antibiotics will do? Will they reduce postoperative wound infection, or other outcomes such as endometritis or urinary tract infection (UTI), or other measures of febrile or infective morbidity such as length of hospital stay? Are there adverse effects?

An example of a focused question is: 'For women having emergency caesarean section, does co-amoxiclav reduce the postoperative endometritis compared with amoxicillin?'. This is a question about treatment, so we would look for the following study designs:

- systematic reviews (with or without meta-analysis) of RCTs,
- RCTs,
- well-designed controlled studies without randomization.

STEP 2. FINDING THE BEST EVIDENCE

Research evidence is often categorized into either primary (RCT, cohort, case control, cross-sectional or case series) or secondary (systematic review with or without meta-analysis, guidelines). If you are attempting to find out what is the right thing to do, one option would be to conduct a systematic review and to identify all the relevant primary research, appraise the quality of the research and summarize the results.[4] However, this would not be a practical solution every time you had a clinical question, nor would it be a good use of resources to repeat a review that has already been done. It is therefore necessary to know where to find good-quality, synthesized information such as systematic reviews or clinical guidelines. Reviews and clinical guidelines are made up of primary research, so it is important that you are able to appraise both the review and the studies on which it is based, so that you can judge whether it is a valid review or guideline.

Clinical guidelines

Clinical guidelines are systematically produced statements to assist practitioners and patients in making decisions about specific clinical situations. Only guidelines that use well-recognized and accepted methodology should be considered. The key features of such guidelines are:

- a multidisciplinary working group,
- a well-described systematic review of the literature,
- graded recommendations with explicit links to the evidence,
- quality control, e.g. input by an independent advisory board or by independent peer review.

Often, guidelines are not published in peer-reviewed journals and therefore will not be indexed in either MEDLINE or EMBASE. Searching for guidelines on the following databases via the Internet will allow you to access those for which the methodological quality can be appraised.

- National Electronic Library for Health (NeLH):
- National Guidelines Clearinghouse: <www.guideline.gov/index.asp>
- OMNI: <www.omni.ac.uk> (click advanced search and specify Practice Guidelines in Resource Type)
- Canadian Medical Association (CMA) Infobase: <www.cma.ca/cpgs/>
- Guidelines and Guidelines in Practice: <www.eguidelines.co.uk>
- Turning Research Into Practice (TRIP):
- Royal College of Obstetricians and Gynaecologists (RCOG): <www.rcog.org.uk>

The RCOG website provides a guide to searching for evidence;[3] a number of National Institute for Clinical Excellence (NICE) evidence-based guidelines.[5-7] *Greentop Guidelines* can also be found on the site. Further information on appraising guidelines is available via the NeLH.[1,8]

Searching for systematic reviews

If no relevant guidelines can be found, the next stage is to search for other forms of pre-synthesized evidence, e.g. systematic reviews (of RCTs) with or without meta-analysis. A systematic review (as opposed to a traditional review) involves clearly defined questions, extensive search of the literature, appraising the quality of studies located by the search with explicit criteria, and analysing the research findings using appropriate methods. Data from each of the individual studies may be pooled and analysed using a technique known as meta-analysis. The best resource for systematic reviews (and RCTs) is the Cochrane Library, which contains the following components for searching for systematic reviews:

- Cochrane Database of Systematic Reviews (CDSR)
- Database of Reviews of Effectiveness (DARE)
- Health Technology Assessment Database (HTA) (this includes UK and international HTA assessments).

Clinical evidence is another source of systematic reviews: <www.nelh.nhs.uk/clinical_evidence.asp>. Fellows and Members can also access Evidence Based Medicine Reviews, the British Medical Journal (BMJ), MEDLINE from 1993, Best Evidence from 1991, and the Cochrane Library.

Searching for primary research evidence

There are numerous different library databases; different databases index different journals and may be general or topic specific. There is a variety of interfaces for the electronic databases, for example OVID, Silverplatter or Pubmed; most are available online. MEDLINE is produced by the US National Library of Medicine and is widely available free of charge. EMBASE has a greater European emphasis in terms of the journals it indexes and has a high level of pharmacologic content. Much of the nursing and midwifery research is not indexed by MEDLINE or EMBASE. To find such research, databases such as MIDIRS, BNI and CINAHL should be searched. Psychological literature is indexed on Psychinfo or Psychlit.

Citation searching ISI Web of Science will locate research papers that have referenced papers you intend to include in your research.

There are methodological filters that identify study designs, for example RCTs; these are designed to make your search more precise, though this may be at the expense of sensitivity, i.e. a high proportion of citations retrieved by your search may be relevant, but it might not include all relevant citations on the topic if these have not been indexed in a way that the filters would pick up. For further information about and examples of filters, visit CASPfew Filters at <wwwlib.jr2.ox.ac.uk/caspfew/filters/>.

Developing a search strategy

Developing a search strategy usually involves combining free text and controlled text terms. Using the components of your clinical question (population, intervention, comparison, outcomes and study design), make a list of the synonyms, abbreviations and spelling variations (e.g. labor or labour) that might have been used by the authors to describe the concept. If you already know of relevant papers, scan them for more possible search terms. This list can be your free text terms.

The next stage is to list useful controlled text terms or subject headings. In MEDLINE, these are known as MeSH (Medical Subject Headings). In most databases they will be found in the thesaurus or index. If you know of a relevant paper, check the subject headings under which it is indexed.

Having developed a focused four-part question (population, intervention, comparison, outcome – PICO), create a separate search strategy for each component. The next stage is to combine these searches. Combination is achieved by 'Boolean Logic' and works in a manner similar to combining numbers in algebra. Boolean Logic uses the terms 'and', 'or' and 'not' to create a set of results that should contain papers relevant to the clinical question.

For example, combining cervical *and* cancer will retrieve all the papers that contain both terms. Combining cervical *or* cancer will retrieve all papers in which either one or both terms are found. To find papers relating to postoperative infection, it would be necessary to combine both the lists of controlled and free text terms above with *or*. Combining induction *not* labour will retrieve all papers that contain the word induction but do not also include the term labour. Care should be used when combining terms with *not*, as it will exclude any papers that discuss both the term of interest and the one to be excluded.

All databases also have useful search commands and symbols, however, these vary amongst databases. If you are conducting a systematic review or hope to publish the findings of your review, you need to keep your search strategies and record how many articles were found and which were included or excluded.

STEP 3. APPRAISING THE EVIDENCE

Critical appraisal is the process of deciding if the research you have found can help you in answering your clinical question. The first filter is: 'Does this paper address my clinical question?' (i.e. are the population, intervention, comparisons and outcomes the same or similar to those in your question?).[1]

The second stage is to look at the study design (the methods section of a paper). The acceptable study design is determined by your clinical question. For questions about therapy, RCTs or systematic reviews of RCTs provide the least biased estimate of effectiveness; for diagnostic test accuracy, studies that compare the 'new' test to a 'gold standard' test are needed; for questions about prognosis, studies that follow up groups of patients for a specified period of time (cohort studies) are needed. A systematic review summarizes the results from a body of research, usually RCTs. Quality assessment is an essential part of the process of systematic review. If the 'constituent studies' are flawed, the conclusions of systematic reviews may also not be valid.[1,4]

Bias

Bias is a systematic difference between groups that distorts the comparison between groups so that the 'true' effect is either exaggerated or reduced. The quality of a study is the degree to which the study design, conduct and analysis have minimized bias. External validity examines the extent to which the results of a study are applicable to other clinical circumstances, i.e. its generalizability. Internal validity examines the extent to which systematic error (or bias) is minimized within the study. The biases include:

- selection bias – the difference in the patient characteristics (such as prognosis) between comparison groups,
- performance bias – differences in the provision of care apart from the treatment under evaluation,
- detection bias – differences in the measurement or assessment of outcomes,
- attrition bias – the occurrence and handling of patient withdrawals or attrition.

Different study types are prone to different biases; therefore, there are different validity checklists for different studies based on the conduct, design and analysis.[1] Appraising the quality of a study is dependent on how the study is reported. To ensure more consistency of study reporting in journals, a number of reporting standards have been introduced in the last decade, for example the CONSORT statement for reporting RCTs,[9] QUOROM for systematic reviews of RCTs,[10] and STARD for diagnostic tests.[11]

Understanding RCTs

For the MRCOG, you need to understand the design of an RCT; therefore, the rest of this section deals only with appraising RCTs. The RCT is the 'gold standard' method for evaluating the effectiveness of therapeutic interventions as it gives the least biased estimate of effect of treatment interventions. A confounder is a factor (such as disease severity) that may influence the choice of treatment and the outcome of care.

Confounding is one reason for the tendency of non-randomized trials to overestimate treatment effects when compared with RCTs. With a well-conducted RCT, randomization will create groups that are comparable with respect to any known or unknown potential confounding factors (providing the sample size is sufficiently large).

There are two common methods used to assess the quality of RCTs: a component approach (assess answers to each question – or quality domain) or assigning a 'score' to answers to each question and creating a composite quality score. Using different quality scores can impact on the conclusions of a review and introduce a 'quality score bias'. There are more than 39 different quality scores for RCTs alone. Many of the items assessed within individual composite scores examine features of trials not known to be associated with bias. The key questions to ask when appraising an RCT are outlined below, with an explanation of why these are important.[1] The first four questions relate to study validity, the fifth to interpreting the results.

1. Was the assignment of treatment randomized?

The process of randomization requires that those recruiting to a trial or participating in the trial cannot predict which group they will be allocated to. The process of randomization involves two stages:

(i) generation of an unpredictable allocation sequence (random number),
(ii) concealment of this sequence from those enrolling participants in the trials.

Failure to secure the concealment of the sequence may allow selective enrolment depending on prognostic factors. A trial in which it is possible to predict the treatment allocation is more likely to be biased. The 'gold standard' for randomization used in large multi-centre trials is 'central computer' randomization. The use of sealed envelopes may be subverted (for example by holding the envelope up to the light); methods that could be predictable are date of birth, alternate days and hospital number.

2. Were the groups similar at the start of the trial?

The aim of randomization is the creation of groups that are comparable with respect to any known or unknown potential confounding factors (providing the sample size is sufficiently large). Randomization reduces bias in those selected for treatment and guarantees treatment assignment is not based on patients' prognosis. RCTs will have eligibility criteria, but within this trials report the characteristics of the patients according to the treatment received in Table 1 of the results section. The characteristics (such as age, parity) of the two groups should not be different.

3. Were the groups treated equally?

Apart from the intervention being studied, the groups should be treated identically – differences in treatment between groups may occur if treatment allocation is known. This is called performance bias and can be minimized by standardization of care protocol and by 'blinding'. RCTs may blind patients and therapists. Therapists may not treat both patient groups in a similar manner or patients may deviate from protocols because of awareness of allocation.

Detection (or measurement) bias applies to the measurement or assessment of the outcome. This should be standardized across all patients. Again, knowledge of treatment allocation may influence assessors. For an objective outcome (such as death), this may be less important, but for outcomes that are subjective, interpretation may differ if the assessor has prior knowledge of allocation. This bias can be minimized by using objective outcomes and by ensuring those assessing outcomes are not aware of treatment allocation. This approach is used in surgical RCTs: the surgeon undertaking the treatment has to be aware of the treatment allocation, identical surgical dressings are used for all patients, and the assessment of recovery is done by another person who is not aware of treatment allocation.

4. Are all the patients accounted for at the conclusion?

The process of randomization gives us comparable groups at the start of a trial, but results are only valid if we can account for all these patients at the end of the trial. Therefore, once randomized, a patient should be included in the analysis of that group even if he or she discontinues therapy, crosses over or never receives treatment. Loss of patients to follow-up or exclusion of patients from the analysis can lead to bias. Some losses may occur even in the best quality studies, but this should not differ between groups, should be of similar types of patients and should not exceed the outcome event rate. Loss to follow-up of more that 20 per cent of recruits poses a serious threat to the validity of a study.

Intention to treat (ITT analysis) of RCTs ensures that comparisons of effects of care are made only between patients in the groups to which they were originally randomly allocated. ITT analysis includes all patients regardless of the treatment actually received or subsequent withdrawal or deviation from the protocol. Some treatments may result in large numbers of drop-outs, for example if side effects are unpleasant. Failure to account for these when examining interventions may cause false conclusions to be reached. These attritional issues are central to the generalizability of a treatment's final effect in clinical practice.

5. Are these findings important?

The analysis of RCTs is often a simple comparison of percentages. The difference in the event rate (outcome of interest) in the treatment group compared to that in the comparison group is:

Control event rate (%) − experimental event rate (%)
= absolute risk reduction or risk difference (%)

If an effect is seen in a trial, the final question is: 'Could this difference have arisen by chance?'. In general, it is accepted that there is a 5 per cent chance of our concluding that there is a difference when in fact there is not – a 5 per cent chance of making a type 1 error, and hence we use a 95 per cent confidence interval (95% CI). Also by convention we accept an 80 per cent chance that we will detect a difference if one exists (this is the 'power' of a study). Increasing the number of patients in a study will reduce the chance of either error or increase the certainty of our estimates. The chance of these errors is also related to the size of difference we want to detect (we will need a larger study to detect a small difference between the two groups) and the frequency of the event (evaluating a very rare outcome such as occurs in 1:1000 people will need more people than an outcome that occurs in 1:100 or 1:10 people).

Confidence intervals can be calculated for this risk difference. The CI estimates the range of values likely to include the 'true' value. Usually, we use 95% CIs.

Finally, if you have a result that suggests a significant difference in outcome between two groups, you may want to consider what this means in practice. An alternative way of expressing this difference is the 'number needed to treat' (NNT). The NNT is simply 1 divided by the absolute risk reduction.

STEP 4. INTEGRATING THE EVIDENCE

If you have found valid research with important findings that address your clinical question, the next step is to consider if these results apply to your individual patient.[1] Two questions to consider are:

- is your patient so different from those in the trial that the results cannot help you?
- do the findings fit with your patient's preferences and values?

One of the consistent findings of health services research is the gap between research evidence and practice.[12] It is a challenge for clinicians to keep up to date, but perhaps even harder is the challenge to alter established patterns of care. This can be a challenge for individuals, but also for the organizations they work in. If the change required is complex or involves change in the organization and/or patients' attitudes, it is harder to achieve. There is no single strategy for getting research into practice that is sufficient on its own or significantly better than alternative strategies. Therefore a number of approaches are needed.

Research evidence is more likely to influence practice if it confirms our preconceptions.[13] In interpreting research evidence, we also need to be aware of our own biases; we may be less questioning of research evidence that affirms our own beliefs or practice, while scrutinizing more closely the evidence that challenges them.[12]

STEP 5. AUDIT

This includes two concepts of audit.

(i) Audit of your practice of evidence-based medicine – keeping a record of your clinical questions and findings and evaluating how you could do this more efficiently.
(ii) Clinical audit – measuring whether you are putting the research evidence into practice.

Clinical audit is a process that seeks to improve patient care and outcomes through systematic review of care against explicit criteria and the implementation of change.[14] Whereas research is concerned with discovering the right thing to do, audit is concerned with ensuring that the right thing is done. A recent review of the evidence has concluded that audit is an effective method of improving the quality of care.[15] The same review also describes the audit methods associated with successful audit projects.

Audit may evaluate the structure (organization or provision) of services, the process of care or the outcome of care against an agreed standard. For example, research evidence suggests that the outcome for patients with ovarian cancer is better if they are operated on by an appropriately trained gynaecologist and managed within the framework of a multidisciplinary team. An audit of the referral and management of patients with ovarian cancer can provide an overview of service provision in this area.

Process measures are clinical practices that have been evaluated in research and been shown to have an influence on outcome. For example, the use of antenatal steroids has improved perinatal outcome; evaluation of this process of care would entail measuring the proportion of appropriate cases that received antenatal steroids.

An *outcome measure* is the physical or behavioural response to an intervention, for example the health status (dead or alive), cure following surgery for stress incontinence, level of knowledge or satisfaction (e.g. users' views on the care they have received). Outcomes can be desirable, for example improvement in the patient's condition or quality of life, or undesirable, e.g. side effects of a treatment. The assessment of outcomes such as cancer survival rates is fundamental to measuring quality of care. Outcomes are not a direct measure of the care provided (e.g. social and health inequalities may contribute to variation in mortality rates); therefore, mechanisms to account for these differences are required (e.g. case-mix adjustment for co-morbidity). Outcomes may be delayed, and not all patients who experience substandard care will have a poor outcome. Outcome measures such as mortality and morbidity are nevertheless important, and this is a major justification for regular monitoring. 'Critical incident' or 'adverse event' reporting involves the identification of patients who have experienced an adverse event (e.g. Confidential Enquiries into Maternal Deaths [CEMD], Confidential Enquiry into Stillbirths and Deaths in Infancy [CESDI] and National Confidential Enquiry into Peri-operative Deaths [NCEPOD]).

Undertaking audit

Audit can be considered to have five principal steps (commonly referred to as the audit cycle):

(i)   selection of a topic,
(ii) identification of an appropriate standard,
(iii) data collection to assess performance against the pre-specified standard,
(iv) implementation of changes to improve care, if necessary,
(v)   data collection for a second, or subsequent, time to determine whether care has improved.

Audit projects require a multidisciplinary approach, with involvement of stakeholders (including consumers or users of the service provided) and the local audit department at the planning stage. Good planning and resources are also necessary to ensure their success.

It is essential to establish clear aims and objectives when choosing what to audit, so that the audit is focused towards addressing specific issues within the selected topic. A key consideration is: 'How will we use the results of this audit to change or improve practice?'. Priority should be given to common health problems, areas associated with high rates of mortality, morbidity or disability, and those for which good research evidence is available to inform practice or aspects of care that use considerable resources. It is important to involve those who will be implementing change at this stage of the audit process.

In audit, review criteria are generally used for assessing care. The criterion is the reference point against which current practice is measured. The first four steps above should be the starting point for developing criteria. Review criteria should be explicit rather than implicit and need to lead to valid judgements about the quality of care, and relate to aspects of care that are important to patients or impact on clinical outcomes.

The standard/target level of performance is defined as 'the percentage of events that should comply with the criterion' (e.g. the proportion of women delivered by caesarean section who received thromboprophylaxis, or the proportion of women with dysfunctional uterine bleeding who were offered TCRE or endometrial ablation). 'Benchmarking' is defined as the 'process of defining a level of care set as a goal to be attained'. There is insufficient evidence to determine whether it is necessary to set target levels of performance in audit.

Data collection

Data collection in criterion-based audit is generally undertaken to determine the proportion of cases in which care is in accordance with the criteria. In practice, the following points need to be considered.

Consideration needs to be given to which data items are needed in order to answer the audit question. For example, if undertaking an audit on caesarean section rates, collecting information on the number of caesarean sections alone will not give sufficient information to measure the caesarean section rate. Data on the number of other births that took place are also required. Definitions need to be clear so that there is no confusion about what is being collected. For example, if collecting data on rupture of membranes, it may need to be specified whether this is spontaneous or artificial.

Data collectors should always be aware of their responsibilities to the Data Protection Act and any locally agreed guidelines. Under the current Data Protection Act, it is an offence to collect personal details of patients such as names, addresses or other items that are potentially identifiable for the individual without consent. There seems to be consensus that clinical audit is part of direct patient care and therefore consent to the use of data for audit can be implied through consent to treatment provided patients are informed that their data may be used in this way. It is rarely acceptable to use patient identifiers such as names and addresses; however, some form of pseudoanonymized identifiers should be used. Audit project protocols should be submitted to the local Research and Development Committee and Ethics Committees to seek approval, if necessary. Guidance on how to do this can be obtained from the respective bodies.

Routinely collected data can be used if all the data items required are available. It will be necessary to check the definitions for data items that are used within the routine database to ensure its usefulness for the aims of the audit. Also, the completeness and coverage of the routine source need to be known. Where the data source is clinical records, the training of data abstractors and the use of a standard proforma can improve the accuracy and reliability of data collection. The use of multiple sources of data may also be helpful; however, this can also be problematic, as it will require linking of data from different sources with common unique identifiers.

Questionnaires

Questionnaires are often used as a tool for data collection. Questions may be open or closed. Generally, questionnaire design using open questions (e.g. 'What was the indication for caesarean section?', followed by space for free text response) is easier, but analysis of these data is difficult, as there will be a range of responses and interpretation can be problematic. Open questions may be more difficult and time consuming to answer and can lead to non-response resulting in loss of data.

Questionnaires can be composed entirely of closed questions (i.e. with all possible answers predetermined). More time needs to be spent in developing this type of questionnaire, but the analysis is generally easier. The following is an example of this.[16]

Which of the following statements most accurately describes the urgency of this caesarean section?

A Immediate threat to the life of the fetus and the mother.
B Maternal or fetal compromise that is not immediately life threatening.
C No maternal or fetal compromise but needs early delivery.
D Delivery timed to suit the woman and staff.

Closed questions assume that all possible answers to the question are known but not the distribution of responses. Time and consideration need to be given to the options available for response, because, if a desired response is not available, the question may just be missed out and it may put people off completing the rest of the questionnaire. The 'other' category can be used with the option 'please specify', which gives an opportunity for the respondent to write in a response. However, if this is used, thought must be given a priori as to how these free text responses will be coded and analysed. In some situations, not having an 'other' category may lead to the question not being answered at all, which means data will be lost.

If questionnaires are developed for a specific project, they need to be piloted and refined to ensure their validity and reliability before use as a tool for data collection. While those who developed the questionnaire understand the questions being asked, the aim of piloting is to check that those who have to fill in the questionnaire are able to understand and respond with ease. Questionnaires that are not user friendly are associated with lower response rates, the quality of data collected will be poor, and hence the results will be of little value.

Who collects the data?

Thought also needs to be given to who is going to collect the data, as well as to the time and resources that will be involved. In small audit projects, it may be feasible for the principal investigators to go through clinical notes for data abstraction. However, for larger projects, e.g. a prospective audit on induction of labour practices within a maternity unit, it may be more appropriate for those involved in the care of the women giving birth (e.g. midwives or obstetricians) to fill in standard data collection sheets. Where available, audit support staff should be involved.

Analysing the data

Data that are collected on paper forms are usually entered onto electronic databases or spreadsheets such as Microsoft Access, Epi Info or Excel for cleaning and analysis. Data entry may be done by Optical Character Recognition (OCR) software, Optical Mark Readers (OMR) or manually. OCR is most accurate for questionnaire data using tick boxes but less accurate for free text responses. The method of data entry needs to be taken into account when designing the questionnaire or data collection sheet. For manual data entry, accuracy is improved if double data entry is used. However, this can be a time-consuming exercise. If the facilities and resources are available, electronic collection of data can be considered. In this case, data are entered immediately at source into a computer and saved onto disks. While this is quick and requires minimal storage space, it can be difficult to handle unexpected responses. As information is entered directly into a computer, it cannot be verified or double-entered.

Consideration also needs to be given to the coding of responses on the database. For ease of analysis of closed questions, it is generally better to have numeric codes for responses. For example, yes/no responses can be coded to take the value 0 for no and 1 for yes. Missing data will also need to be coded, for example with the number 9. The code assigned for missing data should be distinguished from the code used when the response is 'not known' (if this was an option on the questionnaire). It is advisable to incorporate consistency checks as data are being entered to minimize errors.

Simple statistics are often all that is required. Statistical methods are used to summarize data for presentation in the form of summary statistics (means, medians or percentages) and graphs. Statistical tests are used to find out the likelihood that the data obtained have arisen by chance, and how likely it is that a real difference exists between two groups. Before data collection has started, it is essential to know what data items will be collected, whether comparisons will be made, and the statistical methods that will be used to make these comparisons.[17]

Data items that have categorical responses (e.g. yes/no or A/B/C/D) can be expressed as percentages. Some data items are collected as continuous variables, for example mother's age, height and weight. These can either be categorized into relevant categories and then expressed as percentages or, if they are normally distributed (bell-shaped curve), the mean and standard deviations may be reported. If they are not normally distributed, a median and range can be used. These summary statistics (percentages and means) are useful for describing the process, outcome or service provision that was measured.

Comparisons of percentages between different groups can be made using a χ^2 test. T tests can be used to compare means between two groups, assuming these are normally distributed. Non-parametric statistical methods can be used for data that are non-normally distributed. These comparisons are useful in order to determine if there are any real differences in the observed findings, for example when comparing audit results obtained at different time points or in different settings. In some situations, a sample size calculation may be necessary to ensure that the audit is large enough to detect a clinically significant difference between groups if one exists. In this situation, it is important to consult a statistician during the planning stages of the audit project. These simple statistics can be easily done on Microsoft Excel spreadsheets and Access databases. Other useful statistical software packages include Epi Info, SAS, SPSS, STATA and Minitab.

Implementation of findings

Data analysis and interpretation will lead to the identification of areas of clinical practice that need to change. Several methods may be needed to ensure this change takes place, but simple strategies such as feeding back findings are sometimes effective. Change does not always occur in audit, and consideration of the reasons for failure may take place after the second data collection. Resistance to change among local professionals or in the organizational environment or team should be considered. Patients themselves may have preferences for care that make change difficult.

GLOSSARY OF TERMS

Auditable standard An agreed standard against which practice can be assessed.

Case-control study The study reviews exposures or risk factors, comparing the exposure in people who have the outcome of interest, for example the disease or condition (i.e. the cases), with patients from the same population who do not have the outcome (i.e. controls).

Cohort study The study involves the identification of two groups (cohorts) of patients, one of which has received the exposure of interest and one of which has not. These groups are followed forward to see if they develop the outcome (i.e. the disease or condition) of interest.

Confounder A factor that may offer an alternative explanation for the observed association between an exposure and the outcome of interest.

Cross-sectional study The observation of a defined population at a single point in time or time interval. Exposure and outcome are determined simultaneously.

Denominator data Data describing the population within which a study group has been identified (e.g. in a hospital study of caesarean section the denominator data refer to every birth that occurred within the unit during the audited period, irrespective of the type of delivery that was undertaken).

Mean This is the summary statistic used when the data follow a normal distribution. It is the sum of all the values divided by the number of values. The standard deviation gives a measure of the spread of individual values about the mean.

Median If the data are arranged in an increasing order, the middle value is the median. The range is the difference between the largest and smallest values. The interquartile range (IQR) is the difference between the bottom quarter and top quarter of the data. This is the summary statistic used when the data are not normally distributed.

Meta-analysis An overview of a group of studies that uses quantitative methods to produce a summary of the results.

Number needed to treat This is the number of patients who need to be treated to prevent one outcome.

Odds ratio This describes the odds that a case (a person with the condition) has been exposed to a risk factor relative to the odds that a control (a person without the condition) has been exposed to the risk. The crude odds ratio describes the association without taking into consideration the possible effect of any confounders. Adjusted odds ratios describe the association having been adjusted for the effect of confounders.

Positive predictive value This describes the percentage of people who have a positive test who really have the condition. The predictive value is dependent upon the prevalence of the disease in the population being tested, i.e. if the disease is rare, the predictive value is low, due to the greater influence of false-positive tests.

Randomized, controlled trial A group of patients is randomized into an experimental group and a control group. These groups are followed up for the variables and outcomes of interest. This study is similar to a cohort study, but the exposure is randomly assigned. Randomization should ensure that both groups are equivalent in all aspects except for the exposure of interest.

Risk difference The difference in risk of developing the outcome of interest between the exposed and control groups.

Risk ratio Risk is a proportion or percentage. The risk ratio is the ratio of risk of developing the outcome of interest in an exposed group compared with the risk of developing the same outcome in the control group. It is used in RCTs and cohort studies.

Sensitivity The ability of a test to detect those who have the disease, i.e. the proportion (percentage) of people with the condition who are detected as having it by the test.

Specificity The ability of the test to identify those without the disease, i.e. the proportion of people without the condition who are correctly reassured by a negative test.

Systematic review A literature review that aims to minimize bias and random errors by using a system that is documented in a materials and methods section, and which may or may not include meta-analysis.

KEY REFERENCES

1. Sackett DL, Straus S, Scott Richardson W, Rosenburg W, Haynes RB. *How to Practice and Teach Evidence Based Medicine*, 2nd edition. Churchill Livingstone, 2000.
2. EPIQ (Effective Practice, Informatics and Quality Improvement). Professor Rod Jackson, Head of the Section of Epidemiology and Biostatistics, University of Auckland: <www.health.auckland.ac.nz/comhealth/epiq/epiq.htm>.
3. Royal College of Obstetricians and Gynaecologists. *Searching for Evidence*. Clinical Governance Advice No. 3. London: RCOG Press, 2001.
4. Khan KS, Kuntz R, Kleijnen J, Antes G. *Systematic Reviews to Support Evidence Based Medicine. How to Review and Apply Findings of Healthcare Research.* London: Royal Society of Medicine Press, 2003.
5. Royal College of Obstetricians and Gynaecologists: Clinical Effectiveness Support Unit. *Induction of Labour.* National Evidence Based Clinical Guideline No. 9. London: RCOG Press, 2001.
6. Royal College of Obstetricians and Gynaecologists. *The Use of Electronic Fetal Monitoring: the Use and Interpretation of Cardiotocography in Intrapartum Fetal Monitoring.* National Evidence Based Clinical Guideline No. 8. London: RCOG Press, 2001.
7. Thomas J, Paranjothy S, and Royal College of Obstetricians and Gynaecologists: Clinical Effectiveness Support Unit. *The National Sentinel Caesarean Section Audit Report.* London: RCOG Press, 2001.
8. <http://rms.nelh.nhs.uk/guidelinesfinder/guideAppraisal.asp>.
9. Moher D, Schulz KF, Altman D; CONSORT Group (Consolidated Standards of Reporting Trials). The CONSORT statement: revised recommendations for improving the quality of reports of parallel-group randomized trials. *J Am Med Assoc* 2001; 285(15):1987–91.
10. Moher D, Cook DJ, Eastwood S, Olkin I, Rennie D, Stroup DF. Improving the quality of reports of meta-analyses of randomised controlled trials: the QUOROM statement. Quality of Reporting of Meta-analyses. *Lancet* 1999; 354:1896–900.
11. Bossuyt PM, Reitsma JB, Bruns DE et al. Towards complete and accurate reporting of studies of diagnostic accuracy: the STARD initiative. Standards for Reporting of Diagnostic Accuracy. *BMJ* 2003; 326:41–4.
12. Grol R, Grimshaw J. From best evidence to best practice: effective implementation of change in patients' care. *Lancet* 2003; 362:1225–30.
13. Kaptchuk EJ. Effect of interpretive bias on research evidence. *BMJ* 2003; 326:1453–5.
14. Royal College of Obstetricians and Gynaecologists. *Understanding Audit.* Clinical Governance Advice No. 5. London: RCOG Press, 2003.
15. NHS, National Institute for Clinical Excellence, Commission for Health Improvement, Royal College of Nursing, University of Leicester. *Review of the Evidence. Principles for Best Practice in Clinical Audit.* London: National Institute for Clinical Excellence, 2002.
16. Thomas J, Paranjothy S; Royal College of Obstetricians and Gynaecologists: Clinical Effectiveness Support Unit. *The National Sentinel Caesarean Section Audit Report.* London: RCOG Press, 2001.
17. Brocklehurst P, Gates S. Statistics. In: O'Brien PMS, Broughton PF (eds), *Introduction to Research Methodology for Specialists and Trainees.* London: RCOG Press, 1999,147–60.

Chapter 2

The General Principles of Surgery

Fiona M. Reid and Anthony R.B. Smith

INTRODUCTION

'Choose well, cut well, get well'. Surgery has three phases. In the preoperative phase, the correct operation should be chosen for a patient, who should be in an optimal condition. A well-trained, competent surgeon should then perform the surgery in a safe environment. During the postoperative phase, the patient should be monitored, encouraged and advised. Each phase is equally important. These are the basic principles of surgery, and this chapter examines how they may be achieved.

THE PREOPERATIVE PHASE

There is always more than one treatment option and it is the role of a gynaecologist to counsel the patient about the appropriate options. The process of selecting the best procedure for a patient is inseparable from that of obtaining informed consent. A booklet of guidelines to obtaining consent is available from the General Medical Council or on the internet at <www.gmc-uk.org/standards>.

When counselling patients about treatment options, effective communication is imperative. This may necessitate the use of written material or visual aids. It may require the use of interpreters for foreign or sign language. Preferably, interpreters should be independent professionals and not family members, who could have a vested interest in a particular treatment.

Patients should be informed of the advantages and disadvantages of each procedure, the success rates, failure rates, side effects and common complications. Risk should be quantified rather than being described subjectively with terms such as 'slight' or 'rare'.

Increasingly, the adequacy of consent is assessed legally by the concept of 'material risk'. A risk is material if:

In the circumstances of the case, a reasonable person in the patient's position, if warned of the risk, would be likely to attach significance to it or if the medical practitioner is, or should reasonably be aware that the particular patient if warned of the risk, would be likely to attach significance to it.[1]

In practice, this implies that even rare complications that are serious or that carry significance to an individual's social life or employment should be addressed.

Patients should have adequate time to reflect on the information they have been given prior to making a decision. It should not be assumed that a patient understands the general risks of surgery such as anaesthetic complications.

The General Medical Council's guidelines on informed consent state that ultimately it is the responsibility of the person performing the procedure to ensure informed consent has been obtained.

Optimizing preoperative health

Although most gynaecological surgery is performed on relatively healthy women, it is imperative that all patients undergoing surgery are in their optimum condition. Smokers should be encouraged to stop at least 24 hours before surgery to reduce the level of carboxyhaemoglobin in the blood and minimize the cardiovascular effect of nicotine.[2] Screening for sexually transmitted diseases or bacterial vaginosis prior to pelvic procedures should be considered.[3]

Basic preoperative screening involves a detailed history and a general examination. Routine screening blood tests have not been shown to influence cancellations or perioperative complications, and the majority of abnormal results could have been predicted from the history and examination.[4] A study by Golub et al.[5] in the USA demonstrated that avoiding batteries of routine preoperative tests could save US $397 per patient.

Ideally, preoperative investigations should be specific to each individual. Even routine sickle testing of at-risk adults has been challenged because patients with sickle cell disease would already have been detected as children due to chronic haemolytic anaemia. Also no sickling complications have been reported in sickle cell trait patients for the past 15 years.[6]

Table 2.1 Medical conditions most commonly associated with increased surgical morbidity

Ischaemic heart disease
Congestive cardiac failure
Arterial hypertension
Chronic respiratory disease
Diabetes mellitus
Cardiac arrhythmia
Anaemia

Table 2.2 The American Society of Anesthesiologists' (ASA) physical status classification system

ASA 1	Normal healthy patient
ASA 2	Patient with mild controlled systemic disease which does not affect normal activity
ASA 3	Patient with severe systemic disease which limits activity
ASA 4	Patient with severe systemic disease which is incapacitating and is a constant threat to life
ASA 5	Moribund patient not expected to survive 24 hours with or without operation

Table 2.3 Thromboprophylaxis risk assessment for gynaecological patients

Risk	Prophylaxis
Low	
Minor surgery (<30 min); no risk factors other than age	Early mobilization
Major surgery (>30 min); <40 years old; no other risk factors	Good hydration
Moderate	
Major surgery: >40 years old or other risk factors	Anticoagulation Early mobilization Good hydration
Minor surgery: previous history of thrombosis or thrombophilia	Graduated elastic compression stockings
High Major surgery for cancer	Intermittent pneumatic compression

The morbidity and mortality of surgery and anaesthesia are increased in patients with co-existing disease (Table 2.1).[7]

Elective surgery should be delayed for 6 months after a myocardial infarct because 35 per cent will re-infarct before 3 months and this risk falls to 4 per cent after 6 months.[8] Of the deaths reported in the National Confidential Enquiries into Perioperative Deaths (CEPOD) Report 2001, 60 per cent of patients had ischaemic heart disease.[9] The history is as important as the investigations: a preoperative electrocardiogram (ECG) on patients with proven ischaemia will be normal in 20–50 per cent of cases.[10]

Protocols should be available on the ward for the management of common conditions such as diabetes mellitus.

It is the surgeon's responsibility to liaise with the anaesthetist and other specialties if patients have concurrent illness. At times it can be difficult to convey the complexity of a patient's condition, and the American Society of Anesthesiologists' (ASA) scoring system[11] can be a useful communication tool (Table 2.2).

Venous thrombosis is one of the most serious complications of surgery, and all units should have clear protocols for thromboprophylaxis. Most will be derived from the Thromboembolic Risk Factors (THRIFT) Consensus Group,[12] which recommends that the risk of thromboembolism should be assessed in all patients and prophylaxis should be prescribed according to risk (Table 2.3).

Other risk factors include major concurrent illness, preoperative immobility and obesity (body mass index (BMI) >30). Women taking the combined oral contraceptive pill have twice the normal risk of postoperative thrombosis after major pelvic surgery, and should be advised to stop

it 1 month prior to surgery. There is no increased risk following minor surgery.[13] Hormone replacement therapy appears to be associated with a general overall increased risk of venous thrombosis, but no studies on the risk of thrombosis after surgery have been performed in a normal population.[14]

KEY POINTS

Consent
- Selecting the best procedure is inseparable from gaining informed consent.
- It is the operator's responsibility to ensure that informed consent has been obtained.
- Effective communication is imperative: interpreters or visual aids may be necessary.
- Patients should receive detailed information on benefits and risks.
- Patients should have adequate time to reflect on this information.

Optimizing preoperative health
- Smoking should be stopped 24 hours before surgery.
- Combined oral contraceptives should be stopped 1 month before major surgery.
- Preoperative screening should be by history and examination; routine blood tests are rarely helpful.
- Routine surgery should be delayed for 6 months after myocardial infarction.
- If there is concurrent illness, liaison with the anaesthetist and other specialists is essential.
- All units should have clear protocols for thromboprophylaxis.

INTRAOPERATIVE CARE

A full knowledge of abdominal and pelvic anatomy is essential for gynaecological surgery. In cases in which the anatomy is distorted, the surgeon should attempt to restore normal anatomy and work from first principles. Tissue planes should be utilized and tissues should be handled gently. Many gynaecologists gain most of their early surgical experience in the obstetric theatre, where speed tends to be valued above all else. Technique should be valued above speed.

Adequate access is essential. A senior surgeon called to a difficult case often first improves access. This includes good bowel packing.

Asepsis is obviously important; however, some aseptic practices are traditions and are not based on evidence. Pre-operative shaving, for example, is aesthetic to the surgeon and allows for the painless removal of the dressing postoperatively, but it does not appear to alter wound infection rates.[15] The use of a single dose of prophylactic antibiotics to prevent wound infection or septicaemia is now widely accepted.[16]

Facemasks in general abdominal surgery and certainly in laparoscopic procedures do not appear to affect infection rates. However, eye protection or face shields to protect the surgeon's mucous membranes from the patient's bodily fluids are sensible. Without serum testing it is impossible to know if a patient has hepatitis or human immunodeficiency virus (HIV) and therefore all patients are a potential risk. All healthcare workers should be immunized against hepatitis B. Cotton gowns provide protection of one's nakedness only!

Drains may be used if clinically indicated and not as an alternative to good haemostasis. There is no robust evidence to support their use. A drain is probably advisable when a urinary tract injury has been repaired, in case of urinary leakage. Possible complications of drains include trauma during insertion, blockage, infection, erosion of adjacent tissue and retention of a foreign body.

TECHNICAL EQUIPMENT FOR SURGERY

Surgeons should have an understanding of the principles of the equipment they use.

Diathermy involves the passage of electrical current through the patient's body. Electrocution does not occur because the frequency of current used in diathermy is much higher than that of mains electricity. Mains electricity is a low-frequency alternating current (50 Hz in the UK). Low-frequency currents cause depolarization and neuromuscular stimulation. Diathermy utilizes a very high frequency (400 kHz to 10 MHz) alternating current. It does not cause depolarization but it does excite ions, and this causes heat, particularly when in a high-density form.

In monopolar diathermy, the active electrodes and the return electrode are some distance apart. In bipolar diathermy, the two electrodes are only millimetres apart.

Factors that influence the diathermy effect are current density, the resistance of the tissue, the waveform and the duration of activation.

At high current density, heat is produced. The size of the electrode influences current density. At the tip of an active electrode the current density is high, and therefore heat is generated. The return electrode's surface area is large, so the current density is low and no heating occurs.

The resistance of tissues is indirectly proportional to their water content: higher water content reduces resistance. Tissues with high resistance require a higher output (watts), from the diathermy generator, to generate heat.

Cutting is achieved by using a low voltage but a high frequency current that is constantly flowing. The current is concentrated in a very small area and the high energy level causes so much ion excitation that the cells explode, releasing steam. If coagulation is required, an intermittent high-voltage current is used, with current flowing for only 6 per cent of the time. Thus a cutting current is inherently safer because of the lower voltage reducing the risk of inadvertent current discharge.

The safety of diathermy systems is continually improving. Initially, grounded generators were used, whereby current could return to ground via the path of least resistance. Since 1968, solid-state isolated generators have been used. These avoid burns at other sites such as drip stands because current will not flow unless current is returning to the generator. However, return electrode burns can still occur if the pad is not attached completely. Systems of contact quality monitoring have been available since the 1980s to prevent return electrode burns.

There are some specific hazards related to electrosurgery in laparoscopic procedures.

Direct coupling is the inadvertent flow of current from one instrument to another and may be secondary to insulation failure. Insulation failure can result from damaged equipment or the use of excessive voltage with coagulation current. **Capacitance coupling** can occur if a capacitor is created. Two conductors separated by an insulator form a capacitor, for example an insulated laparoscopic instrument passing through a metal port. The current stored in the capacitor can discharge into the patient, causing burns. The higher the current passing through the instrument, the greater will be the capacitance current. Plastic ports do not eliminate the risk of capacitance coupling because the patient's bowel or omentum can act as the second conductor. Capacitance coupling can be avoided with active electrode monitoring systems.

Other causes of diathermy burns are careless technique, not checking the dial setting before use, the use of spirit-based skin preparation near diathermy, or someone other than the surgeon activating the current flow.

More detailed explanations of the principles of diathermy are available at an interactive website: <www.valleylabeducation.org>.

KEY POINTS

- Technique should be valued above speed.
- Adequate access is essential.
- Asepsis is important but some practices are not evidence based.
- Single-dose antibiotic prophylaxis is now widely accepted.
- All patients are a potential risk and all healthcare workers should be immunized against hepatitis B.
- Drains should be used only when clinically indicated.
- Surgeons should understand the principles of the equipment they use: this applies particularly to diathermy.

Minimal access surgery

Diseases that harm call for treatments that harm less.

William Osler (1849–1919)

The most common endoscopic techniques used in gynaecology are laparoscopy and hysteroscopy.

Laparoscopy

The possible benefits of laparoscopy are shown in Table 2.4. Many of these purported benefits have not undergone robust analysis. In a randomized trial of open versus laparoscopic colposuspension, in which the patients were blinded to the type of surgery, there was no significant difference in the length of hospital stay, but the laparoscopic group returned to normal activities significantly earlier than the open group.[17]

Many complications specific to laparoscopic surgery are related to the method of entry into the peritoneal cavity. The risk is as great for a diagnostic laparoscopy as it is for a major operative laparoscopic procedure. The risk of bowel injury is 0.4–3 per 1000 and of vascular injury 0.2–1 per 1000 laparoscopies.[19] Bowel adhesions to the anterior abdominal wall occur in 0.5 per cent of patients with no previous surgery, increasing to 20 per cent if they have had a previous pfannenstiel incision and to 50 per cent if they have had a midline incision.[20] To minimize this risk, safe entry techniques have been recommended (Table 2.5). Open laparoscopy has been advocated, particularly by general surgeons, because it appears to reduce the risk of vascular injury, but it does not reduce the risk of bowel injury. Microlaparoscopy at Palmers point can also be used. Published recommendations on safe entry are formed from expert opinion,[19] not clinical trials, because the number of subjects required to perform trials to investigate entry techniques is prohibitively large.

Table 2.4   Benefits of laparoscopy

Patients
Less pain[17]
Less blood loss[17,18]
Less scarring
Quicker recovery[17]
Surgeon
Safer 'closed/no touch surgery'
Better display of anatomy
Healthcare providers
Reduced in-patient stay
Reduced social cost

Table 2.5   A safe entry technique for laparoscopy

The patient should be lying flat
Ensure the bladder is empty and check the abdomen for masses
Make the primary incision at the base of the umbilicus
Insert the Veress needle through the base of the umbilicus, sensing a double click
Insert 2–3 mL of saline through the Veress: it should run in freely
Aspirate back: nothing should be aspirated
Fill with CO_2 to a pressure of 25 mmHg
Repeat the saline test
Insert the primary trocar

Hysteroscopy

This common procedure has specific safety issues. Distension media for hysteroscopy include carbon dioxide, normal saline or glycine. Water is not used as a distension medium because it is hypo-osmolar and, once absorbed, causes haemolysis.

If intrauterine electrosurgery is to be performed using monopolar equipment, the solution must be non-conductive so that the electrical current is not dissipated. Solutions containing electrolytes can be used with recently developed bipolar electrosurgery equipment.

The complications of hysteroscopy include uterine perforation and fluid absorption. Uterine perforation can be associated with damage to the bowel or intraperitoneal haemorrhage. A high index of suspicion and early recourse to diagnostic laparoscopy are advisable.

Fluid may be absorbed at the time of hysteroscopy. If excessive, it can result in hyponatraemia and hypo-osmolality, clinically characterized by nausea, vomiting, seizures, coma and even death. The amount of fluid absorbed is dependent on the volume infused and the infusion pressure. Owing to the short duration of a diagnostic procedure, excessive fluid retention is unlikely to be a problem.

Large-volume fluid absorption is most likely when large vessels are opened at endometrial resection. The main precaution to avoid excessive absorption is accurate measurement of the fluid deficit throughout the procedure.

Fluid absorption increases significantly when the intrauterine pressure exceeds the mean arterial pressure (MAP). When gravity (the height of the bag) is used to drive the fluid, the lowest pressure (height) to distend the cavity should be used. It should not exceed the MAP (pressure cmH_2O = pressure $mmHg \times 0.74$). If the giving set contains a drip chamber, the height of the fluid is taken from the drip chamber, but if this fills, the pressure is calculated from the fluid level in the bag.

KEY POINTS

Laparoscopy
- Many of the purported benefits have not undergone robust analysis.
- Many of the complications relate to the method of entry into the peritoneal cavity: safe entry techniques, formed from expert opinion, have been published.

Hysteroscopy
- Non-conducting distension media must be used for intrauterine electrosurgery with monopolar equipment.
- Uterine perforation may occur: a high index of suspicion is needed, with early recourse to laparoscopy.
- Excessive fluid absorption may lead to seizures and even death.
- Accurate measurement of fluid deficit is needed throughout the procedure.

Local anaesthetic

Two common complications to consider when using local anaesthetic are systemic toxicity and delayed haemorrhage if it is combined with adrenaline. The duration of action and safe dosages are shown in Table 2.6.

Initial symptoms of toxicity are peri-oral paraesthesiae, tinnitus or visual disturbance. These may be followed by convulsions or cardiotoxicity, arrhythmia, complete heart block or cardiac arrest.

Sedation

A trained doctor should administer sedation. This doctor should be responsible only for administering the sedation and cardiorespiratory monitoring. He or she should not perform the surgery.

The objective is to produce a level of sedation at which the patient is relaxed, calm and rational, and verbal communication is continuously possible. Sedation can result in unconsciousness or general anaesthesia. Facilities must be available to manage an anaesthetized patient.

All patients should be monitored with a pulse oximeter during sedation. Reversal agents should be avoided as their half-life may be shorter than the sedative, leading to delayed respiratory depression. Patients should be observed for at least 2 hours prior to discharge.

Table 2.6   Properties of local anaesthetic agents

Agent	Duration of action (hours)	Maxium dosage (mg/kg)	
		Plain solution	With adrenaline
Lignocaine	1–3	3	7
Bupivicaine	1–4	2	2
Prilocaine	1–3	4	8

KEY POINTS

- Common complications of local anaesthetic are systemic toxicity and (if combined with adrenaline) delayed haemorrhage.
- Sedation should be administered by a trained doctor who is not performing the surgery.
- Facilities must be available to manage an anaesthetized patient.
- Patients should be observed for at least 2 hours prior to discharge.

POSTOPERATIVE CARE

This can be divided into three phases:

1 immediate: theatre recovery
2 early: until discharge from hospital
3 late: home.

Theatre recovery

Airways, breathing and circulation (ABC) are the important parameters immediately after the operation. All staff should maintain life support skills. Up-to-date resuscitation guidelines are available on the internet (www.resus.org.uk). Patients should be stable when they leave the recovery area. This includes the relief of pain.

Ward care

A doctor should review postoperative patients at least daily. A useful acronym for daily postoperative assessments is SOAP (subjective, objective, assessment, plan) (Table 2.7).

Adequate analgesia should be prescribed. Units can rationalize prescribing using guidelines, for example an analgesic ladder – paracetamol, non-steroidal anti-inflammatory drugs (NSAIDs), patient-controlled analgesia (PCA)/opioid and epidural.

Fluid balance is important. Most gynaecological patients will tolerate a 'standard fluid recipe of 2500 mL per day'. Careless prescribing can lead to hyponatraemia or pulmonary

Table 2.7 Daily postoperative assessment

SOAP
Subjective: how does the patient feel?
Objective: blood pressure, temperature and fluid balance
Assessment: physical examination
Plan: plan of care for the next 24 hours

Table 2.8 Follow-up clinics

Advantages
Audit
Proactive detection of complications
Provide ongoing treatment
Completeness of treatment episode
Disadvantages
Delay in reviewing complication
Anxiety waiting for results
Time spent seeing well people
Cost to the health service
Cost to the patient in travel and time off work

oedema. Evidence-based practice of postoperative fluid management is sparse and equivocal. Agreement exists that the daily requirements of sodium and potassium are 1 mmol/kg. However, the effects of stress hormones associated with surgery are poorly understood, and electrolytes should be checked every 24–48 hours, if a patient remains on intravenous fluids, to guide fluid prescription.

Oliguria is a urine output of less than 20 mL/h, in each of two consecutive hours. Oliguria due to hypovolaemia may result from:

- active haemorrhage
- unreplaced blood loss
- ileus: fluid loss into the gastrointestinal tract
- loss of plasma into the abdomen
- oedema.

If fluid balance is difficult, it may require central venous pressure monitoring and transfer to a high dependency unit (HDU) or intensive care unit (ICU). The National CEPOD 2001 enquiry found that 16 per cent of patients were not admitted to ICU/HDU despite there being a demonstrable need.[9]

Fluids for volume expansion should be blood or colloids. Studies have demonstrated that stable patients with a haemoglobin of $\geqslant 8$ g/dL do not require blood transfusion; they should receive oral iron.[21]

DISCHARGE

Discharge should be planned. The patient should be aware of normal recovery rates, and be given advice about when to return to work, social activities and sexual intercourse. However, this information is usually based on traditional practice rather than evidence.

The general practitioner (GP) should be informed of the patient's treatment. An effective way to inform GPs is to give a brief discharge letter to the patient to take to the GP, followed by a formal letter. It may be necessary for social services, Macmillan nurses or district nurses to be involved in discharge procedures.

The need for follow-up visits is dependent on the surgery performed. The advantages and disadvantages are listed in Table 2.8.

KEY POINTS

Immediate
- All staff should maintain life support skills.

Early
- A doctor should review patients at least daily.
- Analgesia and fluid balance are important.

Discharge
- Patients should be given full advice about recovery rates and activities.
- The GP and, if necessary, other services should be promptly informed.
- Not all procedures require routine follow-up.

DAY CASE SURGERY

There are special considerations to be accounted for in day case surgery, including patient selection and discharge arrangements.

Day surgery units should have clear protocols for patient selection to minimize cancellations (Table 2.9): patients should be generally fit and ambulant; they should be able to climb one flight of stairs; they should not be grossly obese (BMI <35).[22]

Day surgery units should have written criteria for patients' discharge.[23,24] Patients should have stable vital signs, be orientated in time and place and able to tolerate oral fluids; they should be able to dress and walk unaided; they must have a responsible and physically able adult to collect them and care for them overnight; they should have adequate analgesia and be aware of the action to take in the event of complications. A contact telephone number should be given for advice after discharge.

KEY POINTS

There should be:
- clear protocols for patient selection
- written criteria for discharge.

Table 2.9   Common conditions that require further assessment

Uncontrolled hypertension, BP >170/100 mmHg
Cardiac failure
MI/TIA/CVA in past 6 months
Severe asthma/respiratory disease
Diabetes – IDDM or poorly controlled NIDDM (BG >11 mmol/L)
Renal or hepatic disease
Alcoholism or narcotic addiction
Advanced multiple sclerosis or myasthenia
Severe cervical spondylosis
Severe psychiatric disease
Drugs: MAOIs, digoxin, steroids, anticoagulants, GTN, diruetics and anti-dysrhythmics

BP, blood pressure; MI, myocardial infarction; TIA, transient ischaemic attack; CVA, cerebrovascular accident; IDDM, insulin-dependent diabetes mellitus; NIDDM, non-insulin-dependent diabetes mellitus; BG, blood glucose; MAOIs, monoamine oxidase inhibitors; GTN, glyceryl trinitrate.

RISK MANAGEMENT

Risk management is the process of examining procedures to prevent accidents and assessing incidents to prevent recurrence. Some of the most serious mistakes occur from the most simple system errors.

The introduction of simple protocols can avoid common mistakes such as retained swabs and ensure that the correct operation is performed on the correct patient.

Examining 'near misses' is as important as examining actual 'incidents'. Hospitals should have a reporting procedure that is accessible to all staff.

KEY POINTS

- Risk can be reduced by simple protocols.
- There should be reporting systems for incidents and 'near-misses'.

CONCLUSIONS

Technicians can perform procedures, whilst surgeons should orchestrate care.

Surgeons have a responsibility to ensure they are adequately trained, have counselled the patient preoperatively and are performing the correct operation, and to provide post-operative care.

Audit is important to review practice and should be part of a surgeon's remit. Surgeons must be provided with the time and resources required to audit their practice. League tables of surgical care will only be informative when all aspects of care are included in the assessment. The National Confidential Enquiry into Perioperative Deaths is a national surgical audit that can be found at <www.ncepod.org.uk>.

KEY REFERENCES

1. Rogers vs Whitaker. *CRL*, 1992:479.
2. Jones R. Smoking before surgery: the case for stopping. *BMJ* 1985; 290(6484):1763–4.
3. *National Strategy for Sexual Health and HIV*. London: Department of Health, 2001.
4. Johnson H, Knee-Iloi S, Butler T, et al. Are routine pre-operative laboratory screening tests necessary to evaluate ambulatory surgical patients? *Surgery* 1988; 104:639–45.
5. Golub R, Cantu R, Sorrento J, et al. Efficacy of preadmission testing in ambulatory surgical patients. *Am J Surg* 1992; 163:565–71.
6. Wong E-M, Tillyer M, Saunders P. Pre-operative screening for sickle cell trait in adult day surgery; is it necessary? *Ambulatory Surg* 1996; 4:41–5.
7. Campling A, Devlin H, Hoile R, Lunn J. The Report of the National Confidential Enquiry into Perioperative Deaths, 1991/1992. London: NCEPOD, 1993.
8. Portal R. Elective surgery after myocardial infarction. *BMJ* 1982; 284:843–4.
9. Changing the way we operate: National Confidential Enquiry into Perioperative Deaths. London: NCEPOD, 2001.
10. Jones R. Influence of coexisting disease. In: Kirk R, Mansfield A, Cochrane J (eds). *Clinical Surgery in General*. London: Churchill Livingstone, 1996, 67–83.
11. Robinson P, Hall G. Preoperative assessment. In: *How to Survive in Anaesthesia*. London: BMJ Publishing Group, 1997, 98.
12. (THRIFT) Thromboembolic Risk Factors Consensus Group. Risk of and prophylaxis for venous thromboembolism in hospital patients. *BMJ* 1992; 305:567–74.
13. Guillebaud J. Surgery and the pill. *BMJ* 1985; 291:498–9.
14. Daly E, Vessey M, Hawkins M, Carson J, Gough P, Marsh S. Risk of venous thromboembolism in users of hormone replacement therapy. *Lancet* 1996; 348:977–80.
15. Leaper D. Surgical access, incisions and the management of wounds. In: Kirk R, Mansfield A, Cochrane J (eds). *Clinical Surgery in General*. London: Churchill Livingstone, 1996, 201–7.
16. Pollock A. Surgical prophylaxis – the emerging picture. *Lancet* 1988; 1:225–30.
17. Carey M, Rosamilla G, Maher C, et al. Laparoscopic versus open colposuspension: a prospective multicentre randomised single blind trial. *Neuro & Urodyn* 2000; 19(4):389–90.
18. Fatthy H, El Hao M, Samaha I, Abdallah K. Modified Burch colposuspension: laparoscopy versus laparotomy. *J Am Assoc Gynecol Laparoscopists* 2001; 8(1):99–106.

GENERAL

19. A consensus document concerning laparoscopic entery techniques: Middlesborough, March 19–20. *Gynae Endo* 1999; **8**:403–6.

20. Audebert A, Gomel V. Role of microlaparoscopy in the diagnosis of peritoneal and visceral adhesions and the prevention of bowel injury associated with blind trocar insertion. *Fertil Steril* 2000; **73**(3):631–5.

21. Tate J. Postoperative care. In: Kirk R, Mansfield A, Cochrane J (eds). *Clinical Surgery in General.* London: Churchill Livingstone, 1996, 267–74.

22. Millar J, Rudkin G, Hitchcock M. *Practical Anaesthesia and Analgesia for Day Surgery.* Oxford: BIOS Scientific Publishers, 1997.

23. Korttila K. Recovery from outpatient anaesthesia. *Anaesthesia* 1995; **50**(Suppl.):22–8.

24. Chung F. Discharge criteria – a new trend. *Can J Anaesth* 1995; **42**:1056–8.

Chapter 3

Communication and Counselling

Richard Porter

> Everything in this chapter is – or should be – self-evident. Communication is the foundation stone of our clinical practice.

INTRODUCTION

Communication takes very many forms. (Counselling is the application of communication skills in a specific area.) This chapter does not presume to cover all aspects of this vast subject, but it will focus on some of those that impinge on the postgraduate trainee.

It is possible to be a proficient diagnostician or a highly competent surgeon, or both, and to be a poor communicator with patients. But I would argue that it is not possible to be a good doctor in the modern world without being a good communicator. After all, communication with patients is what principally distinguishes us from veterinary surgeons – with all due respect to veterinary surgeons.

Medical schools teach many things well, but the teaching of communication skills has until relatively recently lagged behind. However, in postgraduate hospital medical training the subject has not so much been poorly addressed as totally ignored, and the challenge is for new generations to change this.

COMMUNICATION WITH PATIENTS

In obstetrics and gynaecology, good communication with patients generally requires:

- *Respect for the patient as an individual.* Even if she holds opinions and beliefs that may not be the same as ours.
- *Respect for women.* In cultures where this is not automatic, it is frequently observed that communication is at a lamentably low level. At its most extreme,

women will simply avoid contact with medical services, with dire consequences for health outcomes such as maternal and perinatal mortality. If an obstetrician/gynaecologist does not respect patients as women, it is difficult to understand why such a doctor remains in this specialty.

- *The ability of the doctor to understand the patient, and the patient to understand the doctor.* Language barriers are not a justification for sub-standard clinical care on either a medico-legal or a moral level. You may require the use of interpreters, but remember that the problem may not just be with the words used. Even when a doctor and a patient ostensibly speak the same language, they may not be using the words in the same way, and this can be a cause of major and potentially dangerous misunderstanding.
- *The ability to listen.* This is not an open-ended commitment: some patients will want to tell us far more than we need, want or have time to hear. But achieving the right balance is essential.
- *Flexibility.* Any doctor who says that he or she takes a history in the same way under all circumstances is being either extraordinarily naïve or economical with the truth. A good doctor is constantly looking for nuances in the nature of the communication with the patient that will show the way forward.

Verbal communication with patients

Assuming that you and the patient are speaking (literally) more or less the same language:

- *Are you using a vocabulary that is appropriate to her?* I well remember watching a brilliant researcher explaining in detail to a totally bemused mother the physics of Doppler wave forms. This was in response to her anxious question – while being scanned at 34 weeks' gestation – 'Whassat doing then?'. This was (to be honest) hilarious to watch – but a tragic illustration of the limitations of intelligence.

- *Are you going too fast?* How often do we see colleagues checking with patients, after imparting manageable (bite-sized?) chunks of information, whether or not they have understood? Not nearly often enough, I would predict. If we wait until the end of a long discussion, with masses of pieces of information, can we be surprised if the patient surrenders and says that she has understood – just to make us go away? In fact, I cherish the lesson I learnt from a patient who, after I had explained that she needed her urodynamics repeating (I assumed that she knew what I was talking about because she had had the test before), was asked by the Sister when leaving the room, 'So, did you understand all that?', and said loudly (she was a bit deaf), 'Not a word dear'.
- *Are you 'talking down' to her?* In this new era of patients surfing the web, few things are more likely to raise hackles than giving the impression that you assume that they are uneducated imbeciles.
- *Are you giving her more information than she wants?* This is one of the most difficult areas in current practice (see 'Obtaining consent', below). How much is enough, and how much too much? In oncology care, this is a particularly important issue, and is beyond the scope of this chapter. The problem is compounded by perceptions about a litigious environment. Yet we must recognize that we have a duty of care to our patients, and that may mean that we should make judgements about the appropriateness or otherwise of imparting every iota of information.
- *Do you recognize the cultural sensitivities influencing her decisions?* In our multi-cultural society, we are becoming better at not trampling on the sensitivities of, for example, Muslim women, but it is still incumbent upon us to be alert to the possibility of unexpected beliefs and taboos.

Non-verbal communication with patients

A patient is more often than not in a state of some unease when meeting a doctor, and she will be responding to far more than what is said or not said. The nature of the space where the meeting takes place, the smells of the environment, the extraneous noises – all will influence both her perception of the event and the way in which she takes the information on board. A doctor cannot often immediately influence these factors, but can certainly add to or detract from the experience by means of non-verbal communication. Much of this is a matter of common courtesy, but it is easy to let our standards slip on occasion – and patients notice it, you can be sure. Surely the guiding principle here is that you should act towards your patients exactly as you would wish to be acted towards yourself – and the use of the word 'act' is not accidental, for every contact with a patient is to a degree a theatrical event.

The following are some examples.

- *How do you greet the patient?* Do you stand up? Do you have your back to her when she comes in? Do you shake her hand? Do you invite her to sit? I suspect that we have all seen 'eminent' doctors greet a patient by continuing to talk to medical students. What sort of an impression does that give?
- *What is your facial expression?* A smile, a furrowed brow, a scowl, a dead-pan expression – all will convey some message to the patient. Is the message the one you want to convey? The problem can, of course, get slightly out of hand: the phoney facial expression is just as unsettling as the unthinking one. Think of a politician delivering an unpalatable message with a sanctimonious look. None of us would like to be compared to politicians, I assume.
- *Do you look her in the eye when talking to her, or do you stare at the floor?* This again may reflect your cultural background, or even perhaps your innate modesty, but it may lead to unintended inferences by the patient. Would you propose marriage whilst looking at the floor? (Of course some might: I am reminded of the schoolmaster who did so by asking his intended if she wanted his surname on her gravestone. Tastes differ…)
- *How do you sit during a consultation?* Are you leaning forward in an attentive pose, or slouching in the chair? Body language is powerful, and can be deeply unsettling for your patient.
- *When you stand (e.g. in a bedside consultation), how far away are you?* Are you too close for the patient's comfort, or are you so far that you give the impression that you regard the patient as another life form? Remember that differences in height – e.g. when you stand over a patient who is lying on a bed – can result in, to put it mildly, unintended distortions in communication.
- *Have you ensured that she is at her ease?* Is she embarrassed (more than is usual) by her state of undress? As ever, the question is: would you or your nearest and dearest want to be treated like this?

COMMUNICATION WITH OTHER STAFF

Although communication with patients is of paramount importance, the issue of communication with other professionals is also crucial. In hospital medicine there is no such thing as a single-handed department, and dysfunction all too easily follows from poor interprofessional communication.

Any trainee who has worked in a department where rivalries pollute the atmosphere will know how destructive that can be. Many of these problems themselves arise from poor communication skills, but poor communication will surely follow from these rivalries.

The areas of importance are as follows:

Doctor–doctor communication

Juniors need to communicate with more senior doctors (and vice versa), and doctors of the same grade with each other. Now that trainers are themselves being more commonly trained to train, and in the increasingly informal atmosphere in which we work in hospital practice, it should follow that this 'vertical downward' communication will be better handled. This is also assisted by the reduction in 'patronage' over the last few years, which makes for a far more healthy training environment. However, that is beyond the scope of this chapter.

Yet, strangely perhaps, few if any trainees have been taught how to communicate ('upwards') with their trainers. Does this need to be taught? I would suggest that it does. Consider the 2 a.m. phone call to the consultant on call. Does the trainee have any idea what this feels like for the recipient of the call, roused from sleep? Possibly the best advice I received about this was the suggestion that the caller should be taught immediately to communicate the status of the call. Was it a call that: (a) required the consultant's presence, (b) required the consultant's advice, or (c) was merely to inform the consultant? This is an example of learned communication that hugely enhances the transfer of information, almost certainly to the advantage of the patient.

The most formal type of doctor–doctor communication is case presentation. This is a skill and, like many others in postgraduate training, it is at the moment barely, if at all, taught. Yet without this skill there can be serious difficulties within the clinical team.

The simplest advice is, I believe, the best: present cases in three parts – the synopsis, the detail, and the summary (or, in other words, tell them what you are going to say, tell them what you want to say, and then remind them what you have just told them).

All trainees should practise these skills as often as possible, and should learn to teach them to the next generation.

Doctor–midwife/nurse communication

The other area of inter-professional communication – doctor–midwife/nurse communication – is just as important. Gone, thankfully, are the days of the presumed superiority of doctors. Instead we now respect the professional contributions of each other for what they are: interdependent and worthy of mutual respect. Nevertheless, all have to work to maintain the best possible level of communication at all times. Examples of departments where communication has failed abound – and the overall departmental dysfunction that ensues is massive, detrimental to patient care, and wholly unnecessary. Like any relationship, this one will have ups and downs. The mark of maturity is when the system can tolerate these, and learn from them.

Written communication

The two areas are clinical records and letters to other professionals. The skills required are similar, but different in detail.

CLINICAL RECORDS

The quality of your clinical records is of vital importance. Well-constructed clinical records communicate with other professionals and protect patients. They also may protect the writer from future medico-legal attack. Poor quality clinical records, by contrast, confuse other professionals and endanger patients. Records should be (as far as possible for those of us whose handwriting is only marginally more decipherable than Egyptian hieroglyphs) legible. They must also be dated, timed and signed (identifiably), if referring to an in-patient. There should be no exceptions to this.

The thicker clinical records become, the less useful they are as modes of information transfer. Thought must therefore be given to what and how much you write. Write only what is necessary and sufficient. Historically, midwives have written more than is necessary, and doctors far less than is necessary. Fortunately, that gap has recently narrowed considerably. Nevertheless, all those involved in medico-legal practice express continuing concern about the quality of note keeping.

LETTERS

A generation ago, letters between doctors were more stylish, idiosyncratic and interesting. Unfortunately they were also far less useful in transferring medical information. We live in an era in which letters are increasingly computer generated. Whether these letters are more effective in transferring information is yet to be determined, but I would suggest that the best letters are a compromise. If they are too short, they will be easily read, but they may omit relevant and necessary detail. If they are needlessly long, they risk losing the attention of the reader, and remaining unread. Your letter should be relevant to the recipient. I remain astonished by some letters in clinical practice, written by highly intelligent clinicians, which seem not to recognize what the aim of the exercise is (it is communication, not intellectual gratification). You must also remember that letters are crucially important medico-legal documents: you must ensure that what is typed is what you intended.

OBTAINING CONSENT

This is an area in which communication skills are sorely tested. How much information is required to enable a patient to give truly informed consent? All surgery could, for example, lead to death, but is it necessary to include that in the discussion? As it stands today, it is probably fair to say that today's practice will appear wrong within a short time. Even the test of 'how much would you like to know if it were you signing the consent form?' is probably an unreliable yardstick. The sensitive clinician will increasingly need to enter into the discussion with an open mind and sensitive antennae.

COUNSELLING

As obstetricians and gynaecologists, we become involved in counselling in several types of difficult circumstances (e.g. malignant disease, prenatal screening dilemmas, preconception counselling). As stated above, counselling is the application of the full range of communication skills in a specific area of professional expertise. There is no added magic in the process.

KEY POINTS

The guiding principles are:
- Strive not to give any opinion that is not based on evidence.
- Admit ignorance – or absence of professional knowledge – where that pertains.
- Empathy and sympathy are welcome, but professional objectivity is highly valued.
- Involve whatever other professionals are necessary – our patients no longer expect omniscience from us; indeed, they probably distrust those who seem to claim it.

CONCLUSIONS

This is an area where common sense rules. Integrity and respect for others are 'all' that is required.

Always ask yourself if you, or your closest relatives, would want to be communicated with in this manner. It really is that simple.

Chapter 4

The Law, Medicine and Women's Rights

Sheila McLean

INTRODUCTION

It is probably true to say that the relationship between law and medicine in the past has been characterized by confrontation, even hostility. Increasingly, however, doctors are turning to the law themselves as a way of obtaining guidance as to what is and what is not permissible in their practice. Thus, rather than law being seen simply as a mechanism for judging allegations of negligence, it has taken on the role of standard setter, particularly in some areas of medicine such as obstetrics and gynaecology.

Perhaps most obviously, this change has arisen as a consequence of medicine's capacities in managing pregnancy. The ability to monitor fetal development in particular has radically altered the way in which physicians perceive their role in respect of the pregnant woman, and has in some cases led to legal action. It has been said that, in the past, women told their doctors about their pregnancies, but now doctors tell women. The ability to visualize the fetus in the womb means that it becomes endowed, however subconsciously, with the characteristics of a child much earlier in pregnancy than would previously have been the case. The temptation therefore is to treat the fetus as a separate and unique patient. As Harrison says:

> The fetus has come a long way – from biblical 'seed' and mystical 'homunculus' to an individual with medical problems that can be diagnosed and treated. Although he cannot make an appointment and seldom even complains, this patient will at times need a physician.[1]

In some countries, this has led to a growing recognition of the alleged 'rights' of the fetus, which may on occasion conflict with the rights and interests of the pregnant woman. So common is this problem that it has been given a descriptive name of its own – maternal/fetal conflict – yet, as Hubbard says:

> It makes no sense, biologically or socially, to pit fetal and maternal 'rights' against one another. Indeed, legal 'rights' do not offer a proper framework for assessing the situation of a pregnant woman and her fetus. As long as they are connected, nothing can happen to one that does not affect the other.[2]

However, one thing must be made clear at the outset. In law, the fetus has no rights, and therefore to talk about fetal rights is misleading. Nonetheless, it is generally conceded that the embryo or fetus of the human species is worthy of some respect.[3] To say this, however, is quite different from asserting that it is a rights holder and worthy of equal consideration with the pregnant woman.

Most pregnant women will find no difficulty in behaving throughout their pregnancy in ways which maximize the potential health and safe delivery of their child. But not all women feel this way, or act this way, and this may be for reasons which appear to third parties unintelligible – even downright offensive or callous. However, the fact that women are free, autonomous actors means that their decisions – however unpalatable – must be given respect. This is not always easy for clinicians to accept, particularly when the woman's behaviour threatens the survival of an otherwise viable fetus. Indeed, a number of cases have reached courts in which doctors have asked that the choices of women should be overturned in the interest of fetal survival, and often also in the interests of saving the woman's life.

However, the basic legal position is clear. If a woman is otherwise legally competent, then her wishes must be respected, even if they result in her death or in the death of an otherwise viable fetus. No matter how harsh this sounds, it is the law, and there are good reasons for the law to adopt this position. However, the general rule is to offer benefit to the embryo or fetus wherever possible (without e.g. breaching the rights of others). So, for example, once born alive, children are entitled to sue for damage they sustained prenatally. This is based on the assumption that where a benefit *should* accrue, it is for the law to ensure that it does. But this is not to say that the law recognizes the fetus as a rights holder before birth. Rather, it accepts that the injury arises at the moment the fetus becomes a child, and therefore is entitled to have rights attributed to it.

A BRIEF ANALYSIS OF CASE LAW

It is in the grey areas that problems have arisen, and an analysis of some of the leading cases will help to explore both the content of and the rationale for the law's attitude. Although the law is clear that the fetus has no rights, this does not mean that women's autonomous decisions about the management of their pregnancy and labour have always been respected. The first case to arise in the UK was that of *Re S*.[4] In this case a woman refused a caesarean section on religious grounds. Her doctors believed that both her life and the life of her fetus were at risk and sought court authority to proceed with the section, even in the face of her objections. A judge heard the case as a matter of urgency (the hearing took about 20 minutes) and authorized the carrying out of the operation. This happened in 1992.

Perhaps unsurprisingly, this judgement was widely criticized for a number of reasons. First, the speed of the hearing was felt to prevent the nuances of the case being properly considered. Sir Stephen Brown's judgement, which is extremely brief, merely comments that:

The consultant is emphatic. He says it is absolutely the case that the baby cannot be born alive if a Caesarian operation is not carried out. He has described the medical condition. I am not going to go into it in detail because of the pressure of time.[5]

Second, it is most unusual to interfere with people's religious commitments in this way and, given the passing of the Human Rights Act 1998, it is fairly certain that this judgement would not now be made. Article 9 of the European Convention on Human Rights requires states to permit freedom of thought, conscience and religion, with the implication that this also includes the freedom to act on religious commitments. Manifestly, this right would be limited if, for example, X's freedom of religion threatened the life of Y. However, since the fetus – even at full term – is not a person for legal purposes, then this cannot apply. Equally, it is possible that Article 8 of the Convention – the right to respect for private and family life – could be called into play in such situations.

Third, the woman was at no time represented at the hearing, which would also fall foul of Article 6 of the Convention on Human Rights. Finally, the woman was the victim of an assault on her person (again in breach of the Convention, Article 5 – the right to liberty and security of the person) in the interests, in large part, of saving her fetus. Of course, the court was also concerned with the danger to the life of the woman, but as courts have said on numerous occasions, a person is free to decline even life-saving treatment, no matter the reason for that choice, as long as they are competent.[6]

Subsequent cases, such as *St George's Healthcare NHS Trust v S, R v Collins and others, ex parte S*,[7] showed the lengths to which doctors and the law were prepared to go in forcing women to accept medical treatment deemed to be essential to save the fetus. S was diagnosed as suffering from severe pre-eclampsia, and was advised that an early delivery would be needed. She understood that both she and the fetus might die if surgery was not undertaken, but nonetheless refused it. On 26 April 1997 an order had been made which dispensed with her consent to the treatment. She had also been made subject to an order under the Mental Health Act 1983 to be admitted for 'assessment'. No treatment for her alleged depression was offered. S continued to record her extreme objections to the caesarean section. During her time in hospital, '... it was still believed by the psychiatrist who had played a significant part in the decision to admit her to hospital under s 2 that her capacity to consent was intact'.[8] It has already been indicated that a competent adult is free to refuse consent to life-saving treatment. As Lord Mustill said in the case of *Airedale NHS Trust v Bland*:[9]

If the patient is capable of making a decision on whether to permit treatment and decides not to permit it his choice must be obeyed, even if on any objective view it is contrary to his best interests. A doctor has no right to proceed in the face of objection, even if it is plain to all, including the patient, that adverse consequences and even death will or may ensue.[10]

Given that the psychiatrist was willing to state that her competence was not in issue, the decision of the lower court to authorize the section flies in the face of the general rule of law, and was criticized by the Court of Appeal. However, one case had suggested that the only situation in which the law might be different was where '... the choice may lead to the death of a viable fetus'.[11] This, of course, lies at the heart of this matter. As the court in *St George's NHS Trust v S* noted, it is not sufficient simply to ignore the interests of the fetus. But as they also said, in this case there was no conflict between the interests of the mother and the fetus, because '... the procedures to be adopted to preserve the mother and her unborn child did not involve a preference for one rather than the other'.[12]

In addition, the court in this case took a look into the future, noting that it may soon be the case that relatively minor medical intervention on an adult might save the life of an unborn fetus. In contemplating a refusal of consent in such a case, the court said:

The refusal would rightly be described as unreasonable, the benefit to another human life would be beyond value, and the motives of the doctor admirable. If, however, the adult were compelled to agree, or rendered helpless to resist, the principle of autonomy would be extinguished.[13]

Finally, in the context of obstetrical intervention, it is worth restating the words of Butler-Sloss LJ in the case of *Re MB*.[14] In this case she made an obiter explanation of the law as it currently stands:

The fetus up to the moment of birth does not have any separate interests capable of being taken into account when a court has to consider an application for a declaration in respect of a caesarean section operation. The law does not have the jurisdiction to declare that such medical intervention is lawful to protect the interests of the unborn child even at the point of birth.[15]

It would seem, therefore, taking each of these cases into account, that the law is now clear that a competent refusal by a pregnant women of treatment designed to save the life of her fetus (and/or herself) must be respected. This conclusion doubtless will sit uncomfortably with those whose mission is to save life, and particularly uncomfortably given the tendency to view the fetus as a separate entity from the woman. However, there are, as I have suggested, good reasons for the law to adopt this position.

The principle of autonomy permeates our law and our ethics. It is a principle that can be freely exercised as part of our citizenship, subject only to the caveat that it may be restricted when its exercise threatens others. But as courts agreed in the case of *Paton v Trustees of BPAS*[16] – a case in which a man attempted to prevent his wife from terminating a pregnancy – and in *Re F (in utero)*[17] – a case in which an attempt was made to make a fetus a ward of court – the fetus does not have independent legal standing, and its interests cannot serve to outweigh the right of a woman to make autonomous decisions. In the latter case, Balcombe LJ made it clear that it was not for the courts to make such decisions. As he said:

If the law is to be extended in this manner, so as to impose control over the mother of an unborn child, where such control may be necessary for the benefit of that child, then under our system of parliamentary democracy it is for Parliament to decide whether such controls can be imposed and, if so, subject to what limitations or conditions.[18]

That Parliament has declined to do this is a reflection of the interest which we all have in protecting autonomy, even when to do so is emotionally difficult. Just as it is not for judges to change the law, neither is it for doctors to do so.

But it is not just the protection of autonomy which mandates the current legal response. In jurisdictions beyond those of the United Kingdom, decisions – generated by doctors and handed down by courts – have served to demonstrate clearly the dangers of attributing rights to fetuses – and these can arise before the point of labour. Medical understanding of the potential harm that can be caused to developing embryos and fetuses in the course of pregnancy has also resulted in what has been called the aggressive policing of pregnancy. In the USA, for example, Kolder et al.[19] found that of 21 applications for court orders by public hospitals, 86 per cent were successful. Interestingly – and arguably ominously – 81 per cent of the women affected were black, Hispanic or Asian and 24 per cent did not have English as a first language. In addition, 46 per cent of heads of maternal medicine thought that women should be detained when they refused to follow medical advice and thereby endangered their fetuses.

In addition, as Sherman notes:

Pregnant drug abusers have been jailed to keep them free of illegal substances that might harm fetuses. And laws have been expanded so that pregnant women who do ingest drugs harmful to the fetus can be charged with or investigated for child abuse.[20]

Also, of course, medical judgements can be wrong. In *Jefferson v Griffin Spaulding County Hosp. Auth,*[21] a court upheld an order for a forced caesarean section, although in fact the woman delivered naturally. Yet at the time the order was sought, doctors had claimed that vaginal delivery carried a 99 per cent chance of fetal death and a 50 per cent chance of maternal death.

However, perhaps most poignant of all was the case of *In re AC.*[22] It was in fact on this case that the UK judge in *Re S*[23] depended for his authorization of the forced intervention. Interestingly, he appeared to have failed to observe that that case had already been overturned on appeal.[24]

The facts of the case make tragic reading. Angela Carder was a young woman who had suffered from leukaemia as a child. Her condition had gone into remission; she married and became pregnant, but in the course of the pregnancy the leukaemia returned aggressively. It was clear that Angela Carder would die. At about 26½ weeks into the pregnancy, her doctors summoned a judge to the hospital and sought authority to carry out a caesarean section on Mrs Carder, despite her clear refusal to consent. When the case was first heard, the order was granted and the operation proceeded in the face of Mrs Carder's objections. Neither she nor the child survived. In a moving criticism of this judgement, the distinguished American academic George Annas described what had happened as follows:

They [the judges] treated a live woman as though she were already dead, forced her to undergo an abortion and then justified their brutal and unprincipled opinion on the basis that she was almost dead and her fetus's interests in life outweighed any interest that she might have in her own life and health.[25]

Why not intervene?

Despite the temptations to manage pregnancy and childbirth with substantial, if not primary, concern for the welfare of the developing embryo or fetus, it should be clear from consideration of the cases that unthinkingly to adopt such a position is potentially dangerous. In respect of intervening in lifestyle choices during pregnancy, it seems clear that women are being treated differently from other competent adults solely on the basis of their biological capacities. The fact that we generally wish to protect the fetus does not give us a right to do so at the expense of the woman. Equally, since many of the harms likely to be caused will occur in the early stages of pregnancy – when the woman may not even know that she is pregnant – the logical conclusion of this would be that every fertile, sexually active woman would need to behave at all times as if she were pregnant, or run the risk of being accused of harming her fetus, and perhaps even – in the USA at least – of being deprived of her liberty. Equally, as Draper says 'it is one thing to show what a woman ought to do in relation to her unborn child and quite another thing to say that this obligation ought to be enforced'.[26]

Although some authors have suggested that the way forward is through a 'careful balancing of the offspring's welfare and the pregnant woman's interest in liberty and bodily integrity ...',[27] such a balancing act is arguably at best inappropriate and at worst doomed to failure. The very fact of 'balancing' automatically assumes that there are things to be balanced. It has already been agreed that the embryo or fetus of the human species is worthy of some respect, but this is not equivalent to saying that such respect is capable of being weighed in the scales against another person. Even in cases where a born person's life is threatened by the failure of another to undergo medical treatment in their aid, the law is unable to compel submission to treatment. This was clearly seen in one US case. In this case, the defendant refused to consent to a treatment that could have saved the life of the plaintiff. As the judge in that case said:

Morally, this decision rests with the defendant, and in the view of the court, the refusal of the defendant is morally indefensible. For our law to compel the defendant to submit to an intrusion of his body would change every concept and principle upon which our society is founded. To do so would defeat the sanctity of the individual ...[28]

MATERNAL/FETAL CONFLICT

As has been said, the circumstances described above have come to be called maternal/fetal conflict. I have argued elsewhere[29] that this categorization is inherently flawed, not least because it describes the pregnant woman as a 'mother' (which she is not yet) and assumes that conflict is possible. Arguably, conflict implies hostility and yet it is not obvious that a fetus can be hostile to the pregnant women, nor that the pregnant woman's decisions are taken out of hostility for the fetus. Nonetheless, this term has now become an accepted part of the language. Leaving aside these concerns, then, it is worth briefly analysing the implications of this conflict.

As Lew says:

Conflicts between a woman's needs and those of her fetus are vexing because they pit powerful cultural norms against one another; the ideal of autonomy and the ideal of maternal self-sacrifice. Parents who make sacrifices for their children should be encouraged, even lauded, but the law should not require such sacrifices. Self-sacrifice is a gift. Forcing a pregnant woman to sacrifice her health for her fetus is simply slavery.[30]

Nor can it be presumed that it is always possible to measure the risk taken by the woman versus the risk to the fetus of non-intervention. A caesarean section carries risk (albeit that risk is lower given today's standards of medical treatment), but even if the risk is minimal, and the potential benefits to the fetus are considerable, we still do insult to the fundamental principles of law and ethics by compelling women to rescue their fetuses. No such ethical or legal principle is widely recognized and, as has been said, '[e]ven where there is a duty to rescue, the law never requires rescues which jeopardize life and limb'.[31]

CONCLUSION

The developing capacities of modern medicine have served both to enhance the care of pregnant women and to confront them with new dilemmas. The widespread use of prenatal screening makes freedom of reproductive choice both more complex and more intangible. As Gregg has said:

Women's bodies increasingly have become medicalized as fertility testing, techniques of 'assisted conception', prenatal diagnosis, fetal monitoring, induced labor and Cesarean sections have become normal, if not expected, interventions in woman's procreative processes. Procreative technologies can enhance both the range of choices for women and the possibility of greater social control of women's choices.[32]

It is clear that, encouraged by medicine, the law is becoming increasingly intrusive into women's decision-making in the course of their pregnancy. Medicine and the law make powerful allies in this venture, yet their collusion is a direct disavowal of the rights that we otherwise respect. The position in the UK now seems to have been clarified after a decade of highly dubious decisions, at least as far as forced caesarean sections are concerned. However, the impetus that triggered the call for courts to intervene in these decisions has not disappeared. The motivation of those caring for pregnant women is all too intelligible. However, no matter its source – religion, professionalism or whatever – it does violence to other principles which have long been deemed essential to the proper functioning of society. All too often, the motivation for intervention is subliminal, but it is no less a matter of concern for that. As Ikenotos has said:

To the extent that the state invokes the parens patriae *power to prevent harm to the fetus, the state subordinates the interests of the woman to those of the fetus. To the extent that the state regulates pregnant women to promote public health, safety, and morals – an exercise of the police power – it subordinates the interests of the woman to those of the rest of society. In either case, when the state regulates women as childbearers, it legislates the ideology of motherhood.*[33]

It is not necessary to adopt a particular philosophy, such as feminism, to understand the damage done to respect for persons by treating pregnant women with disrespect for their views. To be sure, this does not prevent the legitimate attempt to inform women as to the risks they run both for themselves and for their fetuses if certain decisions are made. However, attempts to enforce the 'right' decision (clinically at least) by resort to the law mark a departure, which should be resisted, from the traditional relationship between doctor and patient. Such a relationship is ideally based on trust, not coercion; on respect, not condemnation. The ability to trace the development of a fetus, and to visualize and monitor it in the womb, is insufficient justification for invading the rights of a live, competent individual, however painful that conclusion may be.

KEY POINTS

- The law is no longer simply a mechanism for judging allegations of negligence, but has taken on the role of standard setter.
- Modern fetal imaging technology has increased the temptation to treat the fetus as a separate patient with unique 'rights'.
- Although the human fetus is worthy of respect, it does not, in law, have rights.
- Occasionally, a woman's decision or behaviour may threaten the survival of an otherwise viable fetus. The law says that if the woman is otherwise legally competent, her wishes must be respected.
- Children are entitled to sue for damage which they sustained prenatally, but this is still not the same as saying that the fetus has rights before birth.
- There have been cases of legally enforced obstetric intervention in the UK but the law has now been made clear: a competent refusal by a pregnant woman of treatment designed to save the life of her fetus (and/or herself) must be respected.
- In the USA, ominously, court-ordered treatment has mainly involved disadvantaged ethnic groups or women who did not have English as their first language.
- Pregnant women should not be treated differently from other competent adults.
- The concept of 'maternal/fetal conflict', in a legal context, is inherently flawed and is best avoided.
- The law and medicine make powerful allies. Attempts by the law to enforce the 'right' clinical decision are a departure from basic legal principles and should be resisted.

KEY REFERENCES

1. Harrison MR. Unborn: historical perspective of the fetus as patient. *The Pharos*, Winter 1982; **19**: 23–4.
2. Hubbard R. Legal and policy implications of recent advances in prenatal diagnosis and therapy. *Women's Rights Law Reporter* Spring 1982; **7**(2):202–15.
3. See, for example, *Review of the Guidance on the Research Use of Fetuses and Fetal Material (Polkinghorne Report)* Cm 762/1989, para. 2.4. 'Central to our understanding is the acceptance of a special status for the living human fetus at every stage of its development which we wish to characterise as a profound respect based on its potential to develop into a fully-formed human being.'
4. Butterworth's Medico-Legal Reports No. 9, p. 69 (1992).
5. Butterworth's Medico-Legal Reports No. 9, p. 70 (1992).
6. See, for example, Re C (adult: refusal of medical treatment) 1994. All England Law Reports No. 1, p. 819: F v West Berkshire Health Authority (Mental health Act Commission intervening) Butterworth's Medico-Legal Reports No. 4, p. 1 (1989).
7. Butterworth's Medico-Legal Reports No. 44, p. 160 (1998).
8. Butterworth's Medico-Legal Reports No. 44, p. 169 (1998).
9. Butterworth's Medico-Legal Reports No. 12, p. 64 (1993).
10. Butterworth's Medico-Legal Reports No. 12, p. 136 (1993).
11. Per Lord Donaldson in Re T (adult: refusal of medical treatment) Butterworth's Medico-Legal Reports No. 9, p. 46 (1992).
12. Butterworth's Medico-Legal Reports No. 9, p. 176 (1992).
13. *id.*
14. Butterworth's Medico-Legal Reports No. 38, p. 175 (1997).
15. Butterworth's Medico-Legal Reports No. 38, p. 186 (1997).
16. All England Law Reports No. 2, p. 987 (1978).
17. All England Law Reports No. 2, p. 193 (1988).
18. All England Law Reports No. 2, p. 200 (1988).
19. Kolder V, Gallagher J, Parsons MT. Court-ordered obstetrical interventions. *N Engl J Med* 1987; **316**:1192.
20. Sherman R. A pyrrhic victory, a court battle: forced Caesarian. *The National Law Journal* January 1989; 16:3.
21. 274 S.E. 2d 457 (Ga 1981).
22. 533 A.2d 611 (D.C. 1987).
23. 533 A.2d 611 (D.C. 1987). Note 4, supra.
24. In re A.C. 573 A.2d 1235 (D.C. 1990).
25. Annas G. She's going to die: the case of Angela C. Volume 18, No 1, Hastings Center Report, 1988, Volume 23, p. 25.

26. Draper H. Women, forced Caesareans and antenatal responsibilities. Working Paper No. 1. Feminist Legal Research Unit, University of Liverpool, 1, 1992, p. 13.

27. Robertson J, Schulman J. Pregnancy and prenatal harm to offspring: the case of mothers with PKU. Volume 17, No. 4, Hastings Center Report, 1987, Volume 23, p. 32.

28. McFall v Shimp (1978) 127 Pitts Leg J 14.

29. McLean SAM. Moral status (who or what counts?). In: Bewley S, Ward RH (eds), *Ethics in Obstetrics and Gynaecology.* London: RCOG Press, 1994, pp. 26–33.

30. Lew JB. Terminally ill and pregnant: state denial of a woman's right to refuse a Caesarean section. *Buffalo Law Review* 1990; 38:619, 621–2.

31. Lew JB. Terminally ill and pregnant: state denial of a woman's right to refuse a Caesarean section. *Buffalo Law Review* 1990; 38 note 30, supra, p. 641.

32. Gregg R. 'Choice' as a double-edged sword: information, guilt and mother-blaming in a high-tech age. *Women and Health* 1993; 20(3):53.

33. Ikenotos LC. Code of perfect pregnancy. *Ohio State Law Journal* 1992; 53:1205, 1284–5.

PART TWO

Obstetrics

PART TWO

Routine Antenatal Care – An Overview

John A.D. Spencer

INTRODUCTION

The antenatal period offers many opportunities to provide targeted health services. Antenatal care became associated with general health evaluation in the UK as a result of the increasing recognition that factors such as nutrition, social conditions and birth spacing influence pregnancy outcome.

The concept of antenatal admission to hospital is attributed to Ballantyne, who was apparently concerned about fetal deformity and stillbirth 100 years ago in Edinburgh. It was after the First World War that interest in maternal well-being

developed. In 1944 the Royal College of Obstetricians and Gynaecologists (RCOG) reported on a National Maternity Service. The National Health Service (NHS) began in 1948 and from then on the pattern of antenatal care – monthly visits to a clinic until 32 weeks, then fortnightly and then weekly visits (see below) – continued broadly unchanged for over 40 years.

A new era in antenatal care began with *Changing Childbirth*, the report of an Expert Maternity Group, published in 1993. At this time, more than 98 per cent of deliveries were in hospital. The main recommendations of the Expert Maternity Group were the need for more choice, better communication and continuity of care. These were accepted as government policy, and so began the first re-organization of antenatal care since its development within the NHS. Not all changes have been evidence based; some have been advocated because of a lack of evidence to support current practice. This chapter describes antenatal care and indicates where evidence is available to support practice.

DEFINITION

Antenatal care embraces:

- maternal health checks,
- evaluation of fetal health and development,
- disease screening,
- analysis of risk for the development of complications, and
- provision of advice and education – antenatal care is intended to facilitate preparation for childbirth and, to some extent, subsequent childcare.

It is now accepted that maternity services should be centred on the woman and her needs. Each woman should be given sufficient help and information to enable her to make an informed decision about her care. In addition to this process of empowerment, communication has become a key factor, not only between health professionals and the woman, but also among the different health professionals providing the service. This is essential for effective team working to provide continuity of care.

COMPONENTS OF ANTENATAL CARE

Table 5.1 lists a number of specific observations and measurements made during pregnancy, along with the reason for

Table 5.1 Components of routine antenatal care in the UK

What and why	When and where	How and who
Prenatal advice Assessment of maternal health Education	Before conception	GP, public awareness, dietician
Diagnosis of pregnancy	Amenorrhoea	Kit, self-testing

First visit
  Education and information
  Identify urgent referral
  Routine referral to maternity services
	GP surgery or clinic	GP or midwife

Early/booking scan
  Confirm dates
  Identify multiple pregnancy
	8–14 weeks	Ultrasound scan

Booking history Assess maternal health Assess risk Education	8–14 weeks Home or clinic	Midwife
Blood pressure Identify hypertension/PET	Booking/early pregnancy and regular intervals	Blood pressure and proteinuria Midwife or healthcare assistant
Midstream urine culture Identify urinary tract infection	Booking/early pregnancy	Midwife
Urinalysis Test for protein and glucose	Booking and regular intervals	Midwife
Down's syndrome test NT/combined/integrated	10–13 weeks (not universally available)	Scan and blood tests
Booking blood tests Infection screen Maternal health screen	10–18 weeks	Blood test
Serum screen for Down's syndrome	16–18 weeks	Blood test
Anomaly scan Fetal anatomy	18–22 weeks	Ultrasound scan
Glucose challenge test Gestational diabetes	24–28 weeks	Glucose tolerance test
Abdominal palpation Uterine size and fetal growth	20–41 weeks, regularly	Symphysis fundal distance Midwife
Fetal movements Fetal hypoxia (chronic)	26–41 weeks	Fetal movements, self-assessment
Blood tests Maternal health screen Fetal risk of Rhesus Isoimmunization Advice on minor symptoms	28 and 34 weeks	Blood test
Abdominal palpation Fetal lie and presentation	36/37 weeks	Midwife

Induction of labour
  Cervical assessment
  Membrane sweep
	41 weeks	Midwife

PET, pre-eclampsia; NT, nuchal translucency.

the task and the application of the method used. It immediately shows the complexity of routine antenatal care, and the overlapping nature of many of the perceived reasons for providing such care.

Antenatal care begins late in the first trimester, at a time when the incidence of miscarriage rapidly declines. Fetal development has already occurred during the first 12 weeks and fetal normality is no longer assumed. Testing strategies aiming to confirm normal fetal development begin at the time of the first (viability) scan and continue until around 20 weeks. Once neonatal viability is reached after 24 weeks, antenatal care focuses more on monitoring maternal and fetal well-being to ensure that deviation from normality is recognized. Blood pressure measurement is the most important maternal observation and is, itself, a diagnostic test as raised blood pressure defines hypertension. Other observations do not give such a clear-cut indication of the problem being looked for.

Screening

Definition of screening

To be effective, screening should lead to identification of a problem in order to allow appropriate intervention. Most tests during pregnancy are considered screening tests and a positive result does not mean the condition is present – rather, a positive result indicates increased risk of the problem being present. The reason for this distinction is that screening tests have a false-positive rate, which means that a proportion of test results are positive when the condition is not present. The effectiveness of a screening test will depend upon whether all the cases with the condition being tested for give a positive result, otherwise some cases will be missed (false-negative result). The detection rate of a screening test describes the proportion of the problem (affected cases) in the population that is actually picked up by the test. It is represented by the proportion of all positive results that are 'true' (ratio of true positives divided by true positives plus false negatives). False-positive results may lead to intervention when the condition is not present.

Information from observations

Recording outpatient cardiotocograph (CTG) traces is an example of an observation commonly used as a test (in this case of fetal well-being) for which benefit has not been shown. However, all practising clinicians are aware of cases in which an outpatient CTG, usually performed in response to maternal concern about fetal activity, has identified chronic fetal hypoxia and resulted in urgent delivery. Thus, as with other observations, confusion has arisen between the true meaning of the observation made versus the clinical predictive value expected – or hoped for. Some observations continue to be used as 'tests' even though the evidence about their routine use either does not exist or does not show benefit.[1,2] Presumably it is believed that not performing such tests would result in greater harm than occurs from the known false positives and false negatives. Many observations have not been studied appropriately to confirm or refute this. Another assumption is that normal observations provide reassurance. This may be the case in the short term, but some studies have shown that 'normal' results may be falsely reassuring.

Maternal health

Social circumstances

Improvements in the standard of living, and general social circumstances, have reduced the need for antenatal care to focus on poor nutrition and poverty. However, poor circumstances still interfere with access to antenatal care, and women with this background still present late for antenatal care. Socially excluded women and their babies are at much higher risk than women in more comfortable circumstances.

Smoking and alcohol (see also Chapters 6.12 and 6.13)

Advice to give up smoking is based on good evidence that doing so is effective [Ia]. If women cease smoking, fewer complications develop during pregnancy. There is less chance of placental abruption, preterm delivery, and fetal cleft lip/palate. The association between maternal smoking and low birth weight is well known. Strategies to reduce maternal smoking during pregnancy have been well studied, and a systematic review is in *The Cochrane Library*.

Alcohol passes across the placenta but there is no good evidence of harm. Although the safe level of alcohol is not known, fetal alcohol syndrome is rare. Women are advised to limit alcohol consumption during pregnancy [II]. The evidence concerning cannabis in pregnancy is insufficient, but it is considered good practice to advise women to discontinue its use during pregnancy.

Supplements and vitamins

Folate supplementation (400 μg up to 3 months before conception) is recommended [Ia] on the basis of strong evidence that the incidence of neural tube defects is reduced (The Cochrane Library). Vitamin A supplements, and liver products, should be avoided in pregnancy. There is insufficient evidence concerning vitamin D (The Cochrane Library), but Asian women are at risk of deficiency.

Food hygiene

Attention to food hygiene is advised in order to avoid food poisoning and the specific effects of some micro-organisms on the pregnancy. Washing salads and fruit (*Toxoplasma*), thorough cooking of meat (*Listeria* and *Salmonella*) and avoiding unpasteurized milk, soft cheese, pâté (*Listeria*) and raw eggs (*Salmonella*) are particularly important. Avoiding cat litter (*Toxoplasma*) and washing hands after gardening (*Toxoplasma*, *Listeria*) are also recommended.

Physical exertion

To continue in employment after 33 weeks of pregnancy, a woman requires a doctor's certificate to indicate that she is fit to do so. Physically demanding work has been associated with poor outcomes, such as preterm birth, pre-eclampsia and low birth weight.[3] Maintenance of normal exercise is encouraged [II] during pregnancy (The Cochrane Library). Sexual intercourse in late pregnancy has not been found to be associated with an increased risk of preterm delivery [Ia].

First antenatal visit (GP or midwife)

This is often a time for confirmation of pregnancy, but general practitioners (GPs) rarely perform pregnancy testing now and women should purchase a testing kit from the chemist. The first day of the last menstrual period, assuming a regular monthly cycle, is used to calculate the estimated date of delivery (EDD) by adding 9 calendar months plus 7 days. Uncertainty about dates or early pregnancy complications are indications for an early ultrasound scan. Antenatal care requires certainty about the EDD in order to determine the timing of routine tests and check-ups.

Urgent referral to maternity services

The main reasons for recommending an early first visit are to check maternal health (see above) and exclude the need for early referral to an obstetrician, usually for prenatal testing. Indications for prenatal testing include sickle cell disease or haemoglobinopathy such as beta-thalassaemia. In such cases the option of chorionic villous sampling (CVS) should be discussed and offered. The point of early testing by 12 weeks is so that suction termination of pregnancy is available if appropriate. If a woman has no intention of terminating an abnormal pregnancy, testing may still be offered for the purpose of obtaining information to reassure her or help her prepare for the delivery of an affected child. However, the risk of miscarriage after CVS may mean that testing is declined, especially if termination is not an option. Such discussions are ideally carried out in a prenatal clinic, before conception, when appropriate blood testing and counselling can occur. Women with some medical conditions, such as diabetes and other conditions requiring medication, should also be referred early.

Routine referral to maternity services

According to the local protocol, the woman is usually directed to a midwife for 'booking' into the local system. The choice of place for delivery and the type of antenatal care available are highly dependent upon local arrangements. Increasingly, a booking history is taken at home, or in the GP surgery. If the GP has identified a pre-existing medical condition, such as insulin-dependent diabetes, asthma, epilepsy or thyroid disease, referral may be directly to a specialist clinic. In some circumstances, midwifery booking can precede attendance at the consultant clinic.

Obstetrics: antenatal

Early pregnancy/booking scan

It is common practice to arrange an ultrasound scan during the late first or early second trimester. This is important for the serum-screening programme for Down's syndrome, which requires an accurate assessment of gestation. The scan is usually arranged before 14 weeks (assessed by dates). Occasionally, gross anomalies will be identified, but the idea of routine scanning in the first trimester for fetal abnormalities is still under research.

Booking (midwife)

History and risk assessment

The primary purpose of the booking history is to identify potential risk factors related to the woman's current or past health. A thorough history, including family history, is essential. Many obstetric units use a family history of diabetes in a first-degree relative as an indication to screen later in pregnancy. Past obstetric history will indicate whether specific risks need to be anticipated. A decision about subsequent care will be governed by the result of this assessment (Table 5.2). A previous normal pregnancy, labour and delivery indicates minimal risk, provided the woman is still under 35 years of age. A pregnancy considered to be at minimal risk is suitable for total midwifery care and may be a candidate for home birth or delivery in a midwife-led unit if these options are available. Currently, however, an evidence base is lacking for risk assessment and the use of selection criteria for booking.[4]

Maternal examination

Assessment of maternal health at booking is guided by the history. General examination needs to note height (short stature is less than 1.50 m) and weight. Obesity should be assessed by body mass index (>29) and is an indication for dietary advice. There is no indication for repeated weighing during pregnancy unless it is part of dietary management. Auscultation of the heart and lungs is not considered necessary in the absence of a relevant medical history.[5] Abdominal examination should look for scars from previous surgery. Pelvic examination is not routine in the absence of complications.

A urine sample should be sent for culture to identify asymptomatic bacteriuria [Ib]. Treatment is effective (The Cochrane Library) and should be offered [Ia]. A history of previous genital tract infection or preterm labour is an indication to culture for pathogenic vaginal flora. Carrier status for group B beta-haemolytic *Streptococcus* is usually an opportunistic finding, and there are insufficient data to recommend routine screening.[6]

Blood pressure
HYPERTENSION
Hypertension – blood pressure (BP) of 140/90 mmHg or above – at booking requires referral to an obstetrician

Table 5.2   Examples of common risk factors at booking and arising during pregnancy

Risk	Suggested action
Maternal health	
Maternal age	
<16 years	Social worker referral
>35 years	Prenatal diagnosis (obstetric clinic)
Short stature	Discuss trial of labour (consultant
(e.g. European <1.5 m)	unit referral)
Obesity (BMI >30 kg/m²)	Dietary advice
Smoking	Reduce
Pre-existing medical condition	Refer to specialist obstetric clinic
and long-term medical treatment	
Hepatitis or HIV positive	Refer to specialist clinic
Past medical history	
Family history of genetic disorder	Refer to specialist clinic
Genital tract surgery or abnormality	
Myomectomy	Obstetric opinion about delivery
Cervical cone biopsy and	Refer by 12 weeks if cervical suture
late termination	to be considered
Anal sphincter surgery	Consider elective casearean section
Past obstetric history	
Five or more previous births	Refer to obstetric unit
Three or more miscarriages	Refer to obstetric unit
Serious complication during:	Refer to obstetric unit
Pregnancy	
Preterm	
Haemorrhage	
Hypertension	
Stillbirth	
Delivery	
Casearean	
Third-degree tear	
Postpartum	
Haemorrhage	
Infection	
Large baby	
Shoulder dystocia	
Neonatal admission	
Neonatal loss	
Present pregnancy	
Hyperemesis gravidarum	Admit
Multiple pregnancy	Refer to obstetric unit
Anaemia (Hb <9 g/dL)	May need transfusion
Any minor symptom persisting	Urgent referral or next clinic as
Significant breathlessness	appropriate
Abdominal pain	
Calf pain/swelling	
Headache	
Vaginal leakage	
Hypertension	Urgent referral to obstetric unit
(BP >140/90 mmHg)	
Haemorrhage after 24 weeks	Admit to obstetric unit
Transverse lie after 36 weeks	Admit to obstetric unit
Concern about fetal movements	Urgent referral to obstetric unit
Not delivered at 41 weeks	Refer to next obstetric clinic

BMI, body mass index; HIV, human immunodeficiency virus; Hb, haemoglobin; BP, blood pressure.

for advice and management; the management of chronic hypertension is discussed in Chapter 6.1. Pregnancy-induced hypertension (PIH) is a benign rise in BP after 20 weeks' gestation (see Chapter 7.6).

Identification of pre-eclampsia requires regular BP checks, use of urinalysis, and measurement of plasma urate (see Chapter 7.6). Oedema no longer forms part of the definition of this condition as it occurs commonly in pregnancy.

Traditional patterns of antenatal care advocated BP testing at 20, 24, 28, 30, 32, 34, 36 weeks and then weekly until delivery. Even with this strategy, some cases of pre-eclampsia are missed; woman may present with symptoms such as headache, epigastric pain, visual disturbance or even eclampsia itself. Recently, models of care with fewer check-ups have been tried, and have shown no increase in adverse outcome (see below). However, the evidence is preliminary. Such practice may lead to an increase in self-testing, of both BP and urine for protein. Urine should be tested for protein whenever BP is measured. Persistent proteinuria is an indication for urgent referral to an obstetric unit.

Booking blood tests

FULL BLOOD COUNT

Haemoglobin is measured [Ib] to assess anaemia (World Health Organization definition <11 g/dL), which, if severe (<7 g/dL), is a risk for maternal morbidity. Referral to an obstetrician is appropriate. Iron deficiency can be confirmed by measuring ferritin. Low values for mean corpuscular volume (MCV), mean corpuscular haemoglobin (MCH) and mean corpuscular haemoglobin concentration (MCHC) are suggestive, but may not occur in the presence of folate deficiency. Alpha-thalassaemia trait may not be distinguishable from mild iron deficiency. Routine iron supplementation has been shown to maintain normal ferritin levels and reduce the likelihood of anaemia, although no benefits during pregnancy have been shown [Ia]. Thrombocytopenia (platelet count $<100 \times 10^9$ L) is also a reason for referral to an obstetrician.

Anaemia complicating pregnancy is discussed further in Chapter 7.1.

BLOOD GROUP AND RED CELL ANTIBODIES

Rhesus status, blood group and red blood cell antibodies should be determined in early pregnancy [Ia]. The presence of red cell antibodies (up to 5 per cent of the population) is a risk factor for haemolytic disease of the newborn. Rhesus-negative blood group is a risk for isoimmunization secondary to contact with rhesus-positive red cells from the fetus. Prophylactic administration of anti-D (currently 1250 IU) is given after potential sensitizing events (delivery, miscarriage, antepartum haemorrhage) and routinely at 28 and 34 weeks of pregnancy [Ia] in non-sensitized women (The Cochrane Library). The presence of atypical red cell antibodies is a reason for referral to an obstetrician (see Chapter 17).

MATERNAL INFECTION SCREENING

Rubella antibodies indicate immunity to infection and therefore negate any risk of congenital rubella syndrome. Seronegative women are identified in order to offer postnatal vaccination. If testing is late (second or third trimester), a positive result may reflect infection in the first trimester of pregnancy.

Syphilis,[7] hepatitis B[8] and human immunodeficiency virus (HIV) screening[9] are advocated because effective treatments are available, either during or after pregnancy. Referral to an obstetric unit is required. There is insufficient evidence to support routine screening for varicella (chicken pox), *Toxoplasma* and human parvovirus B19. A history of possible exposure is an indication for referral to an obstetric unit.

Down's syndrome

Routine screening tests and counselling for anomaly screening are discussed in Chapter 10.

It should be self-evident that appropriate education and counselling about all tests is required during early pregnancy. In particular, the idea of screening for fetal abnormalities with tests that are not diagnostic requires an understanding of the implications of false-negative and false-positive results.

Fetal anomaly scan

An ultrasound scan of the fetus is offered between 18 and 22 weeks to check for major anomalies. This has become known as 'the 20-week scan'. The RCOG[10] has issued guidance with regard to the standard of this scan. About 2 per cent of pregnancies have an abnormality. The detection rate varies between 15 and 80 per cent according to the anomaly present and its severity (see Chapter 10.2).

Glucose tolerance testing

Impaired glucose tolerance occurs in pregnancy, and may be sufficient to merit the term 'gestational diabetes mellitus' (GDM). A number of proposals have been made regarding diagnosis, with advocates for the use of a 75 g or 100 g carbohydrate oral tolerance test (or 'challenge'). After a normal fasting result (upper limit 5.3–5.8 mmol/L), cut-off values of blood glucose at 2 hours are 8.6 or 9.2 mmol/L.[11] Controversy exists over the different proposals for screening, indicating the lack of evidence for routine testing (see Chapter 7.5).

Uterine palpation

Fetal growth monitoring

Fetal growth monitoring is intended to identify cases where the fetus is small or large. Fetal growth restriction (FGR) carries a risk of hypoxia in labour, due to placental insufficiency. A large fetus is at risk of shoulder dystocia. Clinical palpation of the abdomen and measurement of the symphysis – fundal distance are equally effective at predicting the extremes of fetal size at the end of pregnancy. Limited data suggest that there is no difference in outcomes with the use

Obstetrics: antenatal

of either method as routine (The Cochrane Library). Charts exist by which symphysis–fundal measurements can be compared with population data. Use of the value obtained at 20 weeks may help in the interpretation of values later in pregnancy.

Indications for an ultrasound scan

Clinical concern about fetal size or growth is an indication for an ultrasound scan. The risk factors for FGR should be evaluated by an obstetrician. Routine assessment of fetal growth by ultrasound scan in the third trimester of low-risk pregnancies is not effective in identifying differences in pregnancy outcome (The Cochrane Library) and is not recommended [Ia]. Similarly, routine use of Doppler ultrasound examination of the umbilical artery did not alter pregnancy outcome when there were no risk factors present (The Cochrane Library) and is therefore not recommended [Ia].

Abnormal fetal lie and presentation

Ascertainment of a longitudinal lie and cephalic presentation seems appropriate by 36 weeks' gestation, although no testing of this has been reported. Breech presentation prior to 36 weeks is not uncommon. The management of breech presentation after 36 weeks is discussed in Chapter 35. Transverse lie is an indication for admission to an obstetric unit for further investigation and planned delivery.

Fetal movements

Normal fetal activity during the third trimester is an indication of adequate fetal oxygenation. A large trial using movement charts[1] found no reduction in late pregnancy stillbirths when the further management was by CTG. There are a large number of 'false-positive' alarms but the technique is simple. Women who are concerned about inadequate fetal movements will report for further investigation, but the appropriate strategy appears to be lacking. A normal CTG may be falsely reassuring. One trial showed a reduction in stillbirths at the expense of increased operative intervention,[12] but further research is required. Biological variations in fetal activity, including the now well-described fetal 'rest – activity' behavioural cycle, need to be taken into account when interpreting concerns about fetal activity.

Minor symptoms of pregnancy

A number of minor and physiological changes to body function occur during pregnancy. These sometimes cause anxiety and need to be differentiated from more serious conditions.

Gastrointestinal

Early effects of pregnancy on the gastrointestinal system are well recognized. Nausea and vomiting are common, and may be helped by an antihistamine. Hyperemesis gravidarum needs to be identified and requires referral for inpatient assessment and management. Later in pregnancy, gastric reflux and oesophagitis result from relaxation of the gastric sphincter associated with increasing abdominal pressure. Antacids can be helpful, and meals can be smaller and more frequent. Constipation is also common, due to the relaxant effects of progesterone. Fibre supplements and osmotic laxatives such as lactulose may help.

Cardiovascular

Headaches and occasional fainting can occur as the body adapts to the increasing blood volume and fall in vascular resistance. Persistent headache in the late second and third trimesters may be an indication of pre-eclampsia. Palpitations are not common, but short episodes associated with posture change are unlikely to be serious. The supine position should be avoided in the third trimester to prevent supine aorto-caval hypotension. Varicose veins are common, as are haemorrhoids. There are no preventative measures. Support tights may help the symptoms of varicose veins, and frequent short periods of rest, lying laterally, may help.

Respiratory

Dyspnoea of pregnancy may increase during pregnancy, but does not usually cause concern. Significant breathlessness should always be checked in order to exclude infection, asthma, heart failure or pulmonary emboli.

Musculoskeletal

Carpal tunnel syndrome and ulnar nerve compression often cause hand symptoms late in pregnancy, associated with oedema. Analgesia and advice on posture are appropriate. Splinting is not usually required. Backache often develops during the third trimester and should be managed by advice on posture. Pubic symphysis diastasis may require strong analgesia. Leg cramps are common and may indicate overheating of the legs at night. A deep vein thrombosis must be excluded if calf pain persists. Oedema of the lower legs is common.

Genitourinary

Frequency of micturition is common as term approaches, due to pressure of the fetal head on the bladder. Dysuria is an indication for a urine culture. Vaginal discharge is usually mucoid and should not be watery. However, profuse discharge often creates a feeling described as 'being wet', which needs to be distinguished from liquor leakage. Vulval irritation is commonly the result of *Candida* infection and requires appropriate treatment. Vulval ulceration should be checked if there is vulval pain. Herpes is an indication for referral to an obstetrician to discuss mode of delivery.

Skin

Minor rashes and irritations are common, but pruritus is a symptom of cholestasis, and liver function tests should be checked.

Routine induction of labour

By 40 weeks' gestation, less than 60 per cent of women have delivered. Routine induction of labour is not indicated before 41 weeks. By 42 weeks, less than 20 per cent of women remain undelivered, and evidence suggests a rise in the rate of stillbirths. Further evidence has shown that routine induction of labour is less costly and results in a lower caesarean section rate than conservative management with monitoring (The Cochrane Library) [Ia] (see Chapter 25).

ORGANIZATION OF ANTENATAL CARE

Traditional model

Early formalization of antenatal care after the Second World War recommended a minimum of monthly check-ups until 28 weeks, fortnighty check-ups until 36 weeks and then weekly visits until labour. The first visit to the GP would ideally be by 12 weeks. Subsequent care would be according to a risk evaluation performed at the booking clinic. Full (hospital) care, shared care (between hospital and GP) and community care (between community midwife and GP) were the usual options. Community care was often linked to deliveries booked into a 'GP unit', either separate from or co-located with a consultant delivery unit.

New models

One of the earliest changes in recent years was a small reduction in the number of antenatal visits without evidence of an adverse effect (The Cochrane Library). Most studies suggest extending the intervals between check-ups. Whilst there is a suggestion that fewer visits may be associated with a reduction in women's satisfaction with the care received, more women would choose the same care again.[13] Other changes in the provision of antenatal care during recent years include the recognition that uncomplicated pregnancies, and those without risk, do not need to be seen by a consultant obstetrician (The Cochrane Library) [Ia]. Continuity of care provided by a group of midwives is associated with lower intervention rates and beneficial psychosocial outcomes. It is recommended that women carry their own pregnancy record [Ia].

Increasingly, antenatal care for women with uncomplicated pregnancies is being provided in the community, which has resulted in a reduction in the number of women attending hospital antenatal clinics. The quality of care provided to women with complications has increased as a result of the greater time available.

KEY POINTS

- Antenatal care has changed in the last 10 years, with an emphasis on better communication, more care outside hospital, and more care provided by midwives.
- Antenatal care involves checking maternal health and fetal well-being, assessing risk factors, screening for disease and abnormalities and providing education and advice.
- Screening involves false-negative and false-positive results. Some observations have not been fully evaluated in this respect.
- Women are advised about lifestyle matters such as smoking and alcohol use. Social circumstances are still important, and deprived women who book late (or not at all) are at greatest risk.
- At the first visit, women who require urgent referral should be identified.
- An early ultrasound scan for dating can be very helpful.
- Booking involves a detailed history, measurement of weight and height and urine analysis.
- Blood pressure checks are important, but even frequent measurements cannot prevent some unexpected cases of symptomatic pre-eclampsia.
- Full blood count, blood grouping and rhesus status and blood screening for some infections are all recommended.
- Serum screening and ultrasound screening for Down's syndrome are widely available, and research is continuing on combining these methods. Full counselling is essential.
- RCOG guidance has been published concerning the 20-week fetal anomaly scan.
- Controversy exists over the best method of screening for impaired glucose tolerance in pregnancy.
- Abdominal palpation will detect the extremes of abnormal fetal growth. The lie and presentation should be checked at 36 weeks.
- Self-reporting of fetal movements as a test of fetal well-being is simple but has a high false-positive rate.
- Minor symptoms of pregnancy should be treated and should be differentiated from symptoms of serious disease.
- Routine induction of labour at 41 weeks is not justified, but at 42 weeks results in lower rates of casearean section and stillbirth.

ACKNOWLEDGEMENTS

The author wishes to acknowledge assistance from the Clinical Evidence Support Unit, Royal College of Obstetricians and Gynaecologists (Dr Jane Thomas, Director) while he was chairman of the RCOG Multiprofessional Evidence-based Guideline Group looking at Antenatal Care for the Healthy Woman. The group was discontinued in 2002, when production of this guideline was taken over by the National Institute for Clinical Evidence.

KEY REFERENCES

1. Grant A, Elbourne D, Valentin L, Alexander S. Routine formal fetal movement counting and risk of antepartum late death in normally formed singletons. *Lancet* 1989; 2:345–9.
2. Spencer JAD. Assessment of fetal well-being in late pregnancy. In: Edmonds DK (ed.), *Dewhurst's Textbook of Obstetrics and Gynaecology for Postgraduates*. Oxford: Blackwell Science, 1999, 119–33.
3. Mozurkewich E, Luke B, Avni M, Wolf F. Working conditions and adverse pregnancy outcome: a meta-analysis. *Obstet Gynecol* 2000; **95**:623–35.
4. Campbell R. Review and assessment of selection criteria used when booking pregnant women at different places of birth. *Br J Obstet Gynaecol* 1999; **106**:550–6.
5. Hall MH. Prepregnancy and antenatal care. In: Chamberlain G, Steer P (eds), *Turnbull's Obstetrics*. London: Churchill Livingstone, 2001, 105–16.
6. ACOG Committee Opinion (Number 173). Prevention of early-onset group B streptococcal disease in newborns. Committee on Obstetric Practice, American College of Obstetricians and Gynecologists. *Int J Gynecol Obstet* 1996; **54**:197–205.
7. Public Health Laboratory Service. *Antenatal Syphilis Screening in the UK: a Systematic Review and National Options Appraisal with Recommendations*. Report to the National Screening Committee. London: 1998.
8. Department of Health. *Screening of Pregnant Women for Hepatitis B and Immunisation of Babies at Risk*. Health Services Circular Number 127. London: HMSO, 1998.
9. NHS Executive. *Reducing Mother to Baby Transmission of HIV*. Health Services Circular Number 183. London: HMSO, 1999.
10. Royal College of Obstetricians and Gynaecologists *Ultrasound Screening for Fetal Abnormalities*. RCOG Working Party. London: RCOG Press, 1997.
11. Metzger BE and the organizing committee of the Third International Workshop Conference on Gestational Diabetes Mellitus. Summary and recommendations. *Diabetes* 1991; **40**:197–201.
12. Neldam S. Fetal movements as an indicator of fetal well-being. *Dan Med Bull* 1983; **30**:274–8.
13. Carroli G, Villar J, Piaggio G, et al. WHO systematic review of randomised controlled trials of routine antenatal care. *Lancet* 2001; **348**:213–18.

SECTION A

Antenatal complications: maternal

Chronic Hypertension

Andrew Shennan

MRCOG standards

Relevant standards
- Conduct pre-pregnancy counselling to a level expected in independent primary care.
- Conduct booking visit, including assessment of intercurrent disease.
- Diagnose and plan management with appropriate consultation in the following conditions: hypertension.

  In addition, we would suggest the following.

Theoretical skills
- Define chronic hypertension.
- Describe the aetiological causes of chronic hypertension.
- Understand the relationship between chronic hypertension and pregnancy pathology.

Practical skills
- Be able to recognize and diagnose the secondary causes of hypertension.
- Know how to manage moderate hypertension in pregnancy.

INTRODUCTION

Pre-existing hypertension will affect between 1 and 2 per cent of women of reproductive age. Some of these women will be on long-term treatment that may have implications for pregnancy. It is not unusual for hypertension unrelated to the pregnancy to be first diagnosed when these women attend their antenatal clinics. In addition, women who have underlying hypertension are at increased risk of developing pre-eclampsia and its sequelae. Women who present with hypertension in pregnancy must have other causes considered, and an understanding of the aetiology and management is essential to the obstetrician.

DEFINITION

Chronic hypertension is defined as the presence of persistent hypertension, of whatever cause, before the 20th week of pregnancy (in the absence of a hydatidiform mole), or persistent hypertension beyond 6 weeks postpartum.

As hypertension is a continuous variable, there is no standard definition to indicate the point at which adverse events occur. In non-pregnant individuals there is a steady and linear increased risk of future cardiovascular morbid events, directly proportional to both systolic and diastolic blood pressures. Generally, a sustained blood pressure greater than 140/90 mmHg is deemed hypertensive, but the significance of this will depend on the clinical situation, such as the individual's age and other risk factors such as smoking and hyperlipidaemia. Anti-hypertensive treatment is known to reduce the risk of later coronary heart disease (by approximately 16 per cent) and stroke (by 38 per cent) [Ia].

AETIOLOGY

Overall, approximately 95 per cent of hypertension is known as primary or essential hypertension; 5 per cent is secondary, usually related to underlying renal or adrenal disease. However, the incidence of secondary hypertension is increased in the age group of women attending the antenatal clinic. Renal disease may be directly due to glomerulonephritis or tubulo-interstitial disease, such as that due to reflux pyelonephritis or stones. Renal artery stenosis can also cause renal hypertension. Endocrine causes include Cushing's syndrome, Conn's syndrome, phaeochromocytoma and thyroid disease.

MANAGEMENT

Preconception, assessment and counselling

A woman who is found to be hypertensive prior to pregnancy can be advised about appropriate anti-hypertensive therapy suitable for pregnancy and about other life modifications that can be made prior to conception. It is known that a high body mass index (BMI) is associated with increased blood pressure, and that weight loss may reduce hypertension [II]. In addition, it has also been shown that both salt and alcohol intake are associated with high blood pressure, and moderation of both is advised in hypertensive individuals [II]. Generally speaking, hypertensive individuals are asymptomatic, but a careful history needs to be taken in order to identify any relevant symptoms and to exclude possible genetic causes of renal disease, such as autosomal dominant polycystic kidneys.

The type of anti-hypertensive taken should be considered, and it is generally recommended that both diuretics and angiotensin-converting enzyme (ACE) inhibitors be changed to alternative anti-hypertensive agents [III].

A physical examination should include calculation of the BMI as well as fundoscopy to look for evidence of arterial disease. Although rare, possible causes of secondary hypertension should be sought. Bruits in the renal artery or a systolic murmur in association with delayed femoral pulses could indicate coarctation of the aorta. On abdominal examination, polycystic kidneys may be palpable. Retinal changes associated with hypertension include mild vessel tortuousity, silver wiring and arteriovenous nipping. If severe, retinal haemorrhages may be seen in association with hard exudates, cotton-wool spots and papilloedema.

Women who are found to be hypertensive pre-pregnancy or in early pregnancy should have circulating levels of urea and electrolytes checked, urine analysis, and a 24-hour urine collection for protein and creatinine clearance performed. Women with severe hypertension or proteinuria should have a chest X-ray, electrocardiogram (ECG) and antinuclear antibody testing. If there is a long history of severe hypertension, cardiac function should be assessed with an echocardiogram. Investigations of lupus anticoagulant and anticardiolipin antibodies should be performed if there is a history of thromboembolic events or recurrent pregnancy loss.

Glomerulonephritis, polycystic kidney or chronic pyelonephritis may be suggested by haematuria and microscopic proteinuria identified on dipstick testing of the urine. High sodium will be apparent in those individuals with primary hyperaldosteronism (Conn's syndrome). Low sodium can be caused by high doses of diuretics. Potassium is usually low in Conn's syndrome or high in those with renal failure. Some ACE inhibitors or potassium-sparing diuretics can cause hypocalcaemia.

A raised urea or creatinine may indicate renal impairment and a renal cause of hypertension. Chronic renal failure can also result in low serum calcium, although primary hyperparathyroidism can be associated with hypertension and this results in elevated calcium levels.

Young women with chronic hypertension usually require referral for more detailed investigation, which may include baseline ECG and serum lipids to ascertain future risk. Women who have paroxysmal or severe hypertension, particularly associated with sweating or palpitations, need a 24-hour collection for catecholamine metabolites to exclude a phaeochromocytoma. In those cases in which Cushing's syndrome is considered, a 24-hour collection of urinary free cortisol may be taken. Determinations of plasma aldosterone or cortisol and adrenocorticotrophic hormone (ACTH) concentrations are occasionally helpful in identifying particularly uncommon causes of secondary hypertension. If indicated by biochemistry results, renal imaging or angiography may also be performed.

THERAPEUTIC CONSIDERATIONS OF PRE-EXISTING MEDICATIONS
(see also Chapter 8)

Diuretics

Thiazide diuretics are still used (although usually in older patients) as a primary treatment of hypertension in non-pregnant individuals as they are both cheap and easy to use with a once-daily dose. It is generally believed that diuretics should be avoided in pregnancy as they act by increasing renal excretion of sodium and water, which will reduce blood volume, and this is unlikely to be a desirable physiological effect in pregnancy [IV].[1] However, direct evidence of harm is limited.

Angiotensin-converting enzyme inhibitors

These anti-hypertensives act on the rennin–angiotensin–aldosterone system and are increasingly used in individuals with uncomplicated hypertension. However, they are associated with renal toxicity in the fetus[2] and should be avoided in pregnancy [III]. If possible, it is desirable to change to another medication pre-pregnancy or as soon as pregnancy is diagnosed [III].

Other anti-hypertensive agents

There have been some reports that beta-blockers are associated with intrauterine growth restriction [Ib].[3] For this reason, they are usually avoided if an appropriate alternative can be used. Other anti-hypertensives, calcium channel blockers, centrally acting drugs such as methyldopa and labetalol (a combined alpha and beta blocker) have all been used in pregnancy. *There is no significant advantage of one over another* and individuals can continue this therapy into pregnancy, if necessary. The drug with the longest, most established safety profile is methyldopa; both neonatal and longer-term outcome data have been assessed and no detrimental effects have been demonstrated with its use [Ib].[4] As methyldopa can cause depression and tiredness and, very occasionally, liver dysfunction, new anti-hypertensives such as labetalol are increasingly being used [IV].

MATERNAL ASSESSMENT

Once pregnant, the woman with underlying chronic hypertension should be closely monitored for the development of pre-eclampsia. In some studies, as many as one in five women with chronic hypertension have been shown to develop pre-eclampsia [III].[5,6] Uterine artery Doppler velocity waveforms have been used to assess risk in these individuals.[7] It is important to ensure that women have a strict antenatal schedule and that blood pressure and urine analysis are checked at least every 2 weeks [IV]. Even women who do not develop overt signs of pre-eclampsia appear to be at increased risk.[8]

In the chronically hypertensive woman, as in the normotensive woman, pregnancy is associated with a physiological rise in blood pressure, but a sudden and profound increase should alert the clinician to the possibility of pre-eclampsia. For this reason, as blood pressure measurement cannot be relied upon to identify pre-eclampsia, urinalysis is particularly important. Measurement of platelets and uric acid may help identify those individuals who are going to develop the clinical manifestations of pre-eclampsia, as abnormalities may pre-date proteinuria by some weeks [II].

The second commonest complication is a placental abruption (see Chapter 23); the incidence of placental abruptions is 2–10 per cent in women with chronic hypertension.

MANAGEMENT OF MATERNAL HYPERTENSION

There is considerable debate as to whether women who have moderate hypertension (140/90–160/100 mmHg) should have anti-hypertensive treatment. There are 24 randomized control trials evaluating anti-hypertensives in moderate hypertension in pregnancy. However, the total number of women studied is less than 4000. Treatment is associated with a reduction in severe hypertension (by approximately one-half) [Ia].[9] However, there is no significant difference in the incidence of pre-eclampsia or change in perinatal mortality, preterm birth rate or small for gestational age [Ia].

Different drugs have been compared in 17 randomized, control trials with just over 1000 women, and it was shown that no one drug has a clear advantage over another. Therefore, it remains unclear whether anti-hypertensive drug therapy for mild to moderate hypertension during pregnancy is worthwhile [Ia]. Certain investigators have suggested, through careful analysis of data from these trials, that the babies of those individuals who are treated may be slightly smaller [III].[10] This has led certain practitioners to advocate cessation of anti-hypertensive treatment in pregnancy for women with mild/moderate hypertension [IV].[11] If therapy is discontinued, blood pressure should be rigorously monitored (day case assessment units may be the optimal environment for this), and treatment will need to be re-instigated in a substantial minority of women.

Severe hypertension (blood pressure >170/110 mmHg) requires immediate treatment to prevent the risk of stroke and to reduce other morbidity (see Chapter 7.6) [II].[12]

Women with severe chronic hypertension should be carefully monitored for at least 48 hours after delivery, as they are at risk of developing renal failure, pulmonary oedema and hypertensive encephalopathy.

- The treatment of moderate hypertension in pregnancy is associated with a significant reduction in severe hypertension.
- Anti-hypertensive treatment in pregnancy does not influence the perinatal mortality rate or the subsequent development of pre-eclampsia.

KEY POINTS

- Diuretics and ACE inhibitors should be stopped or changed pre-pregnancy or at early gestation.
- Women with hypertension first diagnosed in early pregnancy should be investigated for secondary causes.
- Chronic hypertension is associated with an increased risk of pre-eclampsia.
- Superimposed pre-eclampsia may be diagnosed by identifying proteinuria on urinalysis; raised uric acid levels or falling platelet counts may be the first indication of risk.

KEY REFERENCES

1. Sibai BM, Grossman RA, Grossman HG. Effects of diuretics on plasma volume in pregnancies with long-term hypertension. *Am J Obstet Gynecol* 1984; 150:831–5.

2. Thorpe-Beeston JG, Armar NA, Dancy M, Cochrane GW, Ryan G, Rodeck CH. Pregnancy and ACE inhibitors. *Br J Obstet Gynaecol* 1993; **1000**(7):692–3.

3. Butters L, Kennedy S, Rubin PC. Atenolol in essential hypertension in pregnancy. *BMJ* 1990; **301**:587–9.

4. Cockburn J, Moar VA, Ounsted M, Redman CW. Final report of study on hypertension in pregnancy: the effects of specific treatment on the growth and development in children. *Lancet* 1982; **1**(8273):647–9.

5. Rey E, Couturier A. The prognosis of pregnancy in women with chronic hypertension. *Am J Obstet Gynecol* 1994; **171**:410–16.

6. Sibai BM, Lindheimer M, Hauth J et al. Risk factors for preeclampsia, abruptio placentae, and adverse neonatal outcomes among women with chronic hypertension. National Institute of Child Health and Human Development Network of Maternal–Fetal Medicine Units. *N Engl J Med* 1998; **339**:667–71.

7. Frusca T, Soregaroli M, Zanelli S, Danti L, Guandalini F, Valcamonico A. Role of uterine artery Doppler investigation in pregnant women with chronic hypertension. *Eur J Obstet Gynecol Reprod Biol* 1998; **79**:47–50.

8. McCowan LM, Buist RG, North RA, Gamble G. Perinatal morbidity in chronic hypertension. *Br J Obstet Gynaecol* 1996; **103**:123–9.

9. Abalos E, Duley L, Steyn DW, Henderson-Smart DJ. Antihypertensive drug therapy for mild to moderate hypertension during pregnancy (Cochrane Review). In: *The Cochrane Library*, Issue 2. Oxford: Update Software, 2002.

10. Magee LA, Ornstein MP, von Dadelszen P. Management of hypertension in pregnancy. *BMJ* 1999; **318**:1332–6.

11. Sibai BM. Diagnosis and management of chronic hypertension in pregnancy. *Obstet Gynecol* 1991; **78**:451–61.

12. Sibai BM. Treatment of hypertension in pregnant women. *N Engl J Med* 1996; **335**:257–65.

Diabetes Mellitus

Justin C. Konje

INTRODUCTION

Diabetes mellitus is defined as a carbohydrate disturbance characterized by hyperglycaemia and either peripheral insulin resistance or insulin deficiency. There are two types of diabetes mellitus – insulin-dependent diabetes mellitus (IDDM) and non-insulin-dependent diabetes mellitus (NIDDM). The former is also known as type-1 diabetes, the latter as type-2 diabetes. Patients with IDDM (type-1 diabetes) have an absolute deficiency of insulin, whereas type-2 diabetics have a peripheral resistance to insulin and are unable to compensate for this resistance by increasing insulin production. Whereas there may be serological evidence of autoimmune destruction of the pancreatic islets and genetic markers in type-1 diabetics, type-2 diabetics may be hyperglycaemic for long periods without clinical symptoms. This is because although there is hyperglycaemia, high circulating insulin may prevent the early development of complications of hyperglycaemia. This type of diabetes may therefore be identified for the first time during pregnancy as the diabetogenic effects of pregnancy increase the hyperglycaemia and its consequences. The symptoms of diabetes mellitus are closely related to the degree of hyperglycaemia. These include polydipsia, polyuria, weight loss, recurrent vulval boils and blurred vision. These symptoms are more common outside pregnancy.

Diabetes mellitus complicates about 1–2 per cent of all pregnancies. It is associated with a high perinatal morbidity and mortality. Prior to the introduction of insulin, perinatal mortality from this complication was of the order of 65 per cent. This has, however, fallen drastically with the introduction of medical obstetric clinics – to a level almost equal to that in non-diabetics provided glycaemic control is good and tight.

CARBOHYDRATE METABOLISM IN PREGNANCY

During pregnancy, there is a significant alteration in glucose homeostasis secondary to the complex hormonal changes and increased metabolic demands of the gravid uterus, its contents and the mother. The rise in the hormones that alter this metabolism is largely responsible for the altered homeostasis. These hormones include oestrogens, progesterone, human placental lactogen and cortisol.

Human placental lactogen, a polypeptide produced by the syncytiotrophoblast, induces lipolysis in the adipose tissue. This results in the production of glycerol and fatty acids, which are used as a source of energy by the mother. Consequently, glucose uptake into the cells is inhibited and the spared glucose is made available to the fetus. During pregnancy, human placental lactogen production rises with gestation, and the diabetogenic effects of this hormone increase progressively. Most pregnant women will counteract this antagonistic action by increasing the production of insulin. However, in those with peripheral resistance or deficient production, the compensatory mechanism is inadequate. The placenta not only produces diabetogenic hormones, but also breaks down insulin. This degradation hastens the elimination of available insulin for glucose homeostasis. As a consequence of these diabetogenic hormones, the insulin production during pregnancy has been demonstrated to increase significantly from the second trimester through to term, so that the levels at the end of pregnancy are twice those in the early second trimester.

During pregnancy, there is an increase in glomerular filtration rate as a result of increased renal blood flow. This increase results in an increase in the amount of glucose delivered to the kidneys. Associated with this is a reduction in the renal threshold for glucose. In the non-pregnant woman, the total urine glucose excretion rarely exceeds 0.55 mmol/24 hours, but during pregnancy, about a third of women excrete more than 5.5 mmol/24 hours [II].[1] Since most commonly available commercial glucose oxidase/peroxide paper strips have a sensitivity of approximately 5.5 mmol/L, they will identify glycosuria in between 5 and 50 per cent of the pregnant population, depending on the timing and frequency of testing. The routine use of urinalysis for the monitoring of glycaemic control during pregnancy is therefore unreliable.

Physiological changes that may affect diabetes mellitus in pregnancy

- Reduced threshold for glucose and increased glomerular filtration rate results in glycosuria occurring in 5–50 per cent of women.
- Glycose homeostasis is altered by:
  - human placental lactogen-induced lipolysis,
  - placental degradation of insulin.

CLASSIFICATION OF DIABETES

Although the most commonly accepted classification of diabetes mellitus in pregnancy is that described above, the historical classification of White[2] [IV] is still used by some experts.

White classified diabetes into six categories:

A Asymptomatic, but abnormal glucose tolerance test (the WHO equivalent of impaired glucose intolerance).

B Onset age ≥20 years, duration <10 years, no vascular complications.

C Onset age 10–19 years, duration 10–19 years, no vascular complications.

D Onset age <10 years, duration ≥20 years, vascular disease, benign retinopathy and leg artery calcification.

E Nephropathy.

F Proliferative retinopathy.

DIAGNOSIS OF DIABETES MELLITUS IN PREGNANCY

The onset of IDDM is commonly between the ages of 11 and 14 years and therefore, for most IDDM patients, the diagnosis will have been made prior to pregnancy. In some cases, however, the diagnosis may not have been made; screening may not have been performed despite the presence of symptoms. In this group of women, the diagnosis is often suspected on clinical symptoms, significant hyperglycaemia and not uncommonly ketoacidosis.

Screening strategies for identifying diabetes in pregnancy are described in Chapter 10.1. Where diabetes is suspected, extreme care must be exercised before subjecting the patient to a glucose tolerance test. This is because of the risk of inducing hyperglycaemia, with its attendant complications. In such patients, therefore, serial blood glucose estimation and a glycosylated haemoglobin estimation will be useful in making the diagnosis.

In 1997, an Expert Committee on the Diagnosis and Classification of Diabetes Mellitus defined the criteria for the diagnosis [IV].[3] These criteria are summarized below.

Diagnosis of diabetes mellitus

- Symptoms of diabetes plus casual plasma glucose of ≥11.1 mmol/L. Casual is defined as any time of the day without regard to the time since the last meal.
- Fasting plasma glucose of ≥7.0 mmol/L. Fasting is defined as no caloric intake for at least 8 hours.
- 2-hour plasma glucose of ≥11.1 mmol/L during an oral glucose tolerance test. The test should be performed following a 75 g glucose load.

PREGNANCY COMPLICATIONS OF PRE-EXISTING DIABETES

Various physiological and hormonal changes of pregnancy have a significant effect on diabetes in pregnancy, and can exacerbate complications of diabetes such as nephropathy and retinopathy. Deteriorations in these conditions tend to revert to normal after delivery.

Complications of pregnancy consequent upon pre-existing diabetes are commonly separated into maternal and fetal.

Maternal effects

Exacerbation of pre-existing disease
RETINOPATHY

During pregnancy, the risk of progression of the retinopathy is more than doubled [II].[4] Although the progress of the retinopathy may be influenced by diabetic control, progression may still occur despite a tight control [II].[5] The changes that may occur include neovascularization, streak-blob haemorrhages, soft exudates and vaso-occlusive lesions associated with the development of macular oedema. During pregnancy, all women with IDDM should have an ophthalmic assessment, as some of these changes may occur in patients without prior retinopathy. Fortunately, most of these changes revert soon after delivery.

NEPHROPATHY

Approximately 5–10 per cent of people with IDDM suffer from nephropathy and present with reduced creatinine clearance and proteinuria. In pregnancy, proteinuria may represent diabetic nephropathy or may occur in pre-eclampsia. There is very little evidence for a permanent deterioration of diabetic renal disease as a result of pregnancy [II].[6]

CARDIAC DISEASE

Pregnancy exacerbates the problem of women whose diabetes is complicated by ischaemic heart disease. For those with a previous myocardial infarction, the mortality in pregnancy exceeds 50 per cent [II].[7] Circulatory and cardiovascular changes in pregnancy are responsible for the deterioration in the cardiac function in these patients. It is therefore important to undertake a careful assessment of the cardiac function in such cases, in conjunction with a cardiologist – ideally, before they embark on a pregnancy.

Late pregnancy complications
Pregnancy-induced hypertension and pre-eclampsia are discussed in Chapter 7.6.

Intrapartum complications
The major risks are related to operative morbidity, consequent on fetal macrosomia and obstructed labour.

Maternal complications of diabetes mellitus

- Retinopathy
- Nephropathy
- Cardiac disease
- Pregnancy-induced hypertension including pre-eclampsia
- Recurrent vulvo-vaginal infections (thrush, boils)
- Increased incidence of operative deliveries (forceps, ventouse and caesarean section)
- Obstructed labour

Fetal effects

Congenital malformations
These depend on the degree of glycaemia and its timing. Where there is optimal control pre-pregnancy, at conception and in the first trimester, the rate approximates to that of uncomplicated pregnancies [II].[8] However, the malformation rate in pregnancies complicated by diabetes is typically about five to ten times that in non-diabetics [II].[9–11] These malformations characteristically affect the central nervous, cardiovascular, skeletal, gastrointestinal and genitourinary systems. The common malformations include transposition of the great vessels, ventricular septal defects, atrial septal defects, hypoplastic left ventricle and situs inversus (cardiovascular); neural tube defects, holoprosencephaly and microcephaly (central nervous); caudal regression or sacral agenesis (skeletal); renal agenesis, polycystic kidneys and double ureters (renal) and tracheo-oesophageal fistula, bowel atresia and imperforate anus (gastrointestinal).

Late pregnancy complications
These are related to the degree of glycaemic control and include polyhydramnios, stillbirths, preterm labour and fetal macrosomia. *Polyhydramnios* is thought to be related to the size of the placenta and diabetic control. The incidence of polyhydramnios in diabetes is 5–13 per cent where the control is good, but may be as high as 22–26 per cent where it is poor. Fetal polyuria has been advanced as the main source of the excessive liquor, secondary to osmotic diuresis. *Macrosomia* occurs as a result of an unsatisfactory metabolic environment. The definition of macrosomia is not universal and typically varies from >4000 g to >4500 g. Perhaps the best definitions are those based on birth weight centiles for the relevant population and gender (for example babies weighing above the 95th centile for the gestational age), ethnic origin, parity, infant sex and maternal size (height, weight), race and gender. The risk of delivering a baby weighing above 4500 g is ten times greater in a diabetic pregnancy than in an uncomplicated pregnancy. Although there is generally a greater adiposity and muscle mass in macrosomic babies, the head tends to be spared. Recent evidence supports the concept that being macrosomic predisposes to the development of obesity and carbohydrate intolerance in

later life. The explanation for this may be found from autopsies of babies of diabetic mothers: pancreatic islet hyperplasia and an increase in beta-cell mass has been demonstrated. These changes occur as early as the second trimester. Fetal macrosomia is accompanied by organomegaly and it is not unusual for these neonates to suffer from cardiomyopathy.

The risk of *preterm labour* is three-fold higher than that in non-diabetics. This is mainly attributable to iatrogenic deliveries. Risk factors for the occurrence of *stillbirths* include poorly controlled diabetes, fetal macrosomia, co-existing vasculopathy or pre-eclampsia and hydramnios. With better and tighter control, the incidence of stillbirths falls dramatically, although it is still higher than in non-diabetic pregnancies. Stillbirths are most common after the 36th week of gestation. Various mechanisms have been advanced for the occurrence of stillbirths in IDDM. Chronic intrauterine hypoxia has been suggested as one possible mechanism, based on the frequently observed findings of extramedullary haemopoiesis. However, this is not recognized in all diabetic pregnancies complicated by stillbirths. In cases complicated by vasculopathy, a reduction in uterine blood flow is a possible cause of the hypoxia that results in stillbirth. Hyperinsulinaemia has been described as a cause of fetal hypoxia; it increases the fetal metabolic rate and oxygen requirements. Frequent fluctuations in random glucose levels have also been described as being responsible for the stillbirths. Other recognized causes include ketoacidosis, which is likely in hyperglycaemia, and infections.

Intrapartum complications

These are related to macrosomia and include shoulder dystocia, increased risk of caesarean delivery, fractures of the long bones, especially the humerus and clavicle, Erb's and Klumpke's palsies.

Fetal complications

- Congenital anomalies
- Miscarriage
- Polyhydramnios
- Preterm labour
- Respiratory distress syndrome
- Unexplained intrauterine fetal death
- Trauma – fetus and mother
- Neonatal complications – jaundice, polycythaemia, tetany, hypocalcaemia, hypomagnesaemina, hypoglycaemia

---

MANAGEMENT OF DIABETES MELLITUS IN PREGNANCY

This is best achieved by a team consisting of a physician, an obstetrician, a diabetic midwife/nurse and the patient's general practitioner.

Pre-pregnancy

Ideally, pre-pregnancy glycaemic control should be optimal before pregnancy. The tighter the control, the better the outcome of pregnancy; where pre-pregnancy control is good, the perinatal morbidity and mortality rates approximate to those in non-diabetic pregnancies. Pre-pregnancy clinics ensure that women are educated regarding the need for tight control, and are screened and treated (if necessary) for complications such as retinopathy, nephropathy and cardiac dysfunction. In addition, general advice can be given concerning diet (especially the need for folic acid pre-pregnancy and during the first trimester), smoking and exercise during pregnancy. Ideally, the glycosylated haemoglobin should be below 6.5 per cent before conception.

Pregnancy

Glucose control

Most patients with pre-pregnancy diabetes are taking insulin, and this therapy must be maintained during pregnancy. Over the last few years, new insulin analogues have been introduced and it is likely that an increasing number of women with IDDM will become pregnant on these newer preparations. Diamond and Kormas[12] [III] reported two cases of congenital malformations in women taking the analogue Lispro; however, a study of 42 women on Lispro indicated that the incidence of malformations was not increased (and there were fewer hypoglycaemic attacks) [III].[13] For those on oral hypoglycaemic agents, it is advisable to convert to insulin therapy, as there are possible teratogenic effects and insulin facilitates a more effective manipulation of requirements as pregnancy progresses.

In the first trimester, insulin requirements fluctuate as a result of many factors such as nausea, vomiting and the hormonal changes of early pregnancy. Insulin requirements increase in the second and third trimesters. Insulin is commonly administered as a combination of short-acting and medium-acting insulin, although occasionally long-acting insulin may be used. The short-acting insulin (e.g. Human Actrapid) is administered pre-meals; the medium-acting insulin (Insulatard) is administered pre-bedtime. In a randomized, controlled trial, Nachum *et al.* demonstrated that a four-dose regimen was better that a two-dose regimen [Ib].[14] As detailed in Chapter 7.5, glycaemic control should be monitored by regular capillary glucose measurements. These are ideally performed four times during the day – fasting, and 2 hours post-prandial (breakfast, lunch and dinner). The aim is to maintain glucose levels below 5.5 mmol/L (fasting) and 7.0 mmol/L (post-prandial). In addition to insulin therapy, dietary advice is essential, as it will make glycaemic control with insulin easier. Glycosylated haemoglobin (HbA1c) should be used with glucose monitoring (see Chapter 7.5). The value of fructosamine (glycosylated albumin) in the monitoring of glycaemic control is limited. While HbA1c measures control

2–3 months prior to the sampling, fructosamine measures control 2 weeks prior to sampling.

Hypoglycaemia is more common in women with IDDM than with NIDDM. Women should be educated regarding the symptoms of hypoglycaemia and advised about appropriate treatments. Severe hypoglycaemia may present with dizziness, hypotension, light-headedness, confusional states, coma or seizures. If the patient is able to eat/drink, oral dextrose therapy may suffice; if not, intramuscular or subcutaneous glucagon and 50 mL of 50 per cent dextrose should be given. Pregnant diabetics are more prone to ketoacidosis because of physiological lipaemia, increased metabolic requirements and lowering of blood bicarbonate. This complication is more likely in women who have had diabetes for more than 5 years, and is associated with a high fetal mortality (reported to be in the order of 30 per cent, or higher if the mother becomes comatosed). Ketoacidosis has been reported to occur in about 2 per cent of diabetic pregnancies. In most of these patients, it occurs in association with a precipitating factor – the most common of which are viral or bacterial infections. Women presenting in preterm labour who are prescribed drugs that induce hyperglycaemia (e.g. dexamethasone and β-agonists) are also at an increased risk.

Glycaemic control should aim:

- for fasting blood glucose ≤5.5 mmol/L
- for post-prandial glucose ~7.0 mmol/L
- for HbA1c <7%
- to avoid hypoglycaemia and hyperglycaemia

Fetal surveillance

An early dating ultrasound scan is important to confirm gestational age. A mid-trimester detailed ultrasound scan should also be performed. Fetal echocardiography will exclude congenital cardiac malformations. Prenatal diagnosis in diabetics presents unique problems. Women with IDDM have lower maternal serum alpha-fetoprotein (MSAP) levels. Obesity is also common in diabetics, and maternal weight affects MSAP. Serum screening for chromosomal abnormalities must be undertaken with caution. The role of nuchal translucency and the fetal nasal bone may prove to be of value in this group of patients. Regular ultrasound scanning for fetal growth and amniotic fluid index will identify fetal macrosomia and polyhydramnios. For fetuses weighing more than 4000 g, ultrasound estimations of fetal weight are subject to errors of up to 15 per cent.

The occurrence of unexplained intrauterine deaths (particularly after the 36th week of gestation) is largely responsible for the need for close fetal surveillance in the third trimester. The value of fetal kick charts, amniotic volume monitoring and umbilical artery Doppler velocimetry in the monitoring of these pregnancies is uncertain; in a randomized, controlled trial, Tyrrell et al.[15] demonstrated that the value

of umbilical artery Doppler in the monitoring of diabetic pregnancies was questionable [Ib].

A sensible approach to the monitoring of these patients will therefore include:

- fetal biometry and amniotic fluid quantification at regular intervals from 28 weeks' gestation
- fetal kick chart
- non-stress cardiotocography
- biophysical profilometry
- umbilical and middle cerebral artery Doppler velocimetry

Maternal surveillance

The potential maternal complications (see above) necessitate increased hospital-based antenatal attendances at multidisciplinary clinics; these visits will include frequent renal function testing and blood pressure monitoring, regular ophthalmic examinations and, where indicated, peripheral neurological examination.

Labour and delivery

Timing of delivery

The timing of delivery in diabetic pregnancies remains controversial. There is little evidence from randomized trials to support either elective delivery or expectant management at term. However, many units adopt the policy of elective induction at 38–39 weeks provided the diabetes is well controlled and there are no associated fetal or maternal complications. Kjos et al.[16] attempted to address this issue and randomized women with uncomplicated insulin-treated diabetes into expectant management or elective delivery at 38 + 5 weeks' gestation. They reported an increased prevalence of large for dates (23 vs 10 per cent) and shoulder dystocia (3 vs 0 per cent) in the expectant management group. They concluded that labour should be induced at 38 weeks unless ultrasound biometry excluded fetal macrosomia [Ib]. Unfortunately, ultrasound is unreliable in identifying macrosomic fetuses. The decision about when to deliver should be based on the individual patient. Where the diabetes has been well controlled throughout pregnancy, the evidence for delivery before 39 weeks' gestation is equivocal. In the presence of complications (either maternal of fetal), delivery should be expedited when the risks of continued intrauterine existence are thought to exceed those of premature delivery – particularly the risk of respiratory distress syndrome. It has been suggested that where insulin requirements suddenly fall, careful consideration must be given to delivery, as this may be suggestive of a 'failing' placenta. There is, however, no robust evidence to support this management strategy.

Caesarean section

The rate of caesarean section in diabetic pregnancies is significantly higher than that in non-diabetic pregnancies, and may be as high as 50 per cent. This is partly due to fetal macrosomia with a consequent fear of shoulder dystocia complicating macrosomic vaginal deliveries, and also due to failed induction of labour. There is no universal agreement about the criteria for delivering by caesarean section, but since macrosomia is more common and shoulder dystocia is more likely at a given birth weight in pregnancies complicated by diabetes than in non-diabetics pregnancies, it is reasonable to recommend caesarean section to women at a particular fetal weight threshold. Unfortunately, because of the poor accuracy of fetal weight estimation by ultrasound (up to 15 per cent at estimations >4000 g), the application of this approach may be difficult. One advocated strategy is therefore to counsel regarding elective caesarean delivery when the estimated fetal weight is 4500 g or more [IV]. When the estimated fetal weight is between 4000 g and 4500 g, additional factors such as the past obstetric history should be taken into consideration.

Insulin requirements

The insulin requirements fluctuate considerably during labour and fall quickly after delivery. To avoid these fluctuations and their consequences, a continuous intravenous infusion of glucose and insulin is recommended [IV]. In general, long labours should be avoided and epidural analgesia encouraged. The following is an example of a recommended regimen for women undergoing induction of labour, and can be modified for patients in spontaneous labour.

On the day before induction
- Normal diet.
- Normal insulin on evening before induction.
- Overnight fast not required.

On the day of induction
- Give half the morning dose of insulin before a light breakfast.
- Insert prostaglandin pessaries or gel as early as possible (e.g. 07.30 a.m.).
- Commence intravenous infusion of insulin and 10 per cent dextrose once labour is established. Insulin infusion should be given through an infusion pump and consists of 50 units of Human Actrapid in 49.5 mL of normal saline (to produce 1 unit of insulin/mL).
- Commence 500 mL of 10 per cent dextrose and 20 mmol of potassium chloride at a rate of 100 mL/hour.
- Measure capillary glucose (from finger prick every 30 minutes for the first hour and then hourly thereafter).
- Continuous cardiotocography.

- Manage the labour as per unit protocol – performing amniotomy when possible and instituting oxytocin augmentation when indicated. This should be in 5 per cent dextrose and via an infusion pump.
- Use the sliding scale to determine the rate of insulin infusion.
- Adjust insulin infusion rate to maintain blood glucose readings of 4.0–7.0 mmol/L. If the blood glucose is <4.0 mmol/L, stop the infusion, but continue the 10 per cent dextrose infusion and repeat the blood glucose levels after 15 minutes. Restart the insulin infusion when blood glucose levels are >7.0 mmol/L.
- Monitor glucose levels every 15 minutes during the second stage.

Caesarean section – elective
- The usual dose of insulin and food should be given on the evening before surgery and the patient fasted from 12 midnight.
- On the morning of the delivery, commence on insulin infusion and dextrose infusion.
- The rest of the management is similar to that after a vaginal delivery.

Postpartum
- Half the rate of insulin infusion in women with type 1 and 2 diabetes.
- Adjust the insulin requirements to maintain a blood glucose level of 4–9 mmol/L.
- Continue with the insulin infusion until the patient is eating.
- 30–60 minutes before stopping the insulin, administer subcutaneous insulin.
- Recommence the patient on her pre-pregnancy insulin dose or 30–50 per cent less than the dose at the end of pregnancy. Those who are NIDDM need to continue with insulin until they revert to oral hypoglycaemic agents.
- Monitor the blood glucose hourly for 2 hours and then post-prandially for 48 hours.
- Contraception: this will depend on whether the patient wishes to breastfeed or has other contraindications to different forms of contraception. Options to be discussed include the combined oral contraceptive pill, the progestrogen-only pill, barrier methods and sterilization.

NEONATAL COMPLICATIONS

Neonatal complications include hypoglycaemia, respiratory distress syndrome, hyperbilirubinaemia, hypocalcaemia, hypo-magnesaemia, polycythaemia and hypothermia.

Diabetes mellitus

- Optimal pre-conceptional glycaemic control is associated with a risk of congenital malformations similar to that in non-diabetic pregnancies.
- A combination of insulin types for glycaemic control is associated with a better outcome than when control is with a single insulin type.
- Induction of labour at 39 weeks is associated with less macrosomia and shoulder dsystocia.
- There are no reliable means of fetal surveillance (antenatal and intrapartum).

KEY POINTS

- Diabetes mellitus complicates 1–2 per cent of all pregnancies.
- Management should start pre-conception and good control should be achieved on insulin.
- Ideal care should be under a combined team consisting of an obstetrician, a physician, a dietician, a diabetic nurse/midwife and the GP.
- Glycaemic control in pregnancy should aim for a fasting blood glucose of <5.5 mol/L, a post-prandial glucose of <7.0 mmol/L and a HbA1c of <7 per cent.
- Induction of labour at approximately 39 weeks where glycaemic control is good is associated with a reduced risk of shoulder dystocia.
- Fetal surveillance is important but there is no reliable method for this. A combination of methods must therefore be employed.
- All neonates of diabetic pregnancies must be monitored for complications such as hypoglycaemia.

KEY REFERENCES

1. Lind T, Hytten FE. The excretion of glucose during normal pregnancy. *J Obstet Gynaecol Br Commonwlth* 1972; **79**:961–5.
2. White P. Pregnancy and diabetes, medical aspects. *Med Clin North Am* 1965; **49**:1015–24.
3. Report of the Expert Committee of the Diagnosis and Classification of Diabetes Mellitus. *Diabetes Care* 1997; **7**:1183–97.
4. Klein BEK, Moss SE, Klein R. Effect of pregnancy on the progression of diabetic retinopathy. *Diabetes Care* 1990; **13**:34.
5. Phelps RL, Sakol P, Metzger BE et al. Changes in diabetic retinopathy during pregnancy: correlations with regulation of hyperglycaemia. *Arch Ophthalmol* 1986; **104**:1806–10.
6. Reece EA, Coustan DR, Hayslett JP et al. Diabetic nephropathy: pregnancy performance and fetomaternal outcome. *Am J Obstet Gynecol* 1988; **159**:56–66
7. Gordon MC, Landon MB, Boyle J, Stewart KS, Gabbe SG. Coronary artery disease in insulin-dependent diabetes mellitus of pregnancy (Class H): a review of the literature. *Obstet Gynecol Surv* 1996; **51**:437–44.
8. Fuhrmann K, Reiher H, Semmler K et al. Prevention of congenital malformations in infants of insulin-dependent diabetic mothers. *Diabetes Care* 1983; **6**: 219–23.
9. Carsoon IF, Clarke CA, Howard CV et al. Outcomes of pregnancy in insulin dependent diabetic women: results of a five year population cohort study. *BMJ* 1997; **315**:275–8.
10. Hawthorne G, Robson S, Ryall EA, Sen D, Roberts SH, Ward Platt MP. Prospective population based survey of outcome of pregnancy in diabetic women: results of the Northern Diabetic Pregnancy Audit, 1994. *BMJ* 1997; **315**: 279–81.
11. Mill JL, Knopp RH, Simpson JP et al. Lack of relations of increased malformation rates in infants of diabetic mothers to glycaemic control during organogenesis. *N Engl J Med* 1988; **318**:671–6.
12. Diamond T, Kormas N. Possible adverse fetal effect of insulin lispro. *N Engl J Med* 1997; **337**:1009.
13. Jovanovic L, Ilic S, Pettitt DJ et al. Metabolic and immunologic effects of insulin lispro in gestational diabetes. *Diabetes Care* 1999; **22**:1422–7.
14. Nachum Z, Ben-Shlomo I, Weiner E, Shalev E. Twice daily versus four time daily insulin dose regimens for diabetes in pregnancy: randomised controlled trial. *BMJ* 1999; **319**:1223–7.
15. Tyrell SN, Lilford RJ, Macdonald HN, Nelson EJ, Porter J, Gupta JK. Randomised comparison of routine vs highly selective use of Doppler ultrasound and biophysical scoring to investigate high risk pregnancies. *Br J Obstet Gynaecol* 1990; **97**:901–16.
16. Kjos SL, Henry OA, Montoro M, Buchanan TA, Mestman JH. Insulin requiring diabetes in pregnancy: a randomized controlled trial of active induction of labor and expectant management. *Am J Obstet Gynecol* 1993; **13**:293–6.

Cardiac Disease

Catherine Nelson-Piercy

MRCOG standards

Relevant standards

- Conduct pre-pregnancy counselling to a level expected in independent primary care.
- Conduct booking visit, including assessment of intercurrent disease.
- Diagnose and plan management with appropriate consultation in the following conditions: heart disease.

  In addition, we would suggest the following.

Theoretical skills

- Revise cardiovascular physiology and know the changes in pregnancy.
- Know which cardiac conditions are contraindications to pregnancy.
- Be able to counsel a woman with a valve replacement about the maternal and fetal risk/benefits of anticoagulation.

Practical skills

- Be confident in ability to recognize the common symptoms and signs of heart failure.
- Be able to diagnose and treat pulmonary oedema.

INTRODUCTION

Cardiac disease in pregnancy is rare in the UK, but common in developing countries. This chapter covers the most important conditions relevant to pregnancy, including Eisenmenger's syndrome, Marfan's syndrome, mitral stenosis and mechanical heart valves. Peripartum cardiomyopathy is included as it is specific to the pregnant or postpartum state.

PHYSIOLOGICAL CHANGES IN PREGNANCY

Cardiac output increases by 40 per cent, reaching a maximum by the mid-second trimester. There is peripheral vasodilatation, an increase in heart rate, and a fall in systemic and pulmonary vascular resistance. Labour and delivery are associated with further increases in cardiac output. Palpitations, extrasystoles and ejection systolic murmurs are common in pregnancy but rarely represent underlying pathology. The electrocardiogram (ECG) changes associated with normal pregnancy include atrial and ventricular ectopics, a 'left shift' in the QRS axis, a small Q wave and inverted T wave in lead III, and ST segment depression and T wave inversion in the inferior and lateral leads.

INCIDENCE

Although rare in the UK, cardiac disease was the second most common cause of maternal death in the 1994–96 Confidential Enquiries[1] [III] and equal leading cause in 1997–99.[1a] Ischaemic heart disease is becoming more common in pregnancy, and congenital heart disease is encountered more frequently as those who have received corrective surgery as children reach child-bearing age. Rheumatic heart disease is less common in the UK, but may be encountered in women from developing countries.

AETIOLOGY

The aetiology of heart disease may be divided into congenital and acquired causes. The commonest congenital heart diseases encountered in pregnancy are ventricular and atrial septal defects (ASD, VSD) and patent ductus arteriosus. These are mostly diagnosed before pregnancy and are usually either haemodynamically insignificant or corrected. Acquired causes of cardiac disease include ischaemic heart disease, rheumatic heart disease, cardiomyopathies, and aneurysms and dissection of the aorta or its branches.

GENERAL PRINCIPLES

When assessing or counselling a pregnant or potentially pregnant woman with heart disease, it is important to remember that the outcome and safety of pregnancy are related to the presence and severity of pulmonary hypertension, the presence of cyanosis, the haemodynamic significance of the lesion and the functional class [III].[2] The functional class is determined by the level of activity that leads to dyspnoea. In addition, women with previous transient ischaemic attacks or heart failure, and those with left-sided lesions (e.g. aortic or mitral stenosis) or myocardial dysfunction are at risk in pregnancy. Women with congenital heart disease are at increased risk of having a baby with congenital heart disease, and should therefore be offered detailed scanning for cardiac anomalies. During pregnancy, women with heart disease require multidisciplinary team care, with regular antenatal visits and judicious monitoring to avoid or treat expediently any anaemia or infection. There should be early involvement of obstetric anaesthetists and a carefully documented plan for delivery.

EISENMENGER'S SYNDROME

This results when pulmonary hypertension develops secondary to a large left-to-right shunt such as a VSD, and the shunt is reversed to become right to left, with consequent cyanosis. Pulmonary hypertension is dangerous and may be primary or secondary to lung disease or Eisenmenger's syndrome. Maternal mortality is 40 per cent [III].[3] The danger relates to fixed pulmonary vascular resistance and an inability to increase pulmonary blood flow, with refractory hypoxaemia. Most deaths can be attributed to thromboembolism, hypovolaemia or pre-eclampsia.

Management

Women with severe pulmonary hypertension or Eisenmenger's syndrome should be advised to avoid pregnancy or, in the event of unplanned pregnancy, to have a therapeutic termination [III].[3] If such advice is declined, multidisciplinary care and elective admission for bed rest, oxygen and thromboprophylaxis are recommended [III].[4]

- Most published evidence relating to Eisenmenger's syndrome comes from retrospective cohorts and case series.
- All the literature supports a high risk of maternal death sufficient to make this condition one of the absolute contraindications to pregnancy.
- There is no evidence that monitoring the pulmonary artery pressure prepartum or intrapartum improves outcome.

MARFAN'S SYNDROME

The importance of this autosomal dominant condition in pregnancy is the risk of aortic rupture or dissection. Progressive aortic root dilatation and an aortic root dimension >4 cm are associated with increased risk [III].[5] Conversely, in women with minimal cardiac involvement and an aortic root <4 cm, pregnancy outcome is good [II].[6]

Management

Women with aortic roots >4–4.5 cm should be advised to delay pregnancy until after aortic root repair. Recommendations include monthly echocardiograms, beta-blockers for those with hypertension or aortic root dilatation, vaginal delivery for those with stable aortic root measurements, but elective caesarean section with epidural if there is an enlarged or dilating aortic root [III].[5]

- Most published evidence relating to Marfan's syndrome comes from retrospective cohorts and case series.
- The literature supports a higher risk of aortic rupture and maternal death if the aortic root is >4 cm.

MITRAL STENOSIS

This is the most common rheumatic heart disease and is important in pregnancy because women may deteriorate secondary to tachycardia, arrhythmias or the increased cardiac output. The commonest complication is pulmonary oedema secondary to increased left atrial pressure and precipitated by increased heart rate or increased volume (such as occurs during the third stage of labour) [II].[7] The risk is increased with severe mitral stenosis, moderate or severe symptoms prior to pregnancy, and in those diagnosed late in pregnancy [II].[7]

Antenatal complications: maternal

Management

Women with severe mitral stenosis should be advised to delay pregnancy until after balloon, open or closed mitral valvotomy. Beta-blockers decrease heart rate and the risk of pulmonary oedema [III],[8] but if medical therapy fails or for those with severe mitral stenosis, balloon mitral valvotomy may be safely and successfully used in pregnancy [III].[7] Women with mitral stenosis should avoid the supine and lithotomy positions as much as possible for labour and delivery. Fluid overload must be avoided [IV]. Pulmonary oedema should be treated in the usual way with oxygen and diuretics.

- Most published evidence relating to mitral stenosis comes from retrospective cohorts and case series.
- The literature supports a higher risk of pulmonary oedema in severe mitral stenosis.
- Both beta-blockers and balloon valvotomy are safe in pregnancy.

MECHANICAL HEART VALVES

The problem for women with metal heart valve replacements is that they require life-long anticoagulation, and this must be continued in pregnancy because of the increased risk of thrombosis. Warfarin is associated with warfarin embryopathy[9] and increased risks of miscarriage, stillbirth and fetal intracerebral haemorrhage.[10] Heparin, even in full anticoagulant doses, is associated with increased risks of valve thrombosis and embolic events [II].[9,10]

Management

The safest option for the mother is to continue warfarin throughout pregnancy [II].[9,10] Other management strategies include replacing the warfarin with high-dose unfractionated or low-molecular-weight heparin, either from 6 to 12 weeks' gestation to avoid warfarin embryopathy or throughout pregnancy. Since the risk of thrombosis is less with the newer bileaflet valves (e.g. Carbomedics), it may be that high doses of heparin throughout pregnancy are appropriate in women with these valves [IV]. Whichever management option is chosen, warfarin should be discontinued and substituted with heparin for 10 days prior to delivery to allow clearance of warfarin from the fetal circulation. For delivery itself, heparin therapy is interrupted. Warfarin is recommenced 2–3 days postpartum [IV]. In the event of bleeding or the need for urgent delivery in a fully anticoagulated patient, warfarin may be reversed with fresh frozen plasma (FFP) and vitamin K, and heparin with protamine sulphate.

- Most published evidence relating to mechanical heart valves comes from retrospective cohorts and case series of women with Starr–Edwards valves.
- The literature supports a lower risk of thromboembolic events if warfarin is continued throughout pregnancy.

ISCHAEMIC HEART DISEASE

Myocardial infarction (MI) in pregnancy is becoming more common as maternal age increases. The risk is increased in multigravid women, in those who smoke and in women with diabetes, obesity, hypertension and hypercholesterolaemia [II]. Infarction most commonly occurs in the third trimester and affects the anterior wall of the heart [II].[11] The maternal death rate is 20 per cent. In pregnancy, the underlying aetiology is more likely to be due to non-atherosclerotic conditions (such as coronary artery thrombosis or dissection) than in the non-pregnant [II].[1,11]

Management

Management of acute MI is as for the non-pregnant woman [III]. Intravenous and intracoronary thrombolysis and percutaneous transluminal coronary angioplasty have all been successfully performed in pregnancy [III]. For secondary prevention in women with known ischaemic heart disease, both aspirin and beta-blockers are safe in pregnancy [Ia]. Lipid-lowering drugs are usually discontinued for the duration of pregnancy [IV].

ENDOCARDITIS PROPHYLAXIS

Antibiotic prophylaxis is mandatory for those with prosthetic valves and for those with a previous episode of endocarditis [Ia].[12] Many cardiologists recommend that women with structural heart defects (e.g. VSD) also receive prophylaxis [IV]. Recommendations of the American Heart Association stratify cardiac conditions into high, moderate and negligible (not requiring antibiotic prophylaxis) risk (Table 6.3.1) [Ia].[12] Fatal cases of endocarditis in pregnancy have occurred antenatally, rather than as a consequence of infection acquired at the time of delivery.[1]

The current UK recommendations (see under 'Published guidelines') are amoxycillin 1 g i.v. plus gentamicin 120 mg i.v. at the onset of labour or ruptured membranes or prior to caesarean section, followed by amoxycillin 500 mg orally (or i.m/i.v. depending on the patient's condition) 6 hours later.

Table 6.3.1 Stratification of cardiac conditions according to risk of bacterial endocarditis

High risk	Prosthetic valves (metal, bioprosthetic and homografts)
Endocarditis prophylaxis recommended	Previous bacterial endocarditis
	Complex cyanotic congenital heart disease (Fallot's, transposition of great arteries)
	Surgical systemic/pulmonary shunts
Moderate risk	Other congenital cardiac malformations
	Acquired valvular disease
Endocarditis prophylaxis recommended	Hypertrophic cardiomyopathy
	Mitral valve prolapse with mitral regurgitation
Negligible risk	Isolated secundum atrial septal defects
	Surgically repaired ASD, VSD, PDA
Endocarditis prophylaxis not recommended	Mitral valve prolapse without regurgitation
	Physiological heart murmurs
	Cardiac pacemakers

Adapted from reference 12.
ASD, atrial septal defect; VSD, ventricular septal defect; PDA, patent ductus arteriosus.

For women who are penicillin allergic, vancomycin 1 g i.v. or teicoplanin 400 mg i.v. may be used instead of amoxycillin.[12]

HYPERTROPHIC CARDIOMYOPATHY

Most cases of hypertrophic cardiomyopathy (HOCM) are familial, inherited as autosomal dominant. Women may be asymptomatic, especially if diagnosed because of family screening, or may experience syncope or 'angina-like' chest pain. The danger relates to left ventricular outflow tract obstruction that may be precipitated by hypotension or hypovolaemia. Provided these are avoided, pregnancy is usually well tolerated. Beta-blockers should be continued in pregnancy or initiated for symptomatic women [III].[13]

PERIPARTUM CARDIOMYOPATHY

This pregnancy-specific condition is defined as the development of cardiac failure between the last month of pregnancy and 5 months postpartum, the absence of an identifiable cause, the absence of recognizable heart disease prior to the last month of pregnancy, and left ventricular systolic dysfunction demonstrated by classic echocardiographic criteria [II].[14] Risk factors include multiple pregnancy, hypertension, multiparity, increased age and Afro-Caribbean race [III].

Diagnosis should be suspected in the puerperal patient with breathlessness and signs of heart failure. It is confirmed with echocardiography showing left ventricular dysfunction

and often dilatation of all four chambers of the heart. Treatment is as for other causes of heart failure, with oxygen, diuretics, vasodilators, angiotensin-converting enzyme (ACE) inhibitors if postpartum, and inotropes if required. Prognosis and recurrence depend on the normalization of left ventricular size within 6 months of delivery [II].[14]

ARRHYTHMIAS

A sinus tachycardia requires investigation for possible underlying pathology such as blood loss, infection, heart failure, thyrotoxicosis or pulmonary embolus, but no treatment is required if such causes are excluded. The commonest arrhythmia encountered in pregnancy is supraventricular tachycardia (SVT). An SVT that does not respond to vagal manoeuvres may be safely terminated in pregnancy with adenosine [III].

KEY POINTS

- Heart disease is a common cause of maternal mortality.
- Eisenmenger's syndrome, other causes of pulmonary hypertension, severe mitral stenosis, Marfan's syndrome with aortic root dilatation and severe cardiomyopathy are contraindications to pregnancy.
- The safest option for women with mechanical heart valves is to continue warfarin in pregnancy, notwithstanding the associated fetal risks.
- Women with prosthetic heart valves or previous episodes of endocarditis require antibiotic prophylaxis to cover delivery.

PUBLISHED GUIDELINES

Endocarditis Working Party of the British Society for Antimicrobial Chemotherapy. *Lancet* 1982; 2:1323–6.
British National Formulary. London: British Medical Association/Royal Pharmaceutical Society of Great Britain, 2003.

KEY REFERENCES

1. Department of Health, Welsh Office, Scottish Home and Health Department and Department of Health and Social Services, Northern Ireland. *Confidential Enquiries into Maternal Deaths in the United Kingdom 1994–96.* London: HMSO, 1998.

Antenatal complications: maternal

1a. Department of Health, Welsh Office, Scottish Home and Health Department and Department of Health and Social Services, Northern Ireland. *Confidential Enquiries into Maternal Deaths in the United Kingdom 1997–99.* London: RCOG Press, 2001.

2. McCaffrey FM, Sherman FS. Pregnancy and congenital heart disease: The Magee Women's Hospital. *J Matern Fetal Med* 1995; **4**:152–9.

3. Yentis SM, Steer PJ, Plaat F. Eisenmenger's syndrome in pregnancy: maternal and fetal mortality in the 1990s. *Br J Obstet Gynaecol* 1998; **105**:921–2.

4. Avila WS, Grinberg M, Snitcowsky R et al. Maternal and fetal outcome in pregnant women with Eisenmenger's syndrome. *Eur Heart J* 1995; **16**:460–4.

5. Lipscomb KJ, Clayton Smith J, Clarke B, Donnai P, Harris R. Outcome of pregnancy in women with Marfan's syndrome. *Br J Obstet Gynaecol* 1997; **104**:201–6.

6. Rossiter JP, Repke JT, Morales AJ et al. A prospective longitudinal evaluation of pregnancy in the Marfan syndrome. *Am J Obstet Gynecol* 1995; **173**:1599–606.

7. Desai DK, Adanlawo M, Naidoo DP, Moodley J, Kleinschmidt I. Mitral stenosis in pregnancy: a four-year experience at King Edward VIII Hospital. *Br J Obstet Gynaecol* 2000; **107**:953–8.

8. al Kasab SM, Sabag T, al Zaibag M et al. Beta-adrenergic receptor blockade in the management of pregnant women with mitral stenosis. *Am J Obstet Gynecol* 1990; **163**:37–40.

9. Chan WS, Anand S, Ginsberg JS. Anticoagulation of pregnant women with mechanical heart valves. *Arch Intern Med* 2000; **160**:191–6.

10. Sadler L, McCowan L, White H, Stewart A, Bracken M, North R. Pregnancy outcomes and cardiac complications in women with mechanical, bioprosthetic and homograft valves. *Br J Obstet Gynaecol* 2000; **107**:245–53.

11. Roth A, Elkayam U. Acute myocardial infarction associated with pregnancy. *Ann Int Med* 1996; **125**:751–7.

12. Dajani AS, Taubert KA, Wilson W et al. Prevention of bacterial endocarditis. Recommendations by the American Heart Association. *J Am Med Assoc* 1997; **277**:1794–801.

13. Oakley GD, McGarry K, Limb DG, Oakley CM. Management of pregnancy in patients with hypertrophic cardiomyopathy. *BMJ* 1979; **1**:1749–50.

14. Pearson GD, Veille JC, Rahimtoola S et al. Peripartum cardiomyopathy. National Heart, Lung and Blood Institute and Office of Rare Diseases (NIH). Workshop Recommendations and Review. *J Am Med Assoc* 2000; **283**:1183–8.

Thyroid Disease

Andrew Shennan

INTRODUCTION: PHYSIOLOGY OF THYROID FUNCTION

Maternal physiology

Thyroid disease occurs in more than 1 per cent of the population and is the commonest pre-existing endocrine disorder in pregnant women. A fundamental understanding of thyroid function in pregnancy is essential. Thyroid-stimulating hormone (TSH) is released from the anterior pituitary in 1–2-hourly cycles. It increases both the synthesis and release of thyroxine (T4) and triiodothyronine (T3). The T3 and T4 are mostly protein bound – to thyroid-binding globulin (TBG), albumin and transthyretin. Although the concentration of TBG is low, the binding affinity is high, and TBG binds 75 per cent of thyroid hormones. The unbound thyroid hormones have biological activity; only 0.04 per cent of T4 and 0.05 per cent of T3 are free.

Iodide is essential for the synthesis of thyroid hormones, and the thyroid gland actively traps iodine, ultimately releasing thyroglobulin molecules. Each molecule carries three or four molecules of T4. Circulating T3 is produced principally by peripheral deiodination of T4 and is three times more potent than T4. Although the production of T3 is lower than that of T4, more T3 is available as a free, inactive compound.

In pregnancy, there is altered TBG production as a result of increased oestrogen synthesis. TBG increases in the first 2 weeks of pregnancy, and reaches a plateau by 20 weeks. The increase in TBG leads to an increase in the serum concentrations of total T4 and T3, but there are no changes in the amount of free circulating (unbound) thyroid hormones. There is iodine deficiency in pregnancy as a result of loss through increased glomerular filtration. This results in increased uptake by the thyroid gland, which can result in enlargement and the appearance of a goitre. Fetal thyroid activity also depletes the maternal iodide pool from the second trimester, probably via diffusion along a concentration gradient.

As human chorionic gonadotrophin (hCG) and TSH share a common alpha subunit and have similar beta subunits, TSH receptors are prone to stimulation by hCG. In conditions such as molar pregnancy, with high levels of hCG, increased thyroid activity has been noted. Even in normal pregnancy, a fall in TSH levels is associated with peak hCG concentrations, and there is a correlation between levels of T4 and hCG. In pregnancy, there is also placental conversion of T4 to T3. Low levels of T4 will increase this activity, producing more active thyroid hormone. Deiodination also occurs in trophoblasic and placental tissue, preventing excess thyroid hormone exposure to the baby and perhaps explaining the fall in T4 found in the mother in later pregnancy.[1]

Fetal thyroid function

During the first trimester, the fetus requires maternal T4 for normal fetal brain development. It is likely that T4 crosses the placenta in small amounts before 12 weeks' gestation to facilitate this (otherwise, T3, T4 and TSH do not cross the placenta). From 10 weeks' gestation, the fetal thyroid gland produces both T4 and T3. From this point onwards, the fetal thyroid axis is independent and there is little relationship between maternal and fetal levels. Fetal levels reach those of the adult by 36 weeks' gestation. Although fetal TSH concentrations are greater than maternal TSH levels, T3 is lower in the fetus, probably as a result of little peripheral conversion and a good placental barrier.

Both thyrotropin-releasing hormone (TRH) and iodine freely cross the placenta. (TRH has unsuccessfully been investigated as a method of stimulating thyroid function to enhance fetal lung maturity.)

Congenital hyperthyroidism can occur through TSH receptor stimulating antibodies which cross the placenta. Very rarely, mutations of the TSH receptor result in either congenital hyperthyroidism or hypothyroidism.

Thyroid function tests in pregnancy

In pregnancy, it is important to measure free T4 and T3 and to base management decisions principally on these levels [II]; TSH levels are often suppressed, and can only be detected with new, ultrasensitive assays.

As T4 levels fall during pregnancy, the lower limit of normal for free T4 is below that of non-pregnant women. As there is more conversion of T4 to T3, low levels of T4 are not necessarily indicative of hypothyroidism.[2]

Thyroid hormones are involved in the metabolism of alpha-fetoprotein (aFP), and there has been some concern that aFP measurements may be unreliable. However, in women suspected of having thyroid disease, the available evidence suggests aFP measurements can still be used for Down's serum screening [III].

AETIOLOGY AND MANAGEMENT OF THYROID DISEASE

Iodine

Women in areas of iodine deficiency may have goitres and reduced reproductive success.[3] In iodine deficiency, the maternal thyroid gland has a greater affinity for iodide than the placenta and the fetuses are thus prone to cretinism – the leading preventable cause of mental retardation worldwide. The fetal cochlea, cerebral neocortex and basal ganglia are particularly sensitive to iodine deficiency.[4] Iodine administration prior to conception and up to the second trimester will improve neurological outcome by protecting the fetal brain. Iodination of water, salt or flour or even annual injections for reproductive age women can easily achieve this.

Although the introduction of iodine supplementation in certain areas of the developing world has reduced both the miscarriage and stillbirth rates, high levels of iodine intake

can cause fetal hyperthyroidism. Therefore some cough medicines and eye drops containing iodine should be avoided, as should radiological procedures utilizing iodinated contrast dyes. Similarly, amiodarone, which is rich in iodine, should be avoided in pregnancy unless absolutely necessary for life-threatening arrhythmias. In these cases, neonatal assessment must be made regarding thyroid function. Radioactive iodine, which destroys the fetal thyroid, must never be used, even in early pregnancy, as damage can occur before there is active fetal tissue.

Hyperemesis gravidarum

In women with hyperemesis, T4 levels may be elevated with suppression of TSH. These changes probably result from high levels of hCG, which stimulate the TSH receptors[5] and occur in approximately 40 per cent of hyperemesis cases (particularly in those with more severe disease). The clinical signs of thyrotoxicosis are generally absent and, as the condition improves, T4 levels only remain elevated if true hyperthyroidism ensues.

Antithyroid medication should not be used in hyperemesis as the thyroid abnormality is biochemical and self-limiting and is not related to an overactive thyroid [III]. When used, this type of medication is generally ineffective or required in unacceptably high doses.

Hyperthyroidism

Hyperthyroidism occurs in approximately 1 in 500 pregnancies and is usually due to Graves' disease (autoimmune thyrotoxicosis). Less than 5 per cent of cases result from a toxic nodule, thyroiditis or a carcinoma. If pregnant women present with hyperthyroidism, hyperemesis or a molar pregnancy must be considered.

Graves' disease is associated with a hyperplastic goitre and often with exophthalmos. Disease severity is correlated to immunoglobulin G (IgG) thyrotropin receptor stimulating antibody levels. The disease typically remits in the last two trimesters,[6] and in approximately a third of cases treatment may be discontinued, although a flare may occur following delivery. First trimester disease may be exacerbated by high hCG levels.

Typical signs of thyroidism are difficult to elicit in pregnancy, but poor weight gain in the presence of a good appetite or a tachycardia >100 beats per minute (bpm) that is unresponsive to a Valsalva manoeuvre may indicate the disease. Onycholysis does reflect disease activity, unlike the eye signs and pretibial myxoedema. Unfortunately, many other symptoms, such as fatigue and heat intolerance, are common in pregnancy and are not useful.

It is essential to maintain euthyroidism in pregnancy, as uncontrolled disease is associated with maternal and fetal complications, including thyroid storm, heart failure and maternal hypertension. Observational studies have reported increased rates of premature labour, growth restriction and stillbirth. Treatment is similar to that for non-pregnant women, although radioactive iodine must not be given [III]. Surgery may be considered if medical treatment fails or there is a clinical suspicion of cancer or compressive symptoms due to a goitre.

Medical treatment involves blocking thyroid hormone synthesis. Propylthiouracil (PTU) and carbimazole both reduce the titre of TSH receptor antibodies, directly influencing the aetiology of Graves' disease. PTU was previously the preferred therapy, as it not only inhibits T4 synthesis by blocking the incorporation of iodine into tyrosine, but also inhibits the peripheral conversion of T4 to T3. However, both drugs probably cross the placenta in the same proportion and there is no need to change from carbimazole to PTU [III]. Both drugs are equally beneficial and the dose of either can be titrated against maternal well-being and biochemical status [III].[7] Neither PTU nor carbimazole is thought to be teratogenic, and the relationship previously found between aplasia cutis of the scalp and these drugs is unlikely to exist. Antithyroid drugs can cause agranulocytosis and so a sore throat should be thoroughly investigated.

It is recommended that thyroid function tests be performed every 4–6 weeks. When Graves' disease is stable, betablockers can be used to control the symptoms of tachycardia or tremor, and propranolol is the recommended therapy [III].

As both PTU and carbimazole cross the placenta, both may influence the fetus.[8] The minimal dose required in the mother should therefore be used, and it is usual to aim for free T4 levels at the upper limit of normal [IV]. Even if the fetus does become hypothyroid, neurodevelopmental status is preserved, although careful control can still lead to neonatal hypothyroidism and even neonatal goitre. The goitres are generally small, clinically unimportant and tend to resolve within 2 weeks. No long-term fetal side effects of antithyroid drugs have been demonstrated, although the studies performed have been small and retrospective.

Both drugs are expressed in breast milk, but have little effect on thyroid function.

Fetal hyperthyroidism

When maternal thyrotropin receptor stimulating antibodies cross the placenta, they can cause fetal or neonatal thyrotoxicosis. The fetal thyroid is capable of responding to these antibodies after 20 weeks' gestation, and potential effects should be monitored in the second half of pregnancy. Assessment should include maternal perception of fetal movements, standard growth assessments (symphyseal – fundal height) and measurement of the fetal heart rate, which, if >160 bpm, may be indicative of fetal thyrotoxicosis. An ultrasound scan can be used to exclude a fetal goitre or clinically undetected fetal growth restriction. In suspected cases, cordocentesis for free T4 and TSH determination can be performed and is preferable to amniocentesis [III].

Premature delivery is associated with fetal hyperthyroidism. Hydrops fetalis and death can occur and a fetal goitre can cause polyhydramnios and an obstructed delivery. The condition is also associated with craniosynostosis and intellectual impairment. The fetus can be effectively treated in one of two ways, either by maternal administration of antithyroid agents, which cross the placenta, or by delivery. The fetal heart rate can be used to titrate the dose of antithyroid drugs. The mother can be treated with T4 to offset any hypothyroid effects, as T4 will not cross the placenta [II]. As thyroid TSH receptor stimulating antibodies have a long half-life (3 weeks), they can cause neonatal hyperthyroidism. The symptoms may therefore only present in the baby after a week and tend to be non-specific, such as poor weight gain, feeding and sleeping. A goitre may also cause problems with breathing and feeding. Fetal/neonatal hyperthyroidism is responsible for substantial mortality.

Women who have had Graves' disease treated by surgery may be euthyroid, but still have active antibodies. Therefore TSH receptor antibodies should be measured in these women and in women with active Graves' disease. As long as antibody levels are low, involvement of the fetus is unlikely. If antibody levels are high, fetal/neonatal thyroid function should be checked, both in cord samples and in peripheral samples taken approximately a week after delivery.

Hypothyroidism

Hypothyroidism occurs in nearly 1 per cent of pregnant women and is usually due to autoimmune Hashimoto's thyroiditis or idiopathic myxoedema; the condition can also occur following treatment of hyperthyroidism. Direct pituitary causes are rare.

In pregnancies complicated by hypothyroidism, babies are normally grown and do not seem to have an increased risk of congenital anomalies. Large studies have not yet confirmed this apparent lack of adverse events. (Recent studies suggest that hypothyroidism may be associated with gestational hypertension and thus iatrogenic delivery.) Aberrant thyroid function has been implicated in the aetiology of recurrent miscarriage, but the evidence for this is week, and the current Royal College of Obstetricians and Gynaecologists' (RCOG) guidelines suggest abandoning routine testing of thyroid function in the investigation of recurrent miscarriage.

There is a reduced intelligence quotient (IQ) in babies of women with hypothyroidism that is not adequately treated, or that goes unrecognized. The insult is likely to occur in the first trimester, and therefore pre-conceptual optimization of T4 therapy is important [III].[9,10] Referral to a physician interested in the field would seem prudent.

As hypothyroidism is associated with subfertility, it is rare to make a new diagnosis in pregnancy. The classical symptoms of hypothyroidism such as tiredness, constipation, anaemia, weight gain, carpal tunnel syndrome and hair changes are common in pregnancy and cannot be relied upon to discriminate onset or worsening of the disease. The management is therefore based principally on biochemical measures. Thyroxine is titrated against biochemical results and is safe in pregnancy and lactation [II]. As long as the patient is clinically euthyroid, thyroid function tests should be performed every 2–3 months. More frequent measurements are made if the clinical or biochemical condition is deranged [IV]. Most pregnant women do not need any increase in therapy [II].[11,12] A low free T4 level indicates a need for increased therapy, rather than a raised TSH [III].

Fetal hypothyroidism

Although Hashimoto's hypothyroidism results in the autoantibodies crossing the placenta, it does not affect fetal thyroid development. However, very rarely, TSH receptor blocking antibodies can cause a transient hypothyroidism in either a fetus or baby.

Postpartum thyroiditis

Postpartum thyroiditis can occur up to a year following delivery and can manifest as high or low T4 levels. The incidence varies widely and, when diagnosed biochemically, has been reported as to be as low as 2 per cent in New York and as high as 17 per cent in Wales. Most women will not have clinically apparent disease, and may present with depression or be diagnosed as having Hashimoto's hypothyroidism as they tend to present to general practitioners, who may be unaware of the condition. Women on long-term T4 treatment following an onset soon after pregnancy should have this diagnosis considered.

The condition is thought to be autoimmune and presents postpartum following a return to normal immunity after delivery. Ninety per cent of women will have thyroid antiperoxidase antibodies (compared with 10 per cent of the normal population). Histology from thyroid biopsies suggests a chronic thyroiditis with lymphocytic infiltration but not fibrosis (which is a typical feature of Hashimoto's thyroiditis).

The disease may present initially between 1 and 3 months postpartum with thyrotoxicosis and later with hypothyroidism. Radioactive iodine or technetium uptake tests can help distinguish between postpartum thyroiditis (low uptake) and Graves' (high uptake), but lactation should not continue during testing [III]. If symptomatic with hyperthyroidism, beta-blockers can be used; antithyroid drugs are inappropriate, as T4 production is not increased [III]. Hyperthyroidism is due to destruction of thyroid follicles and the release of preformed hormones. The destruction of thyroid follicles ultimately leads to the hypothyroid phase, which is more likely to be associated with symptoms such as tiredness and cold intolerance and even a goitre. At this stage, the differential diagnosis includes Hashimoto's thyroiditis and Sheehan's syndrome. A course of T4 may be necessary. If the symptoms of hypothyroidism are due to Hashimoto's thyroiditis, withdrawing treatment will result in relapse, but cessation of T4 is probably the only way to avoid unnecessary long-term treatment.

The period of hypothyroid state is variable, and permanent hypothyroidism can result (approximately 5 per cent of antibody-positive postpartum thyroiditis sufferers). The condition will recur in 70 per cent of future pregnancies and women with postpartum thyroiditis should be followed up to ensure that permanent hypothyroidism does not occur [IV]. This would usually involve annual TSH and T4 measurement.

THYROID CANCER IN PREGNANCY

Thyroid cancer is two to three times more common in women than men, and 50 per cent of cases occur within the reproductive age group. Pregnancy itself does not appear to influence the survival rates of women diagnosed with thyroid cancer. It is recommended that pregnancy should be delayed after treatment with radioactive iodine, probably for a period of a year [III], in view of the higher incidence of congenital anomalies that follow this treatment.

If a pregnant woman presents with a thyroid nodule, thyroid function tests and an ultrasound are indicated. Thyrotoxicosis occurring with cystic nodules is unlikely to be malignant, but other nodules should be investigated with a fine-needle aspirate. Cellular cytology from a fine-needle aspirate may suggest an underlying malignancy, and serial ultrasound should be performed. Removal of nodules that are increasing in size should be considered. A thyroidectomy can be performed, usually in the second trimester of pregnancy. If radioactive iodine is required, this should not be administered during breastfeeding [III].

Thyroid globulin concentration cannot be used to detect a relapse of thyroid cancer in pregnancy, as it is already elevated. Women on suppressive doses of T4 may continue this therapy, with the usual aim of reducing TSH to undetectable levels.

KEY POINTS

- Management decisions should be based on free T4 and T3 measurements in pregnancy; T4 is found at the lower limits of normal in pregnancy.
- Forty per cent of women with hyperemesis gravidarum have elevated T4 (and suppressed TSH); they do not require antithyroid treatment.
- Graves' disease is the most common cause of hyperthyroidism, and euthyroidism should be maintained in pregnancy with antithyroid drugs. Thyroid status should be checked every 4–6 weeks.
- Women with hypothyroidism should be euthyroid prior to conception to avoid intellectual impairment in the baby.

KEY REFERENCES

1. Koopdonk-Kool JM, de Vijlder JJM, Veenboer GHM et al. Type II and type III deiodinase activity in human placenta as a function of gestational age. *J Clin Endocrinol Metab* 1996; 81(6):2154–8.
2. Kortaba DD, Garner P, Perkins SL. Changes in serum free thyroxine, free tri-iodothyronine and thyroid stimulating hormone reference intervals in normal term pregnancy. *J Obstet Gynecol* 1995; 15:5–8.
3. Dillon JC, Milliez J. Reproductive failure in women living in iodine deficient areas of West Africa. *Br J Obstet Gynaecol* 2000; 107:631–6.
4. Cao XY, Jiang XM, Dou ZH et al. Timing of vulnerability of the brain to iodine deficiency in endemic cretinism. *N Engl J Med* 1994; 331(26):1739–44.
5. Kimura M, Amino N, Tamaki H. Gestational thyrotoxicosis and hyperemesis gravidarum: possible role of HCG with higher stimulating activity. *Clin Endocrinol* 1993; 38:345–50.
6. Kung AWC, Jones BM. A change from stimulatory to blocking antibody activity in Graves' disease during pregnancy. *J Clin Endocrinol Metab* 1998; 83:514–18.
7. Wing DA, Miller LK, Cunnings PP, Montoro MN, Mestman JH. A comparison of propylthiouracil versus methimazole in the treatment of hyperthyroidism in pregnancy. *Am J Obstet Gynecol* 1994; 170:90–5.
8. Momotani N, Noh JY, Ishikawa N, Ito K. Effects of propylthiouracil and methimazole on fetal thyroid status in mothers with Graves' hyperthyroidism. *J Clin Endocrinol Metab* 1997; 82:3633–6.
9. Haddow JE, Palomaki GE, Allan WC et al. Maternal thyroid deficiency during pregnancy and subsequent neuropsychological development of the child. *N Engl J Med* 1999; 341(8):549–55.
10. Pop VJ, Kuijpens JL, van Baar AI et al. Low maternal free thyroxine concentrations during early pregnancy are associated with impaired psychomotor development in infancy. *Clin Endocrinol* 1999; 50(2):149–55.
11. Girling JC, de Swiet M. Thyroxine dosage during pregnancy in women with primary hypothyroidism. *Br J Obstet Gynaecol* 1992; 99:368–70.
12. Mandel SJ, Larsen PR, Seely EW, Brent GA. Increased need for thyroxine during women with primary hypothyroidism. *N Engl J Med* 1990; 323:91–6.

Haematological Conditions

Joanna C. Gillham

ANAEMIA

Acquired anaemias are discussed in Chapter 7.1. This chapter deals with the pre-existing anaemias.

Aplastic/hypoplastic anaemia

This is secondary to a failure of the bone marrow to produce erythrocytes. It may be pre-existing or develop during pregnancy (and can be recurrent). It is thought that the pregnancy further depresses the bone marrow and exacerbates the condition. In the past, termination of pregnancy was recommended, but supportive measures have improved and, as long as the maternal condition is satisfactory, the pregnancy should be allowed to proceed. Pure red cell aplasia is rare but can be managed with transfusion.

Haemolytic anaemias

These disorders are rare, but the outlook in pregnancy is generally good. Management depends on the underlying pathology. In inherited conditions (congenital spherocytosis, pyruvate kinase deficiency etc.), treatment is with transfusion. Many of these patients will have had a splenectomy, and penicillin prophylaxis should be given. Iron overload should be screened for, because of the chronic haemolysis, and cardiac assessment performed as necessary. In autoimmune haemolytic anaemias, the prognosis has improved significantly with the use of steroids and immunosuppressants. Close monitoring is required to ensure rapidly developing profound anaemia is avoided. Any underlying cause should be treated optimally (e.g. systemic lupus erythematosus, SLE).

HAEMOGLOBINOPATHIES

The haemoglobinopathies are inherited disorders of haemoglobin synthesis (thalassaemias) or structure (sickle cell syndromes) that are responsible for significant morbidity and mortality on a worldwide scale. They have distinct ethnic preponderance, but, secondary to the increased mobility of the world's population and interethnic mixing, these conditions are no longer unusual within the UK, although the prevalence varies enormously from region to region.

There are two pairs of globin chains in each haemoglobin molecule. There are three normal haemoglobins, all of which have one pair of alpha-globin chains and one pair of gamma-chains (HbF), beta-chains (HbA) or delta-chains (HbA2). As alpha-chains are essential for all three types of haemoglobin, alpha-chain production is under the control of four genes, two inherited from the mother and two from the father. The majority of adult haemoglobin (>95 per cent) is HbA, and beta-chain production is under the control of two genes, one from the mother and one from the father. If all four alpha-globin genes are defective (and therefore there is no alpha-globin chain production), the outcome is Hb Bart's hydrops, which results in fetal hydrops and is incompatible with survival. One defective gene results in alpha-thal⁺ trait, and two defective genes result in either alpha-thal⁰ trait (both defective genes from one parent) or homozygous alpha-thal⁺ trait (one defective gene from each parent). In all three of these situations, the patient is asymptomatic. If three defective genes are inherited (one from one parent and two from the other), this results in HbH disease, which causes a moderate haemolytic anaemia. In contrast, if one beta-globin gene is defective, this causes beta-thalassaemia trait or minor, which is associated with mild anaemia. If both beta-globin genes are defective, no beta-globin chains are produced, and this results in beta-thalassaemia major, the majority of affected individuals being transfusion-dependent for life, with all the consequences of iron overload.

In the sickle cell syndromes, it is the structure of the globin chains rather than the production that is abnormal. Many different forms exist, but the commonest and clinically most important is HbS, in which there is a single amino acid substitution in the beta-globin chain which renders it insoluble in the deoxygenated state. This alters the shape of the red blood cell into a sickle shape, hence the name. Sickle cell trait (HbAS) is much commoner than sickle cell disease (HbSS). Other haemoglobin variants exist (e.g. HbC, HbE), but are less common. If both partners carry a haemoglobin variant (i.e. trait), there is a 1:4 chance of the child inheriting both the abnormal genes, and thus sickle cell disease. This risk increases to 1:2 if one partner has two abnormal genes (i.e. disease) and the other has trait.

Screening

The implications of the major haemoglobinopathies (beta-thalassaemia major and sickle cell disease) are such that the introduction of universal antenatal and neonatal screening is being considered by the UK government, as selective screening is proving to be ineffective [IV]. It is suggested that universal antenatal screening should be employed in high-prevalence areas and effective selective screening in other areas.[1] As the major haemoglobinopathies are autosomal recessive conditions, with carrier status having little implication for health, many people are completely unaware that they are carriers. With regard to neonatal screening, it is

proposed to incorporate this into universal blood spot screening, as there is a proven reduction in morbidity and mortality in sickle cell disease with early diagnosis and prophylactic treatment [II].[1]

Screening for the thalassaemias is by examining the red cell indices and the HbA2 levels. With thalassaemia traits, there is a reduced mean corpuscular volume (MCV <75 fL), reduced mean corpuscular haemoglobin (MCH <27 pg), and a normal or near-normal mean corpuscular haemoglobin concentration (MCHC). In addition, in beta-thalassaemia trait there is an elevated HbA2 (>3.5 per cent). In alpha-thalassaemia traits, the changes may be minimal in alpha-thal⁺ trait. DNA analysis is required to confirm the diagnosis. Screening for sickle cell variants is done by HPLC or electrophoresis. Anything other than HbAA is regarded as a variant (e.g. HbAS, AC, SC etc.).

If a woman is found to be a haemoglobinopathy carrier, her partner should be screened as early as possible and, if there is a risk of the fetus having a major haemoglobinopathy, urgent expert counselling should be given to allow the couple to make an informed choice regarding prenatal diagnosis and termination of pregnancy [IV]. Ideally, this screening and counselling should be done pre-pregnancy, as the optimal method of prenatal diagnosis is chorionic villous sampling in the first trimester [IV], which also allows surgical termination of pregnancy should the fetus be affected. Unfortunately, this rarely happens, and there is therefore some urgency to effective antenatal screening to allow optimal care.

Thalassaemias in pregnancy

Alpha-Thalassaemias

Those with trait may become anaemic during pregnancy, and iron and folate supplementation should be given, although parenteral iron should be avoided. Those with HbH disease have a chronic haemolytic anaemia and require 5 mg folic acid daily. They are often not iron deficient because of the chronic haemolysis, and transfusion is often indicated to treat the anaemia. It must be remembered that the maternal complications when a fetus has Hb Bart's hydrops include early-onset severe pre-eclampsia, and intrapartum problems secondary to the delivery of a grossly hydropic fetus and placenta, including primary postpartum haemorrhage.

Beta-Thalassaemia

Those with trait are often anaemic. These women should take 5 mg folic acid daily, and oral iron supplements if the ferritin is low (never parenteral iron). If the anaemia does not respond, transfusion may be indicated.

Pregnancy is rare in transfusion-dependent beta-thalassaemia major, although with aggressive iron chelation programmes the rate is increasing. Some women with beta-thalassaemia major are not truly transfusion dependent, and pregnancies have been reported. In all cases of beta-thalassaemia major, iron overload is a major concern, particularly in terms of myocardial function, and a cardiology assessment should be performed. Iron supplementation should always be avoided, and the anaemia treated with transfusion. Folate supplementation (5 mg/day) is required. All women with beta-thalassaemia major should be looked after in pregnancy by a team consisting of a haematologist and an obstetrician with the relevant expertise [IV].

KEY POINTS

Thalassaemias

- These are inherited disorders of haemoglobin synthesis.
- Normal-structure haemoglobin has one pair of alpha-globin chains and one pair of alpha-, beta- or gamma-globin chains.
- The majority of adult haemoglobin is HbA – alpha- and beta-globin.
- If two defective alpha-globin chains are present = alpha-thalassaemia trait.
- If three defective alpha-globin genes are present = HbH disease.
- If four defective alpha-globin genes are present = Hb Bart's hydrops – incompatible with survival.
- Screening is by examining the red cell indices and the HbA2 levels.
- Thalassaemia traits possess ↓ MCV, ↓ MCH and a normal or near-normal MCHC.

Sickle cell variants in pregnancy

Those with trait are not at increased risk of adverse maternal or fetal outcome other than the risks to the mother if severe hypoxia develops – of which the anaesthetist should be aware and general anaesthesia avoided if possible – and the risks to the fetus of inheriting major disease if the father also has trait.

Sickle cell disease in pregnancy

It is very unusual to diagnose sickle cell disease during pregnancy, as the vast majority of affected individuals are aware of the diagnosis from childhood. The clinical features of sickle cell disease include:

- chronic haemolytic anaemia
- painful crises
- hyposplenism
- increased risk of infection
- avascular bone necrosis
- increased risk of cerebrovascular accidents (CVA)
- chest syndrome.

During pregnancy, crises may become more frequent and close attention must be paid to optimal management. Women with sickle cell disease are at increased risk of:

- miscarriage
- infection
- intrauterine growth restriction (IUGR)
- pre-eclampsia
- stillbirth
- prematurity
- thromboembolic disease
- perinatal mortality
- maternal mortality.

Ideally, women should be seen in a joint clinic by an obstetrician and a haematologist with expertise in haemoglobinopathies [IV]. Pre-pregnancy counselling is optimal, but often women present when already pregnant. Partner screening and counselling regarding prenatal diagnosis should be given if these aspects have not already been addressed. Iron chelation should be stopped prior to conception, as the agents used are contraindicated in pregnancy. A ferritin level should be checked and, if elevated or there is a history of significant iron overload, an echocardiograph and cardiac assessment should be performed to exclude cardiomyopathy. The need for folic acid supplementation (5 mg/day) and penicillin prophylaxis throughout pregnancy should be emphasized. Renal and hepatic function should be assessed regularly, as both can be compromised. Haemoglobin and HbS level should be monitored regularly, and a programme of top-up or exchange transfusion implemented as indicated. These patients have often had multiple transfusions in the past, and may have multiple blood group antibodies that can cause problems with cross-matching. Venous access can also be significantly compromised. Any signs of infection should be treated aggressively, and dehydration and exposure to cold avoided, as in the non-pregnant state.

In the event of a crisis or chest syndrome, good oxygenation and hydration are essential, as well as adequate pain relief. The patient must be kept warm and any infection promptly treated. In severe cases, top-up transfusion or even exchange transfusion may be required. Careful consideration should be given to the use of thromboprophylaxis.

From the fetal perspective, regular assessment of fetal growth and placental function is indicated with ultrasound and Doppler assessment. Caesarean section should only be performed for obstetric indications, and general anaesthesia should be avoided.

In labour, intravenous fluids must be given to avoid dehydration, and oxygen used to prevent hypoxia. Attention should be paid to analgesia, and continuous electronic fetal monitoring is recommended. Consideration should be given to the use of thromboprophylaxis; the use of prophylactic antibiotics remains controversial.

Haemoglobinopathies

- Universal antenatal and neonatal screening for the inherited haemoglobinopathies is being considered as selective screening is not effective.
- Neonatal screening for inherited haemoglobinopathies reduces morbidity and mortality by early diagnosis and prompt treatment.
- If a woman is found to be a haemoglobinopathy carrier, her partner should be screened to allow pre-pregnancy genetic counselling, if necessary, or prenatal diagnosis and the option of a termination of pregnancy.
- Pregnant women with any haemoglobinopathy (if not trait) should be looked after by a haemotologist and an obstetrician with relevant expertise.

KEY POINTS

Sickle cell syndrome

- This is an inherited disease of haemoglobin structure.
- In sickle cell, HbS is secondary to a single amino acid substitution in the beta-globin chain.
- HbS is insoluble in the deoxygenated form – altering the red blood cell shape to a sickle.
- Sickle cell syndrome is inherited as an autosomal recessive disease.
- Screening is via electrophoresis.
- In sickle cell trait, there is no increased maternal or fetal adverse outcome, unless there is severe hypoxia in the mother or the risk of disease to the fetus should the father be a haemoglobinopathy carrier.
- Women with sickle cell syndrome have an increased risk of adverse outcome in pregnancy.

KEY POINTS

Sickle cell disease in pregnancy

- The women should be seen in a joint obstetric/haematology clinic.
- Pre-pregnancy counselling is the gold standard.
- If not, partner screening and counselling regarding prenatal diagnosis are required.
- Folic acid supplementation (5 mg/day) and penicillin prophylaxis should be continued for the duration of the pregnancy.

- Haemoglobin, ferritin and HbS levels and renal and hepatic function tests need to be assessed monthly.
- Top-up or exchange transfusion may be warranted antenatally.
- Any signs of infection or dehydration should be managed aggressively.
- Ultrasound scans for fetal assessment are required from 28 weeks of pregnancy.
- Caesarean section should be for routine obstetric reasons and general anaesthesia avoided if at all possible.

PLATELET DISORDERS

Multinucleated cells in the bone marrow (megakaryocytes) produce platelets. They have a critical role in normal haemostasis and in thrombotic disorders, and circulate for 7–10 days. Bleeding can result from abnormal platelet function or a reduced count of normal platelets.[2] The normal platelet count is $150–350 \times 10^9$/L. The maternal platelet count decreases between 20 and 40 weeks' gestation by approximately 12 per cent.[3] Platelets are removed by the spleen, and an elevated platelet count is found in those patients who have had a splenectomy. There are other, rare, causes of increased platelet counts that are not usually seen in pregnancy. The main concern is that of an increased risk of thromboembolic disease, which can be minimized by low-dose aspirin (75 mg or 150 mg/day).

Thrombocytopenia

Thrombocytopenia, defined as a platelet count of $>150 \times 10^9$/L, occurs in up to 15 per cent of pregnancies. A falsely low platelet count may occur due to platelet agglutination in a blood sample, caused by the anticoagulant EDTA. Thus thrombocytopenia should be confirmed by examination of a peripheral blood film. If clumping is seen, a citrated sample should be sent; if this gives a normal platelet count, all samples should be sent in citrate rather than EDTA, and no other action is required. Patients with severe thrombocytopenia often have petechiae and mucocutaneous bleeding, resulting from small, unsealed endothelial lesions. By contrast, patients with the inherited bleeding disorders do not have petechiae or excessive bleeding from small cuts as their platelet adhesion and aggregation tend to be sufficient.[2]

If mild thrombocytopenia is discovered, a repeat full blood count (FBC) is required in 1 month to ensure there has been no further fall. If the platelet count is falling, or on initial testing is found to be $<100 \times 10^9/L$, the following tests should be performed.

- FBC, clotting profile, renal and liver function tests, urate.
- Examination of peripheral blood film.
- Lupus anticoagulant, anticardiolipin antibodies, antinuclear antibodies.
- Virology screen.
- Platelet autoantibodies. Because of the complexity of platelet membranes, the precise identification and measurement of such antibodies have been difficult. These antibodies can be present in both gestational and immune thrombocytopenia.
- Bone marrow aspiration may need to be considered in severe thrombocytopenia.

Causes of thrombocytopenia in pregnancy

- Pregnancy-associated thrombocytopenia (PAT) – 74 per cent.
- Hypertensive disorders of pregnancy – 21 per cent.
- Immune disorders – 4 per cent.
- Others (disseminated intravascular coagulation (DIC), thrombotic thrombocytopenic purpura (TTP), HELLP syndrome, acute fatty liver) – 2 per cent.

Pregnancy-associated thrombocytopenia

Up to 4 per cent of pregnant women develop PAT. This is a benign, symptomless condition. The mother is at no increased risk of haemorrhagic problems and there is no effect on the fetus, and no treatment is required. Resolution tends to occur within 6 weeks of delivery. The platelet count will be normal at the booking visit if this is in the first or early second trimester. The platelet count usually remains above $100 \times 10^9/L$. If the platelet count is lower than this initially, continues decreasing rapidly or the thrombocytopenia occurs early on in the pregnancy, other diagnoses must be considered.[2] If the woman books late in pregnancy and is already thrombocytopenic, idiopathic thrombocytopenic pupura (ITP) often cannot be excluded and, because of the fetal implications, should be treated as such until the diagnosis can be clarified, often after delivery.

Familial thrombocytopenia

This is an autosomal dominant condition that causes profound thrombocytopenia, with platelet counts of around $20 \times 10^9/L$, although spontaneous bleeding is rare. There is no effective drug therapy and management is supportive when required. The fetus has a 50 per cent chance of being affected, and the same measures apply regarding delivery as with ITP (see below).

Storage pool disease

In this condition, the platelet count is normal but platelet function is abnormal, and a significant bleeding history as well as a family history are usually present. It is unlikely that this diagnosis will be made during pregnancy, and most cases seen are already known about and under the care of a haematologist. Diagnosis is confirmed by platelet function tests, and management is supportive. The condition is autosomal dominant, and the fetus therefore has a 50 per cent risk of being affected. Traumatic delivery should thus be avoided.

AUTOIMMUNE DISEASE

Idiopathic immune thrombocytopenic purpura

This is isolated thrombocytopenia with no clinically apparent associated disorders. The diagnosis is largely after exclusion of the other causes of thrombocytopenia. It is the most common autoimmune disorder, affecting 1–3 in 1000 pregnancies, and the platelet count may well be decreased at the initial booking visit. Antibodies, usually IgG, are directed against the platelet membrane. Often patients are asymptomatic and pregnancy does not always (but can) exacerbate the disease. If the platelet count is $>50 \times 10^9/L$, no treatment is necessary. Major bleeding is rarely seen unless the platelet count is $<10 \times 10^9/L$. Patients with clinical bleeding or a count $<50 \times 10^9/L$ are treated with oral corticosteroids; 70–90 per cent of women will respond within 3 weeks. Corticosteroids act by inhibiting platelet antibody production and increasing bone marrow platelet production. Patients who fail to respond to steroids are treated with intravenous immune globulin, which prolongs the clearance time of circulating immune complexes. The length of effect is variable, but in the order of 2–3 weeks. Steroids should always be tried in the first instance, as immune globulin is a blood product, requires hospital admission for administration, although usually as a day case, and is very expensive. Splenectomy in pregnancy is rarely required. Platelet transfusions are used only in the acute situation, to deal with haemorrhage or to cover delivery. The decision to use platelet transfusions should be made in conjunction with a consultant haematologist.

Maternal antibodies may cross the placenta and affect the fetus, causing thrombocytopenia; 4–10 per cent of neonates are at risk of having severe thrombocytopenia at birth or during the first week of life.[2] The maternal platelet count does not correlate with the fetal platelet count, and it is not predictive of any adverse fetal outcome.[4] Administration of corticosteroids or immune globulin does not affect the fetal platelet count. In labour, fetal blood sampling and invasive fetal monitoring should be avoided, as should ventouse extraction, because of the risk of cephalhaematoma. If an instrumental delivery is unavoidable, low cavity forceps only should be used by an experienced operator, but traumatic delivery must be avoided [III]. There appears to be no benefit conferred by delivery by caesarean section [III]. The management of the baby in the neonatal period is most important; platelet counts and paediatric assessments are indicated (the nadir of the neonatal platelet count occurs on day 4–7).

Acquired Glanzman's disease

Rarely, in some cases of ITP, the circulating immune complexes can bind to the platelets and inhibit their function. In this situation, the haemorrhagic history is in excess of that expected from the platelet count, and patients may give a history of excessive bruising or bleeding, even with a platelet count $>50 \times 10^9/L$ (i.e. platelet function is inadequate). Diagnosis is by platelet function tests and a bleeding time, and treatment consists of immune suppression with steroids etc., as well as supportive measures in the form of platelet transfusion when required. Close liaison with the haematology department is advised.

Antiphospholipid syndrome/systemic lupus erythematosus

The thrombocytopenia found in these conditions can be profound. The presence of IgG antibodies prolongs the partial thromboplastin time and, very rarely, the prothrombin time. Paradoxically, these patients are at a greater risk of thrombosis than of bleeding. Treatment is with aspirin and heparin. The fetus is not at risk of thrombocytopenia. (See Chapter 6.7 for further details.)

Pre-eclampsia

Pre-eclampsia is associated with the activation of the coagulation system. Thrombocytopenia in varying degrees is found in 30 per cent or more of patients.

Between 4 and 12 per cent of women with pre-eclampsia may have haemolysis, increased liver enzymes and low platelets (HELLP syndrome). (See Chapter 7.6 for further details.)

Infection

Many infectious diseases, for example viruses – human immunodeficiency virus (HIV), cytomegalovirus (CMV) and Epstein–Barr virus (EBV) – mycoplasma, bacterial infection

and malaria, can be associated with thrombocytopenia. There are no fetal effects of the thrombocytopenia; however, the underlying disease may have further implications. (See Chapter 7.4 for further details.)

Drugs

Heparin, quinine, rifampicin and trimethoprim are some of the drugs that can cause thrombocytopenia. This usually resolves fairly quickly on stopping the causative agent.

THE HAEMOSTATIC MECHANISM

The factors involved in the cessation of bleeding are:

1 *Haemostasis.* There is obliteration of the injured vessel, with vasoconstrictors released from platelets and external pressure from haematoma formation or contraction of the surrounding smooth muscle. There is an additional contribution via platelet aggregation.
2 *Coagulation*
   - *Stage 1.* Intrinsic mechanism – activation of factors XII, XI and IX by vessel wall damage; then factor VIII activation in the presence of calcium causes activation of factor X.
   Extrinsic mechanism – tissue damage releases factors III and VII, causing activation of factor X.
   - *Stage 2.* Activated factor X, with factor V and calcium, convert factor II (prothrombim) to thrombin.
   - *Stage 3.* Thrombin converts factor I (fibrinogen) to a fibrin monomer, which forms a fibrin polymer and eventually fibrin.

MATERNAL PHYSIOLOGICAL CHANGES IN PREGNANCY

(The changes in the blood volume and red cell mass in a normal pregnancy are discussed in Chapter 7.1.) The total white cell count increases in pregnancy, with counts as high as $16 \times 10^9/L$ observed in the third trimester. Counts up to 30×10^9 have been observed in a normal labour. Lymphocytes and monocytes remain at pre-pregnancy levels; the rise is in polymorphonuclear leucocytes.

Pregnancy is a pro-thrombotic physiological state. There is a marked increase in the level of fibrinogen and factor VIII. Factors V, VII, X, XII and von Willebrand factor (vWF) also increase, but to a lesser extent. There is little increase in factor IX. The anticoagulants antithrombin III and protein C remain at a steady level, and protein S level is decreased by 40 per cent. Acquired activated protein C resistance is present and fibrinolysis is inhibited with decreased plasminogen activator inhibitor.

KEY POINTS

Haematological changes in normal pregnancy

- ↑ white cell count
- ↑ factors V, VII, VIII, IX, X, XII, fibrinogen, vWF
- ↓ antithrombin III, protein C
- ↓ protein S, plasminogen activator inhibitor
- ↓ platelets

VENOUS THROMBOEMBOLIC DISEASE

The major predisposing factors to venous thromboembolic disease (VTE) are the activation of blood coagulation, venous stasis and endothelial injury (Virchow's triad). The risk of VTE is increased with pregnancy to approximately 1/1000 pregnancies,[5] and is greater in the postpartum compared to the antepartum period. The pregnancy-associated increase in clotting factors is discussed above. With advancing gestation, the enlarging uterus diminishes the venous return from the legs, with increasing venous stasis ensuing. These factors, often combined with antenatal immobilization, prolonged labour, dehydration, excessive blood loss and possible surgery, explain the risk of VTE being increased approximately fivefold with pregnancy and the puerperium. Other general risk factors are prolonged immobilization, malignancy, chronic inflammatory disease, oestrogens and the combined oral contraceptive pill/hormone replacement therapy (HRT), nephrotic syndrome, major surgery, particularly orthopaedic and pelvic, antiphospholipid syndrome and sepsis. The presentation of VTE is complicated in that the symptoms of lower limb oedema and dyspnoea are common complaints of the normal pregnant woman. Any clinical suspicion of VTE must be investigated immediately to avoid the risks and costs of inappropriate anticoagulation [II]. VTE disease is the leading cause of maternal mortality in the UK,[6] with the majority of deaths from pulmonary embolism following caesarean section, and occurring after the first week of the puerperium, hence after discharge from hospital. All those involved with the care of these women should be alert to this fact.[6] Many of the guidelines for the management of VTE in the non-pregnant patient are based on level Ia evidence. However, similar evidence for the management of VTE during pregnancy is lacking and, in general, guideline recommendations for management during pregnancy are extrapolated (rightly or wrongly) from these studies.[7]

KEY POINTS

Risk factors for VTE

- Pregnancy
- Malignancy
- Prolonged immobilization
- Chronic inflammatory disease
- Inherited/acquired thrombophilia
- Oestrogen – combined oral contraceptive pill/HRT
- Nephritic syndrome
- Major surgery
- Sepsis

Deep vein thrombosis

Symptoms and signs

The majority of deep vein thromboses (DVTs) occurring during pregnancy are in the left leg. Symptoms include pain in affected calf/leg, swelling, fever, erythema and increased heat of the affected leg. A positive Homan's sign is unreliable.

Investigation

In clinically suspected VTE, treatment with low-molecular-weight heparin should be given until the diagnosis is excluded by objective testing [Ia].[7]

1 D-*dimers*. VTE is associated with increased levels of blood D-dimer, and this is often now used as a screening test in non-pregnant individuals. However, elevations in D-dimer level are found in uncomplicated pregnancy, with levels increasing with advancing gestation. A positive D-dimer screen is of no prognostic significance in VTE in pregnancy, but a low level of D-dimer in pregnancy suggests there is no VTE.

2 *Duplex ultrasound*. This has a high sensitivity and specificity in proximal DVTs and is non-invasive. It is unreliable for calf DVT as it has a much lower sensitivity. If the initial ultrasound scan is negative and there is a low level of clinical suspicion, anticoagulant treatment can be stopped. If the ultrasound is negative and there is a high level of clinical suspicion, the patient should be anticoagulated and the ultrasound repeated in a week, or venography performed [IV].[7] Isolated below-knee DVT is uncommon in pregnancy, but if identified, treatment should be given.

3 *Venography*. This adequately visualizes calf and deep veins. Disadvantages include the use of radiation, an allergic reaction to the dye used and a 5 per cent risk of causing thrombosis.

Management

Graduated compression stockings (TEDS) should be worn in the acute period and it is recommended that they should be worn on the affected leg for 2 years after the event to reduce the incidence of post-thrombotic syndrome [Ia].[7] Compliance is often a problem in pregnancy, mainly secondary to poor fit of the stockings; therefore careful measurement and fitting are essential. Hot weather and not having enough pairs also affect compliance.

Before commencing anticoagulant treatment, blood should be taken for a FBC, clotting, renal and liver function tests, and there should be a thrombophilia screen to screen for both inherited and acquired thrombophilia.[7] Thrombophilia screens can be difficult to interpret with the physiological changes in pregnancy and should only be interpreted by a clinician with expertise in this area, but this is not a reason not to perform them.

Low-molecular-weight heparin (LMWH) by subcutaneous injection is the treatment of choice in both the pregnant and non-pregnant population. A recent Cochrane review concluded that LMWH was at least as effective as unfractionated heparin in preventing recurrent VTE, and significantly reduced the occurrence of major haemorrhage during the initial treatment and overall mortality at the end of follow-up [Ia].[8] Treatment for VTE occurring in relation to pregnancy should continue for at least 6–12 weeks after delivery or 6 months after the initial episode – whichever is the longer [II].[9]

Heparin does not cross the placenta, is not teratogenic and does not cause an anticoagulant effect in the fetus. Complications of long-term heparin treatment are osteopenia, thrombocytopenia and allergic skin reactions at the site of injection.

Osteopenia is less common with LMWHs compared to unfractionated heparins, although it can still occur, especially if other risk factors are present. Early heparin-induced thrombocytopenia (HIT) occurs 1–5 days after the start of therapy and is usually mild. Late heparin-induced thrombocytopenia is due to IgG-mediated platelet activation and usually occurs 5–15 days after commencement. This can produce a rapid fall in the platelet count and is highly prothrombotic. HIT should be screened for by checking the maternal platelet count weekly for the first 4 weeks of treatment. HIT is less common with LMWH compared to unfractionated heparin. Most cases respond rapidly to changing LMWH to danaparoid. If an allergic response develops at the injection sites, changing the brand of heparin (and thus the vehicle) may lead to resolution.

The advantage of the LMWHs in the non-pregnant state is their longer plasma half-life, allowing once-a-day dosing. During pregnancy, however, evidence is emerging that the pharmacokinetics are altered compared to the non-pregnant state, suggesting that monitoring is required [IV], and dose alterations are not infrequent throughout pregnancy, with many women requiring twice-daily dosing in the second half of pregnancy. Any woman on heparin during pregnancy must have a carefully documented care plan for labour and delivery. Induction of labour is often employed to facilitate dose adjustment in a planned way, and to try to minimize exposure to heparin because of the potential bone effects. Women should be advised that if there are any signs of labour, they should omit their heparin until they are seen and assessed. Anaesthetic input may be required when devising the care plan with respect to regional blockade. If prophylactic doses are being used, the heparin can usually be omitted for the course of labour, and if the last dose was taken at least 12 hours previously, regional blockade is not contraindicated. The risk of haemorrhage is low with prophylactic doses. When full therapeutic doses are employed, a decision must be made antenatally as to whether the risk of VTE is such that the heparin cannot be stopped, in which case the dose should be reduced to a prophylactic level for the duration of labour. In this case, regional blockade is contraindicated. In some cases, the risk is low enough to allow heparin to be stopped for the duration of labour. In both cases, heparin should be restarted after delivery. It should be remembered that in an emergency, protamine sulphate can be used to reverse the effects of heparin, but usually only achieves 60 per cent reversal.

Warfarin is an oral coumarin, and is the most commonly used anticoagulant. It acts in the liver by inhibiting the synthesis of four vitamin K-dependent coagulant proteins (factors II, VII, IX, X) and at least two vitamin K-dependent anticoagulant factors, proteins C and S. Warfarin crosses the placenta freely and is teratogenic, causing chondrodysplasia punctata (nasal hypoplasia, saddle nose, frontal bossing, short stature, mental retardation, cataract and optic atrophy; see Chapter 8). The teratogenic effects are avoided if warfarin is stopped prior to 6 weeks' gestation, and patients on long-term warfarin should be fully counselled regarding this and have direct access to either the haematology department or obstetric unit to be converted to heparin as soon as they have a positive pregnancy test. Warfarin also causes anticoagulation in the fetus, with risks of gross retroplacental or intracerebral bleeding, and microcephaly has been described in these fetuses. There is no agent available which can rapidly reverse the effects of warfarin, and reversal by stopping therapy and giving vitamin K takes up to 5 days. Women on warfarin are converted to heparin towards the end of pregnancy to allow more control of the haemorrhagic risk associated with delivery in the anticoagulated patient. Certain patients, those with metal heart valves or heparin allergy, may still require treatment with warfarin in pregnancy despite the risks, although with close heparin monitoring, patients with metal heart valves have been managed successfully throughout pregnancy on LMWH, and newer anticoagulants with less risk to the fetus may be available soon. Warfarin is not excreted in significant quantities in breast milk, and is thus safe in breastfeeding mothers.

KEY POINTS – DEEP VEIN THROMBOSIS

- Symptoms and signs: pain, swelling, fever, erythema, positive Homan's sign.
- The majority in pregnancy are in the left leg.
- Investigation: D-dimer, duplex ultrasound, venography.
- Treatment: TEDS, LMWH.
- Treatment until 6 weeks postpartum or 3 months after VTE – whichever is the longer.

Antenatal complications: maternal

PULMONARY EMBOLISM

This can occur with or without preceding DVT. Symptoms range from minimal disturbance to sudden collapse and death, depending on the size, number and site of the emboli.

Signs and symptoms

These include dyspnoea, chest pain, cough, haemoptysis, pyrexia, tachycardia, tachypnoea, cyanosis, raised jugular venous pressure (JVP), pleural rub, pleural effusion and right ventricular failure.

Investigations

- Arterial blood gas analysis – hypoxia and hypercapnia.
- Electrocardiogram (ECG): inverted T waves and atrial arrhythmia are suggestive. In pregnancy, normal ECG findings can be a right axis deviation and T wave inversion and a Q wave in lead III, which in the non-pregnant patient would be suggestive of a pulmonary embolism (PE).
- Chest X-ray (CXR): an abnormal CXR is found in 69–80 per cent of patients with a PE.
- Ventilation-perfusion scan: in cases of suspected PE, both a V/Q scan and a bilateral Doppler ultrasound of the leg veins should be performed [IV].[7] This is a sensitive but not specific test. Interpretation of a V/Q scan is given as a probability rating. As anticoagulant therapy is a greater health risk to the mother than the radiation dose to the fetus (which does not cause fetal abnormality, but slightly increases the risk of childhood malignancy), diagnosis should be aggressively pursued with the use of these imaging techniques. Anticoagulation should be continued when the V/Q scan reports a medium or high probability of a PE. If the scan reports a low probability and Doppler studies of the leg are positive, anticoagulation should be continued. If the leg Doppler studies are also negative, yet there is a high degree of clinical suspicion, continuation of treatment with repeat testing in 1 week should be considered [IV].[7]
- Spiral computed tomographic (CT) scanning: this is gaining in popularity as a diagnostic tool. It can visualize the blood clot, if present. Other advantages include the ability to identify other disease states that can mimic PE. The radiation risks to the fetus are considered minimal.
- Pulmonary angiogram: the gold standard for the diagnosis of PE. This is invasive, with a mortality rate of 0.5 per cent and associated morbidity of 2–4 per cent.

Treatment

- With massive PE, intravenous unfractionated heparin remains the initial treatment of choice in the acute situation.
- For smaller, minimally symptomatic clots, LMWH may be used in the acute phase, and certainly in the further treatment for the PE after this phase. The initial drug dosage is based on the patient's early pregnancy weight. If the diagnosis of VTE is confirmed, peak anti-Xa activity should be measured 2–4 hours post-injection. The target therapeutic range for LMWH is somewhat arbitrary, but 0.6–1.0 IU/mL appears satisfactory.
- When using long-term treatment doses of thromboprophylaxis during pregnancy, it is recommended to perform regular anti-factor Xa levels and adjust the dose accordingly. However, the frequency of monitoring has not yet been clearly established. There is also evidence to support this approach in prophylactic doses.
- Warfarin has a minimal place in the treatment of the pregnant woman, but is suitable in the postpartum period.
- Inferior vena caval (IVC) filters are reserved for those cases with recurrent PE despite adequate anticoagulation or for patients who cannot receive anticoagulation.
- There is limited information on the use of thrombolysis for a PE in the pregnant woman. Streptokinase is most commonly used and does not cross the placenta. The major side effect can be severe genital tract bleeding, and its use should therefore be reserved for those patients who are haemodynamically unstable.
- Surgical embolectomy: a specialist clinician should follow up women who have experienced a thrombosis during pregnancy. Once they are at least 6 weeks postpartum, and have discontinued anticoagulant therapy, a thrombophilia screen should be performed if this has not already been done or the results are difficult to interpret (e.g. low protein S). This allows assessment of future risk, management decisions to be made regarding future pregnancies and discussion of appropriate contraception.[10]

KEY POINTS – PULMONARY EMBOLISM

- Symptoms and signs: chest pain, dyspnoea, haemoptysis, pyrexia, tachycardia, tachypnoea, cyanosis, ↑ JVP, pleural rub/effusion, right ventricular failure.
- Investigation: arterial blood gas, ECG, CXR, V/Q scan, spiral CT, pulmonary angiogram.
- Treatment: acute phase and a large PE – intravenous unfractionated heparin.
- With smaller, minimal symptom PE or in longer term treatment – LMWH.
- Other treatment: IVC filter, thrombolysis, surgical embolectomy.

Management of venous thromboembolism

- Any clinical suspicion of VTE must be investigated as soon as possible.
- Whilst awaiting investigation, appropriate thromboprophylaxis should be commenced.
- In DVT investigation, if clinical suspicion is high and initial Doppler negative, repeat or more invasive testing should be considered.
- TEDS should be worn for 2 years after a VTE event.
- LMWH by subcutaneous injection is the treatment of choice in DVT in both the pregnant and non-pregnant population.
- If a PE is suspected, a V/Q scan and bilateral leg Doppler ultrasound studies should be performed.

THROMBOPROPHYLAXIS IN NORMAL PREGNANCY

Delivery by caesarean section increases the risk of VTE by two to eight times. The highest risk is with an emergency procedure under a general anaesthetic. In 1995, the Royal College of Obstetricians and Gynaecologists (RCOG) issued guidelines with regard to thromboprophylaxis following caesarean section.[11] These are broad guidelines and in reality most units have a local protocol. Increasingly, many units are giving all patients who are delivered by caesarean section (both elective and emergency) thromboprophylaxis. The most recent Confidential Enquiry into Maternal Deaths in the UK[6] has reported a decrease in the number of deaths from VTE following caesarean section, which they attribute to more widespread use of thromboprophylaxis since the introduction of the RCOG guidelines. However, it still recommends more widespread use of thromboprophylaxis, even after normal delivery.

MANAGEMENT OF THE PREGNANT PATIENT WITH A PREVIOUS VTE

There are no randomized, controlled trials concerning the management of this obstetric problem, and expert advice is conflicting. The RCOG recommends that if a woman has had one previous VTE episode related to pregnancy and has no other risk factors, anticoagulation for 6 weeks postpartum is sufficient, but if any other risk factors are present, anticoagulation throughout pregnancy should be considered.[11] The British Society of Haematologists, however, recommends that all patients with a past history of VTE merit consideration for thromboprophylaxis to cover periods of

increased thrombotic risk (which obviously includes pregnancy) [IV], and highlights the fact that a significant number of thrombotic events occur in the first trimester, and thus recommends thromboprophylaxis from the time that pregnancy is confirmed.[9]

THE THROMBOPHILIAS

A thrombophilia is defined as a predisposition to thrombosis, secondary to any persistent or identifiable hypercoaguable state. This can be inherited or acquired.

A thrombophilia can be identified in up to 50 per cent of those with a history of VTE. Protein C, protein S, antithrombin III, Factor V Leiden (FVL) and the pro-thrombin gene mutation 20210 (PGM) are now the most common causes of hypercoagubility. Others include hyperhomocyteinaemia (HHC), elevated factor VII and the antiphospholipid syndrome.

Protein C deficiency

Protein C circulates in an inactive state. Thrombin 'activates' this vitamin K-dependent protein, and activated protein C with its cofactor protein S inactivates the clotting factors Va and VIIIa. Protein C deficiency is present in approximately 1 in 500 people with an autosomal dominant pattern of inheritance. In patients with protein C deficiency, thrombosis occurs in 25 per cent of pregnancies without anticoagulation. Two-thirds of these are in the postpartum period.

Protein S deficiency

Protein S is a vitamin K-dependent protein, which is a cofactor for activated protein C. Protein S levels decrease in pregnancy, and are reduced in women using the combined oral contraceptive pill and HRT. A definitive diagnosis of protein S deficiency cannot therefore be made until these influences have been removed, which may take several weeks. The prevalence of protein S deficiency in the general population is unknown.

Antithrombin III deficiency

Antithrombin III inactivates thrombin and factors IXa, Xa, XIa and XIIa, and is a naturally occurring anticoagulant. Its activity is amplified by heparin. Deficiency occurs in 1 in 5000 people and its inheritance is autosomal dominant. The risk of thrombosis is up to 70 per cent in untreated patients, thus anticoagulation is recommended.

Factor V Leiden

Activated protein C (APC) resistance has numerous underlying causes, but the vast majority of patients with APC resistance were found to have the same point mutation in the gene for clotting factor V – the Factor V Leiden mutation. Other causes of APC resistance are increased levels of factor VIII or the presence of antiphospholipid antibodies. In Caucasian populations, FVL is the commonest inherited thrombophilia, with a reported prevalence of between 2 and 15 per cent. It is less common in people of African and Asian origin. Depending on patient selection, FVL is found in 20–50 per cent of patients presenting with a first episode of venous thrombosis.[9] Overall, only a small proportion of those who carry the mutation develop a thrombosis, but it is associated with a twenty-fold increased risk of thrombosis during pregnancy. At present routine screening is not advocated, and selective screening should be confined to those with a personal or family history of VTE.

Prothrombin G20210A mutation

The G→A transition at the nucleotide 20210 in the prothrombin gene is associated with elevated plasma prothrombin levels and up to a five times increased risk of venous thrombosis. The prevalence in Northern Europe is around 2 per cent in the healthy population and 6 per cent in unselected cases with a first episode of VTE.[9] It is inherited in an autosomal dominant pattern.

Hyperhomocysteinaemia

Homocysteine is produced solely from the metabolism of the essential amino acid methionine. Inherited HHC results from genetic defects affecting this pathway. Acquired HHC may be secondary to folate, vitamin B6 and B12 deficiencies and antifolate medication such as methotrexate.[10] A fasting value of homocysteine >15 μmol/L is considered to be a raised level. This is associated with both arterial and venous thrombosis.

Antiphospholipid syndrome

This is a thrombophilia characterized by either positive anticardiolipin antibodies or the lupus anticoagulant. It can be primary (no associated autoimmune disease) or secondary. In the latter case it may be secondary to autoimmune conditions (SLE, rheumatoid arthritis), drugs (antibiotics, procainamide), or viral infections (HIV, hepatitis C, syphilis). Clinical manifestations include arterial and venous thrombosis, recurrent pregnancy loss, thrombocytopenia, livedo reticularis and neurological symptoms.

Testing for thrombophilia

Testing of unselected patients is inappropriate and there should be clear guidelines as to which patients should be tested (IV). Some tests for heritable thrombophilia are affected by pregnancy, the post-thrombotic state and by anticoagulant use, thus careful timing of investigation and interpretation of results are required.[9]

Initial assessment

This should include a detailed personal and family history, ideally with any history of VTE objectively confirmed. Any additional risk factors should be identified. A comprehensive thrombophilia screen encompasses the following.

- Activated partial thromboplastin time (APTT)/prothrombin time (PT)/thrombin clotting time.
- Functional assays to determine antithrombin III and protein C levels, antiphospholipid antibodies.
- Immunoreactive assays for protein S antigen.
- The modified APC:SR test can be used to identify causes of APC resistance other than FVL.
- PCR-based testing for PGM and FVL.

Management of pregnancy

Preconception

Thrombophilia clinics looking after young women must have close liaison with the obstetric unit. Women with identified heritable thrombophilias should be given information about the perceived risk of pregnancy-associated venous thrombosis. Women on long-term anticoagulant therapy (warfarin) need to understand the risk of fetal complications (see above).

Antenatal

The management of pregnant women with known thrombophilic defects and no prior venous thromboembolism remains controversial, because of the lack of knowledge of the natural history of the various thrombophilias. Women on long-term anticoagulation and women with antithrombin III deficiency (whether or not they have had a previous VTE) are considered at high risk of pregnancy-associated VTE. Women with a previous history of VTE and who have a thrombophilic defect are at a moderate risk, as are those without prior VTE history but with a protein C deficiency, homozygous for FVL or PGM. The general consensus is that these groups should receive both antepartum and postpartum thromboprophylaxis [IV]. Those at a perceived slight increased risk are women with no personal history of VTE but who have been screened for thrombophilia because they have a family history (protein S deficiency, heterozygous for FVL or PGM). In general, this group of women do not require LMWH antenatally, but consideration should be given to prophylaxis post-delivery [IV].[9] Some would advocate low-dose aspirin in the antenatal period.[10] If a patient does not want to continue injections throughout the puerperium, she may change to warfarin. Generally, oral anticoagulants may be introduced on the first or second postpartum day and the heparin withdrawn when the INR is in the recommended range.

KEY POINTS

VTE prophylaxis and inherited thrombophilia

Table 6.5.1

Previous VTE	Inherited thrombophilia	Antenatal prophylaxis	Postnatal prophylaxis
Yes	Antithrombin III deficiency	Yes – LMWH	Yes – LMWH
No	Antithrombin III deficiency	Yes – LMWH	Yes – LMWH
No	Protein C deficiency	Yes – LMWH	Yes – LMWH
No	Homozygous factor V Leiden	Yes – LMWH	Yes – LMWH
No	Homozygous prothrombin gene	Yes – LMWH	Yes – LMWH
No	Protein S deficiency	No – ? consider aspirin	? – consider
No	Heterozygous factor V Leiden	No – ? consider aspirin	? – consider
No	Heterozygous prothrombin gene	No – ? consider aspirin	? – consider
Yes	Any other thrombophilic defect – e.g. APS	Yes – LMWH	Yes – LMWH

MWH, low-molecular-weight heparin; APS, antiphospholipid syndrome.

Thrombophilia and pregnancy outcome

Maternal thrombophilias are now recognized to be associated with pregnancy complications, including recurrent miscarriage, intrauterine growth restriction, pre-eclampsia, placental abruption and intrauterine fetal death.[12] The proposed pathophysiology is logical, namely that the thrombophilia encourages placental thrombosis, causing placental infarction, which ultimately affects placental function. In view of this, many women with recurrent pregnancy loss, history of intrauterine death, severe or recurrent pre-eclampsia or IUGR are screened for an underlying thrombophilia. In patients with APA syndrome and recurrent miscarriage, a combination of low-dose aspirin and heparin is effective in reducing miscarriage rates [Ia]. No data are available about whether antithrombotic prophylaxis is beneficial in these other conditions. It has therefore been suggested that women with a history of poor pregnancy outcome should not be screened for thrombophilias, as there is no evidence that intervention is beneficial,[12] but unless suitable patient groups are identified for therapeutic interventions, the required randomized, controlled trials will not take place.

KEY POINTS

Pregnancy outcome and inherited thrombophilia

There is an increased association with:

- recurrent miscarriage
- IUGR
- pre-eclampsia
- placental abruption
- intrauterine fetal death

- There is no good evidence available regarding the management of the pregnant women with a previous VTE or with an inherited thrombophilia. Guidelines are based on expert opinion.

INHERITED BLEEDING DISORDERS

Haemophilia

The haemophilias are inherited deficiencies of factor VIII or factor IX. The genes for both factors are located on the X chromosome; thus the haemophilias are X-linked conditions. The daughters of a man with haemophilia are obligate carriers, while his sons are unaffected. The daughters of a haemophilia carrier have a 50 per cent risk of also being carriers, while 50 per cent of the male offspring of a carrier will be affected (the other 50 per cent inheriting no abnormal genes). Genetic counselling should be available before, during and after the process of haemophilia screening [IV], and a fully documented pedigree study should be carried out for each family. The haemophilias are categorized according to plasma levels of factor VIII or IX coagulant into mild (>5 per cent to <40 per cent), moderate (1–5 per cent) and severe (<1 per cent).[13] Severity breeds true in the same kindred. Up to one-third of newly diagnosed infants with haemophilia have no family history and are the result of a spontaneous mutation, often in the mother (>90 per cent). Prenatal diagnosis by chorionic villous sampling in the first trimester is available if the genetic mutation is known (there are >200 known mutations in the factor VIII and IX genes that result in haemophilia), and by fetal sexing only if the mutation is not known. Alternatively, direct fetal blood sampling may be carried out at 18 weeks' or more gestation. This procedure is more technically difficult and is reserved for those cases in whom it is not possible to carry out DNA-based family studies in time or because such studies were carried out and were not informative. If the fetus is found to be female on invasive testing, no further testing is performed. As carriers have one affected gene, it is often assumed that their factor levels will be 50 per cent of normal, but because of lyonization, levels vary from 10 to 120 IU/dL. Those with levels <30 IU/dL may have a significant bleeding history, and are at risk of significant haemorrhage when challenged. Bleeding episodes of both haemophilias are treated with intravenous injection of the relevant coagulation factor concentrate. In the past this consisted of pooled plasma of blood donors, and many haemophiliacs were thus exposed to HIV and the hepatitis viruses. Recombinant (i.e. synthetic) factors are now available, but are expensive. However, the government has now funded the use of recombinant factors in all children and new patients, including carriers who require prophylaxis for periods of high risk. This removal of the risk of virally transmitted disease, plus the use of prophylactic factor replacement from childhood and advances in other therapies, have significantly altered the outlook for children with haemophilia and their families, and less than 50 per cent of those at risk now avail themselves of prenatal diagnosis.

Haemophilia A

Haemophilia A is a deficiency of factor VIII and accounts for 80–85 per cent of haemophilia cases. Most cases are caused by the intron 22 inversion, and prenatal diagnosis is often available if requested. The woman's factor VIII should be assessed; if it is low, she may be at risk of bleeding at the time of the invasive procedure and thus require cover with either desmopressin (DDAVP – see later) or recombinant factor VIII.

Antenatal

Management of these cases should always be co-ordinated by a team with the relevant expertise, and preferably in association with a recognized haemophilia centre [IV]. Clear guidelines should be documented for the management of the remainder of pregnancy and labour and delivery in the form of a care plan. The maternal factor VIII level should be checked in each trimester. The levels of factor VIII and vWF normally increase in pregnancy and, if normal levels are attained, the woman is at no increased risk of haemorrhage either during pregnancy or at the time of delivery, and therefore regional blockade is not contraindicated. For those women who do not attain normalization of factor VIII levels during pregnancy, cover is required for delivery or invasive procedures. Recombinant factor VIII, or DDAVP if they are responders, can be used. DDAVP can increase factor VIII levels. This is a synthetic analogue of antidiuretic hormone, and should only be used under the supervision of a haematologist familiar with its use in pregnancy. It is given intravenously or intranasally, a method that is useful in the prevention and treatment of secondary postpartum haemorrhage or prolonged/heavy postnatal bleeding.

Intrapartum

On admission in labour it is necessary to establish the most recent factor VIII level and read the care plan that has been prepared antenatally. If the factor VIII level is normal in the third trimester, no special maternal precautions are indicated. If it is low, DDAVP or recombinant factor VIII should be given as per the care plan. This should ideally be given under the supervision of a haemophilia centre and there is therefore an argument to deliver these women in an obstetric unit that has direct access to a haemophilia centre [IV]. Once adequate factor VIII levels are attained, no other special precautions are necessary – i.e. there is no contraindication to epidural etc. If haemophilia is suspected in the fetus, it is wise to avoid fetal scalp electrodes and fetal blood sampling. With regard to mode of delivery, there is no place for elective caesarean section unless obstetric indications dictate this [III]. Controversy exists regarding the use of instrumental vaginal delivery, but it is recommended that vacuum and forceps should be avoided [IV].[13]

Postpartum

At the time of delivery, cord blood should be sent for all male newborns for an urgent factor VIII level unless haemophilia has been excluded by prenatal diagnosis.[13] If haemophilia is diagnosed, a dose of recombinant factor VIII is given to the neonate to minimize the risk of intracranial haemorrhage [IV]. This may be difficult to achieve in smaller units, and again consideration should be given to delivering these cases in a unit attached to a haemophilia centre [IV]. Intramuscular injections should be avoided until the haemophilia status is known, and vitamin K can be given orally. If the diagnosis is confirmed, referral to the appropriate paediatric haemophilia centre should be made and follow-up arranged prior to discharge home.

From the maternal perspective, factor VIII levels fall dramatically back to the pre-pregnancy levels within 48 hours of delivery, and there is thus an increased risk of secondary postpartum haemorrhage, particularly in low-level carriers. The use of intranasal DDAVP has been described above and can be used safely in breastfeeding mothers. Tranexamic acid, 1 g three times daily, is also useful in minimizing postnatal bleeding. In some cases, recombinant factor replacement may need to be continued for several days after delivery.

Haemophilia B (Christmas disease)

This is factor IX deficiency, and most of the above counselling, diagnosis and management decisions are the same as for haemophilia A. The exceptions are that factor IX levels do not significantly rise in pregnancy, and therefore haemophilia B carriers are much more likely to require factor replacement to cover delivery, and DDAVP does not increase factor IX levels.

Haemophilia

- If a fetus is suspected of having haemophilia, no advantage is conferred by delivery by elective caesarean section.
- Avoid instrumental delivery if possible; if necessary, preference is for the use of forceps rather than the ventouse.
- Regional analgesia/anaesthesia may well be appropriate.

KEY POINTS

Haemophilia

- Haemophilia B: deficiency of factor VIII.
- Haemophilia B: deficiency of factor IX.
- Both are X-linked recessive disease, with females being carriers.
- Pre-pregnancy counselling is important.
- Prenatal testing: chorionic villous sampling, amniocentesis, cordocentesis.
- Check maternal factor levels at booking/28/34 weeks' gestation.
- Intrapartum: FBC, clotting profile, G + S (Group and Save) i.v. access.
- Avoid intramuscular injection, fetal blood sampling, fetal scalp electrodes.

FACTOR XI DISEASE

Factor XI is a serine protease inhibitor. There is a poor correlation between the plasma level of factor XI and the bleeding tendency. Factor XI does not increase in pregnancy. Despite this, many women with known factor XI deficiency do not experience any problems during pregnancy and delivery, without any factor replacement. However, in view of its unpredictable nature, delivery should be in a centre where fresh frozen plasma can be given immediately if required. There is a plasma-derived concentrate of factor XI available. Care needs to be taken with the use of this concentrate, as it contains a number of other proteins and can contribute a thrombotic risk.

Other factor deficiencies

Deficiencies of most of the clotting factors have been described, and the clinical problems can range from insignificant to severe/life-threatening with respect to labour and delivery. In these rare cases there should be close collaboration with the relevant expert centres.

VON WILLEBRAND'S DISEASE

Von Willebrand factor is a plasma protein that has two main functions: stabilization of factor VIII and adherence of platelets to injured vessel walls. Von Willebrand's disease (vWD) is the most common inherited bleeding disorder (prevalence 0.8–1.3 per cent). Both sexes are affected by vWD as the vWF gene is on chromosome 12, and these patients have defective factor VIII and vWF. There are three different types of vWD. Types 1 and 2 are inherited with an autosomal dominant inheritance pattern, and type 3, the most severe, has an autosomal recessive inheritance pattern. Type I vWD is the most common and mildest form, present in approximately 75 per cent of patients. It is associated with a quantitative deficiency of vWF; in type 2 the defect is qualitative. In type 2b there is an associated thrombocytopenia. In these cases there is often a family history of mucocutaneous bleeding, and a personal history of a bleeding tendency – epistaxis, menorrhagia, inappropriate bleeding after dental/surgical procedures. Type 3 vWD is associated with a negligible amount of vWF (both quantity and function) and therefore a significant reduction in factor VIII activity. In these cases the bleeding history is severe, similar to haemophilia. Laboratory diagnosis measures ristocetin cofactor activity (which assesses vWF activity), as well as vWF antigen and factor VIII (a von Willebrand screen). As stress, tissue trauma and pregnancy all increase vWF and factor VIII levels, it can be difficult to confirm the diagnosis in pregnancy if this has not already been established. Also, during pregnancy, secondary to these increases, the bleeding tendency in type 1 improves, although there is no clinical improvement in type 2 despite an increase in the blood parameters. There is no improvement in type 3 with pregnancy.[14] As with haemophilia, because of the rapid decrease in factor VIII and vWF following delivery, the major haemorrhagic risk is postpartum. In type 1 vWD, DDAVP therapy can be useful. It indirectly stimulates the release of vWF from endothelial cells, causing increased levels of vWF for 4–6 hours. The released vWF binds factor VIII in the liver and increases the levels of circulating factor VIII/vWF complex.[15]

Antenatal

Before conception, ideally the vWD subtype should be ascertained and the patient's response to DDAVP should be evaluated.[15] DDAVP response can be undertaken in the second trimester if this has not previously been determined. Genetic counselling should be undertaken pre-pregnancy. Antenatal diagnosis of vWD is usually not required or requested, as the bleeding tendency is relatively mild, and the majority of cases of type 3 are asymptomatic carriers, unless there has already been an affected child born to the couple. The potential risks of pregnancy and delivery should be discussed with regard to the haemorrhagic risk. The majority of cases are type 1, and most will normalize during pregnancy with no haemostatic support being required until the postnatal period, if at all. Other types require specific counselling regarding haemostatic support and factor replacement. As with the haemophilias, these women should be cared for in association with a haemophilia centre [IV], and care patterns are similar to those described above. A von Willebrand screen should be performed in each trimester, and a clear plan documented for care in labour and delivery, as well as the postnatal period.

Labour and delivery

In type 1 vWD, regional anaesthesia can be considered safe if the von Willebrand screen has normalized (the vast majority of cases). This should be avoided in other types of vWD unless the appropriate factor support has been given, as in type 2 the von Willebrand screen can appear normal but the bleeding diathesis remains. Close collaboration with the haematology department and consultant anaesthetist is required. In view of the genetic inheritance, the fetus may be at an increased risk of haemorrhage, and although there is little evidence available in the literature with regard to vWD, the same conditions should apply as with the haemophilias – i.e. avoid fetal blood sampling and invasive monitoring in labour, and avoid episiotomies and instrumental vaginal delivery. As with the haemophilias, caesarean section should be performed for obstetric reasons only.[15] Primary and secondary postpartum haemorrhages are increased compared to both the normal pregnancy population and haemophilia carriers,[14] as the factor VIII and vWF both decrease rapidly following delivery to pre-pregnancy levels. Active third stage management is recommended to reduce the risk of primary postpartum haemorrhage.

Postpartum

If factor replacement has been necessary for delivery, it should be continued postnatally until the risk of haemorrhage has decreased, unless the patient is a known DDAVP responder, in which case this can be administered intravenously or intranasally.

For those in whom factor replacement was not used, prophylactic intranasal DDAVP and oral tranexamic acid can be used as an outpatient to minimize the risk of PPH.

Type 3 vWD can be diagnosed from cord blood after birth, and should be done if the neonate is known to be at increased risk (this applies to very few cases). It is almost impossible to diagnose the commoner, milder forms of vWD in a neonate, as the levels of vWF rise significantly during birth, and therefore can mask these forms of the disease. However, there is no urgency to make the diagnosis at birth, as the risk of bleeding in the neonatal period is very low.

MALIGNANCY

Haematological malignancies are discussed in Chapter 7.3. It must be noted that after patients have received radiotherapy or chemotherapy, there is an anxiety that this may cause increased genetic mutation and abnormality should they subsequently become pregnant. These subtle defects, if they are indeed present, cannot be diagnosed prenatally, and therefore referral for chorionic villous sampling or amniocentesis on this basis is futile.

ACKNOWLEDGEMENT

With acknowledgement to Tracey Johnston's contribution to this chapter.

KEY REFERENCES

1. SMAC Report. *Sickle Cell, Thalassaemia and other Haemoglobinopathies.* 1993. London: Department of Health.
2. George JN. Platelets. *Lancet* 2000; **355**(9214):1531–9.
3. Kaplan C, Forestier F, Dreyfus M, Morel-Kopp MC, Tchernia G. Maternal thrombocytopenia during pregnancy: diagnosis and aetiology. *Semin Thromb Hemost* 1995; **21**:85–94.
4. Shehata N, Burrows R, Kelton JG. Gestational thrombocytopenia. *Clin Obstet Gynecol* 1999; **42**(2):327–34.
5. McColl MD, Ramsey JE, Tait RC et al. Risk factors for pregnancy associated venous thromboembolism. *Thromb Haemost* 1997; **78**:1183–8.
6. The National Institute for Clinical Excellence, The Scottish Executive Health Department, The Department of Health, Social Services and Public Safety, Northern Ireland. *Why Mothers Die 1997–1999.* The Confidential Enquiry into Maternal Deaths in the United Kingdom. London: RCOG, 2001.
7. Greer IA, Thomsom AJ. *Thromboembolic Disease in Pregnancy and the Puerperium.* Clinical Green Top Guidelines. London: RCOG, 2001.
8. Van den Belt AGM, Prins MH, Lensing AWA et al. Fixed dose subcutaneous low molecular weight heparins versus adjusted dose unfractionated heparin for venous thromboembolism (Cochrane Review). In: *The Cochrane Library*, Issue 1. Oxford: Update Software, 2002.
9. Walker ID, Greaves M, Preston FE (on behalf of The British Society of Haematologists). Guideline – Investigation and management of heritable thrombophilia. *Br J Haematol* 2001; **114**:512–28.

10. Girling J. Thromboembolism and thrombophilia. *Curr Obstet Gynaecol* 2001; 11:15–22.

11. *Report of the RCOG Working Party on Prophylaxis (and Management) against Thromboembolism in Gynaecology and Obstetrics.* London: RCOG, 1995.

12. Alfirevic Z, Roberts D, Martlew V. How strong is the association between maternal thrombophilia and adverse pregnancy outcome? A systematic review. *Eur J Obstet Gynecol Reprod Biol* 2002; 101:6–14.

13. Kulkarni R, Lusher J. Perinatal management of newborns with haemophilia. *Br J Haematol* 2001; 112:264–74.

14. Giangrande PL. Management of pregnancy in carriers of haemophilia. *Haemophilia* 1998; 4:779–84.

15. Fausett B, Silver RM. Congenital disorders of platelet function. *Clin Obstet Gynecol* 1999; 42(2):390–405.

Renal Disease

Catherine Nelson-Piercy

INTRODUCTION

Urinary tract infection is a common cause of maternal morbidity and a potential cause of perinatal morbidity and mortality via premature labour. Renal disease is an important predisposing factor for pre-eclampsia and intrauterine growth restriction (IUGR). The combination of hypertension and proteinuria at booking (provided this is in the first or early second trimester) suggests pre-existing renal disease and should prompt further investigation. A serum creatinine is mandatory in such cases to exclude pre-existing renal impairment.

The number of women with renal transplants considering pregnancy is increasing and success rates are high, but case selection is required. Acute renal failure in pregnancy is rare, but renal impairment and oliguria commonly accompany obstetric conditions, particularly haemorrhage and pre-eclampsia.

PHYSIOLOGICAL CHANGES IN PREGNANCY

There is dilatation of the ureters and renal calyces in pregnancy. This must be remembered when interpreting ultrasound scans of the renal and urinary tract systems in pregnancy. Both renal plasma flow and glomerular filtration increase dramatically in pregnancy. This results in an increased urinary protein excretion and increased creatinine clearance. Thus, in the second trimester, the upper limit for serum creatinine falls to around 65 µmol/L, and throughout pregnancy the upper limit for proteinuria is taken as 300 mg/24 hours.

URINARY TRACT INFECTION

Incidence

Urinary tract infection (UTI) is more common in pregnancy because of the physiological dilatation of the upper renal tract. The incidence of asymptomatic bacteriuria in pregnancy ranges from 4 per cent to 7 per cent, and up to 40 per cent of the women affected will develop symptomatic UTI in pregnancy. Cystitis complicates about 1 per cent of pregnancies, and 1–2 per cent of pregnant women develop pyelonephritis. Women who have a history of previous UTI are at increased risk of UTI in pregnancy, as are those with diabetes, those receiving steroids or immunosuppression, those with polycystic kidneys, congenital abnormalities of the renal tract (e.g. duplex kidney or ureter), neuropathic bladder (e.g. spina bifida or multiple sclerosis) or urinary tract calculi.

Presentation

A midstream urine (MSU) specimen performed as part of routine antenatal screening may reveal asymptomatic bacteriuria. Additional MSUs are indicated in pregnancy in those women at increased risk as described above, and those with symptoms of UTI. Typical clinical features are urinary frequency, dysuria, haematuria, proteinuria and suprapubic pain. Fever, loin and/or abdominal pain, vomiting and rigors suggest pyelonephritis.

Diagnosis

Much dipstick proteinuria in pregnancy is erroneously attributed to UTI. Indeed, a diagnosis of pre-eclampsia may not be considered if it is assumed that proteinuria is due to UTI (see Chapter 7.6). Dipsticks for nitrites and leucocyte esterase may be used to help exclude UTI, but their positive predictive value is low and therefore any positive dipstick should be followed up with an MSU. A clinical diagnosis should always be confirmed with culture of an MSU sample. Bacteriuria is considered significant if there are more than 100 000 organisms per millilitre of urine. Urine culture resulting in a non-significant or mixed growth should be repeated on a fresh MSU specimen.

Management

All bacteriuria in pregnancy requires treatment to prevent pyelonephritis and preterm delivery (Cochrane guideline Ia) (Table 6.6.1). Treatment for 3 days is sufficient for asymptomatic bacteriuria [IV].[1] Regular urine cultures should be taken following treatment to ensure eradication of the organism. About 15 per cent of women will have recurrent bacteriuria during the pregnancy and will require a second course of antibiotics. The choice of antibiotic depends on the sensitivities of the causative organism, but in suspected pyelonephritis, treatment should begin before the results of culture are available. Penicillins (amoxycillin, augmentin) and cephalosporins are safe and appropriate antibiotics in pregnancy. Cefadroxil 500 mg bd is effective against the majority of urinary pathogens. Nitrofurantoin should be avoided in the third trimester and trimethoprim in the first trimester because of their respective haemolytic and antifolate actions. For acute cystitis, a 7-day course of antibiotics is

Table 6.6.1 Suggested treatment regimens for urinary tract infection (UTI) in pregnancy

Oral antibiotics
Amoxycillin 500 mg tds
Cefadroxil 500 mg bd
Cephalexin 250 mg tds
Nitrofurantoin 100 mg tds (not third trimester)
Trimethoprim 200 mg bd (not first trimester)

Intravenous antibiotics for pyelonephritis
Cefuroxime 750 mg tds
Augmentin 1 g tds
Gentamycin 2–5 mg/kg daily in divided doses 8 hourly (for organisms resistant to, or women allergic to, penicillins and cephalosporins)

Duration of treatment
Asymptomatic bacteriuria: 3 days
Acute cystitis: 7 days
Pyelonephritis: 10–14 days

Prophylaxis of UTI
Cephalexin 250 mg od
Amoxycillin 250 mg od

recommended and antibiotics should be continued for 10–14 days for pyelonephritis [IV].[1]

In pyelonephritis with vomiting or pyrexia, antibiotics should be given intravenously until the pyrexia settles; intravenous fluids may also be required. Renal function should be checked. Ultrasound examination of the renal tract is indicated in those with pyelonephritis or two or more proven UTIs. This is to exclude hydronephrosis, congenital abnormalities and renal calculi. Continuous prophylactic antibiotics are only usually recommended for those with two or more *confirmed* (with a positive culture) UTIs and one of the above risk factors.

RENAL IMPAIRMENT

Aetiology

In women of childbearing age, the commonest causes of renal impairment are reflux nephropathy, diabetes, systemic lupus erythematosus (SLE), other forms of glomerulonephritis and polycystic kidney disease. Conventionally, renal impairment is classified as mild, moderate or severe, depending on the serum creatinine. However, it must be remembered that the creatinine level is also dependent on the muscle mass, so a figure that represents moderate impairment in an 85-kg woman may represent severe impairment for a 50-kg woman.

Presentation

If renal disease is not diagnosed pre-pregnancy, it is usually first recognized because of hypertension and proteinuria ± haematuria in early pregnancy, prompting blood tests for urea and creatinine. However, a common caveat is to attribute hypertension and proteinuria to underlying renal disease rather than to the much more common pre-eclampsia, which may rarely present before 20 weeks' gestation. If there is no record of blood pressure or urinalysis in the first trimester to allow the hypertension and proteinuria to be designated 'new onset', a differentiation between pre-eclampsia and renal disease is more difficult.

Effect of pregnancy on renal impairment

In general, those with mild impairment (creatinine <125 μmol/L) tolerate pregnancy well and do not usually suffer deterioration in renal function as a result of the pregnancy. The serum creatinine will follow a trend similar to that in normal pregnancy, i.e. it will fall to a nadir in the second trimester and then rise again but remain below non-pregnant levels in the third trimester. Conversely, those with severe impairment of renal function (creatinine >250 μmol/L) are at increased risk of permanent loss of function during and after the pregnancy and even end-stage renal failure [II].[2]

Effect of renal impairment on pregnancy outcome

All women with renal impairment are at increased risk of pre-eclampsia, IUGR and spontaneous and iatrogenic premature delivery [II].[3] Again, outcome depends on the level of impairment and the level of any pre-existing hypertension [II].[4] Those with severe renal impairment and hypertension have a less than 50 per cent chance of successful pregnancy, often developing severe, early-onset pre-eclampsia with marked fetal growth restriction. Even in the absence of pre-eclampsia or uteroplacental dysfunction, one may be faced with the need to deliver a woman with rapidly worsening renal function in order to avoid dialysis, resulting in a pre-viable or extremely premature infant. For these reasons, it is usual to counsel woman with severe renal impairment against pregnancy [II].[2–4] Women with severe renal impairment may also develop polyhydramnios and the risk of cord prolapse. This is probably the result of fetal polyuria in response to the high osmotic load from increased maternal urea. Those with nephrotic syndrome and heavy proteinuria also develop worsening hypoalbuminaemia in pregnancy, with the associated risks of pulmonary oedema and thrombosis.

Management

This should begin with pre-pregnancy counselling and should involve multidisciplinary care by clinicians with expertise in the management of these high-risk pregnancies. It is important to document baseline (pre-pregnancy and early pregnancy)

values for creatinine, uric acid, albumin and protein excretion. Some increase in proteinuria is inevitable in pregnancy and does not necessarily indicate superimposed pre-eclampsia or worsening renal disease. Deterioration in renal function at any stage in pregnancy should prompt a search for reversible causes such as UTI or dehydration.

Tight control of any hypertension is important to minimize the risk of deterioration in renal function. Many clinicians recommend the treatment of even mild hypertension in women with underlying renal disease. The choice of anti-hypertensive agents is no different in women with renal disease [IV]. Many renal patients are receiving angiotensin-converting enzyme (ACE) inhibitors prior to pregnancy. These should be discontinued once pregnancy is confirmed [II]. Diuretics are also usually discontinued unless there is severe hypoalbuminaemia and insipient pulmonary oedema [III].

Not only are these woman at high risk of pre-eclampsia, but it is also often difficult to diagnose in the presence of pre-existing hypertension and proteinuira. Admission should be considered with worsening hypertension, increasing serum creatinine, and large increases in proteinuria. Useful alternative features to support a diagnosis of pre-eclampsia include IUGR, thrombocytopenia and abnormal liver function. The use of prophylactic low-dose (75 mg/day) aspirin may be appropriate to decrease the risk of pre-eclampsia in those with renal impairment and hypertension [Ia].[5] Serial scans for fetal growth and liquor volume, and serial haematology and biochemistry are essential in the monitoring of these pregnancies [III].

If renal impairment is discovered for the first time in pregnancy, and is not readily attributable to pre-eclampsia, investigation should include blood glucose (for diabetes), antinuclear antibodies (for SLE) and a renal tract ultrasound (e.g. for polycystic kidneys or to demonstrate small kidneys suggestive of chronic renal failure) [III].

Postpartum, continued close monitoring is necessary to ensure the renal function returns to pre-pregnancy levels. ACE inhibitors may be safely used in breastfeeding women. Those with newly suspected underlying renal disease should be referred to a nephrologist.

Renal impairment

- The risks of obstetric complications such as pre-eclampsia, IUGR and iatrogenic prematurity increase with increasing baseline serum creatinine.
- The chances of successful pregnancy decrease with increasing baseline serum creatinine.
- The risks of temporary and permanent deterioration in renal function increase with increased baseline serum creatinine.
- Women with severe renal impairment (creatinine >250 μmol/L) are usually advised against pregnancy.

RENAL TRANSPLANTS

The rates of successful pregnancy outcome in women with well-functioning renal transplants are similar to those of the general population. Women are usually advised to delay pregnancy for 1–2 years after transplantation to allow graft function to stabilize and immunosuppression to reach maintenance levels [IV]. The risks in pregnancy are the same as for women with renal impairment (see above) and relate to the pre-pregnancy level of function of the allograft and the presence of hypertension [II].[6]

In addition, these women are immunosuppressed and therefore more prone to infection. There are substantial data regarding the safety of immunosuppressive drugs in pregnancy. Prednisolone [II], azathioprine [II], cyclosporin[6] [II] and tacrolimus [II] are all considered safe. However, women receiving cyclosporin or tacrolimus are generally advised not to breastfeed [IV]. Mycophenolate mofetil has caused toxicity in animal studies.

DIALYSIS

Because women with end-stage renal failure have markedly reduced fertility, pregnancy on dialysis is unusual. The chances of a successful pregnancy outcome are sufficiently low, and the attendant risks sufficiently high, to counsel women on dialysis against pregnancy [IV]. Anaemia and haemorrhage are common, and the risks of miscarriage, fetal death, pre-eclampsia, preterm labour, preterm rupture of the membranes, polyhydramnios and placental abruption are increased [II].[7] Women who decide to continue with pregnancy require increasing dialysis in order to maintain the pre-dialysis urea <15–20 mmol/L [II].[7] The incidence of poor obstetric outcome is similar with both haemodialysis and peritoneal dialysis.

ACUTE RENAL FAILURE IN PREGNANCY

Acute renal failure is rare in pregnancy, the commonest causes being pre-eclampsia and related syndromes, haemorrhage, infections, drugs, particularly non-steroidal anti-inflammatory drugs, and obstruction due to ureteric damage or stones. Conversely, mild degrees of renal impairment are more common, and again are usually related to pre-eclampsia or blood loss. Acute renal failure most commonly complicates the early postpartum period. It is characterized by oliguria, a rising urea and creatinine, a metabolic acidosis and hyperkalaemia. In the obstetric situation there may be an associated coagulopathy. An isolated rise in urea (without concomitant rise in creatinine) is often observed following antenatal corticosteroid administration. A rare cause of renal failure that is most commonly encountered postpartum is haemolytic uraemic syndrome (HUS). The hallmark of this condition is a microangiopathic haemolytic anaemia (diagnosed with a blood film) associated with renal failure and thrombocytopenia.

Pre-eclampsia and renal failure

Oliguria is an almost universal finding in pre-eclampsia and is excerbated by Syntocinon and caesarean section. It does not alone indicate renal failure, but should prompt measurement of serum urea and creatinine. Renal failure is more common in acute fatty liver (see Chapter 6.8), HELLP syndrome (7 per cent) [II][8] and eclampsia (6 per cent) than in 'straightforward' pre-eclampsia. HELLP syndrome is the commonest cause (50 per cent) of acute renal failure in the context of pre-eclampsia.

The management of acute renal failure depends on the cause: blood volume replacement for haemorrhage, delivery for pre-eclampsia, cessation of nephrotoxic drugs. Postpartum management is largely conservative and supportive. Accurate assessment of fluid balance with the use of a central venous pressure (CVP) line is important. Provided blood loss and volume depletion have been excluded as causes (CVP high or normal), fluids are only given to replace insensible losses and the previous hour's urine output. Iatrogenic fluid overload must be avoided in pre-eclampsia because these women are often hypoalbuminaemic and particularly susceptible to pulmonary oedema. Overzealous fluid administration is far more dangerous than oliguria. Dialysis may rarely become necessary, but a need for long-term renal replacement therapy is extremely unusual.

Antenatal complications: maternal

PUBLISHED GUIDELINES

Smaill F. Antibiotics for asymptomatic bacteriuria in pregnancy (Cochrane Review). In: *The Cochrane Library*, Issue 1. Oxford: Update Software, 1999.

KEY REFERENCES

1. Cattell WR. Urinary tract infection in women. *J R Coll Physicians Lond* 1997; 31:130–3.
2. Epstein FH. Pregnancy and renal disease. *N Engl J Med* 1996; 335:277–8.
3. Jones DC, Hayslett JP. Outcome of pregnancy in women with moderate or severe renal insufficiency. *N Engl J Med* 1996; 335:226–32.
4. Jungers P, Chauveau D. Pregnancy in renal disease. *Kidney Int* 1997; 52:871–85.
5. Knight M, Duley L, Henderson-Smart DJ, King JF. Antiplatelet agents for preventing and treating pre-eclampsia (Cochrane Review). In: *The Cochrane Library*, Issue 3, Oxford: Update Software, 2000.
6. Armenti VT, Ahlswede KM, Ahlswede BA et al. Variables affecting birth weight and graft survival in 197 pregnancies in cyclosporin treated female kidney transplant recipients. *Transplantation* 1995; 59:476.
7. Hou SH. Pregnancy in women with chronic renal insufficiency and end stage renal disease. *Am J Kidney Dis* 1999; 33:235–52.
8. Sibai BM, Villar MA, Mabie BC. Acute renal failure in hypertensive disorders of pregnancy. *Am J Obstet Gynecol* 1990; 162:777–83.

Autoimmune Conditions

Catherine Nelson-Piercy

INTRODUCTION

This chapter covers the autoimmune connective tissue diseases, including rheumatoid arthritis (RA), systemic lupus erythematosus (SLE) and rheumatoid arthritis, antiphospholipid syndrome (APS), Sjogren's syndrome and scleroderma. Autoimmune thrombocytopenia is discussed in Chapter 6.5, myasthenia gravis in Chapter 6.10 and autoimmune thyroid disease in Chapter 6.4.

In pregnancy, many of the issues for women with connective tissue disease relate to the safety of the drugs used to control their disease and to the degree of any systemic involvement of their disease.

RHEUMATOID ARTHRITIS

This is a chronic, inflammatory, symmetrical arthritis causing joint pain, stiffness and deformity. Systemic features include rheumatoid nodules, pulmonary granulomas, vasculitis, Sjogren's syndrome (see below) and scleritis. Haematological abnormalities include a normocytic anaemia and raised erythrocyte sedimentation rate (ESR). Rheumatoid arthritis is usually associated with rheumatoid factor and 30 per cent of cases are antinuclear antibody (ANA) positive. Up to 20–30 per cent are Ro/La positive (see below) and 5–10 per cent are antiphospholipid antibody (aPL) positive (see below), although APS is rare. Pregnancy is associated with a decrease in T-cell immunity that is reversed postpartum.[1] This may explain why three-quarters of women with RA experience improvement in their symptoms during pregnancy and why those who improve usually flare postpartum.[2] Rheumatoid arthritis has no adverse effect upon pregnancy outcome. Limitation of hip abduction is rarely severe enough to preclude vaginal delivery, and atlantoaxial subluxation is a rare complication of general anaesthesia for caesarean section. Severe joint deformity and disability may rarely necessitate the need for help with care of the infant.

Management

Assessment of disease activity is usually clinical. The ESR is raised in normal pregnancy and does not therefore provide a reliable marker of disease activity. As arthritis often improves in pregnancy, some reduction in analgesia may be possible.

Table 6.7.1   Safety in pregnancy of drugs used for autoimmune conditions

Safe to continue or start in pregnancy	Discontinue or avoid in pregnancy
Paracetamol	Non-steroidal anti-inflammatory drugs
Hydroxychloroquine	Cyclophosphamide
Sulfasalazine	Gold
Corticosteroids	Penicillamine
	Methotrexate
	Chlorambucil

DRUGS FOR AUTOIMMUNE CONDITIONS

Paracetamol is safe in pregnancy and may be instituted or continued in maximal doses if required. The commonly used drugs for connective tissue disease are summarized in Table 6.7.1.[3,4]

Non-steroidal anti-inflammatory drugs (NSAIDs), such as ibuprofen and diclofenac, are often used in women with RA and SLE as well as over-the-counter analgesics in the general population. They are normally avoided in pregnancy because they are detrimental to the fetal kidney, causing oligohydramnios, and they may cause premature closure of the ductus arteriosus, leading to pulmonary hypertension and fetal haemorrhage, in large doses. Neither aspirin nor the other NSAIDs are teratogenic, so it is not necessary to discontinue these drugs prior to conception [II]. However, there is an association between NSAIDs and infertility due to luteinized unruptured follicle syndrome.[5] They should therefore be withdrawn if there is a history of infertility [III]. Occasionally, they are used in pregnancy when alternatives such as paracetamol, codeine or corticosteroids are inadequate or inappropriate. In such cases they should be discontinued by 32 weeks' gestation, as the effects on the fetal renal function and the ductus are reversible prior to delivery.[3] The more recently introduced selective cyclooxygenase-2 (COX-2) inhibitors are also currently contraindicated in pregnancy.

Corticosteroids are the first-line anti-inflammatory drugs in pregnancy.[3] They are used for many connective tissue diseases, not only for the arthritis manifestations, but also to treat vasculitis, skin involvement, renal lupus and thrombocytopenia. There is no evidence to support the premise that steroids will prevent flare, either antenatal or postnatal, but they remain the mainstay of management for these disorders in pregnancy. They must never be withheld because of erroneous fears concerning their effects on the fetus. Many women are understandably reluctant to use any drugs, but particularly steroids, in pregnancy and therefore, if they are used, this must be with adequate counselling regarding their safety in pregnancy to ensure concordance with therapy [IV]. Any possible small risk of teratogenesis

(which is unlikely) is dwarfed by the beneficial effects to the fetus of controlling the maternal disease process [II]. Caution is needed because the use of steroids in pregnancy is associated with an increased risk of infections and gestational diabetes. Large doses of steroids are associated with an increased risk of premature rupture of the membranes.

Azathioprine is also safe in pregnancy. The fetal liver lacks the enzyme that converts azathioprine to its active metabolites. Azathioprine is used as a 'steroid-sparing' agent and there are reassuring data regarding a lack of adverse effects on babies born to mothers receiving this drug for renal transplants, inflammatory bowel disease and connective tissue diseases [II].[3] Although women taking azathioprine are normally advised not to breastfeed, this is only because of theoretical risks of immunosuppression of the neonate that are not born out by cases in which women elect to breastfeed. The benefits of breastfeeding may outweigh any risk [IV].

Anti-malarials such as hydroxychloroquine have a good pregnancy safety record when used for malarial prophylaxis. The doses used in connective tissue disorders are higher and may rarely cause sight-threatening pigmentary retinopathy after long-term use in adults. Reported series of use in pregnancy are reassuring and do not suggest an increase in congenital abnormalities or fetal adverse effects. A recent study of 21 children exposed in utero to anti-malarials for maternal SLE or RA showed no ophthalmic abnormality.[6] Hydroxychloroquine may therefore be safely continued or instituted in a pregnant woman [II]. Discontinuation of this drug is associated with a risk of SLE flare.

Sulfasalazine is safe in pregnancy and breastfeeding. It is a dihydrofolate reductase inhibitor and therefore associated with an increased risk of neural tube, oral cleft and cardiovascular defects. Therefore folate supplementation (5 mg per day) is advised [Ib].

Gold and d-penicillamine used in RA are usually avoided in pregnancy, although the risk of abnormalities is probably low. Cytotoxic drugs such as cyclophosphamide, methotrexate and chlorambucil are all highly teratogenic and must be discontinued prior to pregnancy.

SYSTEMIC LUPUS ERYTHEMATOSUS

This is a relapsing and remitting multisystem connective tissue disorder that predominantly affects women of childbearing age. The diagnostic criteria are shown in Table 6.7.2. It most commonly affects the joints (symmetrical non-erosive peripheral arthritis and arthralgia), the skin (malar rash, photosensitivity, discoid lupus, alopecia, vasculitis, Raynaud's phenomenon), and the kidneys (glomerulonephritis). There may be anaemia, lymphopenia, thrombocytopenia, hypocomplementaemia and a raised ESR. The C-reactive protein (CRP) is not raised. Systemic lupus erythematosus is associated with ANA and anti double-stranded DNA (dsDNA) antibodies.

Table 6.7.2 American College of Rheumatology criteria for systemic lupus erythematosus (SLE)

Malar rash	Renal disorder
Discoid rash	Neurological disorder
Photosensitivity	Haematological disorder
Oral ulcers	Immunological disorder
Arthritis	Antinuclear antibody
Serositis	

For a diagnosis of SLE, four of these criteria are required simultaneously or serially

There may be antibodies to extractable nuclear antigens (ENA) including Ro and La, or aPLs.

Effect of pregnancy on SLE

Pregnancy is associated with an increased risk of SLE flare, which may occur at any stage of the pregnancy or postpartum. Neither the severity nor the type (e.g. renal or skin) of flare is altered by pregnancy. Flares may be harder to diagnose in pregnancy because many features, such as fatigue, erythema, anaemia and hair fall, are common to both.[7] Pregnancy does not alter the antibody profile but increases the ESR and may exacerbate thrombocytopenia.

Effect of SLE on pregnancy outcome

In women who have quiescent SLE, have no renal involvement, and are Ro/La and aPL negative, there is no adverse effect of their disease on pregnancy.[8] Active disease at conception, renal involvement and APS increase the risks of miscarriage, pre-eclampsia, IUGR, premature delivery and stillbirth.

Management

This should begin with pre-pregnancy counselling enabling an accurate risk assessment for individual women. Women should be advised to conceive during periods of disease remission. Once pregnancy is confirmed (or pre-pregnancy if there is a delay in conception), NSAIDs are discontinued. Hydroxychloroquine is continued because it is safe, because withdrawal may precipitate flare, and because it has a very long half-life such that the fetus remains exposed for up to 3 months after the mother discontinues the drug.[8] Prednisolone and azathioprine are also continued. During pregnancy, SLE flares are treated with new or increased doses of steroids [II].[7] Not only are women with renal lupus at increased risk of pre-eclampsia, but also pre-eclampsia may be harder to diagnose in such woman, who already have hypertension and proteinuria. Low platelets, renal impairment, oedema, worsening hypertension and proteinuria may be

attributable to either. Pointers to a renal lupus flare include red cells or red cell casts in the urine, hypocomplementaemia (falling levels of C3 and C4), and a rising anti-DNA titre. Pointers to a diagnosis of pre-eclampsia include raised transaminases and hyperuricaemia. Those at high risk of pre-eclampsia and IUGR should be offered serial growth scans and tests of fetal well-being as indicated. Regular visits to the joint clinic are important to screen for pre-eclampsia and SLE flare.

NEONATAL LUPUS SYNDROMES

These are caused by anti-Ro or anti-La antibodies and manifest as cutaneous neonatal lupus, affecting 5 per cent of babies of Ro-positive women, and congenital heart block, affecting 1–2 per cent of babies of Ro-positive women. If the first child is affected, the risk to the second child is about 16 per cent, and once two children are affected the risk rises to about 50 per cent. Neonatal cutaneous lupus develops in the first 2 weeks of life and is a geographical skin lesion of the face or scalp. It may be precipitated by exposure to ultraviolet light and usually regresses spontaneously without scarring within 6 months. Congenital heart block develops in utero at 18–30 weeks. There is no treatment, and one in five affected babies die as neonates. About half of those surviving require pacemakers in early infancy and the rest by their teens.[8] Ro-positive women should be offered fetal cardiology screening [II].

ANTIPHOSPHOLIPID SYNDROME

This describes the association of aPL (either anticardiolipin antibodies or lupus anticoagulant) with the classical clinical features shown in Table 6.7.3.

Additional clinical features include thrombocytopenia, livedo reticularis, epilepsy, migraine, heart valve disease and pulmonary hypertension. Antiphospholipid syndrome may be primary or found in association with SLE, RA or other connective tissue disease. Therefore women with primary APS, even if based on a positive lupus anticoagulant, do not have 'lupus' unless there are features of SLE (see Table 6.7.1).[8]

The pathogenesis of APS involves a co-factor, β_2-glycoprotein. Antiphospholipids (aPLs) reduce human chorionic gonadotrophin (hCG) release and inhibit trophoblast invasion in vitro – a potential explanation for the association with miscarriage. However, the 'typical APS' fetal loss occurs in the second trimester and is associated with severe growth restriction, oligohydramnios and early-onset pre-eclampsia.[9] The common feature is defective or abnormal placentation, possibly related to thrombosis.

Table 6.7.3 3-Classification criteria for antiphospholipid syndrome

Clinical criteria	
Thrombosis	Venous Arterial Small vessel
Pregnancy morbidity	• Three or more consecutive miscarriages (<10 weeks) • One or more fetal death (>10 weeks) • One or more premature birth (<34 weeks) due to severe pre-eclampsia or placental insufficiency
Laboratory criteria	
Anticardiolipin antibody	IgG or IgM Medium/high titre Two or more occasions >6 weeks apart
Lupus anticoagulant	Two or more occasions >6 weeks apart

Table 6.7.4 Management recommendations for antiphospholipid syndrome pregnancies

Antiphospholipd antibody – no thrombosis or pregnancy loss	Aspirin 75 mg or nothing
Previous thrombosis	LMWH and aspirin
Previous recurrent (≥3) miscarriages (<10 weeks)	Aspirin ± LMWH (? stop LMWH at 13-20 weeks)
Fetal loss or severe PET/IUGR/NND	Aspirin + LMWH

LMWH, low-molecular-weight heparin; PET, pre-eclampsia; IUGR, intrauterine growth restriction; NND, neonatal death.

Pregnancy in women with APS is associated with an increased risk of thrombosis. This is particularly so for women with previous thrombosis. Antiphospholipd syndrome is a form of acquired thrombophilia. Thrombosis may therefore affect unusual sites such as the axillary or retinal veins. What makes APS particularly dangerous is the fact that thrombosis may also affect arterial and small vessels, causing, for example, stroke or renal disease. In general, those women who have had a previous venous thrombosis are at risk of recurrent venous thromboses, and those with previous arterial thrombosis from recurrent arterial events. Pregnancy also increases the risk of, or may exacerbate, pre-existing thrombocytopenia.

The effect on pregnancy of APS is to increase the risk of early and late miscarriage, stillbirth, placental abruption, IUGR and pre-eclampsia.

Management

Antiphospholipid syndrome should be managed in pregnancy by multidisciplinary teams with expertise of caring for these high-risk pregnancies. Those women with a previous history of arterial or venous thrombosis will usually be on long-term treatment with warfarin. This should be converted to aspirin and low-molecular-weight heparin (LMWH) as soon as pregnancy is confirmed and at least before 6 weeks' gestation to avoid warfarin embryopathy (see Chapter 8). LMWH is continued in prophylactic doses throughout pregnancy and postpartum for 6 weeks or until warfarin is recommenced.

For women without a previous history of thrombosis, there is agreement that low-dose aspirin (75 mg per day) is beneficial, although supportive evidence is mostly from retrospective, non-randomized studies. Indeed, randomized studies do not support a beneficial effect of aspirin, but this is because such studies have included very low risk groups of women, some without any previous history of adverse pregnancy outcome. Low-dose aspirin is safe and all centres with an

interest in APS use aspirin sometimes from pre-conception [III]. The role of LMWH in addition to aspirin is more controversial.[9] Two prospective studies of women with aPL and recurrent miscarriage demonstrated significantly increased live birth rates in groups allocated to aspirin and LMWH versus those receiving aspirin alone, and current Royal College of Obstetricians and Gynaecologist (RCOG) guidelines advocate the use of LMWH in addition to aspirin for women with recurrent miscarriage and aPL (see 'Published guidelines' at the end of this chapter). However, in both studies the increase in live birth rate was due to a decrease in early miscarriages, raising the issue of whether it is possible to discontinue the LMWH after the first trimester or after the 20-week scan if the uterine artery Doppler waveform is normal. A more recent randomized study failed to show any increased benefit of LMWH over and above aspirin alone in women with APS. That said, it is common practice to recommend LMWH for those women who have suffered late fetal losses or neonatal deaths attributable to APS [III].[9]

- Evidence supports the use of heparin throughout pregnancy in women with APS who have had previous thromboses.
- Evidence from retrospective and cohort studies supports a role for low-dose aspirin for fetal indications.
- Evidence regarding the use of LMWH in addition to aspirin for fetal indications is contradictory.

A suggested management plan is given in Table 6.7.4. The risk of pre-eclampsia, abruption IUGR and premature delivery is less for women with APS diagnosed as a result of recurrent early miscarriage compared to those women with APS diagnosed as a result of later pregnancy adverse outcome. Past obstetric history is the best predictor of risk, although success rates for women diagnosed and treated for APS are about 70–80 per cent.[9] All women require careful and regular monitoring for pre-eclampsia, and serial growth scans and tests of fetal well-being as appropriate [III]. Liaison with obstetric anaesthetists is vital prior to delivery in women receiving LMWH for any indication. In those who have had previous thromboses, discontinuation of LMWH peripartum should be minimal, but for those receiving LMWH for purely fetal indications, it may simplify the management of analgesia and anaesthesia for labour and delivery if the LMWH is discontinued prior to delivery.

SJOGREN'S SYNDROME

This typically causes dry eyes and a dry mouth. The dry eyes may be confirmed objectively with the Schirmer tear test. Similar to APS, Sjogren's syndrome may be primary or associated with SLE, RA or other connective tissue disease. This syndrome is typically associated with positivity for Ro and La, and therefore the risk of neonatal lupus and congenital heart block (see above). Primary Sjogren's is associated with the finding of positive rheumatoid factor and positive ANA, and hypergammaglobulinaemia.

SCLERODERMA

Scleroderma may occur as a localized cutaneous form, as systemic sclerosis or as part of the CREST syndrome (calcinosis, Raynaud's phenomenon, (o)esophageal involvement, sclerodactyly and telangiectasia). Skin involvement produces characteristic facies with a beaked nose and limited mouth opening, limiting facial expression. Systemic fibrosis involves the oesophagus, the lungs, the heart and the kidneys. There is no treatment for scleroderma.

Adverse effects on pregnancy relate to the degree of any renal, lung or cardiac involvement. Women with early diffuse disease are at increased risk in pregnancy and therefore women should be advised to postpone pregnancy until the disease has stabilized.[10] Those with severe pulmonary fibrosis or pulmonary hypertension should be advised against pregnancy [IV]. Those with renal involvement and hypertension are at increased risk of hypertension and IUGR. Oesophageal symptoms often increase in pregnancy, but those of Raynaud's may improve secondary to vasodilatation.

Management

Pre-pregnancy counselling is vital to inform women accurately about the potential risks of pregnancy. Formal lung function and echocardiography to assess the extent of systemic involvement are recommended. During pregnancy, regular multidisciplinary assessment is required, with screens of blood pressure, urinalysis, renal function and maternal symptoms. Scleroderma renal crises are extremely dangerous and ACE inhibitors should not be withheld (IV). Raynaud's phenomenon may be ameliorated with heated gloves and calcium antagonists. Corticosteroids should be

avoided because they may precipitate a renal crisis. Beta-agonists cause vasoconstriction and should also be avoided. Assessment by an obstetric anaesthetist prior to delivery is essential. In women with scleroderma, there are often problems with blood pressure measurement, venous access, capillary oxygen saturation monitoring and difficult airways.

KEY POINTS

- Rheumatoid arthritis usually improves in pregnancy and deteriorates postpartum.
- SLE is more likely to flare in pregnancy.
- Adverse pregnancy outcome in SLE is related to the presence of APS, renal involvement, disease activity and the presence of anti-Ro and La antibodies.
- Ro and La antibodies are associated with Sjogren's syndrome and may cause congenital heart block and neonatal lupus.
- APS may cause thrombosis, miscarriage, late fetal loss, early-onset pre-eclampsia and severe IUGR.
- APS is treated in pregnancy with low-dose aspirin ± LMWH.
- Steroids are safe to treat connective tissue disease in pregnancy and are used in preference to NSAIDs.

PUBLISHED GUIDELINES

RCOG guidelines for recurrent miscarriage/APS. Guideline No. 17. RCOG.

KEY REFERENCES

1. Nelson JL, Ostensen M. Pregnancy and rheumatoid arthritis. *Rheum Dis Clin North Am* 1997; 23:195–212.
2. Barrett JH, Brennan P, Fiddler M et al. Does rheumatoid arthritis remit during pregnancy and relapse postpartum? Results from a Nationwide Study in the United Kingdom performed prospectively from late pregnancy. *Arthritis Rheum* 1999; 42:1219–27.
3. Ostenson M, Ramsey-Goldman R. Treatment of inflammatory rheumatic disorders in pregnancy. *Drug Saf* 1998; 19:389–410.
4. Janssen NM, Genta MS. The effects of immunosuppressive and anti-inflammatory medications on fertility, pregnancy, and lactation. *Arch Intern Med* 2000; 160:610–19.
5. Mendonca LLF, Khamastha MA, Nelson-Piercy C, Hunt BJ, Hughes GRV. Non-steroidal anti-inflammatory

drugs as a possible cause for reversible infertility. *Rheumatology* 2000; **39**:880–2.

6. Klinger G, Morad Y, Westall CXA et al. Ocular toxicity and antenatal exposure to chloroquine or hydroxychloroquine for rheumatic disease. *Lancet* 2001; **358**:813–14.

7. Khamashta MA, Hughes GRV. Pregnancy in systemic lupus erythematosus. *Curr Opin Rheumatol* 1997; 8:424–9.

8. Nelson-Piercy C. Connective tissue disease. In: *Handbook of Obstetric Medicine*, 2nd edn. London: Martin Dunitz, 2001, 135–55.

9. Shehata H, Nelson-Piercy C, Khamastha MA. Management of pregnancy in antiphospholipid syndrome. In: Khamastha MA (ed.), *Antiphospholipid (Hughes) Syndrome*. Rheumatic Disease Clinics of North America, 2001; **27**:643–59.

10. Steen VD. Pregnancy in women with systemic sclerosis. *Obstet Gynecol* 1999; **94**:15–20.

Liver and Gastrointestinal Disease

Catherine Nelson-Piercy

MRCOG standards

Relevant standards
- Conduct pre-pregnancy counselling to a level expected in independent primary care.
- Manage or refer appropriately nausea, vomiting, hyperemesis, gastric reflux.
- Diagnose and plan management with appropriate consultation in the following conditions: liver disease, inflammatory bowel disease.

In addition, we would suggest the following.

Theoretical skills
- Revise basic gastrointestinal and liver physiology.
- Know the obstetric risks associated with chronic liver disease.
- Be able to counsel a woman with obstetric cholestasis about the maternal and fetal risks.
- Understand the risk/benefit issues for a pregnant woman with inflammatory bowel disease requiring drug treatment/immunosuppression.

Practical skills
- Be able to interpret liver function tests in pregnancy.
- Be able to diagnose and manage obstetric cholestasis.

INTRODUCTION

Liver disease in pregnancy is encountered relatively rarely, but gastrointestinal problems, including nausea, vomiting, oesophageal reflux and constipation, are almost universal. Liver disease can be dangerous for both the mother and the fetus. This chapter considers the liver conditions specific to pregnancy – obstetric cholestasis and acute fatty liver of pregnancy – and those that pre-date or coincide with pregnancy – viral hepatitis and chronic liver disease. HELLP syndrome is discussed in Chapter 7.6. Gastrointestinal diseases usually pre-date the pregnancy; inflammatory bowel disease and irritable bowel syndrome are the commonest. Gastrointestinal problems exacerbated or brought on by pregnancy such as gastro-oesophageal reflux and hyperemesis are also discussed.

PHYSIOLOGICAL CHANGES IN PREGNANCY

Pregnancy causes decreased lower oesophageal pressure, decreased gastric peristalsis and delayed gastric emptying. Gastrointestinal motility is reduced, with increased small-bowel and large-bowel transit times. There is a 20–40 per cent fall in serum albumin concentration, partly due to dilution resulting from the increase in total blood volume. Total serum protein concentration also decreases. The alkaline phosphatase concentration more than doubles due to production by the placenta, which increases with gestation. Levels of alanine transaminase (ALT); serum glutamic pyruvic transaminase (SGPT); aspartamine transaminase (AST) and serum glutamic-oxaloacetic transaminase (SGOT) fall and there is a fall in the upper limit of the normal ranges for both enzymes (Table 6.8.1).[1] Thus a mildly abnormal level

Table 6.8.1 Normal ranges for liver enzymes in non-pregnant and pregnant populations

Liver enzyme	Non pregnant	Trimester		
		1st	2nd	3rd
AST (IU/L)	7–40	10–28	10–29	11–30
ALT (IU/L)	0–40	6–32	6–32	6–32
Bilirubin (μmol/L)	0–17	4–16	3–13	3–14
Gamma GT (IU/L)	11–50	5–37	5–43	3–41
Alkaline phosphatase (IU/L)	30–130	32–100	43–135	133–418

AST, aspartamine transaminase; ALT, alanine transaminase; GT, glutamyl transpeptidase.

for transaminases that may be significant in the diagnosis of obstetric cholestasis or in the assessment of pre-eclampsia may be overlooked unless pregnancy-specific ranges are used. The concentrations of other liver enzymes are not substantially altered and there is no significant change in bilirubin concentration during normal pregnancy.

NAUSEA, VOMITING AND HYPEREMESIS

Nausea and vomiting are common symptoms in early pregnancy, affecting over half of pregnant women. The onset of symptoms is usually early in the first trimester at around 5–6 weeks' gestation. Hyperemesis is less common, but causes much morbidity and repeated hospital admissions and can be dangerous if inadequately or inappropriately treated. Nausea and vomiting in pregnancy become hyperemesis if the woman is unable to maintain adequate hydration and nutrition, either because of severity or duration of symptoms. This is associated with marked weight loss, muscle wasting, ketonuria, dehydration and electrolyte disturbance, including hypokalaemia and a metabolic hypochloraemic alkalosis. A common associated symptom is ptyalism – the inability to swallow saliva. The risks associated with hyperemesis include fetal growth restriction, maternal hyponatraemia leading to central pontine myelinolysis, and thiamine deficiency leading to Wernicke's encephalopathy.[2] Markers of severity include weight loss >10 per cent, abnormal thyroid function tests with raised free thyroxine (T4) and suppressed thyroid-stimulating hormone (TSH), and abnormal liver function tests with raised transaminases.

Management

Other possible causes of nausea and vomiting should be excluded (Table 6.8.2). These include urinary tract infection (which often coincides with hyperemesis), thyrotoxicosis (where symptoms of weight loss, diarrhoea and tachycardia precede the pregnancy) and cholecystitis. An ultrasound scan of the uterus is important to exclude hydatidiform mole and to diagnose multiple pregnancy, both of which increase the risk of hyperemesis. The most important component of management is to ensure adequate rehydration. This should be with normal saline with added potassium chloride sufficient to correct tachycardia, hypotension and ketonuria and return electrolyte levels to normal. Dextrose-containing fluids are avoided except in women with diabetes. High concentrations of dextrose in particular may precipitate Wernicke's encephalopathy. This is prevented by routine administration of oral or intravenous thiamine. Anti-emetics may be liberally and safely used in pregnancy [II, Ia].[2,3] Women with severe hyperemesis may require regular parenteral doses of more than one anti-emetic to control their symptoms. Even for women with nausea and vomiting in pregnancy that does not require hospital admission but interferes with work and home life, anti-emetics may be appropriate. For women with severe hyperemesis who do not improve despite conventional treatment with intravenous fluids and electrolytes and regular anti-emetics, a trial of corticosteroids may be considered [Ib].[4] Iron supplements may induce nausea and vomiting and should be withheld until symptoms resolve.

Hyperemesis

- There are substantial data from systematic reviews[3] and cohort studies[2] to support the safety of conventional anti-emetics in pregnancy, including the first trimester.
- Several randomized, controlled trials[4] support a beneficial effect of corticosteroids.

GASTRO-OESOPHAGEAL REFLUX

About two-thirds of women experience heartburn in pregnancy, commonly in the third trimester. This is partly because of increased reflux due to the decreased lower oesophageal pressure, decreased gastric peristalsis and delayed gastric emptying, and partly due to the enlarging uterus. Reflux of acid or alkaline gastric contents into the oesophagus causes inflammation of the oesophageal mucosa, leading to pain, waterbrash and dyspepsia.

Management

Postural changes, such as sleeping in a semi-recumbent position, may help, especially in late pregnancy. Avoiding

Table 6.8.2   Protocol for the management of hyperemesis

Investigations	U + E, FBC, LFTs, TFTs
	MSU
	US scan uterus
Fluid therapy	Normal saline 1 L + 20–40 mmol KCl 8 hourly
Vitamin therapy	Thiamine orally 25–50 mg tds *or*
	Thiamine intravenously 100 mg in 100 mL normal saline weekly
Anti-emetic therapy	Possible regimens include:
	Cyclizine 50 mg p.o./i.m./i.v. tds
	Promethazine 25 mg p.o. nocte
	Stemetil 5 mg po tds; 12.5 mg i.m./i.v. tds
	Metoclopramide 10 mg p.o./i.m./i.v. tds
	Domperidone 10 mg p.o. qds; 30–60 mg p.r. tds
	Chlorpromazine 10–25 mg p.o.; 25 mg i.m. tds

US, ultrasound.

food or fluid intake immediately before retiring may also prevent symptoms. Antacids are safe in pregnancy and may be used liberally. Liquid preparations are more effective and should be given to prevent and treat symptoms. Aluminium-containing antacids may cause constipation, and magnesium-containing antacids may cause diarrhoea. Metoclopramide increases lower oesophageal pressure and speeds gastric emptying and may help relieve reflux. Sucralfate and histamine$_2$-receptor blockers (e.g. ranitidine) are both safe throughout pregnancy. Omeprazole, a proton-pump inhibitor and more powerful suppressor of gastric acid secretion, appears safe from limited data. It should be reserved for reflux oesophagitis when histamine$_2$-receptor blockers have failed.

PEPTIC ULCER

Peptic ulceration is rare in pregnancy. Presentation is usually with epigastric pain rather than with complications such as haemorrhage or perforation. Prostaglandins induced by pregnancy have a protective effect on the gastric mucosa, thus explaining the reduced incidence compared to non-pregnant women. Gastrointestinal endoscopy is safe in pregnancy and should be used to investigate all but minor haematemesis.

Management

Antacids, sucralfate and histamine$_2$-receptor blockers are all safe in pregnancy. *Helicobacter pylori* has a causal role in peptic ulceration, but eradication therapy is usually deferred until after delivery. Misoprostol, a prostaglandin analogue, protects the gastric mucosa, but is contra-indicated during pregnancy because of the risk of miscarriage.

CONSTIPATION

This is another common symptom of normal pregnancy, probably due to reduced colonic motility. Poor dietary intake associated with nausea and vomiting, dehydration, opiate analgesia and iron supplements exacerbate constipation. Management includes advice regarding increased fluid intake and dietary fibre. Temporary cessation of oral iron supplements may help, and laxatives should only be used if the above measures fail. Osmotic laxatives, such as lactulose and magnesium hydrochloride, are safe. Stimulant laxatives, such as glycerol suppositories, and senna (Senokot®) tablets are also safe in pregnancy.

> **Gastro-oesophageal reflux, dyspepsia, constipation**
>
> - There are substantial data from systematic reviews[3] to support the safety of antacids, anti-emetics, sucralfate, histamine$_2$-receptor blockers and proton pump inhibitors in pregnancy.
> - Misoprostol should be avoided.
> - Osmotic and stimulant laxatives are safe to use in pregnancy.

INFLAMMATORY BOWEL DISEASE

Both Crohn's disease and ulcerative colitis tend to present in young adulthood. Ulcerative colitis is more common in women and is encountered more commonly in pregnancy. The course of inflammatory bowel disease (IBD) is not usually affected by pregnancy. The risk of flare in pregnancy is reduced if colitis is quiescent at the time of conception. Most exacerbations occur early in pregnancy and cause abdominal pain, diarrhoea and passage of rectal mucus and blood. Women with Crohn's disease may experience postpartum flare. Pregnancy outcome is usually good in women with IBD, although active disease at the time of conception is associated with an increased risk of miscarriage, and active disease later in pregnancy may adversely affect pregnancy outcome, with an increased rate of prematurity.[5] Prior surgery, including ileostomy, proctocolectomy and pouch surgery, does not preclude successful pregnancy.

Management

Women with IBD should be encouraged to conceive during periods of disease remission. Management is not substantially affected by pregnancy. Oral or rectal sulfasalazine (Salazopyrin), mesalazine (Asacol) and other 5-aminosalicylic acid drugs may be safely used throughout pregnancy and breastfeeding, although as sulfasalazine is a dihydrofolate reductase inhibitor, 5 mg daily folic acid should be used pre-conceptually and in pregnancy to reduce the increased risk of neural tube defects, cardiovascular defects, oral clefts and folate deficiency. Oral and rectal preparations of corticosteroids may be required for acute treatment or maintenance and are safe in pregnancy. Azathioprine may be needed to maintain remission and this should continued in pregnancy (see Chapter 6.7).

Clinicians must remain alert to the possible dangerous surgical complications of IBD, including intestinal obstruction, haemorrhage, perforation or toxic megacolon. Caesarean section may be indicated in the presence of severe peri-anal Crohn's disease with a deformed, inelastic or scarred rectum and perineum. Active perianal Crohn's may prevent healing of an episiotomy.

Inflammatory bowel disease

- Evidence from cohort studies[5] supports an association between conception during periods of active disease and adverse pregnancy outcome.
- Sulfasalazine and related drugs are safe in pregnancy, but folic acid 5 mg/day should be given concomitantly.
- Corticosteroids and azathioprine may safely be used for maintenance or acute management of disease flares.

ACUTE AND CHRONIC VIRAL HEPATITIS

The course of most viral hepatitis is not altered by pregnancy. Pregnant women may contract acute hepatitis in the same way and with the same clinical features as non-pregnant women (see Chapter 7.4). Thus fever, malaise, anorexia, jaundice and possible recent exposure should alert the clinician to the diagnosis. The implications of acute hepatitis infection in pregnancy are discussed in Chapter 7.4. As with acute hepatitis B infections, neonates born to women with chronic hepatitis B virus (HBV) should be given hepatitis B immune globulin and HBV vaccine within 24 hours of birth. Immunization is 85–95 per cent effective at preventing both HBV infection and the chronic carrier state. There is a significant risk (60–80 per cent) of hepatitis C infection progressing to chronic infection, and about 20 per cent of those with chronic infection develop slowly progressive cirrhosis over a period of 10–30 years. Detection of hepatitis C virus (HCV) antibody implies persistent infection rather than immunity. The risk of progressive liver disease with hepatitis C is lower in women and in those aged <40 years who do not abuse alcohol. Women with hepatitis C are at increased risk of obstetric cholestasis (see below).[6]

CHRONIC LIVER DISEASE

Severe hepatic impairment is associated with infertility. Liver disease may decompensate during pregnancy, and pregnancy should be discouraged in women with severe impairment of hepatic function. Those with portal hypertension and oesophageal varices are at risk from variceal bleeding, especially in the second and third trimesters.

OBSTETRIC CHOLESTASIS

This is a liver disease specific to pregnancy, characterized by pruritus affecting the whole body but particularly the palms and soles, and abnormal liver function tests. It is more common in women from South America, the Indian subcontinent and Finland. The prevalence in the UK is about 0.7 per cent.[7] The aetiology is unknown, but relates to a genetic predisposition (one-third of patients have a positive family history) to the cholestatic effect of oestrogens.

Obstetric cholestasis most commonly presents in the third trimester at around 30–32 weeks' gestation.[7] Women with pruritus but without a rash other than excoriations should have liver function tests. These must be interpreted with reference to the normal ranges for pregnancy[1] since often in obstetric cholestasis the hepatic transaminases are only mildly elevated. The most usual abnormality is raised ALT or AST, although a small proportion of women have only a raised gamma GT or raised bile acids.[8] Although raised bile acids are not necessary to confirm the diagnosis, they are useful, especially in those women with typical clinical features but normal standard liver function tests.[8] There may be associated dark urine, pale stools, steatorrhoea and malaise. Obstetric cholestasis is a diagnosis of exclusion, and the differential diagnosis includes extrahepatic obstruction with gallstones, acute or chronic viral hepatitis, primary biliary cirrhosis (PBC) and chronic active hepatitis (CAH). Investigations should therefore include a liver ultrasound, serology for hepatitis A, B and C, Ebstein–Barr virus and cytomegalovirus, and liver autoantibodies (anti-mitochondrial antibodies to exclude PBC and anti-smooth muscle antibodies to exclude CAH).

The risks with obstetric cholestasis include postpartum haemorrhage (related to vitamin K deficiency secondary to malabsorption of fat), premature labour, meconium-stained liquor, fetal distress (cardiotocograph (CTG) abnormalities) in labour and, rarely, intrauterine death (IUD). The cause of the adverse effects on the fetus is unknown. The risk of IUD increases towards and beyond term but does not correlate with either symptoms or liver function tests. Therefore it is not correct to assume that the fetus of a mother with markedly abnormal liver function tests is at higher risk of IUD than that of a mother with only mildly abnormal liver function tests.

Obstetric cholestasis

- Evidence from prospective studies[7,8] supports the need for a high index of clinical suspicion, and therefore serial measurement of liver function tests, in women with onset of pruritus affecting predominantly the palms and soles in the third trimester.
- This evidence also highlights the trade-off between reduced fetal mortality and increased rates of induction, prematurity and caesarean section.

Management

This should involve counselling the woman regarding the above risks. Liver function tests and clotting times should be monitored regularly. Current guidelines suggest that in the absence of premature labour, delivery should be induced at 37–38 weeks. Vitamin K should be given to the mother (10 mg orally daily) from the time of diagnosis to reduce the risk of postpartum haemorrhage. There are few data to support the current practice of fetal surveillance with regular CTGs and ultrasound scans. Although such monitoring may serve to reassure the mother and her carers, delivery is rarely indicated earlier than 37 weeks on the basis of such monitoring. Management strategies that involve elective early (by 38 weeks) delivery and fetal surveillance have shown a decreased risk of IUD compared to earlier studies, but also result in increased rates of caesarean section, prematurity and admissions to neonatal intensive care units.[7]

Control of symptoms may be achieved with a combination of antihistamines and emollients or, if these are insufficient, ursodeoxycholic acid (UDCA). This drug usually leads to rapid reduction in liver function tests and pruritus, but there is as yet no evidence for a reduction in fetal risk.

Following delivery, liver function tests return to normal and there is no permanent detrimental effect on maternal liver function. Symptoms may recur with menstruation (cyclical itching) or with oestrogen-containing oral contraceptives, which should therefore be avoided. Recurrence of obstetric cholestasis in subsequent pregnancies exceeds 90 per cent.

KEY POINTS – OBSTETRIC CHOLESTASIS

- Liver function tests should be requested in any pregnant woman with pruritus without obvious rash.
- Liver function tests should be repeated serially if the itching involves the palms and soles.
- Other causes of pruritus and abnormal liver function tests, including viral hepatitis and gallstones causing extrahepatic obstruction, should be excluded.
- Retrospective studies support active management with elective delivery by 38 weeks.
- Active management increases the risk of caesarean section and prematurity.
- UDCA improves symptoms and liver function tests.

ACUTE FATTY LIVER OF PREGNANCY

This is another pregnancy-specific liver disease. It is rare. Acute fatty liver of pregnancy (AFLP) is closely related to and shares many features and probably pathophysiology with pre-eclampsia. It usually presents in the third trimester with abdominal pain, nausea, vomiting, anorexia and sometimes jaundice. It is associated with markedly deranged liver function tests, renal impairment, a markedly elevated uric acid, a raised white cell count, hypoglycaemia and coagulopathy.[9] Clinical features of pre-eclampsia may be mild or absent. It may come to light only after delivery when coagulation is checked because of excessive bleeding. It is also associated with diabetes insipidus and may present with polyuria. Perinatal and maternal mortality and morbidity are increased.

Management

This should involve a high-dependency or intensive care unit and a multidisciplinary team. Delivery should be expedited following adequate correction of any hypoglycaemia or coagulopathy with 50 per cent dextrose, intramuscular vitamin K and fresh frozen plasma. Management after delivery is conservative, although early referral to a liver unit should be considered if liver function does not improve or if there are any features of hepatic encephalopathy.

PUBLISHED GUIDELINES

British Liver Trust – Obstetric Cholestasis, web link: <www.britishlivertrust.org.uk/publications/obstetric_cholestasis.html>.
Kelly A, Nelson-Piercy C. Obstetric cholestasis. PACE review for RCOG. *The Obstetrician and Gynaecologist* 2000; 2:29–31.

KEY REFERENCES

1. Girling JC, Dow E, Smith JH. Liver function tests in pre-eclampsia: importance of comparison with a reference range derived for normal pregnancy. *Br J Obstet Gynaecol* 1997; **104**:246–50.
2. Nelson-Piercy C. Treatment of nausea and vomiting in pregnancy: when should it be treated and with what? *Drug Saf* 1998; **19**(2):155–64.
3. Mazzotta P, Magee LA. A risk–benefit assessment of pharmacological and non-pharmacological treatments for nausea and vomiting of pregnancy. *Drugs* 2000; **59**:781–800.
4. Nelson-Piercy C, Fayers P, de Swiet M. Randomized, placebo-controlled trial of corticosteroids for hyperemesis gravidarum. *Br J Obstet Gynaecol* 2001; **108**:1–7.

Antenatal complications: maternal

5. Kornfeld D, Crattingnuis S, Ekbom A. Pregnancy outcomes in women with IBD – a population-based cohort study. *Am J Obstet Gynecol* 1997; 177:942–6.

6. Locatelli A, Roncaglia N, Arreghini A et al. Hepatitis C virus infection is associated with a higher incidence of cholestasis of pregnancy. *Br J Obstet Gynaecol* 1999; 106:498–500.

7. Kenyon AP, Nelson-Piercy C, Girling J, Williamson C, Tribe RM, Shennan AH. Obstetric cholestasis, outcome with active management: a series of 70 cases. *Br J Obstet Gynaecol* 2002; 109:1M–7.

8. Kenyon AP, Nelson-Piercy C, Girling J, Williamson C, Tribe RM, Shennan AH. Pruritus may precede abnormal liver function tests in pregnant women with obstetric cholestasis: a longitudinal analysis. *Br J Obstet Gynaecol* 2001; 108:1190–2.

9. Nelson-Piercy C. Liver disease. In: *Handbook of Obstetric Medicine*, 2nd edn. Martin London: Martin Dunitz, 2001, 199–217.

Respiratory Conditions

Alec McEwan

There is no established standard for this topic, but the following points are suggested for guidance:

Theoretical skills
- Recognize the physiological changes occurring in the respiratory system during normal pregnancy.
- Understand the impact that pregnancy may have on pre-existing chest disease and the influence the illness may have on pregnancy.

Practical skills
- Liaise appropriately with other specialists.
- Manage a pregnancy complicated by pre-existing respiratory disease.
- Request and interpret investigations with reference to the pregnancy.

INTRODUCTION

Articles concerning medical disorders and their interaction with pregnancy normally follow a particular format. Physiological changes in pregnancy are described first as these may confuse the presentation of co-existing disease and influence the interpretation of investigations. The effect of the pregnancy on the disease is then considered, followed by the effect of the disease on the pregnancy: are the medications safe, what antenatal complications can be expected and are there likely to be any neonatal ramifications?

The understanding and recollection of this information is also aided by considering the management of medical disorders in pregnancy in a temporal way. Pre-pregnancy issues are considered first, followed by individualized planning for antepartum, intrapartum and postpartum care.

RESPIRATORY DISEASE IN PREGNANCY

The physiological changes occurring within the respiratory system are summarized in Tables 6.9.1 and 6.9.2. Symptomatically, pregnant women may complain of new-onset rhinitis, which may result from oestrogen-induced oedema, hyperaemia and hypersecretion of the upper airways. Although mostly harmless, this contributes to the greater difficulties encountered during intubation of pregnant women. Much

Table 6.9.1 Normal arterial blood gas values and the effect of pregnancy

	Pre-pregnancy	By term
PaO_2	11–13 kPa (83–98 mmHg)	>13 kPa (>98 mmHg)
$PaCO_2$	4.8–6.0 kPa (36–45 mmHg)	3.7–4.2 kPa (28–32 mmHg)
HCO_3^-	24–30 mmol/L	18–21 mmol/L
pH	7.35–7.45	7.4–7.45

Table 6.9.2 The effect of pregnancy on lung function

Lung function	Change by term	Actual volume change
Total lung capacity	4% decrease	200–400 mL
Functional residual capacity	10–20% decrease	300–500 mL
Expiratory reserve volume	15–20% decrease	100–300 mL
Tidal volume	30–50% increase	200 mL
Minute ventilation	30–50% increase	3 L/min
Residual volume	20–25% decrease	200–300 mL
Respiratory rate	No change	
Vital capacity	No change	
Peak flow	No change	
Metabolic rate	15% increase	
Oxygen consumption ($\dot{V}_{O_2}$)	20–33% increase	

more common is the complaint of shortness of breath or 'air hunger'. This dyspnoea is experienced by approximately half of all pregnant women by 20 weeks' gestation and by three-quarters by 30 weeks'. It rarely occurs at rest and does not significantly impair normal activities. The postulated mechanism is high progesterone levels acting via the hypothalamus to increase respiratory drive.

Anatomically, the lower chest wall circumference increases by 5–7 cm, the diaphragm is elevated 4–5 cm by term and the costal angle widens. These changes occur due to the pressure from the expanding uterus and the relaxation of thoracic ligaments. Diaphragmatic excursion is not reduced; however, the accessory muscles contribute proportionally more than the diaphragm to the increase in tidal volume found in pregnancy.

The metabolic rate becomes elevated in pregnancy, as demonstrated by a rise in resting oxygen uptake ($\dot{V}_{O_2}$) and carbon dioxide output ($\dot{V}_{CO_2}$). This extra oxygen turnover is of course necessary for the feto-placental unit and the extra demands made by maternal physiology. Minute ventilation ($\dot{V}_E$) and alveolar ventilation ($\dot{V}_A$) are both increased to meet this demand by an increase in tidal volume (T_V) rather than by a change in respiratory rate, which remains constant. This state of relative hyperventilation causes a fall in $PaCO_2$, which results in a chronic respiratory alkalosis. Blood pH is kept within the normal range by a reactionary increase in renal bicarbonate excretion.

Airway function is maintained and peak expiratory flow rate (PEFR) and forced expiratory volume in 1 second (FEV_1) measurements are not affected by pregnancy.

Investigating respiratory disease in pregnancy

The physiological changes occurring in pregnancy must also be considered when interpreting the results of investigations. The effect on arterial blood gas analysis is clear from Table 6.9.1. The chest X-ray must also be interpreted with caution. The cardiothoracic ratio is elevated, vascular markings may become more prominent, and small pleural effusions are even possible in normal pregnancy. Peak flow and spirometry tests can be interpreted in the usual manner.

Concern is often raised about the safety of various radiological examinations during pregnancy. For a fuller description of risks to the fetus, see Chapter 7.3. Five rad (or 50 000 µGy) is often considered the maximum safe exposure for the fetus, although this is gestation dependent [III]. Chest X-ray, venography, pulmonary angiography and ventilation perfusion scanning all expose the fetus to significantly lower levels than this, and the potential benefits of all these investigations are usually thought to outweigh the risks. However, exposure should be minimized where possible. For example:

- lateral chest X-rays are often unnecessary and carry a greater exposure risk than an AP erect chest film; they can mostly be avoided;

- a mobile chest X-ray carries greater exposure than a departmental film, so the patient should be moved where possible;
- the 'ventilation' component of $\dot{V}/\dot{Q}$ scanning can be omitted in women with no previous history of chest disease;
- pulmonary angiography carries less fetal risk if a brachial route is used in preference to the femoral.

Shielding of the fetus should be used where the situation allows. Computed tomography (CT) scanning utilizes much higher energy levels, and safer alternatives are usually available. However, if the indication is strong enough, even CT has its place. Spiral and non-contiguous axial imaging are techniques that may reduce exposure without compromising diagnostic accuracy. Magnetic resonance imaging (MRI) scanning involves no irradiation and is also considered safe.

ASTHMA

Asthma is the respiratory illness most likely to be encountered during pregnancy, with a prevalence of between 1 per cent and 4 per cent.

The true effect of pregnancy on asthma severity has been addressed by a number of prospective case-controlled studies which suggest that approximately two-fifths will deteriorate, two-fifths will stay the same and one-fifth will improve.[1] The potential benefits of pregnancy-induced immune system alterations and progesterone-mediated bronchodilatation may be opposed by the reluctance of patients and physicians to treat asthma appropriately for fear of harming the fetus through drug exposure. Women with severe asthma seem more likely to deteriorate, whilst those showing improvement during pregnancy are more likely to suffer postpartum relapse.[2] Approximately 1 in 10 asthmatics will suffer an acute attack in labour [II].

The precise effect that the asthma has on the pregnancy is unclear. Almost every conceivable obstetric complication has been found to be more common in pregnant asthmatics by one case-control study or another. However, the pattern of antenatal complications varies greatly among studies and this lack of consistency has cast doubt over the findings. Poor controls, varied case mixes and different treatment regimes make resolution of the data very difficult.

Prospective and retrospective studies suggest that pregnancy outcome is usually extremely good.

A prospective case-controlled study by Schatz in 1995 found no increase in the incidence of any obstetric complications amongst almost 500 asthmatics.[3] These women were managed by an obstetrician and an interested physician and this may explain the normal outcomes. However, only a quarter of the women used steroids of any kind, and the overall mild nature of the condition in this group may have contributed to the favourable outcomes.

It is still accepted that severe and poorly controlled asthma does have a detrimental effect on pregnancy, so closer surveillance for hypertensive disorders, intrauterine growth restriction and preterm rupture of membranes/labour can be justified [IV].

Management of asthma in pregnancy

Asthma will usually have been diagnosed prior to pregnancy and treatment already instituted. However, this is not always the case, and the initial presenting signs and symptoms of asthma are the same as those of asthma that is inadequately treated:

- chest tightness and wheeziness
- cough
- breathlessness, especially in the early hours of the morning.

The management of asthma in pregnancy is essentially the same as in non-pregnant patients.

Prevention is the key, and known triggers of exacerbations should be eliminated or avoided in the home and at work (Table 6.9.3).

Pharmacological treatment of asthma

This follows a step-by-step approach, more clearly outlined in the *British National Formulary*.

- **Step 1: occasional relief bronchodilators** (up to once per day): short-acting inhaled beta$_2$-agonist, e.g. salbutamol, terbutaline, fenoterol.

Table 6.9.3 Triggers and provocative stimuli for exacerbations of asthma

Allergens	Pollen (seasonal) Dust mites, animal danders, moulds (non-seasonal)
Occupational	Industrial chemicals, metal salts, wood and vegetable dust
Infection	Viral and/or bacterial
Environmental pollution	Tobacco smoke, ozone
Pharmacological	Aspirin and non-steroidal anti-inflammatory drugs, beta-blockers
Emotional stress	
Exercise and cold air	

- **Step 2: regular inhaled preventative:** inhaled short-acting beta$_2$-agonist as required (see above) *plus* regular inhaled standard dose corticosteroid (beclomethasone, budesonide or fluticasone), cromoglycate or necrodomil.
- **Step 3: high-dose inhaled corticosteroid:** inhaled short-acting beta$_2$-agonist as required (see above) *plus* regular high-dose inhaled corticosteroid.
- **Step 4: high-dose inhaled corticosteroids plus regular bronchodilators:** inhaled short-acting beta$_2$-agonist as required (see above) *plus* regular high-dose inhaled corticosteroid *plus* one of the following regular long-acting bronchodilators:
  - long-acting inhaled beta$_2$-agonist
  - modified-release oral theophylline
  - inhaled ipratropium or oxitropium
  - cromoglycate or nedocromil.
- **Step 5: regular corticosteroid tablets:** inhaled short-acting beta$_2$-agonist as required (see above) *plus* regular high-dose inhaled corticosteroid *plus* one of the regular long-acting bronchodilators (see step 4) *plus* regular prednisolone tablets.

Short-acting and long-acting beta$_2$-agonists, inhaled steroids and theophylline can all be used with confidence in pregnancy. Neonatal irritability and apnoea have been reported with theophylline; however, this uncommon side effect should not prohibit use of the drug if indication exists. These drugs will suffice for most mild to moderate asthmatics. Women with more severe asthma who have been stabilized on leukotriene receptor anatgonists may continue them throughout the pregnancy. It is less likely that pregnant patients will be using antimuscarinic bronchodilators, sodium cromoglycate or nedocromil; however, no adverse effects have been reported in pregnancy. Prednisolone is the oral steroid of choice for pregnancy, as 88 per cent of it is metabolized by the placenta, limiting fetal exposure. Initial worries about an association with isolated cleft lip have been allayed by a recent case-control study which did not support the original animal experimental work [II].[4] However, a subsequent meta-analysis has once again confused the debate with a statistically significant three-fold increase in oral clefting risk for steroid use in the first trimester.[5] Neonatal adrenal suppression has proven to be a theoretical risk rather than a real practical concern. Newer anxieties have arisen about associations with intrauterine growth restriction, neuronal development, long-term hypertension and preterm labour. If real, these complications are likely to occur in the long-term users of higher doses, i.e. those women with more severe asthma. Corticosteroids are usually only prescribed for good medical reasons, and usually outside of the teratogenic period. Most agree that if a need for steroids exists, pregnancy should not be considered a contraindication. In the recent Confidential Enquiry into Maternal Deaths (1997–1999), five women died from asthma. One of these women stopped maintenance steroid therapy on becoming pregnant.

The teratogenic risk and possible harmful fetal effects of maternal steroid treatment remain an area of controversy. However, the Committee on Safety of Medicines has concluded that 'there is no convincing evidence that systemic corticosteroids increase the incidence of congenital abnormalities such as cleft lip and palate', but that 'prolonged or repeated doses increase the risk of intrauterine growth restriction'.[6]

Specific guidelines also exist for the management of acute asthma attacks and these should also be adhered to in pregnancy.[7] The severity of acute exacerbations is divided into three groups.

1   **Uncontrolled asthma in adults.** Speech must be normal, with a pulse of <110 beats/min and respiratory rate of <25/min. Peak flow should be >50 per cent of predicted or personal best. Treatment involves nebulized salbutamol or terbutaline. Failure to respond should prompt referral to hospital. Otherwise, normal treatment can be stepped up and a course of oral steroids may be prescribed.
2   **Acute severe attack.** These patients will not be able to complete sentences, will have a pulse ≥110 beats/min, a respiratory rate of ≥25/min and a peak flow of ≤50 per cent predicted or personal best. Acute treatment involves oxygen, nebulizers and oral prednisolone. Those not responding well should be transferred to hospital with an aminophylline infusion.
3   **Life-threatening asthma.** This most serious of asthma exacerbations is characterized by a 'silent chest', cyanosis, bradycardia or a peak flow of ≤33 per cent of predicted or personal best. Immediate hospital treatment is necessary with oxygen, nebulizers, intravenous aminophylline, oral steroids or intravenous hydrocortisone.

It is useful for all clinicians to remember these guidelines. However, there should be a low threshold for the involvement of appropriate physicians in cases of deteriorating asthma in pregnancy. Possible precipitating factors should be addressed with all acute exacerbations. For example antibiotics are often prescribed for presumed chest infection.

Managing pregnancy in asthmatic patients

- Well-controlled mild or moderate asthmatics will have a normal outcome with standard antenatal care [II]. For those with poorly controlled or severe asthma, care should be multidisciplinary, preferably through a high-risk antenatal clinic with general medical input [IV].
- Baseline investigations, such as peak flow measurements, should be obtained at booking [IV].

- Medical treatment should be optimized by following the above protocol, with repeated reassurance about the use of these drugs in pregnancy. A recent study has demonstrated that physicians are still reluctant to prescribe oral steroids during pregnancy.[2]
- In view of the uncertainty over the true impact of severe asthma on pregnancy outcome, the maternity team should remain vigilant for signs of preterm labour and follow fetal growth and well-being with ultrasound [IV].
- Induction of labour and caesarean section will mostly be reserved for obstetric indications, although delivery may need to be expedited in the most severe cases [III].
- No form of analgesia is contraindicated, although regional anaesthesia is preferable rather than general for major operative procedures.
- Women taking prednisolone should be screened for glucose intolerance and measures taken to control this if it is found. Those taking prednisolone at the onset of labour should be given supplementary doses of 100 mg hydrocortisone 6–8 hourly until oral intake is resumed. Advice should also be sought for those women who have had a recent course finishing in the week prior to labour, or for those who have intermittent repeated courses of high-dose steroids [II].
- Ergometrine, prostaglandin $F_{2\alpha}$, aspirin and non-steroidal anti-inflammatory drugs should be avoided where possible, as all have been reported to cause bronchospasm [IV].
- The risk of postnatal deterioration should be discussed with the woman.
- Breastfeeding is not contraindicated with any of the medications used, although high-dose oral steroid use (≥40 mg/day) carries a risk of neonatal adrenal suppression.

CYSTIC FIBROSIS

The reporting of pregnancies in women with cystic fibrosis began in the 1960s and the initial outcomes seemed unfavourable. However, with improvements in the care of both individuals with cystic fibrosis and high-risk pregnancies in general, the outlook is more favourable. Although men with cystic fibrosis are usually infertile, this is not the case for women. Menarche is delayed by an average of 2 years and the incidence of anovulatory cycles and secondary amenorrhoea is indeed higher. Cervical mucus may be more tenacious. However, fertility is the general rule rather than the exception. Average life expectancy for those with cystic fibrosis continues to lengthen and many women are now choosing to start a family and employing specialist assistance where subfertility exists.

The spectrum of disease phenotype and severity is highly varied and only loosely correlated to genotype. Individual counselling, preferably prior to conception, is vital and it must be clearly understood that outcome predictors are imprecise.

Outcomes

Outcomes needing consideration are both the effect of the pregnancy on the cystic fibrosis and, conversely, the effect of the cystic fibrosis on the pregnancy. A number of different markers of disease severity have been proposed as predictors of maternal and fetal outcome (Table 6.9.4). Only two women with cystic fibrosis feature in the most recent Confidential Enquiry into Maternal Deaths. One had a pre-pregnancy FEV_1 of 36 per cent and the other had severe nutritional difficulties, with a body mass index (BMI) of 18.

Two recently published series are in general agreement with one another, although the Canadian series from Toronto ($n = 92$)[6] includes cases from as long ago as 1961. The patients in this group had slightly milder disease overall than those in Edenborough's UK group ($n = 22$)[9] (%FEV_1 <50 per cent in 12 per cent and 18 per cent respectively, and pancreatic insufficiency in 60 per cent and 100 per cent respectively).

Effect of pregnancy on cystic fibrosis

No women in either of these studies died during or within 6 weeks of pregnancy. However, only 79 per cent of the Canadian women were still alive 10 years after the delivery, the earliest death occurring 3 years after the birth. Only three-quarters were still alive 4 years after delivery in the UK study, the earliest death occurring only 6 months postpartum. These mortality rates are, however, no different from those for non-pregnant individuals with cystic fibrosis.

Death is a very crude measure of the effect of pregnancy on cystic fibrosis. Decline in lung function has also been examined. Edenborough found a 13 per cent loss in %FEV_1 during pregnancy, although this was mostly regained in the following year, and a net loss of 5 per cent in FEV_1 overall at 1 year following delivery. Gilljam's prediction of 3 per cent is similar; neither deterioration is significantly greater than that expected for the normal cystic fibrosis population [II]. However, caution must be exercised in women with poor pre-pregnancy lung function (<50 per cent predicted %FEV_1). There is evidence suggesting that they do suffer a permanent pregnancy-associated decline in lung function,[10] although this, too, is disputed.[8]

The anatomical and physiological changes in cardiorespiratory function during pregnancy might be thought to impair mucus clearance, increase atelectasis and predispose to pulmonary infections. However, serious medical events would appear to be no more common in pregnancy than would be expected from the pre-pregnancy lung function tests.

> Retrospective studies suggest that pregnancy only accelerates the loss of respiratory function in 'severe' cases of cystic fibrosis.

Effect of cystic fibrosis on pregnancy

Studies have not shown an increase in miscarriage or anomaly risk over the general obstetric population,[8-10] although cystic fibrosis was diagnosed in two of the Canadian offspring. In one case, the diagnosis of maternal cystic fibrosis was not made until after the child was born, and in the second, prenatal screening had indicated that there was only a very low risk that the child would be affected (see below). The mean gestation at delivery was ≥37 weeks in both studies, although 1 in 3 babies were born preterm in the UK study. The prematurity rate was no higher than for the general population in the Canadian group (8 per cent). Intrauterine growth restriction was not encountered more frequently than would normally be expected. Only one neonate died, sepsis being the cause following delivery at 31 weeks' gestation.

The average maternal weight gain of 10–12 kg during pregnancy demands an extra 300 kcal/day. Pancreatic insufficiency is very common in cystic fibrosis, and enzyme supplements are usually needed to aid digestion. Increasing nutritional intake during pregnancy may be very difficult, especially with confounding factors such as nausea, hyperemesis and indigestion. It is hardly surprising that average maternal weight gain is reduced by approximately half. Furthermore, a compromised pancreas may fail to fulfil its added endocrine responsibilities: gestational diabetes occurred in 8 per cent of those women in the Canadian group who were not pre-existing diabetics.

Caesarean section is normally employed only for obstetric reasons in women with mild to moderate cystic fibrosis. However, 1 in 3 women were delivered by preterm section in the UK group, the most common indication being deteriorating lung function. Instrumental delivery rates do not appear to be increased.

The more recent retrospective reviews do suggest a generally good outcome for mother and baby. Problems such as prematurity and maternal death within 5 years of delivery are mostly confined to cases with poor pre-pregnancy lung function, pancreatic insufficiency (especially glucose intolerance) and lung colonization with *Burkholderia cepacia*. A %FEV_1 of <50 per cent is often considered a relative contraindication to pregnancy. Good outcomes with prolonged maternal survival

Table 6.9.4 Predictors of maternal and fetal outcome in pregnancies complicated by cystic fibrosis

Absolute pre-pregnancy pulmonary function
Stability of pre-pregnancy pulmonary function
Colonization with *Burkholderia cepacia*
Presence of pulmonary hypertension
Degree of pancreatic insufficiency
Glucose intolerance/diabetes (pre-dating pregnancy or gestational)
Body mass index
Maternal weight gain during pregnancy
Presence of liver disease and portal hypertension

afterwards are nevertheless possible, even with values below this. The presence of pulmonary hypertension causes grave concern. Serious consideration should be given to termination of the pregnancy to prevent right-sided heart failure.

Management of cystic fibrosis during pregnancy

Retrospective studies of cystic fibrosis in pregnancy support the same management as that used outside of pregnancy. This is strongly evidence based, but not specified in detail here.

- A chest physician should retain responsibility for the management of the cystic fibrosis, in close consultation with the obstetric team.
- Vigilance must be maintained for the complications of cystic fibrosis: haemoptysis, pneumothorax, atelectasis, respiratory failure and cor pulmonale.
- There should be no hesitation in performing chest X-rays where these are deemed necessary.
- Chest physiotherapy and bronchial drainage should continue.
- Serial lung function tests, e.g. spirometry and arterial blood gases, should be performed at regular intervals throughout pregnancy.
- Careful surveillance for signs of chest infection becomes even more important due to the complications of pneumonia in pregnancy (see below). *Pseudomonas aeruginosa* is the most common cause of chest infection in cystic fibrosis. Penicillins, cephalosporins and aminoglycosides are the most commonly used antibiotics (intravenously, orally or inhaled). All are considered safe in pregnancy, even gentamicin (the risk of fetal ototoxicity can be minimized by ensuring maternal serum levels do not exceed recommended levels). The risks to the mother and fetus of withholding appropriate antibiotics are greater. Some antibiotic dosing schedules will need to be adjusted due to the larger volume distribution and enhanced renal elimination found in pregnancy.
- Cardiovascular status should be observed during pregnancy, preferably by echocardiography.
- Pancreatic enzymes should be continued and insulin levels adjusted appropriately.

Managing a pregnancy complicated by cystic fibrosis

Antenatal care in the presence of cystic fibrosis is mostly based on retrospective and uncontrolled studies or expert opinion.

- Ideally, a full discussion should take place prior to conception. Treatment can be optimized and the risks discussed. Patients with poor lung function or pulmonary hypertension may be advised to avoid pregnancy altogether.
- The average age of survival for women with cystic fibrosis in the UK is approximately 28 years. The effect on a child of losing a parent should be considered before conception.
- The issue of prenatal screening should be raised, although this must be done diplomatically, as the condition being screened for is, after all, present in the mother. As cystic fibrosis is an autosomal recessive condition, the offspring will either be all obligate carriers, if the partner is free of mutations, or 1 in 2 will be affected if he is a carrier himself. Approximately 1 in 25 individuals are cystic fibrosis carriers in the UK. ΔF508 is the most common cystic fibrosis mutation in the UK, accounting for 80 per cent of the total. A 'rare' mutation screen may test for as many as 30 different mutations; however, this will still only detect approximately 90 per cent of all mutations. Hence, even when the partner of the woman with cystic fibrosis has a 'negative' mutation screen, there is still a 1 in 250 chance he is a carrier ($1/25 \times 1/10$) and therefore a 1 in 500 chance that the baby will have cystic fibrosis ($1/250 \times 1/2$).
- Termination of pregnancy should be considered by women with very unfavourable features.
- Advice from dieticians will be essential to maintain caloric intake. Rarely, enteral (and even parenteral) feeding is necessary.
- Regular fetal monitoring with growth scans is advisable, especially in more severe cases of lung disease or poor maternal weight gain.
- Ideally, induction of labour and caesarean section are performed only for obstetric reasons. However, deterioration in lung function may prompt intervention. General anaesthesia should be avoided where possible.
- Facial oxygen may be required in labour, and exhaustion should be prevented by instrumental delivery if necessary. Prolonged Valsalva manoeuvres may predispose to pneumothoraces.

TUBERCULOSIS

Infection with *Mycobacterium tuberculosis* most commonly presents in African and Indian ethnic groups, new immigrant populations, refugees and asylum seekers. Human immunodeficiency virus (HIV) positivity is another well-recognized risk factor and this is one reason cited for the increasing incidence of tuberculosis (TB) since the 1980s. Treatment can be safe and effective in pregnancy and the outcome is normally good. Failure to diagnose the condition and patient non-compliance with medication regimens do put the mother and newborn at increased risk.

> There is no good evidence to suggest that pregnancy is an independent risk factor for infection with *Mycobacterium tuberculosis* or that the course and outcome of TB are altered by pregnancy.

Primary infection is usually asymptomatic, although fever, cough, conjunctivitis and erythema nodosum may all occur. A cellular immune response can be detected 3–8 weeks later by a positive tuberculin test.

Any further clinical manifestations are known as 'post-primary tuberculosis' and include pulmonary disease (apical lung cavitation, pneumonia, pleural effusion), miliary TB (widespread disseminated TB), pericarditis, peritonitis, meningitis, bone and genitourinary TB. These may occur months or years after the primary infection following a period of 'latency'.

Public health policies towards TB prevention and detection have differed on each side of the Atlantic. In the USA, tuberculin testing (the Mantoux test) is used to screen high-risk groups during pregnancy. A positive result combined with specific risk factors may prompt a screening chest X-ray and sputum testing for mycobacteria. Based on the results of these, the patient is either treated for active TB or given prophylaxis with isoniazid, on the assumption that latent infection is present and could reactivate at any time. In the UK, widespread vaccination of schoolchildren with bacille Calmette Guérin (BCG – said to prevent 70 per cent of infections) reduces the value of routine tuberculin testing, which will be positive in those who have been vaccinated. There is no screening programme for TB in pregnancy in the UK and clinicians must remain hypervigilant for signs and symptoms suggestive of the disease.

Pulmonary manifestations are the most common presenting features of TB, and a chest X-ray may show upper lobe densities and cavitation, fibrosis, pleural effusion, empyema or calcifications. Sputum is examined for acid-fast bacilli using a Ziehl–Nielsen stain and subsequently cultured for antibiotic sensitivity testing. Bronchoscopic washings must be obtained if there is no sputum. Extrapulmonary TB is diagnosed using tissue biopsies in a similar way. Although the Mantoux test is considered safe in pregnancy, it is unable to distinguish active disease from previous disease and BCG vaccination.

Active tuberculosis infections are treated with a combination of antibiotics, determined by the results of the culture sensitivities. Although regimens vary, treatment usually includes therapy with rifampicin, isoniazid, pyrazinamide and sometimes ethambutol. Less well-known drugs may be necessary in cases of multi-drug resistance including amikacin, kanamycin and ethionamide.

The relationship between pregnancy and TB

It is generally agreed that pregnancy has no impact on the course of TB and that TB, if diagnosed and treated expeditiously, has no significant impact on the pregnancy [III]. Delayed or inadequate therapy would appear to be detrimental to both maternal and fetal outcomes, however, increasing the risks of prematurity and intrauterine growth restriction [III].

Presentation and diagnosis are unaffected by pregnancy, although misguided reluctance in performing chest X-rays may lead to further diagnostic delay.

Vertical transmission (congenital TB) is extremely rare and usually only occurs where maternal disease has gone untreated. Fewer than 300 cases have been reported, although placental infection is somewhat more common. Lateral transmission from the mother or other close contacts, occurring after delivery, is a much more likely cause of infant infection. Therefore strict criteria exist for the diagnosis of congenital TB. One of the following is necessary:

- lesions in the first week of life,
- a primary hepatic complex or caseating granuloma,
- histological evidence of placental or endometrial involvement,
- absence of TB in other carers of the child.

Congenital TB usually presents with fever, lymphadenopathy, hepatosplenomegaly and respiratory distress. It is fatal in 1 in 5 cases. In only half of all cases has the diagnosis of maternal TB already been made.

Treatment of TB during pregnancy

- TB is most likely to be diagnosed by physicians, even during pregnancy, and the specialist advice of a respiratory consultant is essential along with close involvement by microbiologists [IV].
- Isoniazid, rifampicin and ethambutol are used initially. The ethambutol can be stopped when sensitivities show that the other two drugs are adequate. These are then continued for 9 months in total. The most significant toxic side effect of isoniazid in animal and human studies is demyelination (causing a peripheral neuropathy). This can be prevented by supplementation with pyridoxine (vitamin B_6). Hepatotoxicity may be more common in pregnancy, and liver function tests should be performed monthly [III]. Most studies do not show a significant elevation in the anomaly rate above the background 2–3 per cent in users of rifampicin in pregnancy [II]. Liver enzyme induction, with theoretical vitamin K deficiency, should prompt maternal oral vitamin K supplements in the third trimester to prevent haemorrhagic disease of the newborn. The theoretical risks of fetal ocular toxicity with ethambutol

have not been borne out in practice. Although pyrizinamide is usually avoided in pregnancy, there are no data to suggest a harmful effect and it should be used if needed as a second-line agent. Streptomycin, a previous favourite in TB treatment, has well-recognized fetal ototoxicity. Safer alternatives are available.

- Non-compliance with drug regimens outside of pregnancy is a major problem. There is no reason to think that it is any less so during pregnancy. Supervision, encouragement and incentive schemes may be necessary to encourage proper use of the prescribed medications.
- All the anti-tuberculous drugs mentioned in this section are compatible with breastfeeding [III].
- There is often concern over the infectious nature of TB in a maternity setting. Provided that the prescribed drugs have been taken properly, an active TB sufferer will become non-infectious within 2 weeks of commencing treatment. If the mother is still sputum positive, specialist infection control nursing will be necessary. The newborn should be immunized with BCG and also given prophylactic antibiotics (usually isoniazid). Separation of the infant from its mother is not necessary unless she is non-compliant or another carer or family member is highly infectious.
- It would seem prudent to send the placenta for microbiological investigation. Evidence of acid-fast bacilli should increase surveillance of the newborn.

PNEUMONIA

Pneumonia, in otherwise healthy individuals, is no more common in pregnancy than in an age-matched population as a whole, and the maternal outcome, in the main, is no better or worse. The incidence of pneumonia in pregnancy would appear to be on the rise, but this may be accounted for by an increase in the number of pregnancies in women with co-existing problems such as HIV and cystic fibrosis. Only two women in the 1994–96 Confidential Enquiry into Maternal Deaths died from pneumonia without other risk factors, and this mortality rate is in line with that of young adults with community-acquired pneumonia. The other five had cystic fibrosis or HIV or were substance abusers. Fetal outcome may be affected however, and prompt recognition and treatment of pneumonia in pregnancy are essential if this is to be avoided. The main risk would appear to be preterm labour, although growth restriction has also been reported (Table 6.9.5).

Diagnosis of pneumonia in pregnancy

The symptoms and signs of pneumonia are not altered by pregnancy, but may be confused with physiological changes

Table 6.9.5   Risk factors for pneumonia

History of recent upper respiratory tract infection
Chronic respiratory disease (e.g. asthma, cystic fibrosis)
Smoking
Immunocompromise (HIV, substance abuse, alcoholism, recurrent courses of antenatal steroids)
Anaemia
Farm workers (*Coxiella burnetii*)
General anaesthesia (aspiration pneumonitis)

HIV, human immunodeficiency virus.

common to pregnancy. Reluctance to perform a chest X-ray may further delay the diagnosis. Obstetricians have a responsibility in educating other physicians that the fetal radiation exposure with appropriate shielding is minimal and that this examination is safe. This message is even more important if risk factors for pneumonia are present.

Sputum should be sent for microbiological examination and culture. Blood can be taken for serological testing for *Mycoplasma* and viral antibodies.

Treatment of pneumonia in pregnancy

Common organisms

Frequently, no infectious agent is found and the pneumonia is treated empirically. The most common bacteria causing community-acquired pneumonia are *Streptococcus pneumoniae* and *Haemophilus influenzae*, often occurring after a viral infection. Atypical pneumonias caused by *Mycoplasma* and, less commonly, *Legionella* must also be considered. Penicillins, macrolides and cephalosporins are the treatments of choice and none is contraindicated in pregnancy. Higher doses of amoxycillin should be used to counteract the increased renal clearance found in pregnancy. Erythromycin or clarithromycin should be added if there is suspicion of an atyp-ical pneumonia, and cephalosporins used for penicillin-allergic individuals or hospital-acquired infections. Pneumonias requiring hospitalization are usually treated with a third-generation cephalosporin (e.g. ceftriaxone) with erythromycin.

Common viral causes of pneumonia include the three subtypes of influenza myxovirus. Although amantadine and ribavirin antiviral agents have been used in pregnancy with no obvious harmful effects, their use is not recommended. The generally good outcome of viral pneumonia in pregnancy would support this.

Less common causes of pneumonia in pregnancy

More unusual pneumonias occur when there are underlying risk factors. *Klebsiella* is said to be typical of alcoholics, often associated with abscess formation. *Coxiella burnetii* is found in the aerosols produced by farm animals. Q fever, the pneumonia caused by this organism, is said to cause miscarriage, intrauterine death and stillbirth. *Staphylococcus aureus* is significantly more likely after influenza infections and may have a sudden and rapid course. Pneumonia following aspiration of stomach contents is rare, but carries a significant mortality, with anaerobic and Gram-negative organisms being the most common infectious agents.

S. pneumoniae and *Pseudomonas aeruginosa* are common causes of pneumonia in HIV-positive individuals. *Pneumocystis carinii* is an acquired immunodeficiency syndrome (AIDS)-defining illness that carries a high mortality rate, whether or not it occurs in pregnancy. The theoretical risks of using Septrin (trimethoprim-sulphamethoxazole) in pregnancy include folate antagonism, and kernicterus or haemolysis in the newborn. The latter is extremely uncommon, and folate supplementation minimizes the risks associated with the trimethoprim. Pentamidine can be used as an alternative in pregnancy. Other unusual organisms to be considered in HIV-positive women, or those with other causes of significant immunocompromise, include atypical *Mycobacteria* and *Cryptococcus*.

The true incidence of pneumonia in adult chickenpox infections is unclear, but mortality from varicella pneumonitis has been quoted as 11 per cent. Whether the depressed cell-mediated immunity of pregnancy truly influences the incidence and mortality of varicella pneumonia in pregnancy is unclear, although many reports suggest it worsens outcome, with mortality rates quoted as being as high as 1 in 3. Certainly it was the cause of death for one woman in the 1994–96 maternal death enquiry, and care was considered substandard because acyclovir was not prescribed when she first presented with the rash, despite the absence of respiratory symptoms at that time. Varicella Zoster virus infections in pregnancy are discussed further in Chapters 7.4 and 13.

KEY REFERENCES

1. Stenius-Aarniala B, Piirila and Teramo K. Asthma and pregnancy: a prospective study of 198 pregnancies. *Thorax* 1988; **43**:12–18.

2. Cydulka RK, Emerman CL, Schreiber D, Molander KH, Woodruff PG, Camargo CA. Acute asthma among pregnant women presenting to the emergency department. *Am J Resp Crit Care Med* 1999; **160**:887–92.

3. Schatz M, Zeiger RS, Hoffman CP et al. Perinatal outcomes in the pregnancies of asthmatic women: a prospective controlled analysis. *Am J Resp Crit Care Med* 1995; **151**:1170–4.

4. Czeizel AE, Rockenbauer M. Population-based case-control study of teratogenic potential of corticosteroids. *Teratology* 1997; **56**:335–40.

5. Park-Wyllie L, Mazzotta P, Pastuszak A et al. Birth defects after maternal exposure to corticosteroids: prospective cohort study and meta-analysis of epidemiological studies. *Teratology* 2000; **62**:385–92.

6. Committee on Safety of Medicines/Medicines Control Agency. *Current Problems in Pharmacovigilance* 1998; **24**:5–10.

7. British Thoracic Society. The British guidelines on asthma management. *Thorax* 1997; **52**(Suppl.):S1–21.

8. Gilljam MD, Antoniou M, Shin J, Dupuis A, Corey M, Tullis E. Pregnancy in cystic fibrosis. Fetal and maternal outcome. *Chest* 2000; **118**:85–91.

9. Edenborough FP, Stableforth DE, Webb AK, Mackenzie WE, Smith DL. Outcome of pregnancy in women with cystic fibrosis. *Thorax* 1995; **50**:170–4.

10. Edenborough FP, Mackenzie WE, Conway SP et al. The effect of pregnancy on maternal cystic fibrosis vs nulliparous severity matched controls. *Thorax* 1996; **51**(Suppl. 3):A50.

Neurological Conditions

Alec McEwan

MRCOG standards

Relevant standards

- Conduct pre-pregnancy counselling to a level expected in independent primary care.
- Conduct booking visit, including assessment of intercurrent disease.
- Diagnose and plan management with appropriate consultation in the following conditions: epilepsy in pregnancy.

In addition, we would suggest the following.

Theoretical skills

- Conduct a differential diagnosis for the causes of headache and seizures during pregnancy.
- Be able to recognize risk factors for stroke during pregnancy.
- Understand the impact pregnancy may have on the natural history of neurological conditions and, conversely, the effect of the disease and its treatments on the fetus and neonate.
- Understand the role of genetic diagnosis and prenatal counselling and testing.

Practical skills

- Be able to liaise with other healthcare professionals to optimize standards of care.
- Be able to manage, in broad terms, a pregnancy complicated by neurological disease.

The focus of this section is mostly on pre-existing medical conditions and how they interact with pregnancy. Neurological disease is fortunately rare. The details of each and every neurological condition are well beyond the bounds of this textbook, and also of the MRCOG. Candidates sitting this examination are not expected to be obstetric physicians. The aspects of neurological disease chosen for this discussion have been selected for a number of reasons.

Epilepsy and 'headache' are not uncommon problems in the antenatal clinic. Multiple sclerosis demonstrates clearly how pregnancy can alter the clinical course of a disease. The use of anticonvulsant drugs in pregnancy represents a model example of how benefits of treatment to the fetus and mother must be weighed against the risks. Myasthenia gravis illustrates how maternal conditions can continue to cause harm, even after delivery, and the 'triplet repeat diseases' highlight the need for specialized pre-pregnancy counselling and prenatal diagnostic services.

Strictly speaking, stroke need not be included here as it tends to feature more as a problem arising during pregnancy. However, in other respects it fits well with this discussion and it is important to recognize those women presenting with risk factors for stroke at booking, when the possibility of prevention exists.

EPILEPSY

Approximately 6 in every 1000 pregnancies are complicated by a past or current history of epilepsy, making it the most common pre-existing neurological condition complicating antenatal care. This chapter deals with medical conditions recognized and diagnosed prior to pregnancy. Every obstetrician must, however, have a working differential for the causes of seizure during pregnancy (Table 6.10.1). Familial, cryptogenic and trauma-related epilepsy accounts for the vast majority of cases with an established diagnosis at the onset of pregnancy. A minority of cases are caused by brain tumours, congenital abnormalities and vascular problems and these may require even more specialized care during the pregnancy. Seizure frequency may increase, decrease or stay the same in pregnancy (37 per cent, 13 per cent and 50 per cent respectively),[1] with labour being a particularly high-risk time for convulsions. A recent prospective study in the UK demonstrated no major differences in obstetric outcomes (excluding fetal abnormalities); however, an Icelandic retrospective study found a caesarean section rate almost double that of the control population.[2] A proportion

Table 6.10.1 A differential diagnosis of seizures during pregnancy and the postpartum period

Idiopathic epilepsy

Epilepsy secondary to a specific cause
   Previous trauma
   Antiphospholipid syndrome
   Intracranial mass lesions
   Gestational epilepsy (seizures secondary to pregnancy)

Intracranial infection
   Meningitis
   Encephalitis
   Brain abscess/subdural empyema
   Cerebral malaria

Vascular disease
   Cerebral infarction
   Subarachnoid and cerebral haemorrhage
   Hypertensive encephalopathy
   Eclampsia
   Cerebral vein thrombosis
   Thrombotic thrombocytopenic purpura

Metabolic
   Hyponatraemia/hypoglycaemia/hypocalcaemia
   Liver and renal failure
   Anoxia
   Alcohol withdrawal

Drug toxicity
   Local anaesthetics, e.g. lignocaine
   Tricyclic antidepressants
   Amphetamines
   Lithium

'Pseudoepilepsy' (factitious)

Table 6.10.2 Effects of anti-epileptic drugs on the fetus and newborn

Teratogenicity
   Major and minor congenital malformations
   Characteristic dysmorphic syndrome

Neonatal withdrawal effects

Vitamin K deficiency with haemorrhagic disease of the newborn

Developmental delay or behavioural difficulties

Increase in childhood malignancies

Other points are more controversial. No evidence grade is given for these points in view of this uncertainty.

- Women with a history of seizures who are not taking AEDs have a higher risk of congenital anomalies in their offspring than those with no history.
- Women with regular and severe seizure activity during pregnancy carry a higher congenital abnormality risk.
- Lower doses of AED carry a lower risk.
- The use of high-dose folic acid reduces the congenital anomaly risk.
- AED levels should be checked during each trimester as altered pharmacokinetics may disrupt seizure control.

Congenital abnormalities

The reported incidence of congenital abnormalities amongst the offspring of epileptic women varies among studies, mainly due to variations in case ascertainment and definition. Major abnormalities (which are less likely to go unreported) are found in 5–10 per cent of women who have taken AEDs [II].[2–4] The incidence of anomalies may actually be determined by a number of different factors:

- an inherent added risk associated with epilepsy, independent of AEDs,
- genetically inherited tendencies,
- the number and severity of seizures during pregnancy,
- the use of AEDs during pregnancy.

Until recently, it was generally agreed that whether treated or not, women with a history of seizures had a higher fetal anomaly rate than those without such a history. A recent prospective study from Newcastle has supported this assertion, finding *major* abnormality rates amongst treated epileptics, untreated epileptics and controls to be 4.6 per cent, 8 per cent and 2.4 per cent respectively.[3] However, equivalent figures from the USA published in 2001 have suggested differently (5.7 per cent, 0 per cent and 1.8 per cent respectively),[4] as did a study from Milan, which found severe structural anomalies in 5.3 per cent of AED-exposed pregnancies and none in the 25 pregnancies with a history of seizure but no treatment.[5] There is similar disagreement over the impact that first and second trimester seizure activity has on congenital anomaly rates. These studies found

of emergency caesarean sections were performed for seizures occurring during labour.

Therapeutic aspects

Anti-epileptic drugs (AEDs) may affect the fetus and newborn in a number of ways (Table 6.10.2).

The evidence is confusing and often contradictory. There are no randomized, controlled trials and studies are mostly retrospective with ascertainment bias. This makes patient counselling very difficult. However, a number of points are generally accepted.

- The incidence of congenital anomalies is increased significantly amongst the offspring of epileptic mothers [II].
- AEDs are responsible for most or all of this increase [II].
- The benefits of seizure control during pregnancy outweigh the risks [IV].
- Polytherapy with more than one AED carries greater risks to the fetus than monotherapy [II].
- Although certain AEDs are more strongly linked to particular congenital abnormalities, there is significant overlap, and the first-line agents can all cause the fetal anticonvulsant syndrome [II].

no evidence of increased congenital anomaly rates in the offspring of women with higher level seizure activity.

The medications themselves undoubtedly carry the greatest risk [II]. Non-epileptic women using these drugs for other reasons demonstrate similar anomaly rates.[4] The 'fetal hydantoin syndrome' described by Hanson and Smith in 1975 has been renamed the 'fetal anticonvulsant syndrome' after the realization that AEDs other than phenytoin (carbamazepine, valproate, phenobarbitone, benzodiazepines) could also cause a similar array of abnormalities (Table 6.10.3).

The incidence of this syndrome in AED-exposed pregnancies is two to three times higher than in controls [II]. Behavioural problems, learning difficulties, speech and gross motor delay and features of autism were found in more than 50 per cent of children diagnosed with this syndrome when studied retrospectively [III].[6]

Despite this generic effect seen with most anticonvulsants, certain drugs are more closely associated with particular groups of anomalies. Valproate and, to a lesser extent, carbamazepine are thought to increase the risk of neural tube defects to between 1 and 2 per cent [II]. Doses >1000 mg/day of valproate seem more likely to be associated with this outcome [III]. Valproate may likewise increase the incidence of genitourinary anomalies and, along with phenytoin, cardiac abnormalities also. Prospective studies have estimated a risk as high as 1 in 5 of developmental delay with phenytoin and carbamazepine therapy, although this is disputed.

The various studies do agree on one point: polytherapy carries greater risk than treatment with one drug alone [II].[4,5] Holmes and colleagues, for example, found the incidence of major malformations to be 5.7 per cent in the offspring of women using monotherapy but 8.6 per cent in those using two or more AEDs.[4]

The question is often asked: which anticonvulsant carries least risk of fetal harm? Women presenting already pregnant on AEDs should probably remain on their current regimen, as any teratogenic harm is likely to have occurred already. If a pregnancy is being planned, some have the opinion that valproate should be avoided, as it would appear to carry the greatest teratogenic risk and more recent reports suggest it may also cause developmental delay. Newer drugs such as lamotrigine, gabapentin and tiagabine so far have a good record in animal studies, but experience in human pregnancies is still too limited to assess their safety confidently [IV].

Table 6.10.3   The fetal anticonvulsant syndrome(s)

Major abnormalities	Minor abnormalities
Microcephaly	Hypertelorism
Cleft lip and palate	Distal digital and nail hypoplasia
Neural tube defects	Flat nasal bridge
Congenital heart defects	Low-set abnormal ears
Intrauterine growth restriction	Epicanthic folds
Developmental delay	Long philtrum

Other important drug effects

For reasons that are not entirely clear, carbamazepine, phenytoin, phenobarbitone (and even valproate) cause vitamin K deficiency, perhaps by inducing liver enzymes responsible for its oxidative degradation. Vitamin K is required for the carboxylation of factors II (prothrombin), VII, IX and X, and deficiency in the neonate may cause haemorrhagic disease of the newborn, with catastrophic intracranial and gastrointestinal bleeding occurring in a few. Owing to the extremely low levels of vitamin K in a healthy neonate, deficiency must be measured indirectly by studying 'prothrombin induced by vitamin K absence' (PIVKA) levels. Use of these anticonvulsants has been shown to increase PIVKA levels [II]. This increase can be prevented by maternal therapy with vitamin K supplements in the third trimester [II]. Indeed, some have even postulated that vitamin K deficiency may contribute to some of the structural abnormalities found in the fetal anticonvulsant syndrome, raising the possibility that vitamin K supplements earlier in pregnancy might be warranted.

Neonatal withdrawal effects have been noted with maternal use of phenobarbitone, carbamazepine and valproate, and range from poor feeding to jitteriness and convulsions. Such effects are uncommon now that phenobarbitone is used less frequently.

Phenytoin and carbamazepine *may* also cause an increase in childhood cancers such as neuroblastoma, although the rarity of these makes statistical certainty difficult [III].

Drug pharmacokinetics

A number of factors during pregnancy serve to reduce effective serum concentrations of various AEDs:

- the increased volume distribution of pregnancy,
- the increased renal clearance,
- induction of hepatic enzyme metabolism by pregnancy and high folate levels,
- vomiting and delayed malabsorption.

The reduction in serum protein concentration during pregnancy means that a greater proportion of the drug is found in the free (active) state. This is especially true for those AEDs exhibiting strong protein-binding characteristics (Table 6.10.4).

Table 6.10.4   Protein binding of anti-epileptic drugs

≤50% Protein bound	>50% Protein bound
Clonazepam	Carbamazepine
Gabapentin	Phenytoin
Valproate	Lamotrigine
	Phenobarbitone
	Vigabatrin

Serum levels of AEDs include both the free and the protein-bound components. Keeping the total level in the low 'normal' range is therefore advised during pregnancy to limit the chances of maternal toxic side effects and fetal complications [IV]. In reality, even free levels do not correlate well with seizure control [III] and some authorities disagree with routine testing of serum levels.

However, testing should be performed in a number of special cases [IV]:

- suspected non-compliance (60 per cent of pregnancies in a recent survey),
- increasing seizure activity,
- concerns over toxic side effects,
- polypharmacy with drug interactions.

The enzyme-inducing AEDs may enhance their own metabolism and that of other agents (Table 6.10.5). Valproate may inhibit the enzyme epoxide hydrolase, which metabolizes phenytoin and carbamazepine.

Managing epilepsy and pregnancy

There are no randomized, controlled trials pertinent to the management of epilepsy in pregnancy. Guidelines such as the one given below are based on evidence of grades II, III and IV.[7,8] Retrospective studies highlight how poorly such guidelines are adhered to.

Pre-pregnancy counselling

As with diabetes, there is much to be gained by planning pregnancy carefully following detailed counselling from a joint team including obstetricians and neurologists [IV].

- The diagnosis should be reviewed by a neurologist – this is dubious in a proportion of women using AEDs.
- Consideration should be given to stopping AEDs in those who have been seizure free for more than 2 years. The risk of relapse is 20–50 per cent, being higher for some forms of epilepsy (e.g. juvenile myoclonic epilepsy) than others (e.g. absence or tonic-clonic seizures) [II]. Serious health and social consequences

Table 6.10.5 Enzyme-inducing ability of anti-epileptic drugs

Enzyme-inducing AEDs	Non-enzyme-inducing AEDs
Phenobarbitone	Valproate
Phenytoin	Lamotrigine
Carbamazepine	Gabapentin
	Ethosuximide
	Clonazepam

AEDs, anti-epileptic drugs.

may result from a recurrence of seizures (e.g. driving prohibition). If withdrawal is to be attempted, it should occur in small increments over a prolonged period, supervised by a specialist. The patient should not drive during this period.

- Where possible, treatment regimens should be simplified to a single AED and the lowest effective dose used to minimize the risk of congenital abnormalities [III].
- The risks to the mother and the fetus of non-compliance with prescribed medications, especially status epilepticus, must be discussed along with the AED-associated fetal risks [IV].
- Folic acid 5 mg should be taken each day periconceptually. This is most important for women taking valproate and carbamazepine, although it is still unclear whether this reduces the risk of neural tube defects in this group [IV].
- The risk to the offspring of epilepsy should also be discussed. Few cases of epilepsy exhibit autosomal dominant inheritance. However, having one parent with idiopathic epilepsy confers a 4 per cent risk of epilepsy in the offspring, increasing to 10 per cent when a parent and a sibling are affected, and to 15 per cent when both parents have epilepsy [II].

Antenatal management

- Care should be carried out by an obstetrician with a special interest in epilepsy, jointly with a neurologist [IV].
- All pregnancies occurring in women on anticonvulsant drugs should be notified to the UK Register of Anti-epileptic Drugs in Pregnancy [IV].
- Screening for fetal anomalies should be offered to all women with epilepsy, with particular attention paid to those anomalies more commonly found in this group. A fetal cardiac scan may be warranted at 22 weeks' gestation [IV].
- Drug level monitoring may not need to be carried out as a routine but many clinicians like a 'starting' value and there are other situations that may prompt testing (see above) [III].
- Oral vitamin K supplements should be taken from 36 weeks onwards (10 mg per day) to prevent haemorrhagic disease of the newborn [II].
- If steroids are to be given for the usual obstetric indications, women using enzyme-inducing AEDs should be given 48 mg in total (two lots of 24 mg dexamethasone 24 hours apart) [IV].
- Women should be advised to take showers rather than baths. Of the nine maternal deaths from epilepsy reported in *Why Mothers Die 1997–1999*, three resulted from drowning in the bath at home.

Intrapartum care

- Induction of labour and caesarean section are indicated for the usual obstetric indications. Vaginal delivery should otherwise be the aim [IV].

- Labour carries a higher risk of seizure due to sleep disruption, reduced intake and absorption of AEDs and hyperventilation, which may alter free levels of AEDs. Every effort must be made to administer anticonvulsants as usual. Intravenous phenytoin can be used if necessary, although it may cause arrhythmias.
- Seizures during labour are best controlled with intravenous benzodiazepines (e.g. clonazepam or diazepam). Rectal diazepam can be used in the absence of intravenous access. Provided the fetal heart rate tracing remains reactive, this is not usually considered an indication for emergency caesarean section. However, status epilepticus or recurrent seizures in labour may warrant abdominal delivery for fetal reasons [IV].

Postpartum care

- The serum levels of AEDs may rise in the postpartum period and monitoring may be necessary to prevent maternal toxic side effects. However, sleep deprivation may lower the normal threshold for seizure activity. If doses have been raised during pregnancy, a reduction in the immediate postpartum period may be necessary [IV].
- All anticonvulsants reach breast milk. Neonatal side effects are rare, but sedation and withdrawal effects must be watched for, in particular where phenobarbitone and benzodiazepines have been used. Breastfeeding is to be encouraged [II].
- A single 1 mg intramuscular vitamin K neonatal supplement is advised in order to prevent haemorrhagic disease of the newborn [II].
- Contraceptive advice should be given before discharge home. The enzyme inducers will reduce the contraceptive efficacy of the combined pill, minipill and Depo-Provera injections. A combined oral contraceptive pill containing 50 μg of oestrogen should be used, preferably with a shorter pill-free interval (5–6 days instead of 7). 'Tricycling' will further reduce the chances of ovulation. Depo-Provera should be given every 10 weeks instead of every 12. The Mirena intrauterine system is ideal, as the locally administered progestogen will not be affected by induced liver enzymes [II].
- Special advice should be given to new mothers who also have epilepsy [II].
  - Ask for extra help if you are not getting enough sleep.
  - Ensure that someone else is present when you bath your baby.
  - Surround yourself with cushions and pillows when you are holding your baby.
  - Feed and change your baby on the floor whilst leaning against a wall to prevent you falling onto the baby in the event of a seizure.

Unfortunately, a recent UK prospective study[3] has shown how poorly such recommendations are being followed. Less than 50 per cent of pregnancies were planned and only 1 in 10 epileptic women took folic acid appropriately. Most did not have pre-pregnancy counselling and 1 in 5 were using AEDs despite a fit-free interval of greater than 2 years prior to the pregnancy. Sixty per cent were looked after solely by general practitioners, and vitamin K was given to only a third of those who should have received supplements in the third trimester.

MULTIPLE SCLEROSIS

Multiple sclerosis (MS) is a multifocal autoimmune disease of the central nervous system. Infiltrating lymphocytes and macrophages bring about inflammation, demyelination and axonal damage whilst further activating inherent central nervous system (CNS) immune cells such as astrocytes and microglia. Optic nerve, brain and spinal cord may all be affected and this may manifest as almost any neurological deficit, symptom or sign. Most cases are characterized by a 'relapsing and remitting' natural history, with slow gradual decline. Less commonly, the MS follows a more rapidly progressive pattern. Diagnoses of MS are either 'probable' or 'definite', depending on whether the clinical features (probable) have been supported by the results of specialized investigations (oligoclonal abnormalities in cerebrospinal fluid, white matter lesions on magnetic resonance imaging (MRI) or prolonged latency of evoked potentials on neurophysiological testing). An inheritable genetic element to the disease does exist, but very rarely is a true Mendelian pattern of autosomal dominance seen. Risks to the offspring of women with MS appear to be approximately 1 per cent [III]. Viral infection is likely to be a more important aetiological factor and indeed relapses are more common following non-specific viral illness [III].

Effect of pregnancy on MS

Various studies, both prospective and retrospective, suggest that pregnancy does not accelerate the course of MS, but relapses are more common in the puerperium. Pregnancy may have a protective effect.

The key part that the immune system plays in MS disease activity is highlighted by the effects of pregnancy on this condition. Pregnancy is characterized by a shift from type 1 (pro-inflammatory) to type 2 (anti-inflammatory) T-cell activity. Although various studies have reached slightly different conclusions, the combined evidence suggests that pregnancy itself is associated with a reduction in the number of relapses [II][9] and that this may even reduce the overall progression of the disease in the long term [III].[10] Also, the incidence of MS may be lower in multiparous women than in women who have never been pregnant [III].[10] As with rheumatoid arthritis, however, relapses in the puerperium are more common [II],[9] although this is not influenced by breastfeeding and one recent study has even reported a possible protective effect.[9] It is important to be aware of potential bias in such studies; women with more active disease are less likely to become pregnant for many reasons. However, the most recent reports have tried to avoid such bias and the above effects remain. Confavreux and colleagues[9] found a relapse rate of 0.2 per woman per year during the third trimester, compared to 0.7 in the year before pregnancy. In the first 3 months postpartum this rate increased to 1.2. The overall progression in disability scores was not altered by pregnancy over a 3-year time period. The effect of pregnancy on the course of the chronic progressive variant of MS is less clear.

Management of MS during pregnancy

Multiple sclerosis sufferers experience a wide variety of neurological symptoms and treatment should be tailored to the individual. Non-pharmacological therapy may be sufficient in some cases, but expert help should be requested from a neurologist.

Moderate to severe relapses are traditionally treated with intravenous high-dose methylprednisolone followed by a tapering course of oral steroids. This is not contraindicated in pregnancy. Urinary urgency may be treated with tricyclic antidepressants such as imipramine and this is safe to continue. Spasticity and paroxysmal pain may be treated with baclofen (probably safe in pregnancy) and anticonvulsant drugs (see epilepsy). Mood alterations are also common in MS. Depression and hopelessness are just as typical as the frequently mentioned 'euphoria'. Treatment with tricyclic antidepressants is not contraindicated in pregnancy.

Prophylaxis for MS remains an area of controversy. Although cyclophosphamide and azathioprine have been used, they are not as effective as beta-interferon (β-IFN) and glatiramer (a synthetic amino acid polymer). Currently, a funding issue in the UK is restricting access to β-IFN, a cause of much argument. None of these drugs should be continued through pregnancy for prophylactic reasons, although experience to date suggests that β-IFN is not associated with any specific obstetric complications, and the increased miscarriage risk seen in animal studies with high doses has not yet been confirmed in humans. Trials are underway to assess the role of such treatments in the post-partum period. Breastfeeding is not advised whilst using β-IFN, although harmful effects have not been noted.

Induction of labour and caesarean section are mostly reserved for obstetric indications [IV], although serious disability may make vaginal delivery impractical and an exacerbation of urinary symptoms and limb spasm may warrant earlier planned delivery. The use of epidural anaesthesia is not contraindicated and does not cause an increased rate of disease progression [II].

MYASTHENIA GRAVIS

This relatively rare neurological condition nevertheless deserves mention as it is more common in women of childbearing years and illustrates well how maternal disease can interact with pregnancy in ways not yet covered in this chapter.

Myasthenia gravis (MG) is caused by autoimmune disruption at the nicotinic neuromuscular junction. It may present with double vision, difficulty swallowing, ptosis and respiratory muscle failure. Anti-acetylcholine receptor autoantibodies can be found in 85–90 per cent of patients, and thymic abnormalities (hyperplasia or thymoma) in somewhat fewer. However, these autoantibodies can also be found in women who do not have the disease, and the diagnosis instead is usually made by administration of edrophonium chloride (a short-acting anticholinesterase), which transiently improves symptoms, notably muscle strength, in those with MG (the Tensilon test). Longer acting acetylcholinesterase inhibitors are the mainstay of treatment (neostigmine and pyridostigmine), but immunosuppressive therapy with corticosteroids, azathioprine, cyclosporin A and methotrexate is a second-line option. Plasmapharesis and intravenous immunoglobulin infusions are used for serious exacerbations. Undertreatment and overtreatment both carry their own risks. 'Myasthenic crises' can be precipitated by infection, aminoglycosides, magnesium sulphate, local anaesthetics, beta-blockers, beta-receptor agonists, narcotics and neuromuscular blockers (Table 6.10.6).

Interaction between myasthenia and pregnancy

The effect of the pregnancy on MG is unpredictable. A recent retrospective review found deterioration in 19 per cent, improvement in 22 per cent and no change in 59 per cent.[11] Myasthenic symptoms worsened postpartum in approximately a third of the women in this study [II]. The severity of the pre-pregnancy disease did not predict well

Table 6.10.6 Emergencies in myasthenia gravis

Myasthenic crisis	Cholinergic crisis
Nasal regurgitation	Abdominal 'colicky' pain
Dysphagia	Diarrhoea
Respiratory impairment	Excess salivation and sweating
	Severe weakness (depolarizing block)
	Bradycardia

what would occur during the confinement, although women who have previously undergone thymectomy have been noted in other studies to be less likely to have an exacerbation [III]. Review of further pregnancies in the same women did not show any consistency of effect between pregnancies. Owing to the change in volume distribution of pregnancy, the dose of anticholinesterase inhibitors needed to control symptoms usually increases. Increasing the dosage frequency has been found to be more effective in some cases. Persistent vomiting in the first trimester will necessitate intravenous administration of anticholinesterases. Prolonged labour (associated with delayed gastric emptying and malabsorption) may also be an indication for parenteral drug delivery.

Anticholinesterases are considered safe in pregnancy, although neonatal intestinal tube muscular hypertrophy has been reported following a pregnancy exposed to very high doses. Although there have been concerns regarding the teratogenicity and fetal effects of corticosteroids and azathioprine, their use is not contraindicated [IV] and most clinicians will continue using them through pregnancy if an indication exists. Experience with cyclosporin in pregnancy is growing, although there remains an added possible risk of intrauterine growth restriction. Methotrexate should be avoided before and during pregnancy due to its teratogenic effects. The theoretical reduction in serum hormone levels brought about by plasmapharesis has not caused preterm labour in practice. Miscarriage rates and preterm delivery rates are not significantly different from those of a control population [II].

Transplacental passage of the immunoglobulin G autoantibodies may cause two distinct fetal/neonatal problems.

1 Women with anticholinergic receptor antibodies occasionally deliver infants with arthrogryposis multiplex congenita, a serious congenital syndrome characterized by multiple joint contractures and pulmonary hypoplasia. Although the aetiology of this syndrome is diverse, severely reduced movement in utero is thought to be the basic mechanism. Animal experiments have shown that sera from these women can cause a similar range of anomalies in vivo.

2 Neonatal myasthenia gravis (NMG) is a more common manifestation of these antibodies, affecting 10–50 per cent of newborns delivered to women with MG. The onset is usually within 24 hours and most cases are mild, presenting with generalized hypotonia, poor sucking, difficulty feeding and weak cry. Less commonly, ventilation is required, sometimes for a number of weeks. The newborn is usually treated with anticholinesterases but exchange transfusions, plasma exchange and intravenous immunoglobulins have been used in more resistant cases. The correlation between maternal disease severity, or antibody titres, and the incidence and severity of NMG is not a strong one. However, sero-negative mothers may be less likely to have an affected baby, and affected babies themselves are usually seropositive.

Clearly, the pregnancy should be managed in conjunction with a neurologist. Anaesthetic and paediatric colleagues should be informed [IV]. Regular fetal surveillance is warranted and polyhydramnios should be excluded. Preterm delivery is only necessary in severe crises and a vaginal delivery should be aimed for [IV]. Problems may occur in second stage due to the skeletal muscle fatigue and there should be a low threshold for instrumental delivery. Advice should be taken before any medications are prescribed, as various drugs may precipitate a myasthenic crisis. Magnesium sulphate is contraindicated for the treatment of hypertension or eclampsia. The neonate should be carefully observed for signs of NMG and caution should be exercised with breastfeeding when high doses of anticholinesterases have been used. Drug doses may need to be reduced slowly to pre-pregnancy levels.

INTRACRANIAL VASCULAR EVENTS: 'STROKE'

'Stroke' is a generic term used to describe a cerebrovascular accident, the causes of which are many and varied. Assigning a diagnosis to 'stroke' is vital for appropriate treatment and prevention of further events.

Stroke can be further classified as shown in Table 6.10.7.

Across all age groups, hypertension, diabetes and cigarette smoking are the most common 'causes' of stroke, working through a common atherosclerotic pathway.

> Retrospective studies (Grade III evidence) consistently show that the incidence of stroke is increased during pregnancy, and that this increase is mostly confined to the postpartum period. The aetiology of pregnancy associated stroke is very different from that of stroke in general.

Various studies have estimated a stroke risk of between 5 and 10 per 100 000 deliveries, although a Canadian retrospective review gave a six-fold higher risk than this.[12] Most do not find a significant increase in strokes antenatally compared with a female population of the same age distribution, but the increase in the postpartum period is striking. A US study published in 1996 found a relative risk for stroke in pregnancy of 2.4 overall (95 per cent confidence intervals 1.6–3.6); however, when subdivided into

Table 6.10.7 Stroke classification

Ischaemic	Arterial
	Venous
Haemorrhagic	Subarachnoid
	Intracerebral

antepartum and postpartum periods, the relative risk in the first 6 weeks after delivery was found to be 9 for ischaemic stroke (infarcts) and 28 for haemorrhagic [III].[13] Evidence from other studies supports these findings.

In women under 40 years of age, infarcts are more common than haemorrhagic strokes. However, this predominance of infarcts is less marked in the pregnancy-associated group.

Causes of pregnancy-associated strokes

Below are the causes of pregnancy-associated strokes found in two recent studies.[12,13]

Infarcts
- Pre-eclampsia/eclampsia
- Primary CNS vasculopathy
- Carotid artery dissection
- Cardiac embolic events
- Coagulopathies (e.g. thrombophilias, antiphospholipid syndrome)
- Thrombotic thrombocytopenic purpura (TTP)
- Post-herpetic vasculitis

Haemorrhagic
- Pre-eclampsia/eclampsia
- Disseminated intravascular coagulation
- Arteriovenous malformations
- Ruptured aneurysms
- Cocaine abuse
- Primary CNS vasculopathy
- Sarcoid vasculitis

In a significant number of cases no underlying cause is found. The wide aetiology of stroke in pregnancy presents a diagnostic challenge. The subsequent treatment will depend very much on the diagnosis. Investigations undertaken to determine a cause may include:

- MRI/computerized tomography (CT) scanning
- cerebral angiography
- echocardiogram
- thrombophilia screen
- antiphospholipid testing.

Clearly, treatment and management of the pregnancy will depend on the diagnosis: anticoagulation, for example, may be necessary after a cerebral venous thrombosis. Haemorrhagic strokes caused by bleeding aneurysms or arteriovenous malformations (AVMs) carry a significant risk of re-bleeding if left untreated in pregnancy [III].[14] Ideally, such abnormalities would be diagnosed and treated before conception, but some will present for the first time in pregnancy. AVMs, in particular, may enlarge as pregnancy progresses, perhaps in response to hormonal changes. Outside of pregnancy they are a much less common cause of

subarachnoid haemorrhage than aneurysms. In the two studies cited above, AVM was found to be the cause of subarachnoid haemorrhage in more cases than was a bleeding aneurysm (8 vs 3) [III]. A few will present with recurrent headaches and neurological deficit, but without haemorrhage. Treatment in these cases is the same as in the prepregnant state, with surgery (excision of AVM, clipping of aneurysm) or obliteration with neuroradiological techniques. However, some consideration must be given to fetal radiation exposure. Subarachnoid haemorrhage may present with headache, vomiting, reduced consciousness, neck stiffness and focal neurology. In view of the high risk of rebleeding, most advocate early treatment rather than an initial delay. Nimodipine is used to reduce vasospasm, and hypertension must be controlled. Neurosurgery is normally tolerated well by the pregnancy, although decision-making can be complicated by reduced maternal conscious level. Vaginal delivery is encouraged if there is confidence that the source of the bleeding has been treated adequately, although this can be difficult sometimes with AVMs. A longer passive second stage is usually encouraged to reduce the need for the Valsalva manouevre, with early recourse to instrumental delivery [IV]. If the aneurysm or AVM has not been treated, or this treatment has occurred recently, an elective caesarean section is advocated, as labour is considered by many to be a high-risk time for a first bleed or a re-bleed [IV]. Of note, however, is that only one death has occurred from subarachnoid haemorrhage during labour in the last 6 years in the UK, leading some to believe that this risk has been previously overstated. Poor maternal clinical state (coma, brainstem death) is of course another indication for caesarean section. Epidurals can be used provided there is no evidence of raised intracranial pressure. Special anaesthetic techniques are used to limit the hypertensive responses found with intubation, which carry the risk of precipitating a re-bleed [IV].

Investigation and treatment of the pregnant patient with stroke obviously require significant input from neurologists and neurosurgeons. However, all those in maternity care have an important part to play in stroke prevention. For example, women with antiphospholipid syndrome and thrombophilias can be treated, once recognized, with prophylactic anticoagulation [III]. Optimal management of hypertension in pre-eclampsia and eclampsia will also help to reduce the associated stroke risk [III].

MIGRAINE AND HEADACHE

Tension headaches are more common in pregnancy, and migraines may present for the first time. Clinically they must be differentiated from much less common but far more serious causes of headache (see below). Making a diagnosis may involve special investigations and the help of a neurologist or radiologist. Treatment will depend on the cause.

A classical migraine attack in a woman with a history of migraines does not normally warrant review by a neurologist. Visual disturbance, aphasia and paraesthesia or numbness usually last no more than an hour or so and are followed by a throbbing unilateral headache with associated nausea, vomiting and photophobia. However, as many as 1 in 10 women with migraine in pregnancy have no previous history [III]. In view of the considerable symptom overlap with other diagnoses, a specialized opinion may be warranted. This applies also to women with migraine who suffer a presumed attack with atypical or prolonged neurological deficits. Hemiplegic migraine, for example, may last for many hours and should raise the possibility of an alternative diagnosis.

Causes of headache in pregnancy

- Tension headache
- Migraine
- Pre-eclampsia
- Benign intracranial hypertension
- Cerebral vein thrombosis
- Meningitis
- Subarachnoid haemorrhage (see below)
- Intracranial mass
- Inadvertent dural puncture (spinal headache)

Between 60 and 70 per cent of women with migraine will improve, or be symptom free, during pregnancy [II]. Those women who have cycle-related migraines are most likely to note an improvement. No more than 10 per cent seem to deteriorate in pregnancy. Every effort should be made to avoid precipitating factors, such as chocolate and cheese. Non-drug therapies such as relaxation techniques, sleep, massage and ice packs can be tried. Acute attacks in pregnancy are normally treated with paracetamol (rectal may be better than oral administration) and/or codeine-based drugs along with an anti-emetic such as metoclopramide. Occasional use of non-steroidal anti-inflammatory drugs is permitted, but should be avoided after 32–34 weeks [II]. Stronger opiates are sometimes needed. Ergotamine derivatives should be avoided, although studies have failed to show obvious harm. Sumatriptan, a serotonin antagonist, is in common use outside of pregnancy. Initial data collected by the manufacturers of unintended pregnancy exposures have demonstrated no clear problems, but it is still best avoided at present [IV].

Prophylaxis against migraine attacks in pregnancy is best provided by low-dose aspirin or amitriptyline (commencing with low doses such as 10 mg per day). Propranolol and atenolol have been used, with the awareness of the associated potential for intrauterine growth restriction. The safety of pizotifen and methysergide in pregnancy is still in question.

PRENATAL DIAGNOSIS OF NEUROLOGICAL DISEASES

Although most severe neurological disorders limit life expectancy, many milder problems do not, and women suffering from these conditions may wish to become pregnant, or may present at the booking clinic. Alternatively, a healthy woman with a previously affected child may come under your care. Such individuals may or may not be interested in recurrence risks in their offspring. Good quality information is needed so that an informed choice can be made. The first step is to seek out the true diagnosis. The term 'cerebral palsy', for example, does not give any indication of aetiology. Although cerebral palsy usually occurs as a result of various environmental factors, genetic factors are responsible for a few cases, raising the recurrence risk. 'Muscular dystrophy' is all too often assumed to be Duchenne's muscular dystrophy (an X-linked recessive condition); in fact, there are many different kinds of muscular dystrophy with different inheritance patterns. A careful family history is vital, but help is likely to be needed from neurologists, paediatricians and clinical geneticists.

Once the maternal diagnosis has been established, empiric recurrence risks can often be quoted. In a few cases genetic testing offers the possibility of more precise prenatal prediction. This entire process can take many weeks, and plans should be made before the woman actually becomes pregnant, if possible.

The *triplet repeat diseases* highlight best some of the complexities of prenatal testing. Huntington's chorea, myotonic dystrophy, Friedreich's ataxia and fragile X all share a similar genetic abnormality. A three base pair sequence (the 'triplet') which is repeated a variable number of times in the healthy gene becomes 'expanded', so that many more copies of the triplet are present and gene function becomes disrupted. To a degree, the disease severity may be related to the size of the expansion. Expanded sequences have a tendency to expand further, causing so-called 'anticipation', i.e. the condition becomes more severe in successive generations. Myotonic dystrophy provides the clearest example.

Myotonic dystrophy is the most common muscular dystrophy affecting pregnant women and occurs as a result of the disruption of a gene coding for a protein kinase on chromosome 19. The gene is disrupted by the expansion of a CTG triplet repeat; 5–35 CTG repeats is considered normal. More than 40 is abnormal, and mildly affected individuals will show a degree of expansion beyond this size. Severely affected individuals often have many thousands of repeats. Clinical features include muscle weakness, myotonia of hands and tongue, swallowing and speech disability, cataracts and cardiac arrhythmias, testicular atrophy and peripheral insulin resistance. Mental retardation occurs in those affected severely from a young age.

Myotonic dystrophy is an autosomal dominant condition, affected individuals having one normal and one abnormal allele. Their offspring have a 50 per cent risk of inheriting the mutated allele. Quite how severely affected the child will be is difficult to predict with any degree of accuracy. A woman with moderate to severe disease herself is likely to have a significantly expanded mutation already. If this is inherited by the fetus, further expansion is likely and the neonate will be born with severe congenital myotonic dystrophy. Such a pregnancy may be characterized by polyhydramnios and poor fetal movements. Preterm delivery is more common, and severe hypotonia and respiratory difficulties are evident at birth. Talipes and facial diplegia may be present and survival beyond the neonatal period is followed by significant developmental delay in most cases. A woman with minimal or absent disease (and therefore a shorter expansion) has a risk of approximately 1 in 10 that her child will be severely affected. However, if such a woman has delivered a severely affected newborn in a previous pregnancy, the risk of another badly affected child is higher (approximately 40–80 per cent). This reflects the greater likelihood that she has an inherently unstable mutation.

Inheritance and further expansion of the mutated allele can be detected by molecular testing carried out on placental biopsy material, although precise analysis of expansion size and prediction of outcome can still be difficult.

KEY REFERENCES

1. Tomson T, Lindbom U, Ekqvist B, Sundqvist A. Epilepsy and pregnancy: a prospective study of seizure control in relation to free and total plasma concentrations of carbamazepine and phenytoin. *Epilepsia* 1994; **35**:122–30.
2. Olafsson E, Hallgrimsson JT, Hauser WA, Ludvigsson P, Gugmundsson G. Pregnancies of women with epilepsy: a population-based study in Iceland. *Epilepsia* 1998; **39**(8):887–92.
3. Fairgrieve SD, Jackson M, Jonas P et al. Population based, prospective study of the care of women with epilepsy in pregnancy. *BMJ* 2000; **321**:674–5.
4. Holmes LB, Harvey EA, Coull BA et al. The teratogenicity of anticonvulsant drugs. *N Engl J Med* 2001; **344**(15):1132–8.
5. Canger R, Battino D, Canevini MP et al. Malformations in offspring of women with epilepsy: a prospective study. *Epilepsia* 1999; **40**(9):1231–6.
6. Moore SJ, Turnpenny P, Quinn A et al. A clinical study of 57 children with fetal anticonvulsant syndromes. *J Med Genet* 2000; **37**:489–97.
7. Brodie MJ, French J. Management of epilepsy in adolescents and adults. *Lancet* 2000; **356**:323–9.
8. *The Management of Pregnancy in Women with Epilepsy.* A Clinical Practice Guideline for Professionals Involved in Maternity Care. Aberdeen, 1997. SOGAP (Scottish Obstetric Guidelines and Audit Project).
9. Confavreux C, Hutchinson M, Marie Hours M, Cortinovis-Tourniaire P, Moreau T and the Pregnancy in Multiple Sclerosis Group. Rate of pregnancy-related relapse in multiple sclerosis. *N Engl J Med* 1998; **339**:285–91.
10. Rumarker B, Andersen O. Pregnancy is associated with a lower risk of onset and a better prognosis in multiple sclerosis. *Brain* 1995; **118**:253–61.
11. Batocchi AP, Majolini L, Evoli MD, Lino MM, Minisci MD, Tonali MD. Course and treatment of myasthenia gravis during pregnancy. *Neurology* 1999; **52**:447–52.
12. Jaigobin C, Silver FL. Stroke and pregnancy. *Stroke* 2000; **31**:2948–51.
13. Kittner SJ, Stern BJ, Feeser BR et al. Pregnancy and the risk of stroke. *N Engl J Med* 1996; **335**:768–74.
14. Stoodley MA, Macdonald RL, Weir BK. Pregnancy and intracranial aneurysms. *Neurosurg Clin North Am* 1998; **9**:549–56.

Dermatological Conditions

Alec McEwan

There are no recognized standards, but we would suggest the following.

Theoretical skills
- Be aware of the potential effects that pregnancy may have on skin disease and vice versa.
- Recognize that many skin problems carry a genetic, inheritable, element.

Practical skills
- Be able to provide women with reassurance regarding the normal physiological cutaneous changes in pregnancy.
- Provide detailed information regarding the safety of various dermatological treatments in pregnancy.
- Recognize when to involve specialist help from a dermatologist.

Although this section of the book deals with pre-existing diseases and their interaction with pregnancy, the dermatological conditions of most interest to the obstetrician are the 'dermatoses of pregnancy', i.e. the skin conditions peculiar to pregnancy. These are thus discussed alongside pre-existing conditions.

The skin may be the sole organ affected by a particular condition or it may be just one of many involved in a multi-system disease. Skin disorders occurring as part of multi-system disease (connective tissue disease, infections and malignancies) are considered in the appropriate chapters. It is worth remembering, however, that the skin manifestation of these disorders may be the initial presentation of these conditions.

PHYSIOLOGICAL SKIN CHANGES IN PREGNANCY

Physiological cutaneous skin changes during pregnancy are common and rarely cause major concern. Hyperpigmentation may occur of the nipples and areolae, axillae, linea alba (which becomes the linea nigra), face (melasma or cloasma) and pre-existing pigmented moles and freckles. Oestrogen is probably responsible for cutaneous vascular changes such as an increase in spider naevi, palmar erythema and even the occurrence of head and neck haemangiomas. Oedema is almost universal, and venous varicosities of the legs, vulva and rectum often become more prominent or appear for the first time. Striae gravidarum are pinkish purple linear markings on the lower abdomen and breast, which later fade to white and usually persist after pregnancy is over as depressed, irregular bands. Some women maintain that hair growth and condition improve in pregnancy. Postpartum alopecia, however, is a recognized phenomenon that is usually mild and transient.[1] Sebum secretion increases (see below), but apocrine activity may decline.

PRE-EXISTING CONDITIONS

Women with pre-existing skin problems are likely to present with a diagnosis already established. As with all pre-existing maternal conditions, one must consider the effect both the disease and its therapies will have on the pregnancy, the labour, the fetus and the neonate. Conversely, the pregnancy may influence the course and nature of the condition itself.

The effect of pregnancy on atopic dermatitis (atopic eczema) and psoriasis is unpredictable.[2] The former often improves in pregnancy but may deteriorate postnatally, due to physical factors such as breastfeeding, environmental agents such as detergents or even immune factors. A generalized pustular psoriasis may occur in pregnancy (see below) and is more common in women with previous psoriasis. Sebum secretion increases in pregnancy and may be responsible for the common deterioration of acne during pregnancy. Apocrine gland activity, on the other hand, declines in pregnancy, meaning that the rare conditions affecting these glands (hidradenitis suppurativa and Fox–Fordyce disease) are likely to improve. The pregnancy-associated suppression of cell-mediated immunity is thought to cause the often marked increase in human papilloma virus warty lesions (condylomata acuminata). In rare cases, these may obstruct the vagina. Only then are they an indication for caesarean section.

Impact of pre-existing skin diseases on the pregnancy itself is usually minimal in the absence of any multisystem involvement (clearly, connective tissue disorders and infections with skin involvement are quite different).

Conditions affecting the abdominal wall may interfere with abdominal delivery and delay wound healing. Vulval problems may similarly affect vaginal delivery and the healing of tears and episiotomies. A rare condition called X-linked ichthyosis is associated with steroid sulphatase deficiency and this in turn is said to delay the onset of labour, increasing the need for induction for prolonged pregnancy.

Certain skin conditions have a genetic component and the offspring may be at risk of the condition themselves. A few examples are cited in Table 6.11.1.

One of the most important factors to consider is the potential impact that dermatological drugs and therapies may have on a pregnancy.[3] A number of such treatments are confirmed teratogens and are absolutely contraindicated in pregnancy (Table 6.11.2). The retinoids are used to treat severe acne and psoriasis. Isotretinoin is especially harmful, causing central nervous system, craniofacial and cardiovascular abnormalities in as many as 50 per cent of exposed pregnancies.

Other drug treatments should only be used with careful consideration in pregnancy, including cyclosporin,

Table 6.11.1   Examples of inheritable skin disorders

Autosomal dominant
Ichthyosis hystrix and vulgaris
Palmoplantar hyperkeratosis (tylosis)
Epidermolysis bullosa simplex
Ectodermal dysplasia (some forms)
X-linked recessive
X-linked icthyosis
Hypohidrotic ectodermal dysplasia
Multifactorial
Atopic eczema (the risk of some allergic problems may reach 50% in the offspring of a couple with one affected person; the risks are higher where both parents are eczema sufferers)
Psoriasis (the children of two psoriatic parents have a risk of approximately 50% of being affected themselves)

Table 6.11.2   Dermatological treatments to be avoided during pregnancy

Acitretin and tazarotene (retinoids used in psoriasis)
Isotretinoin (retinoid used to treat severe acne)
Griseofulvin (antifungal treatment)
Methotrexate (antimetabolite used to treat psoriasis)
Podophyllin (used for genital warts)
Tetracycline (used for skin infections/acne)
Thalidomide (leprosy treatment)

hydroxyurea, penicillamine, psoralens and ultraviolet A (PUVA) and rifampicin.

A number of these medications may linger in body tissues for many months after treatment has ended. Great care must be taken that women undergoing such therapies are made aware of the vital role of reliable contraception, which may need to be continued long after the treatment has stopped. The *British National Formulary* advises the following periods of time during which conception should be avoided after the drugs have been stopped [IV]:

- acitretin – 2 years
- methotrexate – 6 months
- griseofulvin – 1 month.

It should be noted that these drugs may also carry potential harm through an effect on the male gametes. Men who have used griseofulvin, for example, are advised against fathering offspring within 6 months of treatment ending.

Emollients, dithranol, coal tar and topical corticosteroids are safe in pregnancy, as is chlorpheniramine.

DERMATOSES PRECIPITATED BY PREGNANCY

This section covers two groups of conditions:

1 skin conditions in which pregnancy is just one of a number of precipitating factors,
2 skin conditions unique to pregnancy.

Acne, erythema multiforme, erythema nodosum and generalized pustular psoriasis form the first group. Pre-existing **acne** may deteriorate during pregnancy, but may also present de novo. **Erythema multiforme** and **erythema nodosum** are both caused by a multitude of other aetiological factors, which must be excluded before it is possible to attribute the onset to pregnancy alone. **Generalized pustular psoriasis** describes a superficial sterile eruption occurring on the background of widespread erythema, which is associated with fever, systemic upset and hypocalcaemia (with tetany) in the more severe cases. It carries significant perinatal mortality and is more common in those with a history of plaque psoriasis. A clinically identical condition called **impetigo herpetiformis** was previously thought to be a pregnancy-specific dermatosis, but the two are now considered the same condition. Pregnancy appears to be one of a number of triggers for generalized pustular psoriasis.

This leaves four reasonably well-defined dermatoses found only in pregnancy (see Table 6.11.3).

A diagnosis can usually be made on clinical grounds alone; however, pemphigoid gestationis can be confused with polymorphic eruption of pregnancy if there are no vesicles present. The two conditions are easily distinguished by immunofluorescence studies of skin biopsies. Pemphigoid

Table 6.11.3 Pregnancy-specific dermatoses

Name	Incidence	Onset	Resolution	Clinical features	Histology	Immunofluorescence	Fetal effects	Recurrence	Management	Associated conditions
Polymorphic eruption of pregnancy (pruritic urticarial papules and plaques of pregnancy, toxaemic rash of pregnancy, toxic erythema of pregnancy)	1 in 250	27–40 weeks (usually late third trimester)	Usually within 2 weeks of delivery	Red urticarial papules and plaques Rarely, vesicles and target lesions Begins abdominally within striae Umbilical sparing May spread to thighs and occasionally limbs	Epidermal/dermal oedema Perivascular infiltration Patchy parakeratosis	Negative	None	Uncommon	Calamine lotion 1% hydrocortisone aqueous cream Antihistamines Systemic steroids	None
Pemphigoid gestationis (herpes gestationis)	1 in 3000–60 000	2nd/3rd trimester (occasionally postpartum)	Few weeks postpartum to 1 year	Erythematous urticarial plaques Vesicles and bullae form at the centre or periphery of plaques Often begins periumbilically Spreads to trunk and extremities	Perivascular inflammation Subepidermal blister	Positive	Possible increased risk of IUGR and preterm labour	Common	Moderate/strong topical steroids Systemic steroids Antihistamines	Graves' disease and other autoimmune conditions
Prurigo of pregnancy	1 in 300	25–30 weeks	Several months	No urticated lesions Multiple excoriated papules Abdomen and limbs	See polymorphic eruption of pregnancy	Negative	None	Recorded	Aqueous cream Topical steroids Antihistamines	Atopy
Pruritic folliculitis of pregnancy	Uncertain	2nd/3rd trimester	Within 2 weeks of delivery	Masses of itchy red follicular papules	Non-specific folliculitis	Negative	None	Uncertain	Topical 10% benzoyl peroxide Mild topical steroids Antihistamines	None

IUGR, intrauterine growth restriction.

gestationis is characterized by C3 deposition along the epidermal/dermal junction. Immunoglobulin G (IgG) deposition is usually another feature, the target protein being a 180 kDa component of hemidesmosomes. Immunofluorescence studies are negative in polymorphic eruption of pregnancy. Clinical distinction is appropriate as pemphigoid gestationis has been linked to increased rates of stillbirth, intrauterine growth restriction (IUGR) and preterm labour [III]. Although this may represent biased reporting of poor outcomes, extra surveillance would seem warranted in these pregnancies [IV].

KEY REFERENCES

1. Schiff BL, Kern AB. A study of postpartum alopecia. *Arch Dermatol* 1963; **87**:609.
2. Winton GB. Skin diseases aggravated by pregnancy. *J Am Acad Dermatol* 1989; **20**:1–13.
3. Perlman SE, Rudy SJ, Carissa P, Townsend-Akpan C. Caring for women with childbearing potential taking teratogenic dermatologic drugs. *J Reprod Med* 2001; **46**(Suppl. 2):153–61.

Drug and Alcohol Misuse

Alec McEwan

MRCOG standards

The Royal Society of Obstetricians and Gynaecologists (RCOG) has published a guideline, *Alcohol Consumption in Pregnancy* (May 2001), and this is referred to where appropriate.

In addition, we would suggest the following.

Theoretical skills
- Revise the pharmacological actions of opioids, cocaine, marijuana, amphetamines, benzodiazepines and alcohol.
- Appreciate the acute and chronic maternal effects and associations of substance abuse to optimize recognition and management during pregnancy.
- Understand the fetal/neonatal effects of in-utero exposure to these substances.
- Recognize the association between substance abuse and other health and social problems.

Practical skills
- Manage a pregnancy complicated by substance abuse.
- Liaise with social and specialist drug services to individualize care.

The incidence of substance misuse in the UK varies widely by geographical location. Three per cent of the under-35s in the UK are said to have a drug problem, although London, Glasgow, Liverpool and Manchester have traditionally been considered the 'hotspots'. However, in the year April 2000–April 2001, the Nottingham Drugs Liaison Service received over 55 referrals for substance-abusing pregnant women and over half of these actually delivered in Nottingham. Clearly the problem is increasing, and maternity services must have local guidelines and action plans in place to manage it.

There is a tendency to focus attention on the medical aspects of substance abuse in pregnancy. Although these drugs may involve actual harm to the pregnancy, the associated social and health problems are as important, if not more so. Throughout this chapter it will become clear that separating the two is very difficult, and the contributions made firstly by the drugs themselves and secondly by the socio-economic environment are almost impossible to disentangle. Separating the two is of greater theoretical than practical importance. Substance-exposed pregnancies are 'high risk', and tailored antenatal care must be provided which tackles all the problems, both social and medical.

Substances of abuse are rarely used in isolation. 'Polydrug' use is the norm, and heavy alcohol consumption and tobacco smoking compound the harm done by street drugs. The discussion below therefore does not tackle each drug independently, but aims to explore their individual contributions to each problem encountered in the pregnancy.

Many studies demonstrating harmful effects of substance abuse in pregnancy are retrospective and little or no effort is made to control for confounding factors. Clearly, there are no randomized studies. Better study design is often associated with negative results or a diminution in the harm reported. There is little doubt, however, that drug use during pregnancy *is linked* to poorer outcomes.

PHARMACOLOGY

It is valuable to revise the basic pharmacological actions of abused substances, as these actions help to explain both the short-term and long-term effects on the pregnancy outcome.

Cocaine

Cocaine is a central nervous system (CNS) stimulant. It prevents the reuptake of neurotransmitters (adrenaline, noradrenaline, dopamine) at nerve terminals, causing an exaggerated response to these chemical messengers. Increased motor activity, tremors, convulsions, tachycardia, generalized vasoconstriction, hypertension and hyperpyrexia may result. The sense of euphoria occurs as a result of dopamine accumulation within the mesolimbic system. Chronic cocaine use brings about dopamine depletion. Use of cocaine with alcohol results in a more powerful vasoconstrictor called cocaethylene.

Opiates

Opiates (heroin, methadone, morphine, buprenorphine) mimic the actions of the endogenous opioid peptides widely distributed throughout the CNS which bind to mu, delta or kappa opioid receptors. These compounds have a wide diversity of physical functions but are intimately linked with pain perception and mood control. The 'reward circuitry' of the mesolimbic dopaminergic system is influenced by endogenous and exogenous opioids and is responsible for both the pleasurable effects and psychological dependence found with opiate abuse.

Amphetamines

Amphetamines similarly enhance the dopaminergic neurotransmitter system. *Ecstasy* (3,4-methylenedioxymethamphetamine – MDMA) is a derivative of metamphetamine. It causes accumulation of synaptic serotonin and dopamine, but direct axonal damage and serotonin depletion can occur with prolonged use.

Alcohol and marijuana

Alcohol and marijuana have fundamental non-specific actions on the neural membrane, in common with the sedative–hypnotic–anaesthetic group of drugs. They differ somewhat in their actions due to differing lipid solubilities, routes of intake, metabolic pathways and different ratios of stimulant and depressant effects. Marijuana, unlike alcohol, has hallucinogenic properties.

Benzodiazepines

The actions of benzodiazepines (diazepam, temazepam) are mediated through the neuroinhibitory gamma-aminobutyric acid type A receptor (GABA-A). GABA and benzodiazepines have anxiolytic, sedative and hypnotic effects and also affect cognition. They bring about muscle relaxation and act as anticonvulsants. GABA has trophic effects and this may be important in neurodevelopment. Excessive benzodiazepine use leads to receptor down-regulation and tolerance.

MATERNAL EFFECTS

The effects of substance abuse on the mother may be acute or chronic and may be specific to the drug used or part of a general pattern of illness found amongst substance abusers. It is vital for obstetricians to have an understanding of these problems, as they may present in the antenatal clinic or as emergencies on the labour suite. Furthermore, they may be confused with complications of pregnancy.

Acute maternal effects

Drug abuse is associated with a wide range of health problems, which may present acutely to various different health-care professionals.

Overdose
Excess alcohol intake causes ataxia, confusion, stupor and eventually coma. Opiates in excess depress respiratory drive and may also cause coma. Cocaine, amphetamines and ecstasy cause tachycardia, hypertension and hyperthermia and predispose to cardiac arrhythmias, myocardial infarction, seizures and stroke. The potential for diagnostic confusion with fulminating pre-eclampsia and eclampsia is clear. Acute presentations also include aggression, paranoia and psychosis, particularly with the CNS stimulants such as amphetamines, ecstasy and cannabis.

Withdrawal
Withdrawal from the physically addictive substances may also present acutely. Alcohol withdrawal may result in blackouts, tremor, hallucinations, delirium and seizures. Opiate withdrawal is characterized by sweating, coryza and lacrimation. Pyrexia, nausea and vomiting, diarrhoea and abdominal pain, tachycardia and hypertension are also common.

Infections
Drug abuse is often associated with poor diet, poor hygiene and generalized immunosuppression. Pneumonia and tuberculosis (TB) may present acutely. Sexual disinhibition and prostitution increase the risk of sexually transmitted diseases (STDs), including human immunodeficiency virus (HIV). Intravenous substance use predisposes to endocarditis, hepatitis and septicaemia (which may be fungal). Local infections such as cellulitis and osteomyelitis are not uncommon.

Other acute presentations
Hypoglycaemia, acute or chronic hepatic failure and Wernicke's encephalopathy may result from excessive alcohol consumption. Aspiration pneumonitis, subdural haematomata and rhabdomyolysis with acute renal failure are further examples of acute complications of substance abuse. All

types of trauma, including road traffic accidents (RTAs) and grievous bodily harm, are more common amongst drug users.

Chronic maternal effects

The effects of HIV infection and chronic hepatitis (whether alcoholic or infectious) are well known. Nutritional deficiencies may cause peripheral neuropathy (vitamin B_1 and vitamin B_{12}), pellagra (niacin), cerebellar degeneration and Wernicke–Korsakoff syndrome (vitamin B_1). Poor venous access is common in intravenous substance users and this may cause difficulty during emergency situations (drug induced or otherwise). Femoral nerve neuropathy may result from frequent trauma during injection into the femoral vein. Obstructive and restrictive pulmonary lesions may occur, as can pulmonary hypertension.

OBSTETRIC PROBLEMS

Substance abuse has been associated with a number of obstetric complications, including:

- miscarriage
- preterm rupture of membranes
- preterm labour
- placenta praevia
- abruption
- pre-eclampsia
- breech presentation
- chorioamnionitis
- intrauterine growth restriction (IUGR) and intrauterine death (IUD).

Although plausible biological explanations exist for why substances of abuse might cause these problems, the exact contribution from the drugs themselves is very difficult to isolate from the confounding factors such as smoking, poor nutrition and general health, lack of antenatal care and low socio-economic status.

Miscarriage

Studies examining rates of miscarriage in substance-exposed pregnancies are often retrospective and poorly controlled. Confirmation by tissue diagnosis is often missing. Opiates, cocaine and CNS stimulants have all been implicated, but good-quality evidence is mostly lacking. Most attention has been paid to the effect of alcohol on miscarriage rates, and large quantities have been shown to have abortive properties in animal experiments. There is general agreement that alcoholics have a higher rate of miscarriage, although it is almost impossible to separate the effect of the alcohol from the

confounding effects of ill-health, poor nutrition and low socio-economic status. Alcohol consumption is closely related to smoking and caffeine use (coffee drinking), both of which have stronger causative relationships with miscarriage. North American studies have linked 'heavy drinking' (more than two drinks per day) with an increase in miscarriage rate, giving relative risk values of between 2 and 3. This association is not, on the whole, confirmed in European and Australian studies, where greater effort has been made to control for confounding factors.[1] Most agree, however, that more than six drinks a day for several days per week is associated with higher miscarriage risk [II].

There is no good evidence to suggest that the other substances discussed in this chapter cause miscarriage.

Teratogenicity

The only confirmed teratogen amongst this group of substances is alcohol. The *fetal alcohol syndrome* (FAS) describes a clearly defined group of problems caused by in-utero alcohol exposure:

- prenatal or postnatal growth restriction/microcephaly,
- nervous system dysfunction (mental retardation, intellectual impairment, ataxia, attention defects),
- characteristic facial appearance (mid-face hypoplasia, narrow palpebral fissures, underdeveloped philtrum, ptosis, rotated low-set ears).

Alcohol-related birth defects (ARBDs) is the term used to describe other alcohol-induced abnormalities which do not qualify for the 'full' diagnosis of FAS.

The relationship between alcohol consumption during early pregnancy and the incidence of FAS is not a simple one. Despite having the highest rates of worldwide alcohol consumption, France has a significantly lower rate of reported FAS than North America, where less alcohol is consumed. A number of reasons have been cited to explain this discrepancy, including a difference in drinking patterns between the two countries and a greater readiness to label newborns with the diagnosis of FAS in the USA. 'Heavy drinking' is defined as more than two drinks per day, or more than 45 per month. This group of women have an approximate incidence of FAS of 4 per cent. Alcoholics, or those drinking more than 18 units per day, carry a risk of 1 in 3 of their offspring having FAS. These figures are altered by socio-economic status, general health, smoking and possibly ethnicity, which all act as confounding factors. There is no clear threshold below which alcohol consumption is considered entirely safe; however, the incidence of ARBDs and FAS increases sharply after three units per day [II].[2] 'Binge drinking' of more than 5 units in one session may be more harmful than taking the same quantity in 'divided doses', although there is no good evidence for this at present. Clearly this practice should be discouraged during pregnancy [IV].

The relationship between benzodiazepine use in the first trimester and congenital anomalies, most notably cleft lip and palate, has been examined many times. A meta-analysis by Dolovich et al.[3] included the 23 most technically robust studies. The cohort studies could not significantly link benzodiazepine use with any fetal abnormalities. The case-control studies, however, gave a three-fold increase in risk for all major anomalies and an odds ratio of 1.79 (1.13–2.82) for oral clefting. They suggest detailed scanning for those pregnancies exposed in the first trimester.

There are good scientific reasons why ecstasy and cocaine might act as teratogens, although the better controlled studies and meta-analyses have not confirmed the effects found in laboratory animals exposed to high concentrations of these drugs in utero. Neurotransmitters can be found in the fetal brain from very early gestations, and it is likely that they are involved in neuronal migration and establishment of synaptic circuitry. It is simple to imagine how these processes could be disturbed by exposure to such drugs and bring about the microcephaly said to be characteristic of cocaine-exposed neonates.

After maturation of the muscularis layer of fetal cerebral vessels, acute vasoconstriction may lead to infarction followed by the subsequent development of cavitary lesions (e.g. porencephalic cysts). Vascular disruption secondary to cocaine use has also been postulated as a cause for the increase in gut, genitourinary and limb defects reported by some authors. Controlled studies have failed to support these findings.

A recent prospective follow-up study[4] of 136 babies exposed to ecstasy in utero has reported a significant increase in the anomaly rate (15.4 per cent); however, almost half the women used other illegal substances or alcohol and most of the abnormalities were 'minor', raising the possibility of ascertainment bias. To reach statistical significance, the background congenital anomaly rate was quoted as 2–3 per cent; in fact, if minor abnormalities are included, it may be closer to 10 per cent.

Although congenital anomalies will undoubtedly complicate a proportion of pregnancies exposed to marijuana and opiates, no consistent pattern of abnormalities has been found. Most studies show no increase in anomaly risk or are uncontrolled and retrospective.

Preterm labour and abruption

The obstetric effects of cocaine have perhaps drawn the most attention. Its vasoconstrictive properties are thought to cause abnormal implantation, hypertensive episodes and abruption. Down-regulation of beta-adrenoreceptors in the myometrium may lead to increased uterine irritability and predispose to preterm labour. Amphetamines and ecstasy may have similar effects, although there are much less data. Studies of cocaine use in pregnancy have confirmed the increased risk of preterm labour and abruption; however,

these are often lost when confounders (alcohol use and smoking) have been accounted for.[5]

Opiate withdrawal is also thought to cause uterine excitability and result in preterm rupture of membranes and preterm labour [IV]. However, smoking is more common amongst opiate abusers, and minimal antenatal care is the norm. Failure to consider the effect of these confounding factors means the effect of opiates per se is often overestimated.

The effect of prenatal alcohol exposure on the length of gestation remains unclear.

In-utero growth and development

Intrauterine growth restriction and stillbirth more commonly occur in pregnancies exposed to high alcohol levels, opiates and cocaine. The vasoconstrictive properties of cocaine and ecstasy may cause placental insufficiency and predispose to abruption, uterine irritability and preterm labour. The high metabolic demands of a fetus alternately exposed to opiate 'highs' and withdrawals might also be responsible for IUGR and even stillbirth [IV].

Fetal growth restriction is one of the three defining criteria for FAS. Although there are many reasons why growth might be restricted in pregnancies exposed to high levels of alcohol, it is generally held that alcohol per se has a growth-retarding action. The RCOG guideline on alcohol consumption in pregnancy gives the following recommendation:

Consumption of 15 units or more per week has been associated with a reduction in birthweight.

The actual decrement in birth weight is affected by many factors but, on average, this level of drinking is seen to be associated with a 66 g deficit per 15 units consumed per week.[6]

Although low birth weight is a consistent finding in opiate-exposed pregnancies, a *causative* link between opiate use and IUGR has been difficult to prove due to the action of the following confounding factors:

- 'polydrug' use
- tobacco smoking and alcohol consumption
- chaotic and reduced attendance for antenatal care
- high rates of HIV and other STDs
- low socio-economic status
- poor nutrition.

Substituting methadone for heroin has a beneficial effect on prenatal growth, but this may have more to do with increased levels of antenatal care than the action of the heroin itself (see below).

The vasoconstrictive properties of cocaine suggest it should cause prenatal growth restriction. The Maternal Lifestyles Study (MLS)[7] demonstrated a 450 g reduction in birth weight in cocaine-exposed pregnancies even after the effects of alcohol and tobacco were controlled for [II]. This growth limitation is thought to occur mostly in the third trimester.

NEONATAL EFFECTS

In the newborn period, substance-exposed infants are more likely to suffer low Apgar scores, infectious complications and CNS disturbance, and *opiates* may also cause neonatal respiratory depression. Prematurity, low birth weight and IUGR contribute as much to the neonatal problems as do the short-term actions of the drugs themselves.

Finnegan was the first to describe the **neonatal abstinence syndrome** (NAS). This results from the acute withdrawal of transplacental opioid which occurs at the delivery of a baby born to an opiate–abusing mother. The onset of the syndrome is normally within 24 hours of birth if the opiate used was short acting (e.g. heroin). It consists of:

- irritability, hypertonicity, tremor, exaggerated startle response and occasionally seizures,
- sweating and sneezing,
- abnormal sleep behaviour, high-pitched cry, poor feeding with weak suck and uncoordinated swallowing.

Methadone maintenance does not prevent NAS, but may delay its presentation until the second day of life due to its longer half-life.

Alcohol, *cocaine* and *amphetamines* have a less marked effect on neonatal behaviour, if any effect at all. Rare events such as neonatal hypertension, arrhythmias and necrotizing enterocolitis are said to be more common in the offspring of cocaine users, although the confounding effects of prematurity are difficult to separate. Abnormal electroencephalogram (EEG) and brainstem auditory-evoked responses have been demonstrated in these neonates, and the use of neonatal behavioural assessment scales has shown dampened arousal, poor orientation and reduced state control.

Amphetamine-exposed newborns occasionally demonstrate hyperactivity, poor feeding and disrupted sleep patterns. The neonatal effects of *marijuana* are debated. Greater irritability, tremors and startle responses have been reported, but a well-controlled Jamaican study[8] has suggested that once again the postnatal environment is more important than drug exposure per se. In fact, neonatal scores were found to be higher in the offspring of heavy marijuana users. In rural Jamaican society, these women tend to be wealthier and more highly educated. *Benzodiazepines* may cause neonatal respiratory depression, reduced tone and poor feeding.

CHILD DEVELOPMENT

Tests of child development are complex and beyond the scope of this chapter. They examine many aspects of behaviour, including language and motor skills, attention and play, cognition and problem-solving and arousal and affective expression. They themselves are open to interpretation and

bias. The Brazleton Neonatal Behavioural Assessment Scale (NBAS) and Bayley Scales of Infant Development (BSID) are examples.

Mothers willing to participate in longitudinal studies may be more highly motivated, and superior parenting skills in cooperative families may make the effects of the substance abuse appear less significant. Children, as they grow up, may find that society's low expectations of their substance-abusing mothers are reflected onto themselves.

Alcohol

Impaired development of the CNS is a key criterion of FAS. Although children with FAS have an average IQ of less than 70, the consequences of alcohol consumption that does not result in the full syndrome are less clear. The RCOG guideline gives the recommendation that:

> *Consumption of 20 units or more per week has been associated with intellectual impairment in children.*

The RCOG consider it a good practice to advise women to drink no more than 1 unit of alcohol per day whilst pregnant.

Opiates

Opiate use in pregnancy is indeed associated with poor developmental outcomes for the offspring; however, it seems that confounding factors are most likely to be responsible, rather than the drug itself. BSID scores have been found to be lower at 1 and 2 years of age by some researchers. However, a clear harmful effect of opioids themselves on child development is not strongly suggested by the literature.

Cocaine

Head circumference is inversely related to cocaine exposure during pregnancy. Along with the reported association with serious fetal/neonatal intracranial pathology, it is unsurprisng that cocaine itself is thought to be directly damaging to neurodevelopment, with or without confounding social factors. Indeed, neurophysiological testing of such children suggests reduced numbers of oligodendrocytes and impaired myelination.

Closer examination of the data on neurodevelopmental outcome has challenged this view, and the two sides of the debate are difficult to reconcile. The meta-analysis performed by Frank and colleagues[9] selected 36 prospective and blinded studies in which polydrug use was uncommon. After controlling for confounding factors, there was no significant overall association between prenatal cocaine exposure and cognition, language and motor skills, behaviour, attention, affect or neurophysiology, up to 6 years of age [II].

This controversy is likely to continue. For practical purposes, cocaine use in pregnancy should be considered a marker of 'high risk'. Independent of any direct actions of the drug, pregnancy and neurodevelopmental outcomes are nevertheless poor and will only improve with better access to healthcare and social support. A judgemental and punitive approach to pregnant cocaine users will not achieve this aim.

SCREENING FOR SUBSTANCE ABUSE IN PREGNANCY

Pregnant women who use drugs may avoid antenatal care for fear of inciting closer scrutiny of their lifestyles, which may often include other criminal activities. They may fear that their child, or children, will be removed from them. Because of this, they may present needing help only at the time of a social, domestic or medical crisis. All those caring for pregnant women should be vigilant for substance abuse and take the opportunity to institute specialized antenatal care whenever presentation occurs. Enquiry about illicit substance use should be routinely made of all pregnant women in a matter-of-fact way. Be prepared to ask more than once. Covert urine testing may confirm substance abuse, but be careful when disclosing this information source, as it may be seen as underhand and untrustworthy and may damage the fragile relationship between the woman and the healthcare services.

Screening for heavy alcohol consumption can be quickly carried out in all pregnant women using the T-ACE questionnaire, as suggested in the RCOG guideline. Only four questions are asked:

T (for Tolerance): *how many drinks does it take to make you feel high*? More than two suggests a degree of tolerance and scores 2 points.
A (for Annoyance): *has anyone annoyed you by criticising your drinking*? Answering 'yes' scores 1 point.
C (for Cutting down): *have you ever thought you needed to cut down your drinking*? Answering 'yes' scores 1 point.
E (for 'Eye opener'): *have you ever had a drink first thing in the morning to steady your nerves or to get rid of a hangover*? Answering yes scores 1 point.

A score of 2 or more points is considered a positive screen and carries a 70 per cent sensitivity for detection of heavy drinkers. Further questioning and assessment are needed of those who screen positive.

MANAGEMENT OF PREGNANCY COMPLICATED BY SUBSTANCE ABUSE

A multidisciplinary team approach is necessary to create a confidential, reassuring and non-judgemental environment in which the pregnancy outcome and childbirth experience can be optimized. This team will include social workers, specialist drug services, drug-liaison midwives, general practitioners (GPs), obstetricians and paediatricians.

'Harm minimization' recognizes the futility of simply telling users to stop using. It aims initially to promote a change in the nature of the drug taking, to stabilize lifestyles and reduce criminal behaviour. Stopping drug abuse altogether is a much longer term aim. Exchanging needles or moving to non-intravenous modes of delivery would be examples of harm reduction. Reducing alcohol and tobacco consumption and establishing methadone maintenance are particularly important aims in pregnancy.

Antenatal care

Significant improvements in pregnancy outcome are achieved by regular antenatal care, which should be tailored to the individual. Points to consider include:

- carefully targetted history taking,
- counselling about the possible effects of the drug abuse on the pregnancy,
- possible urine testing for illicit substances,
- discussion and delineation of achievable aims to reduce harm,
- ultrasound scanning to accurately date the pregnancy,
- screening for hepatitis B and C, HIV and possibly bacterial vaginosis,
- detailed anomaly scanning,
- serial growth scanning and fetal assessments as necessary,
- reflection on the need for a child protection case conference,
- communication with anaesthetic and paediatric services: cocaine and opiate abusers may pose particular problems for obstetric anaesthetists, and admission to a special care baby unit (SCBU) is very likely, even if only for observation.

Focused history taking from the pregnant drug abuser

- Type of drug(s) used, when, how often, how much and mode of administration.
- Does her partner use drugs?
- Has the woman particular fears or concerns of her own?
- Are there specific psychological or health problems leading to, or a consequence of, the drug abuse?
- What are the social/financial circumstances?
- Is she in any legal trouble?
- Does she drink alcohol or smoke tobacco?
- Does she practise safe sex?
- Does she share needles?

Women using street narcotics should be offered **methadone maintenance treatment** (MMT). Methadone has a longer half-life than heroin and blood levels remain more stable. Users are provided with a regular supply, which offers the opportunity to remove themselves from the criminal high-risk behaviours often necessary to fund a street habit and which carry such risk to the pregnancy. Having to attend regularly allows close antenatal surveillance and healthcare. The fetus avoids opiate 'highs' and withdrawals and other possible harmful contaminants of street drugs. Compliance with these regimens can reduce neonatal mortality and increase birth weight, although the benefits are lost if MMT is supplemented with street 'top-ups', which many abusers need for the 'highs' not provided by methadone. Negotiating the dose with the user is a difficult task. Low doses (<60 mg/day) are associated with higher rates of non-compliance. Twice-daily dosing regimens may minimize the trough levels and reduce relapses.

Using methadone during pregnancy (as opposed to no opiates at all) is associated with an approximate doubling of neonatal mortality. Use of both methadone *and* heroin carries a six-fold increase in neonatal mortality risk.

Women established on MMT may consider gradual withdrawal (e.g. a reduction in dose of 2–2.5 mg every 7–10 days). Anecdotal evidence recommends that this should occur in the second trimester, as leaving it until later risks preterm labour [IV]. The greater risk of withdrawal during pregnancy is a subsequent relapse of illegal narcotic use. This is considered to carry the greatest risk of fetal harm, and withdrawal during pregnancy should only be attempted in highly motivated women with a stable, supportive and drug-free environment to which they can return.

Unfortunately, there is no such 'replacement' regimen for cocaine users. Harm reduction must involve a reduction in cocaine use. Without an incentive, it may be very difficult to gain the trust and co-operation of pregnant users who fear reprisals for their substance abuse (especially in the USA).

Intrapartum care

Labour may be the first time a pregnant substance abuser presents to medical services. It should be managed as normal, with a few additional points to bear in mind.

- Recommend continuous cardiotocography (CTG) monitoring in view of the increased risk of placental insufficiency and fetal compromise.
- Be aware that opiates may influence the CTG and interpretation may be more difficult.

- Avoid, as far as possible, fetal blood sampling, scalp electrodes and episiotomies to reduce the vertical transmission risk of hepatitis and HIV.
- Elective caesarean section before membrane rupture reduces HIV vertical transmission and possibly that of hepatitis C[10] (although this needs confirmation).
- Give normal maintenance doses of methadone to prevent withdrawal. These will not provide analgesia, which should be offered in addition. Epidural analgesia may prove most effective if opioid receptors are already saturated by the illegal opiate.
- Those women who have undergone supervised withdrawal from opiates during the pregnancy should avoid systemic opiates in labour. Nitrous oxide and epidural analgesia are preferable.
- Naloxone should not be given to opiate-dependent mothers or their offspring – severe withdrawal effects may occur.
- In cocaine users, ephedrine may be less effective at reversing hypotension secondary to regional analgesia. Phenylephrine is a useful alternative.

Postnatal care

Above all, the new mother should be supported in her first few days, as any new parent should be. Indeed, she is likely to have minimal help when she leaves hospital. Ongoing assistance from the specialist midwife is vital.

- If the baby seems well it should be transferred to the postnatal ward with the mother. NAS usually presents in the first 2 days and the baby must be closely observed for signs of this. Methadone withdrawal may take a little longer, but will usually have begun by 4 days (the minimum time period that women are advised to stay in hospital). If the infant is demonstrating withdrawal symptoms, it will need special care facilities.
- Breastfeeding is encouraged in most women, even those on methadone. Infant weaning should occur gradually; fortunately the quantities of opiates reaching breast milk are small. HIV-positive women, those using large amounts of benzodiazepines and cocaine users are exceptions to this general rule. These women should be advised to bottle-feed. Hepatitis C is not a contra-indication to breastfeeding.[10]
- Babies born to hepatitis-B-positive mothers should be immunized.
- Drug misuse by a parent does not necessarily equate with child neglect or abuse, and automatic child abuse registration will only discourage women from seeking antenatal care. Social services should be informed of the delivery and decisions made about the levels of support needed to ensure child safety.
- Appropriate contraceptive advice must be provided before discharge.

KEY POINTS

- Regardless of the direct harm caused by drug abuse during pregnancy, much of which is still debated, such behaviour is a powerful marker of poor obstetric outcome and should prompt close antenatal surveillance by specialized healthcare workers.
- Alcohol is the only clear teratogen, although benzodiazepines may predispose to oral clefting.
- The effects of these substances on short-term and long-term child development are still in question. Potent cellular actions and devastating complications such as intracerebral haemorrhage are well recognized, but have a less striking impact on the results of larger population studies.
- The aim of antenatal care should be to minimize harm by setting realistic goals.
- All units should have a dedicated team with defined guidelines to optimize outcomes for mother and baby.

KEY REFERENCES

1. Abel EL. Maternal alcohol consumption and spontaneous abortion. *Alcohol* 1997; 32:211–19.
2. Allebeck P, Olsen J. Alcohol and fetal damage. *Alcoholism: Clinical & Experimental Research* 1998; 22:329S–325 (Suppl. 7).
3. Dolovich LR, Addis A, Vaillancourt JM, Power JD, Koren G, Einarson TR. Benzodiazepine use in pregnancy and major malformations or oral cleft: meta-analysis of cohort and case-control studies. *BMJ* 1998; 317:839–43.
4. McElhatton PR, Bateman DN, Evans C, Pughe KR, Thomas SHL. Congenital anomalies after prenatal ecstasy exposure. *Lancet* 1999; 354:1441–2.
5. Sprauve ME, Lindsay MK, Herbert S, Graves W. Adverse perinatal outcome in parturients who use crack cocaine. *Obstet Gynecol* 1997; 89:674–8.
6. Florey C duV, Taylor D, Bolumar F, Kaminski M, Olsen J. EUROMAC – A European concerted action: maternal alcohol consumption and its relation to the outcome of pregnancy and child development at 18 months. *Int J Epidemiol* 1992; 21 (Suppl. 1):S38–9.
7. Bada HS, Verter J, Bauer CR et al. Maternal Lifestyle Study (MLS): Intrauterine growth of infants exposed to cocaine/opiates in utero. *Paediatr Res* 1996; 39:256.
8. Dreher MC, Nugent K, Hudgins R. Prenatal marijuana exposure and neonatal outcomes in Jamaica: an ethnographic study. *Pediatrics* 1994; 93:254–60.
9. Frank DA, Augustyn M, Knight WG, Pell T, Zuckerman B. Growth, development and behaviour in early childhood following prenatal cocaine exposure. A systematic review. *J Am Med Assoc* 2001; 285:1613–26.
10. Gibb DM, Goodall RL, Dunn DT et al. Mother-to-child transmission of hepatitis C virus: evidence for preventable peripartum transmission. *Lancet* 2000; 356:904–7.

Smoking

Andrew Shennan

INTRODUCTION

Smoking-related morbidity and mortality affect millions of individuals throughout the world. Each year, almost a quarter of all deaths of men can be attributed to a smoking-related cause and although far fewer female deaths are related to smoking, the gap is rapidly closing. More women are becoming smokers in industrialized countries. The cause of this morbidity and mortality is largely related to the effects on cardiovascular disease, although smoking is also a cause of cancer, particularly of the lung.

In the Western world, almost a quarter of young women smoke and this affects their risks of developing gynaecological cancers such as cancer of the cervix. Other risks, such as that of thromboembolic disease, are increased. Effects on the menopause and miscarriage as well as low birth weight have been reported. However, in spite of educational programmes to point out these obvious detrimental effects to fetal well-being, it has proved very difficult to introduce preventative strategies. Smoking remains a major preventable cause of low birth weight, preterm delivery and perinatal mortality; this section reviews the relationship between smoking and pregnancy outcome, and discusses management strategies to reduce adverse events.

INCIDENCE IN PREGNANCY

In the developed world, approximately 20–30 per cent of pregnant women report smoking; the figure of 27 per cent in the UK has been stable for some years. As with the non-pregnant population, there is a strong association with socio-economic background, so that those from lower groups have considerably higher smoking rates. Generally, actual smoking rates are about 3 per cent higher than reported rates, as evidenced by cotinine levels.[1]

It has been reported that women who continue to smoke, in spite of knowledge of the detrimental effects, are more likely to have problems at work and, in general, are less well supported on a psychosocial basis. Women without partners and who already have children are less likely to stop.

AETIOLOGY AND CLINICAL EFFECTS

Prematurity

There is good epidemiological evidence that smoking is related to the risk of premature delivery, including early preterm birth. There is also an established relationship with perinatal death [II]. The association is strong and often dose related, which therefore adds considerable evidence that the effect is causative and not related to other associated factors [II].

Women who smoke have approximately double the risk of premature delivery. This is principally due to spontaneous preterm delivery, but it also can increase the risk of the need for iatrogenic delivery through association with placental abruption and placenta praevia [II]. Smoking is also a risk factor for preterm premature rupture of the fetal membranes.[2]

Lower mean birth weight has been associated with a high mean systolic blood pressure in later life in the children of mothers who smoke. Smoking may therefore be contributing to the possible in-utero programming effects with which reduced fetal growth potential is now thought to be associated.

Intrauterine growth restriction

It is established that low birth weight for gestation is more common in women who smoke.[3] On average, babies will be approximately 200 g lighter as a result of smoking. There is a dose relationship to this effect and it is established that women who smoke more than ten cigarettes a day will have lower birth weight than those who smoke less than this number, the effects being greater in male fetuses [II]. Even passive smoking can reduce birth weight.[4]

Intelligent quotient

Cognitive performance is reduced in the children of the mothers who smoke during pregnancy, even after adjustment for other confounding variables.[5] Longer term effects on the children may include influence on respiratory illness over and above that which may be caused by the children living in a family where smoking continues [II].

Smoking and pre-eclampsia

There are many studies that demonstrate an association between a reduced risk of pre-eclampsia and smoking [II].[6] However, it is clear that any possible benefit in this reduction is completely superseded by the harmful effects of smoking [III]. Indeed, women who do show the clinical signs of pre-eclampsia have much more severe disease. In these women, there are increased rates of perinatal mortality, abruption and intrauterine growth restriction.

Infertility, ectopics and miscarriage

There is now evidence that both ovarian function and implantation may be affected by smoking, thus reducing the fertility of these women. There is also an increased incidence of ectopic pregnancy that is apparent from recent meta-analyses. The risk of miscarriage is also increased.

MANAGEMENT: SMOKING CESSATION IN PREGNANCY

A minority of women will stop smoking when they become pregnant. These individuals frequently smoke less and have better support from home, including a partner who gives up or is a non-smoker. Programmes that encourage smoking cessation have been associated with some improved outcome, in terms of less low birth weight and premature delivery [II]. However, these programmes are highly intensive before they are successful, and standard advice from midwives and other clinicians to stop smoking has had little impact on overall quitting rates during pregnancy [II]. Approximately 7 per cent of pregnant women who undergo focused counselling will give up smoking. However, a small number of individuals do stop on brief advice and, as this is inexpensive, it is worthwhile [IV].

Specialist staff are known to be more effective than others, with more than a doubling of cessation rates [Ib].[7] Unfortunately, few women are willing, or have the opportunity, to use these counselling services. Self-help material has some benefit in approximately 4 per cent of smokers. The effectiveness and safety of nicotine replacement therapy in pregnancy have yet to be established.

There is, however, good evidence that stopping smoking will reduce the adverse effects of smoking in pregnancy, and result in an improvement in birth weight [Ib].[8]

Specialist staff trained in counselling women about smoking are more likely to succeed in cessation programmes.

KEY POINTS

- A quarter of pregnant women in the developed world smoke in pregnancy.
- Smoking in pregnancy is associated with prematurity, low birth weight and perinatal death and is the single most preventable cause of these adverse events.
- Smoking in pregnancy is known to increase the risk of sudden infant death syndrome.
- Most adverse events are dose related and reversed if pregnant women stop smoking.
- The children of mothers who smoke have lower intelligence quotients.

KEY REFERENCES

1. Tapen DM, Forward RP, Wilde CJ. Smoking at the end of pregnancy measured by cord blood cotinine assay. *NZ Med J* 1995; **108**:108–9.
2. Harger JH, Hsing AW, Tuomala RE et al. Risk factors for preterm premature rupture of fetal membranes; a multi-center case control study. *Am J Obstet Gynecol* 1990; **163**:130–7.

3. Kramer MS. Determinants of low birthweight: methodological assessment and meta analysis. *Bull WHO* 1987; **65**:663–737.

4. Rubin DH, Krasilnikoff PA, Leventhal JM, Weile B, Berget A. Effect of passive smoking on low birthweight. *Lancet* 1986; ii:415–17.

5. Sexton M, Fox NL, Hebel JR. Prenatal exposure to tobacco: II Effects on cognitive functioning at age three. *Int J Epidemiol* 1990; **19**:72–7.

6. Cnattingiuss S, Mills JL, Yuen J et al. The paradoxical effect of smoking in pre-eclamptic pregnancies. Smoking reduces the incidence with increases of rates of perinatal mortality, abruptio placentae and intra-uterine growth. *Am J Obstet Gynecol* 1997; **177**:156–61.

7. West R. Helping patients in hospital to quit smoking. Dedicated counselling services are effective – others are not. *BMJ* 2002; **324**:64.

8. Sexton M, Hebel JR. A clinical trial of change in maternal smoking and its effect on birthweight. *J Am Med Assoc* 1984; **251**:911–15.

Anaemia

Tracey A. Johnston

MRCOG standards

Relevant standard
- Be able to detect and manage anaemia antenatally.

In addition, we would suggest the following.

Theoretical skills
- Revise the physiological changes of the blood in pregnancy.
- Know the maternal and fetal effects of anaemia.
- Understand the causes of anaemia in pregnancy.

Practical skills
- Be able to detect and manage antenatally.

INTRODUCTION

Anaemia is the commonest medical disorder of pregnancy. Pre-existing bone marrow disorders and inherited haemoglobin (Hb) variants are discussed in Chapter 6.5. This chapter aims to revise the physiological changes in pregnancy, and discusses the maternal and fetal risks of anaemia, diagnosis and management.

PHYSIOLOGICAL CHANGES

- Plasma volume increases by 50 per cent.
- Red cell mass increases by up to 25 per cent.
- There is a consequent fall in Hb concentration, haematocrit and red cell count because of haemodilution.
- Mean cell volume (MCV) increases secondary to erythropoiesis.
- Mean cell Hb concentration (MCHC) remains stable.
- Serum iron and ferritin concentrations decrease secondary to increased utilization.
- Total iron-binding capacity increases.

- Iron requirements increase (due to expanding red cell mass and fetal requirements) from 2.5 mg/day in the first trimester to 6.6 mg/day in the third trimester (700 1400 mg total pregnancy).
- There is a moderate increase in iron absorption.
- Folate requirements increase in pregnancy (due to the fetus, placenta, uterus and expanded maternal red cell mass).
- There is no major effect on B_{12} stores, although levels decrease (preferential active transport to the fetus).

DEFINITION

A pathological condition in which the oxygen-carrying capacity of red blood cells is insufficient to meet the body's needs.

Often the diagnosis is based on blood values, in particular Hb concentration. The World Health Organization (WHO) recommends that the Hb concentration should not fall below 11 g/dL at any time during pregnancy,[1] but many clinicians use the figure of 10.5 g/dL as recommended by the Centers for Disease Control of North America.[2]

INCIDENCE

Around 30–50 per cent of women become anaemic during pregnancy, with iron deficiency being responsible in more than 90 per cent of cases. The incidence of folate deficiency is around 5 per cent (though it is often underdiagnosed) and this is almost always the cause of megaloblastic anaemia in pregnancy, with vitamin B_{12} deficiency being rare.

CLINICAL FEATURES

Anaemia is very often asymptomatic in pregnancy, with the diagnosis being made on routine screening. Clinical features include tiredness, dizziness, fainting and lethargy. Pallor may be apparent.

SCREENING

Anaemia is routinely screened for in pregnancy by estimating the Hb concentration by means of a full blood count at the beginning of pregnancy and again later in pregnancy, often at the start of the third trimester, and again at term. This lacks specificity but has the advantage of being cheap and simple to perform. The presence of a low Hb does not reveal the cause of the anaemia.

IRON DEFICIENCY ANAEMIA

Aetiology

Iron deficiency anaemia is classically described as a microcytic, hypochromic anaemia because of the reduced MCV and MCHC. This is the commonest cause of anaemia in pregnancy, but the diagnosis should still be confirmed. There are significant iron demands during pregnancy, secondary to expanding red cell mass and fetal requirements, which can only be met by a limited increase in iron absorption, and by utilization of iron stores. If iron stores are already depleted because of menstruation, recurrent pregnancies and poor intake, anaemia will develop rapidly. During pregnancy, the total iron-binding capacity (TIBC) increases secondary to the increased plasma volume, and serum iron falls. As iron demands exceed supply during pregnancy, ferritin levels fall. Decreased Hb concentration is a late event in iron deficiency anaemia.

Consequences

The evidence regarding the consequences of iron deficiency anaemia in pregnancy is conflicting. From the maternal perspective, as well as the clinical features described above, it has been suggested that impaired function of iron-dependent enzymes causes alterations in muscle function, neurotransmitter activity and epithelial changes throughout the body.[3] This has been used as the basis for the explanation for the apparent link between iron deficiency anaemia and preterm delivery, infection, medical intervention during labour and postpartum blood loss. It is clear that women with significant anaemia at the time of delivery will not tolerate blood loss as well, and are more likely to receive blood transfusion postnatally. From the fetal perspective, it is widely accepted that there is an increased risk of preterm delivery and intrauterine growth restriction. However, many of the studies have not controlled for other factors, such as smoking, that

may be important.[4] There is also conflicting evidence regarding the neonatal iron status and cognitive development and behaviour of babies born to iron-deficient mothers.[5]

Diagnosis

Iron deficiency can be present in the absence of anaemia, and other parameters of the full blood count that usually give a clue to this (reduced MCV, MCH (mean cell haemoglobin) and MCHC) are not as accurate during pregnancy (Table 7.1.1).

The diagnostic test for iron deficiency is a ferritin concentration. This is not affected by pregnancy, and a concentration of $<12\,\mu g/L$ is diagnostic. This could be used as a screening test as iron deficiency is so common in pregnancy, but requires an extra blood test (although many laboratories now have the facilities to estimate the ferritin concentration from the full blood count sample) and adds cost.

Treatment

Oral iron

The treatment for iron deficiency is oral iron replacement [Ib], which is usually effective if there is enough time (maximum increase in Hb = 0.8 g/dL per week). The recommended dose is 120–240 mg of elemental iron per day. Ferrous salts are absorbed better than ferric salts [Ib] and should be used in preference. There is little to choose between the different ferrous salts in terms of absorption and efficacy, and side effects are related to the amount of elemental iron contained. The choice of preparation should therefore be dictated by cost and patient tolerance, but it should be noted that a reduction in side effects is usually secondary to a reduction in the amount of elemental iron absorbed. Vitamin C taken simultaneously aids absorption [Ib], hence the common advice to take iron with fresh orange juice. There is, however, little to gain, other than increased cost, by using combination preparations with ascorbic acid included.

There is a 40 per cent risk of side effects with oral iron preparations, mainly gastrointestinal, and this can have a direct effect on tolerance and compliance. Slow-release preparations are often associated with a decrease in the incidence of side effects, but this is mainly secondary to decreased

Table 7.1.1 Haematological values

	Non-pregnant	Pregnant	Iron deficiency
Hb (g/dL)	12–15	11–15	<10.5
MCV (fL)	75–99	More	Less
TIBC (mmol/L)	45–72	Increases	Decreases by <15%
Se Fe (mmol/L)	13–27	13–27	<12
Fe (mg/L)	15–300	15–300	<12

Hb, haemoglobin; MCV, mean cell volume; TIBC, total iron-binding capacity; Se Fe, serum ferritin; Fe, ferritin.

absorption of elemental iron, as most is not released from the preparation until it has passed through the first part of the duodenum, where iron absorption is optimal. For those with proven iron deficiency that cannot be managed with oral therapy because of lack of compliance, severe gastro-intestinal side effects, continuing significant blood loss or malabsorption, parenteral preparations exist.

Intramuscular Iron

Iron sorbitol injection has a low molecular weight and thus allows rapid absorption from the injection site, although high levels may be excreted before utilization. It is not suitable for intravenous use. It is administered by deep intramuscular injection and can be associated with pain at the time of injection and tattooing of the skin. The dose is calculated depending on the degree of iron deficiency and patient weight, but requires repeated injections, usually over the course of 2 weeks.

Intravenous iron

There are various intravenous iron preparations that are now available with significantly fewer side effects compared to iron dextran, which has now been withdrawn from use because of the high incidence of anaphylaxis. These newer preparations have all been used successfully in pregnancy in selected cases, and are associated with a greater and more rapid rise in Hb concentration with fewer side effects when compared with oral preparations.[6] This form of therapy can require daily trips to hospital for several days, as well as an intravenous cannula, and is thus more disruptive and invasive than oral therapy, but is a realistic alternative to blood transfusion when oral therapy has failed.

A new preparation of iron sucrose (Cosmofer™) is now licensed for total dose iron replacement in the second and third trimesters. It is given as a single infusion and takes 4–6 hours to complete.

Blood transfusion

Towards the end of pregnancy there may not be the time available to increase the Hb with iron therapy, and blood transfusion may be indicated as well as iron therapy. It should be borne in mind that blood transfusion is not without risk,[7] and effective screening programmes should detect anaemia early enough to allow iron therapy to be utilized. However, transfusion is the most rapid way to increase Hb concentration, but is a relatively slow way to increase iron stores.

Erythropoietin

Recombinant human erythropoietin is mainly used for the anaemia associated with erythropoietin deficiency in chronic renal failure, but can also be used to increase the autologous production of blood in normal individuals. It has been used in cases of severe postpartum anaemia with success, and has been life saving in cases where blood transfusion is declined, for example Jehovah's Witnesses. It has also been used during pregnancy in a small number of renal patients with no adverse maternal or perinatal complications.[8]

Prevention/prophylaxis

Prevention of iron deficiency is usually possible with a good balanced diet in the absence of ongoing blood loss, and identification and treatment of iron deficiency prior to pregnancy are optimal. However, many women enter pregnancy already iron deficient, or become so during pregnancy. Health education by the midwife regarding diet is therefore important.[9]

There has been much work done on the role of routine iron supplementation in pregnancy, and this has been the subject of a Cochrane Review.[10] This meta-analysis of 24 trials concluded that there is clear evidence of improvement in haematological indices in those women who receive iron supplements during pregnancy, but no conclusions could be drawn regarding either harmful or beneficial effects for the mother or baby. The reviewers felt that there was no evidence to advise against a policy of routine iron supplementation in pregnancy, and that such a policy could be warranted in high-prevalence areas [Ia].

Oral iron therapy with ferrous salts is the treatment of choice for iron deficiency anaemia in pregnancy [Ib].

- Vitamin C aids absorption but there is no evidence to support the use of combined preparations [Ib].
- There is no evidence to advise against a policy of routine iron supplementation in pregnancy [Ia].

FOLATE DEFICIENCY

Aetiology

There is a significant increase in folate requirements during pregnancy because of the increased cell replication that is taking place in the fetus, uterus and bone marrow (increase in red cell mass). Plasma folate concentrations decrease throughout pregnancy, reaching half the non-pregnant levels by term. The incidence of folate deficiency is higher in multiple pregnancies. Folate deficiency causes a megaloblastic anaemia, the incidence of which in pregnancy is around 5 per cent, although higher rates are found in other parts of the world and are thought to be secondary to poor diet. In the UK, many foods now have folate supplements added, making the recommended daily intake of 800 μg easier to achieve.

Consequences

There are clear links between periconceptual folate deficiency and neural tube defects,[11] as well as a suggested association with other anomalies,[12] hence the advice that all women planning a pregnancy should take 400 µg/day of folic acid and continue this for the first 12 weeks of pregnancy until the neural tube is closed [Ib]. From the maternal perspective, the consequences of folate deficiency are not just anaemia, but involvement of tissues with high rates of cell turnover, in particular mucous membranes; the effects of folate deficiency can thus be exacerbated by malabsorption if the gut mucosa is affected.

Diagnosis

Outside pregnancy, the macrocytosis of folate deficiency anaemia is diagnosed by an increased MCV. However, during pregnancy the MCV is increased, but the macrocytosis may be masked by co-existing iron deficiency leading to a reduced MCV. Red cell indices are therefore not particularly useful for diagnosis. Examining the blood film may be useful, but in pregnancy the diagnosis often entails examination of a bone marrow aspirate.

Treatment

Severe folate deficiency is extremely rare, but once megaloblastic haematopoiesis is established, treatment is difficult secondary to poor folate absorption from the affected gastrointestinal tract. In this uncommon situation, 5 mg oral pteroylglutamic acid daily or parenteral folate can be used.

Prevention/prophylaxis

The case for routine prophylaxis with 400 µg/day for the prevention of neural tube defects has already been discussed above. However, there are other situations in which folate prophylaxis is indicated. These include women taking anticonvulsant drugs [IV] and those with haemolytic anaemias (see Chapter 8). In these situations the recommended prophylactic dose is 5 mg/day throughout pregnancy.

VITAMIN B$_{12}$ DEFICIENCY

Vitamin B$_{12}$ deficiency is rare during the reproductive years, and is associated with infertility; therefore, vitamin B$_{12}$ deficiency during pregnancy is very uncommon. Absorption is unchanged by pregnancy, and vitamin B$_{12}$ is actively transported across the placenta to the fetus.

Chronic tropical sprue can give rise to megaloblastic anaemia in pregnancy secondary to both vitamin B$_{12}$ and folate deficiencies.

Management

In cases of known B$_{12}$ deficiency, treatment should be optimized prior to conception (and may be necessary to allow

conception). Women on B$_{12}$ replacement therapy should continue this as normal. Virtually all diets that contain animal products will supply enough B$_{12}$ during pregnancy, although strict vegans may become deficient.

KEY POINTS

- Anaemia is the commonest medical disorder of pregnancy, with significant implications for both mother and child.
- Although iron deficiency is the major cause of anaemia in pregnancy, this diagnosis should be established to allow optimal treatment.
- Screening for anaemia in pregnancy is simple, as is treatment of iron deficiency anaemia.
- There is no evidence to support routine iron prophylaxis in the absence of other risk factors.
- The role of periconceptual folate supplementation should be emphasized at pre-conceptual counselling.

FURTHER READING

Why Mothers Die 1997–1999. Confidential Enquiry into Maternal Deaths in the United Kingdom. Chapter 4, Hall MH. Haemorrhage. London: RCOG Press, 2001.

KEY REFERENCES

1. World Health Organization. *Nutritional Anaemias.* Technical Report Series. Geneva: WHO, 1972.
2. Centers for Disease Control. Current Trends: CDC criteria for anaemia in children and child bearing-aged women. *Morb Mortal Wkly Rep* 1989; **38**:400–4.
3. Finch CA, Cook JD. Iron deficiency. *Am J Clin Nutr* 1984; **39**:471–7.
4. Scholl TO, Hediger ML. Anemia and iron deficiency anemia: compilation of data on pregnancy outcome. *Am J Clin Nutr* 1994; **59**(Suppl.):492S–501S.
5. Walter T. Effect of iron-deficiency anaemia on cognitive skills in infancy and childhood. *Baillière's Clin Haematol* 1994; **7**:815–27.
6. Al-Momen AK, Al-Meshari A, Al-Nuaim L et al. Intravenous iron sucrose complex in the treatment of iron deficiency anemia during pregnancy. *Eur J Obstet Gynecol Reprod Biol* 1996; **69**:121–4.
7. *SHOT Annual Report 2000/2001.* London: Serious Hazards of Transfusion Steering Group, 2002.
8. Breymann C, Major A, Richter C et al. Recombinant human erythropoietin and parenteral iron in the

treatment of pregnancy anemia: a pilot study. *J Perinat Med* 1995; **23**:89–98.

9. Watson F. Routine iron supplementation – is it necessary? *Modern Midwife* 1997; **7**(7):22–6.

10. Mahomed K. Iron supplementation in pregnancy. In: *The Cochrane Library*, Issue 3, Oxford: Software Update, 1999, 1–9.

11. Wald NJ. Folic acid and neural tube defects: the current evidence and implications for prevention. In: *Neural Tube Defects* (CIBA Foundation Symposium). Chichester: Wiley, 1994, 192–211.

12. Elwood JM. Can vitamins prevent neural tube defects? *Can Med Assoc J* 1983; **129**:1088–92.

Abdominal Pain

Justin C. Konje

INTRODUCTION

Abdominal pain is a common complaint in pregnancy. The management of this symptom is a challenge to the clinician, who needs to understand the pathologies that may result in pain and the features that will aid in the diagnosis. The causes of abdominal pain in pregnancy vary from those due to the pregnancy, those related to pregnancy but not directly due to it, and those unrelated to pregnancy (Figure 7.2.1). The physiological changes occurring in pregnancy alter the presentation of many conditions, especially those due to extrauterine causes.

The incidences of the different causes of abdominal pain in pregnancy are difficult to estimate. This is because classifying this symptom into 'pregnancy' and 'non-pregnancy' causes is often not possible until after delivery. The investigations that may be performed outside pregnancy are difficult to justify in pregnancy, not least because of the associated complications. For example, a diagnostic laparoscopy is not advisable, especially after the first trimester, because of possible complications.

An effective approach to the management of abdominal pain in pregnancy must include the following:

- an understanding of the physiology of pain
- the nature of pain
- the treatment of pain.

In this chapter, the basic physiology of pain is discussed, followed by the causes of pain, investigations and treatment. As the causes of pain are so varied, each condition is discussed separately, rather than providing a generic description of the management of this symptom.

PHYSIOLOGY

Pain is produced in different tissues and it is a protective mechanism for the body. It occurs whenever any tissues are being damaged, and it causes the individual to react to remove the pain stimulus. Three types of stimuli excite pain receptors: mechanical, thermal and chemical. It has been suggested that pain is chemically mediated and that the stimuli that provoke it have in common the ability to liberate a chemical agent that stimulates nerve endings. This chemical agent might be a kinin or histamine, both of which cause pain on local injection.

The two types of nerve fibres transmitting pain impulses to the central nervous system reflect the two types of pain

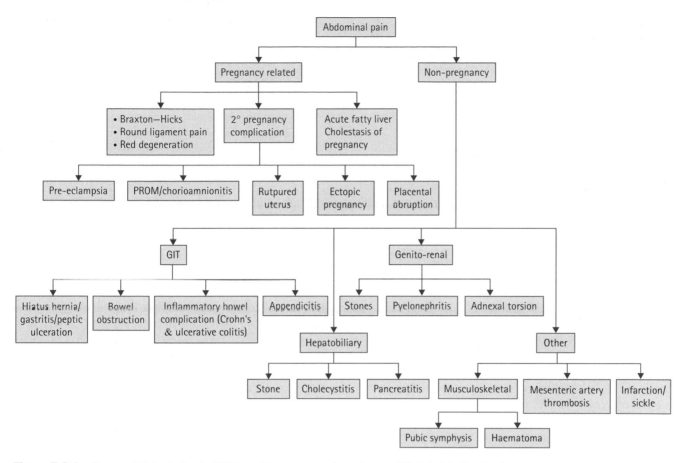

Figure 7.2.1 Causes of abdominal pain. PROM, pre-labour rupture of membranes; GIT, gastrointestinal tract

pathway – fast and slow pathways. Fast pain is typically sharp, pricking, acute, electric, bright and localized, whereas slow pain is dull, intense, chronic, throbbing, nauseous, diffuse and unpleasant. Fast pain is felt when a needle is stuck into the skin, when the skin is cut with a knife or when the skin is burned, while slow pain is associated with tissue destruction.

Deep and superficial pain

Deep pain is poorly localized, nauseating and frequently associated with sweating and changes in blood pressure. Superficial pain, on the other hand, is well circumscribed, tends to be sharp and is not associated with nausea and blood pressure changes.

Muscle pain

Muscle pain results from muscle contraction, which is accompanied by occlusion of blood supply to the muscle. In the absence of this occlusion, there is no pain. Such pain

tends to persist after the contraction until the blood flow has been re-established. The mechanism of the pain is through the release of a chemical agent that causes pain when its local concentration is high enough. Following re-establishment of blood flow, this is washed out or metabolized.

Visceral pain

Visceral pain tends to be deep pain; hence it is poorly localized, unpleasant and associated with nausea and autonomic symptoms. It is not uncommon for this pain to radiate or be referred to other sites, which can make establishing a diagnosis difficult. The reason for the poor localization of this type of pain is the low concentration of pain receptors in the viscera. This type of pain can be very severe; receptors, which may be located on the hollow walls of the viscera, are particularly sensitive to the distension of these organs.

Referred pain

Referred pain is perceived at some considerable distance from the site of initial provocation. Pain is usually referred to a somatic structure, even though it may originate from a viscus. While deep somatic pain may be referred, superficial pain is not. In cases where visceral pain spreads and is localized, it may be perceived as spreading from the original site to the referred site. Adequate knowledge of the common sites of pain referral from each of the viscera is important, as such knowledge will be essential in diagnosing the origin and therefore the likely cause of pain. The most well known example is of the left shoulder tip pain following irritation of the diaphragm. Usually the dermatomal rule applies to referred pain. This states that referred pain is usually to a structure that developed from the same embryonic segment or dermatome as the structure in which the pain originates.

CAUSES/SOURCES OF ABDOMINAL PAIN IN PREGNANCY

The reproductive organs

Round ligament pain

This pain is secondary to stretching of the round ligaments as the uterus enlarges and becomes an abdominal rather than a pelvic organ. It therefore occurs commonly in the late first and early second trimesters of pregnancy. The pain, which may occur in up to 10–30 per cent of pregnancies, is characterized by a dragging, stabbing or cramp-like sensation located in the outer lower abdomen and radiating to the groin. The diagnosis is usually made after excluding other causes of lower abdominal pain. It is more common in multigravidas. The mainstay of treatment is reassurance [IV]; an explanation of the pathophysiology of the pain is often sufficient. Encouragement to reduce physical activity and avoid overstraining should be provided. Local heat application with a hot water bottle to the affected side may be soothing enough to alleviate the pain. Occasionally, ultrasound heat therapy may offer the only means of relief. Where there is a need for additional analgesia, simple analgesics such as paracetamol are adequate. Occasionally, the pain may be so severe as to require opiates and admission to hospital; in this scenario, it is mandatory to exclude other causes of pain.

Braxton–Hicks contractions

During pregnancy, spontaneous uterine contractions occur. These are initially painless and very infrequent, but they become more frequent as pregnancy advances. In the early half of pregnancy, these contractions are easily visualized during ultrasound scanning, when they may be confused with fibroids or the placenta. Most women experience these contractions as vague backache, which is minimally uncomfortable but does not require any form of analgesia. In some women, however, this may be perceived as very severe pain requiring hospital admission or assessment. Primiparas are more likely to present with this type of pain. Simple reassurance is adequate for the management of this type of pain.

However, because of the cyclical nature of the pain, preterm labour and its precipitants, for example urinary tract infection, must be excluded.

Uterine fibroids

Uterine fibroids are benign tumours of the uterus and occur in approximately 20 per cent of women in the reproductive years. They are more common in older women. These fibroids contain oestrogen receptors, and the high circulating levels of oestrogen in pregnancy stimulate their growth. Lev-Toaff et al.[1] demonstrated that smaller fibroids (defined as those <6 cm) increased in size in the second trimester, whereas larger fibroids decreased in size. In the third trimester, a decrease in size was documented regardless of initial size.

The blood supply to the fibroids is mainly from myometrial vessels entering through the false capsule. Whilst most fibroids are asymptomatic, as they enlarge in pregnancy, the central areas can suffer from relative ischaemia and therefore present with pain. This complication is referred to as red degeneration. The cut surface of the fibroid, which has undergone red degeneration, is usually freshly red, suggesting that the ischaemia is of the haemorrhagic type. The pain is typically constant and localized to one side of the uterus, although it may sometimes be diffused. Tenderness is usually confined to the site of the fibroid.

Where the patient is known to have fibroids, the diagnosis is easy. Women with red degeneration may have a low-grade pyrexia and leucocytosis – both of which tend to be absent in placental abruption.

Although ultrasound may be useful in making a diagnosis, the absence of fibroids on ultrasound scan does not exclude the diagnosis. This is because, during pregnancy, not only can fibroids grow larger, but they can become softer and thus more difficult to differentiate from normal myometrium. A diagnosis is therefore commonly made by exclusion. Where the fibroid is pedunculated, torsion may occur. This will present in a similar way to torsion of the ovary (see below).

The treatment for pain secondary to red degeneration is in the form of potent analgesics and reassurance [IV]. Most women are satisfied with a logical explanation, but for those who require treatment, medication should start with simple analgesics and only progress to the opiates if there is no significant improvement in the pain.

Ruptured uterus

This complication is unlikely to occur silently during pregnancy. It can, however, occur in women with previous classical casearean sections – usually from the early third trimester. Other cases occur in labour, especially in women who have had casearean sections or perforated uteri during a termination of pregnancy. The use of misoprostol and cervagem (gemeprost) to terminate pregnancies in the first and second trimesters has been associated with reported cases of ruptured uterus. In those cases in which there are risk factors, the index of suspicion needs to be high.

Rupture of the gravid uterus typically presents with acute abdominal pain. This may be associated with shock, shoulder tip pain or vaginal bleeding. In labour, there may be a severe and persistent bradycardia. The diagnosis is made based on the associated clinical features of maternal tachycardia, hypotension and severe abdominal tenderness. The fetal parts may also be easy to palpate. Once the diagnosis is made, resuscitation should be initiated, blood cross-matched and a laparatomy performed. The definitive treatment will depend on the type of rupture, the ease with which a repair can be effected and the risk of rupture in subsequent pregnancies [III].

Placental abruption

This is a complication that is more likely in the second half of pregnancy. It may present with abdominal pain alone or pain and vaginal bleeding (see Chapter 23). It complicates 0.5–1 per cent of all pregnancies. In those cases in which there is no overt bleeding, the diagnosis may be difficult in mild cases. A high index of suspicion is therefore essential. In these patients, the only symptom may be mild abdominal pain, which may be constant or intermittent, often mimicking labour pains. This cause of pain must be considered as a differential diagnosis in cases in which there is no obvious diagnosis. Since this complication is associated with intrauterine growth restriction and intrauterine fetal death, a diagnosis needs to be followed by close fetal surveillance [III].

Premature labour and chorioamnionitis

These complications may exist together. Premature rupture of fetal membranes may predispose to ascending chorioamnionitis, although the latter can occur with intact membranes. The patient presents with abdominal pain, which may be intermittent or constant. There may be an associated vaginal discharge, abdominal tenderness and maternal and fetal tachycardia. The diagnosis may be difficult, but a high index of suspicion is required, as failure to treat may result in intrauterine fetal death and/or significant pelvic septicaemia that may necessitate a hysterectomy. The treatment consists of a broad-spectrum antibiotic and expedition of delivery.

Premature labour typically presents before 37 completed weeks of gestation. The diagnosis is not difficult; however, when it occurs, the exact cause must be identified and treated as this may arrest the preterm labour. The cause, diagnosis and management of this complication are discussed in Chapter 22.

Ectopic pregnancy

The incidence of this complication is 1:100 in the UK and higher in countries where pelvic infections are common. The clinical presentation is with amenorrhoea and abdominal pain. The pain may be referred to the tip of the shoulder and may also be associated with vaginal bleeding. The diagnosis is confirmed by laparoscopy or a combination of serum beta-human chorionic gonadotrophin (β-hCG) and transvaginal ultrasound. However, ultrasound does not exclude the diagnosis. A high index of suspicion is required if the diagnosis is to be made correctly.

Adnexal accidents

These include haemorrhage, rupture of a cyst or torsion of an ovarian cyst or fibroid.

Corpus luteum cysts are common in early pregnancy and most are asymptomatic. Occasionally, there is bleeding into the cyst and women may present with constant abdominal pain, with the severity of the pain rising to a crescendo and then remaining stable before gradually diminishing in intensity. If the cyst ruptures, the pain may be excruciating and the woman may present in shock. For a large cyst, the diagnosis may be suspected on bimanual examination, but in most cases it is made on ultrasound scan. Where the cyst has not ruptured and the symptoms are not getting worse, conservative management is the preferred option. Where the cyst is large and there are features suggestive of abnormal pathology, it must be removed – usually after the 14th week of gestation [III]. For rupture in early pregnancy, the differential diagnosis of an ectopic pregnancy will make conservative management difficult.

Torsion may be of a pre-existing ovarian cyst (such as a dermoid, cystadenomas, malignancies etc.) or a corpus luteum cyst. The classical history is of intermittent abdominal pain, which later becomes constant. By the time the pain becomes constant, the torsion must be at least twice on its stalk, thus causing ischaemia to the ovary. The pain may be associated with systemic symptoms such as nausea, vomiting and prostration, and there may be low-grade pyrexia. By the time this stage is reached, the ovary is unlikely to be viable. A full blood count will demonstrate a leucocytosis. If ignored, the ovary will gradually become gangrenous. Ultrasound may help in identifying the cyst, but intervention must not be delayed on account of lack of ultrasound scanning facilities. The treatment is laparotomy and a cystectomy and/or fixing of the ovary if viable, or oophorectomy if not viable (see Chapter 7.3).

Torsion of pedunculated fibroids may occur independently of red degeneration. The clinical symptomatology is similar to that of a torted ovarian cyst. The pedunculated fibroid needs to be removed at laparotomy but it is inadvisable to

Causes of abdominal pain from the reproductive organs in pregnancy

- Round ligament pain
- Braxton–Hicks contractions
- Uterine fibroids
- Ruptured uterus
- Placental abruption
- Chorioamnionitis/premature labour
- Ectopic pregnancy
- Adnexal accidents/torsion of fibroids

Antenatal complications: maternal

attempt a myomectomy on other fibroids that are subserous or intramural, as this may result in a hysterectomy.

GASTROINTESTINAL TRACT

Reflux oesophagitis (heartburn)

Reflux oesophagitis is a common cause of upper abdominal pain in pregnancy, with an estimated incidence of 60–70 per cent. It is more common in late pregnancy and in women with multiple pregnancies, polyhydramnios or fetal macrosomia. During pregnancy there is relaxation of the lower oesophageal sphincter, induced by hormones, especially progesterone. In addition, as the uterus enlarges, it pushes the distal oesophagus upwards and distorts the sphincteric mechanism, which prevents reflux into the oesophagus. As a consequence, epigastric pain and discomfort are not uncommon. The delayed emptying of the stomach, which becomes progressively greater with gestation, contributes to the frequency of this complication.

The pain is described as a warm or burning sensation felt in the upper epigastrium and behind the sternum. The pain is made worse by lying flat, bending or straining; it is not unusual for it to be accompanied by flatulence. The diagnosis is easy, provided the history is typical, although the differential diagnosis includes cholecystitis and hiatus hernia. The treatment includes simple preventative measures such as avoiding lying flat, antacids and frequent meals. If the condition is complicated by severe vomiting, an endoscopic assessment may be necessary to exclude other causes. The pathology is usually self-limiting and gradually resolves soon after delivery.

Hiatus hernia

Hiatus hernia presents with symptoms similar to heartburn. It is thought to occur in 7–22 per cent of pregnancies. Radiological examinations have demonstrated that this complication is present in about 62 per cent of cases of severe heartburn in the third trimester. Fortunately, most herniae are small and regress soon after delivery. Very severe cases present with severe vomiting and haematemesis.

The treatment is similar to that of reflux oesophagitis; however, anti-emetics may be used in cases of severe vomiting. Surgery is very rarely indicated.

Peptic ulceration

Peptic ulceration is uncommon in pregnancy, and in most cases there is a pre-existing history. The symptoms are similar to those outside pregnancy, and tend to improve in pregnancy as gastric acid secretion is reduced. Sufferers commonly complain of epigastric/upper right hypochondrial pain, which is made worse by hunger or spicy hot foods. The diagnosis may be difficult if it is occurring for the first time in pregnancy. The treatment consists of antacids, most of which are safe in pregnancy (see Chapter 8). Although rare, complications such as haematemesis and perforation have been described, especially soon after delivery. The patient presents with an acute onset of abdominal pain and peritonitis and is often collapsed. The diagnosis may be challenging; however, a plain abdominal X-ray will demonstrate the presence of gas under the diaphragm. The role of vagotomy and pyloroplasty in the treatment of peptic ulcerations is now very limited, even outside pregnancy, and it is very unlikely to be performed in pregnancy [III].

Gastritis

Gastritis is a very poorly defined cause of abdominal pain in pregnancy. Again, because of reduced acid production, the incidence tends to fall in the first and second trimesters. The presentation is similar to that of reflex oesophagitis. Pain tends to be located in the central epigastrium and is aggravated by spicy foods or hunger. The treatment consists of antacids and avoidance of aggravating factors. Most patients are advised to avoid lying flat. Any antacid will provide some relief for these women.

Cholelithiasis and cholecystitis

During pregnancy, there is biliary stasis and delayed emptying, and these, combined with raised cholesterol levels, predispose women to cholelithiasis. The incidence of this complication is not very well ascertained, purely because of difficulties in making the diagnosis. However, an incidence of about 3.5 per cent was reported in one study of 338 women.[2] Most women are asymptomatic; the small proportion who are symptomatic present with a sudden onset of abdominal pain, nausea and vomiting and in some cases may suffer from intermittent vaso-vagal attacks. The pain tends to be colicky and radiates to the back in the right hypochondrion. The pain may be exacerbated by eating. The only clinical signs may be tenderness and a positive Murphy's sign; these may be difficult to elicit in a gravid abdomen, especially in late pregnancy. The diagnosis is often made on ultrasound scan, which will demonstrate an enlarged gallbladder and stones in the bile duct.

In most cases, the treatment is conservative; however, surgery may sometimes be indicated. Open surgery was previously the treatment of choice, but there is increasing evidence that stones can be dealt with laparoscopically. However, this becomes increasingly difficult with advancing gestation. The main complications of surgery in pregnancy are preterm labour and cholangitis, which may result in septicaemia. In a review of 15 cases of laparoscopic cholecystectomy performed in our unit over a 7-year period, there was one severe complication. The patient, whose surgery was performed at 26 weeks' gestation, developed a Gram-negative septicaemia, adult respiratory distress syndrome and intrauterine fetal death. She had a laparotomy and was ventilated for 1 week.

Acute cholecystitis is uncommon in pregnancy. It presents with acute-onset right hypochondrial pain, nausea, vomiting and pyrexia. The pyrexia helps distinguish this from cholelithiasis, although an ultrasound scan of the gallbladder will usually demonstrate the presence of stones. This complication has been reported to complicate about 1:1000 pregnancies. Like gallstones, it is more common in obese and older women. The treatment consists of antibiotics (intravenous amoxycillin or ceftazidime) and potent analgesics [III]. The analgesia must not stimulate the sphincter of Oddi, and pethidine is the preferred opiate. The differential diagnoses of these conditions include cholestasis of pregnancy, hepatitis and HELLP syndrome. Acute cholecystitis, like any inflammatory condition, may predispose to preterm labour.

Constipation

Constipation may present as severe or chronic abdominal pain. The physiological changes of pregnancy often result in a slowing of bowel peristalsis, and lead to this complication. The presentation is widely varied. The most common is a dull, constant and sometimes colicky pain in the iliac fossae (the left more than the right). Very occasionally, patients may present with associated nausea and vomiting, but this is not typically projectile, as in cases of mechanical bowel obstruction. The treatment includes simple attention to diet (increasing fruit and fibre) and, in severe cases, laxatives (e.g. lactulose) and suppositories (e.g. glycerine). In the treatment of this complaint, it must be remembered that any medication that will result in a significant increase in bowel activity may induce preterm labour.

Bowel obstruction

Bowel obstructions are a rare cause of abdominal pain, and occur in 1:2500 to 1:3500 pregnancies – an increasing incidence being attributable to an increase in abdomino-pelvic surgery in young women. The aetiology includes adhesions (~60 per cent),[3] bands across bowels and, rarely, strangulation of herniae (inguinal or femoral), volvulus, intussusception, Crohn's disease and tumours. Patients with ileostomies have been demonstrated to be at a greater risk of obstruction during pregnancy.

Typically, cases present in the second trimester, when the uterus becomes an abdominal organ, or in the puerperium. Symptoms include acute-onset colicky pain, nausea, vomiting and constipation. Abdominal distension as a symptom may easily be missed in pregnancy, but the presence of hyperactive bowel sounds should make the diagnosis easy. An abdominal X-ray my be necessary to establish the diagnosis, and will demonstrate distended loops of bowel with fluid levels defining the level of the obstruction.

The management in most cases is conservative – withholding feeding, intravenous correction of any fluid and electrolyte imbalances, and antispasmodics such as hyoscine butylbromide (Buscopan). Nasogastric suction may be necessary. With conservative management, most cases of obstruction will be relieved after a few hours; if the symptoms persist or there is deterioration in the clinical condition, a laparotomy should be performed. There are some who advocate laparoscopic exploration of the abdomen and division of adhesions (the laparoscope is introduced by an open method rather than after a pneumoperitoneum). However, this may be technically difficult in the third trimester. Failure to relieve this complication may result in perforation and peritonitis, which may precipitate preterm labour and be associated with high perinatal morbidity and mortality. Similarly, surgery may precipitate preterm labour, and the decision to perform surgery must only be made after careful consideration.

Acute appendicitis

This cause of abdominal pain complicates between 1:1500 and 1:2500 pregnancies, and the incidence approximates to that outside pregnancy.[4] The symptoms and signs of appendicitis may be atypical. The pain may be located in the right lumbar region in early gestation or even in the right hypochondrium in late gestation. This is due to displacement of the caecum and therefore the appendix by the gravid uterus.

In early pregnancy, the pain starts in the central abdomen (para-umbilical region) and then settles in the right iliac fossa. Although it is typically accompanied by systemic symptoms such as anorexia, nausea, vomiting and fever, these symptoms may be absent in late pregnancy. Because of the widely varied presentation, the diagnosis must always be suspected in a pregnant woman presenting with abdominal pain and leucocytosis. There is a physiological leucocytosis in pregnancy, and serial measurements provide a better assessment of this important laboratory finding. Often the only signs are pyrexia, tenderness over the right abdomen and guarding. An inflamed appendix may induce reflex uterine contractions, which will make the diagnosis even more difficult.

The differential diagnoses depend on the location of the pain. These include a torted ovarian cyst, pyelonephritis, a degenerating fibroid, acute cholecystitis, uretric calculi or obstruction, bowel obstruction, preterm labour and placental abruption. The complications of appendicitis in pregnancy include rupture, peritonitis, preterm rupture of fetal membranes and preterm labour. It has been suggested that the displacement of the abdominal organ in pregnancy prevents the walling-off of the inflamed appendix, therefore making it more likely to rupture and cause peritonitis. The mortality from appendicitis in pregnancy varies; although figures as high as 2 per cent have been reported, more recent series quote lower figures. Perforations are associated with maternal and fetal mortalities of 17 per cent and 43 per cent respectively.

The treatment of choice is appendicectomy. The type of incision will depend on the gestation and the location of the appendix. In the first trimester, an appendicectomy may be performed laparoscopically or through a classical McBurney incision [IV]. However, a paramedian incision over the area of maximum tenderness may allow the best access and the option of extension should the need arise. Preterm labour is a recognized complication of surgery, and adequate precaution must be taken to minimize this complication and its consequences. A casearean section should not be performed at the same time as the appendicectomy, even if the fetus is mature [IV]. This is primarily because of the danger of endometritis and a significantly higher morbidity. In most cases, with adequate antibiotic cover, spontaneous vaginal delivery can be achieved.

Pancreatitis

Pancreatitis is uncommon in pregnancy, with an incidence of about 1:5000 pregnancies, but is more common in pregnant than non-pregnant women of similar age. The higher risk of gallstones in pregnancy is thought to be responsible for this higher incidence. In a small study of 20 patients with pancreatitis, McKay et al.[5] found gallstones in 18 cases. Apart from gallstones, high lipids and high alcohol consumption are associated risk factors.

Typical presentation is with central or upper abdominal pain, which may radiate to the back. Associated systemic symptoms include nausea, vomiting and shock. A few patients may present with jaundice, but this is uncommon unless there is accompanying obstruction within the biliary system. Where vomiting has been persistent, there may be dehydration and features of electrolyte imbalance. The diagnosis is confirmed by a raised serum amylase. However, it is important to remember that serum amylase levels may be mildly raised in normal pregnancy. Where there is haemorrhagic pancreatitis with massive necrosis or if the blood sample is taken 24–72 hours after the attack, false-negative results may be obtained. Ultrasonography of the gallbladder should be performed in all patients with suspected pancreatitis, as gallstones will be identified in about 50 per cent of cases with the diagnosis [III].

The treatment of this condition in pregnancy is similar to that outside pregnancy. It must include adequate fluid replacement if there is electrolyte imbalance. Calcium and glucose disturbances should be corrected. Anticholinergics (e.g. hyoscine butylbromide) should be administered to reduce pancreatic activity. In addition, drugs such as steroids, prostaglandins, glucagons, cimetidine and trypsin inhibitors may be used to complement the suppression of pancreatic activity. Potent analgesics (preferably pethidine and not morphine) and prophylaxis against infections with either intravenous amoxycillin (1 g) 6 hourly or ceftazidime (1 g 8 hourly) should be offered. The role of nasogastric suction is unclear; although it is still advocated by some, it may result in an increase in serum amylase activity. Laparotomy should be avoided if possible and only undertaken if conservative treatment fails. However, where there are gallstones, a cholecystectomy may be beneficial. Termination of pregnancy does not improve the outcome of the disease [III]. The above conservative management has led to a marked reduction in mortality.

Inflammatory bowel diseases (Crohn's and ulcerative colitis)

Ulcerative colitis and Crohn's disease are inflammatory bowel conditions that may cause pain and diarrhoea in pregnancy (see Chapter 6.8). The severity of the pain is more marked with Crohn's disease. Both conditions may be associated with weight loss and features of anaemia. It is recognized that in those with pre-existing disease, pregnancy may result in a significant improvement in the symptoms. However, if there is active disease in early pregnancy, there is a greater chance of a flare-up in later gestations. If quiescent disease does relapse, the most likely times are in the first trimester and the puerperium.[6] The treatment is often a combination of analgesics (e.g. 5-aminosalicylic acid), steroids (e.g. prednisolone 30–60 mg daily) and dietary modifications. Opiates and bowel sedatives should be avoided. Occasionally, these conditions may cause pain from adhesions (especially in the case of Crohn's disease).

Hepatic disorders of pregnancy

Liver causes of abdominal pain in pregnancy include acute fatty liver of pregnancy, cholestasis of pregnancy, hepatic pain secondary to pre-eclampsia and hepatitis (see Chapter 6.8). The first three conditions are unique to pregnancy, whereas the fourth is unrelated. Pain is commonly located in the right hypochondrium. If the pain is associated with pre-eclampsia, features of pre-eclampsia will usually be apparent. In acute fatty liver and cholestasis, there are biochemical derangements in liver function tests, which are characteristic of the various pathologies. The management of these conditions will depend on the pathology. The place of analgesics is limited, as in most of these conditions there is some hepatocellular damage; choice of analgesia must therefore exclude those that are metabolized in the liver and may cause further damage (e.g. paracetemol).

Causes of abdominal pain from the gastrointestinal tract in pregnancy

- Reflux oesophagitis (heartburn)
- Hiatus hernia
- Peptic ulceration
- Gastritis
- Cholelithiasis and cholecystitis
- Constipation
- Bowel obstruction
- Acute appendicitis
- Pancreatitis
- Inflammatory bowel disease
- Hepatic disorders

URINARY TRACT

Urinary tract infection

Pyelonephritis is the most common renal cause of abdominal pain, and occurs in 1–2 per cent of pregnant women.[7] Physiological changes in pregnancy (dextro-rotation of the uterus, pressure from the gravid uterus and progestogenic effects on muscle result in ureteric dilatation) increase the risk of pyelonephritis. Pyelonephritis is more common on the right side. The condition is also more common in those with asymptomatic bacteriuria (which is present in 4–7 per cent of women at the onset of pregnancy); about 15 per cent of these women develop pyelonephritis in pregnancy.

Most cases present in the second and third trimesters. The symptoms include severe abdominal pain in the lumbar region, which may radiate to the iliac fossa or vulva. Occasionally, the pain is bilateral. It may be associated with nausea, vomiting, tachycardia, pyrexia and rigors. The physical signs include loin tenderness, generalized abdominal tenderness and uterine irritability. The differential diagnoses include appendicitis, cholecystitis, a torted adnexal mass and degenerating leiomyomas.

The most important investigation is a midstream specimen of urine for urinalysis, and microscopy culture and sensitivity. The most common organism responsible for this infection is *Escherichia coli*. However, other organisms, such as *Proteus mirabilis*, *Pseudomonas* spp. and beta-haemolytic *Streptococcus*, may be responsible for the infection. When *Pseudomonas* sp. is the causative organism, congenital malformations of the urinary system and renal calculi must be excluded by ultrasound scan in pregnancy or an intravenous urogram 3–4 months after delivery. Recently, the resurgence of pulmonary tuberculosis (TB) has been associated with an increase in the incidence of TB pyelonephritis. The diagnosis of TB pyelonephritis is made on an early-morning specimen of urine, which needs to be cultured in a Lowestein–Jensen medium.

Treatment of asymptomatic bacteriuria will reduce the incidence of pyelonephritis in pregnancy from 1–2 per cent to 0.5 per cent. Screening for bacteriuria in pregnancy prevents progression to pyelonephritis but also minimizes the risk of preterm labour (a sequela of pyelonephritis). Once the diagnosis has been confirmed, the most appropriate antibiotics should be administered, preferably intravenously for 48 hours and then orally. Fluid intake needs to be liberal. Where the infection is recurrent, the patient may have to be placed on long-term prophylactic antibiotics [III]. Most potent analgesics will alleviate the pain.

Cystitis

Cystitis presents with abdominal discomfort, frequency, nocturia and dysuria, and affects about 1–2 per cent of pregnant women. This complication is easy to diagnose from a midstream urine sample. The presence of nitrites, leucocytes and or protein in a midstream specimen is suggestive of an infection. The treatment is with liberal intake of fluids, analgesics if required and antibiotics.

Renal stones

Kidney stones affect about 0.03–0.05 per cent of pregnant women; the incidence is similar to that in non-pregnant women.[8] Pregnancy does not predispose to the formation of stones and in fact the dilatation of the ureters may allow small stones to be passed easily without being noticed.

Presentation is with loin pain, which starts in the renal angle and radiates to the suprapubic region. Occasionally, the pain radiates to the back, and patients may present in shock because of excruciating pain. Clinical examination may reveal tenderness over the renal area, but it is not unusual to fail to demonstrate any signs other than vague generalized abdominal discomfort. An ultrasound scan may demonstrate a dilated renal tract and possibly a stone; however, the absence of a stone on an ultrasound scan should not exclude the diagnosis.

Treatment consists of potent analgesics and liberal fluid intake. Anticholinergics may be useful to minimize the pain of renal peristalsis [IV]. If renal obstruction persists, surgical removal will be indicated. However, surgery risks precipitating preterm labour, and a more conservative approach should be adopted unless the symptoms become unbearable. In some women, delivery will resolve the symptoms.

Acute retention of urine

Acute retention of urine is more likely to occur in early pregnancy or in the puerperium. The causes include an incarcerated retroverted gravid uterus or pelvic mass (e.g. fibroid or ovarian cyst), acute herpes infection and a vulval haematoma.

Presentation is with severe pain of sudden onset. The history is classical, and physical examination often reveals a full bladder. Treatment is with catheterization, analgesics and bed rest to remove the cause of the retention. Leaving the indwelling catheter for 24–48 hours will allow a gravid uterus to become intra-abdominal. Treatment of herpes with antiviral drugs will not prevent further retention; however, the use of opiates may be extremely helpful.

Renal causes of abdominal pain in pregnancy

- Urinary tract infections
- Renal stones and ureteric obstruction
- Acute retention of urine

MISCELLANEOUS CAUSES OF PAIN

There are many other causes of abdominal pain in pregnancy that will not be discussed in detail. Among these are:

- musculoskeletal problems of exaggerated lumbar loidosis and pubic symphysis pain (symphyseal diasthesis)
- sickle cell crisis – acute haemolytic crises
- sequestration crises
- porphyria
- aneurysms
- haematomas of the rectus sheet.

Although straining of muscles may be responsible for pain in pregnancy, this is uncommon and is a diagnosis of exclusion. The pain may be related to a variety of muscles, which include the lumboides, rectus abdominis and external and internal oblique muscles of the anterior abdominal wall. There is rarely a clear history of trauma or straining of the muscles, and often examination does not reveal any signs. The treatment is with simple analgesics, physiotherapy and bed rest.

The common skeletal causes of abdominal pain include exaggerated lumbar loidosis and symphysis pubis pain. The features of this type of pain are characteristic: difficulties in walking and tenderness over the symphysis pubis. The treatment is a brace to support the joints of the pelvis; if there is no improvement, a walking frame may be required. In most cases, the pregnancy can be supported to term. There is often no need to interfere in the delivery process, as this may exacerbate the complication. It is important to remember that the pain may cause prolonged hospitalization and therefore increase the risk of venous thromboembolism.

In sickle cell disease (see Chapter 6.5), acute sequestration or splenic infarction may result in severe abdominal pain and organomegaly. This is less likely in adults, as repeated infarction during childhood and early adolescence is likely to have resulted in autosplenectomy. However, in cases of HbSC disease, the complication may occur for the first time in pregnancy. Pain is excruciating and only relieved by very potent analgesics such as opiates. Treatment must involve a haematologist and incorporate potent analgesia, transfusion (in the case of sequestration crises) and antibiotics.

Acute intermittent porphyria is a rare but recognized cause of abdominal pain in pregnancy. It tends to present with abdominal pain, gastrointestinal symptoms and disturbances of the autonomic nervous system. Occasionally there may be exacerbations presenting for the first time in pregnancy and these may mimic various neuropsychiatric disorders. Acute intermittent porphyria presents a diagnostic challenge. In the investigations and treatment of this condition, all drugs that may precipitate an attack must be discontinued. The therapy during pregnancy should include analgesics and anti-emetics.

Amongst the other causes of abdominal pain in pregnancy, which need to be carefully excluded if there are any suggestive symptoms, are: advanced extrauterine pregnancy, aneurysms, haematomas of the rectus muscle, arteriovenous malformations, mesenteric thrombosis (common in sickle cell patients), rupture of the spleen and malignancies.

Abdominal pain in pregnancy

There are no randomized, controlled trials relating to abdominal pain in pregnancy. The evidence for the causes, diagnosis and treatment is from retrospective studies, cohort studies or expert opinions.

KEY POINTS

- Abdominal pain in pregnancy is a common clinical presentation.
- Diagnosis is often difficult and may be obscured by the pregnancy.
- Pregnancy and non-pregnancy causes must be considered in the differential diagnosis.
- Urinary tract infections are the most common non-genital causes of abdominal pain in pregnancy.

KEY REFERENCES

1. Lev-Toaff AS, Coleman BG, Arger PH et al. Leiomyomas in pregnancy: sonographic study. *Radiology* 1987; 164:375–80.
2. Stauffer RA, Adams A, Wygal J, Lavery JP. Gallbladder disease in pregnancy. *Am J Obstet Gynecol* 1982; 144:661–4.

3. Hill LM, Symmonds RE. Small bowel obstruction in pregnancy: a review and report of four cases. *Obstet Gynecol* 1977; **40**:170–3.

4. Tamir IL, Bongard FS, Klein SR. Acute appendicitis in the pregnant patient. *Am J Surg* 1990; **160**:571–2.

5. McKay AJ, O'Neill J, Imrie CE. Pancreatitis, pregnancy and gallstones. *Br J Obstet Gynaecol* 1980; **87**:47–50.

6. Willoughby CP, Truelove SC. Ulcerative colitis and pregnancy. *Gut* 1980; **21**:469–74.

7. Gilstrap LC, Cunningham FG, Whalley PJ. Acute pyelonephritis in pregnancy: an anterospective study. *Obstet Gynecol* 1981; **57**:409–13.

8. Coe FL, Parks JH, Lindheimer MD. Nephrolithiasis during pregnancy. *N Engl J Med* 1978; **298**:324–6.

Malignancy

Alec McEwan

There is no established standard for this topic, but we would suggest the following points for guidance.

Theoretical skills
- Recognize the influence that pregnancy has on the presentation and prognosis of malignant disease.
- Understand the need to balance benefit and harm to the fetus and the mother by delaying or proceeding with treatment.
- Know currently available evidence for guiding management and predicting outcomes for the more common cancers arising in pregnancy.

Practical skills
- Be able to manage a pregnancy with co-existing malignant disease.
- Be able to liaise with surgeons, oncologists, paediatricians and psychologists to create an individualized plan of care.
- Be able to manage a pregnancy complicated by an adnexal mass.
- Be able to manage a pregnancy with an abnormal cervical smear.

Approximately 1 in every 1000 pregnancies is complicated by a new diagnosis of cancer, with cervical and breast cancer being the most common. This figure may rise as more women are choosing to start their families later in life.

Pregnancy does not affect the course of cancer per se. However, diagnosis is often delayed as the presenting symptoms of malignancy may be confused with the common symptoms of pregnancy. Both the investigation and treatment of a malignancy may carry risks for the fetus, and serious conflict may occur between the desire to treat the mother appropriately whilst limiting harm to the pregnancy.[1] Future prospects for childbearing may be subsequently limited by surgery, radiotherapy and chemotherapy. Psychological adjustment to a diagnosis of cancer is likely to be more difficult whilst pregnant.[2]

Managing cancer during pregnancy therefore requires a multidisciplinary approach involving obstetricians, oncologists, paediatricians and counsellors. The role of an individual midwife or oncology nurse should not be underestimated.

Evidence to support management decisions in pregnancies complicated by cancer is derived mostly from retrospective uncontrolled studies [III]. Few case-controlled studies have been performed, but overall the paucity of good-quality evidence must be made clear during patient counselling.

RADIOTHERAPY AND CHEMOTHERAPY DURING PREGNANCY

Fetal exposure to radiation and/or chemotherapeutic agents may potentially have a number of detrimental effects. These include:

- miscarriage and intrauterine fetal death,
- congenital anomalies,
- severe mental retardation (SMR) and microcephaly,
- prenatal and postnatal growth restriction,
- increase in the risk of childhood malignancy,
- infertility in the offspring,
- induction of germ-line genetic abnormalities.

Counselling couples about the fetal risks associated with cancer treatment is complicated by a lack of high-quality evidence. There have been no randomized trials, and publication and ascertainment bias skew the available data. Studies often involve small numbers, are retrospective and unsystematic in their approach and follow-up. Chemotherapy and radiotherapy are often used in combination and the contributory effects of the illness itself on the pregnancy are impossible to isolate from other variables. Data are often out of date and irrelevant to newer management regimes.

Experimental data from animal studies can be helpful, but there are marked interspecies differences and caution must be exercised in extrapolating directly to human pregnancies. Remember also that the background fetal anomaly rate is variably quoted as 3–6 per cent. All studies should be interpreted with this in mind.

Radiation exposure during pregnancy

Radiation dose is measured in Grays and rads.

> 1 Gray (1 Gy) = 100 rad
> 1 centiGray (cGy) = 1 rad

Calculating fetal exposure and radiation absorption during radiotherapy and radiological investigations is complicated and often imprecise. Although the primary radiation beam can be accurately directed and quantified, additional exposure occurs from leakage through the head of the linear accelerator, external scatter from beam modifiers and internal scatter within the patient. With appropriate shielding, fetal exposure can be reduced by as much as 50 per cent, although the effects of shielding also can be difficult to quantify. The gestation at which exposure occurs is also important for two reasons. Most importantly, fetal tissues show differential radiosensitivity throughout the course of the pregnancy (see below). Secondly, a larger fetus is more difficult to shield effectively and may lie closer to the irradiated field. *Tissue equivalent phantoms* are models designed to help predict fetal absorption more objectively as the gestation advances and uterine size increases.

The effects of prenatal exposure to ionizing radiation are described as either **deterministic** or **stochastic**. Deterministic effects are those where loss of function occurs due to cell destruction. The severity of the effect is dose related and a critical threshold exists below which the effect is not seen. Miscarriage, intrauterine death, congenital anomalies and SMR are believed to follow this pattern. Stochastic effects are those where ionizing radiation causes genetic cell modification and loss of cell cycle control, which, after a period of latency, leads to the development of cancer. Stochastic effects also demonstrate a dose–effect relationship, but without a threshold value.[3]

- Very early exposure to radiation during pregnancy (pre-implantation and early organogenesis; 0–2 weeks post-conception) will either result in miscarriage or the pregnancy will continue unaffected.
- Mammalian animal experiments show that congenital abnormalities are more likely when exposure occurs during early organogenesis (3–7 weeks post-conception in a human pregnancy).
- Generalized growth and neurological development continue throughout normal pregnancy. Microcephaly,

SMR and permanent growth restriction remain potential risks for the fetus exposed during the remainder of the pregnancy. The 8–15-week period appears to be time of highest risk and corresponds to a critical stage of cortical formation and organization. There is minimal risk after 25 weeks, unless very high exposures occur.
- An increased predisposition to malignancy later in life appears to be a risk whatever the gestational age at which exposure occurs.

Evidence for the effects of radiation exposure during pregnancy is derived from three sources:

1 animal experiments[4]
2 accidental human exposures
3 the Japanese survivors of the atomic bomb.[5,6]

The high rate of fetal loss occurring with exposure during pre-implantation (conception to day 10) has been confirmed by rodent experiments and epidemiological data from Nagasaki and Hiroshima. Miscarriage and intrauterine death occur with a threshold of 10 rad in these first few weeks; however, this increases steadily towards term, at which time the lower threshold for causing intrauterine death is estimated as >100 rad.[3]

Animal experiments, mostly involving rodents, have shown that exposure during organogenesis causes a variety of congenital anomalies, notably involving the skeleton, eye and urinary tract. The threshold, extrapolating to humans, is possibly as low as 5 rad, with a marked dose–response effect. However, human studies have failed to find this effect, with the exception of microcephaly. Teratogenesis should nevertheless remain a concern. It may be that the critically sensitive time in the human fetus is shorter, or that pregnancies with major anomalies abort spontaneously or have gone unrecorded.

Destruction of neural cells or failure of their migration may lead to microcephaly and/or mental retardation. Data from Japan[6] has estimated a lower threshold for microcephaly of 10 rad, with the 8–15-week period being most crucial. The incidence of microcephaly was 40 per cent with exposures of 50 rad or higher. Severe mental retardation was also found more commonly in the offspring exposed between 8 and 25 weeks, with lower thresholds for SMR of 6 rad (8–15 weeks) and 28 rad (16–25 weeks). Studies of intelligence quotient (IQ) reflect these observations.[7]

There are fewer data on the effect of the radiation exposure on developing germ cells. Delayed menarche has been observed in Japanese girls exposed to radiation in utero with a threshold of 25 rad. No increase in the rates of infertility has yet been demonstrated.

A safe exposure limit of 5 rad during pregnancy has been suggested. However, this does not take account of possible stochastic effects that do not show a lower threshold. An increase in childhood malignancies has been reported in a famous Oxford study of pelvimetry during pregnancy in which exposures were typically 1 rad (The Oxford Survey of

Table 7.3.1　Fetal radiation exposures during various radiological investigations[3]

Background radiation exposure	0.002 rad/week
Chest/skull X-ray	<0.001 rad
Mammogram	0.0004 rad
Ventilation/perfusion scan with ^{99m}Tc	<0.2 rad
Abdominal X-ray	0.26 rad
IVP/lumbar spine	0.32 rad
Bone imaging with ^{99m}Tc	<0.5 rad
Abdominal CT	0.8 rad
Barium enema	1.6 rad
Pelvic CT	2.5 rad

IVP, intravenous pyelogram; CT, computerized tomography.

Childhood Cancers).[5,8] The background rate of childhood malignancy is 1 in 1300 before the age of 15. This study gave a relative risk of 1.4 for those offspring exposed in utero to pelvimetry. A pelvic computerized tomography (CT) scan typically exposes a fetus to approximately 2.5 rad and this is thought to double the risk of a childhood malignancy. Clearly, setting a 5 rad 'safe limit' may be considered simplistic, and the debate continues. Table 7.3.1 lists the mean fetal dose exposures predicted for various investigations. It is important to realize, however, that the actual dose is dependent on many factors and that the true value may be five-fold higher.

In practice, safer alternatives to CT scanning are usually available. Magnetic resonance imaging (MRI) is thought to be safe during pregnancy, as is ultrasound.

It is likely that single exposures carry greater fetal risk than divided doses, adding further to the difficulties in applying the available human data to real diagnostic and therapeutic scenarios [IV].

Chemotherapy and pregnancy

Prior to implantation, the blastocyst is immune to the effects of chemotherapy. The period of organogenesis between 5 and 10 weeks is, however, a critically sensitive time. Exposure to chemotherapy during this period may be associated with malformations in 10–20 per cent of cases [III].[9] After 12 weeks' gestation, malformations should be less common, although growth and neurological development remain potentially vulnerable throughout pregnancy.

A number of retrospective studies support these generalizations regarding the importance of the timing of chemotherapy during pregnancy. Congenital malformations seem no more likely if chemotherapy is given only during the second and third trimesters [III].[10] First-trimester exposure does indeed seem more hazardous, and this is somewhat dependent on the agents used [III].[9]

Antimetabolites carry the greatest risks to a first-trimester pregnancy. Although miscarriage is the most common outcome, aminopterin may cause neural tube, skeletal and clefting abnormalities. This anti-neoplastic agent has been replaced by methotrexate, which is structurally similar and has the same effects on the early fetus. Both should be avoided in the first trimester and later in the pregnancy where possible. A 14 per cent congenital anomaly risk has been quoted for **alkylating agents** (e.g. cyclophosphamide) if given in the first trimester. This risk falls to near background levels for administration in the second and third trimester. The **antibiotics** such as doxorubicin and bleomycin do not have clear teratogenic effects, although they are still to be avoided in the first trimester where possible. **Vinca alkaloids**, such as vincristine and vinblastine, are harmful in animal pregnancies but this effect is not obvious in the few human pregnancies so far exposed in the first trimester [III]. Information is constantly updated with regard to the use of these drugs during pregnancy and it is wise to consult a drug information bureau before deciding management.

Other effects of fetal exposure to chemotherapy in the second and third trimesters are even less clear. Studies are conflicting with regard to prenatal and postnatal growth restriction, although one review concluded that intrauterine growth restriction occurred in 40 per cent of exposed pregnancies [III].[9]

The longer term effects of fetal exposure to chemotherapy are also unclear. Survivors of cancer who received chemotherapy as children have been followed up closely with the assumption that late complications of treatment in this group might also be expected to occur in individuals exposed in utero. Investigators have looked for evidence of impaired intellect, reduced gonadal function (delayed puberty and reduced fertility), visceral damage and mutagenesis within germ cells.

There is some evidence to suggest that future fertility may be affected and there are certainly concerns over the potential cardiotoxicity of doxorubicin and the pulmonary damage associated with bleomycin. There is no good evidence to suggest any intellectual impairment or increase in the genetic problems in the next generation. However, to directly apply these findings from individuals treated during childhood to those exposed to chemotherapy in utero makes the assumption that fetal cells behave in the same way as those of a child. This may not be the case, and fetal germ cells, for example, might be more susceptible to genetic damage than those of an older child.

A more consistent effect of chemotherapy on the fetus is myelosuppression. A third of newborns delivered to women who received treatment for leukaemia during their pregnancy showed evidence of bone marrow suppression in one study [III].[11] Fortunately, this is rarely of clinical importance, and sepsis, serious anaemia and haemorrhage are uncommon in the neonate. However, it is good practice to avoid myelosuppressive agents in the 3 weeks prior to delivery, if possible [IV].

Despite the lack of evidence for major harm from chemotherapy in the second and third trimesters, breast-feeding is usually discouraged if treatment continues into the puerperium [IV]. This reflects unresolved uncertainties about the true safety of these agents and the knowledge that significant quantities do reach breast milk.

SYMPTOM CONTROL IN THE PREGNANT PATIENT WITH CANCER

The symptoms of cancer and of normal pregnancy overlap and can easily be confused. Early satiety, nausea and vomiting, constipation, dyspnoea, fatigue and depression are all common during a normal pregnancy but can also be significant symptoms of malignancy. Every effort should be made to determine symptom aetiology when a known cancer coexists with pregnancy. Shortness of breath, for example, may simply be the effect of high progesterone levels and expanded tidal volume typical of the third trimester. However, in the cancer patient it may be a sign of pleural effusions, significant anaemia or lung metastases. Similarly, nausea and vomiting may have a more sinister cause, such as hypercalcaemia, electrolyte imbalance, uraemia and even intracranial metastases. Early advice from an oncologist should be sought when new symptoms arise.

Pain should be managed with paracetamol and opiates. Non-steroidal anti-inflammatory drugs are best avoided, especially in the third trimester. Tricyclic antidepressants can be safely used for neuropathic pain, but carbamazepine should not (see Chapter 8) [II].

Poor appetite may be secondary to depression, pain and nausea and vomiting. Treatments for nausea include metoclopramide, prochlorperazine and cyclizine. Ondansetron and haloperidol can be used if necessary. Prednisone is effective for a number of symptoms, including nausea, anorexia and fatigue. Cannabis seems to be beneficial in a number of ways but is not advised during pregnancy [III]. Constipation is effectively treated with docusate, magnesium hydroxide and senna, all of which are safe in pregnancy.

The psychological adjustment to a diagnosis of cancer is always difficult, seldom more so than during pregnancy. Fears of limited life expectancy deprive couples of future hopes and plans for themselves and their family. Focusing on short-term goals and enjoying the present are so much harder to do during pregnancy. More specifically, there may be anxieties regarding the effect of the disease or its treatment on the fetus. The question of termination of a wanted pregnancy will be extremely distressing. There may be conflict over what is best for the woman herself and what will do least harm to the pregnancy. Concern for other children and anxieties about future fertility add further to the crisis. There is remarkably little research or evidence to guide practice, but the involvement of a mental health team or counselling service should be offered at the very least.

SPECIFIC EXAMPLES

Breast cancer

Breast cancer accounts for a quarter of all cancers diagnosed in pregnancy, occurring in approximately 1 in 3000 pregnancies. Stage for stage, the outcome is no different from that for breast cancers diagnosed outside of pregnancy [II].[12] Continuing the pregnancy certainly does not seem to have a deleterious effect on outcome, and termination of pregnancy is not indicated for this reason [III]. However, at diagnosis, pregnancy-associated breast cancer tends to be larger in size, more advanced and more likely to have metastasized to local lymph nodes. This, in part, may be due to the 6-month average delay in its diagnosis. This is thought to increase the risk of nodal metastases by at least 10 per cent.

Breast masses are common in pregnancy. Lactational adenomas, galactoceles, mastitis and infarction of hypertrophied breast tissue are all benign pregnancy-induced breast lumps that may masquerade as malignancy. Breast enlargement, greater vascularity and increased tissue density add to the diagnostic difficulty. Mammography is safe with appropriate shielding but has a lower sensitivity in pregnancy. Fine-needle aspiration or excisional biopsy should be performed if there is any suspicion of malignancy. Once carcinoma has been diagnosed, a chest X ray may be needed for staging, and once again this is safe with shielding. CT scanning for metastases should be replaced by ultrasound and MRI. If necessary, technetium bone scans can be employed, exposing the pregnancy to <0.5 rad.

A common surgical option for breast cancer is lumpectomy followed by postoperative chest-wall radiotherapy to reduce local recurrence risks. Radiotherapy for breast cancer might typically be 50 Gy (5000 rad). With appropriate shielding, fetal exposure may be as little as 4 rad at very early gestations (<5 weeks), rising to 14–18 rad in the second trimester when the uterus is larger. This is above the 'accepted' threshold of safety, and a modified radical mastectomy, which does not necessitate postoperative radiotherapy, should normally be advised during pregnancy instead [IV]. The surgery itself carries minimal risk, if any, to the fetus. Conservative breast surgery can sometimes be performed in the third trimester, with adjunctive radiotherapy delayed until the puerperium.

Chemotherapy for breast cancer in the second and third trimesters is not associated with obvious fetal harm,[13] although there are still concerns about the longer term effects [III]. Where possible, the last dose should be given 3 weeks prior to delivery to limit the effects of fetal bone marrow suppression [IV]. Tamoxifen use in pregnancy has previously been discouraged. Experiments in rodents have demonstrated anomalies similar to those found with in-utero diethylstilboestrol (DES) exposure and an increased intrauterine fetal death rate. Although these effects appear to be species specific, there are only minimal human data testifying to the safety of tamoxifen in pregnancy and its use is not currently recommended.

Fetal surveillance by regular growth scanning is warranted, although a clear link with prenatal growth restriction has not been established. Placental metastases are found very rarely and there are no reports of breast cancer spreading to the fetus. Some authors suggest delivery at 34 weeks' to limit the fetal exposure to chemotherapeutic agents. Others await spontaneous labour if fetal growth is normal. Neonatal blood sampling is necessary to exclude clinically relevant pancytopenia.

Pregnancy after breast cancer

With the high background incidence of breast cancer and progressive delay in childbearing, it is not uncommon now to be asked for advice on this matter. Indeed, the Royal College of Obstetricians and Gynaecologists (RCOG) has published an evidence-based guideline to help clinicians. Four studies are cited which have failed to show any effect on survival if pregnancy occurs after breast cancer [II].[14–17] Although it can be argued that women with a more favourable prognosis are more likely to consider a pregnancy, the survival amongst node-positive patients was not affected by pregnancy either. It has been suggested that becoming pregnant soon after breast cancer may affect long-term survival and that a delay should be advised. Studies that demonstrate a survival advantage with such a delay may simply be highlighting the improved prognosis for women who remain alive 2–5 years after the diagnosis. For younger women (who have a worse prognosis anyway), a delay of 2–5 years will have minimal impact on fertility. Allowing more time will help to give a more individualized prognosis. Such a delay may be more difficult to justify in women in their late thirties and forties.

The use of tamoxifen during pregnancy is not recommended (see above). Breastfeeding is not contraindicated, but previous surgery and radiotherapy may impair subsequent lactation.

The following five points are the recommendations given in the RCOG guideline.

- Some women will not be fertile after treatment for breast cancer, depending on the use of radiotherapy or chemotherapy. However, choice of appropriate treatment for breast cancer should not at the present time be compromised by thoughts of future fertility [IV].
- Women planning pregnancy or who become pregnant after breast cancer should consult their clinical oncologist, surgeon and obstetrician, and it is important that there is good communication between these members of the clinical team in the management of the woman [IV].
- There is no evidence that the survival of women who have had breast cancer and subsequently become pregnant is compromised. However, an interval of at least 2 and preferably 3 years between treatment and conception is recommended [II].

- There is no indication that termination of pregnancy will improve the prognosis, and this should only be considered if there are further indications [II].
- There is no evidence that previous treatment for breast cancer affects the welfare of the offspring, although the situation for women who become pregnant while taking tamoxifen remains unclear [II].

Cervical cancer

Cervical cancer is the most common pregnancy-related cancer, although the quoted incidence varies from 1 in 1200 to 1 in 10 000 pregnancies. It commonly presents with vaginal bleeding but discharge and pain may also occur. A high proportion of cases are detected by cervical screening and are otherwise asymptomatic.

Cervical screening in pregnancy

False-positive cervical smears are more likely during pregnancy for a number of reasons:

- eversion of the squamocolumnar junction occurs as a consequence of high oestrogen levels and exposed columnar epithelium undergoes squamous metaplasia;
- cervical infiltration by leucocytes occurs in pregnancy;
- decidualization of the cervix is a frequent finding;
- trophoblasts may be present in the cervical canal;
- relative immunosuppression may allow greater human papilloma virus (HPV) activity.

It is vital that the cytologist reading the smear is aware that it has been taken from a pregnant woman if false positives are to be kept to a minimum. In the UK it is not usual for routine cervical screening to be carried out in pregnancy, and smears are normally deferred until the postnatal appointment. However, if there is clinical concern regarding the cervix, or if it seems unlikely that the individual will return after the pregnancy for a smear to be carried out, there should be no hesitation in performing it whilst the woman is pregnant.

Most studies show a high degree of concordance between cytology (smears) and colposcopy [II][18] during pregnancy but the possibility of false-positive or false-negative results must always be considered.

Management of an abnormal smear in pregnancy

A reluctance to perform cervical smears during pregnancy may also arise from anxieties over the subsequent management of the abnormal smear. How safe and reliable are the usual techniques in the context of pregnancy? One study of colposcopy during pregnancy found concordance, overestimation and underestimation of the final diagnosis (based on cone histology) in 73 per cent, 17 per cent and 10 per cent respectively, and this did not differ significantly from the non-pregnant control group.[19] Indeed, unsatisfactory colposcopy is less common during pregnancy due to eversion of the squamocolumnar junction. Squamous metaplasia is more common and the cervix will usually look larger and have increased vascularity. Colposcopy during pregnancy therefore requires experience and careful judgement. Hacker and colleagues demonstrated a 99.5 per cent diagnostic accuracy for colposcopy, with only a 0.5 per cent false-negative rate (with no missed invasive lesions) amongst 1064 pregnant women.[20]

If a smear taken in pregnancy has suggested low-grade cervical intraepithelial neoplasia (CIN) and the colposcopic impression agrees, these women can be managed by repeat colposcopy in each trimester, with a further evaluation in the postpartum period. There is no evidence that CIN progresses more rapidly in pregnancy, and indeed regression rates of 25–70 per cent have been documented for high-grade CIN first detected in pregnancy.[21]

If the colposcopic impression is of a higher grade lesion, it is vital that microinvasive and invasive cancers are excluded. Older studies recorded an unacceptably high rate of complications with knife conization during pregnancy, principally a >500 mL blood loss in 7–13 per cent of cases (mostly in the third trimester).[22] Any causative association with miscarriage, preterm rupture of membranes, preterm delivery and chorioamnionitis remains uncertain, but concerns do exist. These concerns have seen a shift away from conization in pregnancy towards the use of directed punch biopsies, which carry less morbidity. Concordance between directed biopsies and the final diagnosis is complete or within one degree of severity in over 95 per cent of cases [II].[19] Missed invasive lesions are extremely uncommon. Treatment of CIN II and III should be delayed to the postpartum period, but colposcopy every 8 weeks antenatally is advised to monitor for progression of the lesion [IV].

An even less invasive alternative approach uses directed brush cytology in combination with colposcopy. This is not widely practised, but results have been encouraging.[23]

Despite this discussion, cervical conization may still be warranted during pregnancy. If invasive cancer cannot be excluded by directed punch biopsies, or colposcopy is inadequate, a cone biopsy may be necessary. Also, 'microinvasion' can only be confirmed on a cone specimen. Although diathermy loop conization has been used in pregnancy, the little evidence there is would suggest that cold knife conization gives fewer positive margins and higher quality biopsy specimens.[24]

Postpartum evaluation is extremely important for women who have antenatal colposcopy, even those who have undergone cone biopsy. Lesions may regress, persist or progress, and the diagnosis made during pregnancy may need to be upgraded. High rates of residual intraepithelial neoplasia and cytological abnormalities have been found following conization, which should not necessarily be considered adequate treatment for CIN during pregnancy.[25]

Management of cervical cancer in pregnancy

Cervical cancer is normally staged clinically by chest X-ray, cystoscopy, pyelogram and CT or MRI scanning. MRI is the investigation of choice for pelvic imaging during pregnancy.

Cervical cancer is usually treated surgically in its early stages. Chemoradiotherapy is reserved for more advanced disease due to the effects this treatment has on ovarian, bladder, bowel and sexual function. Knife conization may be sufficient treatment for Ia1 (microinvasive) cervical cancer outside of pregnancy due to the low risk of recurrence or lymph node (LN) metastases. If this diagnosis is made during pregnancy and the cone biopsy margins are clear, the pregnancy should be allowed to continue, with vaginal delivery [IV]. However, the significant rate of positive margins and residual disease found with conization in pregnancy make further evaluation in the postpartum period imperative.[25] For women who have completed their families, a postpartum simple hysterectomy with ovarian conservation is recommended [IV].

Higher grade lesions (Ib1–IIa) are usually treated by simple or radical hysterectomy with lymph node sampling. Cancers presenting at less than 20 weeks' gestation have traditionally been treated immediately [IV]. The hysterectomy can usually be performed with the fetus in situ; however, a hysterotomy, avoiding the lower part of the uterus, can be employed to remove the pregnancy and improve access if necessary. Delaying treatment until after delivery becomes an increasingly favourable option after 20 weeks' gestation for stage I cancers.[26] Nine studies involving 63 patients with stage I cervical cancer have examined the effect of a delay, varying between 1 and 32 weeks. Only one outcome was possibly affected by the delay. However, these studies are clearly nonrandomized and the decision to delay should be made with oncologists and neonatologists after careful patient counselling. Steroids should be given to promote fetal lung maturation. Delivery at 32–34 weeks can now be justified with advances in the care of the preterm infant. Caesarean section is normally advised, due to theoretical concerns of haemorrhage from cervical lesions and increased malignant cell dissemination with vaginal delivery [IV]. Local recurrence within episiotomy sites is well documented and is associated with a high mortality rate. Radical hysterectomy at the time of caesarean section is associated with greater blood loss, but the rate of other complications is not increased [III].

Consideration should also be given to the use of neoadjuvant chemotherapy in the second and third trimesters. This may limit progression of disease and more confidently allow delay in surgical treatment, although its safety also remains in question.

Radiotherapy is employed with more advanced lesions (stage IIb and above) and usually takes the form of external beam *teletherapy* and intracavitary *brachytherapy*. The external beam alone employs 40–50 Gy. Most pregnancies will spontaneously abort after such high doses, usually within 5 weeks [III]. Occasionally, the fetus must be removed surgically. Preterm delivery of the fetus may be necessary at later gestations.

Where a lesion is very advanced, and the maternal prognosis poor, the woman may prefer to compromise her own treatment if this means limiting the risks to the fetus. Careful, sensitive counselling is clearly very important in this situation.

Ovarian cancer

The incidence of ovarian tumours in pregnancy is quoted as 1 in 1000 deliveries, although ovarian cancer is much less common (1 in 5000–18 000). Adnexal masses are found in approximately 1 in 100 pregnancies; 50 per cent measure <5 cm, 25 per cent are 5–10 cm and the remaining quarter are >10 cm in size. Table 7.3.2 lists various causes of adnexal mass found in pregnancy, in decreasing order of incidence.

There are various non-neoplastic ovarian lesions which are unique to pregnancy and which will resolve spontaneously after delivery. These include:

- luteoma of pregnancy
- follicular cyst of pregnancy
- hyperreactio luteinalis
- granulosa cell proliferations
- hilus cell hyperplasia
- ectopia deciduo.

With the extensive use of ultrasound for dating and assessing pregnancies, the recognition of adnexal masses in pregnancy has increased. Although most remain asymptomatic, 10–15 per cent will rupture, bleed or cause adnexal torsion [III], and these acute events are thought to increase the risk of miscarriage and preterm labour [III]. Occasionally, an ovarian mass may cause dystocia during labour or virilization. As 1 in 20–50 ovarian lesions in pregnancy will be malignant[27] and as many as 1 in 6 may become symptomatic, a careful management decision has to be made when they are first recognized. Symptomatic adnexal lesions may need to be operated on immediately. Small (<6 cm) unilocular cysts are likely to resolve spontaneously before 16 weeks without causing harm and should be left alone [III].[28] A further ultrasound should be performed at 16 weeks' gestation. A persistent complex mass should prompt a laparotomy. Miscarriage is said to be less likely if intervention occurs at this point in the second trimester. Persistent simple cysts that are not associated with ascites and have no solid areas or thick septae within them can be treated conservatively. Dermoid cysts are often confidently diagnosed by ultrasound. These, too, can be left although the risk of a cyst accident must always be considered, as this may increase the risk of miscarriage. MRI may help with diagnosis in selected cases.

Tumour markers such as Ca 125, alpha-fetoprotein (aFP) and human chorionic gonadotrophin (hCG) are helpful for diagnosis and treatment monitoring outside of pregnancy. These substances may all be elevated during a normal pregnancy and do not usually feature in the diagnosis or management of the adnexal mass antenatally. Of note, however, an extremely high maternal serum aFP value, performed for fetal anomaly screening, has led to the diagnosis of endodermal sinus tumours on a number of occasions.

Surgery for an adnexal mass in pregnancy usually involves a lower midline incision, which allows adequate access with minimal uterine manipulation. Peritoneal washings should be taken and omental and peritoneal biopsies. Where appropriate, a simple cystectomy with ovarian conservation is attempted. Otherwise, a unilateral salpingo-oophorectomy should be performed. Frozen sections of the contralateral ovary can be taken to help intraoperative management, but bilateral oophorectomy should normally be avoided at the initial operation, as even malignant cases are usually early stage, chemosensitive or of low malignant potential. Para-aortic lymph node sampling and debulking should be considered in more complex cases, although it would be unusual for the uterus to need to be removed.

If an ovarian cyst is removed in the first trimester, it may have arisen from the corpus luteum and may have been providing hormonal support to the early pregnancy. It is accepted practice in this situation to provide progesterone supplementation until the second trimester is reached [IV].

Management of ovarian cancer in pregnancy

The histopathological nature of ovarian cancer in pregnancy reflects the younger age of the affected population. Germ cell and epithelial cell cancers each account for 30–40 per cent of cases, but two-thirds of the epithelial group are of 'low malignant potential'. The remainder are mostly sex cord stromal tumours. Dysgerminomas are the most common malignant ovarian tumours found in pregnancy.

Stage I epithelial cancers, tumours of low malignant potential and Stage Ia dysgerminomas do not require adjunctive treatment with chemotherapy. Other forms of germ cell tumour and more advanced epithelial cancers would normally be treated with chemotherapy postoperatively. Beyond the first trimester, the use of bleomycin, etoposide, cisplatin and vincristine/vinblastine has not been clearly linked with fetal harm, with a number of successful outcomes having been reported in the literature.[29] However, until more data have been collected, concerns will remain over the use of antineoplastic drugs during pregnancy, especially during the first trimester (see above).

Table 7.3.2 The most common causes of adnexal mass in pregnancy

Functional cyst
Mature teratoma (dermoid)
Cystadenoma (serous and mucinous)
Para-ovarian cyst
Endometrioma
Leiomyoma
Malignancy (3–6 per cent of all cases)

Other malignancies

The principles of managing cancer in pregnancy can be illustrated by further examples.

- Older, uncontrolled studies suggested a poorer outcome stage for stage when melanoma presented during pregnancy. More recent, case-controlled studies show no difference in 3-year and 5-year survival rates [II].[30] Although melanoma is the malignancy most likely to metastasize to the placenta and fetus, this nevertheless rarely occurs. However, the placenta should be examined at delivery and sent for histopathology. The fetus will have metastases in 30 per cent of cases where placental involvement is found. Biopsy of the sentinel or draining node may be useful in predicting spread of malignant melanoma. A blue dye can be used to locate this lymph node, as an alternative to technetium-labelled sulphur colloid, avoiding fetal radiation exposure [III].
- Radiotherapy for head, neck and brain tumours usually carries a fetal dose exposure of <10 rad due to the distance between the field and the uterus. Abdominal shielding can reduce this to <2 rad.
- The treatment for Hodgkin's lymphoma and chronic myeloid leukaemia can often be delayed until after the pregnancy. Acute leukaemias and non-Hodgkin's lymphoma must be treated immediately, as the risks to the woman and her pregnancy from haemorrhage, anaemia and sepsis outweigh the possible fetal harm from chemotherapy, even in the first trimester [III].

KEY POINTS

- Pregnancy does not alter the course of cancer but may cause a delay in diagnosis.
- Sensitive methods of investigation can be safely employed during pregnancy.
- Safe treatments are available during pregnancy for dealing with all symptoms caused by cancer.
- Chemotherapy in the first trimester is associated with a significantly increased risk of fetal abnormalities. Treatment during the second and third trimesters of pregnancy would seem to be safer, but the data are limited.
- Radiation exposure must be restricted to the very low levels found with investigative X-rays. Radiotherapy for pelvic, abdominal or chest malignancies usually carries excessive fetal risk, even with shielding.
- Management requires a multidisciplinary approach.

KEY REFERENCES

1. Iseminger KA, Lewis MA. Ethical challenges in treating mother and fetus when cancer complicates pregnancy. *Obstet Gynecol Clin North Am* 1998; **25**:273–85.
2. Schover LR. Psychosocial issues associated with cancer in pregnancy. *Semin Oncol* 2000; **27**:699–703.
3. Fattibene P, Mazzei F, Nuccetelli C, Risica S. Prenatal exposure to ionising radiation: sources, effects and regulatory aspects. *Acta Paediatr* 1999; **88**:693–702.
4. Tribukait B, Cekan E. *Developmental Effects of Prenatal Irradiation*. Dose–effect relationship and the significance of fractionated and protracted radiation for the frequency of fetal malformations following X-irradiation of pregnant C3H mice. Stuttgart: Gustave Fischer, 1982, 29–35.
5. Muirhead CR, Kneale GW. Prenatal irradiation and childhood cancer. *J Radiol Prot* 1989; **9**:209–12.
6. Otake M, Schull W. Radiation-related small head sizes among prenatally exposed A-bomb survivors. *Int J Radiat Oncol Biol Phys* 1992; **63**:255–70.
7. Mole RH. Irradiation of the embryo and fetus. *Br J Radiol* 1987; **60**:17–31.
8. Gilman EA, Kneale GW, Knox EG, Stewart AM. Pregnancy X rays and childhood cancers: effects of exposure age and radiation dose. *J Radiol Prot* 1988; **8**:3–8.
9. Partridge AH, Garber JE. Long-term outcomes of children exposed to anti-neoplastic agents in utero. *Semin Oncol* 2000; **27**:712–26.
10. Doll DC, Ringenberg S, Yarbo JW. Antineoplastic agents and pregnancy. *Semin Oncol* 1989; **16**:337.
11. Reynosa E, Shepherd F, Messner H et al. Acute leukaemia in pregnancy: The Toronto Leukaemia Study Group experience with long-term follow-up of children exposed in utero to chemotherapeutic agents. *J Clin Oncol* 1987; **5**:1098–106.
12. Lethaby AE, O'Neill MA, Mason B et al. Overall survival from breast cancer in women pregnant or lactating at or after diagnosis. *Int J Cancer* 1996; **67**:751–5.
13. Berry DL, Theriault RL, Holmes FA et al. Management of breast cancer during pregnancy using a standardised protocol. *J Clin Oncol* 1999; **17**:855–61.
14. Harvey JC, Rosen PP, Ashikari R et al. The effect of pregnancy on the prognosis of carcinoma of the breast following radical mastectomy. *Surg Gynecol Obstet* 1981; **153**:723–5.
15. Mignot L, Morvan F, Berdah J et al. Pregnancy after breast cancer. Results of a case-control study. *Presse Med* 1986; **15**:1961–4.
16. Ariel I, Kempner R. The prognosis of patients who become pregnant after mastectomy for breast cancer. *Int Surg* 1989; **74**:185.

17. von Schoultz E, Johansson H, Wilking N, Rutquist LE. Influence of prior and subsequent pregnancy on breast cancer prognosis. *J Clin Oncol* 1995; 13:430–4.

18. Guerra B, De Simone P, Gabrielli S, Falco P, Montanari G, Bovicelli L. Combined cytology and colposcopy to screen for cervical cancer in pregnancy. *J Reprod Med* 1998; 43:647–53.

19. Baldauf JJ, Dreyfus M, Ritter J, Philippe E. Colposcopy and directed biopsy reliability during pregnancy: a cohort study. *Eur J Obst Gynecol Reprod Biol* 1995; 62:31–6.

20. Hacker NF, Berek JS, Lagasse LD et al. Carcinoma of the cervix associated with pregnancy. *Obstet Gynecol* 1982; 59:735–46.

21. Yost NP, Santoso JT, McIntire DD, Iliya FA. Postpartum regression rates of antepartum cervical intraepithelial neoplasia II and III. *Obstet Gynecol* 1999; 93:359–62.

22. Hannigan EV, Whitehouse HH, Atkinson WD, Becker SN. Cone biopsy during pregnancy. *Obstet Gynecol* 1982; 60:450–5.

23. Lieberman RW, Henry MR, Laskin WB, Walenga J, Buckner SB, O'Connor DM. Colposcopy in pregnancy; directed brush cytology compared with cervical biopsy. *Obstet Gynecol* 1999; 94:198–203.

24. Robinson W, Webb S, Tirpack J et al. Management of cervical intraepithelial neoplasia during pregnancy with LOOP excision. *Gynecol Oncol* 1997; 64:153–5.

25. Connor JP. Noninvasive cervical cancer complicating pregnancy. *Obstet Gynecol Clin North Am* 1998; 25:331–42.

26. Duggan B, Muderspach LI, Roman LD, Curtin JP, d'Ablaing G, Morrow P. Cervical cancer in pregnancy: reporting on planned delay in therapy. *Obstet Gynecol* 1993; 82:598–602.

27. Creasman WT, Rutledge F, Smith JP. Carcinoma of the ovary associated with pregnancy. *Obstet Gynecol* 1971; 38:111.

28. Thornton JG, Wells M. Ovarian cysts in pregnancy: does ultrasound make traditional management inappropriate? *Obstet Gynecol* 1987; 69:717.

29. Boulay R, Podczaski E. Ovarian cancer complicating pregnancy. *Obstet Gynecol Clin North Am* 1998; 25:385–99.

30. MacKie RM, Bufalino R, Morabito A. Lack of effect of pregnancy on outcome of melanoma. *Lancet* 1991; 337:653–5.

Infection

Joanna C. Gillham

MRCOG standards

- Conduct booking visit, including assessment of intercurrent disease.
- Diagnose and plan management with appropriate consultation in the following conditions: intercurrent infection and infectious disease.

  In addition, we would suggest the following.

Theoretical skills
- Have general knowledge of the immune system.
- Understand how the immune system may be changed in pregnancy.
- Have comprehensive knowledge of the common infectious diseases.
- Know the microbiology of the underlying disease.
- Understand epidemiology, aetiology, clinical symptoms/signs, investigations and treatment of each disease and how these can change in pregnancy.

Practical skills
- Recognize the clinical presentation of disease and perform the necessary investigations.
- Be able to treat infectious disease appropriately, with multidisciplinary team involvement.
- Be able to conduct pre-pregnancy counselling if needed; be aware of the maternal and fetal implications of the disease.
- Understand the requirement for antenatal, intrapartum and postnatal intervention.

INTRODUCTION

The body has a natural resistance to infection, with the ability to 'acquire' resistance to pathogens through natural exposure and vaccines. Immune defences at the body surface are the epithelial barriers of skin and the mucous membranes. Secretory immunoglobulin (Ig) A is found on the mucosa and provides the ability to resist proteolytic enzymes. Chemical factors, for example gastric acid, are active against certain gut pathogens and the low pH maintained in urine and vaginal secretions helps to inhibit their growth. Natural antibodies are present in extracellular fluids. Organisms may be carried by the lymphatics and trapped in lymph nodes, where they may become a target for phagocytosis by macrophages. Alternatively, they can enter the circulation, where they may be ingested by neutrophils or phagocytic cells in the liver (Kupffer's cells), spleen, bone marrow, pituitary or adrenal gland.

Acquired resistance occurs when the presence of foreign antigens stimulates production of antibodies by plasma cells. The primary response is production of IgM. This is a large molecule that does not cross the placenta. Within 10–14 days, production of IgG begins; this smaller molecule becomes prominent, with the ability to cross the placenta.

Immunity is not always acquired by antibody production. Cell-mediated immunity via T-lymphocytes is important in fungal, viral and some bacterial infections (tuberculosis, syphilis, leprosy, brucellosis). T-lymphocytes possess the ability themselves to be cytotoxic or to produce lymphokines that activate and attract macrophages to the site of infection.

Pregnancy represents a relatively immunocompromised state, with hormonal and immunological changes. Various hormones made by the trophoblast have been shown to interfere with the induction of the immune response. These include progesterone and oestrogen, which inhibit cytotoxic T-cells and natural killer cells. These physiological alterations in immunoregulation may help support the feto-placental allograph, but may expose the mother to increased susceptibility to various pathogens.

VIRAL INFECTIONS

Relevant viral infections

- Herpes viruses: herpes simplex, varicella zoster, cytomegalovirus, Epstein–Barr
- Parvoviruses: parvovirus B19
- Togaviruses: rubella
- Paramyxoviruses: measles
- Retroviruses: human immunodeficiency virus (HIV)
- Hepatitis viruses: hepatitis A, hepatitis B, hepatitis C, hepatitis D, hepatitis E.

Herpes viruses

All of the herpes virus group are composed of DNA.

Herpes simplex virus infection

This virus is classified into types 1 and 2. Type 1 herpes simplex virus (HSV) is classically associated with the oro-facial infections and encephalitis, HSV-2 with the genital manifestations. In reality, there is a great amount of overlap with these subtypes.[1]

EPIDEMIOLOGY AND AETIOLOGY

The virus is transmitted through close physical contact and sexual intercourse. HSV must contact mucosal surfaces or abraded skin to initiate infection. HSV type 1 is often contracted in childhood, with 80–90 per cent of the adult population having positive serology. Antibodies to both subtypes are thought to offer some cross-protection. The prevalence of type 1 HSV increases with decreasing socio-economic class. HSV-2 infections are acquired sexually, so their incidence begins to increase in adolescence. Both viruses establish latent infections in sensory neurons. In the oro-facial form, the virus can remain latent in the trigeminal nerve; in the genital disease, it remains in the sacral ganglia. There are many reactivation triggers: trauma, febrile illness, stress, menstruation and ultraviolet radiation. Immunocompromised patients can develop severe disseminated HSV infection involving multiple viscera.

PRESENTATION AND DIAGNOSIS

Primary infection in the facial area is often asymptomatic. If lesions appear, they can involve the lips, eyes and face. Most characteristic are painful lesions of the oral mucosa. A first attack of genital herpes is usually more severe and symptomatic, presenting with multiple painful genital ulcers after a short incubation period. In 80–90 per cent of cases, primary genital herpes involves the vulva and cervix. All the skin lesions start with erythema, progressing to vesicles, then ulcers and finishing with crusting. These lesions can last up to 2 weeks.

Inguinal lymphadenopathy is associated with most primary cases. Fever, malaise and headaches are present in approximately 30 per cent patients. Retention of urine is a rare symptom. Recurrent infections tend to be less severe. Patients infected with HSV type 2 tend to suffer more frequent episodes. Local tingling and paraesthesiae are often noted 1–2 days before recurrent attack. Some viral carriers may be permanently asymptomatic.

Diagnosis is suggested by clinical history and examination. Swabs of the affected area for viral culture and isolation of the organism give definitive diagnosis. ELISA enables serological testing of HSV-specific IgG and IgM antibodies. This has limited value due to extensive cross-reactivity between HSV-1 and HSV-2; this makes it impossible to differentiate between primary, past and recurrent infection. Primary HSV infection can be shown if seroconversion can be demonstrated with paired sera. Polymerase chain reaction (PCR) detection of HSV DNA may be utilized.

Full sexually transmitted disease screening by a genitourinary clinic with appropriate contact screening and a cervical smear should be performed.

MANAGEMENT

This is an unpleasant disease with no cure. It is recurrent, which can lead to relationship and psychosexual problems, making specialist advice and counselling support mandatory. The patients need to be informed that when lesions are noted they are infectious, thus the need to refrain from sexual intercourse.

Treatment involves bathing lesions in warm saline, and simple analgesics. Initial genital or oral HSV infection can be treated with topical, oral or intravenous acyclovir. Topical therapy is less effective. Although intravenous acyclovir is the most effective treatment, oral acyclovir is normally preferable and adequate [II].[1] Secondary bacterial infection is treated with antibiotics. Rarely, hospital admission is needed for stronger analgesia, parenteral acyclovir or catheterization.

In relation to pregnancy

Antepartum   The relevant history should be appropriately documented, and the suggested mode of delivery should be discussed. There is no value in performing antepartum maternal viral cultures as they do not predict the infant's risk of exposure to HSV at delivery [II].[2]

Primary HSV infection has been associated with spontaneous abortion, stillbirth, intrauterine growth restriction (IUGR) and preterm labour. Owing to the increased susceptibility of the pregnant immune system, earlier recourse to intravenous acyclovir in suspected primary genital HSV infection is suggested. Management should involve a genitourinary physician. Acyclovir is tolerated in pregnancy and there is no clinical or laboratory evidence of maternal or fetal toxicity.[1]

If primary genital herpes occurs during pregnancy, treatment with daily suppressive acyclovir in the last 4 weeks of pregnancy may prevent recurrence at term. This could decrease the need for delivery by caesarean section [II].[3]

Intrapartum   The vulva and cervix should be carefully examined for herpes lesions when women present in labour. Caesarean section is recommended for all women presenting with first-episode genital herpes at the time of delivery. If the first episode is in the first or second trimester and there is no recurrence, a vaginal delivery is permitted. If the first episode is within 6 weeks of the due date, elective caesarean should be considered [II].[3]

There is no agreement on the use of caesarean section in the management of patients with a history of recurrent HSV. If a patient presents in early labour with a visible herpetic lesion, caesarean section is recommended. If a patient has frequent symptomatic recurrences during pregnancy, the use of acyclovir from 36 weeks is recommended, and vaginal delivery is not contraindicated [IV].[3]

Postpartum   If any oro-facial lesions are present, parents should be advised to refrain from close contact with the baby in that region. Breastfeeding is recommended unless the mother has lesions around the nipples. Acyclovir is excreted in breast milk but its use is not contraindicated and there are no harmful effects to the infant.

Fetal infection   The implications to the fetus of HSV infections are discussed in Chapter 13.

- There is no value in performing viral cultures in the antenatal period, as they have no predictive value for potential neonatal infection.
- There may be a role for treatment with daily suppressive acyclovir in the last 4 weeks of pregnancy. This may decrease the need for delivery by caesarean section.
- If the first episode of HSV is within 6 weeks of the due date, delivery by caesarean section should be considered.

KEY POINTS

- Management of these patients should be in conjunction with a genitourinary physician.
- Acyclovir is considered appropriate to use in pregnancy.
- Careful inspection of the vulva and vagina should be performed when a woman presents in labour. If there are any visible herpetic lesions, delivery by caesarean section is recommended.

Varicella zoster virus

Varicella zoster virus (VZV) has two distinct diseases: varicella (chickenpox) and herpes zoster (shingles).

EPIDEMIOLOGY AND AETIOLOGY

The primary infection is chickenpox, which commonly occurs in childhood. The virus enters through the mucosa of the upper respiratory tract and then remains latent in sensory and motor nerve cells. Recurrence tends to occur localized to one dermatome. Patients with both diseases are infective, the virus being spread by direct contact or airborne transmission.

PRESENTATION AND DIAGNOSIS

The incubation period for varicella is 14–21 days. Following a prodromal illness of fever and malaise, a florid pruritic rash erupts. Initially, a maculopapular rash, this rapidly turns to vesicles and then crusts over. The rash is commonly most extensive on the face and trunk, being minimal on the extremities. Patients are contagious from approximately 2 days before the onset of the rash until the vesicles have crusted over.

Primary varicella infection in adults is associated with more complications: pneumonia, encephalitis and hepatitis are the most common.

Shingles presents with painful and pruritic vesicles along a single sensory or motor nerve. Rarely, there can be systemic involvement with this reactivation, involving multiple visceral inflammation. This tends to be associated with significant immunosuppression.

In both manifestations the clinical presentation of the disease is classical enough to make a confident diagnosis clinically. Laboratory tests are available, and measure IgM and IgG anti-varicella antibodies.

MANAGEMENT

Although available, VZV vaccination is not routinely used in the UK.

Chickenpox in childhood is usually a self-limiting illness, with both anti-pruritic and anti-pyretic measures being taken to alleviate the symptoms. The non-pregnant adult needs to be more closely monitored, with evidence of any systemic symptoms needing prompt evaluation and treatment by a specialist medical team. Antibiotics may be required for subsequent secondary infection of the vesicles. Routine oral antivirals are not required, but intravenous antiviral agents are utilized with systemic VZV.

In relation to pregnancy

More than 90 per cent of the antenatal population is seropositive for VZV IgG antibody. Thus potential contact with affected individuals in pregnancy is high, but primary VZV is uncommon – affecting approximately 3/1000 pregnancies.

Antepartum   A past history of chickenpox should be sought. If there is no positive history, pregnant women should be advised about avoidance of contact with the disease and to contact healthcare personnel immediately if exposure occurs. If a suspected non-immune pregnant woman has contact with VZV, her VZV antibody status should be investigated. This can usually be performed within 24–48 hours on either a current blood sample or serum stored from blood tests performed at the antenatal booking visit.

As pregnancy may confer a mildly immunocompromised state, if the mother is not immune to VZV, she should be given VZV immunoglobulin (VZIG). This is effective up to 10 days after contact, but does not absolutely preclude development of the disease [IV].[4]

The UK Advisory Group on Chickenpox recommends that oral acyclovir be prescribed for pregnant women if they present within 24 hours of the onset of the rash and are over 20 weeks' gestation. VZIG is of no benefit once chickenpox has developed. Hospital assessment and intravenous acyclovir are required for those patients with varicella pneumonia, those over 36 weeks' gestation and patients with clinical deterioration after day 6 of the rash [IV].[4]

The obstetrician, the infectious disease team and the virologist should manage pregnant women with chickenpox. A neonatologist is required to be involved should the disease onset coincide with the delivery period.

The risk of developing secondary complications is increased in cigarette smokers and in patients with chronic lung disease, immunosuppression, and prolonged courses of steroids.

Intrapartum   Delivery during the viraemic period can be hazardous to both the mother and baby. Thus treatment with acyclovir is recommended and delivery postponed, if appropriate, until 5 days after the onset of maternal illness. Delaying delivery decreases the maternal complications of bleeding, thrombocytopenia and disseminated intravascular coagulation. It also allows time for transfer of protective antibodies from the mother to the fetus, thus decreasing the incidence of varicella of the newborn, which has high associated morbidity and mortality [IV].[4]

Maternal shingles at the time of delivery is not a risk to the neonate, as transplacentally acquired antibodies will already be in the fetal system.

Fetal infection   The implications to the fetus of VZV infections are discussed in Chapter 13.

- If a confirmed non-immune pregnant women has contact with chickenpox, she should be offered VZVIG.
- If a pregnant woman presents within 24 hours of onset of VZV rash, oral acyclovir should be administered.
- Delivery in the viraemic period should be avoided if at all possible. Ideally, delivery should be delayed until 5 days after the onset of the maternal illness. This allows transplacental transfer of antibodies.

KEY POINTS

- If a suspected non-immune pregnant woman has contact with VZV, her immunological status should be ascertained.
- If infection with VZV occurs in pregnancy, management should involve a physician with a specialist interest in infectious diseases.
- Consider admission to hospital and intravenous acyclovir if the woman is >36 weeks' gestation, has any signs of varicella pneumonia or has any clinical deterioration.

Cytomegalovirus
EPIDEMIOLOGY AND AETIOLOGY
Transmission can be horizontal via direct human-to-human contact and with sexual activity. Cytomegalovirus (CMV) is excreted in saliva, urine, semen, cervical secretions, stool and tears. It can be transmitted via blood transfusion and organ transplantation. Vertical transmission can occur during pregnancy, delivery and breastfeeding. Viral shedding from the cervix increases as the pregnancy advances in gestation. The lungs, liver, kidney and salivary glands are the most commonly affected organs.

PRESENTATION AND DIAGNOSIS
In healthy adults, the presentation is indistinguishable from infectious mononucleosis. Fever and malaise are typical, with lymphadenopathy. The blood picture shows a lymphocytosis, with atypical lymphocytes. Haemolytic anaemia, thrombocytopenia and deranged liver function tests may be present. This disease runs a benign course.

Disseminated, sometimes fatal, infection occurs in the immunocompromised, particularly transplant recipients and patients with acquired immunodeficiency syndrome (AIDS). The varied manifestations include encephalitis, retinitis, pneumonitis and involvement of the gastrointestinal tract. Virology of the urine, saliva, blood, cerebrospinal fluid or nasopharynx secretions is diagnostic. Serological tests can identify past or current infection. Other less utilized tests are detection of monoclonal antibodies to CMV antigens and PCR. However, IgM levels rise with reactivation and cannot therefore be used as a marker for first infection.

MANAGEMENT
In the normal adult population, infection with CMV will largely go unrecognized. Treatment is directed at alleviation of the symptoms.

In relation to pregnancy
There are no implications from a maternal health point of view.

Fetal infection

The implications to the fetus of CMV infections are discussed in Chapter 13.

Epstein–Barr virus

EPIDEMIOLOGY AND AETIOLOGY

This virus causes infectious mononucleosis, commonly referred to as 'glandular fever'. The commonest affected age groups are adolescents and young adults. Transmission is via saliva and aerosol droplets. Epstein–Barr virus (EBV) is considered to be the aetiological agent for Burkitt's lymphoma and nasopharngeal carcinoma.

PRESENTATION AND DIAGNOSIS

The predominant symptoms are fever, malaise, sore throat and headache. A petechial rash on the soft palate and a macular rash are common. These rashes typically occur in 90 per cent of patients who have been treated with ampicillin for their sore throat. Characteristic features are cervical lymphadenopathy and splenomegaly. Mild hepatitis is common. Rare complications include meningitis, myocarditis and mesenteric adenitis. In the majority of cases, this is a self-limiting illness, but it can run a protracted course, with the patient feeling debilitated for several months.

Peripheral blood film shows atypical mononuclear cells. Serological tests for specific EBV IgM antibodies can demonstrate recent infection. The two classical tests for the virus are the monospot test and the Paul–Bunnell reaction. The latter detects antibodies that agglutinate sheep erythrocytes. False-positive results can occur in hepatitis, Hodgkin's disease and acute leukaemia.

MANAGEMENT

In the majority of cases, no specific treatment is required, although corticosteroid treatment may be necessary if there is neurological involvement.

In relation to pregnancy

There are no special features involving the pregnant woman, and no known effects of vertical transmission.

Parvoviruses

Human parvovirus B19

The virus is a single-stranded DNA virus. This is a common infection, particularly in infants and younger children, alternatively known as erythema infectiosum or 'Fifth's disease'.

EPIDEMIOLOGY AND AETIOLOGY

Aerosol droplets and exchange of bodily fluids transmit this virus. Fifty to eighty per cent of adults are seropositive.

PRESENTATION AND DIAGNOSIS

Children typically have a fever and a bright erythematous, photosensitive malar rash – the 'slapped cheek rash'. Most adult infections are asymptomatic. The rash is less prominent but more widespread, involving the face, trunk and extremities. Chronic bone marrow failure can occur in the immunocompromised. Those patients with hereditary blood dyscrasias, for example sickle cell anaemia, are susceptible to aplastic crises.

Serological testing is required for diagnosis, as the clinical presentation is similar to that of a number of viral syndromes. The presence of IgG to parvovirus B19 can confirm immunity. If this is not confirmed, paired rising titres 10–14 days after exposure or the presence of specific IgM antibody can indicate those at risk of fetal infection. PCR can detect parvovirus B19 DNA in maternal sera.

MANAGEMENT

In healthy individuals this is normally a self-limiting illness, with no specific therapy being warranted.

In relation to pregnancy

Spontaneous abortion and intrauterine fetal death have been associated with parvovirus B19 infection. All pregnant women presenting with a non-vesicular rash compatible with a viral infection should be investigated for rubella and parvovirus B19 infection [IV]. When serology shows potential for early infection with parvovirus B19, the patient should be referred to a fetal medicine unit capable of fetal blood sampling and intravascular transfusion [IV].[5]

Fetal infection

The implications to the fetus of parvovirus B19 infections are discussed in Chapter 13.

Togaviruses

Rubella

EPIDEMIOLOGY AND AETIOLOGY

This is a fragile, single-stranded RNA virus, easily killed by heat and ultraviolet light. Spread is via respiratory droplets or in-utero transmission.

PRESENTATION AND DIAGNOSIS

The incubation period varies between 14 and 21 days. Malaise and fever are the common clinical features, with conjunctivitis and lymphadenopathy (particularly post-auricular and suboccipital). The classical rash is a pink/red macular type, starting on the forehead and spreading to the trunk and limbs. Rare complications are secondary pulmonary bacterial infection, arthralgia, encephalitis and haemorrhagic manifestations due to thrombocytopenia.

The diagnosis is usually clinical, but can be confirmed by culturing the virus from urine, nasopharynx or cerebrospinal fluid. Serological testing for rubella IgG and IgM is available.

MANAGEMENT

This disease is usually self-limiting, and treatment is symptomatic.

In relation to pregnancy

Rubella infection in pregnancy does not confer increased risk to the mother; it is the devastating teratogenic effects of this virus that are of concern (see Chapter 13). Human Ig can decrease the symptoms of the disease, but does not prevent the teratogenicity.

All children are offered the vaccine in the form of the MMR (measles, mumps and rubella) injection at approximately 15 months of age. All susceptible women who are receiving healthcare should ideally have their serological state tested. Opportunistic testing for this can be performed, for example family planning clinics, infertility investigation. If immunity to rubella is not confirmed, the vaccine should be offered. It is recommended that pregnancy should be avoided for 1 month after the vaccine is administered.

Antepartum   The routine booking bloods taken in the antenatal period include serological testing for the presence of rubella antibodies. If not immune, the patient should be counselled about avoidance of any affected persons.

All pregnant women presenting with a non-vesicular rash compatible with a viral infection should be investigated for rubella and parvovirus B19 infection, irrespective of a prior history of rubella vaccination or previous positive rubella antibody tests [IV].

Postpartum   For non-immune individuals, the opportunity should be taken to administer the vaccine in the post-delivery period. With hospital delivery, the vaccine is given on discharge from the hospital.

Fetal infection   The implications to the fetus of rubella infections are discussed in Chapter 13.

Paramyxoviruses

Measles

This is a highly contagious virus, mostly occurring in childhood. Immunization in early infancy is with the MMR vaccine. This acute febrile illness is associated with high morbidity and mortality, particularly in developing countries.

EPIDEMIOLOGY AND AETIOLOGY

The virus is spread by respiratory droplets.

PRESENTATION AND DIAGNOSIS

The incubation period varies from 8 to 14 days. The viraemic phase is prior to the classical measles rash developing. This is characterized by fever, malaise, rhinorrhoea, cough, conjunctivitis and small greyish spots on the buccal mucosa (Koplick's spots). A maculopapular rash then occurs, initially on the face, then spreading to the rest of the body. Complications include otitis media, bacterial pneumonia, myocarditis, hepatitis and encephalomyelitis. Infection in the adult is rare, but often a more severe illness.

Diagnosis is made on clinical symptoms and signs. Rarely used serological tests include a haemagglutination inhibition antibody that is present by the onset of the rash and remains positive for life.

MANAGEMENT

Treatment is symptomatic.

In relation to pregnancy

As with any acute febrile illness, measles can precipitate spontaneous miscarriage or premature labour. No teratogenic effects of this virus are recognized.

Retroviruses

Human immunodeficiency virus

This virus affects the normal immune cells of the body. AIDS occurs when the immune system is so depleted that unusual infections from bacteria and viruses develop. On average, it takes 8–10 years from infection with HIV to the development of AIDS.

EPIDEMIOLOGY AND AETIOLOGY

Infection with HIV occurs through sexual contact and contact with infected blood. Women are more likely to be infected through sexual contact than men. Risk factors are frequent unprotected sexual intercourse with different partners and intravenous drug abuse. The presence of other sexually transmitted infections increases shedding of HIV. Perinatal transmission can occur in utero, intrapartum or through breastfeeding. In the majority of cord blood samples, HIV is not detected, thus suggesting that the majority of transmission is not in the antenatal period.[6]

In relation to pregnancy

Antepartum   Voluntary testing for HIV should be an integral part of antenatal care, offered and recommended to all pregnant women, irrespective of their risk factors. Joint care is required from the beginning of pregnancy with a physician expert in HIV.

In HIV-positive women, the initial booking visit should include a thorough history and physical examination. Baseline examination should include fundoscopy, neurological and pelvic examination. The initial visit should include counselling about the perinatal transmission of HIV and the importance of compliance with antiretroviral regimens. All treatment should be performed in a multidisciplinary setting, with involvement of other relevant health professionals. If appropriate, patients should be referred for drug treatment and/or detoxification programmes.

The implications of serum screening need to be discussed due to the recommended avoidance of invasive sampling procedures. Otherwise, screening should be undertaken as for all pregnant individuals, with the addition of screening for hepatitis C, tuberculosis, bacterial vaginosis and other sexually transmitted diseases. Baseline antibody titres of *Toxoplasma gondii* and CMV should be obtained. Liver function tests need to be performed. HIV viral load and CD4⁺ lymphocyte count should be measured at the initial visit and repeated each trimester to follow response to therapy or to detect indications for therapy.

Prophylaxis of opportunistic infections during pregnancy should be based on criteria similar to those for non-pregnant women with HIV. These opportunistic infections are *Pnemocystis carinii* pneumonia, *Mycobacterium avium* infection, toxoplasmosis, tuberculosis and herpes simplex virus.

It is estimated that approximately 6000 women of child-bearing age worldwide acquire HIV infection each day. Approximately 98 per cent of HIV-infected children have acquired the virus from their mothers – during pregnancy, at delivery or through breastfeeding. Thus prevention of mother-to-child transmission is a major health priority. Varying mother-to-child transmission rates have been quoted, ranging from 13–25 per cent in Europe to 35 per cent in developing countries. Risk factors for transmission include maternal viral load, maternal clinical and immunological status, mode of delivery, prematurity and breastfeeding. Possible strategies to decrease the risk of mother-to-child transmission of HIV infection are delivery by elective caesarean section, lavage of the birth canal, vitamin A supplementation and antenatal/intrapartum/neonatal antiretroviral therapy.[7]

The presence of the virus in blood and mucus in the vagina may increase the risk of transmission in vaginal delivery. Thus the benefits of vaginal cleansing with antiseptic and virucidal agents during delivery have been investigated in several developing countries. The efficacy of chlorhexidine solution in reducing transmission was evaluated in a large controlled trial conducted in Malawi.[6] Although this study failed to reduce mother-to-child transmission overall, two positive results were obtained: in women with premature rupture of membranes, chlorhexidine disinfection was associated with reduced transmission, and overall neonatal and maternal morbidity and mortality from infectious causes were statistically reduced with the medical intervention [Ib].[6]

Vitamin A deficiency was proposed as a possible factor increasing the vertical transmission rate. Vitamin A has a stimulatory effect on the immune system and helps to maintain the integrity of mucosal surfaces. Both pregnancy and HIV are risk factors for vitamin A deficiency. Unsurprisingly, a study in Malawi showed a high proportion of the women had vitamin A deficiency, which was associated with a three-to-four-fold increased risk of vertical transmission.[8] Nutritional intervention is practical, inexpensive and applicable for developing countries [II].

HIV-positive pregnant women should receive the same antiretroviral treatment as non-pregnant women. Antiretroviral therapy should not be withheld unless clear maternal or fetal contraindications to standard therapy exist. The choice of therapy should be individualized, based on the woman's

clinical, virological and immunological status, as well as the gestational age of the fetus. Women with stable CD4⁺ counts and undetectable viral loads who are already on an antiretroviral regimen prior to pregnancy should continue on the same therapy, even during the first trimester. For women diagnosed with HIV infection during the first trimester, treatment should be delayed until the second trimester.

The AIDS Clinical Trial Group (ACTG) 076 trial of zidovudine (ZDV) administered this drug to mothers in pregnancy (14–34 weeks' gestation) and delivery and to the newborn for 6 weeks. They showed that transmission could be reduced by as much as two-thirds, reducing to 8.3 per cent [Ib].

Currently, the ZDV regimen is not suitable for developing countries, due to its long, expensive and complicated administration schedule. ZDV needs to be taken orally from the second trimester. It should be administered by intravenous infusion at the time of delivery and then taken by the child during the first 4–6 weeks after birth.

Pregnancy has not been shown to have an adverse affect on the natural history of HIV. No benefit to maternal health from termination of pregnancy has been demonstrated.

HIV is non-teratogenic.

The issue of associated drug abuse is discussed in Chapter 6.12.

Intrapartum   A meta-analysis of six observational, prospective studies showed a reduction of approximately 30 per cent in transmission with delivery by caesarean section.[9] However, this analysis was based on a crude comparison of transmission rates and was unable to control for potential confounding factors [Ia]. The European Collaborative Study suggested a reduction of HIV transmission by up to 50 per cent.[10] However, any potential protective benefit of caesarean section has to be balanced against its risks and costs. Morbidity is more common and severe in HIV-infected women. The implications of caesarean section for the health of the mother and child are particularly fraught in developing countries. If there is longer than 4 hours between rupture of the membranes and delivery, the value of caesarean section is decreased.

The current American College of Obstetricians and Gynecologists guideline on HIV states that the additional benefit of caesarean section in women who have an undetectable viral load and who are on combination antiretroviral therapy is likely to be very marginal. This guideline recommends vaginal delivery when the viral load is <1000 copies. The current UK guidelines continue to recommend caesarean section for everybody.

Factors that increase the risk of vertical transmission of HIV are advanced stage of HIV infection, low CD4⁺ count, high viral HIV RNA load, invasive needling procedures (amniocentesis, artificial rupture of membranes), prolonged interval between rupture of membranes and delivery, use of fetal scalp electrode in labour, ascending bacterial infection of the placental–fetal unit during the peripartum period, and vitamin A deficiency.

Factors that decrease the risk of vertical transmission of HIV are undetectable maternal HIV RNA, ZDV administration [Ia],[11] nevirapine administration [Ia],[11] caesarean section, treatment of associated sexually transmitted diseases, and highly active antiretroviral therapy (HAART).

Fetal infection   A high serum viral load significantly increases the likelihood of newborn infection. The avoidance of breastfeeding is recommended.

- Vaginal lavage in labour does not decrease the overall mother-to-child transmission rate of HIV. However, transmission in premature rupture of membranes is reported to be decreased with this intervention, as is overall neonatal and maternal morbidity and mortality from infectious causes.
- Vitamin A deficiency appears to be associated with an increase in mother-to-child HIV transmission.
- The ACTG trial, showed a decrease in HIV transmission by two-thirds with the administration of ZDV in the antepartum and intrapartum periods.
- In HIV-positive women, delivery by elective caesarean section is recommended.
- There is an increase in the vertical transmission once the membranes have been ruptured for 4 hours. However, if a woman presents with this history, delivery by caesarean section is still recommended.
- Breastfeeding is contraindicated.

KEY POINTS

- Testing for HIV in the antenatal period should be offered to all women, irrespective of their supposed risk for the virus.
- If HIV positive, the care of the pregnant woman is managed jointly with a physician with a specialist interest in infectious disease.
- Increased mother-to-child transmission occurs with:
  - a low maternal CD4$^+$ count
  - high maternal HIV RNA load
  - invasive needling procedures in the antenatal period
  - invasive procedures during labour – artificial rupture of membranes (ARM), fetal blood sampling (FBS) and fetal scalp electrode (FSE)
  - prolonged interval between rupture of membranes and delivery
  - concurrent ascending bacterial infection
  - vitamin A deficiency.

- Decreased vertical transmission occurs with:
  - undetectable maternal HIV RNA
  - ZDV/nevirapine/HARRT administration
  - delivery by elective caesarean section
  - avoidance of breastfeeding.

Hepatitis viruses

Hepatitis A
EPIDEMIOLOGY AND AETIOLOGY
The virus is most commonly transmitted by the fecal–oral route by either person-to-person contact or ingestion of contaminated food or water. Hepatitis A is endemic in developing countries due to poor hygiene and sanitation.

PRESENTATION AND DIAGNOSIS
Acute hepatitis A infection is clinically indistinguishable from other causes of acute viral hepatitis. Most infected children under the age of 6 years are asymptomatic. In the older child and adult, clinical manifestations can vary from a mild, non-specific, anicteric infection to fulminant hepatic failure. Symptoms include fever, malaise, anorexia, nausea, vomiting and abdominal discomfort. Jaundice may be present, with dark urine and hepatomegaly. A raised serum alanine transaminase indicates acute hepatic injury. Infection can be diagnosed by the presence of anti-hepatitis A IgM.

MANAGEMENT
Treatment is supportive, and complete recovery with no long-term illness is the usual outcome. Administration of human serum immunoglobulin protects against hepatitis A by either preventing infection or attenuating symptoms. Protection is short lived, so injections needed to be repeated every 3–6 months. A vaccine is available and gives up to 10 years' protection.

In relation to pregnancy
Antepartum   Advice on travelling to areas where hepatitis A is endemic should be available. The safety of the hepatitis A vaccine in pregnancy has not been determined, although the theoretical risk to the fetus of an inactivated vaccine is low.

Fetal infection   There are no long-term fetal consequences of hepatitis A infection.

Hepatitis B
This is a blood-borne, double-stranded DNA virus. The virus has three major structural antigens: surface antigen (HbsAg), core antigen (HbcAg) and e antigen (HbeAg).

EPIDEMIOLOGY AND AETIOLOGY
This is an extremely infectious virus; the UK prevalence may be as high as 1 per cent in inner city areas, with high

proportions of immigrant women. Transmission of the virus is by bodily secretions (principally blood) and thus with sexual contact, blood transfusions, intravenous drug abuse and perinatal transmission.

CLINICAL PRESENTATION AND DIAGNOSIS

Infection with hepatitis B is often asymptomatic, except in intravenous drug abusers, of whom 30 per cent will develop jaundice. Non-specific symptoms and signs include nausea and vomiting, fatigue and malaise, photophobia and headache, right upper abdominal pain and diarrhoea. Physical examination of patients often shows no abnormality, although hepatomegaly (10 per cent of patients), splenomegaly (5 per cent) and lymphadenopathy (5 per cent) may be present.[12] Hepatitis B virus causes acute and chronic hepatitis and the chances of becoming chronically infected vary with age. Infected neonates and young children are more likely to develop chronic infection.

Acute hepatitis B is usually self-limiting and most patients who contract the virus will clear it completely. Fulminant hepatic failure occurs in about 1 per cent of cases. All cases must be notified and sexual and close household contacts screened and vaccinated.

Non-specific haematological tests commonly show a leucopenia, and may show anaemia and thrombocytopenia. Biochemistry reveals elevated serum aminotransferase.

Diagnosis is by the presence of HbsAg. The presence of HbeAg shows disease is active with viral shedding into the bloodstream. Antibodies to e begin to appear in the serum at the time HbeAg is disappearing. The presence of the e antigen indicates a period of high patient infectivity, as the presence of e antibodies indicates low infectivity. Complete resolution of the disease is indicated by the disappearance of HBsAg and the appearance of surface antibodies. These antibodies provide immunity, whether obtained from resolution of infection or vaccination with HbsAg.

MANAGEMENT

Patients should be monitored to ensure fulminant liver disease does not develop, and should have serological testing 3 months after infection to check the virus is cleared from the blood.

About 5–10 per cent of patients will remain positive for HbsAg at 3 months and a smaller proportion will have ongoing viral replication. These patients require follow-up by a hepatologist.[12]

Some individuals with chronic hepatitis B will have clinically insignificant or minimal liver disease and never go on to develop complications. Long-term sequelae can be the development of cirrhosis/hepatocellular carcinoma.

In relation to pregnancy

Antepartum   All women are routinely offered testing for hepatitis B antibodies at their antenatal booking visit. If testing positive for the first time, the infectious state of the patient should be ascertained by serology. Relevant issues include testing of the partner, testing for other sexually transmitted disease including HIV, and safe sexual practice.

The presence of hepatitis B does not seem to pose additional risk for the pregnancy.

Intrapartum   Fetal scalp electrodes and fetal blood sampling should be avoided. The use of forceps rather than ventouse has been suggested as most appropriate for instrumental delivery.

Postpartum   Neonates infected at birth have a >90 per cent chance of becoming chronic carriers of hepatitis B virus, with the associated risks of subsequent cirrhosis and hepatocellular carcinoma. Management plans should thus include administration of passive immunoglobulin in the first 24 hours after birth to those neonates with mothers of high infectivity, and administration of the active hepatitis B vaccine to those neonates whose mothers have a low infectivity or those deemed to be going to an 'at-risk' household.

Provided babies are immunized, there is no contraindication to breastfeeding.

- There is limited research on the most appropriate mode of delivery for hepatitis-B-positive women. Thus, vaginal delivery is considered appropriate.
- Breastfeeding is permitted.

KEY POINTS

- If the patient tests positive for hepatitis B, her infectious state should be ascertained.
- Screen also for hepatitis C, HIV and all other sexually transmitted diseases.
- This disease appears to confer no increased risk on fetal well-being during pregnancy.
- Vertical transmission, usually at the time of delivery, is high, reaching 95 per cent in mothers who are both HBsAg positive and HbeAg positive.
- In labour, aim to keep the membranes intact for as long as possible. Avoid FBS/FSE use.
- Deliver in a way that confers least trauma to the baby. Forceps delivery is favoured over ventouse by many clinicians, although this is not evidence based.
- Administer hepatitis B immunoglobulin to those neonates born to high-infectivity mothers. Administer hepatitis B vaccine to those neonates born to low-infectivity mothers.

Hepatitis C
EPIDEMIOLOGY AND AETIOLOGY
As with hepatitis B, this virus can be transmitted sexually and perinatally. However, the main group of hepatitis-C-positive individuals is within the intravenous drug culture. A new injection drug user has an 80 per cent chance of becoming positive for hepatitis C antibody within 1 year.[13]

CLINICAL PRESENTATION AND DIAGNOSIS
The clinical features of hepatitis C are non-specific. It is often diagnosed when patients have vague symptoms and are revealed to have abnormal alanine transferase levels. Cirrhosis develops in 20–40 per cent of patients, and in these there is up to 3 per cent annual development of hepatocellular carcinoma.[13]

Early identification and referral of cases of acute hepatitis C infection are important, as there is strong evidence to suggest that early treatment with alpha-interferon reduces the risk of chronic infection. The rate of chronicity in untreated patients is approximately 80 per cent.[12] Antibodies to hepatitis C appear relatively late in the course of the infection and if clinical suspicion is high, the patient's serum should be tested for hepatitis C RNA to establish a diagnosis.

MANAGEMENT
In relation to pregnancy
Antepartum   Systematic screening for HCV is not indicated. Screening is indicated in high-risk groups or if a women tests positive for hepatitis B virus or HIV. Antenatal care should involve a physician with a specialist interest in hepatitis C. With a positive hepatitis C virus test, the woman should be counselled about the risk of giving birth to an infected newborn and about the higher infection rate if there is co-existent HIV. Hepatitis C virus RNA determination is useful because, if negative, these patients can be counselled about the lower transmission rate.

Intrapartum   This management is the same as for hepatitis B. Further research is required into whether delivery by caesarean section will reduce transmission.

Postpartum   There is no contraindication to breastfeeding.

Fetal infection   Vertical transmission rates vary greatly in reported studies, although most rates are in the range 10–15 per cent.[12] Increased perinatal transmission occurs in women who have high titres of hepatitis C virus RNA or who are co-infected with HIV.

- There is limited knowledge about the appropriate mode of delivery in hepatitis-C-positive women. Thus vaginal delivery is permitted.
- Breastfeeding does not appear to increase the risk of mother-to-child transmission.

KEY POINTS
- Screening for hepatitis C is not routinely offered in the antenatal period.
- There is increased mother-to-child transmission with detectable maternal hepatitis C virus RNA and if there is co-existent HIV infection.
- Intrapartum management is the same as for hepatitis B individuals.
- There is no neonatal immunoprophylaxis available.

No immunoprophylaxis is available at this time.

Hepatitis D
This is a single-stranded RNA virus that requires co-infection with hepatitis B virus. It often increases the severity of the illness. It is usually confined to intravenous drug abusers in the UK.

Hepatitis E
This virus is transmitted by the fecal–oral route and produces a self-limiting illness similar to hepatitis A. It is common in the developing world. Pregnant women with acute hepatitis E infection have a risk of fulminant liver failure of around 15 per cent, with a mortality of 5 per cent.

BACTERIAL INFECTIONS

Gonorrhoea

Epidemiology and aetiology
The bacterium *Neisseria gonorrhoeae* is a Gram-negative, intracellular diplococcus that can be found in the epithelium of the genitourinary tract and in the rectum, pharynx and eye. *N. gonorrhoeae* can ascend, causing uterine and tubal infection. It is a sexually transmitted disease. Risk factors include multiple or casual sexual contacts, 20–24 years of age, past or current history of illicit drug use and low socioeconomic status.

Presentation and diagnosis
The incubation period is approximately 10 days. The commonest symptom is an increased vaginal discharge, classically a purulent yellow-green. Other symptoms are vaginal itching or burning, bleeding during or after intercourse, urethritis, dysuria and tender Skene's or Bartholin's glands. Between 30 and 60 per cent of infected women will have asymptomatic or subclinical infection.

Infections that are not treated or are treated inadequately may spread from the lower genital tract to the endometrium and fallopian tubes – pelvic inflammatory disease. Silent episodes of pelvic inflammatory disease can occur, grossly affecting the reproductive capacity of the woman, increasing the risk of tubal infertility/ectopic pregnancy and causing chronic lower abdominal pain.

Disseminated gonococcal infection is rare, involving fever, arthritis and skin disorders. It is reported to be more common in pregnancy.

The diagnosis is culture of the gonococcal organism from endocervical, urethral, anal or pharyngeal swabs. A quicker, less sensitive method is the demonstration of the Gram-negative diplococci on direct microscopy. PCR can demonstrate gonoccocal DNA, and is an accurate but expensive test.

Management

Management of the patient should involve a genitourinary physician. Classical treatment of gonorrhoea was by penicillin, but large-scale resistance is occurring by the organism. In the non-pregnant, treatment is with a quinolone, for example ciprofloxacin/ofloxacin. Concomitant treatment for chlamydia should be given, as these infections co-exist in 45 per cent of cases.

Management plans should include avoidance of sexual intercourse until treatment is completed, eradication of the organism (confirmed with follow-up cultures), contact tracing with treatment of affected partners, and advice on safe sex practices.

IN RELATION TO PREGNANCY
Antepartum
Acute gonococcal infection is associated with miscarriage, premature labour, pre-labour rupture of membranes, chorioamnionitis and small for gestational age fetus. It has also been associated with stillbirth.

During pregnancy, recommended treatment is with a cephalosporin or spectinomycin. Dilatation and curettage after a miscarriage or for a termination of pregnancy has an increased risk of endometritis if the organism is present. Thus, ideally, vaginal swabs are performed prior to this surgery.

Intrapartum
Neisseria gonorrhoeae can be transmitted from the mother's genital tract to the neonate during labour. The usual manifestation of neonatal infection is gonococcal ophthalmia neonatorum, which has a risk of transmission of 30–50 per cent, which is increased with premature rupture of membranes and premature delivery. It occurs in the first few days of life, presenting as a bilateral, purulent, conjunctivitis. Prompt identification and treatment are necessary, as resulting blindness can occur.

Postpartum
Gonorrhoea can cause endometritis and pelvic sepsis.

Meningococcal disease

This is any clinical condition caused by Gram-negative aerobic bacterium *Neisseria meningitidis*. The most prevalent subtypes in Europe are B and C. The conditions include purulent conjunctivitis, septic arthritis, meningitis, and septicaemia with or without meningitis.

Epidemiology and aetiology
In the UK, the incidence varies from 2 to 8 cases/100 000 people. Outbreaks may occur among family contacts, school children and students. It is transmitted by close contact, by exchange of upper respiratory tract secretions. The age peaks are under 2 years and between 15 and 24 years of age. Carriage of meningococcus in the nasopharynx has been reported to be 10–15 per cent.

Presentation and diagnosis
Meningitis typically presents with headache, fever, neck stiffness, nausea, vomiting and photophobia. Meningococcaemia is characterized by a petechial or purpuric rash. When meningococcus reaches the bloodstream, there is massive production of endotoxin, and shock and disseminated intravascular coagulation are induced. This can lead to hypotension and multi-organ failure. The mortality rate of fulminant meningococcal septicaemia is approximately 30 per cent. Classical diagnosis is culture of the organism, but this has a low sensitivity, especially if antibiotics have been administered prior to the sample. Gram staining or methods detecting polysaccharide antigen can obtain rapid results. Serological testing and PCR can also be utilized.

Management

Prompt recognition and treatment are essential, as the case fatality is 10–20 per cent. Treatment is with penicillin or cephalosporin, for example ceftriaxone. Antibiotics are recommended in people exposed to someone with meningococcal disease – rifampacin, ceftriaxone or ciprofloxacin. There are vaccines available for the serogroups A and C; these are only effective in older children and adults.

IN RELATION TO PREGNANCY

The presentation and treatment of the disease are the same in the pregnant woman. As with any acute febrile illness, miscarriage and premature labour are associated complications. There are no teratogenic effects of the pathogen.

Listeria

Listeria monocytogenes is a Gram-positive bacterium. Unusually for a bacterium that does not form spores, it is very resistant to the effects of freezing, drying and heat.

Epidemiology and aetiology

Up to 10 per cent of humans may carry *Listeria* in their intestinal tract. The infective consequences depend on both the strain of the pathogen and the susceptibility of the victim. Most healthy people are unaware of an infection with *Listeria*. The vulnerable groups are the immunocompromised, pregnant women and the newborn. *Listeria* has been associated with ingestion of various contaminated foods, including raw milk, soft cheese, ice cream, raw meat and vegetables, and is associated with ready-to-eat meals.

Presentation and diagnosis

The symptoms of listeria can be non-specific, with influenza-like symptoms and fever, nausea and vomiting. Complications are septicaemia and meningo-encephalitis.

Diagnosis is by culture of the organism from blood, cerebrospinal fluid or stool or from serological testing.

Management

Treatment is with penicillin.

IN RELATION TO PREGNANCY
Antepartum

Listeria infection predisposes to miscarriage, premature labour and stillbirth, thus advice pertaining to the avoidance of danger foodstuffs during pregnancy should be given.

Meconium presence in liquor at very premature gestation has been associated with *Listeria* infection.

Other bacterial infections are discussed in relevant chapters elsewhere in this book: urinary tract infections/pyelonephritis in Chapter 6.6, bacterial vaginosis in Chapter 21 and group B *Streptococcus* in Chapter 21.

MYCOBACTERIUM INFECTION

Tuberculosis

The causative organism is *Mycobacterium tuberculosis*. This is a widespread disease, more common in the developing world.

Epidemiology and aetiology

Upper respiratory tract droplets spread the bacilli. Risk factors for infection are poor living conditions, overcrowding and poor nutrition. People are more susceptible at the extremes of age and if immunocompromised. There is an increased incidence in the immigrant population in the UK.

Presentation and diagnosis

There are two major patterns of disease with tuberculosis (TB). Primary TB is seen as an initial infection, usually in children. This is a non-specific illness, with a cough and wheeze. The initial focus of infection is a small subpleural granuloma accompanied by hilar lymph node infection. In nearly all cases these granulomas resolve and there is no further spread of the infection.

Secondary TB, seen mostly in adults, is a re-activation of previous disease, particularly if the health status of the person declines. The granulomatous inflammation is much more florid and widespread. In pulmonary TB there is typically a gradual onset of symptoms over weeks/months. Malaise, anorexia, weight loss, night sweats and purulent or blood-stained sputum predominate.

Miliary TB is the result of acute diffuse dissemination of tubercle bacilli via the bloodstream.

Sputum is positive for acid-fast bacilli when stained with Ziehl–Nielsen and cultures grown. The tuberculin skin test is based on the type 4 hypersensitivity reaction, i.e. with previous TB infection there will be sensitized lymphocytes that can react to another encounter with antigens from TB organisms. Injection with tuberculin will then produce a wheal and red induration. This test will also be positive if a person has been vaccinated with bacille Calmette–Guérin (BCG). A chest X-ray is required.

Management

Treatment and drug regimens are given by a specialist chest physician. Contact tracing is vital. BCG vaccination is traditionally given at approximately 13 years of age. In high-risk populations the vaccine is given in the neonatal period.

IN RELATION TO PREGNANCY
Antepartum

Tuberculosis discovered during pregnancy should be treated without delay, with immediate involvement of a chest physician. Isoniazid, rifampacin and ethambutol can be used in pregnancy. Pyridoxine is recommended for pregnant women taking isoniazid. No increase in morbidity and mortality from TB has been noted during pregnancy and there does not appear to be an increase in the relapse rate in pregnancy.[14] The one exception is in pregnant women with HIV infection previously infected with TB.

Intrapartum

Any patient with active disease should be isolated. Inhalational anaesthesia should be avoided.

Postpartum

The small concentration of anti-TB drugs in breast milk does not produce toxicity, so breastfeeding is permitted.[14] The neonate needs to be vaccinated with BCG and may need anti-tuberculous drugs.

Fetal infection

Congenital tuberculosis is rare.

TOXOPLASMOSIS

Toxoplasma gondii is an intracellular protozoan parasite.

Epidemiology and aetiology

The definitive host of this organism is the domestic cat. Transmission may occur transplacentally, by ingestion of raw or undercooked meat containing protozoan cysts, or by exposure to oocysts in soil/cat litter contaminated with cat faeces.

Presentation and diagnosis

Asymptomatic infections are common, and up to 80 per cent of some populations are infected. The disease mostly has no clinical consequences. Those at risk for severe disease are the developing fetus and the immunocompromised. Serological testing can demonstrate antibodies to *Toxoplasma gondii*, IgM antibody or significant changes in the IgG antibody titre, indicating recent infection.

Management

Treatment is with spiromycin.

IN RELATION TO PREGNANCY

Antenatal

Routine testing for immunity to toxoplasmosis is not undertaken in the UK. To minimize the risk, pregnant women should not eat undercooked meat or handle cat litter and should wear rubber gloves if gardening. Frequent hand washing is advised.

If testing is performed, present and past infection need to be carefully distinguished. Old toxoplasmosis infection does not pose a fetal risk.

It is not known whether antenatal treatment in women with toxoplasmosis reduces the congenital transmission of *Toxoplasma gondii* [Ia].

Fetal infection

The implications to the fetus of *Toxoplasma* infections are discussed in Chapter 13.

CHLAMYDIA

Chlamydia is the most prevalent bacterial sexually transmitted disease. It is an obligatory intracellular bacterium – *Chlamydia trachomatis* – that contains DNA and RNA. There are numerous serotypes, D–K being responsible for the oculogenital and sexually transmitted strains of the disease.[15]

Epidemiology and aetiology

Risk factors include multiple sexual partners, young age, history of other sexually transmitted diseases and low socio-economic class.

The cost-effectiveness of the screening and treatment of chlamydia has long been a subject of debate. The greatest rise in chlamydial infection over the past 10 years has been in the younger sexually active population – 16–19-year-old females. Although professional awareness of the infection is rising, genitourinary clinics remain the only setting in which nationwide screening of this often symptomatic but devastating disease is undertaken. Screening is recognized to significantly reduce the prevalence of genital tract infections and pelvic inflammatory disease. The prevalence of chlamydia varies considerably in different populations (1–29 per cent); restricted screening would be unlikely to have a great effect on its prevalence, as the general population makes limited use of genitourinary clinics.

After identifying demographic and behavioural risk factors, the Chlamydia Advisory Group concluded that, in addition to testing symptomatic patients and those in higher risk groups (people attending genitourinary clinics or those seeking termination of pregnancy), the evidence supported opportunistic screening. Recommendations were that screening should be offered to all sexually active women below the age of 25 years and to those over the age of 25 years with a new sexual partner or who have had two or more partners in the past year. Recommended screening is by the ligase reaction test on a first-catch urine sample, rather than the more invasive endocervical swabs of older, less accurate, tests such as ELISA.

Presentation and diagnosis

The incubation period is 7–21 days.

Infection with chlamydia can be asymptomatic in up to 75 per cent of cases. Symptoms are increased/unusual vaginal discharge, dyspareunia, intermenstrual bleeding, abdominal pain or dysuria.

The complications of inadequately treated or untreated chlamydia are pelvic inflammatory disease, chronic pelvic pain and salpingitis, thus increasing the risk of future ectopic pregnancies and/or tubal infertility. A perihepatitis can occur, the Fitz–Hugh–Curtis syndrome.

An endocervical swab and/or first void urine are suitable specimens for establishing the diagnosis. Cell culture of the organism is too expensive in non-endemic regions. The most commonly employed diagnostic tests are PCR and

Antenatal complications: maternal

ligase chain reaction. These amplification assays possess higher sensitivities than previously used enzyme immuno-assay tests.[15]

Management

These patients should be managed with input from the genitourinary clinic.

Contact tracing and treatment are essential – failure to treat partners is probably the commonest cause of 'treatment failure'. First-line agents for treatment outside pregnancy are doxycycline (for 1 week) or a single dose of azithromycin (better compliance but more expensive).

IN RELATION TO PREGNANCY

Antepartum

Antibiotic therapy in pregnancy reduces the number of women with positive cultures following treatment by approximately 90 per cent compared with placebo [Ia].[16]

Classical treatment of chlamydia is with tetracyclines, which are contraindicated in pregnancy. Erythromycin is an acceptable alternative, but can have gastrointestinal side effects and needs a full 7-day course. A recent Cochrane Review cites amoxicillin as an acceptable alternative therapy to erythromycin in pregnancy if the drug is not being tolerated. If amoxicillin/erythromycin are contraindicated or not tolerated, clindamycin or azithromycin (single dose/ fewer side effects compared to erythromycin) may be prescribed [Ia].[17]

Preterm labour, premature rupture of the membranes and low birth weight have also been associated with chlamydial infection.

Intrapartum

Perinatally transmitted *Chlamydia trachomatis* can cause conjunctivitis and pneumonitis. In untreated mothers, the incidence of conjunctivitis is 35–50 per cent and of pneumonitis 11–20 per cent. Conjunctivitis occurs earlier, typically between the fifth and twelfth postnatal days, with a mucoid discharge that becomes purulent, followed by oedema of the eyelids and conjunctival erythema. Pneumonia occurs later, at 2–3 weeks of age, with symptoms including tachypnoea and cough.

Postpartum

Chlamydia can cause postpartum endometritis.

- Antibiotic therapy decreases the number of pregnant women with positive cultures following treatment by 90 per cent.
- Typical treatment of this disease is with tetracyclines. These are contraindicated in pregnancy. Acceptable alternatives are amoxicillin or erythromycin.

KEY POINTS

- Screening for this disease is recommended for all those aged <25 years who are sexually active and all those aged >25 years who have had a new sexual partner in the last year or who have had two or more different partners.
- Screening should be performed on first-catch urine samples and analysed by the ligase chain reaction.
- This disease is asymptomatic in up to 75 per cent of cases.
- Classical symptoms are increased vaginal discharge, intermenstrual bleeding and dyspareunia.
- Pelvic complications are the same as for gonorrhoea.
- Management should be in conjunction with a genitourinary clinic.
- Contact tracing and treatment are vital.

SPIROCHAETES

Syphilis

This disease is caused by the spirochaete *Treponema pallidum* and is usually transmitted by sexual contact. It is a complex systemic disease with multiple clinical manifestations.

Epidemiology and aetiology

Humans are the natural hosts of *T. pallidum*. The organism usually penetrates abraded or damaged skin or mucous membrane, although intact membrane can be penetrated. Dissemination rapidly occurs. The average incubation period is 28 days.[18] There is an association between syphilis and HIV; it is not known whether syphilis predisposes individuals to HIV acquisition, or whether transmission of either disease is potentiated by the presence of the other.

Presentation and diagnosis

Infection with syphilis is characterized by several stages. Initial disease development is usually denoted by the appearance of a chancre (ulcer). This is the classical primary syphilis lesion at the site of inoculation, which is usually small, firm, round and painless. Most patients then develop secondary syphilis 3 weeks to 3 months after the primary stage. This is a systemic illness, with fever, malaise, lymphadenopathy, non-pruritic rash and mucosal lesions. Without treatment, these clinical manifestations usually resolve spontaneously. There is then a latent period.[18] In about one-third of untreated patients, latent syphilis develops subsequently into tertiary syphilis, with neurosyphilis, cardiovascular involvement or gummatous disease 3–10 years after the initial stages.

Unlike most bacterial infections, syphilis cannot be cultured quickly or cheaply. Visualization of *T. pallidum* can be made by darkfield microscopy, but this is very sensitive to the method of sample collection. Serological testing is the mainstay of screening and diagnosis. There are two main types of test: the non-treponemal and the treponemal tests. Non-treponemal tests detect antibodies to reagin (a cholesterol–lecithin–cardiolipin antigen). The usual tests are the Venereal Disease Research Laboratory (VDRL) and the rapid plasma reagin (RPR), which are positive within about 4–7 days of onset of primary syphilis. However, there is lack of sensitivity in primary syphilis, with 13–41 per cent of affected individuals testing negative. These tests are usually positive in people presenting with secondary syphilis. The tests become negative between 3 and 12 months after treatment.[18] Advantages of non-treponemal tests are that they are inexpensive, easy to perform and sensitive, and therefore good for screening. The disadvantages are consequent upon false-positive results, which may be caused by acute viral infection (such as hepatitis and measles), malaria, TB, advanced malignancy, pregnancy and various autoimmune conditions. The diagnosis of syphilis needs to be confirmed by a treponemal serological test, such as the FTA-ABS (fluorescent-treponemal antibody–absorbed test). These tests remain positive whether or not treatment has been administered.[18]

Management

Treatment is with a single intramuscular dose of penicillin for patients who have had syphilis for less than a year; greater doses are needed for patients infected for longer. Contact tracing and counselling should be performed through the genitourinary clinic.

IN RELATION TO PREGNANCY
Antepartum

Syphilis is screened for in the routine antenatal booking bloods by the non-treponemal tests. If positive, confirmatory treponemal tests should be performed.

Treatment during pregnancy is with the penicillin regimen appropriate for the stage of syphilis [II]. A complication of treatment is the Jarisch–Herxheimer reaction, a systemic reaction that may occur a few hours after the administration of penicillin, with fever, myalgia and vasodilatation. Women who are treated in the second half of pregnancy need to seek medical help, as they are at risk of premature labour or fetal distress. Pregnancy does not affect the course of the disease in the mother.

Syphilis has been associated with spontaneous abortion, stillbirth, non-immune hydrops, intrauterine growth restriction and perinatal death as well as serious sequelae in live-born affected children.

Fetal infection

The implications to the fetus of syphilis infections are discussed in Chapter 13.

KEY POINTS

- Non-treponemal tests are used for syphilis screening.
- False-positive results on non-treponemal tests can occur with:
  - acute viral infection
  - malaria/tuberculosis
  - advanced malignancy
  - pregnancy
  - autoimmune conditions.
- Treponemal tests are used for the diagnosis of syphilis.
- Management should be in conjunction with the genitourinary clinic.
- Contact tracing and treatment are essential.

PROTOZOA

Trichomonas

Trichomoniasis vaginalis is the vaginal infection caused by this flagellated protozoon. It prefers a high vaginal pH (>4.5) and is transmitted by sexual contact.

Epidemiology and aetiology

Risk factors for trichomoniasis are smoking, Afro-Caribbean/African race, decreased educational level and increased number of sexual partners. There is a high co-infection rate with other sexually transmitted diseases.

Clinical presentation and diagnosis

Symptoms vary widely, but common presenting complaints are pruritis, frothy copious yellow/green discharge, dyspareunia and vulvovaginal soreness. Signs of the infection are the typical odour of the discharge and erythema of the vulva and cervix. Diagnosis is made on a saline wet preparation and motile flagellated trichomonads can be seen on the periphery of clumps of epithelial cells. More sensitive techniques such as culture, immunofluorescence and enzyme immunoassay are available, although these are more expensive and time consuming.

Management

Metronidazole is the treatment of choice. Partners must also be treated.

IN RELATION TO PREGNANCY
Antepartum

Owing to the increased pelvic blood supply in pregnancy, trichomoniasis may result in vaginal bleeding, particularly postcoital.

Trichomoniasis has been associated with preterm birth and other pregnancy complications. Metronidazole treatment provides a parasitological cure but it is not known whether this treatment has any effect on pregnancy outcome; it is only recommended after the first trimester.

FUNGAL INFECTION

Candida

Superficial and subcutaneous fungal infections affect the skin, keratinous tissues and mucous membranes. Systemic infection can occur by opportunistic infection in the at-risk host or with more invasive organisms. These systemic infections are associated with a high morbidity and mortality. *Candida albicans* alone is the cause of vaginitis in approximately 85–90 per cent of cases. Other non-albicans species are *Candida glabrata* and *Candida tropicalis*, which are increasing in frequency.

Epidemiology and aetiology
The normal vaginal flora, lactobacilli, are the most important barrier to candidal infection.

Factors predisposing to an increased colonization by *Candida* are pregnancy, uncontrolled diabetes, oral contraceptives, antibiotic usage, intrauterine contraceptive devices and increased frequency of sexual intercourse.

Most women will suffer from a symptomatic candidial infection ('thrush') at some time, and up to 20 per cent of women in the reproductive age group can be found to have asymptomatic candida. This shows a dramatic decrease after the menopause. It is not a sexually transmitted disease. Approximately 5 per cent of women are inflicted with candida as a chronic condition. Sources of the recurrence can be vaginal inoculation or from a gastrointestinal reservoir.

Recurrent infections are associated with increased candidal virulence, *Candida* non-albicans and host factors such as decreased secretory local immunity or IgE-mediated hypersensitivity reaction.

The incidence of fungal infections is increasing rapidly, in relation to the growing number of immunocompromised individuals in the population – on chemotherapy, on immunosuppressive drugs and HIV positive.

Presentation and diagnosis
Presentation is with itching and pain in the vulval and vaginal area, which may be associated with an increased vaginal discharge and dysuria. Erythema and excoriation can be seen around the vulval area. The vaginal epithelium and cervix may be reddened. There may be a thick, curd-white discharge. A high vaginal swab should be taken to confirm the clinical diagnosis, with microscopy of both the cells and mycelia being stained Gram positive, and subsequent culture of the organisms.

Management
Self-treatment with anti-mycotics is available in the form of vaginal creams, pessaries and oral tablets. Recurrent self-medicating is not recommended, and microbiological diagnosis of the disease is necessary. Preventative measures, such as avoiding tight synthetic underwear, avoidance of heavily perfumed bath products and perfumes, application of live yoghurt to the affected area and avoiding sweet foods, may decrease the recurrence.

IN RELATION TO PREGNANCY
Antepartum
Vaginal candida infections are more common in pregnancy. Owing to the higher oestrogen stimulation, there is more glycogen available in the vaginal cells, which provides nutrients promoting candidal multiplication.

Clinical symptoms should have the diagnosis confirmed with a high vaginal swab, and topical treatment is appropriate in pregnancy.

Fetal infection
There is no risk to the fetus from candidal infection.

KEY REFERENCES

1. Whitley RJ, Roizman B. Herpes simplex virus infections. *Lancet* 2001; **357**:1513–18.
2. Arvin AM, Hendsleigh PA, Prober CG et al. Failure of antepartum maternal cultures to predict the infant's risk of exposure to herpes simplex virus at delivery. *N Engl J Med* 1986; **315**:796–800.
3. Low-Beer NM, Smith JR. *Management of genital herpes in pregnancy.* Royal College of Obstetricians and Gynaecologists. Clinical 'Green Top' Guidelines. London: RCOG, 2002.
4. Byrne BMP, Crowley PA, Carrington D. *Chicken pox in pregnancy.* Royal College of Obstetricians and Gynaecologists. Clinical 'Green Top' Guidelines. London: RCOG.
5. Brown T, Anand A, Ritchie LD. Intrauterine parvovirus associated with hydrops fetalis. *Lancet* 1984; **2**:1033–4.
6. Biggar RJ, Miotti PG, Taha TE et al. Perinatal intervention trial in Africa: effect of a birth canal cleansing intervention to prevent HIV transmission. *Lancet* 1996; **347**:1647–50.
7. Giaquinto C, Ruga E, Giacomet O, Rampon R. HIV: mother to child transmission, current knowledge and ongoing studies. *Int J Gynaecol Obstet* 1998; **63**(Suppl. 1):S161–5.
8. Semba RD, Miotti PG, Chiphangwi JD et al. Maternal vitamin A deficiency and mother-to-child transmission of HIV-1. *Lancet* 1994; **343**:1593–7.
9. Villari P, Spino C, Chalmers TC, Lau J, Sacks HS. Caesarean section to reduce perinatal transmission of

human immunodeficiency virus. A metaanalysis. Online J Curr Clin Trials. 1993 Jul 8; Doc no 74.

10. The European Collaborative Study. Caesarean section and risk of vertical transmission of HIV-1 infection. The Lancet; 343(8911):464–7.

11. Brocklehurst P, Volmink J. Antiretrovirals for reducing the risk of mother to child transmission of HIV infection (Cochrane Review). In: The Cochrane Library, Issue 1, 2002. Oxford: Update Software.

12. Ryder SD. Acute hepatitis. *BMJ* 322 (7279):151–3.

13. Maddrey WC. Update in hepatology. *Ann Int Med* 134 (3):216–23.

14. Lazarus A, Sanders J. Management of Tuberculosis. Postgraduate Medicine; 108(2), 2000.

15. Guaschino S, De Seta F. Update on Chlamydia Trachomatis. Annals of the New York Academy of Sciences; 900:293–300 (2000).

16. Brocklehurst P, Rooney G. Interventions for treating genital chlamydia trachomatis infection in pregnancy (Cochrane Review). In: The Cochrane Library, Issue 1, 2002. Oxford: Update Software.

17. Turrentine MA, Newton ER. Amoxycillin or erythromycin the treatment of antenatal chlamydial infection: a meta-analysis. *Obstet Gynecol* 1995; 86(6):1021–5.

18. Walker GJA. Antibiotics for syphilis diagnosed during pregnancy (Cochrane review). In: The Cochrane Library, Issue 1, 2002. Oxford: Update Software.

Gestational Diabetes

Justin C. Konje

DEFINITION AND PREVALENCE

Gestational diabetes mellitus (GDM) is defined as carbohydrate intolerance that begins or is first recognized during pregnancy and in most cases resolves after pregnancy. In the broader sense of this definition, therefore, women with previously unrecognized (i.e. pre-gestational diabetes mellitus) Type 2 (non-insulin-dependent) diabetes mellitus (NIDDM) and newly presenting type 1 (insulin-dependent) diabetes mellitus (IDDM) during pregnancy ought to be considered as GDM.

In most cases, the diagnosis is made in the late second and early third trimesters after screening for various indications. The prevalence of GDM in a given population is thought to vary in direct proportion to that of type 2 diabetes mellitus. This depends on the various demographic characteristics of the specific geographic population, including age and ethnic group, and is generally reported as 2–5 per cent. As many as 50 per cent of women developing GDM will go on to develop overt (type 2) diabetes.[1]

SCREENING FOR GESTATIONAL DIABETES

The occurrence of GDM may go unrecognized throughout pregnancy unless complications arise and some of these may occur very late. Because GDM is associated with adverse effects on the pregnancy and a significant number of patients subsequently develop overt diabetes, it is important to screen for the condition.

There are two approaches to screening:

- universal glucose tolerance tests
- selective glucose tolerance tests.

Universal glucose tolerance test screening provides the most effective means of identifying most cases of GDM and therefore of preventing perinatal morbidity and mortality. Despite this theoretical advantage, there are no data to support this population-based approach [IV],[2] which is considered by some to be too expensive. On the other hand, *selective* screening targeting a high-risk population, based on various historic risk factors, will miss approximately 50 per cent of women with GDM. The lack of evidence and the cost implications of universal glucose tolerance test screening have resulted in the provision of selective screening in many populations.

The following methods can be used to determine whether selective glucose tolerance test screening should be performed:

- history
- clinical risk factors
- urine testing
- laboratory tests for blood glucose levels.

Selective screening can be based on the traditional risk factors that have been demonstrated to be associated with an increased risk of GDM. These include:

1 glycosuria in the first trimester,
2 glycosuria on two occasions in either the second or third trimester,
3 polyhydramnios in the current pregnancy,
4 macrosomia (abdominal circumference above the 95th centile) in the current pregnancy,
5 large for gestational age (LGA) fetus – estimated fetal weight above the 95th centile,
6 previous unexplained stillbirth,
7 family history in a first-degree relative,
8 obesity – body mass index (BMI) >25 or weight >85 g,
9 age >35 years,
10 Indo-Asian race,
11 previous GDM,
12 recurrent miscarriages,
13 previous macrosomic baby (weighing above the 95th centile for gestational age, race and sex).

For factors 1–5, the oral glucose tolerance test (OGTT) should be performed at any stage up to 32 weeks' gestation; whereas for factors 6–13, the OGTT should be performed between 26 and 28 weeks' gestation. The value of an OGTT after 32 weeks' gestation or in women with polyhydramnios is debatable as the interpretation is difficult and there is variable absorption of glucose from the gastrointestinal tract after this gestation. In these patients, capillary blood glucose profiles (fasting and post-prandial) are recommended, which can be done at home or in hospital [IV], and glycosylated haemoglobin estimations (discussed below) should be performed.

A history should be taken from all pregnant women, and urinary dipstick testing should also be performed.

Controversy abounds with regard to the laboratory screening methods: both random blood glucose and fasting blood glucose measurements have been advocated, but there are no data to support the effectiveness of either of these as a screening method for GDM.[3] The timing of blood glucose sampling also varies: some authorities advocate it at the initial booking visit, others at 28 weeks' gestation, and others suggest that blood glucose levels should be checked whenever there is >+glycosuria on dipstick testing. For those who advocate blood glucose measurements as a screening method prior to a formal OGTT, an upper limit (see box at top of next column) should be defined relative to the time the patient last ate:

within 2 hours: >7 mmol/L
2–6 hours: >5.5 mmol/L
fasting: >4.8 mmol/L

Values above the thresholds should lead to a full OGTT.

An alternative to this random glucose testing is the 50 g 1-hour glucose test (following an overnight fast) that is commonly used in the USA. A recent recommendation from the American Diabetic Association is to offer a full OGTT if a 1-hour value >7.8 mmol/L is obtained [IV].[4]

If an OGTT is performed, either as part of universal screening or following the identification of increased risk during selective screening, the test should be performed after an overnight fast, with a 75 g glucose load. Pure glucose may induce nausea and vomiting, so Lucozade® may be used as a more patient-friendly alternative. The woman should be seated throughout the procedure and only *two* blood samples are required. If a 75 g OGTT is performed prior to 24 weeks' gestation and does not demonstrate GDM, a repeat OGTT should be considered and undertaken in higher risk patients. During a standard OGTT, venous blood glucose is measured. Venous and capillary fasting blood glucose levels are usually similar; however, after a meal or a glucose challenge, capillary levels are higher than venous levels. Therefore, when interpreting glucose levels, the source of the sample must be taken into consideration.

Indications for selective OGTT screening for gestational diabetes

- Risk factors (personal medical, family and past obstetric history)
- Race
- Abnormal random glucose
- Persistent glycosuria in pregnancy
- Abnormal 50 g 1-hour glucose load after overnight fast

DIAGNOSIS OF GESTATIONAL DIABETES: WHO AND BDA CRITERIA

The diagnosis of GDM is dependent on an OGTT. The World Health Organization (WHO) recommends that the 75 g glucose load is used (although there are still many units in the USA in which 100 g is used).

Historically, an OGTT was performed over a 3-hour period. Recently, however, the WHO has recommended that only fasting and 120-minute values should be used in the diagnosis of GDM. The British Diabetic Association (BDA) [III][5] also recommends that the 2-hour screening test be used.

The WHO recommends the following cut-off values for the diagnosis GDM:[6]

- fasting plasma glucose ⩾5.5 mmol/L,
- 2-hour plasma glucose ⩾8 mmol/L (this is the most important).

It is not necessary for both values to be abnormal.

According the BDA,[5] GDM may be further classified into impaired glucose tolerance and overt diabetes. The criteria for diagnosing gestational impaired glucose tolerance and overt diabetes are considered to be useful in determining when to commence the patient on insulin [III].

For impaired glucose tolerance:

- fasting plasma glucose = 5.5–6 mmol/L,
- 2-hour plasma glucose = 8–11 mmol/L.

For overt diabetes:

- fasting plasma glucose >6 mmol/L,
- 2-hour plasma glucose >11 mmol/L.

Glycosylated haemoglobin (HbA1C) has no role in the diagnosis of GDM. It is, however, useful in the monitoring of effective control of glucose homeostasis.

COMPLICATIONS OF GESTATIONAL DIABETES

In untreated or poorly controlled GDM, the perinatal mortality is about four times that in uncomplicated pregnancies. Where there is early recognition and adequate control, this can be significantly reduced. The complications listed below are discussed in Chapter 6.2.

Maternal

- Pre-eclampsia
- Pregnancy-induced hypertension
- Recurrent vulvo-vaginal infections (thrush, boils)
- Increased incidence of operative deliveries (forceps, ventouse and caesarean section)
- Obstructed labour
- Long term – development of diabetes mellitus.

Fetal

- Macrosomia
- Polyhydramnios
- Preterm labour
- Respiratory distress syndrome
- Unexplained intrauterine fetal death
- Traumatic delivery

- Neonatal complications – jaundice, polycythaemia, tetany, hypocalcaemia, hypomagnesaemia, hypoglycaemia.

MANAGEMENT

Monitoring of glycaemic control

Blood glucose

The only effective means of monitoring glycaemic control in patients with GDM is by regular blood glucose measurements. The frequency of these measurements and whether to perform capillary or venous estimates vary from one unit to another, and the optimum frequency of blood glucose testing has not been established. The frequency of monitoring has varied from weekly to up to seven times daily. However, it is generally acknowledged that more frequent monitoring is associated with a lower perinatal morbidity and mortality and a lower operative delivery rate for the mother.

In non-pregnant diabetic patients, the timing of glucose sampling is preferably pre-prandial. In the gravid patient, because the fetus is more sensitive to hyperglycaemia than to nadirs of glucose values at various times of the day, post-prandial glucose values are preferable. A randomized trial comparing pre-prandial and 1-hour post-prandial glucose measurements in the monitoring of GDM severe enough to require insulin therapy demonstrated that the incidence of macrosomia, neonatal hypoglycaemia and caesarean deliveries for shoulder dystocia were significantly higher in the group managed on the basis of pre-prandial values.[6] *It therefore appears that post-prandial measurements are more effective* [Ib]. Whether such measurements should be made 1 or 2 hours post-prandially remains unresolved, although most authorities advocate the use of 2-hour post-prandial glucose levels [IV].

For the mild forms of GDM, such monitoring may be undertaken by the patient twice a day, but in the more severe forms, it is preferable to measure four readings (fasting, and 2 hours after breakfast, lunch and dinner). The minimum goals for glycaemic controls are a fasting glucose of <5.5 mol/L and a 2-hour post-prandial capillary blood glucose value of <7.0 mmol/L.

Glycosylated haemoglobin (HbA1c)

This is considered by some as the gold standard for the monitoring of glycaemic control, as it overcomes the problems of patients falsifying self-monitoring readings, especially before attending clinics. However, this measurement only provides a retrospective assessment of glycaemic control. It should be performed monthly, and excellent control would yield values below 7 per cent. The disadvantages of HbA1c include the need to have laboratory quantification and the fact that glycaemic control is only assessed over the 6–8 weeks before the measurement. Serum fructosamine was introduced to provide a shorter retrospective time-scale, but has not proved to be useful due to the low sensitivity of the test.

Fetal monitoring

Irrespective of the type of diabetes, all patients with poorly controlled diabetes are at an increased risk of fetal demise. In those with well-controlled diabetes, this risk is minimal, although it is still higher than that in pregnancies uncomplicated by diabetes. There are no randomized, controlled trials of antepartum fetal monitoring of patients with GDM. However, various case series reporting on various testing methods report good outcomes and therefore recommend the adoption of their fetal monitoring protocols. For example, Kjos et al.[7] recommend an approach of twice-weekly non-stress testing and amniotic fluid determinations following their case series in which no stillbirths were reported (the caesarean rate was 4.9 per cent for non-reassuring fetal status) [II]. In another study in which a daily record of fetal movements from 28 weeks' gestation was combined with the non-stress test after 40 weeks, no stillbirths or neonatal deaths were reported [II].[8] It was concluded that such an approach should be adopted in all women with GDM on dietary therapy. There is a need to undertake randomized, controlled trials to provide robust support for the adoption of any given monitoring protocol.

While the value and nature of antepartum fetal monitoring in well-controlled GDM remain poorly defined, it is generally accepted that antenatal fetal monitoring to minimize the risk of adverse outcome is essential in the following groups:

- poorly controlled diabetics,
- diabetics requiring insulin,
- women who have suffered a previous stillbirth,
- women with chronic hypertension,
- women with pregnancy-induced hypertension,
- women with other complications of pregnancy.

There are no universally agreed monitoring methods; the chosen method will depend on the local practice. Methods include regular ultrasound scan, biophysical profilometry, non-stress testing and Doppler velocimetry (see Chapter 14).

Glucose control

The aim of control is to maintain normoglycaemia, which is associated with good perinatal and maternal outcomes. This can be achieved through:

- dietary control,
- insulin therapy.

Dietary control

Although there are no randomized trials comparing dietary to medical therapy in patients with GDM, nutritional interventions are commonly recommended. These must be designed to achieve normoglycaemia and at the same time avoid ketoacidosis. This is best achieved through a multidisciplinary team, which includes a dietician. The American Diabetic Association recommends counselling by a dietician, if possible [IV].[4] The dietary recommendation must take into consideration the patient's height and weight. Severe calorie-restricted diets are not recommended, as they can predispose to ketosis.

In a randomized, controlled trial of women with an abnormal 1-hour glucose challenge test (but normal OGTT), Bevier et al.[9] demonstrated that dietary interventions significantly decreased the prevalence of fetal macrosomia [II]. Patients with GDM are often advised to consume 50 per cent or more of their energy from carbohydrates and less than 30 per cent from fat. However, Anderson et al.[10] in a study of the food actually eaten by pregnant diabetics and non-diabetics, showed that despite personalized dietary advice, this recommendation was never achieved. The dietary restriction most often advised is 30–35 kcal/kg per day for non-obese and 25 kcal/kg body weight daily for obese individuals with GDM. This equates to about 2000–2400 kcal/day (assuming an average weight of 70 g for non-obese woman). The composition of this diet should be 40–60 per cent carbohydrate (no more than 200 g per day), 20–30 per cent protein and the remainder fat. It is essential to individualize meals to the patient's eating habits, thus maximizing compliance and limiting the extent of hyperglycaemia. During pregnancy, there is accelerated starvation, therefore at least three meals and four snacks (with the last snack at bedtime) should be recommended to minimize the overnight complications of hypoglycaemia and starvation ketosis.

Insulin control (see Chapter 6.2)

Insulin has an important role in the treatment of GDM. Although Persson et al.[11] in a comparative evaluation of two treatment regimens for GDM, concluded that insulin was not required for all patients, some prospective trials have demonstrated that insulin treatment of all women with GDM can reduce the likelihood of delivering a macrosomic baby [II].[12,13] The approach that is generally adopted by most physicians is one of selective treatment, for which clear criteria must be defined for the initiation of insulin treatment. These criteria include the following.

- Fasting blood glucose: the traditional approach has been to treat those with fasting blood sugar (FBS) levels >5.8 mmol/L [IV]. This recommendation emanated from extrapolations in the management of women with pre-pregnancy diabetes; women with higher fasting levels are more likely to require insulin therapy to achieve optimum glycaemic control. The value of this criterion is increased if it is combined with 1-hour post-prandial glucose monitoring.
- Post-prandial glucose: patients with 1-hour post-prandial glucose levels >7.2–7.8 mmol/L should be started on insulin [III].

- Fetal macrosomia in the third trimester: the presence of an abdominal circumference above the 95th centile between 29 and 33 weeks' gestation despite apparently good glycaemic control should be considered as an indication for initiating insulin treatment [II]. Using this criterion for insulin therapy, Buchanan et al. reduced fetal macrosomia at birth from 45 per cent to 14 per cent.[14]
- Failed dietary treatment: where diet has failed to control the blood glucose levels, insulin should be instituted. The issue is how long to persist with the diet before commencing insulin. Although there is no consensus, many practitioners will attempt to attain control using dietary methods for 2 weeks prior to switching to insulin [IV].

Insulin regimes are discussed further in Chapter 6.2.

Oral hypoglycaemic agents

These are not recommended in pregnancy as they cross the placenta, may have teratogenic effects, and may stimulate the fetal pancreas leading to hyperinsulinaemia. (In GDM, teratogenicity is not a major problem, as the complication tends to develop in the late second and third trimesters.) Moreover, achieving a tight glycaemic control with these agents is often extremely difficult. However, a recent randomized, controlled trial comparing the efficacy of a second-generation sulphonylurea (Glyburide, more commonly known in the UK as glibendamide) with insulin in the attainment of glycaemic control amongst patients who failed to respond to diet alone showed that glycaemic control and pregnancy outcome were similar in both groups.[15] Until further evidence is available, these agents must be avoided in pregnancy. Nevertheless, in third world countries where insulin may not be readily available, treatments such as Glyburide may have much potential [Ib].

Delivery

The timing of delivery in patients with GDM remains debatable. Where glycaemic control is good and there are no supervening complications (e.g. abnormal fetal growth), there is no reason to deliver the fetus before 40 weeks' gestation. It has been argued that such women may be allowed to go beyond 40 weeks' gestation, but most authorities agree that once maturity is achieved, there is little value in delaying delivery [III].

Where the patient is on insulin, the timing of delivery is more contentious. In a randomized, controlled trial at 38 weeks' gestation into elective induction at 39 weeks' or expectant management, there was no difference in the incidence of caesarean delivery, but the percentage of large for gestational age babies in the expectant group was higher than in the induction group.[16] In another study that compared the outcome in women induced at 38–39 weeks' gestation with those managed expectantly, Lurie et al.[17] demonstrated that although there were more cases of shoulder dystocia in the

expectant group (10 per cent vs 1.4 per cent), there were no differences in caesarean rates between the two groups. The overall conclusion from these studies is that in well-controlled GDM, delivery should be considered at 38–40 weeks' gestation [Ib]. This is based on the fact that the risk of respiratory distress syndrome is minimal in well-controlled GDM by the 39th week. Since pulmonary maturity in the presence of high glucose levels is lessened by as much as 2 weeks, the use of steroids to accelerate pulmonary maturity should be considered in all deliveries before 36–37 weeks' gestation.

The rate of fetal shoulder dystocia and the incidence of caesarean section are much higher in women with GDM. Although fetal macrosomia is partly responsible for this, it is not the only explanation. It may be that obstetricians are more likely to offer caesarean sections to women with GDM because of concerns about shoulder dystocia. There are no data to support a generalized policy of caesarean section to overcome the complication of dystocia. Since macrosomia is more common in women with GDM and shoulder dystocia is more likely at a given birth weight in pregnancies complicated by diabetes than in non-diabetic pregnancies, it is reasonable to recommend caesarean section to women at a particular fetal weight threshold. Unfortunately, because of the poor accuracy of fetal weight estimation by ultrasound (up to 15 per cent at estimations >4000 g), the application of this approach may be difficult. One advocated strategy is therefore to recommend that women with GDM be counselled regarding elective caesarean delivery when the estimated fetal weight is 4500 g or more [III]. When the estimated fetal weight is between 4000 g and 4500 g, additional factors, such as the past obstetric history and the progress of labour, must be taken into consideration before determining the mode of delivery.

Induction of labour

Gestational diabetics on diet therapy do not require any specific measures during labour, other than ensuring that hypoglycaemia does not occur. This is achieved by the measurement of hourly glucose levels. If labour is to be induced, there is no need to omit breakfast. However, a prolonged induction–delivery interval should be avoided, as this may lead to diabetic ketoacidosis [III].

Women with GDM on insulin should be managed in a similar way to pre-pregnancy insulin-dependent (pre-gestational) diabetics (see Chapter 6.2). However, those receiving small doses of insulin (<10 i.u. per day) do not require infusions of insulin and 10 per cent dextrose with potassium chloride. Nevertheless, if two consecutive hourly glucose levels >7 mmol/L are obtained, parallel infusions of insulin and dextrose should be instituted [IV].

Caesarean section

Women undergoing an elective caesarean section should be commenced on an infusion of dextrose and insulin on the morning of surgery. A sliding scale should be used, but once the placenta is delivered, the insulin requirements fall (as detailed below).

Puerperium

Insulin requirements after delivery usually return to pre-pregnancy levels soon after the placenta has been delivered. In women with GDM on diet therapy, there is no need to control the diet. However, women using insulin must reduce their insulin requirements. If they are breastfeeding, insulin should not be discontinued immediately, but should be reduced by 75 per cent before being discontinued. In those not breastfeeding, the insulin should be discontinued once the patient can eat and drink.

Contraception should be discussed. In breastfeeding women, whilst the combined oral contraceptive pill is relatively contraindicated, the progestogen-only contraceptive may be a useful option. Other options include intrauterine contraceptive devices and barrier methods of contraception. In women who are not breastfeeding, the combined oral contraceptive is not contraindicated, provided enough time is allowed for uterine involution to occur.

Long-term follow-up of patients with GDM is important, as there is an increased risk for the development of diabetes (generally type 2 diabetes mellitus) later in life [II]. In some women, diabetes will be diagnosed soon after the completion of pregnancy, suggesting that they had pre-existing diabetes that was not diagnosed prior to pregnancy. It would therefore seem reasonable to screen women who had GDM after the puerperium to ensure that normoglycaemia has returned. The issue is not *whether* to screen but *how* to screen. A full OGTT is recognized to be cumbersome and if it is not practicable to undertake this, a fasting plasma glucose level should be estimated and, if this is abnormal, a full OGTT should be undertaken. The exact number of women with GDM who will eventually develop type 2 diabetes is unknown. However, in a 28-year follow-up of patients, O'Sullivan showed that 50 per cent of women developed type 2 diabetes, compared to 7 per cent of controls.[18]

- Post-prandial 1-hour glucose values are more effective in monitoring glycaemic control.
- Umbilical Doppler velocimetry is of no proven value in the monitoring of fetuses.
- Dietary interventions alone improve outcome.
- Induction of labour does not reduce caesarean section rates.
- Shoulder dystocia is more likely when delivery is after 39 weeks in the presence of macrosomia.

KEY POINTS

- Gestational diabetes mellitus is a common medical complication of pregnancy.
- Screening is crucial to early identification and effective control.
- In poorly controlled patients, the perinatal mortality is as high as four times that in non-diabetics.
- With tight control of glucose levels during pregnancy, the perinatal mortality is similar to that in uncomplicated pregnancies.

KEY REFERENCES

1. Report of the Expert Committee on the Diagnosis and Classification of Diabetes Mellitus. *Diabetes Care* 1997; **20**:1181–97.
2. ACOG Practice Bulletin. Gestational Diabetes. Clinical Management Guidelines for Obstetricians/ Gynecologists, Number 30. *Obstet Gynecol* 2001; **98**:525–38.
3. McElduff A, Goldring A, Gordon P, Wyndham L. A direct comparison of the measurement of random plasma glucose and a post 50 g glucose load, in the detection of gestational diabetes. *Aust NZ J Obstet Gynaecol* 1994; **34**:28–30.
4. American Diabetic Association. Gestational diabetes mellitus. *Diabetes Care* 2001; **24**(Suppl. 1):S77–9.
5. British Diabetic Association, 1988.
6. de Veciana M, Major CA, Morgan MA et al. Postprandial versus preprandial blood glucose monitoring in women with gestational diabetes mellitus requiring insulin therapy. *N Engl J Med* 1995; **333**:1237–41.
7. Kjos SL, Leung A, Henry OA, Victor MR, Paul RH, Medearis AL. Antepartum surveillance in diabetic pregnancies: predictors of fetal distress in labor. *Am J Obstet Gynecol* 1995; **173**:1532–9.
8. Rossavik IK, Joslin GL. Macrosomia and ultrasonography: what is the problem? *South Med J* 1993; **86**:1129–32.
9. Bevier WC, Fischer R, Jovanovic L. Treatment of women with abnormal glucose challenge test (but normal oral glucose tolerance test) decreases the prevalence of macrosomia. *Am J Perinatol* 1999; **16**:269–75.
10. Anderson AS, Len MEJ, Pearson DWM, Sutherland HW. A comparison between the diets of pregnant diabetic women and pregnant non-diabetic women. *Diabet Med* 1990; **7**:452–6.
11. Persson B, Stangenberg M, Hansson U, Nordlander E. Gestational diabetes mellitus (GDM). Comparative

evaluation of two treatment regimens, diet versus insulin and diet. *Diabetes* 1985; **34** (Suppl. 2):101–5.

12. Coustan DR, Lewis SB. Insulin therapy for gestational diabetes. *Obstet Gynecol* 1978; **51**:306–10.

13. Thompson DJ, Porter KB, Gunnells DJ, Wagner PC, Spinaato JA. Prophylactic insulin in the management of gestational diabetes. *Obstet Gynecol* 1990; **75**:960–4.

14. Buchanan TA, Kjos SL, Montoro MN, Wu PY, Madrilejo NG, Gonzalez M. Use of fetal ultrasonography to select metabolic therapy for pregnancies complicated by mild gestational diabetes. *Diabetes Care* 1994; **17**:275–83.

15. Langer O, Conway DL, Berkus MD, Xenakis EM, Gonzales O. A comparison of glyburide and insulin in women with gestational diabetes. *New Engl J Med* 2000; **343**:1134–8.

16. Kjos SL, Henry OA, Montoro M, Buchanan TA, Mestman JH. Insulin-requiring diabetes in pregnancy: a randomized controlled trial of active induction of labor and expectant management. *Am J Obstet Gynecol* 1993; **169**:611–15.

17. Lurie S, Insler V, Hagay ZJ. Induction of labor at 38–39 weeks of gestation reduces the incidence of shoulder dystocia in gestational diabetic patients class A2. *Am J Perinatol* 1996; **13**:293–6.

18. O'Sullivan JB. Diabetes mellitus after GDM. *Diabetes* 1991; **29** (Suppl. 2):131–5.

Pre-eclampsia and Non-proteinuric Pregnancy-Induced Hypertension

Andrew Shennan

MRCOG standards

- Conduct pre-pregnancy counselling to a level expected in independent primary care.
- Manage severe pre-eclampsia/eclampsia.

  In addition, we would suggest the following.

Theoretical skills

- Distinguish between the different causes of hypertension in pregnancy.
- Understand the principles underlying the pathophysiology of pre-eclampsia.
- Describe and quantify the risk factors for pre-eclampsia.
- Know the principles of management of the woman who presents with pre-eclampsia.
- Advise a woman with a previous history of pre-eclampsia.

Practical skills

- Know how to manage the woman with severe pre-eclampsia; this will involve detailed knowledge of fluid management, hypertension control and anaesthetic issues.
- Be able to treat eclampsia.

INTRODUCTION

Women who are hypertensive and pregnant must be subdivided into those with:

- chronic hypertension (see Chapter 6.1),
- pregnancy-induced or gestational hypertension (PIH).

Women with PIH are subdivided further: the majority have non-proteinuric PIH, a condition associated with minimal maternal or perinatal mortality/morbidity, whereas a minority have the major pregnancy complication of pre-eclampsia.[1]

It is imperative that every effort is made to accurately classify women with hypertension in pregnancy as having chronic hypertension, non-proteinuric PIH or pre-eclampsia. The aetiology and management of the three conditions are very disparate. The aetiology and management of chronic hypertension in pregnancy are discussed in Chapter 6.1. Women with non-proteinuric PIH need to be monitored to ensure that proteinuria does not develop and pre-eclampsia become apparent; non-proteinuric PIH is not an indication for admission, induction of labour or anti-hypertensive treatment.[2] This chapter focuses on pre-eclampsia.

Even in developed countries, women still die from pre-eclampsia and eclampsia.[3] In the UK, fewer than ten women die each year, but eclampsia has an associated mortality of 2 per cent.[4] Worldwide, however, maternal mortality from hypertensive disease accounts for approximately 100 000 deaths per year.

Because of concerns about the potential adverse effects of pre-eclampsia, many women who have a normal outcome require intensive surveillance; up to a quarter of antenatal admissions are as a direct result of monitoring and managing women with hypertension. Antenatal care is directed towards identifying women with hypertension and proteinuria. Day units reduce the need for inpatient management, but current methods for screening women at risk are poor and the onset and progression of the disease are unpredictable.

Perinatal mortality is also increased with pre-eclampsia. Early-onset pre-eclampsia is associated with intrauterine growth restriction (IUGR). Placental involvement also explains the association with placental abruptions. As delivery is the only cure, the hypertensive diseases of pregnancy have become the commonest cause of iatrogenic prematurity. They account for 15 per cent of all premature births, but up to a quarter of very low birth weight infants. There is strong evidence linking size at birth to health in adulthood, i.e. that there are fetal origins of adult disease.[5] Thus the small babies resulting from pregnancies affected by pre-eclampsia have health implications in adult life, including an increased risk of hypertension, heart disease and diabetes when they become adults. Additional and significant longer term health service resource implications result from subsequent learning disabilities and low intelligence quotient (IQ). Maternal disease severity and fetal involvement do not always correlate; for example, the babies of women who have eclampsia at term have normal birth weight.[4]

CLASSIFICATION AND DEFINITION

The term pregnancy-induced hypertension usually implies hypertension caused by but unrelated to other pathology associated with the pregnancy, a diagnosis that is difficult to make until after the pregnancy has ended.

Blood pressure and proteinuria define pre-eclampsia, but they are not fundamental to the aetiology and are more indicative of end-organ damage. In clinical practice, the threshold of abnormality is set low to identify at-risk cases, but this results in many women being identified with hypertension and/or proteinuria who are not at increased risk.

Table 7.6.1 The International Society for the Study of Hypertension in Pregnancy (ISSHP) classification (modified and abbreviated)

A. Gestational hypertension and/or proteinuria developing during pregnancy, labour or the puerperium in a previously normotensive non-proteinuric woman
  1. Gestational hypertension (without proteinuria)
  2. Gestational proteinuria (without hypertension)
  3. Gestational proteinuric hypertension (pre-eclampsia)
B. Chronic hypertension (before the twentieth week of pregnancy) and chronic renal disease (proteinuria before the twentieth week of pregnancy)
  1. Chronic hypertension (without proteinuria)
  2. Chronic renal disease (proteinuria with or without hypertension)
  3. Chronic hypertension with superimposed pre-eclampsia (new-onset proteinuria)
C. Unclassified hypertension and/or proteinuria
D. Eclampsia

Definitions

Hypertension in pregnancy:

- Diastolic BP ≥110 mmHg on any one occasion *or*
- Diastolic BP ≥90 mmHg on two or more consecutive occasions ≥4 hours apart

Proteinuria in pregnancy:

- One 24-hour collection with total protein excretion ≥300 mg/24 hours *or*
- Two 'clean-catch – midstream' or catheter specimens of urine collected ≥4 hours apart with ≥2+ on reagent strip

Adapted from Davey and MacGillivray.[6]

The International Society for the Study of Hypertension in Pregnancy (ISSHP), based on the recommendation of Davey and MacGillivray,[6] uses the term 'gestational hypertension' to include all women with PIH whether proteinuric or not, as long as they had been previously normotensive and not proteinuric. Once proteinuria has developed, this is assumed to be pre-eclampsia (Table 7.6.1).

If any organ system known to have the potential to be affected by pre-eclampsia is involved, the possibility of the disease must be suspected; hypertension and proteinuria cannot be relied upon to define the disease. However, for pragmatic reasons, these signs must remain hallmarks for definition. Tests for liver, kidney, blood and placental involvement should always be sought if pre-eclampsia is suspected (see below).

INCIDENCE

The prevalence of pre-eclampsia varies with the definition used and the population studied; however, pre-eclampsia occurs in less than 5 per cent of an average antenatal population. In some recent prospective studies, the incidence has been as low as 2.2 per cent, even in a primigravid population, in which the condition is known to have the highest prevalence.[7] The incidence of non-proteinuric PIH is approximately three times greater. In the USA, the incidence of pre-eclampsia has been reported to be slightly higher, possibly because of the high-risk status of the populations studied (usually primiparous women at large teaching centres).

AETIOLOGY

Although the primary events leading to pre-eclampsia are still unclear, it is now widely believed that a cascade of events leads to the clinical syndrome (summarized in Figure 7.6.1).

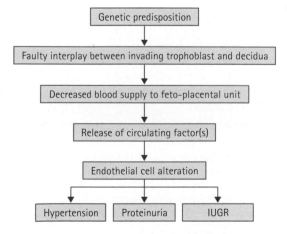

Figure 7.6.1   Aetiology of pre-eclampsia. IUGR, intrauterine growth restriction

Although the inheritance of pre-eclampsia has yet to be char-acterized, there is a strong familial predisposition: a family history in either mother or sister increases the risk of pre-eclampsia four–eight-fold. This genetic predisposition leads to a faulty interplay between the invading extravillous tropho-blast cells (of fetal origin) and the maternal immunologically active decidual cells.

The faulty interplay results in a failure of trophoblast invasion into the myometrium and the maternal spiral arteries do not undergo their physiological vasodilatation.[8] Only the most superficial decidual portion of the spiral artery is invaded by the trophoblast. This inadequate tropho-blast invasion is also seen in pregnancies complicated by fetal growth restriction (without pre-eclampsia), demon-strating that the maternal syndrome of pre-eclampsia must be related to additional factors.

The diminished dilatation of the spiral arteries, associated increased resistance in the utero-placental circulation and an impaired intervillous blood flow probably result in an inad-equately perfused placenta. Ischaemia or ischaemia/reperfu-sion in the second half of gestation produces reactive oxygen species and oxidative stress in the placenta.

The placental hypoperfusion is also postulated to result in the secretion of a factor(s) into the maternal circulation that causes 'activation' of vascular endothelium.[9]

Endothelial cell activation explains the widespread manifestations of the disease, as the vascular endothelium supplies all organ systems involved. Many markers of endothelial damage are raised. Pre-eclampsia is associated with lipid changes (there is a two-fold increase in triglyc-erides and free fatty acids), and an increase in lipid peroxi-dation, both in the placenta and systemically, suggests that oxidative stress (an imbalance between free radical synthesis and antioxidant defence) may be involved in the endothelial cell changes.

MANAGEMENT

Screening for pre-eclampsia

History

More than a third of pre-eclampsia occurs in women with risk factors; a careful history will allow the clinician to assess risk.

A family history in a first-degree relative increases the risk of pre-eclampsia four–eight-fold, illustrating the strong genetic influence [III]. A woman has double the risk of pre-eclampsia if pregnant by a partner who had previously fathered an affected pregnancy [III].

An immunological element to the disease process is evidenced by the effect of exposure to the paternal antigen, via either the fetus or the partner. Pre-eclampsia occurs more commonly in first pregnancies; miscarriages or termi-nations of pregnancy provide some reduction in risk in subsequent pregnancies [III]. A new partner increases risk,

whereas non-barrier methods of contraception and increased duration of sexual cohabitation reduce risk [III]. Exposure to a partner's 'foreign' antigens is common to these phenomena. Teenage mothers and pregnancies con-ceived by donor insemination have increased risk of pre-eclampsia, presumably due to the lack of exposure to such antigens [III].

Underlying medical disorders, particularly those involving vascular disease – such as chronic hypertension – increase the risk of pre-eclampsia; this highlights the importance of the maternal susceptibility as well as the placental aetiology in the disease process. All forms of glucose intolerance, includ-ing gestational diabetes, are associated with an increased risk [III]. This may be related to obesity, which is an independent risk factor. Women with antiphospholipid syndrome and multiple pregnancies are at increased risk. Risk may be related to the size of the placenta; molar preg-nancies have been associated with pre-eclampsia, as have pregnancies complicated by hydrops fetalis (mirror syn-drome) or trisomy chromosomal complement.

Women with a history of pre-eclampsia, particularly those requiring delivery before 37 weeks, all have about a 20 per cent chance of developing pre-eclampsia again [III].

Biophysical tests

The detection of raised blood pressure in early gestation is related to the subsequent risk of pre-eclampsia, even within the normal blood pressure range (i.e. the lower the blood pressure, the lower the risk). Ambulatory automated moni-toring removes many of the errors of standard sphygmo-manometry, but is only a weak indicator of risk, and these monitors may under-read in pre-eclampsia [III].[7] Two other biophysical tests have been investigated but are not useful: isometric exercise testing and the roll-over test. Problems with reproducibility and poor predictor values mean that these have not been introduced into clinical practice. The angiotensin II sensitivity test, involving assessing the blood pressure response to infusion of the vasoconstrictor angiotensin II, has also shown poor predictor values in larger studies and is invasive, time consuming and costly [Ib].

In contrast, Doppler analysis of the uterine artery wave-form has reasonable sensitivity and specificity, and is rela-tively quick, non-invasive and relatively inexpensive if performed at the same time as other ultrasound scans. Poor placental perfusion is a characteristic feature of pregnancies destined to develop pre-eclampsia and therefore it would seem logical to identify those women who have increased resistance in this circulation. In pregnancies at increased risk of pre-eclampsia, there is persistence of a relatively high resistance circulation with a notch. The later this test is per-formed, the better the predictive values [III]. At 20 weeks' gestation in a low-risk population, approximately one in five women will develop pre-eclampsia[10] if they have an abnormal waveform; the prediction value is considerably greater at 24 weeks' [III]. This screening test does allow women to be targeted for increased surveillance and possible prophylactic therapies. The importance of screening tests will escalate if an adequate treatment to prevent pre-eclampsia is established.

Biochemical tests

The simple measurements of plasma volume, haemoglobin concentration and haematocrit all have a weak association with the development of pre-eclampsia but poor prediction values [III]. Uric acid and platelets are sometimes measured in women with chronic hypertension to predict superimposed pre-eclampsia, but are lacking in sensitivity and specificity. The measurement of second trimester human chorionic gonadotrophin and maternal serum alpha-fetoprotein is associated with a two-fold increase in pre-eclampsia, and is likely to reflect the disease process that occurs at the utero-placental interface [III]. This increase in risk is not sufficient to significantly alter clinical practice. Many markers of endothelial activation have been shown to be increased in pre-eclampsia. Some will rise before the clinical manifest-ations of the disease, but there is invariably overlap between the women who are subsequently normal and those who develop pre-eclampsia, again limiting clinical usefulness. Urinary excretion of calcium, microalbuminuria and prosta-cyclin metabolites have been investigated, as well as urin-ary kallikrein:creatinine ratios, and further work may eventually establish a combination of tests that could be clinically useful, perhaps by combining endothelial and placental markers of the disease.

The role of prophylaxis

Surveillance and timely delivery are the essence of current antenatal management in order to prevent the conse-quences of pre-eclampsia. Preventing the manifestation of the disease would be highly preferred. There are a number of potential therapies that have been investigated in an effort to prevent the occurrence of pre-eclampsia. Aspirin, calcium and fish oils have gained the most focus in this regard, although other substances such as magnesium, zinc and even rhubarb have been investigated. Aspirin, a cyclo-oxygenase enzyme inhibitor, reverses the imbalance between the vasoconstrictor thromboxane A2 and the vasodilator prostacyclin that is known to occur in pre-eclampsia. The Cochrane Collaboration reported that there have been 42 randomized trials that have studied the use of aspirin in pregnancy. These demonstrated a 15 per cent relative risk reduction in the risk of pre-eclampsia associated with the use of aspirin or other antiplatelet agents [Ia].[11] Overall, an 8 per cent significant reduction in the risk of preterm deliv-ery and a 14 per cent significant reduction in the risk of death to the baby have also been demonstrated in these trials. Aspirin should be seriously considered in the management of very high-risk women and is likely to be safe. The dose, timing and the populations to be targeted are still being thoroughly investigated.

In the ten trials (6864 women) that investigated the role of calcium as prophylaxis, there was a moderate reduction in the incidence of pre-eclampsia [Ia]. However, in the four trials of women who had an adequate calcium intake prior to the study, this effect was not apparent. The role of cal-cium supplementation in developed countries is uncertain, and is the subject of an ongoing World Health Organization (WHO) trial.

Fish oils containing n-3 fatty acids are thought to inhibit platelet thromboxane A2. The four trials that have investigated their use have not shown any reduction in pre-eclampsia [Ia].

The potential role of oxidative stress in the aetiology of the maternal syndrome of pre-eclampsia has resulted in the study of the antioxidants vitamin C and E supplementation from the second trimester of pregnancy. In a high-risk popu-lation (selected on the basis of abnormal uterine artery Doppler waveform analysis), vitamin C and E supplementa-tion reduced the likelihood of developing pre-eclampsia by at least 50 per cent [Ib].[12] One thousand milligrams of vitamin C and 400 IU of vitamin E were used and acted synergistically. Thus far, there has been one study of 283 women, and further work is required to determine whether the potential benefit extends to other populations, particu-larly to the low-risk primigravid population.

Maternal and fetal assessment

Before any management decisions are made, the first task is to confirm the diagnosis of pre-eclampsia (see above), in order to ensure that iatrogenic morbidity does not ensue [IV].

The gestation at which women present with hypertension is an important factor in establishing risk: late-onset hyper-tension after 37 weeks' gestation rarely results in serious morbidity to mother or baby [III]. However, hypertension that presents early, particularly before 28 weeks', will result in pre-eclampsia developing in almost half of women.

Care in assessing blood pressure will prevent misdiag-nosis; blood pressure measurement is poorly performed in clinical practice, for example digit preference (the practice of rounding the final digit of the blood pressure to 0) occurs in more than 80 per cent of antenatal measurements. The antenatal population within the UK has a significant proportion of obese women. The standard bladder used in sphygmomanometer cuffs (23×12 cm) under-cuffs about a quarter of the antenatal population, resulting in the over-diagnosis of hypertension, usually by more than 10 mmHg. Over-cuffing underestimates measurements, but usually by less than 5 mmHg, and is preferable in cases of doubt. Keeping the rate of deflation during measurement to 2–3 mm/s will prevent overdiagnosing diastolic hypertension. A similar effect is achieved by using Korotkoff 5; fewer women will be diagnosed as hypertensive than when Korotkoff 4 is used. Korotkoff 4 is also less reproducible [II], and randomized, controlled clinical trials have confirmed that all healthcare providers should be using Korotkoff 5 when measuring blood pressure in pregnancy [Ib]. Repeating the blood pressure or obtaining a series of readings in the day unit will limit the overdiagnosis of hypertension [IV].

Errors in the interpretation of proteinuria are also common with dipstick urine analysis, and 24-hour collections of urine are necessary to confirm the diagnosis [IV]. More than 300 mg in 24 hours is considered abnormal. Newer automated devices that can be used by the bedside relate the proteinuria to creatinine, and closely equate to 24-hour collections.

Every effort should be made to identify women at risk of life-threatening complications. Most women who present with eclampsia will not have had a recent blood pressure or urine analysis that was sufficiently abnormal to have identified them as at risk. Only just over half of women who presented with eclampsia had had prior hypertension and proteinuria diagnosed together.[4] Blood pressure and proteinuria cannot be relied upon alone. The syndrome of pre-eclampsia is multisystemic and it is the ease of measurements of hypertension and proteinuria that has led to their adoption in the diagnosis of pre-eclampsia. Other organ involvement must be considered, such as fetal involvement, or other signs such as epigastric tenderness. For pragmatic reasons, other signs have not been introduced to define the disease, but they are equally important.

Management remote from term

Early-onset pre-eclampsia is frequently associated with placental insufficiency, which can result in IUGR, abruption of the placenta and fetal death [II]. Fetal well-being must be carefully considered in all cases. A symphyseal–fundal height should be carefully measured in all women who present with pre-eclampsia, in addition to an enquiry as to fetal movements [IV]. At early gestations, or in pregnancies with suspected IUGR, it is usual to confirm fetal growth with ultrasound, and to assess the amniotic fluid volume and umbilical artery Doppler waveform [IV]. Suspected fetal compromise is a frequent cause for delivery in pre-eclampsia.

Involvement of other organ systems in the affected women must be sought.

- *Platelets* are consumed due to the endothelial activation. A platelet count $>50 \times 10^9/L$ is likely to support normal haemostasis [IV]; however, a falling platelet count, particularly to $<100 \times 10^9/L$, may indicate a need to consider delivery [IV].
- Hypovolaemia results in an increased *haematocrit* and the *haemoglobin* may also be raised.
- If delivery or induction of labour is likely to be imminent, or if the platelet count is low, it is also sensible to screen for *clotting abnormalities* [IV]. Pre-eclampsia can cause disseminated intravascular

coagulation, and clotting must be adequate for regional anaesthesia.

- *Uric acid*, a measure of fine renal tubular function, is used to assess the disease severity, although severe disease can still occur with a normal uric acid level. Spuriously high levels of uric acid are associated with acute fatty liver of pregnancy.
- Raised *urea* and *creatinine* are associated with late renal involvement, but are not useful as an early indicator of disease severity (serial measurements may identify renal disease progression) [IV].
- Pre-eclampsia can cause subcapsular haematoma, liver rupture and hepatic infarction, and liver *transaminases* should be measured. Aspartate aminotransferase (AST) and other transaminases indicate hepatocellular damage, and elevated levels may again indicate a need to consider delivery. It should be remembered that the normal range for transaminases is approximately 20 per cent lower than the non-pregnant range [II].

When liver involvement is associated with haemolysis and low platelets, this is known as HELLP syndrome, which is a severe variant of pre-eclampsia. If proteinuria excretion is high (usually >3 g/24 hours), circulating albumin may fall, increasing the risk of pulmonary oedema. A raised AST can be associated with either haemolysis or liver involvement; lactate dehydrogenase levels are also elevated in the presence of haemolysis.

Corticosteroids should be given to enhance fetal lung maturity and are safe in pre-eclampsia [III]. Steroid therapy may assist in the recovery from HELLP syndrome and has been used in the postpartum period. It is not unusual to see a slight improvement in biochemical parameters in the antenatal period associated with corticosteroid use [III].

The treatment of moderate hypertension may be detrimental to fetal growth [III].[13] However, severe hypertension should be avoided, and blood pressures $>170/110$ mmHg require urgent therapy (see below) [IV].[13]

In women with an established diagnosis of pre-eclampsia, delivery should be considered once fetal lung maturity is likely (approximately 32 weeks' gestation), particularly if either maternal multi-organ involvement or fetal compromise is apparent. However, women with pre-eclampsia presenting between 28 and 32 weeks' can often be managed conservatively without substantial risk to the mother, as long as close inpatient supervision is maintained (IV). In such cases, conservative management reduces neonatal morbidity without significantly increasing maternal morbidity.

Maternal indications for delivery include an inability to control hypertension, deteriorating liver or renal function, progressive fall in platelets or neurological complications. A non-reactive cardiotograph (CTG) with decelerations or a fetal condition that is clearly deteriorating often warrants delivery.

Labour ward management of pre-eclampsia

A set protocol should be followed when a women has severe pre-eclampsia [IV]. All staff working on the labour ward must be familiar with the protocol in use. Typical entry criteria for such a protocol would be:[14]

- eclampsia, or
- severe hypertension (>170/110 mmHg) with + or >1 g/24 hours proteinuria, or
- hypertension (>140/90 mmHg) with ++ or >3 g/24 hours proteinuria with an additional complication such as headache, visual disturbance, epigastric pain, clonus (more than three beats) or a platelet count <100 × 10^9/L or AST >50 IU/L.

The two main reasons why women die, as evidenced by the Confidential Enquiry, are cerebral haemorrhage and adult or acute respiratory distress syndrome,[3] and the two most important aetiological factors for these are severe hypertension and excess fluid intake. Control of blood pressure and fluid balance is therefore crucial.

Intrapartum blood pressure control

Blood pressure should be measured frequently (every 15 minutes) [IV]. To facilitate this, automated sphygmomanometers may be used, but these oscillometric devices underread the blood pressure in pre-eclampsia. Large changes in blood pressure should therefore be confirmed with a mercury sphygmomanometer [IV].

Intracerebral haemorrhage complicated 7/15 deaths in the last Confidential Enquiries into Maternal Deaths (CEMD).[3] Mean arterial pressures (MAPs) are used to guide management, and most protocols recommend the instigation of intravenous anti-hypertensive therapy at MAP >125 mmHg [IV]. Labatolol or hydralazine is the usual first-line treatment [II]. Regimens vary (although there is an increasing trend towards regional protocols), for example:

- Labetolol: bolus of 20 mg i.v. if the MAP remains >125 mmHg, followed at 10-minute intervals by 40, 80, 80 mg boluses, up to a cumulative dose of 220 mg. Once the MAP is <125 mmHg, an infusion of 40 mg/hour is commenced, doubling (if necessary) at 30-minute intervals, until a satisfactory response or a dose of 160 mg/hour is attained.
- Hydralazine: bolus of 5 mg i.v. if the MAP remains >125 mmHg, followed by further boluses of 5 mg up to a cumulative dose of 15 mg. Once the MAP is <125 mmHg, an infusion of 10 mg/hour is commenced, doubling (if necessary) at 30-minute intervals, until a satisfactory response or a dose of 40 mg/hour is attained. Colloid should be infused prior to treatment if the baby is undelivered, to protect the utero-placental circulation and prevent hypotension and fetal distress [IV].

If one agent is ineffective, or if side effects occur (e.g. tachycardia with hydralazine), the other agent can be used. Third-line agents include sodium nitroprusside and nifedipine.

Fluid management

As women with pre-eclampsia can have a reduced intravascular volume, leaky capillary membranes and low albumin levels, they are prone to pulmonary oedema. Renal failure is a rare complication of pre-eclampsia that usually follows acute blood loss, when there has been inadequate transfusion, or as a result of profound hypotension. *Oliguria without a rising serum urea or creatinine is a manifestation of severe pre-eclampsia and not of incipient renal failure. Administration of intravenous fluid in response to oliguria must be performed with caution* [IV].

Most protocols limit fluid intake (in the form of intravenous crystalloid) to approximately 1 mL/kg per hour [IV]. A Foley catheter should be inserted and fluid balance recorded.

In a well-perfused women, oliguria (<400 mL/24 hours) requires no treatment per se. A low threshold for central venous pressure (CVP) assessment is recommended; in the absence of invasive monitoring, repetitive fluid challenges are to be avoided. If the CVP is high (>8 mmHg) with persistent oliguria, a dopamine infusion can be considered (1 μg/kg per minute) [IV]. If the creatinine or potassium rises, haemodialysis or haemofiltration may be necessary, and the advice of a renal physician should be sought. The administration of diuretics temporarily improves urine output, but further decreases the circulating volume and exacerbates electrolyte disturbances; frusemide should only be given if there are signs of pulmonary oedema [IV]. In particularly difficult cases, pulmonary artery catheterization should be considered.

Anticonvulsant therapy

Magnesium sulphate can be used to control an eclamptic fit (up to 8 g). Alternatively, diazepam (10 mg) can be used [IV]. An eclamptic fit is usually self-limiting, and prolonged fitting warrants a brain scan to rule out other pathology such as an intracerebral bleed [IV].

If an eclamptic fit occurs, magnesium sulphate is the prophylaxis of choice, as demonstrated by the Eclampsia Trial [Ib].[15] In addition to reducing the incidence of further fits, the benefits of magnesium sulphate over both diazepam and phenytoin include a significantly lower need for maternal ventilation, less pneumonia and fewer intensive care admissions. Magnesium sulphate acts as a membrane stabilizer and vasodilator and reduces intracerebral ischaemia. It is usually given as a 2 g intravenous loading dose and a maintenance infusion at 1–2 g/hour. In cases of oliguria, care must be taken, as magnesium sulphate is renally excreted. Toxicity is detected by the absence of patellar reflexes, but ultimately respiratory arrest and muscle paralysis or cardiac arrest will occur. The antidote is 10 mL of 10 per cent calcium gluconate.

Even with severe pre-eclampsia, eclamptic fits are rare (<1 per cent). However, the Magpie Trial evaluated magnesium sulphate versus placebo in women with pre-eclampsia and demonstrated a clear benefit of prophylactic therapy [Ia]. Magnesium sulphate halved the risk of eclampsia and probably reduced the risk of maternal death. There did not appear to be any substantive harmful short-term effects to either the mother or baby.[15]

Anaesthesia

A general anaesthetic can be dangerous, as endotracheal intubation can cause severe hypertension. Regional blockade is the preferred method of analgesia for labour and of anaesthesia for operative deliveries [IV], but a coagulopathy must be excluded. Platelet levels of $>80 \times 10^9$/L should ensure haemostasis, and most obstetric anaesthetists will insert a regional block under these circumstances. Care must be taken to avoid arterial hypotension (particularly following postpartum haemorrhage) in view of the vasoconstriction and reduced intravascular volume. A low threshold for central invasive monitoring is necessary in women who require a caesarean section [IV].

Postpartum care

As a third of eclamptic fits occur postpartum, intensive monitoring is required, usually for 48 hours after delivery. Although eclampsia has been reported beyond this time, it is unlikely to be associated with serious morbidity. Blood pressure is frequently at its highest 3–4 days after delivery. Anti-hypertensive therapy may therefore need to be continued after discharge home; in the absence of fetal considerations, the most effective therapy can be used – and drugs such as methyldopa discontinued.

All women who have suffered severe pre-eclampsia should be reviewed at a hospital postnatal clinic 6–12 weeks after delivery [IV]. In addition to blood pressure and urine testing, tests of renal and liver function should be instigated; residual disease may merit referral to a physician. Underlying predispositions to pre-eclampsia, such as an inherited thrombophilia or antiphospholipid syndrome, should be excluded (multiparous women are more likely to have an underlying cause). The postnatal visit is also an excellent opportunity to discuss complications of the pregnancy and the planned management of any future pregnancy.

- The use of anti-hypertensive therapy in moderately hypertensive women demonstrates a significant reduction in severe hypertension only; there are no other proven additional benefits.
- Low-dose aspirin in pregnancy results in a small (15 per cent) but significant reduction in pre-eclampsia; there is an associated reduction in fetal death and preterm delivery.

- Magnesium sulphate is the anticonvulsant of choice following an eclamptic fit, resulting in fewer fits and less maternal morbidity compared to diazepam and phenytoin. There is also a clear benefit to prophylactic magnesium sulphate therapy – the risk of eclampsia is halved.

KEY POINTS

- Pre-eclampsia is a multisystem disorder involving the placenta, liver, kidneys, blood, and neurological and cardiovascular systems; hypertension and proteinuria are diagnostic signs.
- Both maternal and fetal morbidity and mortality are more likely to occur with early-onset disease.
- Despite the many tests being investigated, pre-eclampsia cannot be accurately predicted. An abnormal uterine artery Doppler at 20 weeks will increase risk approximately six-fold in both high-risk and low-risk women.
- Cerebral haemorrhage and adult respiratory distress are common causes of death in pre-eclampsia; therefore acute management focuses on controlling blood pressure and restricting fluid intake.

KEY REFERENCES

1. Hayman R, Baker PN. *Hypertension in Pregnancy: Definition, Diagnosis and Investigation.* A CME Self-assessment Test. London: RCOG Press, 1997.
2. Hayman R, Baker PN. *Hypertension in Pregnancy: Management.* A CME Self-assessment Test. London: RCOG Press, 1997.
3. Department of Health. *Why Mothers Die, 1997–1999.* Report on Confidential Enquiries into Maternal Deaths in the United Kingdom. London: RCOG Press, 2001.
4. Douglas KA, Redman CWG. Eclampsia in the United Kingdom. *BMJ* 1994; 309:1395–400.
5. Barker DJP, Bull AR, Osmond C. Fetal and placental size and risk of hypertension in adult life. *BMJ* 1990; 301:259–61.
6. Davey DA, MacGillivray I. The classification and definition of the hypertensive disorders of pregnancy. *Am J Obstet Gynecol* 1988; 158:892–8.
7. Higgins JR, Walshe JJ, Halligan A, O'Brien E, Conroy R, Darling MR. Can 24-hour ambulatory blood pressure measurement predict the development of hypertension in primigravidae? *Br J Obstet Gynaecol* 1997; 104:356–62.

8. Brosens IA. Morphological changes in the utero-placental bed in pregnancy hypertension. *Clin Obstet Gynecol* 1977; **77**:573–93.

9. Roberts JM, Taylor RN, Musci TJ, Rodgers GM, Hubel CA, McLaughlin MK. Pre-eclampsia: an endothelial cell disorder. *Am J Obstet Gynecol* 1989; **161**:1200–4.

10. Mires GJ, Williams FL, Leslie J, Howie PW. Assessment of uterine arterial notching as a screening test for adverse pregnancy outcome. *Am J Obstet Gynecol* 1998; **179**:1317–23.

11. Duley L, Henderson-Smart D, Knight M, King J. Antiplatelet drugs for prevention of pre-eclampsia and its consequences: systematic review. *BMJ* 2001; **322**:329–33.

12. Chappell LC, Seed PT, Briley AL et al. Prevention of pre-eclampsia by antioxidants: a randomized trial of vitamins C and E in women at increased risk of pre-eclampsia. *Lancet* 1999; **354**:810–16.

13. Von Dadelszen P, Ornstein MP, Bull SB, Logan AG, Koren G, Magee LA. Fall in mean arterial pressure and fetal growth restriction in pregnancy hypertension: a meta-analysis. *Lancet* 2000; **355**:87–92.

14. North West Pre-eclampsia Care Group. Regional Guidelines for the Management of Severe Pre-eclampsia. In: Baker PN, Kingdom J (eds). *Pre-eclampsia: Aetiology and Management.* London: Parthenon, 2004, in press.

15. Which anticonvulsant for women with eclampsia? Evidence from the Collaborative Eclampsia Trial. *Lancet* 1995; **345**:1455–63.

16. The Magpie Collaborative Group. Do women with pre-eclampsia, and their babies, benefit from magnesium sulphate? The Magpie Trial: a randomised placebo-controlled trial. *Lancet* 2002; **359**:1877–90.

Medication in Pregnancy

Justin C. Konje

INTRODUCTION

Drug administration in pregnancy is unique for two reasons: first, the physiological changes associated with pregnancy affect drug metabolism and, second, the presence of the fetus has a significant bearing on the type of drugs that can be prescribed. This is largely because some of these drugs may cross the placenta and affect the fetus in several ways, depending on the drug and the gestational age. In this chapter, attempts have not been made to treat individual drugs separately; instead, a generic presentation is made, with some examples where applicable.

Physiological changes in pregnancy that may affect drug metabolism

- Gastrointestinal
- Pulmonary
- Skin/mucous membrane
- Central nervous system
- Plasma and blood volume
- Plasma proteins
- Urinary

PHYSIOLOGICAL CHANGES IN PREGNANCY THAT MAY AFFECT DRUG METABOLISM

Drug therapy in pregnancy is linked closely with the problem of pharmacokinetics and drug disposition in the maternal–placental–fetal interphase. Pharmacokinetics is concerned with drug absorption, distribution, metabolism and excretion. Continuous morphological and physiological changes in pregnancy affect drug pharmacokinetics and make it difficult to predict the time course of drug concentrations. These changes must be recognized when prescribing in pregnancy; failure to do so may result in errors in the prediction of drug interactions and effects. The physiological and morphological changes that occur in pregnancy and that may affect drug pharmacokinetics involve various systems in the body.

Gastrointestinal system

In early pregnancy, most women suffer from nausea and vomiting, and later heartburn – all of which may result in poor compliance. During pregnancy, the acid content of the stomach is reduced and gastric emptying slows. Drugs which are absorbed in the stomach or which need to pass into the small bowel for absorption may therefore be affected. Salicylates (absorbed from the stomach) may therefore remain longer in the stomach and may fail to attain therapeutic serum levels at the anticipated time; there may also be side effects from the prolonged time spent in the stomach. During labour, narcotic analgesia may further delay gastric emptying and result in an accumulation of repeated medications, such that toxic levels ensue. An understanding of these physiological mechanisms may result in modification of the route of administration.

The reduction in intestinal activity during pregnancy prolongs the drug transit time. Prolonged contact with the intestinal surface may result in a more complete absorption. In contrast, if a drug is metabolized in the gut wall, less of the parent drug may reach the systemic circulation and therefore bioavailability will be reduced. The prolonged time spent in the bowel may also interfere with absorption of other therapies, for example iron supplementation chelates and interferes with the absorption of other drugs.

Pulmonary system

Changes in the pulmonary system are of limited importance, as most drugs are not administered through this route in pregnancy. However, drugs for asthma and analgesia in labour may be administered through this route.

Highly lipid-soluble substances cross the alveolar membranes almost instantaneously and are rapidly removed from the lungs. Alveolar air is almost completely cleared of such substances with each breath and therefore, with a pregnancy-induced increase in respiratory rate, diffusion will be increased. This type of diffusion is described as respiration-limited diffusion and is characteristic of substances such as nitrous oxide used for analgesia in labour.

For compounds of lower lipid solubility, equilibration occurs at a slower rate and therefore only a proportion of the drug is absorbed from the alveolae with each breadth. Increasing the cardiac output in pregnancy will increase the removal rate of such compounds from the lungs, as the pulmonary blood immediately removes all that has crossed the alveolar membrane. This effect is of limited importance in pregnancy, as few aerosols likely to be used in pregnancy actually reach the alveolae before absorption – they tend to be absorbed from the upper airways.

Skin and mucous membranes

The skin and mucous membranes serve as the site for metabolism of various drugs. In pregnancy, blood flow to the skin is increased significantly, and this results in a more rapid absorption of drugs from the skin surfaces. Absorption of drugs such as glyceryl trinitrate (GTN) patches may be enhanced in pregnancy. The same changes occur in the nasal and oral mucous membranes. Although similar changes occur in the vagina, there is no evidence to indicate that absorption from the vagina is improved.

Central nervous system

There is an increase in the vascularity of the epidural space. Opiates placed in this space are more rapidly absorbed in pregnant than in non-pregnant women [II].[1] This facilitates the rapid establishment of analgesia in labour.

Plasma and blood volume

Body water increases by 6–8 L during pregnancy. Most of this is extracellular, although a significant proportion is incorporated into the products of conception (fetus, placenta, amniotic fluid and uterus). Plasma volume increases by 50 per cent by the third trimester. Red cell volume increases by 18 per cent in pregnancy. These physiological changes increase the area of distribution for water-soluble drugs.

Plasma proteins

The concentration of plasma albumin falls in the first half of pregnancy from about 35 g/L to 25 g/L. For drugs which are highly bound to albumin, this results in a decrease in the bound fraction – with a corresponding increase in the free drug concentration. An inverse relationship between free (unbound) drug fraction and albumin concentration in the plasma of pregnant women has been demonstrated for drugs such as phenytoin, diazepam, phenobarbitone and sodium valproate.

The urinary system

The kidneys are an important route for the metabolism and excretion of drugs. Physiological changes in pregnancy such as an increase in the renal plasma blood flow and the glomerular filtration rate may therefore affect the concentration and elimination of these drugs from the body and consequently alter their efficacy.

TERATOGENICITY

When a drug is administered to the mother and crosses into the embryo or fetus, it may have severe consequences. Drugs administered during the critical period of intrauterine development may induce harmful effects to the embryo and/or fetus. The fetus is most vulnerable during the embryonic period, which is between the second and eighth week post-conception. Organogenesis, which occurs at this time, may be either interrupted or altered, with a resulting abnormality or fetal death. Drugs that affect organogenesis are described as teratogenic. When administered after the second to eighth weeks, the consequences of teratogenic agents on the fetus are often limited, although structural consequences may still occur, especially in those organs still undergoing organogenesis (such as the brain and kidneys). There are certain drugs with well-recognized teratogenicity. In addition, there are others with known teratogenic effects in animals but with uncertain safety in humans. This uncertainty has resulted in extreme caution being exercised in the prescription of some of these drugs in pregnancy – even when there are proven benefits. Most women are reluctant to take medication during pregnancy for fear of teratogenicity, and thus compliance with prescribed medication is also affected. Such a decision to refuse medication may increase the risk of disease complications.

Table 8.1 contains examples of therapies with known teratogenic effects and also details non-teratogenic fetal side effects.

Thalidomide teratogenicity increased awareness of the potential adverse effects of drugs on the fetus. This drug was used to treat nausea and vomiting in early pregnancy and was reported to be associated with malformations, which included phocomelia, amelia and other abnormalities such as heart and external ear defects.[2] When this drug was withdrawn, there was a significant fall in the incidence of these malformations. Very recently, however, there has been a resurgence, especially in South America where thalidomide is being used to treat leprosy and acquired immunodeficiency syndrome (AIDS)-related complications.

Examples of teratogenic and/or other fetal side effects are discussed below.

Anticonvulsants

Controversy remains over the effect of pregnancy on the frequency of epileptic seizures (see Chapter 6.10). Because of the significant consequences of repeated seizures in pregnancy on the fetus and mother, adequate control is considered paramount. Unfortunately, most of the anti-epileptic drugs are teratogenic. The most common groups of drugs include the hydantoin agents, carbamazepine, and sodium valproate. It has been estimated that approximately one-third of children born to mothers on phenytoin have minor anomalies and 10 per cent have major anomalies.[3]

Carbamazepine, hitherto considered one of the safest anti-epileptic drugs in pregnancy, is associated with a pattern of malformations similar to those induced by the hydantoin group. In addition, carbamazepine induces neural tube defects in about 1 per cent of cases.

The malformations associated with the hydantoin group of drugs include cranio-facial abnormalities (e.g. cleft palate and lip, hypertelorism, broad nasal bridge), hypoplasia of the distal phalanges and nails, and cardiac defects. There is also an increased risk of intrauterine growth restriction and mental abnormality. A deficiency of the enzyme epoxide hydrolase is thought to be responsible for the defects induced by hydantoin and carbamazepine.

Sodium valproate is associated with a risk of neural tube defects of 1–2 per cent. It is also associated with some of the malformations associated with the other anti-epileptic

Table 8.1   Examples of drugs and their teratogenic consequences

Drug family	Specific drugs	Teratogenic consequences	Non-teratogenic fetal consequences
Anti-epileptics	Sodium valproate (Epilim)	Spina bifida, cleft lip and palate, dental hypoplasia	
	Phenytoin, trimethadone, carbamazepine and other hydantoins	Cleft lip and palate, dental hypoplasia	IUGR, mental deficiency
Anti-emetics	Thalidomide	Phocomelia, amelia, external ear defects, cardiac defects	
Antidepressants	Lithium	Cardiovascular	
Anti-hypertensives	ACE inhibitors	Skull defects	Fetal renal impairment
Antibiotics	Tetracycline		Yellowish coloration of the teeth
	Aminoglycosides		Damage to the eighth cranial nerve
Anti-metabolites	Cyclophosphamide, methotrexate, cisplatin, busulphan, aminopterin	Multisystemic including skeletal, CNS, CVS	IUGR
Steroids	Androgens, e.g danazol, diethylstilbestrol	Virilization of a female fetus Ambiguous external genitalia Clear cell carcinoma of the vagina or cervix, vagina adenosis, uterine hyopoplasia, T-shaped uterus, incompetent cervix, hypoplastic testes, cryptorchidism	
Anticoagulants	Warfarin	Dental hypoplasia, hypoplastic nails, upturned nose, low-set ears, chondrodysplasia punctata, dental hypoplasia	Intracranial haemorrhage, IUGR
Retinoids and other vitamin A derivatives	Vitamin A, liver extracts, isoretinoin	Micrognathia, cleft lip and palate, CVS, CNS and limb defects	IUGR, IUFD

ACE, angiotensin-converting enzyme; CNS, central nervous system; CVS, cardiovascular system; IUGR, intrauterine growth restriction; IUFD, intrauterine fetal death.

Antenatal complications: maternal

drugs. The newer anti-epileptics such as lamotrigine and gabapentin are thought to be less teratogenic, and therefore appear to be safer in pregnancy. It is important to caution that the experience with these newer preparations is still limited, and long-term consequences must be observed and documented carefully.

Anticoagulants

Heparin is a large molecular weight compound and does not cross the placenta. It therefore has no teratogenic effects. In contrast, coumarin derivates cross the placenta and have significant teratogenic and fetal effects. Warfarin can cause a broad spectrum of anomalies, reported to occur in 15–25 per cent of children born to women exposed to warfarin in the first trimester. The warfarin embryopathy syndrome includes nasal hypoplasia, stippled bone epiphyses, hydrocephaly, microcephaly, malformations of the vertebral bodies,[4] intrauterine growth restriction and neurodevelopmental delay.

Steroids

Steroid use in early pregnancy is uncommon. Occasionally, a woman taking steroids may become pregnant and only realize after the period of organogenesis is complete. The most common drug in this category is danazol (used to treat endometriosis or other ovarian cycle-related pathologies). As an androgen, danazol induces virilization of the external genitalia of female fetuses, causing labioscrotal fusion and hypertrophy of the clitoris. These defects are mainly cosmetic and tend to resolve spontaneously during infancy.

Diethystilbestrol (DES) was used in the past to treat nausea and vomiting in pregnancy. The offspring of women exposed to this non-steroidal synthetic oestrogen are at an increased risk of clear cell carcinoma of the cervix and vagina, vaginal adenosis, T-shaped uterus and/or hypoplasia of the uterus.

The association between other steroids and malformations is weak. Prolonged use of steroids as therapy for various medical conditions has been associated with a variety of malformations described by the acronym VACTERAL (vertebral, analatresia, cardiac, tracheo-oesophageal, renal and limb). The true incidence of the association between steroids and these malformations is uncertain.

Psychotropic drugs

This family of drugs is used to treat various psychiatric disorders in pregnancy. Although most of these drugs will cross the placenta, the only well-recognized member with significant teratogenic effects is lithium. Lithium therapy is associated with an increased incidence of cardiac malformations, particularly Ebstein's anomaly. A meta-analysis revealed an incidence of this anomaly in 1–12 per cent of the offspring of mothers exposed to lithium.[5] This is significantly greater than the population incidence of 1:20 000 live births. There is no increase in other non-cardiovascular defects, although exposure in late pregnancy has been associated with polyhydramnios and diabetes insipidus.

Sedatives or tranquillizers are not known to be associated with major malformations. However, they may have effects on the fetus such as intrauterine growth restriction and reduced fetal movements. Benzodiazepines, such as diazepam and chlordiazepoxide, may induce transient hypotonia, hypothermia and respiratory depression when administered in late pregnancy and close to delivery.

There are no robust data to suggest that antidepressants such as fluoxetine (Prozac) are teratogenic. Large case series have failed to demonstrate any association of Prozac with congenital malformations. Although there are isolated reports linking the tricyclic antidepressant amitriptyline with limb reduction defects, the association is unproven.

Phenothiazine derivates are used in pregnancy for the treatment of hyperemesis gravidarum, and chlorpromazine is used to treat schizophrenia. There is no recognized association between this family of drugs and congenital malformations. When used in late pregnancy, especially in the peripartum period, they may induce transient extrapyramidal effects on the neonate.

Antimicrobials

Antifungal agents

The most common indication for prescribing antifungal agents in pregnancy is vaginal candidiasis. In most cases antifungal agents are applied vaginally, although systemic therapy may occasionally be offered. The most frequently prescribed therapies are clotrimazole, nystatin, amphotericin B and miconazole. There is no evidence to link these agents with teratogenicity or fetal effects.[6] A few reports have linked griseofulvin (used to treat mycotic infections of the skin and nails) with an increased incidence of abnormalities of the central nervous and musculoskeletal systems, but the evidence is minimal and limited to animals; the only case-control study in human pregnancy did not demonstrate any association.[7] Although topical and systemic antifungal agents do not appear to be associated with teratogenicity in human pregnancy, caution must be exercised, especially when these agents are prescribed in high doses or for prolonged periods.

Antiviral agents

The two most commonly prescribed antiviral agents in pregnancy are acyclovir and zidovudine (AZT). Others include ramantadine, idoxuridine and vidarabine. Zidovudine is the primary agent for the treatment of human immunodeficiency virus (HIV) infection in pregnancy. Although this drug has been very widely used in this condition, there are currently no large epidemiological studies of its effects on the embryo/fetus. However, it is generally regarded as safe and indeed if there were any associated teratogenic effects, the risk:benefit ratio would be beneficial.

Amongst the other antiviral agents, amantadine has been reported to be associated with an increased incidence of malformations. Ribavirin, used for the treatment of respiratory syncytial virus, is associated with an increased incidence of congenital malformations in animals at doses similar to those used in humans. These agents should therefore be avoided in pregnancy, especially during the period of organogenesis [III].

Acyclovir is the antiviral agent of choice in the treatment of herpes and varicella infections. It is administered systemically. This drug has been prescribed for pregnant women at all gestations and there are no reported malformations attributable to it. It is therefore considered safe and has been recommended as the primary treatment of women with active genital herpes and those with overwhelming varicella [III]. Case reports of neonatal mitochondrial toxicity have been noted in mothers treated with AZT or Neviparine for HIV. Ongoing reporting of all HIV cases in the UK should help to clarify the situation.

Antibacterial agents

Bacterial infections, especially of the urinary tract, are common in pregnancy. Fortunately, most appropriate antimicrobial agents are safe in pregnancy. The families of antimicrobials that are associated with either teratogenic or fetal effects include the tetracyclines, aminoglycosides, sulphonamides and fluoroquinolines.

Penicillin and its derivatives are some of the safest antimicrobials in pregnancy. Although they may cross the placenta, they are not teratogenic. They should therefore be considered the drugs of choice whenever possible. The combination of the penicillins with the beta-lactamase inhibitor clavulanic acid (Augmentin) has been demonstrated to induce significant side effects in the fetus, although these may not be associated with congenital malformations.[8] It is therefore advisable to avoid Augmentin in pregnancy [Ib].

Macrolides are large molecules and do not cross the placenta. These agents are also considered to be safe in pregnancy. The most common member of this family is erythromycin – the drug of choice for infections which are not sensitive to penicillin derivatives. The main disadvantage of these agents is that if the fetus needs treatment, they will be ineffective. For example, patients with syphilis treated with erythromycin have had offspring with congenital syphilis. Erythromycin is the drug of choice in patients with premature rupture of fetal membranes (see Chapter 22) [Ia].

Second-generation and third-generation cephalosporins contain the N-methylthiotetrazole (MTT) side chain that has been associated with testicular hypoplasia in animals. Although no similar effect has been demonstrated in humans, these drugs should be used with caution in pregnancy, especially in the first trimester. Cefatoxin is a second-generation cephalosporin that does not contain this MTT

side chain and is therefore the cephalosporin of choice in pregnancy [III].

Aminoglycosides are teratogenic. When administered to the pregnant woman, they cross into the embryo/fetus at significant levels. Streptomycin, a member of this family, has been reported to be associated with sensorineural deafness (eighth cranial nerve damage). This risk of ototoxicity is thought to be of the order of 2 per cent (20-fold higher than the background risk). Although no similar effects have been reported with other aminoglycosides, they should be avoided if possible [IV].

Tetracycline and its derivatives are effective in the treatment of chlamydial infections. They are broad-spectrum antibiotics, which are cheap and affordable in most developing countries. Their use in pregnancy is associated with well-recognized effects, including the discolouration of the deciduous teeth. This group of antimicrobials is therefore best avoided in pregnancy [II].

Sulphonamides cross the placenta and may compete with the binding of bilirubin in the fetus, resulting in neonatal jaundice. Trimethoprim, which is a weak folate antagonist and may be used in combination with a sulphonamide (e.g. in the form of Septrin), has not been associated with congenital malformations, although there is a theoretical risk (secondary to its antifolate action). Chloramphenicol should be avoided in pregnancy [II]; although it is not recognized to cause specific congenital malformations; it is associated with the neonatal grey baby syndrome.

Among the antimicrobial agents that have not been demonstrated to have congenital malformations are nitrofurantoin and the fluoroquinolones (e.g. ciprofloxacin). However, the latter has been associated with congenital arthropathy in dogs (not demonstrated in humans) and the manufacturers caution against its use in pregnancy.

Antiprotozoal agents

The three most common protozoal infections in pregnancy are *Trichomonas vaginalis*, *Plasmodium* sp. and *Toxoplasma gondii*. Others include *Entamoeba histologica*, *Giardia lamblia*, leishmaniasis, *Trypanosoma haematobium* (which is more common in developing countries) and *Pneumocystis carinii*.

Trichomonas vaginalis is a flagellate, which causes a vaginal discharge. Metronidazole is the treatment of choice, and should be used in pregnancy with caution, although there are no data to suggest teratogenicity or fetal effects [IV]. During breastfeeding, it may alter the taste of breast milk and affect breastfeeding. Where metronidazole is ineffective, tinidazole could be used. During treatment with metronidazole, alcohol should be avoided.

Antiprotozoal agents for *Plasmodium* include those used for prophylaxis and for therapy. Prophylactic agents include mefloquine, chloroquine, proguanil hydrochloride, pyremethamine and sulfadaxone. Although there are no human data suggesting teratogenicity, mefloquine has been demonstrated to be teratogenic in animals. The manufacturers therefore caution against the use of all of these agents in pregnancy. However, when the consequences of malaria infection are considered, the benefits of prophylaxis outweigh any theoretical risks [IV]. (It may also be advisable not to travel to an endemic area in the first trimester.) Any recommendation for prophylaxis must consider the type of malaria prevalent in the area. It is inadvisable to use drugs to which the *Plasmodium* sp. may be resistant; although the use of chloroquine has not been demonstrated to be associated with congenital malformations, the protozoon has become resistant to chloroquine in many parts of the world.

Toxoplasmosis infection in non-pregnant women is commonly self-limiting and treatment is not necessary. However, in pregnancy, toxoplasmosis may be associated with teratogenic and fetal effects following transplacental infection. Treatment may therefore theoretically reduce the risk of transmission to the fetus. The drug of choice is spiramycin, which is available on a named-patient basis. There are no reports of associated malformations with spiramycin. Pyremethamine (an anti-malarial agent) may also be used to treat toxoplasmosis.

Treatment for the other uncommon protozoal infections include metronidazole or tinidazole for amoebiasis; metronidazole or mepacrine hydrocholoride for giardiasis; sodium stibogluconate, amphotericin B or pentamidine isetionate for leishmaniasis and co-trimoxazole, pentamidine isotionate, atovaquone or trimetrexate for *Pneumocystis carinii*. For most of these drugs, there are no data linking them with congenital malformations, but their use in pregnancy must be with extreme caution.

Anthelmintics

Helmintic infections that may be acquired in pregnancy include threadworms/pinworms (enterobiasis), roundworms (ascarides), hookworms (necatoriasis), strongyloides, whipworms (trichuriasis), tapeworms, cutaneous larva migrans, schistosomicides and filariacides. The common infections are hookworms, threadworms and roundworms. Mebendazole and piperazine are effective against all these common infestations. They should be used with caution in pregnancy. Although mebendazole has been shown to be toxic at high doses to rat embryos, no such effect has been described in humans.

Analgesics

The analgesics used in pregnancy can be subdivided into narcotics and non-narcotics. The narcotics include morphine and its derivatives and pethidine. The non-narcotics can be further subclassified as salicylates and the non-steroidal anti-inflammatory agents (NSAIDs).

Narcotic analgesics are used more commonly intra-partum; however, in cases of severe pain in early pregnancy, they may be the only effective option. The two most common agents are pethidine and morphine and its derivatives. There is no increase in the incidence of malformations

with these drugs, but there are considerable fetal effects depending on the duration of use. When used over a prolonged period, they may be associated with neonatal withdrawal symptoms. Chronic use should therefore be avoided [IV]. Large doses used in labour may cause respiratory depression in the neonate.

Although aspirin is also a NSAID, it is the prototype of the salicylates. As a NSAID, it may cause premature closure of the patent ductus arteriosus and pulmonary hypertension in the newborn. When used in large doses, it may be associated with haemorrhagic disorders in both the mother and fetus due to reduced platelet activity. It is most likely that the usual adult dose is not sufficiently high to cause malformations; however, aspirin at standard doses should only be used in pregnancy if there are no alternatives [IV]. Low-dose aspirin is currently used to treat women with antiphospholipid syndrome and may be considered for women with significant risk of developing pre-eclampsia and intrauterine growth restriction. At these very low dosages, there is no evidence to suggest an association with congenital malformations or fetal effects.

Acetaminophen (paracetamol) is considered the analgesic of choice in pregnancy. Although no malformations or fetal effects have been reported with therapeutic doses, larger doses may cause significant liver damage in the mother and the fetus. Acetaminophen is not associated with premature closure of the ductus arteriosus or oligohydramnios.

The most common NSAIDs available for use as analgesics in pregnancy include indomethacin, ibuprofen and naproxen. These agents inhibit prostaglandin synthetase inhibitors and, like aspirin, may be associated with premature closure of the patent ductus arteriosus and pulmonary hypertension in the neonate. In large doses, they may cause fetal renal failure.

Cardiovascular drugs

Cardiovascular disorders include some of the common medical complications of pregnancy, and affect approximately 3–5 per cent of all gravidas (see Chapter 6.3). The most common are valvular and hypertensive disorders. Although rarely indicated, anti-arrhythmic drugs may be used not only to treat the mother but also to treat dysrrhythmic conditions in the fetus. For the valvular disorders, thromboprophylaxis and antibiotics (especially in labour) are the common medications.

Cardiac glycosides increase the force of myocardial contraction and reduce conductivity within the atrioventricular (AV) node. The most commonly used agent is digoxin. The indications for use in pregnancy include cardiac failure and supraventricular tachycardia, especially due to atrial fibrillation. Digoxin is effective in treating maternal supraventricular tachycardia and also in the correction of fetal supraventricular tachycardia. The side effects include nausea, vomiting, diarrhoea, abdominal pain, visual disturbances, fatigue, drowsiness and hallucinations. It is important to avoid hypokalaemia during therapy, as this may precipitate severe side effects. There are reported associations between cardiac glycosides and teratogenicity, but the exact nature of these malformations is unclear.

> **Cardiovascular drugs which may be used in pregnancy**
>
> - Cardiac glycosides
> - Diuretics
> - Anti-arrhythmic drugs
> - Beta-adrenoceptor-blocking drugs
> - Drugs affecting the renin–angiotensin system
> - Nitrates, calcium channel blockers and potassium channel activators

Other examples of anti-arrhythmic drugs include adenosine, amiodarone hydrochloride, flecainide acetate, procainamide hydrochloride, lidocaine hydrochloride and quinidine. The indications for these drugs include ventricular ectopics, atrial fibrillation, paroxysmal supraventricular tachycardia, arrhythmias after myocardial infarction and ventricular tachycardia. There are no reported associations with fetal malformations; however, these agents should only be prescribed in hospital and with the advice of a physician [IV].

Diuretics are rarely used in pregnancy except in the treatment of severe pulmonary oedema. They should be avoided as first-line drugs in the treatment of hypertensive disorders of pregnancy (see Chapters 6.1 and 7.6). When used, they may cause a transient thrombocytopenia and a decreased uterine blood flow, which could potentially be associated with intrauterine growth restriction. Spironolactone, the potassium-sparing diuretic, is a competitive inhibitor of aldosterone and has mild anti-androgenic effects, which could theoretically cause feminization of a male fetus if given in large doses.

Beta-adrenoceptor blocking drugs (beta-blockers) block the beta-adrenoceptors in the heart, peripheral vasculature, bronchi, pancreas and liver. Some beta-blockers, such as oxprenolol, pindolol and acebutolol, have intrinsic sympathomimetic activity and are not recommended in pregnancy [IV]. Examples of beta-blockers that may be used to treat hypertension in pregnancy include labetalol (alpha-blocker and beta-blocker), propranolol and atenolol (see Chapter 6.1). These drugs are not contraindicated in diabetes, although they can lead to a deterioration of glucose tolerance and interfere with metabolic and autonomic responses to hypoglycaemia. When used in pregnant diabetics, glycaemic control must be monitored very closely. Although beta-blockers are not associated with a greater incidence of congenital malformations, they have been linked with a greater incidence of intrauterine growth restriction [II].[9]

Hydralazine and diazoxide are vasodilators that may be used to reduce hypertension rapidly in pregnancy. They are very potent when used in combination with beta-blockers. When administered in pregnancy, the dangers of a very rapid fall in blood pressure must always be considered, as this may result in significant hypotension and fetal compromise. Less commonly used vasodilators in pregnancy include minoxidil and sodium nitroprusside. Important side effects of these drugs include tachycardia, palpitations, fluid retention and, for hydralazine, gastrointestinal disturbances and systemic lupus-like symptoms after long-term therapy. The use of hydralazine in pregnancy has not been reported to be associated with teratogenicity, but the use of diazoxide has been associated with transient neonatal hypoglycaemia and alopecia in the mother.

Methyldopa is the most commonly prescribed centrally acting anti-hypertensive in pregnancy, and is not a recognized teratogen. Side effects include gastrointestinal disturbances, dry mouth, stomatitis, bradycardia, postural hypotension, headaches, dizziness, nightmares, depression, mild psychosis, hepatitis, jaundice, pancreatitis and anaemia. In a few cases, it may cause Bell's palsy, bone marrow depression, leucopenia and thrombocytopenia. Where there is hypersensitivity, therapy may result in systemic lupus erythematosus-like symptoms.

The adrenergic neurone blocking (such as debrisoquine and guanethidine monosulphate) and the alpha-adrenoceptor blocking drugs (e.g. prazosin, terazosin, indoramin) are not commonly prescribed in pregnancy. Occasionally, women being treated for essential hypertension conceive while taking these drugs. While there are no recognized teratogenic or fetal effects, the manufacturers advise caution with their use in pregnancy.

The newer generation of anti-hypertensives include the angiotensin-converting enzyme (ACE) inhibitors. These agents inhibit the conversion of angiotensin I to angiotensin II. Although they are well tolerated, in general they are contraindicated in pregnancy [III]. They are associated with skull defects and oligohydramnios secondary to impairment in renal function in fetuses and, in addition, adversely affect neonatal blood pressure control and renal function. Angiotensin-II receptor inhibitors such as losartan and valsartan should also be avoided in pregnancy.

Nitrates are used to treat angina. Although they are potent coronary vasodilators, the principal benefit results from a reduced venous return, which decreases left ventricular work. Unwanted side effects include headaches and postural hypotension. Glyceryl trinitrate is one of the most effective in this group, and there are no reported teratogenic or fetal effects.

Calcium channel blockers interfere with the inward displacement of calcium ions through the slow channels of active cell membranes. Myocardial and vascular smooth muscle cell contractility is therefore reduced, and the formation and propagation of electrical impulses within the heart may be depressed. Examples include nifedipine, which can be administered sublingually or swallowed. Nifedipine is not recognized to cause congenital malformations, but must be used with caution as it can lead to a rapid drop in blood pressure and can cause significant fetal compromise [IV].

Respiratory drugs

The most common respiratory problem requiring medication during pregnancy is asthma (see Chapter 6.9). Although in most cases the condition pre-dates pregnancy, in a few cases the diagnosis may be made in pregnancy. Bronchodilators and steroids are the most common drugs used to treat this condition. Compliance with medication in pregnancy is variable, mainly because women are inclined to discontinue medication for fear of teratogenicity and fetal effects.

Bronchodilators administered orally (theophylline) or parenterally (aminophylline) are not associated with any adverse effect on pregnancy. Salbutamol is commonly used and is not associated with teratogenicity. It is therefore important that women on these drugs are reassured about their safety and advised to continue with medication throughout pregnancy, as deterioration in the disease may have significant consequences. An increase in the frequency of heterogeneous, non-major malformations has been reported with the use of ephedrine, and ephedrine is only recommended therapy for acute asthma attacks.

Steroids are used primarily as immunosuppressants in the treatment or prevention of deterioration of asthma. They prevent airway inflammation and hence reduce the oedema and secretions of mucus within the airway. Disodium cromoglycate is used to inhibit mast cell histamine release. It is given via the nasal route and is used primarily for prophylaxis in chronic asthmatics. There are no reported teratogenic effects of this drug. Beclomethasone dipropionate (Becotide) is the most commonly used steroid in the UK. It is administered by inhalation. In most cases, the dose of the steroids is low and therefore there is no adrenal suppression. However, if high and/or parenteral doses are needed, adrenal suppression may occur; therefore management must include the avoidance and prevention of adrenal failure following stressful conditions such as labour and infections. In these circumstances, parenteral hydrocortisone should be administered [IV].

Anti-neoplastics

The common types of malignancy that will require treatment include Hodgkin's lymphoma, malignant melanoma and breast carcinoma (see Chapter 7.3). Chemotherapeutic agents used in the treatment of these conditions may be grouped into alkylating agents, anti-metabolites, plant alkaloids, antibiotics and carboplatin derivatives. Most of these agents interfere with cell division and are therefore associated with a spectrum of malformations. These agents are best avoided in pregnancy, although normal pregnancies have resulted after chemotherapy.

Endocrine medication

Thyrotoxicosis and diabetes mellitus are the most common endocrine disorders of pregnancy. Oral hypoglycaemic agents used in the control of diabetes in the non-pregnant woman should be avoided during pregnancy because of the risk of poor glycaemic control. In addition, there are reported teratogenic effects in animals. The newer agents have been tried in a small number of cases but the results are not convincing (see Chapter 6.2).

Treatment of thyrotoxicosis may involve ^{131}I, carbimazole or propylthiouracil. Both carbimazole and propylthiouracil cross the feto-placental barrier and in high doses may cause fetal goitre or hypothyroidism. The lowest dose that controls maternal hyperthyroidism is therefore advisable. On very rare occasions, the use of carbimazole may be associated with aplasia cutis. Because these drugs cross the placenta, attempts should be made to reduce therapy to a maintenance dose at the time of delivery. These drugs also cross into breast milk, but are not contraindicated in breastfeeding. Radioactive iodine should be avoided in pregnancy because of potential fetal side effects. In hypothyroid states, the use of thyroxine is not associated with any malformations as it does not cross the placenta.

Vaccines

It is not uncommon for women travelling abroad to seek advise on vaccination. Such vaccines include yellow fever, tuberculosis and typhoid. In general, all live vaccines should be avoided during pregnancy [IV]. These vaccines have a more significant effect when administered in the first trimester. Vaccinia virus multiplication may lead to fetal infection, miscarriages and perinatal deaths.[10] Rubella vaccine in the first trimester poses a significant risk to the fetus; the risks diminish with increasing gestational age. Rubella immunization in non-immune gravidae should be delayed until after delivery and pregnancy should be avoided for at least 1 month after immunization. Other live vaccines that should be avoided in pregnancy include yellow fever vaccine, poliomyelitis oral vaccine, bacille Calmette–Guérin (BCG) vaccine and hepatitis B vaccine.

Killed vaccines such as those for typhoid, cholera, plague and typhus can, if indicated, be given to pregnant women without risk to the fetus. Other viral vaccines such as influenza and poliomyelitis (non-live) are also considered safe in pregnancy.

Drugs and breastfeeding

The administration of some drugs to nursing mothers may cause toxicity in the infant. Other drugs may inhibit lactation and therefore be unsuitable to the nursing mother. The effect of the drug on the infant can only occur if the drug enters into the milk in pharmacologically significant quantities. The concentrations of some drugs, for example iodides, in the infant may exceed those in the mother. Drugs that may sedate the infant, although not associated with any significant toxic effects, may result in failure to breastfeed, especially if the infant is repeatedly drowsy. Even drugs that cross into the breast milk in small quantities can cause hypersensitivity reactions in the infant.

The list of drugs that cross into breast milk in significant quantities can be found in each formulary. There are very few drugs that are contraindicated in nursing mothers, but the list of those that have to be administered with caution is important and should be studied carefully before prescribing.

Medication in pregnancy

- There are no randomized studies of the safety of drugs in pregnancy.
- Augmentin is unsafe to the fetus when administered in pregnancy.
- Terotogenicity induced by drugs at higher dosages in animals is difficult to prove in humans because of the ethical debate such exposure raises.

KEY POINTS

- The fetus is most vulnerable to drug teratogenicity at 2–8 weeks.
- Physiological changes in pregnancy alter the metabolism of drugs.
- Live vaccines should be avoided during pregnancy.
- Very few drugs are absolutely contraindicated in breastfeeding.
- Anti-neoplastic drugs should be avoided in pregnancy unless absolutely necessary.

KEY REFERENCES

1. Husemeyer RP, Cummings AJ, Rosankiewicz JR, Davenport HT. A study of pethidine kinetics and analgesia in women in labour following intravenous, intramuscular and epidural administration. *Br J Clin Pharmacol* 1982; 13:171–6.
2. McBirdie WG. Thalidomide embryopathy. *Teratology* 1977; 16:79–82.
3. Kelly TE. Teratogenecity of anticonvulsant drugs. I. Review of the literature. *Am J Med Genet* 1984; 19:413–34.
4. Barker DP, Konje JC, Richardson J. Warfarin embryopathy. *Acta Paediatr Scand* 1994; 83:411.
5. Cohen LS, Friedman JM, Jefferson JW et al. A re-evaluation of risk of in utero exposure to lithium. *J Am Med Assoc* 1994; 271:146–50.
6. Rosa FW, Baum C, Shaw M. Pregnancy outcomes after first trimester vaginitis drug therapy. *Obstet Gynecol* 1987; 69:751–5.
7. Cunningham FG, MacDonald PC, Grant NF et al. Medication use during pregnancy. Part I. Concepts of human teratology. In: *Williams Obstetrics*, 20th edn, Supplement 10. Norwalk, CT: Appleton & Lange, 1997, 943–67.
8. Kenyon SL, Taylor DJ, Tarnow-Mordi W, for the ORACLE Collaborative Group. Broad spectrum antibiotics for preterm, prelabour rupture of fetal membranes: the ORACLE I randomised trial. *Lancet* 2001; 357:979–88.
9. Rubin PC. Current concepts: beta-blockers on pregnancy. *N Engl J Med* 1981; 305:1323–6.
10. Levine MM. Live-virus in pregnancy. Risks and recommendations. *Lancet* 1974; 2:34–8.

Chapter 9

Maternal Mortality

James Drife

INTRODUCTION

The death of a woman in pregnancy is now uncommon in developed countries. Nevertheless, in the UK the long-established Confidential Enquiries into Maternal Deaths have a high profile among obstetricians. Their reports have been called 'the obstetrician's bible' and are frequently quoted in clinical and research papers. There is also widespread awareness of the global problem of maternal mortality.

INCIDENCE

Worldwide

The World Health Organization (WHO) estimates that there are over 600 000 maternal deaths annually, equivalent to one death every minute of every day. Most are in developing countries. In some parts of Africa, maternal mortality rates are over 1000/100 000 live births, and when this is combined with high fertility rates, the result is disastrous. For example, in Ethiopia a young woman enters the reproductive phase of her life with a 1 in 10 chance that she will die as a result of pregnancy or delivery (Figure 9.1).[1]

UK

In the UK, maternal death occurs in around 1 in 10 000 pregnancies. The maternal mortality rate rose from 9.9/100 000 pregnancies in 1985–87 to 11.4/100 000 in 1997–99, possibly due to more complete reporting of *indirect* deaths, which now outnumber *direct* deaths, as shown in Table 9.1.

The number of late deaths has also risen due to better reporting. The rise in the total in 1994–96 was due to a new computer program linking birth and death registration, which identified deaths that might previously have been missed. The Confidential Enquiry consistently identifies more maternal deaths than the Registrar General, and this high ascertainment in the UK makes comparisons with other countries potentially misleading.

Confidential enquiries into maternal deaths

Since 1952, every maternal death in England and Wales has been the subject of a detailed enquiry, conducted by clinicians – doctors and, nowadays, midwives. Any death during pregnancy or within a year after delivery is reported to the local director of public health, who sends a form, requesting all relevant details, to all staff involved, including the general practitioner (GP), midwife, obstetrician and anaesthetist. The completed form is sent to regional assessors and then to

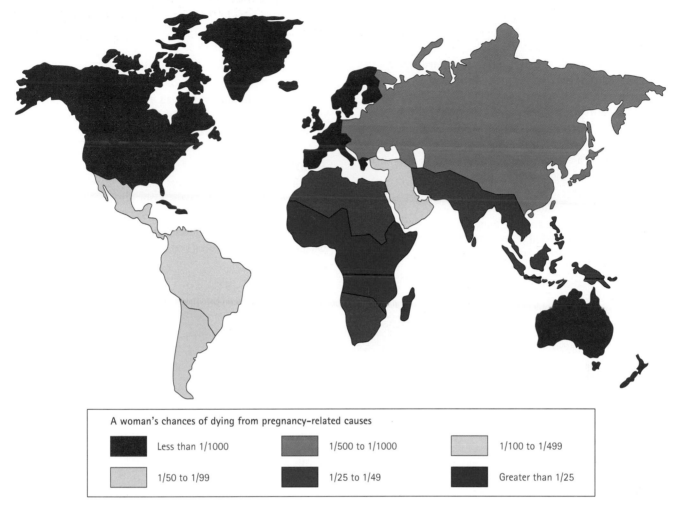

A woman's chances of dying from pregnancy-related causes

■ Less than 1/1000	■ 1/500 to 1/1000	■ 1/100 to 1/499
■ 1/50 to 1/99	■ 1/25 to 1/49	■ Greater than 1/25

Figure 9.1   World map of maternal mortality

Table 9.1   Number of maternal deaths in the UK

	1988–90	1991–93	1994–96	1997–99
Direct	145	129	134	106
Indirect	93	100	134	136
Coincidental	39	46	36	29
Late	48	46	72	107
Total	325	321	376	378

the Department of Health, where it is anonymized before being seen by national assessors in obstetrics, pathology, anaesthetics, general medicine, intensive care, midwifery and psychiatry.

Anonymity allows those involved to comment frankly and make their own suggestions for improvements. No blame is attached to individuals, and the forms are destroyed as soon as the national report is produced. Similar systems exist in Scotland, Wales and Northern Ireland and the final reports are UK-wide, making it more difficult for individual cases to be identified. The reports, which are published every 3 years, list the causes of death, draw attention to substandard care and make recommendations for improving practice.[2]

DEFINITIONS

The definitions given here are those used by the Confidential Enquiries.

- *Maternal death*: death of a woman while pregnant or within 42 days of termination of pregnancy, from any cause related to or aggravated by the pregnancy or its management, but not from accidental or incidental causes.
- *Direct death*: death resulting from obstetric complications of the pregnant state (pregnancy, labour and puerperium), from interventions, omissions, incorrect treatment or from a chain of events resulting from any of the above.
- *Indirect death*: death resulting from previous existing disease or disease that developed during pregnancy and was not due to direct obstetric causes, but was aggravated by the physiological effects of pregnancy.

- *Late death*: death occurring between 42 days and 1 year after abortion, miscarriage or delivery, due to 'direct' or 'indirect' maternal causes.
- *Coincidental death*: death from an unrelated cause which happens to occur in pregnancy or the puerperium. The word 'coincidental' has replaced the term 'fortuitous'.
- *Maternal mortality rate (MMR)*: this expressed in the UK as the number of deaths per 100 000 maternities. A 'maternity' is a clinical pregnancy ending in live birth, stillbirth, miscarriage or abortion.
- The WHO, however, defines the maternal mortality *rate* as 'the number of maternal deaths per 100 000 women of reproductive age', and the maternal mortality *ratio* as 'the number of maternal deaths per 100 000 live births'. Close attention needs to be paid to definitions and denominators.

AETIOLOGY

The causes of maternal mortality are similar all over the world, although overall rates and the relative contribution of each cause vary from country to country.

Worldwide

The WHO has published the estimates shown in Table 9.2.

The *underlying causes* in many developing countries include lack of access to contraception, unsafe abortion, lack of primary care or transport facilities, and inadequate equipment and staffing in district hospitals. Only 55 per cent of deliveries within the developing world are attended by a trained attendant and only 37 per cent of deliveries occur within health facilities.

Education of women is important. In India, the states with high rates of female literacy also have high rates of contraceptive use and low maternal mortality rates. In all countries, safer care could be provided to illiterate women if there were the political will to do so.

UK

Direct deaths

The specific causes of direct death in the UK are shown in Table 9.3.

Too much should not be read into the differences between two triennia, but deaths from some causes appear to have fallen while others have not.

THROMBOEMBOLISM
This has been the leading direct cause of maternal death in the UK since 1985. The 31 deaths from pulmonary embolism in 1997–99 (there were also four deaths from cerebral embolism) were almost equally divided between antepartum and postpartum deaths. Eight occurred before 12 weeks of pregnancy.

HYPERTENSIVE DISEASE
In 1952–54, there were 246 deaths from hypertensive disease in England and Wales. In 1997–99 in the UK, the total was 15. The condition is no less common, but care is now better. Of the 15 deaths in 1997–99, five were from HELLP syndrome (haemolysis, elevated liver enzymes and low platelets).

HAEMORRHAGE
Haemorrhage is treated well in the UK. Out of almost 2 million deliveries in the triennium 1997–99, there were only seven deaths from this cause. Three were from placenta praevia and three from abruption. Postpartum haemorrhage (PPH) caused only one death, even though there must have been about 2000 cases of life-threatening PPH in 1997–99, as it occurs in 1 in 1000 deliveries.

AMNIOTIC FLUID EMBOLISM
Formerly, amniotic fluid embolism (AFE) was diagnosed only when the pathologist confirmed fetal squames in the lungs. From 1991–93, clinically obvious cases have also been included, but there were no such cases in 1997–99. The number of histologically confirmed cases has remained at 8–10 per triennium over the last 15 years.

Table 9.2 Causes of maternal mortality worldwide (WHO)

Causes of maternal death	Estimated number of deaths worldwide per year
Haemorrhage	150 000 (25%)
Indirect (including HIV/AIDS)	120 000 (20%)
Sepsis	90 000 (15%)
Unsafe abortion	78 000 (13%)
Eclampsia	72 000 (12%)
Obstructed labour	48 000 (8%)
Other direct causes	48 000 (8%)

HIV, human immunodeficiency virus; AIDS, acquired immunodeficiency syndrome.

Table 9.3 Causes of direct deaths in the UK[2]

Cause	1994–96	1997–99
Thromboembolism	48	35
Hypertensive disease	20	15
Haemorrhage	12	7
Amniotic fluid embolism	17	8
Early pregnancy deaths	15	17
Genital tract sepsis	14	14
Other	7	7
Anaesthetic	1	3
Total	134	106

From reference 2.

EARLY PREGNANCY DEATHS

Deaths before 24 weeks' gestation now fall in this category (formerly the upper limit was 20 weeks). There were 13 deaths from ectopic pregnancy (out of an estimated 32 000 cases) in 1997–99, and two deaths from miscarriage. There were two deaths from termination, but neither was due to criminal abortion, which has caused no maternal deaths in the UK since 1982. Before the Abortion Act of 1967, there were around 30 maternal deaths every year from criminal abortion.

SEPSIS

Until 1935, streptococcal puerperal sepsis was the leading cause of maternal death in the UK. The 1982–84 report included this modest sentence: 'No deaths could be directly attributed to puerperal sepsis'. The abolition of this cause of death was one of the great medical achievements of the twentieth century. Since 1985, however, there has been a small but steady rise in the number of deaths from sepsis, to 16 in 1997–99, with two of these (and two late deaths) being due to puerperal sepsis.

GENITAL TRACT TRAUMA AND OTHER DIRECT CAUSES

Two deaths were due to genital tract trauma – one from a vaginal wall haematoma in a woman who delivered spontaneously unattended, and the other being a uterine rupture in a woman who had labour induced after a previous caesarean section. 'Other' causes included four deaths from acute fatty liver of pregnancy.

ANAESTHESIA

Despite the rising caesarean section rate, the number of maternal deaths from anaesthesia has fallen steadily from 37 in 1970–72 to only one in 1994–96, and three in 1997–99.

Indirect deaths

The 136 indirect deaths were divided into 35 cardiac and 15 psychiatric cases, 11 cases of malignancy possibly affected by pregnancy, and 75 'other' cases.

CARDIAC DISEASE

The total of 35 deaths makes this the joint leading cause of maternal death (alongside thromboembolism) in 1997–99. Formerly, the major problem in Britain was rheumatic heart disease, as it still is in many developing countries, but now there is a wider spectrum, as shown in Table 9.4.

Table 9.4 Deaths from cardiac disease in the UK, 1997–99[2]

Cardiac disease	Deaths
Congenital heart disease	10
Cardiomyopathy	12
Ruptured aortic aneurysm	5
Myocardial infarction	5
Endocarditis/heart failure	3

PSYCHIATRIC

In 1997–99, 13 women committed suicide (usually by violent means) within 6 weeks of delivery and another 15 suicides were late indirect deaths. There were 42 cases in which psychiatric disorder caused or contributed to the death. In the past, not all psychiatric deaths have been reported to the enquiry, but in 1997–99, a study by the Office of National Statistics, linking birth certificates and death certificates, found another 40 deaths from suicide or violent causes, plus eight in which the coroner had recorded an open verdict and 11 of accidental drug overdose. It is now clear that when late deaths are included, suicide is the leading cause of pregnancy-related death in the UK.

CANCER

In most countries, death from cancer during pregnancy is classed as 'coincidental', but in the UK, cases of cancer are classed as indirect deaths if it appears that the pregnancy may have masked the disease or affected the diagnosis or outcome. Central nervous system (CNS) tumours in particular fall into this category.

OTHER INDIRECT DEATHS

There were 75 'other indirect' deaths in 1997–99. The main ones were diseases of the central nervous system (34 deaths), infectious diseases (13) and respiratory diseases (9). Among diseases of the CNS, nine deaths were due to epilepsy, and among respiratory diseases, five were due to asthma. It is not known whether the number of sudden deaths from epilepsy is greater than in a similar group of non-pregnant women.

Coincidental deaths

Formerly called 'fortuitous' deaths, the 29 coincidental deaths included six cases of neoplasia unaffected by the presence of pregnancy, eight road traffic accidents and eight cases of homicide – in each case by the woman's partner or close relative. Domestic violence is now a major concern to the maternity services. In 1997–99, of the 378 women whose deaths were reported to the enquiry, 45 (12 per cent) had reported domestic violence during the pregnancy. Of the young women under 18 years old who died, 80 per cent had suffered violence in the home.

PREVENTION

Worldwide

Many agencies are promoting initiatives to reduce the global toll of maternal death. These include the WHO and the World Bank. As well as the individual human tragedies, there are also major economic consequences of losing women who are productive members of society. Several countries – such as South Africa and Malaysia – have set up confidential enquiries similar to the UK model. These have identified

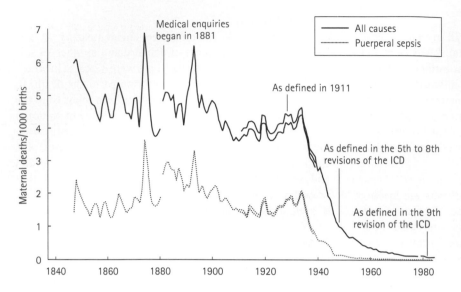

Figure 9.2   Maternal mortality rate in England and Wales, 1847-1984 (reproduced from *Report on Confidential Enquiries into Maternal Deaths in England and Wales 1982-84*, published by HMSO, 1989)

the major problems, but implementing their recommendations requires commitment from politicians, doctors, other healthcare workers and the population as a whole.

Postpartum haemorrhage can be reduced by routine oxytocics at delivery, and unsafe abortion by contraceptive services and legal termination of pregnancy. Otherwise, the main need is less for prevention than for prompt treatment of pregnancy complications. This requires transport, trained healthcare workers, drugs and equipment. The importance of medical care in pregnancy and childbirth was underlined by a comparative study in the USA, which showed that a religious group that had good general health but refused all modern medical care had a maternal mortality rate similar to those in developing countries.[3]

Past experience in the UK

Until 1935, the UK's maternal mortality rate was around 400/100 000 (one death in 250 births), but it fell steadily between 1936 and 1985 (Figure 9.2). Other indicators of public health, such as infant mortality, fell slowly and steadily during the twentieth century, but maternal mortality, by contrast, fell rapidly during the Second World War, when social conditions could hardly be said to be improving. This strongly suggests that the fall was due to specific factors, such as:

- antibiotics: sulphonamides were introduced in 1937 and penicillin in 1944; death rates from puerperal sepsis quickly fell;
- blood transfusion became safe during the 1940s;
- ergometrine, for the treatment and prevention of postpartum haemorrhage, was introduced in the 1940s;
- better training of midwives and obstetricians: Midwives Acts were passed in 1902 and 1936, and the Royal College of Obstetricians and Gynaecologists was founded in 1929;

- reduced parity: the average family size began to fall long before the pill was introduced in 1961;
- legalization of abortion in 1967 was followed by elimination of criminal abortion as a cause of maternal death (Figure 9.3).

The current picture in the UK

Preventing maternal deaths involves targeting the women most at risk. Using denominator data collected by the Office of National Statistics, general risk factors can be identified.

General risk factors

- *Age and parity.* The 'grande multipara' has long been recognized as a high-risk case. In 1997–99, the maternal mortality rate was 6.2 among primigravidae and 35 among women of parity 4 or more. Age and parity go together, but as high parity is now uncommon, the importance of maternal age is becoming clearer. In 1985–99, the maternal mortality rate was 7.2 at age 20–24 and 35.5 among women aged over 40.
- *Ethnicity.* A higher risk among black women has been found in the USA, France and Holland, and was documented in the UK for the first time in 1994–96, when black women were found to have three times the risk of white women, with Asian women in between. In 1997–99, Asian women had three times the risk of white women, with black women in between. The main reason identified by the enquiry was poor communication between maternity services and the woman and her family. There may be language difficulties, problems with the organization of services, failure of the woman or her family to access services, or failure of the services to appreciate the seriousness of symptoms.
- *Social class.* The 1997–99 report identified for the first time the high risk among the lowest social class in Britain, whose maternal mortality rate is similar to the

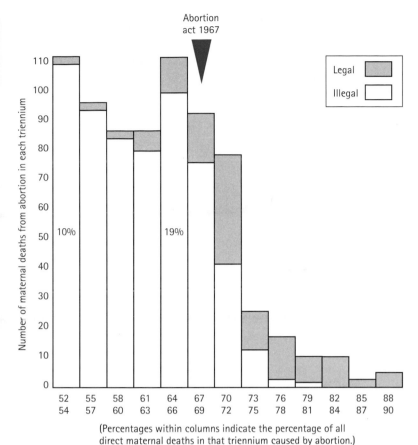

(Percentages within columns indicate the percentage of all
direct maternal deaths in that triennium caused by abortion.)

Figure 9.3 Maternal deaths from abortion, 1952–90.
Reproduced with permission from *Maternal and Child
Health* 1994; **19**:348

rate in a developing country (Table 9.5). This group
includes itinerant people ('travellers'), who tend to turn up
at the wrong time or day at the antenatal clinic or fail to
keep appointments. It is all too easy to overlook their
needs in a service that caters for the wishes of more
articulate and better organized women.

Forty per cent of the maternal deaths in the UK
occur in social class 9. The 1997–99 report includes
some tragic case histories – for example a homeless
teenager who was discharged from hospital after a
miscarriage and froze to death in a front garden.

- *Other risk factors* include infertility and multiple
pregnancies. This is relevant to couples undergoing
assisted conception.

Direct deaths

The Confidential Enquiries also identify substandard care
(Table 9.6). This may involve only a minor aspect of the treatment and does not necessarily mean that the death could have
been avoided. Standards are rising all the time and are very
high in anaesthesia.

Identifying substandard care helps to indicate how deaths
may be avoided.

THROMBOEMBOLISM

Most women who died from thromboembolism had obvious
risk factors which were disregarded. Obesity, a personal or

Table 9.5 Maternal deaths and social class in the UK, 1997–99[2]

Social class	Direct and indirect deaths	MMR/100 000 maternities
1	5	2.94
2	25	4.19
3	31	15.21
4	33	5.32
5	26	8.31
6	12	11.35
7	7	23.81
8	5	38.96
9	97	135.46

MMR, maternal mortality rate.

Table 9.6 Contribution of substandard care to direct deaths in the
UK, 1997–99[2]

	Total	Number (%) with substandard care
1. Thromboembolism	35	20 (57%)
2. Hypertensive disease	15	12 (80%)
3. Haemorrhage	7	5 (71%)
4. Amniotic fluid embolism	8	2 (25%)
5. Early pregnancy deaths	17	11 (65%)
6. Genital tract sepsis	14	7 (50%)
7. Other	7	4 (57%)
8. Anaesthetic	3	3 (100%)
Total	106	64

Table 9.7   Puerperal deaths from thromboembolism

Mode of delivery	1994–96	1997–99
Vaginal delivery	10	10
Caesarean section	15	4
Total	25	14

family history of thromboembolism, and age over 35 can be identified early in pregnancy. Women should be routinely weighed at booking to identify those with a body mass index (BMI) >30 kg/m². During pregnancy, immobilization and long-haul air travel are also risk factors.

An important factor is caesarean section. In 1995, the Royal College of Obstetricians and Gynaecologists produced a guideline[4] with recommendations on thromboprophylaxis after caesarean section (but not after vaginal delivery). In 1997–99, the first full triennium after its publication, deaths from thromboembolism after caesarean section fell dramatically, while those after vaginal delivery did not change (Table 9.7).

Similar guidelines are now needed for all pregnant women. Prophylaxis involves early mobilization of all women after delivery, and compression stockings for those at higher risk. Women with a personal or family history of thromboembolism and those with thrombophilia should receive heparin prophylaxis.

The other type of substandard care occurs when symptoms are not taken seriously. Most deaths from thromboembolism were preceded by chest pain, cough or leg pain. These require prompt investigation, especially in high-risk women.

HYPERTENSIVE DISEASE

In 1994–96, almost 50 per cent of the 20 deaths from this cause were due to fluid balance problems during treatment. In 1997–99, none was due to oedema, but seven were due to intracranial haemorrhage, i.e. failure of anti-hypertensive therapy. Twelve of the 15 women who died received substandard care, in the form of inadequate monitoring, delay in treatment, or lack of multidisciplinary care. In hospital, pregnancy-induced hypertension is often managed at too junior a level, and symptoms are not taken seriously enough. Recommendations include:

- investigation of symptoms such as headache or abdominal pain,
- clear protocols for hospital treatment,
- the use of magnesium sulphate as the anticonvulsant of choice, and
- early collaboration with intensive care specialists.

HAEMORRHAGE

Placenta praevia carries particular dangers when the placenta is implanted over a uterine scar. The reports have repeatedly emphasized the importance of caesarean section for placenta praevia being carried out by an experienced surgeon. Abruptio placentae is usually complicated by

coagulopathy, which may be extremely difficult to treat. Three women died from this cause in 1997–99 despite satisfactory or even exemplary care.

As severe obstetric haemorrhage becomes less frequent, teams become less experienced in treating it. A multidisciplinary massive haemorrhage protocol should be available in all units and updated and rehearsed regularly in conjunction with the blood bank. Women at known higher risk of haemorrhage should be delivered in a consultant unit with an on-site blood bank.

Guidelines have also been produced for the management of haemorrhage in women who refuse blood transfusion for religious reasons.

AMNIOTIC FLUID EMBOLISM

Amniotic fluid embolism is rare when there has been no obstetric intervention at all. Of the eight deaths in 1997–99, labour had been induced or augmented in five, and another had a previous caesarean section. Nevertheless, there is no clear link with a specific intervention. In six of the cases, the interval between collapse and death was less than 4 hours, but if death does not occur quickly, the woman may be saved by prompt transfer to an intensive care unit. A register of women who survive is now being kept, in the hope that it will shed some light on how best to prevent or treat this enigmatic condition.

EARLY PREGNANCY DEATHS

With modern tests, diagnosing pregnancy is easy, but only if the doctor thinks of the possibility and arranges the test. Ectopic pregnancy is notoriously deceptive, and GPs and casualty officers should perform a urinary pregnancy test on any woman of reproductive age with unexplained abdominal pain. Gastrointestinal symptoms may mask the diagnosis.

SEPSIS

Streptococci can still produce overwhelming sepsis in a relatively short time, even after the woman has left hospital. Now that puerperal sepsis has become rare, doctors and midwives have little experience of the fulminating disease, but it is essential to be alert to the early signs.

Controlled trials have shown that prophylactic antibiotics should routinely be given for caesarean section. In 1997–99, sepsis caused only one death after caesarean section. There were, however, 13 antenatal deaths. When infection develops during or after pregnancy, urgent and repeated bacteriological specimens should be taken and a microbiologist's advice should be sought, but in severe cases parenteral antibiotics should be given before the diagnosis is confirmed.

GENITAL TRACT TRAUMA AND OTHER DIRECT CAUSES

Obstetricians in the UK rarely attempt difficult forceps deliveries now, preferring caesarean section. Vacuum extraction

Table 9.8 Contribution of substandard care to indirect deaths in the UK, 1997-99[2]

	Cases	Number (%) with substandard care
Cardiac disease	35	3 (9%)
Psychiatric	43*	17 (39%)
Other indirect	75	13 (25%)

*This total of psychiatric deaths includes late deaths, mainly from suicide.

is used more often than forceps for instrumental deliveries. These factors have all but abolished death from genital tract trauma in this country.

ANAESTHESIA

The fall in maternal deaths from anaesthesia, despite a rising caesarean section rate, has been achieved by a shift towards regional anaesthesia (avoiding the danger of inhalation associated with general anaesthesia in labour), and by ensuring that only appropriately trained staff give anaesthetics in the labour ward (with the exclusion of the most junior grades from obstetric anaesthesia).

Indirect deaths

Although the proportion of cases with substandard care is lower among indirect deaths than among direct deaths, there is nevertheless potential for improvement (Table 9.8).

CARDIAC DISEASE

Multidisciplinary care is important. Women who are known to have heart disease should be managed by a cardiologist in co-operation with an obstetrician. At delivery, oxytocin must be used with great care.

The possibility of endocarditis should be considered in a pregnant woman with an obscure febrile illness. The possibility of aortic aneurysm should be borne in mind when a woman has severe chest pain, and appropriate imaging should be carried out.

Women with congenital cardiac disease may desperately want a child, but the risk of dying in pregnancy with Eisenmenger's syndrome is 30 per cent. Women with pulmonary vascular disease should be strongly advised against getting pregnant, but should not be alienated from seeking care if pregnancy occurs.

PSYCHIATRIC DISEASE

Ten per cent of new mothers suffer from a depressive illness, which is severe in up to half of cases. Two per cent see a psychiatrist within 1 year of delivery and 2/1000 suffer from puerperal psychosis. The term 'postnatal depression' (PND) should no longer be used, as it may mask the difference between mild and severe depressive illness. Women with a past history of severe mental illness complicating pregnancy have a 33–55 per cent chance of recurrence, which cannot be prevented by hormonal treatment.

Maternal death from suicide shows no social class gradient: professional women and unemployed women are at the same risk. The booking history should include sensitive enquiry about past history and, when appropriate, psychiatric assessment should be arranged during pregnancy. Each unit should have a protocol for the management of women at high risk. There is a need for assessment and management of psychiatric illness by a specialist perinatal mental health team, and every region should have a mother and baby unit to which women may be admitted.[5]

OTHER INDIRECT DEATHS

Women with epilepsy need specific specialist advice in pregnancy, if possible from a combined clinic run by an obstetrician, a physician and a specialist nurse or midwife. Relatives should be informed about the risks and educated to place patients in the recovery position once the fit is over.

Pregnancy is not a reason for withholding plain X-rays of the chest or abdomen, some computed tomography films or magnetic resonance imaging from sick women.

Coincidental deaths
ROAD TRAFFIC ACCIDENTS

Pregnancy is not a contraindication to the use of seat belts, and women should be advised that the belt is placed 'over and under the bump'.

DOMESTIC VIOLENCE

Domestic violence may begin or worsen during pregnancy and may be the reason for late booking or poor attendance, or conversely for repeated attendance with minor injuries or non-existent complaints. Other warning signs include drug or alcohol abuse, or the constant presence of a partner at examinations. Staff need sensitivity and ingenuity to help an affected woman to communicate with them. There should be local strategies for referral, routine enquiries about violence to be included when a social history is taken, and the need for every woman to be seen on her own at least once during the pregnancy.[6]

THE FUTURE

As maternal mortality has fallen in Britain, attention has turned to 'near misses' – incidents that might have resulted in a maternal death but for prompt and effective treatment. Local 'near miss' studies have used criteria such as admission to an intensive care unit,[7] and a comprehensive survey in Pretoria, South Africa, developed a full list of criteria for 'near misses'.[8] One of the main findings of these investigations is that haemorrhage is much more common among 'near misses' than in mortality enquiries.[9]

In England, the four Confidential Enquires, into Maternal Deaths, Stillbirths and Deaths in Infancy, Perioperative Deaths, and Suicides and Homicides, are now grouped together under the National Institute for Clinical Excellence (NICE), which recognizes that for conditions that occur infrequently, observational studies provide essential information.

SUMMARY

The worldwide total of 600 000 maternal deaths every year is largely preventable, as treatment is already available for most of the causes. Ensuring that such treatment reaches the women who need it is a matter of political will, and obstetricians have a duty to act as advocates for the women at risk.

In the UK, the maternity services have been very successful in making pregnancy safe for most women. Nevertheless, sub-standard care still occurs, and the number of maternal deaths has by no means reached an irreducible minimum. Women from ethnic minorities are at increased risk, as are the most deprived sections of the community in Britain. Across all social classes, the leading cause of death in association with pregnancy is suicide.

> Because maternal deaths are rare events, it is very difficult to organize randomized, controlled trials of methods of prevention or treatment.

KEY POINTS

- Maternal death is the death of a woman while pregnant or 42 days after the end of pregnancy. *Direct* deaths result from obstetric complications and *indirect* deaths from disease aggravated by, but not directly due to, pregnancy.
- In developed countries the MMR is around 10 per 100 000 maternities. In many developing countries it is still around 400 per 100 000. More than 600 000 women die during pregnancy every year, mainly in developing countries.
- In Britain, the MMR fell after 1936 due to antibiotics, safe blood transfusion, ergometrine for the prevention of postpartum haemorrhage, better training of midwives and obstetricians and the introduction of the Abortion Act of 1967.
- The commonest direct causes in the UK are thromboembolism, cardiac disease, hypertensive disease and ectopic pregnancy.
- Risk factors include age, parity, low social class and being of an ethnic minority.
- Including late deaths and deaths not reported to the Confidential Enquiry, psychiatric disease is now the leading cause of maternal death in the UK.
- Many of the deaths are preventable, both in Britain and worldwide.

KEY REFERENCES

1. Brundtland GH. Perinatal mortality and morbidity – a global view. Speech delivered at the XVIII European Congress of Perinatal Medicine, Oslo, 19 June 2002: <www.who.int/director-general/speeches/2002>.
2. Lewis G (ed.). *Why Mothers Die 1997–1999*. The Fifth Report of the Confidential Enquiries into Maternal Deaths in the United Kingdom. London: RCOG Press, 2001.
3. Kaunitz AM, Spence C, Danielson TS, Rochard RW, Grimes DA. Perinatal and maternal mortality in a religious group avoiding obstetric care. *Am J Obstet Gynecol* 1994; 150:826–31.
4. RCOG Working Party. *Thromboprophylaxis in Obstetrics and Gynaecology, Report of a Working Group*. London: RCOG Press, 1995.
5. Royal College of Psychiatrists. *Perinatal Mental Health Services*. Council Report CR88. London: Royal College of Psychiatrists, 2000.
6. Bacchus L, Bewley S, Mezey G. Women's perceptions and experiences of routine enquiry for domestic violence in a maternity service. *Br J Obstet Gynaecol* 2002; 109:9–16.
7. Baskett TF, Sternadel J. Maternal intensive care and near-miss mortality in obstetrics. *Br J Obstet Gynaecol* 1998; 105:981–4.
8. Mantel GD, Buchmann E, Rees H, Pattinson RC. Severe acute maternal morbidity: a pilot study for a definition of a near-miss. *Br J Obstet Gynaecol* 1998; 105:985–90.
9. Waterstone M, Bewley S, Wolfe C. Incidence and predictors of severe obstetric morbidity: case-control study. *BMJ* 2001; 322:1089–94.

SECTION B

Antenatal complications: fetal

SECTION B

Biochemical Screening

Michele P. Mohajer

INTRODUCTION

Over the last 40 years, many biochemical substances produced by the feto-placental unit have been identified. A number of these have been found to be associated with certain fetal conditions and have been incorporated into national screening programmes. This section aims to describe those programmes, along with their advantages and disadvantages.

In 1956, the first biochemical marker identified in maternal serum was alpha-fetoprotein (AFP); the association between a raised serum AFP and open spina bifida was not demonstrated until 1974.[1]

BIOCHEMICAL SCREENING FOR NEURAL TUBE DEFECTS

Alpha-fetoprotein is produced by the fetal liver. It crosses into the maternal serum from the amniotic fluid or via the placenta. Maternal serum AFP (MSAFP) rises throughout most of pregnancy (from 12 to 32 weeks), hence accurate determination of gestational age is mandatory. To allow for the increase in concentration in the second trimester, it is convenient to express all AFP values as a multiple of the normal median (MoM) at the relevant gestational age. The separation between the distribution of MSAFP levels in pregnancies with open fetal defects and normal pregnancies is greatest at 16–18 weeks' gestation, and therefore screening is optimum at this stage.

Alpha-fetoprotein screening was intended for the detection of open spina bifida, and not closed spina bifida. Using a cut-off level of 2.5 MoM, 79 per cent open spina bifida and 88 per cent anencephaly can be detected [II]. If all neural tube defects (NTDs) are considered, the detection rate is 72 per cent, with a false-positive rate of 0.001 per cent.[2]

Raised MSAFP is also associated with other fetal malformations or conditions, including:

- multiple pregnancy
- abdominal wall defects (gastroschisis, exomphalos, bladder extrophy)
- congenital nephrosis
- spontaneous fetal loss.

There is also some degree of association between a raised MSAFP and the following conditions:

- pre-eclampsia
- preterm delivery
- low birth weight
- underestimated gestation
- low maternal weight
- Afro-Caribbean ethnic origin
- male fetus
- raised MSAFP in a previous pregnancy
- smoking.

Levels of MSAFP may be lowered in association with other conditions, including:

- Down's syndrome (trisomy 21)
- Edward's syndrome (trisomy 18)
- insulin-dependent diabetes
- overestimated gestation
- high maternal weight.

Alpha-fetoprotein screening now has a relatively minor role in the detection of fetal defects due to the widespread use of sophisticated ultrasound techniques. Using ultrasound to demonstrate the characteristic cranial signs of spina bifida (the 'lemon and banana' sign), the detection rate of all NTDs is 81 per cent (II), with a false-positive rate of 0.0003 per cent (see Chapter 10.2).[3] This detection rate exceeds that of AFP screening programmes. However, AFP screening is still used in areas of high NTD prevalence, or where high-resolution ultrasound is not routinely available.

The role of amniocentesis in MSAFP screening

Prior to high-resolution ultrasound, amniocentesis was routinely performed to detect increased levels of AFP and acetylcholinesterase (AChE) in the amniotic fluid in an attempt to diagnose open fetal defects. The risk of fetal loss may be eight times higher when amniocentesis is performed in these circumstances [Ia], and it therefore should not be performed as an initial investigation.[4]

Many more biochemical substances have been identified that are produced during pregnancy. Many of these have been investigated for their usefulness in detecting pregnancy complications. Two notable hormones, human placental lactogen (hPL) and oestriol (E3), were used widely to assess placental function. These have now been abandoned due to the development of better biophysical methods.

BIOCHEMICAL SCREENING FOR DOWN'S SYNDROME

The main area of development of other biochemical markers in pregnancy has been in screening for Down's syndrome (trisomy 21).

Down's syndrome is still the commonest cause of severe mental retardation. The natural birth prevalence increases with maternal age, from 1 in 1500 under the age of 25, to 1 in 1000 at age 30, and to 1 in 100 at age 40. The overall incidence of the condition has increased due to women having their babies at an older age.

In the early 1980s, antenatal screening relied on identifying women above a specified age (e.g. 35 years) and offering them amniocentesis. In 1984, low MSAFP levels in the mid-trimester were found to be associated with Down's syndrome.[5] Later, human chorionic gonadotrophin (hCG) was found to be raised in Down's syndrome, and unconjugated oestriol (uE3) was found to be reduced. Division of hCG into its free subunits (alpha-hCG and beta-hCG) provided additional value in screening. More recently, a fourth biochemical marker, inhibin-A, has been found to be raised in Down's syndrome pregnancies.[6]

Subsequently, measurement of biochemical substances in the first trimester of pregnancy has also demonstrated an association with Down's syndrome. The two markers used are free beta-hCG and pregnancy-associated plasma protein A (PAPP-A).

Accurate gestational age assessment is vital to the utility of these biochemical markers. Screening is only applicable to singleton pregnancies, so ultrasonic assessment is again mandatory. All markers vary with gestation, and so MoMs are used to determine abnormal values.

Second trimester screening

Second trimester screening is carried out between 15 and 22 weeks of pregnancy. Serum screening programmes incorporate:

- two components (MSAFP and total hCG or free beta-hCG): the double test;
- three components (MSAFP, hCG and uE3): the triple test; or
- four components (MSAFP, hCG, uE3 and inhibin): the quadruple test.

The screening performance of these markers improves with the addition of markers, such that for a false-positive rate of 5%, the detection rates for the double, triple and quadruple tests are 59 per cent, 69 per cent and 76 per cent, respectively.[7] However, the extra cost of using additional serum markers must be considered.

Certain factors can influence serum markers.

- Insulin-dependent diabetes and increased maternal weight lower all markers.
- Twin gestation produces approximately twice the level of all serum markers.
- Minor variations occur with ethnic differences and in smokers.
- Other conditions in which serum screening may be unreliable include maternal renal failure and severe dehydration (e.g. severe hyperemesis gravidarum).

The aim of screening is to maximize the detection rate with a low false-positive rate, in order that invasive testing is minimized.

First trimester screening

Two biochemical markers, namely free beta-hCG and PAPP-A, when measured between 8 and 14 weeks in combination with maternal age, can detect 62 per cent of Down's syndrome pregnancies, with a 5 per cent false-positive rate.[8] Data suggest that this method of screening is as effective as those serum markers in established use at 15–20 weeks [Ib].

These serum markers, when combined with maternal age and nuchal translucency (NT) measurement (see Chapter 10.2), comprise the triple test or combined test, which has an estimated detection rate of 85 per cent for a 5 per cent false-positive rate.[9] This test is usually performed in a single visit, which reduces the anxiety of waiting for a result.

First trimester screening provides the opportunity to establish a diagnosis in early pregnancy (if chorionic villus sampling is utilized). To introduce this method of screening on a nationwide basis would require enormous financial support for the training and education of health professionals, the provision of information and counselling services, and the expansion of expertise in diagnostic ultrasound and invasive tests such as chorionic villus sampling [II].

Integrated/hybrid screening

Simultaneously using markers from both trimesters yields a better screening performance than using markers in either trimester alone. Thus, if the first trimester triple test is combined with the second trimester quadruple test, the detection rate for Down's syndrome has been estimated at 94 per cent for a 5 per cent false-positive rate.[10] If the false-positive rate is fixed at 1 per cent, the detection rate will be 85 per cent. This approach therefore yields a higher detection rate than any other screening test at a given false-positive rate. However, the logistics of introducing such a screening system need to be considered. The result of the first trimester screen would need to be concealed from the woman, and thus would negate the advantage of early pre-natal diagnosis. If ultrasound facilities are not sufficiently developed to perform reliable NT measurement, the full, integrated test cannot be provided. In the absence of NT, the detection rate for the integrated test is 85 per cent for a 5.5 per cent false-positive rate.[10] In addition, the infrastructure necessary for the organization and counselling of integrated/hybrid screening far exceeds that required for the present screening programmes. Nevertheless, the enormous financial and emotional advantage of a test with a 1 per cent false-positive rate cannot be denied.

BIOCHEMICAL SCREENING FOR OTHER ABNORMALITIES

A number of other chromosomal abnormalities have been shown to be associated with biochemical markers.

- *Trisomy 18*. Trisomy 18 (Edward's syndrome) is the second most common aneuploidy surviving to birth. In the second trimester, MSAFP, hCG and uE3 levels are all low. Risk assessment for trisomy 18 has been incorporated into some screening programmes.

- *Triploidy*. This chromosomal abnormality is inconsistent with survival. Affected pregnancies may be identified in the mid-trimester, as there are very high or very low levels of AFP and hCG, and low levels of E3.

- *Turner's syndrome (45, X)*. In Turner's syndrome associated with hydrops, the serum markers show a pattern similar to that of Down's syndrome pregnancies. In those without hydrops, the hCG level is low.

- *Smith–Lemlie–Opitz syndrome*. This is an autosomal recessive condition associated with moderate to severe mental retardation. In these pregnancies, uE3 is very low or undetectable, and MSAFP and hCG tend to be low. The risk of a pregnancy affected with this condition can thus be calculated, and the diagnosis is confirmed by measuring 7-dehydrocholesterol (7-DHCO) in the amniotic fluid.

HEALTH ECONOMICS OF SCREENING

A major challenge in the delivery of Down's screening services is the need to set up an adequate organizational structure. This not only means dedicated laboratory facilities with computer-assisted test interpretation and expertise to provide invasive prenatal testing, but also a team of experienced co-ordinators to undertake the enormous workload of counselling. This counselling is essential, both prior to undertaking the test and in the event of a screen-positive result when invasive testing is contemplated. It is this last service provision that has poor structure in many screening programmes, and fiscal implications are generally underestimated. In the ideal structure, each unit should have a clear screening policy agreed centrally. A screening co-ordinator would be responsible for reporting results to women and co-ordinating the local screening service. A local director of screening, of consultant status, would guide and support the service, and be attentive to advances in screening and their controlled introduction into practice.

- High-resolution ultrasound has a better detection rate for open fetal defects than a high MSAFP [II].
- With accurate ultrasound dating, second trimester biochemical screening using four markers can detect 76 per cent of Down's syndrome pregnancies [Ib].
- First trimester serum screening is as effective as mid-trimester serum screening [Ib].

KEY POINTS

- A raised MSAFP has good sensitivity but poor specificity for open fetal defects, but is still used in areas of high NTD prevalence.
- Mid-trimester serum screening for Down's syndrome is widely available in the UK.
- Detection rates vary depending on the number of markers used.
- Counselling before and after testing accounts for the bulk of the workload.

PUBLISHED GUIDELINES

Grudzinskas JG, Ward RHT (eds). *Screening for Down's Syndrome in the First Trimester. Recommendations arising from the Study Group.* London: RCOG Press, 1997.

KEY REFERENCES

1. Wald NJ, Brock DJH, Bonnar J. Prenatal diagnosis of spina bifida and anencephaly by maternal serum alpha-fetoprotein measurement. A controlled study. *Lancet* 1974; I:765–7.
2. Report of UK Collaborative Study on Alpha-fetoprotein in Relation to Neural Tube Defects. Maternal serum alpha-fetoprotein measurement in antenatal screening for anencephaly and spina bifida in early pregnancy. *Lancet* 1977; I:1323–32.
3. Papp Z, Toth-Pal E, Papp CS, Torok O. Impact of prenatal mid-trimester screening on the prevalence of fetal structure anomalies: a prospective epidemiological study. *Ultrasound Obstet Gynecol* 1995; 6:320–6.
4. Morrow RJ, McNay MB, Whittle MJ. Ultrasound detection of neural tube defects in patients with elevated maternal serum AFP levels. *Obstet Gynecol* 1991; **78**:1055–7.
5. Cuckle HS, Wald NJ, Lindenbaum RH. Maternal serum alpha-fetoprotein measurement. A screening test for Down's syndrome. *Lancet* 1984; I:926–9.
6. Wald NJ, Densem JW, George L, Muttukrishna S, Knight PG. Prenatal screening for Down's syndrome using Inhibin-A as a serum marker. *Prenat Diagn* 1996; 16:143–53.
7. Wald NJ, Densem JW, Smith D, Klee GG. Four marker serum screening for Down's syndrome. *Prenat Diagn* 1994; 14:707–16.
8. Wald NJ, George L, Smith D, Densem JW, Petterson K, on behalf of the International Prenatal Screening Group. Serum screening for Down's syndrome between 8 and 14 weeks of pregnancy. *Br J Obstet Gynaecol* 1996; **103**:407–12.
9. Wald NJ, Hackshaw AK. Combining ultrasound and biochemistry in first trimester screening for Down's syndrome. *Prenat Diagn* 1997; **17**:821–9.
10. Wald NJ, Watt HC, Hackshaw AK. Integrated screening for Down's syndrome based on tests performed during the first and second trimesters. *N Engl J Med* 1999; 341:461–7.

Ultrasound Screening

Michele P. Mohajer

INTRODUCTION

The incidence of major structural abnormality is 2–3 per cent, and far exceeds all chromosomal abnormalities or single gene defects. As a result of the technological development in high-resolution ultrasound equipment, the prenatal diagnosis of most major structural malformations is possible. As a consequence, there has been a significant fall in perinatal mortality rates due to the termination of affected fetuses. In addition to this role, ultrasound scanning is vital in determining gestation, viability and number of fetuses. The advent of such technological development has provided the foundation for the subspecialty of fetal medicine.

WHAT IS SCREENING?

The purpose of screening for fetal malformation is not simply to terminate the fetus prior to viability in order to reduce perinatal mortality rates. Although screening does reduce perinatal mortality rates, the identification of fetal malformation allows parents to make informed choices regarding their pregnancy. This facilitates physical and psychological preparation for the delivery of an infant with a birth defect, which may even take place in another centre. In addition, identification of certain abnormalities may allow parents to avail themselves of in-utero treatments that can improve the infant's condition prior to birth. Ultrasound screening can also be used to identify some fetuses with chromosomal disease in which case invasive diagnostic procedures can be performed.

WHO SHOULD BE SCREENED?

Certain conditions increase a woman's chance of having a malformed fetus. So-called 'high-risk' groups can be identified, such as women with insulin-dependent diabetes, maternal drug ingestion (e.g. anticonvulsants, warfarin), or a positive family history. However, 95 per cent of abnormalities occur in fetuses born to mothers who have no risk factors at all.[1] Therefore, routine ultrasound scanning of all pregnancies has been suggested as the preferred method to identify structural malformations [Ia]. Evidence to support this recommendation is unsatisfactory. Vast differences exist in detection rates, from 16 per cent[2] to 85 per cent.[3]

The reasons for these differences are unclear. The skill and training of the operator are important, but perhaps an important variable is the gestational age at which the scan is done. The optimum time for the identification of structural fetal anomalies is 18–20 weeks [Ib].[4]

Prior to performing the ultrasound scan, it is vital that the parents understand the objectives, the limitations and also the detection rates for the major malformations. This is ideally done by the provision of information leaflets [II].

TIMING OF SCREENING

The detailed fetal anomaly scan at 18–20 weeks

The scan initially checks viability and number of fetuses, as well as placental site and amniotic fluid volume. Standard views of the fetus are then taken. These are:

1 transverse section through the fetal head, assessing head shape and internal structures;
2 fetal spine: sagittal, coronal and transverse views;
3 fetal abdomen: longitudinal and transverse; identifying intra-abdominal organs: stomach, kidneys, bladder and ventral wall integrity and cord insertion;
4 transverse section through fetal thorax to examine four-chamber view of the heart;
5 limbs: identify three long bones in each limb.

Inability to obtain the standard images may occur due to fetal position or maternal size.

MAJOR STRUCTURAL MALFORMATIONS

Central nervous system malformations

Many major structural defects of the central nervous system (CNS) may identified at the 20-week scan, and certain malformations can be identified at earlier gestations.

Neural tube defects

These malformations occur when there is a failure of dorsal fusion in early embryological life, such that neural tissue is exposed. Neural tube defects (anencephaly, cephaloceles and spina bifida) are the commonest CNS malformations in the UK, and much energy has been applied to the screening and prevention of these anomalies. Anencephaly is characterized by the absence of the cerebral hemispheres and cranial vault, and can be identified from as early as 11–12 weeks. The prognosis is uniformly fatal within the first hours or days of life. Cephalocele is a protrusion of the intracranial contents through a bony defect of the skull. These contents may include only meninges (cranial meningocele) or brain tissue (encephalocele). Ultrasound examination can identify a solid or cystic paracranial mass. The prognosis depends on the presence of brain tissue within the sac and other associated intracranial features. Spina bifida, in which the defect

exists in the vertebral fusion, is the commonest CNS malformation. Demonstration of the lesion itself by ultrasound may be difficult. However, the intracranial signs associated with spina bifida, the Arnold–Chiari malformation (herniation of the cerebellum and brainstem through the foramen magnum), are more easily identifiable.[5] This demonstration of the 'lemon and banana' sign has displaced maternal serum alpha-fetoprotein (MSAFP) as the main screening test for spina bifida in some units. The detection rate for open spina bifida on ultrasound screening is 81 per cent, with a false-positive rate of 0.0003 per cent.[6]

Hydrocephalus

This condition arises when there is an abnormal accumulation of cerebrospinal fluid (CSF), resulting in enlargement of the ventricular system. It is commonly associated with other intracranial and extracranial abnormalities. Diagnosis on ultrasound examination is achieved by demonstration of enlarged lateral ventricles and anterior displacement of the choroid plexus. The three major forms are aqueduct stenosis, communicating hydrocephalus and Dandy–Walker syndrome. This last syndrome is characterized by the addition of a cyst in the posterior fossa and defect in the cerebellar vermis, both of which are detectable on ultrasound. The prognosis is variable, again depending on the severity of the hydrocephalus and presence of additional malformations.

Other less common CNS malformations may be identified on ultrasound. These include holoprosencephaly, iniencephaly, arachnoid cysts, porencephalic cysts, agenesis of the corpus callosum, hydrancephaly, microcephaly, intracranial tumours and aneurysm of the vein of Galen.

Cardiac malformations

Systematic examination of the fetal heart has enabled the prenatal diagnosis of many congenital heart defects. Since the fetal heart is almost horizontal, a transverse section through the fetal chest will demonstrate a four-chamber view. This standard view provides information about the position and size of the fetal heart, the cardiac chambers and the atrioventricular connections. Congenital heart abnormalities associated with an abnormal four-chamber view include:

• hypoplastic left heart
• hypoplastic right heart
• atrioventricular canal defect
• large ventricular septal defect
• large atrial septal defect
• single ventricle
• valve stenosis or atresia
• Ebstein's anomaly
• cardiac tumour
• cardiac situs abnormalities.

However, there is a wide variation in the ability of ultrasound screening for cardiac abnormalities, with detection rates varying from 6 per cent to 77 per cent.[1] These differences may be related to the gestational age at which the scan is performed, the type of congenital heart abnormality, as well as the experience of the operator. Several cardiac defects are associated with a normal standard four-chamber view. These include:

- tetralogy of Fallot
- transposition of the great arteries
- small atrial and ventricular septal defects
- mild pulmonary or aortic valve stenosis
- mild coarctation of the aorta.

With the improvements in paediatric cardiac surgery, prenatal diagnosis of cardiac conditions has become much more important. Parents can make informed choices, if given the realistic expectations of the problem.

Thoracic malformations

By obtaining transverse and longitudinal views of the fetal chest, space-occupying lesions, solid or cystic, may be diagnosed. The fetal lungs are uniformly echogenic. Fluid within the pleural cavity (pleural effusions) may be identified as a result as certain fetal conditions. Chylothorax, a relatively common cause of pleural effusion in neonatal life, is an accumulation of chyle in the pleural cavity. Bronchogenic cysts may appear as sonolucent areas within the fetal chest.

Congenital cystic adenomatous malformation of the lung (CCAML) is a condition whereby there is overgrowth of terminal bronchioles at the expense of saccular spaces. The ultrasound appearance varies according to the type: either macrocystic, with large cystic structures within the chest, or microcystic, where there is increased echogenicity of the lung tissue. Lung sequestrations may also appear as an echogenic mass. Cystic structures within the chest may also be demonstrated in the fetus with congenital diaphragmatic hernia. When there is a defect, the stomach or other abdominal contents may be demonstrated above the level of the diaphragm.

Gastrointestinal and abdominal wall malformations

Demonstration of the integrity of the abdominal wall is made on transverse and longitudinal views. Ventral wall defects, gastroschisis and exomphalos may be identified.

Gastroschisis is a para-umbilical defect, and can be diagnosed by the presence of herniated organs floating freely within the amniotic cavity. An exomphalos is a central defect surrounded by a membrane on which the umbilical cord is inserted. These defects may also be associated with an elevated MSAFP. In isolation, the prognosis for both of these malformations is good with surgical correction, but karyotyping should be considered in the case of exomphalos, as an association with aneuploidy exists. Rarer defects in the abdominal wall may be diagnosed, known as bladder and cloacal extrophy.

Intra-abdominal pathology may be diagnosed on ultrasound such as:

- fetal ascites
- small and large bowel obstruction
- meconium peritonitis
- mesenteric, omental and retroperitoneal cysts.

Many of the obstructive malformations may be associated with polyhydramnios.

Urogenital malformations

The fetal kidneys and bladder are relatively easily identified structures in the mid-trimester. Many fetal renal problems are associated with a disturbance in amniotic fluid volume. By 16 weeks, the majority of the amniotic fluid is produced by the fetal kidneys. If oligohydramnios is diagnosed in the mid-trimester, in the absence of a history of ruptured membranes, fetal renal malformation must be suspected.

Renal agenesis may be bilateral or unilateral. If bilateral, there is associated anhydramnios, and the condition is fatal. Visualization of the fetal kidneys in this situation is difficult due to loss of the acoustic window and may be facilitated by an amnio-infusion.

Infantile polycystic kidney disease is an autosomal recessive disease. Ultrasound diagnosis is made by the demonstration of bilateral enlarged hyperechogenic fetal kidneys, absent fetal bladder and associated oligohydramnios. The prognosis is poor.

Obstructive uropathy may occur due to an obstruction at the urethra or ureter. Urethral obstruction, due either to urethral atresia or posterior urethral valves, may be demonstrated by the presence of a distended fetal bladder, hydroureter and hydronephrosis. Ureteric obstruction, which may be unilateral or bilateral, can be diagnosed by ultrasound by the demonstration of hydronephrosis.

In multicystic dysplastic kidney disease (MDKD), ultrasound examination of the fetal kidneys shows the presence of multiple cysts, and increased echogenicity of the surrounding parenchyma. The kidneys are enlarged and where there is bilateral disease, the prognosis is fatal.

Tumours of the kidney and adrenal gland, if present in fetal life, can also be diagnosed on ultrasound scans.

Skeletal malformations

Diagnosis of skeletal abnormalities requires a full examination of the fetus, with a skeletal survey. This involves both morphological and biometric examination of the skull, vertebrae, ribs, long bones and digits of the hands and feet. Measurement of the femur length at a dating scan may be the first clue to a skeletal problem.

Skeletal malformations may affect the whole skeleton and may be lethal, such as:

- achondrogenesis
- thanatophoric dysplasia
- short-rib polydactyly syndromes
- fibrochondrogenesis
- homozygous achondroplasia
- osteogenesis imperfecta (perinatal type)
- hypophosphatasia (perinatal type).

Lethality is usually dependent on thoracic cage involvement and subsequent development of pulmonary hypoplasia.

Other skeletal problems, such as radial anomalies, talipes equinovarus, femoral hypoplasia, facial clefts and digital anomalies, may be identified and may form part of another syndrome, including chromosome anomalies.

The prognosis depends on the involvement of other, non-skeletal, malformations.

The overall detection rate of skeletal problems is 90 per cent.[7]

Hydrops fetalis and cystic hygroma

This is a condition in which fluid accumulates within the body cavities and soft tissues of the fetus. The aetiologies of this condition are numerous (see Chapter 17).[8] Visualization of fluid within the fetus is relatively easy, and the commonest area of fluid accumulation is at the fetal neck, the cystic hygroma. This is usually due to lymphatic obstruction, and is recognized as a cystic structure adjacent to the fetal neck. Cystic hygromas are frequently associated with chromosomal abnormalities. Smaller degrees of fluid in this area are referred to as nuchal oedema or nuchal translucency. As detailed below, it is this latter anomaly that has been identified at earlier gestations (11–14 weeks), and has now been incorporated into screening programmes for aneuploidy.

Screening for chromosomal disease

Many structural malformations identified on scan may be associated with chromosomal disease, such as:

- cystic hygroma
- cardiac defects
- exomphalos
- holoprosencephaly
- microcephaly
- diaphragmatic hernia
- oesophageal/duodenal atresia

- renal anomalies
- radial aplasia
- micrognathia
- clinodactyly of the fifth finger
- polydactyly
- talipes.

At the time of the 20-week scan, minor ultrasound abnormalities may be seen that may also be associated with aneuploidy. These are known as 'soft markers'. They may not constitute a structural defect, but when seen along with another risk factor for chromosomal disease, karyotyping may be considered. Soft markers include:

- nuchal oedema
- mild renal pyelectasis
- hyperechogenic bowel
- echogenic intracardiac foci
- strawberry-shaped skull
- mild ventriculomegaly
- shortened long bones
- choroid plexus cysts
- clenched fists
- rocker bottom feet
- sandal gap.

These soft markers have been included in some screening programmes for Down's syndrome. However, apart from nuchal oedema, there is no strong evidence at present that the other soft markers are helpful in identifying Down's syndrome [Ia].[9]

FIRST TRIMESTER SCREENING

Ultrasound scanning in the first trimester was primarily introduced for viability and accurate dating. With improved resolution, a number of fetal defects may also be seen, such as:

- anencephaly
- holoprosencephaly
- encephalocele
- Dandy–Walker syndrome
- univentricular heart
- gastroschisis
- exomphalos
- multidysplastic kidney.

Using a combination of transabdominal and transvaginal ultrasound, up to 59 per cent of major structural defects may be diagnosed at the 11–14-week scan.[10]

An important component of the first trimester scan is the NT measurement, which is the maximum thickness of the subcutaneous translucency between the skin and the soft tissue overlying the cervical spine. It has not only been shown to be an effective screening test for aneuploidy, but also may identify a fetus at risk of cardiac defects, skeletal dysplasias and genetic syndromes.[11] There are sufficient data to suggest that NT screening for Down's syndrome at 10–14 weeks is similar, if not superior, to serum screening with multiple markers at 15–20 weeks' gestation [Ib]. Although it appears to be useful, the availability of nuchal screening in the UK is limited. The counselling, expertise and training required to successfully implement such a national screening test would be difficult to achieve.

HAZARDS OF ULTRASOUND SCAN

Many epidemiological and laboratory studies have been performed to search for evidence of possible biological effects of diagnostic ultrasound. Childhood cancer, dyslexia, non-right handedness, delayed speech development and reduced birth weight have all been implicated, but as yet there is no good evidence to establish a firm link between ultrasound and these endpoints.[1]

Although a sophisticated investigation, there are limitations to ultrasound. Adequate visualization of the fetal anatomy may not be possible due to the fetal position or maternal habitus. In situations of gross maternal obesity, confirmation of fetal viability may be extremely difficult.

Visual confirmation of fetal normality appears to promote a positive attitude towards the pregnancy, with improved compliance on healthcare issues such as smoking and alcohol.[12] However, the detection of fetal defects and, in particular, soft ultrasound markers may generate immense anxiety and rejection, even if the subsequent invasive testing proves the fetus is healthy. Hence, for the successful maintenance of ultrasound screening programmes, a framework of skilled midwives, sonographers and counsellors is necessary. This is not only to deal with parents in whom a fetal abnormality has been diagnosed, but also to ensure that prior to the ultrasound scan, women have a clear idea about what the test is likely to achieve and its reliability in doing so.

- Screening the whole population rather than selective scanning is the only reliable way to identify fetal abnormality [Ia].
- A scan undertaken between 18 and 20 weeks is the most effective method to identify a wide range of fetal abnormality [Ib].
- Screening for fetal abnormality reduces the perinatal mortality rates through identification and termination of affected pregnancies [Ia].

KEY POINTS

- Detailed ultrasound at 18–20 weeks is an important screening examination in which most life-threatening malformations can be diagnosed.
- Pregnant women should receive clear information regarding the objectives of the ultrasound examination and the likelihood of finding an abnormality.
- Success of the ultrasound examination depends on the operator, the ultrasound equipment, the fetal position and the maternal habitus.
- When an abnormality is detected on ultrasound, the parents should have ready access to skilled counsellors who are able to provide them with full information, options and support in order to allow them to make an informed choice.

PUBLISHED GUIDELINES

Grudzinskas JG, Ward RHT (eds). *Recommendations Arising from the Study Group on Screening for Down's Syndrome in the First Trimester.* London: RCOG Press, 1997.

KEY REFERENCES

1. Whittle M. *Ultrasound Screening for Fetal Abnormalities.* Report of the RCOG Working Party. London: RCOG Press, 1997.
2. Crane JP, LeFevre ML, Winborn RC et al. and the RADIUS Study Group. A randomized trial of prenatal ultrasonographic screening: impact on the detection, management and outcome of anomalous fetuses. *Am J Obstet Gynecol* 1994; **171**:392–9.
3. Luck C. Value of routine ultrasound scanning at 19 weeks: a four year study of 8849 deliveries. *BMJ* 1992; **304**:1474–8.
4. Drife JO, Donnai D (eds). *Antenatal Diagnosis of Fetal Abnormalities.* London: RCOG Press, 1991, 354–5.
5. Nicolaides KH, Campbell S, Gabbe SG, Guidetti R. Ultrasound screening for spina bifida: cranial and cerebellar signs. *Lancet* 1986; ii:72–4.
6. Papp Z, Toth-Pal E, Papp CS, Torok O. Impact of prenatal mid-trimester screening on the prevalence of fetal structure anomalies: a prospective epidemiological study. *Ultrasound Obstet Gynecol* 1995; **6**:320–6.

7. Whittle MJ. *Routine Ultrasound Screening in Pregnancy.* Report of the RCOG Working Party. London: RCOG Press, 2000, 7–12.

8. James D. Fetal hydrops. In: *The Yearbook of Obstetrics and Gynaecology,* Vol. 9. London: RCOG Press, 2001, 277–87.

9. Smith-Bindman R, Hosmer W, Feldstein VA, Deeks JJ, Goldberg JD. Second-trimester ultrasound to detect fetuses with Down's syndrome. A meta-analysis. *J Am Med Assoc,* 2001; **285**(8):1044–55.

10. Whitlow BJ, Chatzipapas IK, Lazanakis ML, Kadir RA, Economides DL. The value of sonography in early pregnancy for the detection of fetal abnormalities in an unselected population. *Br J Obstet Gynaecol* 1999; **106**:929–36.

11. Nicolaides KH, Heath V, Liao AW. The 11–14 week scan. *Clin Obstet Gynaecol* 2000; **14**(4):581–94.

12. Reading AE, Campbell S, Cox DN, Sledmere CM. Health beliefs and health care behaviour in pregnancy. *Psychol Med* 1982; **12**:379–83.

Invasive Prenatal Diagnosis

Michele P. Mohajer

MRCOG standards

Theoretical skills
- Understand the indications for an invasive test.
- Know the advantages and disadvantages of each test.

Practical skills
- Be able to counsel a woman about the procedure and its risks.
- Have assisted in the procedure of amniocentesis.
- Have observed other procedures such as chorionic villus sampling, placental biopsy, cordocentesis, intrauterine transfusion.

INTRODUCTION

High-resolution ultrasound imaging has enabled direct access to the different constituents of the gestational sac from the middle of the first trimester of pregnancy. An ever-increasing range of invasive techniques is being developed to facilitate the diagnosis of chromosomal and single gene defects, metabolic disorders, intrauterine infection, fetal anaemia, thrombocytopenia and some structural problems.

All invasive procedures carry a small risk of fetal loss. Early prenatal testing provides the opportunity for surgical termination of the pregnancy if required, but the earlier invasive testing tends to increase the fetal loss rate. Non-invasive techniques for identifying fetal cells in maternal blood and cervical mucus are the focus of current research.[1]

The routinely used invasive procedures are amniocentesis, chorionic villus sampling (CVS) and fetal blood sampling (FBS).

AMNIOCENTESIS

Amniocentesis involves the aspiration of amniotic fluid from the amniotic sac via a needle inserted through the maternal abdomen. It is the commonest prenatal diagnostic procedure in the UK. It was first introduced in the 1966 for the diagnosis of genetic disease[2] and subsequently used to confirm open neural tube defects the presence of a raised maternal serum alpha-fetoprotein (see Chapter 10.1).[3] It is usually performed between 15 and 16 weeks' gestation.

Method

Using an aseptic technique, a 22-gauge needle is inserted through the maternal abdomen under direct real-time ultrasound control with continuous needle-tip visualization. This method is more successful than blind techniques [Ib]. Fifteen to 20 mL of fluid containing fetal cells is aspirated into a syringe. The cells are then cultured for 2–3 weeks before further testing can be performed.

Indications for amniocentesis

The main indication for amniocentesis is for fetal karyotyping. In view of the risk of miscarriage, the procedure is offered when there is an increased risk of aneuploidy, such as for:

- women with positive serum screening for Down's syndrome;
- women of advanced maternal age (traditionally >35 years);
- ultrasound detection of an abnormality or soft marker;
- parental balanced translocation;
- a previous history of chromosomal abnormality.

One of the major disadvantages for the woman is the long wait for the result, which may take from 2 to 4 weeks.

Molecular genetics has developed two techniques, which have permitted the rapid diagnosis of the many major chromosomal abnormalities. These two tests, fluorescence in-situ hybridization (FISH) and polymerase chain reaction (PCR), can provide results in 24–48 hours.[4] FISH relies on the unique ability of a portion of single-stranded DNA (known as a probe) to hybridize with its complementary target DNA sequence. By attaching a fluorescent label to the appropriate probe, diagnosis of autosomal trisomies for chromosomes 13, 18, 21 and X and Y chromosomes can be made in 6–8 hours by direct fluorescent microscopy. PCR uses highly polymorphic small tandem repeat markers, which allow distinction between normal and trisomic DNA samples. Diagnosis of the major chromosomal abnormalities can be performed in 24 hours. Both techniques share the same diagnostic dilemma in that conventional chromosomal analysis is required to detect other chromosomal disorders.

Amniocentesis is also used for the diagnosis of single gene disorders. However, culture of the cells and extraction of the DNA often means a significant delay in receiving the result.

Using PCR techniques, amniocentesis can also be used to facilitate the diagnosis of certain congenital infections (see Chapter 13), such as cytomegalovirus and toxoplasmosis.

Amniocentesis has a role to play in isoimmunized pregnancies. PCR techniques can be used to identify the blood group of the fetus and, later on, the optical density difference at the wavelength 450 nm (AOD450) provides an indirect measurement of the bilirubin. However, in view of the increased likelihood of further sensitization, many other non-invasive methods for estimating the degree of fetal anaemia are in routine use.

Amniocentesis is no longer routinely used to estimate the alpha-fetoprotein and acetylcholinesterase for the diagnosis of neural tube defects. Amniocentesis performed in the presence of raised maternal serum alpha-fetoprotein is associated with a significant increase in fetal loss [Ia].

Complications

The fetal loss rate from the procedure varies, but the only randomized, controlled trial of low-risk women reports a rate of 1 per cent [Ia].[5] Many units report their own miscarriage rate based on their own individual audit data. Operator experience has been shown to be important [Ib]. Adequate levels of training (>30 procedures per year) are necessary to maintain success and reduce complications. Cell culture may fail in 0.5 per cent of amniocenteses, necessitating a further invasive test.

Early amniocentesis

Owing to the relative ease of the procedure, amniocentesis at earlier gestations was performed in order to provide women with the advantages of early prenatal diagnosis. Early amniocentesis can be performed from 10 weeks' gestation, but the technique has been largely abandoned due to the increased fetal loss rates, fetal talipes and reduced amniocyte culture rate [Ia].[6]

CHORIONIC VILLUS SAMPLING AND PLACENTAL BIOPSY

These procedures refer to the sampling of placental tissue. Placental biopsy is the term used when the procedure is performed after the first trimester. Placental tissue can be obtained by catheter, needle aspiration or biopsy forceps. Transabdominal and transcervical methods are both used. The procedure can be performed from 10 weeks' gestation. Early diagnosis allows the woman the option of termination before 13 weeks' gestation.

Transabdominal CVS

Using aseptic techniques, an 18–20-gauge needle is inserted through the maternal abdomen to the placental site under direct ultrasound guidance. Placental tissue is aspirated into a syringe attached to the needle. Similarly, a fine biopsy forceps can be used through an outer guide needle. If the placenta is completely posterior and low lying, access via the transabdominal route may not be possible.

Transcervical CVS

This method is ideal for the posterior low-lying placenta. The cervix and vagina are visualized through a speculum and cleaned with sterile solution. Transabdominal ultrasound is performed to visualize the cervical canal. The needle, catheter or biopsy forceps is then introduced through the cervix towards the placenta under ultrasound guidance, and a sample is taken.

The choice of a transabdominal or transcervical approach should be dependent on operator experience, the placental site and the axis of the uterus. Transcervical CVS is associated with less discomfort than the transabdominal approach, but the potential risk of infection and then procedure-related loss is higher with the transcervical route.

Indications for CVS

Chorionic villus sampling has the advantage of yielding a large amount of tissue and is therefore the method of choice when large amounts of DNA are required in the diagnosis of monogenic disorders. With the increasing use of early screening tests for Down's syndrome, and with high-resolution ultrasound detecting abnormalities in the first trimester, CVS is more frequently requested.

Direct chromosome preparations and other rapid cell culture techniques allow rapid karyoptying within 24–48 hours. This is advantageous to parents who do not wish to wait for results and who wish to avail themselves of early termination if an affected fetus is found.

Complications

The fetal loss rate has always been considered to be higher with CVS than with amniocentesis. However, randomized comparisons of the two procedures have not shown a significant difference in fetal loss rates [Ib]. The procedure-related loss above the individual background risk is considered to be 1 per cent.[7]

Placental mosaicisms can occur in about 2 per cent of cases. This presents counselling difficulties and necessitates further invasive testing to obtain fetal cells.

There has been concern regarding the association of CVS and limb defects. This complication appears to be related to the procedure being performed at earlier gestations. Subsequent studies have shown no association when the procedure is performed after 10 weeks.[8]

FETAL BLOOD SAMPLING

Sampling of blood from the fetal circulation has now been used for a variety of diagnostic purposes. It requires expertise, and should be performed by clinicians with extensive experience in all other ultrasound-guided procedures.

Method

The procedure can be performed from 16 to 18 weeks' gestation. A 20-gauge needle is introduced through the maternal abdomen under direct ultrasound control. Fetal blood can be aspirated from either the placental insertion or fetal insertion of the umbilical cord. Cardiac puncture or intrahepatic vessels may also be sampled.

Indications for FBS

Rapid high-quality karyotyping can be obtained with this method within 48–72 hours. This is particularly useful when an abnormality is detected late in the pregnancy.

Fetal blood sampling is also vital in the diagnosis of fetal haematological problems such as anaemia and thrombocytopenia. It has also been used to assess the acid–base status of the fetus in growth restriction, but non-invasive biophysical methods and Doppler studies are more routinely used.

Complications

Bleeding at the site of the needle and fetal bradycardia may occur as a result of the procedure, especially in association with the umbilical artery site. The overall procedure-related fetal loss is 1–2 per cent. Introduction of infection may occur and, more importantly, if the mother is carrying human immunodeficiency virus (HIV) or other viruses, transmission to the fetus may occur.[9]

FETOSCOPY

With improvement in fibreoptic technology, direct in-utero visualization of the fetus can now be achieved. This may be useful for identifying small structural abnormalities and facilitating direct organ biopsy, such as skin and muscle biopsy. Organ biopsy can also be performed under ultrasound control.

COUNSELLING

The decision as to which invasive test is required must be tailored to the individual mother. It is imperative that she is given full details of the range of tests available, the procedures, advantages and disadvantages, and risk of fetal loss or damage. This information should be given well before the procedure is attempted, allowing her to make her decision, and should be non-directive. The discussion should be followed up with written information.

CONCLUSIONS

These invasive procedures allow the diagnosis and assessment of a large number of abnormalities, so that parents can make choices about the continuation or otherwise of their pregnancies. Early diagnostic procedures provide the advantage of early termination, if sought, but must be balanced against the increased fetal loss, or the possibility of terminating a fetus that may have miscarried spontaneously. Rapid molecular tests have improved the waiting time for results but have limitations. Further developments in the identification of fetal cells in maternal tissues may reduce the necessity of invasive diagnostic tests.

- The rate of miscarriage following amniocentesis is approximately 1 per cent [Ia].
- Early amniocentesis has a higher complication rate than CVS and mid-trimester amniocentesis [Ia].
- Amniocentesis performed under direct ultrasound visualization is associated with higher rates of success [Ib].

Antenatal complications: fetal

KEY POINTS

- Amniocentesis is the most commonly performed prenatal diagnostic procedure.
- CVS should not be performed at less than 10 weeks' gestation because of the association of limb defects.
- Most invasive tests other than amniocentesis are generally performed in a tertiary referral centre.
- The specific invasive test should be tailored to the individual woman's circumstances and wishes.
- A team of specialist counsellors should be available for the parents both before and after invasive techniques are performed.

PUBLISHED GUIDELINES

Whittle MJ. *Amniocentesis*. RCOG 'Green Top' Guideline No. 8, February. London: RCOG Press, 2000.

KEY REFERENCES

1. Lamvu G, Kuller JA. Prenatal diagnosis using fetal cells from the maternal circulation. *Obstet Gynaecol Surv* 1997; **52**:433–7.

2. Steele MW, Breg WR. Chromosome analysis of human amniotic fluid cells. *Lancet* 1966; I:383–5.
3. Bennet MJ. Fetal loss after second trimester amniocentesis in women with raised serum alpha-fetoprotein. *Lancet* 1978; 2:987.
4. Thein AT, Abdel-Fattah SA, Kyle PM, Soothhill PW. An assessment of the use of interphase FISH with chromosome specific probes as an alternative to cytogenetics in prenatal diagnosis. *Prenat Diagn* 2000; 4:275–80.
5. Tabor A, Philip J, Madsen M, Bang J, Obel EB, Norgaard-Pederson B. Randomised controlled trial of genetic amniocentesis in 4606 low-risk women. *Lancet* 1986; 1:1287–93.
6. Nicolaides K, Brizot MdeL, Patel F, Snijders R. Comparison of chorionic villus sampling and amniocentesis for fetal karyotyping at 10–13 weeks gestation. *Lancet* 1994; **344**:435–9.
7. Canadian Collaborative CVS–Amniocentesis Clinical Trial Group. Multicentre randomised clinical trial of chorion villus sampling and amniocentesis. *Lancet* 1989; i:1–6.
8. Froster UG, Jackson L. Limb defects and chorion-villus sampling: results from an international registry, 1992–94. *Lancet* 1996; **347**:489–94.
9. Workman MR, Philpott-Howard J. Risk of fetal infection from invasive procedures. *J Hosp Infect* 1997; 35:169–74.

Management of Fetal Anomalies

Michele P. Mohajer

INTRODUCTION

The management of the pregnancy in which an abnormal fetus is identified involves a whole multidisciplinary team of specialists. This team comprises the sonographer, fetal medicine specialist, geneticist, neonatologist and paediatric surgeon, along with the nurse specialists within each specialty. When the diagnosis is made, clear information should be made available to the parents regarding the condition, prognosis and level of disability, should the baby be born alive. This may be very difficult to achieve. Many conditions have such a wide variation in outcome (e.g. Down's syndrome and spina bifida) that accurate prediction may not be possible. When given an adverse prenatal diagnosis, parents are deeply shocked and experience acute grief. They may not be able to take in the information given to them. Written information, contact numbers and support groups are important, but parents may have great difficulty reaching a decision, especially one that results in the termination of the pregnancy. Therefore, management includes not only the practical aspect of the specific disorder, but also the psychological support for the parents and family involved in the pregnancy.

PRACTICAL MANAGEMENT

Termination of pregnancy

When parents are told of a fetal abnormality, they must make decisions, the most important being whether to continue or terminate the pregnancy. The response to diagnosis will be tempered by the options available to the parents, including in-utero treatment, postnatal treatment or termination. If the condition is lethal, the decision to terminate may be easier, but more often than not, the condition carries a risk of physical or mental impairment, which is difficult to quantify. Once a serious abnormality has been diagnosed, evidence shows that the parents will terminate the pregnancy in 80–90 per cent of cases.[1]

Conditions that are considered lethal include:

- anencephaly
- bilateral renal agenesis
- lethal skeletal dysplasias
- some severe complex cardiac defects
- triploidy
- trisomy 18, 13, 15.

Other conditions are not lethal, but are well documented as being associated with long-term handicap, include:

- spina bifida
- trisomy 21 and other chromosomal abnormalities
- cardiovascular abnormalities
- muscular dystrophies
- phocomelia.

If the decision to terminate is reached, the methods available and associated risks must be discussed with the parents.

METHODS OF TERMINATION

Surgical termination

Surgical termination may be performed by vacuum aspiration or dilatation and evacuation. Vacuum aspiration or suction curettage is the method used until the end of the first trimester. Dilatation of the cervix prior to surgery is achieved by passing graduated metal dilatators or inserting vaginal prostaglandin preparations. Abortion is then performed by the use of a Perspex suction tube connected to vacuum apparatus. The inherent risk associated with abortion relates to the use of general anaesthesia and the invasive nature of the procedure – with complications of haemorrhage, uterine perforation and infection. The incidence of haemorrhage is 1.5/1000, the incidence of uterine perforation is 1–4/1000 and of cervical trauma <1 per cent. Post-abortion infection occurs in up to 10 per cent of cases and is significantly reduced if prophylactic antibiotics are given [Ib]. Suction curettage has been shown to produce lower risks of these complications than sharp curettage.[2] Complications are lessened the earlier the gestation. Couples should also be informed of the risk of failed abortion, which occurs in 2.3/1000 surgical terminations.

Dilatation and evacuation is performed in some areas up until 20 weeks' gestation. Mechanical dilatation of the cervix to 14 mm is performed, and fetal parts are extracted with the use of appropriate instruments. This may be done under ultrasound control. Cervical dilatation may be complicated by cervical tears, uterine perforation and the creation of false passages. The use of cervical priming agents such as mifepristone, misoprostol and gemeprost has improved the safety of the procedure [Ib].[3] It is a very distressing procedure, but safe and effective when undertaken by specialist practitioners with a sufficiently large caseload [Ia]. However, it is not widely available. It also prevents a full post-mortem examination of the fetus being carried out in order to confirm any ultrasound diagnosis.

Medical termination

Medical termination of pregnancy has been revolutionized by the introduction of prostaglandins and the antiprogesterone mifepristone.

Gestations of 9 weeks (63 days) or less can be successfully terminated with mifepristone 600 mg, followed 48 hours later by a prostaglandin (gemeprost or misoprostol). Less than 0.5 per cent will fail to respond to this regimen,[4] which should be the method of choice at these gestations [Ia]. However, the diagnosis of fetal abnormality is extremely rare by 9 weeks' gestation and so medical termination is usually performed in the second trimester. Medical termination has the additional advantage of allowing the opportunity for a post-mortem examination. Pre-treatment with mifepristone (200 mg) sensitizes the myometrium to prostaglandin agents and so reduces the induction–abortion interval [Ib]. Misoprostol is the prostaglandin of choice as it requires specific conditions for storage and transfer. The risk of failure to terminate the pregnancy is 6/1000. The standard regimen is:

mifepristone 200 mg orally, followed 36–48 hours later by misoprostol 800 μg vaginally, then misoprostol 400 μg orally to a maximum of four oral doses.

Third trimester termination and intrauterine fetocide

Since 1990, termination of pregnancy after 24 weeks has become legal if there is a lethal abnormality or sufficient evidence that the infant will be born with serious mental or physical disability.[5] This is an extremely distressing situation to all involved, including the parents, obstetricians and midwives. The safety of medical termination has made late termination much safer, but the law states that the fetus must not be born alive. This requires intrauterine fetocide – which is achieved by fetal intracardiac injection of potassium chloride (KCl) via a 20-gauge transabdominal needle under ultrasound control. This procedure should be performed by an operator experienced in invasive fetal procedures. Fetal sedation may be necessary prior to the fetocide. This is achieved by the administration of diazepam or pethidine into the fetal circulation. An ultrasound should be performed 1 hour after the injection of KCl to ensure cessation of fetal heart pulsation.

The assessment of the level of disability is an extremely difficult area. Although the outcome of some abnormalities is well documented, an accurate prognosis of many prenatally detected anomalies is not possible. Advice from genetic specialists, counsellors and support groups may be sought, but ultimately the decision to terminate the pregnancy will rest with the parents.

The post-mortem examination

Parents may find the prospect of a post-mortem examination of their baby very distressing, but it is a vital part of the management. Although high-quality ultrasound provides an accurate diagnosis of major fetal pathology, post mortem provides more detail, identifies abnormalities that permit a more specific diagnosis and modifies genetic counselling. Important diagnostic refinements are identified in up to 40 per cent of cases.[6]

The issue of post mortem has become further complicated by the legal requirement of consent. Consent is now required for the post-mortem examination of fetuses at all gestations and, additionally, if tissues or organs are retained for later study or research. If parents do not consent to a post mortem, it is important to request photographs, X-rays and a sample of tissue (skin or placenta) for cytogenetic studies, which may provide additional information.

THE CONTINUING PREGNANCY

The pregnancy may continue for many reasons. For example, the condition may be amenable to postnatal treatment. This particularly applies to structural malformations that can be surgically corrected, such as:

- gastroschisis
- exomphalos
- diaphragmatic hernia
- duodenal atresia
- some cardiac defects (Fallot's tetralogy, atrial septal defect, ventricular septal defect, transposition of the great vessels)
- posterior urethral valves
- cleft lip.

It is important that parents receive full information regarding the treatment and long-term outcome of the condition; this is preferably provided by the surgeon performing the procedure. Certain conditions such as gastroschisis will require continued fetal surveillance throughout pregnancy, as there may be growth problems or loops of bowel may become obstructed. Most pregnancies will also require continued surveillance for psychological support. Even though parents have been given optimistic expectations of the outcome, they will be anxious throughout, and need constant reassurance from all members of the team. If paediatric surgical teams are not within the hospital, parents may have to travel to a main centre to receive both prenatal counselling and delivery if their neonatal unit is unable to cope with their situation.

Certain fetal conditions are amenable to intrauterine therapy.

Hydrops fetalis is discussed in Chapter 17. Cases secondary to fetal anaemia may respond to intrauterine fetal blood transfusion. Fetal tachydysrhythmias may also result in fetal hydrops. Maternal administration of antidysrhythmic drugs (digoxin, flecainide, amiodarone) is effective in converting the fetal rate to sinus rhythm and also reversing the hydrops.[7]

If fluid is in a particular cavity, for example a pleural effusion, its presence may compromise normal lung development. Pleural drainage may be performed, as both a diagnostic and a therapeutic procedure. If the fluid accumulates, a pleuro-amniotic shunt can be inserted. This shunt procedure can be applied to other conditions. In the case of posterior urethral valves, outflow obstruction can be so severe as to cause bilateral hydronephrosis and irreversible renal damage. A vesico-amniotic shunt can be inserted into the fetal bladder and so bypass the urethral obstruction.

Sophisticated techniques to perform intrauterine surgery have been developed. If a diaphragmatic hernia is present early in pregnancy, the presence of a mass in the fetal chest compromises fetal lung development such that the infants often die of pulmonary hypoplasia. In-utero repair of the diaphragmatic defect has been performed with some success, but only in extremely specialized units, and not without significant maternal morbidity.[8]

Parents may elect to proceed with the pregnancy because there is not enough certainty or evidence that the malformation will result in a significant degree of mental or physical disability. This decision will vary amongst individuals and depending on their own particular circumstances, for example an infertile couple with a long-awaited pregnancy may accept the risk of potential handicap more than a multigravid mother for whom the risk of a handicapped child may compromise the well-being of her existing family.

Examples of such abnormalities include:

- Dandy–Walker malformation
- agenesis of the corpus callosum
- distal limb abnormalities
- some cardiac defects.

Finally, parents may not want termination, even if the condition has 100 per cent mortality, because of religious or moral beliefs. These wishes must be respected.

The management of these continuing pregnancies requires skilled, personalized care. There are few published data that consider the psychological impact of continuing the pregnancy with a prenatally diagnosed abnormality. There are reasons to hypothesize that women who elect to continue a pregnancy may experience a better psychological outcome than women who terminate: such women are thought to be spared the guilt associated with decision-making. However, some reports suggest that these women would seek early prenatal diagnosis in a subsequent pregnancy. Management of continuing pregnancies includes communication between hospital and community health workers, continuity of care with the same personnel, adequate time and repeated counselling (outside routine clinic hours), written information and contacts with support groups.[9] Serial ultrasound scans may be requested to provide reassurance that the baby is still alive and growing.

The management of the pregnancy with a malformation requires additional considerations as well as emotional support. Parents need to be prepared for:

- how, where and when their baby will be delivered,
- what their baby will look like,
- what will happen to their baby after delivery.

There may also be practical difficulties if delivery is to take place in a tertiary centre. The costs of transport, childcare and subsistence must be considered.

PLAN FOR THE FUTURE

Once the pregnancy is over, carefully planned follow-up is an essential part of the management. In the case of termination or death of the infant, time for grieving must be allowed. Grief reactions will vary amongst individuals depending on different circumstances. Some couples want intensive counselling and contact with the medical team, whereas others want time away from what has become an emotionally painful environment. Post-mortem results may provide additional information as to the precise diagnosis. This could influence the management of a subsequent pregnancy and the choice of a prenatal test.

Referral to a genetic specialist may be required in order to assess the risk of recurrence and possibly to investigate other family members. Follow-up with the paediatric or neonatal team involved is an important part of the bereavement counselling.

Parents will require information on the availability of early, reliable prenatal diagnosis if another pregnancy is contemplated.

Couples may require more than one bereavement counselling session, either because the results are incomplete or because they wish it. Sensitivity to the individual's needs is essential in this situation.

Finally, a letter summarizing the discussion should be sent to the parents. This provides documentation and also allows the information to be assimilated at a later date, away from the hospital environment.

- Termination of pregnancy is more likely if the diagnosis is made earlier in gestation [II].
- The risks of termination of pregnancy are reduced if abortion is performed at earlier gestations [Ib].
- Psychological stress is high after termination, with 40 per cent of women showing symptoms of psychiatric morbidity [Ib].

KEY POINTS

- Parents must have as much access to information as possible before making a choice.
- Referral to a tertiary centre may be necessary for further investigation or treatment.
- Psychological morbidity is high following termination for fetal abnormality using either surgical or medical methods.
- Whether or not they continue the pregnancy, the parents will need long-term support from both hospital specialists and the community.

PUBLISHED GUIDELINES

Penney G. *The Care of Women Requesting Induced Abortion.* (Evidence-Based Clinical Guidelines No. 7. London: RCOG Press, 2000.)

KEY REFERENCES

1. Royal College of Obstetricians and Gynaecologists. *Ultrasound Screening for Fetal Abnormalities.* Report of the RCOG Working Party. London: RCOG Press, 1997, 2–3.
2. Edelman DA, Brener WE, Berger GS. The effectiveness and complications of abortion by dilatation and vacuum aspiration versus dilatation and rigid metal curettage. *Am J Obstet Gynecol* 1974; **119**:473.
3. Schulz KF, Grimes DA, Cates W. Measures to prevent cervical injury during suction curettage abortion. *Lancet* 1983; **i**:1182–4.
4. UK Multicentre Trial. The efficacy and tolerance of mifepristone and prostaglandin in first trimester termination of pregnancy. *Br J Obstet Gynaecol* 1990; **97**:480–6.
5. Gevers S. Third trimester abortion for fetal abnormality. *Bioethics* 1999; **13**(3/4):306–13.
6. Clayton-Smith J, Farndon PA, McKeown C, Donnai D. Examination of fetuses after induced abortion for fetal abnormality. *BMJ* 1990; **300**:295–7.
7. van Engelen AD, Weijtens O, Brenner J et al. Management outcome and follow-up of fetal tachycardia. *J Am Coll Cardiol* 1994; **24**:1371–5.
8. Flake AW. Fetal surgery for congenital diaphragmatic hernia. *Semin Paediatr Surg* 1996; **5**(4):266–74.
9. Chitty LS, Barnes CA, Berry C. Continuing with pregnancy after a diagnosis of lethal abnormality: experience of five couples and recommendations for management. *BMJ* 1996; **313**:478–80.

Chapter 11

Previous History of Fetal Loss

Murray Luckas

MRCOG standards

- Be able to counsel after perinatal death and miscarriage.

In addition, we would suggest the following.

- Understand the causes of late fetal death/stillbirth.
- Understand the investigations of the causes of late fetal death/stillbirth.
- Be able to manage subsequent pregnancies in women with a history of late fetal loss/stillbirth.

INTRODUCTION

The loss of a child at any stage during pregnancy is a devastating event for a woman and her family. The grief reaction following the death of a fetus is severe and similar to that following the death of an adult family member. The process of grieving is now well described; an initial period of shock, anger and disbelief is followed by yearning for the lost child and then gradual adjustment to the loss. The whole process may well be lengthy; however, the majority of parents will have resolved their grief within 12 months.[1] It is important to recognize that the loss of a child during pregnancy is a cause of major protracted psychological morbidity for some women and their families.[2]

The causes of fetal loss are myriad, and many will have implications for future pregnancies. One observational American study reported that women with a previous stillbirth had a ten-fold increased risk of recurrent stillbirth.[3] In contrast, if known aetiological factors that may well have a recurrence risk are excluded, women with so-called 'unexplained stillbirths' were found not to be at increased risk of further stillbirth.[4]

However, any further pregnancy for a woman who has suffered a fetal loss or stillbirth is a time of huge apprehension; indeed, it is associated with high levels of anxiety,

depression and post-traumatic stress disorder,[1,2] and behavioural problems have been noted to be more prevalent in subsequent offspring.[5] Naturally, anxiety levels are high amongst care providers as well. This may result in increased levels of intervention, which in turn may result in increased levels of maternal and perinatal morbidity.[4]

It is therefore essential that the cause of the death of the fetus is determined where possible. Only then can the likely recurrence risk and the possibility of prevention be ascertained and a proper plan of care in subsequent pregnancies made. It is sad to note that in the aftermath of the Alder Hey scandal, inappropriate action by a perinatal pathologist has led to falling post-mortem rates for stillborn infants.[6] One study demonstrated that post mortem provided additional useful information in 26 per cent of cases, and resulted in a complete revision of the clinico-pathological classification in 13 per cent of the cases for which the cause of the demise of the fetus was thought to be known.[7] Many parents are thus missing the opportunity to gain valuable information about the death of their children.

DEFINITIONS

Fetal death is defined as death before delivery at any stage in pregnancy until birth. A late fetal loss is defined as a death occurring between 20 weeks + 0 days and 23 weeks + 6 days.[6] The legal definition of stillbirth in England and Wales is a child delivered after the 24th week of pregnancy, which does not show any signs of life. For the purposes of this chapter, fetal loss is defined as late fetal loss and stillbirth.

INCIDENCE

The Confidential Enquiry into Stillbirths and Deaths in Infancy (CESDI) has collected data on stillbirth and late fetal deaths from England, Wales and Northern Ireland since 1993. Rigorous ascertainment of cases has ensured that the

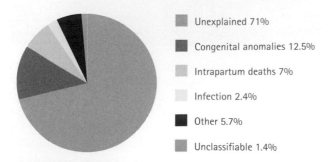

Figure 11.1 Stillbirths according to the Wigglesworth Classification[6]

data collected are accurate. The stillbirth rate in 1999 was 5.4/1000 live births and stillbirths; this rate has remained relatively constant during the period of CESDI data collection. The late fetal loss rate for the same year was 2.5/1000 live births, stillbirths, late fetal losses and legal abortions.[6]

AETIOLOGY

Fetal death can be associated with a multitude of both maternal and fetal factors. Perhaps the most widely used classification in the UK is that devised by Wigglesworth,[8] which is used in an extended form by CESDI (Figure 11.1).

1 *Congenital defects, malformations and serious biochemical abnormalities.* This includes such diverse causes as anencephaly, trisomy and alpha-thalassaemia. Approximately 12.5 per cent of stillbirths will fall into this category.

2 *Deaths from intrapartum asphyxia, anoxia or trauma.* This category covers any baby who would have survived but for some catastrophe occurring during labour (e.g. cord prolapse) and accounts for 7 per cent of stillbirths.

3 *Infection.* This applies where there is clear microbiological evidence of infection sufficient to cause death, such as the TORC infections (toxoplasmosis, rubella and cytomegalovirus). In 1999, 2.4 per cent of stillbirths fell into this category.

4 *Other specific causes.* This category is reserved for cases in which there is a clearly identifiable cause not covered under the other categories, such as abruption, hydrops fetalis and feto-fetal transfusion syndrome. This constituted 5.7 per cent of cases of stillbirth in 1999.

5 *Unexplained stillbirth.* This rather unsatisfactory categorization was made in 71 per cent of stillbirths in 1999. A case falls into this category when no clear cause can be found to account for the fetal demise. Perhaps as many as 40 per cent of these infants are small for gestational age, and it is hypothesized that placental failure may account for fetal demise.[9]

Table 11.1 The Aberdeen Classification of obstetric and fetal causes of stillbirth

Congenital anomaly
  Neural tube defects
  Others
Isoimmunization
  Rhesus disease
  Others
Pre-eclampsia
  Without antepartum haemorrhage (APH)
  With APH
Antepartum haemorrhage
  With placenta praevia (PP)
  Without PP
  Unknown cause
Mechanical
  Cord prolapse
  Other vertex or face presentation
  Breech
  Oblique/compound/transverse lie
Maternal disorder
  Hypertensive disease
  Other maternal disease
  Maternal infection
Miscellaneous
  Specific fetal condition
Unexplained
  More than 2.5 kg
  Less than 2.5 kg

Further subdivision of various obstetric and fetal causes can be made according to the Aberdeen Classification (Table 11.1).[6]

MANAGEMENT

Investigations

Many investigations will have been performed at the time of fetal death. Central to these should be a post-mortem examination of the fetus and placenta by a pathologist with expertise in perinatal pathology [IV].[6] Other investigations should include cytogenetic analysis of the fetus, studies of fetal products for infection, maternal serology for infection, Kleihauer testing of maternal serum, screening for maternal red cell antibodies, maternal glycosylated haemoglobin measurement and thrombophilia screening (including antiphospholipid antibodies) [IV].

It should be remembered that the interpretation of thrombophilia and antiphospholipid antibody syndrome (APAS) screening is difficult in pregnancy. Pregnancy is associated with reduced protein S activity and relative activated protein C resistance. In addition, pregnancy is associated with fluctuating levels of both anticardiolipin antibodies (ACA) and lupus anticoagulant (LA). Many authorities thus recommend that thrombophilia and APAS screening are repeated after the puerperium [IV].[10]

Assessment of risk

Risk assessment is vital for a woman with a history of fetal loss. Ideally, a full set of investigations leading to a diagnosis of causation will have been established. Where the fetal loss remains unexplained, the risk of recurrence would appear to be low. However, these pregnancies do appear to be at increased risk of premature delivery and small for gestational age infants.[4] Increased maternal age and lower socio-economic class appear to be risk factors for recurrent stillbirth.[3]

Where the previous death was associated with complications such as pre-eclampsia, fetal growth restriction or placental abruption, there is a significant recurrence risk. However, causes such as cord prolapse are associated with an extremely low recurrence risk.

Many of these obstetric complications, such as abruption, pre-eclampsia and fetal growth restriction, are associated with thrombophilia or APAS[10] (see Chapter 6.5). Maternal factor V Leiden mutation, protein S deficiency, activated protein C resistance, anticardiolipin IgG antibodies or lupus anticoagulant are independently associated with increased risk of stillbirth,[10] and their presence in a woman with a previous history of fetal loss must be considered ominous.

Monitoring

Even when the recurrence risk of fetal loss is deemed to be low, a past history of fetal loss is associated with higher rates of adverse pregnancy outcome, and thus regular assessment through pregnancy with ultrasound monitoring of fetal growth is recommended [IV]. One small observational study of monitoring from 32 weeks with a combination of biophysical profile scoring and stress testing for 300 women resulted in only one recurrent stillbirth.[11]

Increased levels of anxiety in parents and caregivers is likely to result in high levels of monitoring, which in turn can lead to increased levels of intervention, including early delivery and caesarean section. Although these interventions should be reserved for standard obstetric indications, it is difficult to resist the request for delivery just prior to the gestation at which a woman suffered a term stillbirth, or to offer caesarean section to a woman whose baby previously died in labour. Care providers in subsequent pregnancies should also be alert to the risk of the mother's psychological well-being deteriorating through the pregnancy [IV].

Aspirin and heparin

The combination of aspirin and heparin reduces pregnancy loss in women with APAS and is superior to aspirin alone,[12] mainly by reducing the risk of miscarriage [Ia]. It is not clear if late fetal loss or stillbirth is reduced. Nevertheless, it would seem sensible to treat women with APAS and a past history of fetal loss by a combination of aspirin and heparin throughout their pregnancy [IV]. The use of aspirin alone or in combination with heparin for women with a previous fetal loss and thrombophilia has not been assessed in the context of trials, thus its use in this context is controversial.

Systematic review of 39 randomized, controlled trials has demonstrated that aspirin alone has been shown to reduce the risk of pre-eclampsia and consequent preterm delivery and stillbirth.[13] It is not clear whether aspirin will reduce the risk of stillbirth in the absence of pre-eclampsia, and the use of aspirin should probably be reserved for women at high risk of pre-eclampsia [IV] (see Chapters 6.1 and 7.6).

SUMMARY

Fetal loss in a previous pregnancy leads to high levels of anxiety and intervention in subsequent pregnancies. The risk of recurrent stillbirth depends upon the cause of the first fetal death, but adverse pregnancy outcomes appear to be more common in these women. Their pregnancies should be regarded as high risk and monitored accordingly.

- Systematic review of 16 studies demonstrates that stillbirth is associated with APAS, factor V Leiden mutation, protein S deficiency and activated protein C resistance.
- Observational study suggests that a post mortem results in additional valuable information, even when it is thought that the cause of fetal death is known.
- No randomized trials of aspirin alone, or in combination with heparin, for the management of pregnant women with a history of stillbirth in association with either APAS or congenital thrombophilia have been reported.
- No comparative trials of different monitoring strategies for pregnant women with a history of fetal loss have been reported.

KEY REFERENCES

1. Turton P, Hughes P, Evans CD, Fainman D. Incidence, correlates and predictors of post-traumatic stress disorder in the pregnancy after stillbirth. *Br J Psychiatry* 2001; **178**:556–60.
2. Hughes PM, Turton P, Evans CD. Stillbirth as risk factor for depression and anxiety in the subsequent pregnancy: cohort study. *BMJ* 1999; **318**:1721–4.

3. Samueloff A, Xenakis EM, Berkus MD, Huff RW, Langer O. Recurrent stillbirth. Significance and characteristics. *J Reprod Med* 1993; **38**:883–6.

4. Robson S, Chan A, Keane RJ, Luke CG. Subsequent birth outcomes after an unexplained stillbirth: preliminary population-based retrospective cohort study. *Aust NZ J Obstet Gynaecol* 2001; **41**:29–35.

5. Hughes P, Turton P, Hopper E, McGauley GA, Fonagy P. Disorganised attachment behaviour among infants born subsequent to stillbirth. *J Child Psychol Psychiatry* 2001; **42**:791–801.

6. CESDI. 8th Annual Report, 2001. London: HMSO.

7. Cartlidge PH, Dawson AT, Stewart JH, Vujanic GM. Value and quality of perinatal and infant post-mortem examinations: cohort analysis of 400 consecutive deaths. *Br Med J* 1995; **310**:155–8.

8. Keeling JW, MacGillivray I, Golding J, Wigglesworth J, Berry J, Dunn PM. Classification of perinatal death. *Arch Dis Child* 1989; **64**:1345–51.

9. Gardosi J, Mul T, Mongelli M, Fagan D. Analysis of birthweight and gestational age in antepartum stillbirths. *Br J Obstet Gynaecol* 1998; **105**:524–30.

10. Alfirevic Z, Roberts D, Martlew V. How strong is the association between maternal thrombophilia and adverse pregnancy outcome? A systematic review. *Eur J Obstet Gynecol Reprod Biol* 2002; **101**:6–14.

11. Weeks JW, Asrat T, Morgan MA, Nageotte M, Thomas SJ, Freeman RK. Antepartum surveillance for a history of stillbirth: when to begin? *Am J Obstet Gynecol* 1995; **172**:486–92.

12. Empson M, Lassere M, Craig JC, Scott JR. Recurrent pregnancy loss with antiphospholipid antibody: a systematic review of therapeutic trials. *Obstet Gynecol* 2002; **99**:135–44.

13. Duley L, Henderson-Smart D, Knight M, King J. Antiplatelet drugs for prevention of pre-eclampsia and its consequences: systematic review. *BMJ* 2001; **322**:329–33.

Chapter 12

Multiple Pregnancy

Sailesh Kumar

MRCOG standards

Theoretical skills
- Understand the aetiology and different risks of types of twins.
- Understand the potential problems of multiple pregnancies and the general principles of management.

Practical skills
- Be able to discuss with a patient the differences between monochorionic and dichorionic placentation.
- Be able to discuss the general complications of multiple pregnancies.
- Be able to discuss the increased perinatal risk of multiple pregnancies.

INTRODUCTION

Dizygous pregnancy rates vary with maternal age, race, nutrition and geography. The highest rates are reported in sub-Saharan Africa (Nigeria) and the lowest in the Far East (Japan). Monozygous twinning rates are, however, fairly constant, at 3–5/1000 births, although there is some anecdotal evidence that the incidence is also increasing. Multiple pregnancies have increased in the UK from 10.4/1000 maternities in 1985 to 14.4/1000 maternities in 1997, with triplets and higher order multiples increasing almost three-fold. This increase is largely due to assisted conception techniques, which result in multiple rates of between 20 and 30 per cent.[1] Though predominantly dizygotic, pregnancies which result from assisted conception techniques are at greater risk of monozygotic division than those spontaneously conceived. Both the British Fertility Society and the Human Fertilisation and Embryology Authority suggest transferring a maximum of two embryos in each treatment cycle, without compromising pregnancy success [IV].

MATERNAL RISKS

The mother is at increased risk for several pregnancy complications, including miscarriage, hyperemesis, premature labour and delivery, anaemia, pre-eclampsia, antepartum and postpartum haemorrhage, polyhydramnios, operative delivery and increased stay in hospital. Women who have twins are also at increased risk of developing postnatal depression and of having problems with breastfeeding.[2]

FETAL RISKS

Multiple pregnancies are associated with an increase in fetal and neonatal mortality compared with singleton pregnancies. The higher the order of multiple pregnancy, the greater the perinatal morbidity and mortality. The majority of perinatal deaths are associated with preterm birth and intrauterine growth restriction. Perinatal mortality rates are 37, 52 and 231 per 1000 births for twins, triplets and higher order multiple births respectively. Each of these contributing factors will be discussed in turn.

Preterm labour

Twins are five times more likely to be born preterm compared with singletons,[3] and delivery before 32 weeks is approximately twice as common in monochorionic compared with dichorionic twins.[4] Almost 15 per cent of triplets deliver prior to 30 weeks' gestation.

Intrauterine growth restriction

Growth restriction of one or all of the fetuses in a multiple pregnancy is very common. The aetiology is not well understood, but the incidence varies between 25 and 33 per cent.[5] Twin birth weight discordance has also been demonstrated to be a risk factor for preterm birth. This effect was found particularly with discordances ≥40 per cent before

32 weeks' gestation and was usually attributable to fetal growth restriction, most often in the second twin.[6]

Single fetal death

This may occur either early in gestation or later as the pregnancy progresses. Fetal death at 20 weeks' gestation or later is relatively uncommon, occurring in 2.6 per cent of twin and 4.3 per cent of triplet gestations.[7] Morbidity to the surviving fetus depends very much on the chorionicity of the pregnancy. When one monochorionic twin dies in utero, there is a 25 per cent risk in the survivor of necrotic neurological and renal lesions, and a similar risk of intrauterine death of the healthy co-twin.[7,8] These complications are usually as a consequence of severe hypotension occurring during the death of the other twin.[8]

The risk of cerebral palsy is increased in the surviving twin after a co-twin death, and same-sex twins are at greater risk than unlike-sex twins. The likely cause, in addition to the consequences of prematurity, is twin–twin transfusion problems associated with monochorionicity.[9]

Twin–twin transfusion syndrome

Twin–twin transfusion syndrome (TTTS) is a condition that complicates up to 15 per cent of monochorionic twin pregnancies.[4] It is characterized by a relative lack of superficial bilateral vascular anastomoses, which protect against haemodynamic imbalances caused by unidirectional deep arteriovenous vessels.[10]

The diagnosis requires the ultrasound demonstration of polyhydramnios around one twin (the recipient) and oligohydramnios around the other twin (the donor), with the separating membrane completely covering this fetus (stuck twin). The recipient twin is usually appropriately grown for gestational age, has a large distended bladder and may, if severely compromised, be hydropic (see Chapter 17). Recipient fetuses may also develop cardiac dysfunction and neonatal hypertension. The donor twin, on the other hand, is frequently severely growth restricted, with abnormal umbilical artery Doppler waveforms. If untreated, the perinatal mortality is extremely high (>80 per cent). Although twin–twin transfusion is usually a gradual process, it can happen suddenly with the death of one twin, usually the recipient.

Twin reversed arterial perfusion (TRAP) sequence

This complication occurs in approximately 1 per cent of monochorionic pregnancies. It is characterized by an acardiac twin, which receives its blood supply via a large arterio-arterial anastomosis from a normal 'pump' co-twin. This results in absent or rudimentary development of the upper body structures. The perinatal mortality of the pump twin is considerable, with death usually occurring from cardiac failure, hydrops or polyhydramnios-induced preterm delivery.

Congenital anomalies

There is an excess of malformations in twins compared to singleton pregnancies.[2,11]

- Malformations arising from the process of development: often midline structural anomalies (i.e. neural tube defects, cardiac and cleft lip anomalies). This also includes conjoined twins (abnormalities of duplication).
- Malformations associated with twins with 'disruption' in a previously normally formed fetus. Disruptions are more common in monochorionic pregnancies and consist of predominantly vascular-type lesions (i.e hydrancephaly, porencephaly, small bowel atresia).
- Structural anomalies associated with the constraints of sharing the uterine cavity (i.e. talipes, congenital dislocation of the hip).

Other fetal risks

These complications comprise for the most part those associated with the third trimester and in particular intrapartum complications. Such risks include intrapartum hypoxaemia, twin entanglement (i.e. collision, compaction and interlocking) and umbilical cord accidents, associated with amniorrhexis (i.e. cord prolapse) or entanglement in monoamniotic twins.[2]

KEY POINTS

- Preterm labour and delivery are the biggest cause of adverse perinatal outcome in multiple pregnancy [II].
- Maternal risks relate mainly to increased uterine distension and the development of pre-eclampsia [II].
- An excess of congenital malformations means that examination of multiple pregnancies by detailed ultrasound scanning is mandatory [II].

MANAGEMENT

Diagnosis and determination of chorionicity

The early establishment of chorionicity is crucial to the management. Twenty per cent of twins are monochorionic and such pregnancies are associated with an almost 26 per cent risk of perinatal mortality. Dizygous twins can only be dichorionic diamniotic, whereas monozygous twins may be dichorionic diamniotic, monochorionic diamniotic or monochorionic monoamniotic, depending on the timing of embryo splitting.

In the first trimester, chorionicity may be determined with almost 100 per cent accuracy. In contrast, mid-trimester assessment is only 80–90 per cent accurate. If two placentae are visualized or if the fetuses are discordant for gender, the pregnancy must be dichorionic. Visualization of the *twin-peak* or *lambda* sign is also useful in the diagnosis of dichorionicity; however, the absence of this sign is not as reliable in the confirmation of monochorionicity. The identification of an arterial–arterial anastomosis by colour Doppler insonation of the chorionic plate may confirm monochorionicity.[10] Membrane thickness has also been used to assign chorionicity. In difficult cases, zygosity studies may need to be performed. However, there is no evidence base (in the form of systematic reviews [Ia]) that such 'triaging' of care improves overall outcome in the monochorionic twins.

Screening for aneuploidy and prenatal diagnosis

Unlike in singleton pregnancies, serum screening in multiple pregnancies is not possible. Therefore the screening method of choice is nuchal translucency, which can be performed in the first trimester and allows calculation of an individual risk for each fetus. It may also be predictive for the development of TTTS if monochorionic pregnancies are discordant for nuchal thickness.[12] The efficacy of nuchal translucency measurement screening in twins might be improved when combined with first trimester maternal serum screening.[13]

Before any invasive procedure is undertaken for karyotyping, careful ultrasound mapping of the different placentae and gestational sacs is mandatory to assist in subsequent management when the karyotype results are available. The pregnancy loss rates for genetic amniocentesis in twins are considered similar to those seen in singletons.[14] No data exist on loss rates with amniocentesis for higher order multiples. Chorionic villus sampling (CVS) is also possible in multiple pregnancy; although CVS carries a higher loss rate, it has the advantage of being performed earlier (see Chapter 10.3). Up to 4 per cent of CVS samples show evidence of co-twin contamination.[15]

Monitoring of fetal growth

Serial growth scans should be performed to evaluate fetal growth velocity and to detect any abnormalities in umbilical/fetal artery Doppler waveform analysis and amniotic fluid volume. The overall frequency of growth restriction in twins is 29 per cent, with 42 per cent of monochorionic twins compared with 25 per cent of dichorionic twins having one or more fetuses above the fifth centile. A sensible policy to monitor twins is 4-weekly scans from 24 weeks in dichorionic pregnancies, with more frequent scans if growth restriction is suggested. Monochorionic pregnancies should be monitored fortnightly from 18 weeks [IV].

The management of growth restriction in twin pregnancies needs to consider the risks to both the fetuses. Severe growth restriction in one fetus in a dichorionic pregnancy might warrant a conservative approach (even allowing the growth restricted fetus to succumb in utero), thus sparing the healthy fetus the risks of iatrogenic prematurity.

Multifetal pregnancy reduction

In pregnancies involving three or more fetuses, multi-fetal pregnancy reduction (MFPR) substantially reduces the risk of perinatal morbidity and mortality. With increasing experience, post-procedure miscarriage rates are now approximately 7.5 per cent,[16] such that reductions from triplets to twins and from quadruplets to twins carry outcomes as good as those of unreduced twin gestations, and the chance of taking home a live baby increases from 80 per cent to 90 per cent.

When offering MFPR, women should be counselled about mortality rates with expectant management (i.e. non-reduction) as well as the mean gestational age at delivery (33 weeks for triplets and 31 weeks for quadruplets)[17] and the risk of severe neurodevelopmental sequelae in the survivors (12 per cent in triplets and 25 per cent in quadruplets).[18]

Preterm labour

Prediction of preterm labour in twin pregnancies is as difficult as in singleton pregnancies. Cervical assessment has been suggested as one method to evaluate the risk of preterm labour. However, the frequency of monitoring/assessment of the cervix is unclear. In twin pregnancies, the mean cervical length is similar to that of singletons (3.8 mm), but a cervical length <25 mm (cf. <15 mm in singletons) at 23 weeks' gestation predicts about 80 per cent of women who deliver spontaneously at ≤30 weeks, with a false-positive rate of approximately 11 per cent.[19]

Home uterine monitoring,[20] fetal fibronectin estimation,[21] prophylactic cervical cerclage[22] and beta-mimetic therapy[23] have not been shown to reduce the incidence of preterm labour in twin pregnancies and have largely been abandoned.

There is currently not enough evidence to support a policy of routine hospitalization for bed rest in multiple pregnancies. No reduction in the risk of preterm birth or perinatal death is evident, although there is a suggestion that fetal growth is improved. Indeed, in uncomplicated twin pregnancies, there is a suggestion that bed rest may be harmful in that the risk of very preterm birth is increased.

Antenatal steroids

The effect of antenatal steroids in twin pregnancies may be limited, with a lesser odds ratio (0.79; 95% CI, 0.33–1.91) for reducing the risk of respiratory distress syndrome than in singleton pregnancies. Whether a larger dose of steroids may be beneficial in multiple pregnancies is at present unclear.

Treatment of TTTS and TRAP

Treatment options include serial amnioreduction, septostomy, selective feticide and laser ablation of the communicating anastomoses. Amnioreduction treats the polyhydramnios and has a success rate of 60–65 per cent. Septostomy aims to equilibrate the discordant amniotic fluid between the two sacs, and in a recent study had an 85 per cent success rate.[24] Selective feticide allows the survival of one twin with a >85 per cent success rate.[25] Laser treatment has a survival rate of 49–67 per cent.[26]

In cases of TRAP, disruption of the acardiac twin's cord is the treatment of choice. However, if this is technically challenging, diathermy or interstitial laser of a central vessel may be attempted.

Treatment of co-twin death

In dichorionic pregnancies, expectant management is indicated. Regular assessment of the pregnant woman's coagulation status is necessary in order to detect changes in the coagulation system that may occur. In monochorionic pregnancies, management depends upon the gestation and on the elapsed time since the fetal death. When death has occurred within 24–36 hours at an early gestation, fetal blood sampling with rescue transfusion may be considered if the surviving fetus is anaemic. At later gestations, delivery may more appropriate.

If a co-twin death has occurred some time previously, consideration should be given to appropriate imaging of the surviving fetus's brain with either ultrasound or magnetic resonance imaging (MRI) to detect cystic changes. If these changes do evolve and are apparent, offering termination of the pregnancy may be an option.

Labour and delivery

Timing of delivery in uncomplicated monochorionic twins is controversial. There is no conclusive evidence as to when delivery should be undertaken. For example, at Queen Charlotte's Hospital in London, the management plan is routinely to deliver monochorionic twins at 36 weeks' gestation, after steroid cover. If there is evidence of TTTS or other complications, delivery is expedited. In dichorionic twins, most obstetricians would recommend delivery by 40 weeks.[2]

The mode of delivery is decided on standard principles based on the presentation of the first twin. Vaginal delivery is preferred in vertex–vertex presentations. The optimal mode of birth for the second twin presenting as non-vertex is controversial. Retrospective reviews in the literature provide support for both caesarean birth and vaginal birth for the second non-vertex twin [II].

For the very low birth weight infant (<1500 g), opinion is divided as to the optimal mode of delivery. Whereas some authors advocate caesarean delivery in all cases,[27] it is not clear that caesarean section improves perinatal outcome.[28]

Although some authors suggest that triplets and higher order multiples may be safely delivered vaginally, caesarean section is frequently practised. This may prevent birth trauma and also allows the delivery to be conducted in a planned manner when the requisite number of paediatric staff is in attendance.

KEY POINTS

- Determination of chorionicity is important to allocate pregnancy risk [IV].
- Serum screening is not suitable for multiple pregnancy, and nuchal translucency is the method of choice for aneuploidy screening [II].
- Prenatal diagnosis using amniocentesis or CVS is suitable in multiple pregnancy.
- The management of TTTS and TRAP necessitates referral to an appropriate fetal medicine unit [II, IV]. Such conditions carry high perinatal mortality, even with treatment.
- Cervical length measurement may be useful in predicting preterm birth in multiple pregnancy [II].

CONCLUSIONS

The management of a multiple pregnancy is a challenge with potential serious complications for the unwary or non-vigilant obstetrician. Maternal and fetal complications require specialized management and these patients are frequently best managed in collaboration with a fetal medicine specialist with a special interest in multiple pregnancy.

KEY REFERENCES

1. Svendsen TO, Jones D, Butler L, Muasher SJ. The incidence of multiple gestations after in vitro fertilization is dependent on the number of embryos

transferred and maternal age. *Fertil Steril* 1996; **65**(3):561–5.

2. Ward RH, Whittle MJ. *Multiple Pregnancy*. London: RCOG Press, 1995.

3. Alexander GR. Reducing preterm and low birthweight rates in the United States: is psychosocial assessment the answer? *Matern Child Health J* 1998; **2**(3):195–9.

4. Sebire NJ, Snijders RJ, Hughes K, Sepulveda W, Nicolaides KH. The hidden mortality of monochorionic twin pregnancies. *Br J Obstet Gynaecol* 1997; **104**(10):1203–7.

5. Houlton MC, Marivate M, Philpott RH. The prediction of fetal growth retardation in twin pregnancy. *Br J Obstet Gynaecol* 1981; **88**(3):264–73.

6. Cooperstock MS, Tummaru R, Bakewell J, Schramm W. Twin birth weight discordance and risk of preterm birth. *Am J Obstet Gynecol* 2000; **183**(1):63–7.

7. Fusi L, Gordon H. Twin pregnancy complicated by single intrauterine death. Problems and outcome with conservative management. *Br J Obstet Gynaecol* 1990; **97M**(6):511–16.

8. Kilby MD, Govind A, O'Brien PMS. Outcome of twin pregnancies complicated by a single intrauterine death: a comparison with viable twin pregnancies. *Obstet Gynecol* 1994; **84**:107–9.

9. Glinianaia SV, Pharoah PO, Wright C, Rankin JM. Fetal or infant death in twin pregnancy: neurodevelopmental consequence for the survivor. *Arch Dis Child Fetal Neonatal Med* 2002; **86**(1):F9–15.

10. Denbow ML, Cox P, Talbert D, Fisk NM. Colour Doppler energy insonation of placental vasculature in monochorionic twins: absent arterio-arterial anastomoses in association with twin-to-twin transfusion syndrome. *Br J Obstet Gynaecol* 1998; **105**(7):760–5.

11. Keeling JW. Anomalous development in twins. In: Ward RH, Whittle MJ (eds). *Multiple Pregnancy*. London: RCOG Press, 1995, 83–99.

12. Nicolaides KH, Heath V, Cicero S. Increased fetal nuchal translucency at 11–14 weeks. *Prenat Diagn* 2002; **22**(4):308–15.

13. Dommergues M. Prenatal diagnosis for multiple pregnancies. *Curr Opin Obstet Gynecol* 2002; **14**(2):169–75.

14. Ghidini A, Lynch L, Hicks C, Alvarez M, Lockwood CJ. The risk of second-trimester amniocentesis in twin gestations: a case-control study. *Am J Obstet Gynecol* 1993; **169**(4):1013–16.

15. Wapner RJ. Genetic diagnosis in multiple pregnancies. *Semin Perinatol* 1995; **19**(5):351–62.

16. Evans MI, Goldberg JD, Horenstein J et al. Selective termination for structural, chromosomal, and mendelian anomalies: international experience. *Am J Obstet Gynecol* 1999; **181**(4):893–7.

17. Collins MS, Bleyl JA. Seventy-one quadruplet pregnancies: management and outcome. *Am J Obstet Gynecol* 1990; **162**(6):1384–91; discussion 1391–2.

18. Lipitz S, Reichman B, Uval J et al. A prospective comparison of the outcome of triplet pregnancies managed expectantly or by multifetal reduction to twins. *Am J Obstet Gynecol* 1994; **170**(3):874–9.

19. Souka AP, Heath V, Flint S, Sevastopoulou I, Nicolaides KH. Cervical length at 23 weeks in twins in predicting spontaneous preterm delivery. *Obstet Gynecol* 1999; **94**(3):450–4.

20. Dyson DC, Danbe KH, Bamber JA et al. Monitoring women at risk for preterm labour. *N Engl J Med* 1998; **338**(1):15–19.

21. Wennerholm UB, Holm B, Mattsby-Baltzer I et al. Fetal fibronectin, endotoxin, bacterial vaginosis and cervical length as predictors of preterm birth and neonatal morbidity in twin pregnancies. *Br J Obstet Gynaecol* 1997; **104**(12):1398–404.

22. Weekes AR, Menzies DN, de Boer CH. The relative efficacy of bed rest, cervical suture, and no treatment in the management of twin pregnancy. *Br J Obstet Gynaecol* 1977; **84**(3):161–4.

23. Ashworth MF, Spooner SF, Verkuyl DA, Waterman R, Ashurst HM. Failure to prevent preterm labour and delivery in twin pregnancy using prophylactic oral salbutamol. *Br J Obstet Gynaecol* 1990; **97**(10):878–82.

24. Saade GR, Belfort MA, Berry DL et al. Amniotic septostomy for the treatment of twin oligohydramnios–polyhydramnios sequence. *Fetal Diagn Ther* 1998; **13**(2):86–93.

25. Taylor MJ, Shalev E, Tanawattanacharoen S et al. Ultrasound-guided umbilical cord occlusion using bipolar diathermy for Stage III/IV twin–twin transfusion syndrome. *Prenat Diagn* 2002; **22**(1):70–6.

26. Ville Y, Hecher K, Gagnon A, Sebire N, Hyett J, Nicolaides K. Endoscopic laser coagulation in the management of severe twin-to-twin transfusion syndrome. *Br J Obstet Gynaecol* 1998; **105**(4):446–53.

27. Chervenak FA, Johnson RE, Youcha S, Hobbins JC, Berkowitz RL. Intrapartum management of twin gestation. *Obstet Gynecol* 1985; **65**(1):119–24.

28. Rydhstrom H. Prognosis for twins with birth weight less than 1500 g: the impact of cesarean section in relation to fetal presentation. *Am J Obstet Gynecol* 1990; **163**(2):528–33.

Antenatal complications: fetal

Fetal Infections

Sailesh Kumar

INTRODUCTION

Congenital infections may cause significant morbidity and mortality through various different mechanisms. Some infectious agents cause a self-limiting maternal illness with minimal or no adverse fetal consequences, whereas others cause major sequelae in the form of malformations, neurodevelopmental delay and even long-term childhood consequences.

Infectious agents may affect the fetus by vertical transmission, which can be either blood borne or at the time of delivery (e.g. varicella, rubella, cytomegalovirus (CMV) infection, toxoplasmosis and listeriosis). Pre-pregnancy or routine antenatal screening for the presence of some of these infections and appropriate management can prevent adverse fetal or perinatal outcomes. If an infection is suspected because of a positive antenatal test result, confirmatory tests for maternal and, if indicated, fetal infection are essential

before intervention is considered. In addition, screening for past infection and immunization to increase herd immunity are also an important public health measure.

The diagnosis of fetal infection is important in order to counsel the mother about the likely sequelae. In some cases the risk of congenital malformations may be so high that an offer of termination of pregnancy may be appropriate (i.e. congenital rubella syndrome). There are numerous infectious agents, and many have either a direct or indirect affect on pregnancy. It is beyond the scope of this chapter to discuss all infectious agents; however, the following are discussed in specific detail: rubella virus, varicella zoster virus (VZV), CMV, toxoplasma, parvovirus B19 and *Treponema pallidum*.

RUBELLA (see also Chapter 7.4)

Rubella (German measles) is a self-limiting, mild viral illness that poses little danger to children or adults. For the developing fetus, however, infection with rubella virus is a grave threat, capable of inducing severe anomalies and permanent disability. In general terms, the earlier the gestational age at which infection occurs, the greater the risk of fetal morbidity. Despite widespread vaccination programmes, populations of susceptible individuals persist, among them women of childbearing age, whose pregnancies remain vulnerable to congenital rubella syndrome. Natural infections of rubella occur only in humans and are generally mild.

The primary public health concern of rubella infection is its teratogenicity. Infection during the first trimester of pregnancy can induce a spectrum of congenital defects in the newborn, known as congenital rubella syndrome (CRS). The mechanism of infection leading to teratogenesis is not clear, but analysis of infected fetal tissues suggests hypoxia, necrosis and/or apoptosis as well as inhibition of cell division of critical precursor cells involved in organogenesis. Although malformations can occur in almost all organ systems, the eyes, heart and ears seem to be preferentially affected. Cataracts, retinopathy, microphthalmia, glaucoma, patent ductus arteriosus, pulmonary valve lesions and sensorineural deafness are common abnormalities seen in early fetal infection.[1] The risk of fetal infection and congenital abnormalities is in excess of 80 per cent if infection occurs in the first trimester,[2] and decreases to approximately 25 per cent in early second trimester [II].[1] The risk of congenital abnormalities continues to decrease as pregnancy progresses.

There is emerging evidence indicating that in-utero exposure to rubella infection may have more long-term consequences, with such individuals being at higher risk of schizophrenia. It is hypothesized that prenatal infection increases the liability to schizophrenia in adulthood by adversely affecting the maturation of critical brain structural and functional components implicated in the aetiology of this disorder.[3]

Although national immunization programmes in many countries have made this disease increasingly rare because of herd immunity, immigrants to the UK may be susceptible and therefore a high index of suspicion is needed for this infection in recent immigrants from countries with no immunization programme. Targeted immunization for such groups should be considered [IV].

Diagnosis

The clinical diagnosis of rubella is difficult, as it is frequently subclinical and the rash is similar to that of other viral infections; therefore serology remains the mainstay of diagnosis. In the mother, acute infection may be diagnosed by isolation of the virus from throat swabs, but it is more common for an acute rubella-specific immunoglobulin (IgM) response to be detected [II] in an individual previously noted to be non-immune using fluorescent immunoassay techniques. Rubella-specific IgG indicates previous infection or immunization. Immunity is usually life long.

Management

Vaccination of children remains the cornerstone of the preventative strategy for this devastating fetal disease. Pre-pregnancy counselling should include evidence of immunity and vaccination should be offered to susceptible individuals [II].

If infection is confirmed in the first trimester, termination of pregnancy should be offered, as the sequelae of congenital infection are devastating. Later in pregnancy, evidence for fetal infection may be sought. Fetal blood sampling to measure levels of rubella-specific IgM[4] may be performed and rubella-specific RNA identified using reverse transcriptase-polymerase chain reaction (RT-PCR) [II, IV].[5]

The rubella vaccine is a live attenuated virus and therefore theoretically should be avoided in pregnancy. However, the Centers for Disease Control in the USA have monitored cases of inadvertent rubella vaccination during

pregnancy (1971–89) and no adverse sequelae have been documented [II].[6]

KEY POINTS

- Early pregnancy infection results in an extremely high fetal transmission rate [II].
- Termination of pregnancy should be discussed with patients if maternal infection occurs in the first trimester, because of the very high risk of congenital malformation [II].

CYTOMEGALOVIRUS (see also Chapter 7.4)

Cytomegalovirus, a member of the herpes virus family, is the most common cause of congenital infection in humans, affecting 0.5–3 per cent of all newborns worldwide. It has a high prevalence in the general population, is unpredictable in its transmission, and causes an asymptomatic disease in otherwise healthy women. Intrauterine infection with CMV remains the most common congenital virus infection in many regions of the world. Although most CMV-infected newborns lack signs of infection, approximately 10 per cent have low birth weight, jaundice, hepatosplenomegaly, skin rash, microcephaly and chorioretinitis. Other fetal consequences of CMV infection include haemolytic anaemia, ventriculomegaly, cerebral atrophy and intracranial calcification. The sequelae of fetal infection are gestation dependent: early fetal infection causes brain anomalies, whereas symptomatic late fetal infection results in hepatitis and thrombocytopenia. Neonates with signs of CMV infection at birth have high rates of audiologic and neurodevelopmental sequelae. Congenital CMV infection is the leading infectious cause of deafness, learning disabilities and mental retardation in children (rubella, measles and mumps have become rare due to vaccination).

Diagnosis

Recent advances in the screening of pregnant women with CMV IgM, CMV IgG and CMV IgG avidity serological tests have led to more accurate diagnosis of CMV infection. When serological screening is performed early in gestation, it is possible to identify those women at risk of intrauterine transmission of the virus (women with a primary CMV infection). The use of quantitative PCR on the amniotic fluid from pregnant women at 21–22 weeks of gestation in prenatal diagnosis is an effective diagnostic tool [II]. Quantitative PCR on peripheral blood leucocytes from CMV-infected newborns can be used to monitor viral load.[7]

Management

There is no effective fetal therapy. Although postnatal therapy with ganciclovir transiently reduces virus shedding and may lessen the audiological consequences of CMV in some infected infants [II, IV], additional strategies are needed to prevent congenital CMV disease.

Some cases of intrauterine infections can be prevented in susceptible women by avoiding contact with the urine or saliva of young children who may be shedding CMV. Vaccines against CMV remain in the experimental stages of development. Termination of pregnancy can be offered to women whose infants have evidence of intrauterine CMV infection and sonographic signs of central nervous system (CNS) damage. Infants who survive symptomatic intrauterine infections have high rates of neurodevelopmental sequelae and require comprehensive evaluation and therapy through centre-based and home-based early intervention programmes.

Women who work in high-risk professions should be given pre-pregnancy advice. If maternal infection is confirmed, consideration should be given to performing an invasive procedure to obtain fetal samples for analysis. Tests can be performed on chorionic villus samples, amniotic fluid or fetal blood [II].[8]

KEY POINTS

- Pre-pregnancy immunity to CMV infection is socio-economically dependent, ranging from 55 to 85 per cent.
- The rate of primary CMV infection is 1–4 per cent and it carries a 40 per cent risk of fetal transmission [II].
- There is no gestation-dependent alteration of fetal risk from primary perinatal infection with gestation.
- The incidence of congenital infection varies between 0.3 and 3 per cent [II].
- Of these, 5 per cent will be symptomatic at birth, with a 30 per cent neonatal mortality and long-term morbidity in the majority of survivors. This includes neurodevelopmental delay in up to 90 per cent and hearing loss in 60 per cent [II].

TOXOPLASMA (see also Chapter 7.4)

Toxoplasma gondii is a unicellular protozoon. The cat is the definitive host and produces oocysts and sporozoites. Ingestion leads to the formation of tachyzoites, which cause parasitaemia and further dissemination, and subsequent bradyzoites, which lead to latent infection with the formation of tissue cysts in skeletal muscle, heart muscle and CNS tissue. Toxoplasmosis can be transmitted to humans by:

- ingestion of tissue cysts in raw or inadequately cooked infected meat or in uncooked foods that have come in contact with contaminated meat;
- inadvertent ingestion of oocysts and sporozoites in cat faeces; or
- transplacentally.

Immunocompetent adults and adolescents with primary infection are generally asymptomatic, but symptoms may include mild malaise, lethargy and lymphadenopathy. Specific treatment for non-pregnant adults and adolescents is not required. Immunosuppressed patients may experience more severe manifestations, including splenomegaly, chorioretinitis, pneumonitis, encephalitis and multisystem organ failure. These patients are also prone to reactivation of latent infection involving the CNS.

Congenital toxoplasmosis is marked by the classic triad of chorioretinitis, intracranial calcifications and hydrocephalus. If congenital infection occurs in the first trimester, spontaneous miscarriage is common. The risk of fetal infection rises throughout gestation, with approximately 65 per cent of fetuses affected in the third trimester. Early first trimester maternal infections are less likely to result in congenital infection, but the sequelae are more severe. Transplacental passage is more common when maternal infection occurs in the latter half of pregnancy, but fetal injury is usually much less severe. The majority of infants are born without any obvious problems. There is no accurate logarithm to predict the severity of fetal infection, although high maternal antibody levels may be weakly correlative.[9]

Diagnosis

All positive screening tests in pregnant women must be confirmed at a toxoplasma reference laboratory using a specific and sensitive ELISA testing [II]. Paired serological titres are important in confirming acute maternal infection. Recent studies have shown that PCR testing of amniotic fluid is useful for identification or exclusion of fetal *T. gondii* infection [II].[10] Ultrasound evidence of intracranial infections can be used as an adjunct to serological screening, but cannot itself definitively diagnose disease because of the relatively low sensitivity and specificity of diagnosis.

Management

Prevention of primary maternal infection is critical in this regard. This is best achieved by adequate public education through health campaigns to ensure that non-immune pregnant women handle and cook meat appropriately, use gloves when handling cat litter, and avoid contact with objects that are potentially contaminated with cat faeces.

If maternal infection is confirmed, spiramycin should be commenced to reduce the likelihood of fetal infection; this treatment reduces the risk of transmission by almost 60 per cent [II].[10] Spiramycin should be started as soon as maternal infection has been confirmed, as the longer the delay the greater the risk of fetal damage [II]. A recent study failed to detect a beneficial effect of early or more potent prenatal anti-toxoplasma treatment (pyrimethamine-sulfadiazine) on the risks of intracranial or ocular lesions in children with congenital toxoplasmosis [II].[11]

Termination of pregnancy is also an option if infection occurs early in gestation or if there is ultrasound evidence of congenital infection.

KEY POINTS

- In the UK, the risk of congenital toxoplasmosis infection is deemed to be relatively low. Health-economic evaluation has indicated that routine screening of pregnant women would not be cost effective [III].
- Both prenatal and antenatal health education of women with regard to the food that may cause vertical transmission is important.
- In women who have been investigated and are positive for an acute toxoplasmosis infection, investigation and management in a fetal medicine centre is advisable, with maternal treatment to reduce transplacental transmisson and minimize acute fetal infection [II].
- If infection occurs in the first or second trimester, the risk of severe congenital disease approaches 25 per cent.

VARICELLA (see also Chapter 7.4)

Varicella zoster virus (chickenpox) is a highly contagious DNA virus of the herpes family that is usually transmitted by respiratory droplets and by direct personal contact with vesicle fluid. The primary infection is characterized by fever, malaise and a pruritic rash that becomes maculo-papular and vesicular and finally crusts over before healing. The incubation period is 10–21 days and the disease is infectious 48 hours before the rash appears and until the vesicles crust over. More than 90 per cent of pregnant women are seropositive for varicella zoster IgG (VZIG).

Spontaneous miscarriage does not appear to be increased if chickenpox occurs in the first trimester.[12] Maternal infection before 20 weeks may result in fetal varicella syndrome. However, only 1–2 per cent of maternal varicella infections that occur before 20 weeks' gestation result in the fetal varicella syndrome.[12] Typical fetal and neonatal manifestations include skin scarring in a dermatomal distribution, eye defects (microphthalmia, chorioretinitis, cataracts), hypoplasia of the limbs and neurological abnormalities (microcephaly, cortical atrophy, mental retardation and dysfunction of bowel and bladder sphincters). Maternal infection after 20 weeks and up to 36 weeks does not appear to be associated with adverse fetal effects.

Diagnosis

Prenatal diagnosis is possible using detailed assessment ultrasound, when findings such as limb deformity, microcephaly, hydrocephalus, soft tissue calcification and intrauterine growth restriction may be detected some weeks after the initial infection.[12] VZV DNA can be detected by PCR in amniotic fluid or fetal blood, but its presence does not necessarily indicate development of the fetal varicella syndrome [IV]. Passive immunization may reduce the risk of fetal infection, but there is no evidence that it prevents fetal viraemia [IV]. There are also no controlled studies concerning the role of antiviral chemotherapy in preventing the fetal syndrome.

Management

The management of women who have either been exposed to or develop chickenpox is discussed in Chapter 7.4. There is no evidence that VZIG given within 24 hours of contact prevents intrauterine infection [II].

PARVOVIRUS B19 (see also Chapter 7.4)

Parvovirus B19 (erythema infectiosum, Fifth disease) is a small, single-stranded DNA virus that can cause fetal infection. Approximately 50 per cent of adults will be seropositive, indicating past infection and immunity. Among non-immune individuals, approximately 1 in 5 carries a risk of acute infection if exposed to erythema infectiosum. There is no evidence that the infection is teratogenic [IV], but in the fetus the virus has a predilection for erythropoietic cells, causing a transient but severe pancytopenia.[13] Parvovirus may cause unexpected stillbirths at term and late miscarriages; however, the main concern with fetal infection is the potential to develop hydrops secondary to fetal anaemia or cardiac dysfunction from acute myocarditis [III, IV].[13]

Diagnosis

The diagnosis of human parvovirus B19 in a hydropic fetus requires the isolation of the virus (by PCR) and/or parvovirus-specific IgM from paired maternal and fetal blood

[II].[13] Hydrops may occur 2–4 weeks after acute fetal infection (see Chapter 17) [II].[13]

Management

The anaemic hydropic fetus may be salvaged by aggressive in-utero transfusions of red cells [II]. Infantile red cell aplasia has been reported following in-utero transfusions, and hence these babies should be followed up to detect this potential complication.

KEY POINTS

- In non-immune pregnant individuals (50 per cent of the population), the presence of an acute infection carries at least 1 in 5 risk of transplacental transmission [II].
- Overall, the fetal death rate associated with acute human parvovirus B19 infection is 9 per cent [II].
- After acute exposure, the interval between maternal infection and fetal consequences is 4–5 weeks.
- The fetal consequences of human parvovirus B19 infection are potentially self-limiting and/or treatable. Investigation and management should take place in a regional fetal medicine centre [II, IV].

SYPHILIS (see also Chapter 7.4)

Syphilis is caused by the spirochaete *Treponema pallidum*. Pregnancy has no known effect on the clinical course of syphilis. The mother can transmit the infection to the fetus either transplacentally or by contact of the newborn with a genital lesion. *T. pallidum* can infect the fetus from as early as 9–10 weeks.[14,15] Untreated syphilis during pregnancy can profoundly affect pregnancy outcome, resulting in spontaneous abortion, stillbirth, non-immune hydrops, growth restriction, preterm delivery, neonatal death, and infant disorders such as deafness, neurological impairment and bone deformities.

Traditionally, congenital syphilis has been divided into two clinical syndromes: early and late congenital syphilis. Early disease refers to clinical manifestations that appear within the first 2 years of life. Late syphilis occurs after 2 years, usually around puberty.

Diagnosis

In routine clinical practice, serological tests on maternal blood such as the VDRL, RPR, FTA-Abs, MHA-TP or TPI assay are used to make the diagnosis (see Chapter 17).

Prenatal laboratory diagnosis of fetal infection is possible. As maternal IgM does not cross the placenta, detection of fetal IgM is indicative of transplacental infection. Fetal blood can be obtained either by cordocentesis or from the intrahepatic vein. *T. pallidum* DNA can also be detected using PCR techniques with amniotic fluid, and this method has been shown to be sensitive and specific [III].[16] Ultrasound can also be used to detect some of the manifestations of syphilis in the fetus. Hydrops, hepatosplenomegaly, placentomegaly and small bowel dilatation have all been demonstrated.[17–19] Hepatomegaly seems to be the most sensitive ultrasound marker of fetal infection [IV].

Management

Treatment of syphilis during pregnancy should be with the penicillin regimen appropriate for the mother's stage of syphilis [II]. Monthly follow-up of serological titres is recommended for the evaluation of the adequacy of treatment. Despite administration of the recommended penicillin regimen to pregnant women, as many as 14 per cent will have a fetal death or deliver infants with clinical evidence of congenital syphilis [II].[20–22]

The major factor accounting for the failure to prevent congenital infection is the lack of adequate antenatal care. This is particularly relevant in underdeveloped countries and amongst the socially deprived in industrialized communities. Routine prenatal screening remains the major line of defence against congenital syphilis [II].

KEY POINTS

- Congenital syphilis is till a major cause of perinatal morbidity and mortality worldwide.
- The risk of perinatal transmission is greatest within the first year of untreated disease.
- If untreated, 30 per cent of infected fetuses will die in utero, 30 per cent will die in the early neonatal period, and the remainder will develop late symptomatic syphilis.
- It is a common cause of poor in-utero growth worldwide.

KEY REFERENCES

1. Miller E, Cradock-Watson JE, Pollock TM. Consequences of confirmed maternal rubella at successive stages of pregnancy. *Lancet* 1982; 2(8302):781–4.
2. Mellinger AK, Cragan JD, Atkinson WL et al. High incidence of congenital rubella syndrome after a rubella outbreak. *Pediatr Infect Dis J* 1995; 14(7):573–8.

3. Brown AS, Susser ES. In utero infection and adult schizophrenia. *Ment Retard Dev Disabil Res Rev* 2002; **8**(1):51–7.

4. Daffos F, Forestier F, Grangeot-Keros L et al. Prenatal diagnosis of congenital rubella. *Lancet* 1984; 2(8393):1–3.

5. Bosma TJ, Corbett KM, O'Shea S et al. PCR for detection of rubella virus RNA in clinical samples. *J Clin Microbiol* 1995; **33**:1075–9.

6. Centers for Disease Control. Rubella vaccination during pregnancy – United States, 1971–1988. *MMWR Morb Mortal Wkly Rep* 1989; **38**:289–91.

7. Maine GT, Lazzarotto T, Landini MP. New developments in the diagnosis of maternal and congenital CMV infection. *Expert Rev Mol Diagn* 2001; 1(1):19–29.

8. Enders G, Bader U, Lindemann L, Schalasta G, Daiminger A. Prenatal diagnosis of congenital cytomegalovirus infection in 189 pregnancies with known outcome. *Prenat Diagn* 2001; **21**(5):362–77.

9. Sever JL, Ellenberg JH, Ley AC et al. Toxoplasmosis: maternal and pediatric findings in 23,000 pregnancies. *Pediatrics* 1988; **82**(2):181–92.

10. Hohlfeld P, Daffos F, Costa JM, Thulliez P, Forestier F, Vidaud M. Prenatal diagnosis of congenital toxoplasmosis with a polymerase-chain-reaction test on amniotic fluid. *N Engl J Med* 1994; **331**(11):695–9.

11. Gras L, Gilbert RE, Ades AE, Dunn DT. Effect of prenatal treatment on the risk of intracranial and ocular lesions in children with congenital toxoplasmosis. *Int J Epidemiol* 2001; **30**(6):1309–13.

12. Pastuszak AL, Levy M, Schick B et al. Outcome after maternal varicella infection in the first 20 weeks of pregnancy. *N Engl J Med* 1994; **330**(13):901–5.

13. Ismail K, Kilby MD. Human parvovirus B19 and pregnancy. *Obstet Gynecol* 2003; 5:4–9.

14. Harter C, Benirschke K. Fetal syphilis in the first trimester. *Am J Obstet Gynecol* 1976; **124**(7):705–11.

15. Nathan L, Bohman VR, Sanchez PJ, Leos NK, Twickler DM, Wendel GD Jr. In utero infection with *Treponema pallidum* in early pregnancy. *Prenat Diagn* 1997; **17**(2):119–23.

16. Zoechling N, Schluepen EM, Soyer HP, Kerl H, Volkenandt M. Molecular detection of *Treponema pallidum* in secondary and tertiary syphilis. *Br J Dermatol* 1997; **136**(5):683–6.

17. Hill LM, Maloney JB. An unusual constellation of sonographic findings associated with congenital syphilis. *Obstet Gynecol* 1991; **78**(5 Pt 2):895–7.

18. Satin AJ, Twickler DM, Wendel GD Jr. Congenital syphilis associated with dilation of fetal small bowel. A case report. *J Ultrasound Med* 1992; **11**(1):49–2.

19. Nathan L, Twickler DM, Peters MT, Sanchez PJ, Wendel GD Jr. Fetal syphilis: correlation of sonographic findings and rabbit infectivity testing of amniotic fluid. *J Ultrasound Med* 1993; **12**(2):97–101.

20. McFarlin BL, Bottoms SF, Dock BS, Isada NB. Epidemic syphilis: maternal factors associated with congenital infection. *Am J Obstet Gynecol* 1994; **170**(2):535–40.

21. Mascola L, Pelosi R, Alexander CE. Inadequate treatment of syphilis in pregnancy. *Am J Obstet Gynecol* 1984; **150**(8):945–7.

22. Conover CS, Rend CA, Miller GB Jr, Schmid GP. Congenital syphilis after treatment of maternal syphilis with a penicillin regimen exceeding CDC guidelines. *Infect Dis Obstet Gynecol* 1998; **6**(3):134–7.

Chapter 14

Tests of Fetal Well-being

Murray Luckas

INTRODUCTION

Assessing fetal well-being should reduce perinatal mortality and morbidity; however, the outcome of pregnancy in the developed world is usually good, with adverse perinatal outcomes being relatively rare. It therefore follows that the majority of fetuses subjected to tests designed to assess fetal well-being will be healthy. Those tests should not only be sensitive in their ability to detect a compromised fetus, but also specific in that they do not give an abnormal result when the fetus is well; poor specificity may lead to unnecessary parental anxiety and rates of intervention.

A major problem in the evaluation of tests of fetal well-being is the absence of useful outcome criteria. Perinatal mortality is now too rare an occurrence and too late an outcome measure to be useful. The condition of the neonate at birth is of little help, because it is difficult to separate the effects of parturition from factors present antenatally.

Long-term neurodevelopment can be assessed, but such an assessment is subject to many influences and is probably best done some 5 years after birth.

The ideal test will be quick and easy to perform and will yield readily interpreted results that are reproducible. It should clearly identify the compromised fetus at a stage at which intervention will improve the outcome, but in turn it should not give an abnormal result for a healthy fetus. Unfortunately, this ideal test does not yet exist!

DEFINITIONS

For the purposes of this chapter, we regard fetal compromise as *a fetus that is at risk of damage from hypoxia*. Energy, in the form of adenosine triphosphate (ATP) and its sister molecules, is vital for the metabolism of cells. In the absence of sufficient quantities of this energy, cells will no longer be able to function and will eventually die. The production of ATP via oxidative phosphorylation from polysaccharides (glucose), fats and proteins requires oxygen – so-called oxidative metabolism. Where oxygen levels are insufficient to support oxidative phosphorylation, anaerobic metabolism occurs. This is an inefficient process, resulting in reduced production of ATP per molecule of glucose compared to aerobic metabolism (2 vs 24 molecules of ATP). Ultimately, the hypoxic fetus will no longer be able to maintain cellular metabolism, with resultant cell damage and death. The developing brain, myocardium and kidneys are the organs most sensitive to this damage, although fetal demise will eventually occur.

In addition, hypoxia leads to build up of by-products such as lactic acid, resulting in metabolic acidaemia, which in itself may exacerbate the effects of hypoxia on cellular metabolism. This is a more chronic process than respiratory acidosis, which occurs because of an inability of the feto-placental unit to rid the fetus of carbon dioxide.

AETIOLOGY

An exhaustive list of the causes of fetal hypoxia is beyond the remit of this chapter. However, the causes include:

- reduced maternal oxygenation such as chronic disease states,
- utero-placental damage (see Chapter 15),
- impaired fetal blood supply to the placenta, as in cord accidents,
- intrinsic fetal conditions resulting in poor tissue oxygenation, such as fetal anaemia.

PHYSIOLOGY

The human fetus demonstrates complex patterns of activity from early pregnancy. These include fetal breathing movements, gross body movements and fine motor movements. The linkage of gross body movements to other behavioural patterns has led to the description of fetal behavioural states.[1] Fetal body movements are frequent during state 2F (periods of activity analogous to rapid eye movement (REM) sleep), whereas in 1F, the fetus is quiescent (analogous to non-REM sleep). A third state, 4F, occurs when the fetus displays frequent and vigorous gross body movements; this appears to represent fetal wakefulness.

Human fetal breathing movements occur 30 per cent of the time and gross body movements 10 per cent of the time during the last 10 weeks of pregnancy.[2,3] Cycling between activity and quiescence occurs over a time span of approximately 60 minutes at term. In most fetuses, activity is highest in late evening. Fetal heart rate variation increases during fetal activity, and accelerations are associated with fetal body movements.[4]

As outlined above, a fetus exposed to hypoxia will become progressively more acidotic and will eventually suffer irreversible damage, leading ultimately to death. During this process, the fetus will demonstrate several adaptations designed to conserve energy and reduce oxygen.

One of the first responses of the fetus is to reduce movements, although the human fetus may well adapt to hypoxia in the absence of acidaemia, with breathing movements, in particular, reverting to normal.[5] It would appear that reduced fetal heart rate reactivity and absence of fetal breathing movements are earlier manifestations of fetal hypoxia. With more severe hypoxia, fetal body movements and tone become abnormal. Blood is distributed preferentially to the brain, myocardium and adrenals at the expense of organs such as the kidney. This renal hypoperfusion results in a reduced glomerular filtration rate, oliguria and hence reduced liquor volume. As fetal growth accounts for a substantial fraction of the total substrate consumption, it

is reduced – leading to fetal growth restriction (FGR). The majority of the currently available tests of fetal well-being are designed to detect these adaptive changes.

TESTS OF FETAL WELL-BEING

Fetal movement counting

Maternal perception of fetal movements occurs from the second trimester. It is well recognized that, on an individual basis, reduced maternal perception of movements may be the harbinger of a sick fetus. However, all too often the mother will present too late, with her fetus already dead. Alternatively, the fetus may well be demonstrating normal activity with the mother failing to recognize those movements.

Structured fetal movement counting (FMC) has been advocated in an attempt to reduce these confounding effects. In the biggest study to date, Grant et al.[6] reported a randomized, controlled trial (RCT) evaluating the effects of FMC involving 68 000 women. The authors concluded that routine daily counting by women followed by appropriate action when movements are reduced seemed to offer no advantage over informal inquiry about movements during standard antenatal care and selective use of formal counting in high-risk cases [II]. Although the study did not rule out a beneficial effect of FMC, the policy would have to be used by 1250 women to prevent one perinatal death, and an adverse effect of FMC was just as likely.

The effect of FMC in high-risk pregnancies is not known; however, it would seem prudent to advise women deemed at high risk of fetal compromise to pay careful attention to their fetal movements. It is recommended that women who report a reduction or an alteration in the movements of their fetus should be offered some form of assessment of fetal well-being [IV].

Fetal heart rate recording

Cardiotocography

Fetal heart rate recording by non-stress test (NST) cardiotocography (CTG) is perhaps the most commonly performed antenatal test of fetal well-being. Although it is quick and simple to perform, interpretation can be difficult; indeed, over 20 studies have demonstrated poor agreement between experts in assessing the various components of the CTG. This reduces the reliability and the predictive value of the CTG. A normal NST would be regarded as a CTG demonstrating two accelerations (15 beats per minute increase lasting for 15 seconds) within a 30-minute trace.[7]

As outlined above, fetal heart rate accelerations are linked closely with fetal movements and are thought to be due to increased sympathetic output. They are strongly indicative of fetal well-being. The long-term variability of the heart rate is produced by a balance between sympathetic and parasympathetic tone, whereas short-term variability (baseline or bandwidth variability) reflects parasympathetic (vagal) tone. Heart rate variability is usually reduced in the compromised fetus and is virtually always absent prior to fetal death. Despite these observations, the predictive value for an abnormal NST for perinatal morbidity and mortality is less than 40 per cent.[7]

Analysis of 13 trials of NST has failed to demonstrate any significant effect on perinatal outcome. Indeed, in a systematic review of four RCTs, NST was associated with a trend towards increased perinatal mortality.[8] It is therefore apparent that NST should not be relied upon as the sole means of establishing fetal well-being [Ia].

In an effort to improve the predictive ability of antenatal CTG, fetal stress testing has been tried. The basis of this test is to invoke uterine contractions, thereby reducing placental perfusion and unmasking fetal compromise. This can be performed by inducing natural oxytocin release (nipple stimulation) or by maternal oxytocin administration, with the appearance of late fetal heart rate decelerations indicating fetal compromise. The role of this technique has yet to be established and it has been associated with reports of fetal death in cases of unrecognized severe fetal compromise [IV].

Stimulation of the fetus by shaking, vibration or even by sound profoundly alters fetal behaviour and heart rate. When used in conjunction with antenatal CTG, vibroacoustic stimulation of the fetus has been found to reduce the number of unreactive traces due to fetal sleep states; however, the effect on the predictive ability of the CTG remains obscure.[9]

Computerized cardiotocography

In an attempt to improve the objectivity of antenatal CTG, computer programs have been developed to analyse the fetal heart rate recoding. The most advanced and widely used is that developed by the Oxford Group utilizing the Dawes Redman Criteria[10] (Table 14.1). This system places major emphasis on the fetal heart rate variability and, unlike conventional CTG, allows the measurement of short-term variability (STV – defined as the variation measured in 3.75 s epochs). Fetal heart rate variability has been found to be a better predictor of fetal compromise than the presence or absence of fetal heart rate acceleration or decelerations.[11] Indeed, the likelihood of metabolic acidaemia or intrauterine death can be calculated according to the STV.[12]

In addition to the promising evidence of observational studies, one RCT comparing conventional and computerized NST concluded that computerized NST is associated with fewer additional fetal surveillance examinations and less time spent in testing. However, the study was not large enough to demonstrate any effect on severe perinatal morbidity or mortality rates [Ib].[13] Results from larger RCTs are awaited.

Biophysical activity

Assessment of fetal activity has been used as a predictor of fetal compromise, with perhaps the best known system being

Table 14.1   The Dawes Redman criteria for a normal antenatal computerized cardiotocogram[10]

- **There must be an episode of high variation that is above the first centile for gestational age**, high variation being defined as a section of trace where the 1-minute peak-to peak variation is above a predefined threshold for 5 out of 6 consecutive minutes. These episodes of high variation must be greater than the first centile for gestation (11 beats/minute at 38 weeks).
- **There must be no large decelerations (>20 lost beats).**
- The basal heart rate must be between 116 and 160 beats per minute. **A slightly lower or higher rate may be acceptable after 30 minutes if all else is normal.**
- **At least one fetal movement or three accelerations.**
- **There should be no evidence of a sinusoidal fetal heart rate (FHR) rhythm.**
- **The short-term variation should be 3 ms or greater.**
- **Either an acceleration or variability in high episodes >the tenth centile and fetal movements >20.**
- **There should be no errors or decelerations at the end of the record.**

Table 14.2   Parameters of biophysical profile scoring[14]

- **Fetal breathing movements** – More than one episode of 30 seconds duration or more within a 30-minute period.
- **Gross body/limb movements** – Four or more discrete body movements (including fine motor movements including thumb sucking etc.).
- **Fetal tone and posture** – Active extension and return to flexion opening and closing of mouth and hands etc.
- **Fetal heart rate reactivity** – Normal non-stress test over 20 minutes.
- **Amniotic fluid volume evaluation** – One pocket >3 cm subjectively normal.

described by Manning in the 1980s.[14] This biophysical profile (BPP) depends on the ultrasonic assessment over 30 minutes of liquor, fetal tone, body and breathing movements and finally NST. Each component is scored discretely as normal (2) or abnormal (0), with a maximum of 10 and scores under 8 being regarded as abnormal (Table 14.2). Observational data based on over 80 000 high-risk pregnancies show that BPP has a negative predictive value of 99.946 per cent and a positive predictive value of 35 per cent for perinatal morbidity including low Apgar scores, acidaemia at birth, fetal distress and fetal growth restriction.[14]

It must be remembered, however, that adverse outcomes are rare, and therefore the false-negative rates of BPP will inevitably be low (1.9/1000 in the series reported by Harman et al.[14] giving a false-negative rate of a *placebo* test of 99.81 per cent). In addition, although there does appear to be a direct relationship between an abnormal BPP and adverse perinatal outcomes, even a borderline score (6) is associated with a six-fold increase in perinatal mortality rates, indicating that the test may not give sufficient warning to allow effective intervention.

The BPP is a difficult and time-consuming test to perform. In addition, cessation of movements can occur for up to 40–60 minutes due to cycling in fetal behavioural states. Systematic review of four RCTs has failed to demonstrate any significant benefit of BPP on pregnancy outcome when compared to conventional assessment (NST). However, these trials have included fewer than 3000 women and therefore the review concluded that the current evidence is insufficient to reach any definite conclusions about the benefit or otherwise of the BPP [Ia].[15] Of concern is the observation in one small RCT that use of the BPP was associated with an increase in obstetric interventions without any benefit in perinatal outcomes when compared with assessment by NST and liquor measurement alone.[16] Indeed, the false-positive rate of BPP is in the order of 70 per cent,[14] and this may well lead to increased rates of unnecessary intervention. The most powerful components of the BPP would seem to be liquor volume assessment and NST and therefore assessment of fetal well-being using these two tools alone may well be as effective as formal BPP [Ib].[16]

Biophysical profile in pregnancies complicated by pre-labour rupture of the membranes

The observation that fetal activity (in particular fetal breathing movements) is reduced in the presence of chorioamnionitis has led to the suggestion that BPP is of benefit in monitoring women with pre-labour amniorrhexis. However, the sensitivity for abnormal BPP in the presence of chorioamnionitis appears to be no greater than 25 per cent [Ib].[17] The value of BPP in this context is thus limited; indeed, absence of fetal breathing movements may correlate more to the onset of labour with intrauterine infection than the infection itself.[5]

Placental grading

Placental grading according to senescent changes seen on ultrasound examination – the Grannum classification – has been demonstrated to reduce perinatal mortality in one RCT.[18] However, this study was small and needs repeating. This technique has been incorporated in the BPP to give an overall score out of 12 rather than 10.

Fetal biometry and Doppler ultrasonography

These are covered in Chapter 15.

SUMMARY

There is a distinct lack of reliable evidence on which to base protocols for assessing fetal well-being. It is likely that those protocols should incorporate some form of CTG, but this must not form the sole basis for the assessment of the fetus. Computerized CTG may well be more effective than standard CTG. Formal assessment of the BPP does not appear to hold any advantage over assessment of liquor volume alone. Where fetal growth restriction is suspected, fetal biometry and assessment of umbilical artery waveforms by Doppler ultrasonography should be incorporated.

- Systematic review of 20 trials has failed to demonstrate any beneficial effect of CTG alone on perinatal outcomes.
- Observational data from 12 studies and one small RCT have demonstrated that computerized CTG is more efficient than standard CTG.
- Systematic review of seven trials demonstrates that vibroacoustic stimulation may well reduce the number of false-positive NST CTGs.
- Although observational data based on 80 000 pregnancies show that formal BPP is effective in monitoring the 'at-risk' fetus, systematic review of four RCTs has failed to demonstrate any advantage over simple methods of fetal assessment.
- One RCT has demonstrated that simple monitoring by CTG and liquor assessment is associated with reduced levels of intervention, with similar perinatal outcome compared to BPP.
- Placental grading has been found to be associated with a reduction in perinatal mortality in one small RCT.
- Systematic review of 11 RCTs indicates that the use of umbilical artery Doppler waveform analysis is of benefit in monitoring high-risk pregnancies.

KEY REFERENCES

1. Nijhuis JG, Prechtl HF, Martin CB Jr, Bots RS. Are there behavioural states in the human fetus? *Early Hum Dev* 1982; **6**:177–95.
2. Patrick J, Campbell K, Carmichael L, Natale R, Richardson B. Patterns of human fetal breathing during the last 10 weeks of pregnancy. *Obstet Gynecol* 1980; **56**:24–30.
3. Patrick J, Campbell K, Carmichael L, Natale R, Richardson B. Patterns of gross fetal body movements over 24-hour observation intervals during the last 10 weeks of pregnancy. *Am J Obstet Gynecol* 1982; **142**:363–71.
4. Timor-Tritsch IE, Dierker LJ, Zador I, Hertz RH, Rosen MG. Fetal movements associated with fetal heart rate accelerations and decelerations. *Am J Obstet Gynecol* 1978; **131**:276–80.

5. Richardson B. Biophysical activity. In: Rodeck CH, Whittle MJ (eds). *Fetal Medicine: Basic Science and Clinical Practice*. London: Churchill Livingstone, 1999, 919–37.

6. Grant A, Elbourne D, Valentin L, Alexander S. Routine formal fetal movement counting and risk of antepartum late death in normally formed singletons. *Lancet* 1989; 2:345–9.

7. Devoe LD, Castillo RA, Sherline DM. The nonstress test as a diagnostic test: a critical reappraisal. *Am J Obstet Gynecol* 1985; 152:1047–53.

8. Pattison N, McCowan L. Cardiotocography for antepartum fetal assessment. *Cochrane Database Syst Rev* 2000; CD001068.

9. Tan KH, Smyth R. Fetal vibroacoustic stimulation for facilitation of tests of fetal wellbeing. *Cochrane Database Syst Rev* 2001; CD002963.

10. Dawes GS, Moulden M, Redman CW. Improvements in computerized fetal heart rate analysis antepartum. *J Perinat Med* 1996; 24:25–36.

11. Dawes GS, Moulden M, Redman CW. The advantages of computerized fetal heart rate analysis. *J Perinat Med* 1991; 19:39–45.

12. Dawes GS, Moulden M, Redman CW. Short-term fetal heart rate variation, decelerations, and umbilical flow velocity waveforms before labor. *Obstet Gynecol* 1992; 80:673–8.

13. Bracero LA, Morgan S, Byrne DW. Comparison of visual and computerized interpretation of nonstress test results in a randomized controlled trial. *Am J Obstet Gynecol* 1999; 181:1254–8.

14. Harman CR, Menticoglou S, Manning FA. Assessing fetal health. In: *High Risk Pregnancy*. London: Elsevier, 1998, 249–89.

15. Alfirevic Z, Neilson JP. Biophysical profile for fetal assessment in high risk pregnancies. *Cochrane Database Syst Rev* 2000; CD000038.

16. Alfirevic Z, Walkinshaw SA. A randomised controlled trial of simple compared with complex antenatal fetal monitoring after 42 weeks of gestation. *Br J Obstet Gynaecol* 1995; 102:638–43.

17. Lewis DF, Adair CD, Weeks JW, Barrilleaux PS, Edwards MS, Garite TJ. A randomized clinical trial of daily nonstress testing versus biophysical profile in the management of preterm premature rupture of membranes. *Am J Obstet Gynecol* 1999; 181:1495–9.

18. Proud J, Grant AM. Third trimester placental grading by ultrasound as a test of fetal wellbeing. *BMJ* 1987; 294:1641–4.

Chapter 15

Fetal Growth Restriction

Murray Luckas

MRCOG standards

Theoretical skills
- Understand the definition of fetal growth restriction and be able to distinguish it from small for gestational age.
- Know the causes of fetal growth restriction.

Practical skills
- Be able to interpret the ultrasound diagnosis of fetal growth restriction by ultrasound.
- Know how to investigate the cause of growth restriction, monitor progress and decide on timing and mode of delivery.

INTRODUCTION

One of the most challenging areas currently facing obstetricians is the detection and management of pregnancies in which the growth of the fetus is poor. There is little doubt that these fetuses experience not only increased rates of perinatal morbidity and mortality but also higher levels of morbidity extending into adult life.

As many as 40 per cent of so-called unexplained stillbirths are small for gestational age (SGA), leading to the suggestion that early detection and timely delivery may well prevent many fetal deaths. Some 30 per cent of sudden infant death syndrome (SIDS) cases were SGA at birth, and the overall infant mortality of infants suffering from fetal growth restriction (FGR) is as much as eight-fold greater than that for appropriately grown infants. These infants are also at high risk of perinatal hypoxia and acidaemia, operative delivery and neonatal encephalopathy. Other neonatal problems include hypoglycaemia, hypothermia, hypocalcaemia and polycythaemia. Paradoxically, these infants

have a slightly reduced incidence of respiratory distress syndrome, presumably because of the intrauterine stress resulting in increased surfactant production.

It is possible that babies who suffer with FGR are at increased risk of early cognitive and neurological impairment and cerebral palsy. Long-term data from the 1970 British Birth Cohort indicate that adults who were born SGA had significant differences in academic achievement and professional attainment compared with adults who were of normal birth weight. It would also appear that the uterine environment to which the fetus is exposed can lead to 'programming', resulting in consequences in adulthood – the so-called Barker hypothesis. SGA is associated with an increased risk of hypertension, glucose intolerance and atheromatous vascular disease in later life.[1]

DEFINITIONS

Traditionally, FGR has been synonymous with SGA based on fetal biometry or birth weight, the latter being one of the few unambiguous measurements made in obstetrics. Being SGA is merely a statistical observation, and the incidence of SGA infants will depend on which cut-off is used. The World Health Organization (WHO) suggests that the cut-off should be made at the tenth centile, thus labelling 10 per cent of all infants as SGA.

This approach would appear to be overly simplistic. Chard et al. argue that there is no evidence of a distinct subpopulation of low birth weight babies amongst the whole population of babies at term, and that the majority of SGA babies are in fact 'healthy but small'.[2] Instead, they suggest that the diagnosis of FGR should be reserved for infants that have failed to reach their genetic growth potential. This definition does not adequately categorize abnormalities such as Edward's syndrome (trisomy 18), which commonly have FGR as a feature of their genetic make-up. A better definition would be fetuses whose growth velocity slows down or stops completely because of inadequate oxygen and nutritional supply or utilization. It is this group of fetuses with FGR that is most at risk of the sequelae associated with poor growth.

It is self-evident that not all infants suffering from FGR will be SGA and that not all infants who are SGA will suffer from FGR. Indeed, as few as 15 per cent of SGA fetuses may be small as a result of FGR. Although FGR can afflict larger infants – indeed, theoretically, some 70 per cent of fetuses suffering from reduced growth velocity will have a birth weight considered appropriate for gestational age – it does not seem to affect neonatal outcomes unless the fetus is also small, with an abdominal circumference under the fifth centile.[3] It is therefore logical to concentrate on the SGA fetus that is suffering from FGR.

Thus, in summary, using the model espoused by Bobrow and Soothill,[3] SGA fetuses can be categorized according to aetiology into:

1 normal SGA: no structural anomalies, with normal liquor, normal umbilical artery Doppler waveforms (UADWs) and normal growth velocity;
2 abnormal SGA: those with structural or genetic abnormalities;
3 FGR: those with impaired placental function identified by abnormal UADWs and reduced growth velocity.

Biometrical measurement of the fetus allows a further categorization of SGA into *symmetrical* and *asymmetrical*. Where the fetus is symmetrically small, both the head and the abdomen are equally affected. This pattern is seen where the fetal insult occurs in early pregnancy, such as with fetal infection, or where the fetus is abnormal. Asymmetrical SGA is seen where the abdomen is small but the head is relatively spared. This pattern is typical of FGR, although it should be remembered that early-onset placental dysfunction can lead to symmetrical SGA.

AETIOLOGY

The determinants of fetal size are multifactorial. Maternal size is of greater importance in determining fetal size than paternal build. In addition, ethnic and socio-economic factors play a role, male fetuses being on average some 200 g heavier than their female counterparts at term. The aetiology of SGA can be divided up into maternal factors, fetal factors and, lastly, placental factors.

Maternal factors

Nutrition

Population studies such as those performed during the Dutch Hunger Winter in 1944 have demonstrated that significant effects were only seen at the extremes of starvation. Even then, the fetus is relatively protected during the first and second trimesters. Anorexic mothers have twice

the risk of having a SGA baby, with a similar level of risk being seen in women whose booking body mass index (BMI) is <19.

Smoking

There is extensive evidence implicating a link between maternal smoking and SGA, infants of women who smoke being some 460 g lighter than the offspring of non-smokers. Of concern is the observation that infants delivered by women exposed to passive smoking are 190 g lighter than babies born to women not exposed to tobacco smoke. The causal mechanism of this effect is not clear but is probably related to increased levels of fetal carboxyhaemoglobin.

Alcohol and drugs of abuse (see Chapter 6.12)

The infants of alcoholic women have a 12-fold increase in their risk of SGA. Consumption of more than 15 units (120 g) of alcohol has been associated with a small reduction (66 g) in birth weight, leading the Royal College of Obstetricians and Gynaecologists to recommend that pregnant women keep their alcohol consumption below this threshold [II]. It is unclear whether marijuana and cocaine are independent risk factors for SGA, but heroin does appear to cause a reduction in fetal size.

Maternal therapeutic drug administration

Maternal ingestion of beta-blockers in the second trimester has been linked to SGA infants, as have anticonvulsants, particularly the hydantoins such as phenytoin.

Maternal disease

Many severe maternal debilitating conditions can lead to a reduction in fetal growth. Severe cardiorespiratory compromise resulting in a failure of adaptation to pregnancy and maternal hypoxaemia can result in reduced fetal growth. Maternal conditions such as sickle cell disease, collagen vascular diseases and the antiphospholipid antibody syndrome, which result in reduced placental bed perfusion, can also result in reduced fetal growth. Meta-analysis shows that women with intrauterine growth restriction had a higher prevalence of heterozygous G20210A prothrombin gene mutation, homozygous MTHFR C677T gene mutation and protein S deficiency than controls [Ia].[4] Although maternal diabetes is usually associated with fetal overgrowth, where it is complicated by microvascular disease (retinopathy or nephropathy) it can result in poor placental bed perfusion. Lastly, maternal chronic hypertension, particularly if associated with renal impairment, is often associated with reduced fetal growth.

Fetal factors

Fetal abnormality

In the second trimester, 20 per cent of SGA fetuses have chromosomal abnormalities, although this rate falls to 1–2 per cent by mid third trimester.[5] Triploidy is the most common

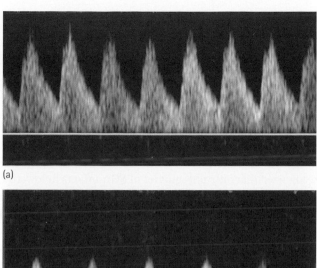

(a)

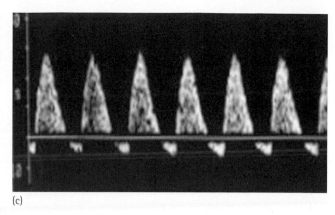

(c)

(b)

Figure 15.1   a Umbilical artery Doppler waveforms (UADW) with normal end diastolic flow **b**   Umbilical artery Doppler waveforms (UADW) with absent end diastolic flow **c**   Umbilical artery Doppler waveforms (UADW) with reversed end diastolic flow

finding under 26 weeks, trisomy 18 being the most common abnormality after this time. Growth restriction is not usually a feature of trisomy 21. Low birth weight is often a feature of non-chromosomal structural anomalies. Major cardiac defects can affect fetal blood flow to the placenta. Gastroschisis is commonly associated with FGR.

Infection

Reduced fetal growth is frequently seen in intrauterine fetal infection. Examples include varicella, cytomegalovirus, rubella, syphilis and toxoplasmosis. Worldwide, the malaria parasites are a common cause of SGA.

Placental factors

Placental mosaicism, often associated with chromosomes 16 and 22, is a frequent finding at chorionic villus sampling. This can be associated with reduced placental bulk and placental dysfunction, resulting in severe FGR.

The adequacy of blood supply to the placenta requires invasions and remodelling of the maternal spiral arteries by fetal extravillous trophoblast cells. The end result is destruction of the smooth muscle in the spiral arteries, converting them from high-resistance vessels to low-resistance circulation, thereby promoting an increase in maternal blood supply to the placental bed.

In pregnancies affected by pre-eclampsia and FGR, there is a failure in the second wave of trophoblast invasion,

resulting in reduced maternal blood supply to the placental bed (see Chapter 7.6). This does not appear to result in hypoxia in the intervillous spaces but in a reduction in oxygen transfer to the fetus.

On the fetal side of the placenta, this reduced oxygen transfer leads to high impedance of the fetal blood supply to the intervillous space. This may be due to obliteration or defective angiogenesis leading to a reduction in the tertiary villi. It is this high-resistance fetal circulation in the placenta which leads to reduced end-diastolic flow (EDF) velocities detected by UADW analysis (Figure 15.1).

PREDICTION

Accurate prediction of those pregnancies destined to be complicated by FGR would allow increased vigilance and fetal monitoring, which in theory would enable intervention to improve outcomes. Currently, such interventions are limited to avoiding certain risk factors, such as smoking, and timely delivery, thereby avoiding the worst sequelae of FGR.

History/examination

As outlined above, several risk factors can be identified at booking, such as a BMI <19 and maternal smoking, which place a pregnancy at high risk of FGR. In addition, a past

Antenatal complications: fetal

history of having an SGA baby increases the risk of recurrence in subsequent pregnancies. Congenital uterine anomalies have been associated with a reduction in fetal growth, as have large maternal fibroids. Babies born to older mothers are significantly smaller than the offspring of younger women, although this effect seems to be largely confined to nulliparous women over the age of 40.

Pregnancy-specific complications are also associated with FGR. Pre-eclampsia is perhaps the best known, and many of the placental abnormalities are common to both conditions. Retroplacental haemorrhage in the second and third trimesters can impair placental function sufficiently to reduce fetal growth.

Maternal serum screening

Several biochemical markers measured in the maternal serum in the second trimester are associated with reduced growth in latter pregnancy. These include alpha-fetoprotein (AFP) oestriol (E3), human placental lactogen (HPL) and human chorionic gonadotrophin (hCG). Of these, the most robust is AFP: if the level is 2.5 or more multiples of the median for gestation in the absence of fetal anomaly, there is a 5–10-fold increase in the risk of FGR.

Ultrasound markers

The best known ultrasonic predictor of subsequent FGR is abnormal uterine artery Doppler velocimetry; this reflects high impedance levels in the maternal arterial blood supply to the placental unit resulting from deficient trophoblast invasion of the maternal spiral arteries. The abnormalities are apparent as either reduced EDF or so-called notching of the waveform. Systematic review of 27 studies involving 12 994 women has shown that abnormal uterine artery Doppler flow velocity is associated with a roughly three-fold increase in the risk of FGR, although the diagnostic accuracy of the technique is limited [Ia].[6] It would appear that the combination of unexplained elevated maternal AFP and uterine artery Doppler velocimetry is a much more power predictor of adverse perinatal outcomes (particularly FGR).

Bright or echogenic fetal bowel in the second trimester is associated with an elevated risk of subsequent FGR. Again, a combination of elevated maternal serum AFP (MSAFP) and this ultrasonic marker provides a more precise estimate of the risk of FGR than either predictor alone.

Scoring systems

Several different scoring systems utilizing various risk factors for reduced fetal growth have been devised to better predict women at particular risk of having an FGR baby. All suffer from poor specificity and sensitivity and are therefore of limited clinical use.

Currently, the mainstay of detection of FGR remains the identification of high-risk groups for increased obstetric vigilance, which in most instances includes serial ultrasound examination of the fetus to measure size and growth velocity. Detection of FGR in low-risk women depends upon the identification of SGA fetuses by clinical assessment. Despite the best efforts of providers of obstetric care, it is recognized that only one-quarter of SGA infants in low-risk pregnancies will be recognized in the antenatal period.

Clinical assessment

Although maternal weight gain in pregnancy has been traditionally recorded, its effectiveness in detecting FGR has never been tested by randomized studies, and observational data give little evidence that it is of benefit. Palpation of the gravid uterus is the standard technique of clinically assessing fetal size; however, it should be remembered that parous women have proven to be more accurate in the estimate of the size of their fetuses than either care providers or one-off fetal measurement by ultrasound. Fundal height measurement (FHM) was introduced as a more objective assessment of the size of the fetus. However, both palpation and FHM to assess the size of the fetus are subject to various factors that reduce their accuracy, such as maternal shape, fetal lie and liquor. A systematic review has recently concluded that FHM measurement held no particular advantage over palpation alone.[7] Interestingly, Gardosi and Francis[8] have demonstrated in a controlled trial that a policy of serial FHM using a standard technique with plotting on customized antenatal growth charts (adjusted for variables such as maternal height, weight and ethnic group) significantly increased the detection rate of SGA babies, as compared to standard clinical assessment (48 per cent vs 29 per cent). Although more work is needed, this technique holds promise for increasing the detection rate of SGA babies in low-risk women.

Ultrasound assessment

Ultrasound examination of the fetus allows biometric measurements; the fetal abdominal circumference is the most accurate predictor of the fetal weight. An estimate of the fetal weight can be made using this measurement, the head circumference, biparietal diameter and the femur length. All these measurements can be plotted on centile charts and should allow the identification of the SGA infant. In addition, comparison of the head and abdominal circumferences will indicate whether the small fetus is symmetrically or asymmetrically small. However, a single set of measurements will not differentiate the normal SGA fetus from the SGA fetus suffering from FGR;[3] this requires serial measurements over time.

Despite the theoretical advantages of screening for FGR by ultrasound, systematic review of seven trials involving some 25 000 low-risk women, comparing a policy of routine ultrasound examination after 24 weeks' gestation with scanning based on standard clinical indications, found no advantage of routine ultrasound examination. Routine scanning did not increase the pick-up rate of SGA babies, nor did it significantly affect the perinatal mortality rate [Ia].[9]

The most effective way of detecting FGR would appear to be by measuring fetal growth over time with serial ultrasound examinations. Serial growth scans are indicated in the woman who is identified as high risk for FGR and/or whose baby is SGA. Although this policy has been universally adopted, it has not been shown to be of benefit in clinical trials [IV]. This method of screening for FGR has a high false-positive rate. Mongelli and Gardosi have demonstrated that the use of customized fetal growth charts (again adjusted for variables such as weight of previous children, maternal height, weight and ethnic group) may reduce this.[10] A 4-week measurement interval was shown to be superior to a 2-week interval, in terms of reducing the false-positive rate.[11] Fortnightly scans should be undertaken where linear growth velocity is not maintained or where the abdominal circumference is below the third centile [IV].

The main problem with this approach of serial fetal measurement is one of practicality: clinical imperatives may demand that a diagnosis of FGR is made within a matter of days rather than weeks. Additional indicators of fetal condition may be given by liquor volume, Doppler analysis of the umbilical artery waveform, a careful history of the maternal perception of movements and cardiotocography (CTG).

Liquor volume

Reduced liquor volumes are a common finding in association with FGR. Progressive fetal hypoxaemia results in blood flow redistribution, with blood being preferentially directed to the brain, with resultant diminished renal perfusion and fetal urine output. The degree of reduction in liquor volume appears to correlate well with the degree of fetal hypoxaemia as reflected by fetal blood PO_2 measured at cordocentesis.

Umbilical artery Doppler studies

Doppler assessment of the umbilical artery waveform demonstrates that, in normal pregnancy, there is forward flow from the fetus to the placenta throughout the cardiac cycle. In the placentae of fetuses suffering from FGR, there is increased vascular resistance, which leads to reduced flow in the diastolic component of the fetal cardiac cycle in the umbilical artery. This reduced flow, together with absent end-diastolic flow (AEDF) or, at the most extreme, reversed end-diastolic flow (REDF), reflects progressive degrees of placental pathology. The degree of abnormality in the UADW correlates well with the risk of fetal hypoxia. In high-risk pregnancies with AEDF, 80 per cent of fetuses will be hypoxic and 46 per cent acidaemic, with the relative risk of perinatal mortality rate being 1.0 where EDF is present, 4.0 with AEDF and 10.6 with REDF.[12]

In a systematic review of 11 randomized, controlled trials conducted in high-risk pregnancies, particularly those complicated by FGR, Neilson and Alfirevic concluded that the use of UADW analysis significantly improved several pregnancy outcomes, including fewer inductions of labour and hospital admissions.[13] In addition, it was associated with a strong trend towards reducing perinatal mortality (odds ratio 0.71, 95 per cent CI 0.5–1.01). It would thus appear that UADW studies are a valuable tool in the assessment of the SGA infant [Ia]. In contrast, the use of UADW studies in low-risk pregnancies seems to hold no advantage [Ia].[14]

Bobrow and Soothill proposed that UADW studies were pivotal in the assessment of the SGA fetus, and allowed the separation of the normal SGA from FGR.[3] Recently, this approach has been challenged by an observational study which concluded that abnormal umbilical artery Doppler studies reflect earlier onset and more severe FGR; however, 'normal' SGA fetuses still had high levels of malnutrition at birth and were not all just normal small babies.[15] Therefore vigilance is still important for SGA fetuses with normal UADW studies.

Thus, in summary, once a SGA fetus is detected, it is important to consider the causation. A careful history must be obtained from the mother and detailed fetal anatomical assessment, exclusion of fetal infection and karyotyping should be considered. The distinction between normal SGA and FGR can only be made by observing the fetal growth velocity over time. Markers such as reduced liquor volume and UADW assessment can aid the distinction.

MANAGEMENT

Prophylaxis and treatment

Several prophylactic and therapeutic interventions have been evaluated, perhaps the best known of which is low-dose aspirin administration. Despite promise from early trials, the Collaborative Low-dose Aspirin Study in Pregnancy (CLASP) trial concluded that the prophylactic or therapeutic administration of low-dose aspirin was of no benefit in women deemed as high risk [Ib].[16] Since then, interventional studies with aspirin have focused on women deemed at high risk not on the basis of history alone but by abnormal maternal uterine artery waveforms. Analysis of these studies indicates that this approach is not justified.[17] The only measures which do seem to be of benefit are smoking cessation, anti-malarial treatment (in high-risk areas) and protein/energy supplementation in poorly nourished women [Ia].[18] Maternal nutrient supplementation in an attempt to increase fetal weight gain in established cases of FGR may well increase adverse outcomes.

Monitoring the normal SGA fetus

For the normal SGA fetus, conservative management by fetal surveillance is appropriate. Intervention by delivery is only appropriate if there is evidence of fetal compromise. Umbilical artery Doppler waveform analysis has proved superior to biophysical profile score and computerized CTG analysis in predicting perinatal morbidity in this group,[19] and its inclusion in monitoring policies for these pregnancies is warranted [Ia].[13]

It must be remembered that AEDF or REDF is unusual in the late third trimester, because the size of the placenta at this stage of pregnancy protects against changes in placental resistance. Fetal compromise is thus possible at this late stage in pregnancy with a normal UADW.

The most important aspect of the biophysical profile would appear to be liquor assessment, and it should also be monitored closely (see Chapter 14). A reduction in the growth velocity of the abdominal circumference often mirrors UADW abnormalities, and continued monitoring of the growth velocity of these fetuses should be performed to detect superimposed FGR [IV].

The optimal frequency for fetal assessment in normal SGA is unclear; however, a recent pilot randomized, controlled trial found twice-weekly surveillance held no advantage when compared to fortnightly review.[20] In the absence of other signs of fetal compromise, it is thus appropriate to monitor normal SGA fetuses on a fortnightly basis [Ib]. The fetal assessment should include biometry, UADW analysis and liquor assessment. Although computerized CTG assessment is superior to conventional CTG assessment, the role of CTGs in the assessment of normal SGA is unclear.

Monitoring the growth-restricted fetus

Once growth restriction is diagnosed, management options are limited to timely delivery, balancing the risks of continuing with the pregnancy against the risks of prematurity. This policy is based on the assumption that timely delivery will improve the outcome; however, this has never been tested (nor is it ever likely to be) by an interventional trial. The Growth Restriction Intervention Trial (GRIT) randomized women to delivery or conservative management where the

clinician was uncertain. This trial found no significant difference between immediate delivery and delayed delivery.[21]

If a diagnosis of FGR in a SGA fetus (on the basis of reduced growth velocity, severely reduced liquor volume or abnormal uterine artery waveform) is made after 34 weeks' gestation, delivery is indicated [IV].

Under 34 weeks' gestation, steroids should be administered prior to delivery if possible; there is no clear evidence to guide management. Between 28 and 34 weeks' gestation, the presence of REDF should prompt delivery [IV]. The management of AEDF under 34 weeks' gestation and indeed REDF under 28 weeks' gestation is more controversial.

It is apparent that the interval between the loss of EDF and fetal demise may vary from days to weeks and that the onset of CTG abnormalities is very late in the process – at which stage fetal damage may well be irreversible. Thus, particularly at the extremes of viability, much interest has been paid to methods of fetal surveillance that would allow pregnancy to be prolonged in cases of FGR with AEDF. In these fetuses, so-called brain sparing can be detected by changes in Doppler waveform indices of the middle cerebral artery (MCA), which represent increased flow. Long-term follow-up of fetuses demonstrating increased MCA flow indicate that it is a benign adaptive mechanism. Although this increase in cerebral blood flow occurs sequentially after reduced growth velocity and loss of umbilical artery EDF, reversal of this adaptation is sudden and is associated with a poor prognosis. Thus serial assessment of the MCA waveform does not give suitable forewarning of deterioration for it to be used in monitoring fetuses with AEDF. Many other arterial waveforms, including those from the fetal aorta and renal arteries, have been assessed, although none seems to be able to predict decompensation in FGR with AEDF. One area of interest is the examination of fetal venous systems. Increased pulsatility in the umbilical veins and vena cava and reversed flow during atrial contraction in the ductus venous do seem to give adequate warning of fetal decompensation, with the latter being particularly promising.

The management of pregnancies complicated by FGR and AEDF in the umbilical artery should be in units capable of providing intensive neonatal care and should be provided by clinicians with a special interest in fetal medicine [IV].

Labour and delivery

Growth-restricted fetuses are at high risk of intrapartum hypoxia and acidaemia. At gestations under 37 weeks, delivery by caesarean section is usually the best option [IV]. It would appear that fetuses with normal UADW tolerate labour well, making induction of labour a possibility at more advanced gestations. It is imperative that adequate plans are made for the management of labour, and these must be clearly documented in the notes. Continual electronic fetal monitoring with early recourse to fetal scalp sampling is strongly advisable. Because of the risk of uterine hypertonicity, prostaglandins and oxytocin must be used with great care [IV].

SUMMARY

The prediction and detection of SGA must be a priority of obstetric care. However, the SGA fetus is not necessarily sick, and efforts should be made to discover why the fetus is small. If FGR is detected, close monitoring and early intervention for suspected fetal compromise are warranted. If the fetus is normal SGA, providing adequate fetal surveillance is undertaken, a conservative approach is appropriate.

- Observational data indicate that only one-quarter of SGA fetuses are detected antenatally.
- One controlled trial has demonstrated that the detection rate is increased using systematic FHM and customized charts.
- Systematic review of seven RCTs shows no benefit of the routine use of ultrasound in late pregnancy in detecting FGR.
- Systematic review of 11 RCTs indicates that the use of UADW analysis is of benefit.
- Observational data support the use of liquor volume assessment in FGR. There is no clear evidence that formal biophysical profiling is warranted.
- Limited evidence is available to demonstrate an improvement in outcome with timely compared to conservative management for FGR.
- Expert opinion advocates delivery for FGR where the fetus is viable and shows signs of significant compromise.
- One observational study concluded that caesarean section is advisable in the presence of significant abnormalities of the UADW.

KEY REFERENCES

1. Barker DJ. The long-term outcome of retarded fetal growth. *Clin Obstet Gynecol* 1997; **40**:853–63.
2. Chard T, Yoong A, Macintosh M. The myth of fetal growth retardation at term. *Br J Obstet Gynaecol* 1993; **100**:1076–81.
3. Bobrow CS, Soothill PW. Fetal growth velocity: a cautionary tale. *Lancet* 1999; **353**:1460.
4. Alfirevic Z, Roberts D, Martlew V. How strong is the association between maternal thrombophilia and adverse pregnancy outcome? A systematic review. *Eur J Obstet Gynecol Reprod Biol* 2002; **101**:6–14.
5. Snijders RJ, Sherrod C, Gosden CM, Nicolaides KH. Fetal growth retardation: associated malformations and chromosomal abnormalities. *Am J Obstet Gynecol* 1993; **168**:547–55.
6. Chien PF, Arnott N, Gordon A, Owen P, Khan KS. How useful is uterine artery Doppler flow velocimetry in the prediction of pre-eclampsia, intrauterine growth retardation and perinatal death? An overview. *Br J Obstet Gynaecol* 2000; **107**:196–208.
7. Neilson JP. Symphysis–fundal height measurement in pregnancy. *Cochrane Database Syst Rev* 2000; CD000944.
8. Gardosi J, Francis A. Controlled trial of fundal height measurement plotted on customised antenatal growth charts. *Br J Obstet Gynaecol* 1999; **106**:309–17.
9. Bricker L, Neilson JP. Routine ultrasound in late pregnancy (after 24 weeks gestation). *Cochrane Database Syst Rev* 2000; CD001451.
10. Mongelli M, Gardosi J. Reduction of false-positive diagnosis of fetal growth restriction by application of customised fetal growth standards. *Obstet Gynecol* 1996; **88**:844–8.
11. Owen P, Maharaj S, Khan KS, Howie PW. Interval between fetal measurements in predicting growth restriction. *Obstet Gynecol* 2001; **97**:499–504.
12. Karsdorp VH, van Vugt JM, van Geijn HP et al. Clinical significance of absent or reversed end diastolic velocity waveforms in umbilical artery. *Lancet* 1994; **344**:1664–8.
13. Neilson JP, Alfirevic Z. Doppler ultrasound for fetal assessment in high risk pregnancies. *Cochrane Database Syst Rev* 2000; CD000073.
14. Bricker L, Neilson JP. Routine Doppler ultrasound in pregnancy. *Cochrane Database Syst Rev* 2000; CD001450.
15. McCowan LM, Harding JE, Stewart AW. Umbilical artery Doppler studies in small for gestational age babies reflect disease severity. *Br J Obstet Gynaecol* 2000; **107**:916–25.
16. CLASP: a randomised trial of low-dose aspirin for the prevention and treatment of pre-eclampsia among 9364 pregnant women. CLASP (Collaborative Low-dose Aspirin Study in Pregnancy) Collaborative Group [see Comments]. *Lancet* 1994; **343**:619–29.
17. Goffinet F, Aboulker D, Paris-Llado J et al. Screening with a uterine Doppler in low risk pregnant women followed by low dose aspirin in women with abnormal results: a multicentre randomised controlled trial. *Br J Obstet Gynaecol* 2001; **108**:510–18.
18. Gulmezoglu M, de Onis M, Villar J. Effectiveness of interventions to prevent or treat impaired fetal growth. *Obstet Gynecol Surv* 1997; **52**:139–49.

Antenatal complications: fetal

19. Soothill PW, Ajayi RA, Campbell S, Nicolaides KH. Prediction of morbidity in small and normally grown fetuses by fetal heart rate variability, biophysical profile score and umbilical artery Doppler studies. *Br J Obstet Gynaecol* 1993; **100**:742–5.

20. McCowan LM, Harding JE, Roberts AB, Barker SE, Ford C, Stewart AW. A pilot randomized controlled trial of two regimens of fetal surveillance for small-for-gestational-age fetuses with normal results of umbilical artery Doppler velocimetry. *Am J Obstet Gynecol* 2000; **182**:81–6.

21. GRIT Study Group. A randomised trial of timed delivery for the compromised preterm fetus: short term outcomes and Bayesian interpretation. *BJOG* 2003; **110**(1):27–32.

Chapter 16

Aberrant Liquor Volume

Sailesh Kumar

INTRODUCTION

Amniotic fluid surrounds the fetus in intrauterine life, providing protected, low-resistance space suitable for growth and development. The total amniotic fluid volume (AFV) arises from secondary partitioning of body water within the fetoplacental extracellular space and reflects fetal fluid balance, which is in a homeostatic state of constant flux. In the first trimester, contributions from the fetal renal system or respiratory tract are minimal in the generation of amniotic fluid. The most likely mechanism is the active transport of electrolytes such as sodium and chloride by the fetal membrane into the amniotic sac, with water passively accompanying the solute flow.

After approximately 20 weeks, when the fetal skin keratinizes, there are several potential mechanisms that allow fluid to either enter or leave the amniotic space. The excretion of fetal urine and swallowing of amniotic fluid by the fetus represent one of the main pathways for the formation and clearance of amniotic fluid. The fetal lungs also contribute significantly to amniotic fluid by secreting large volumes of fluid every day. Other potential mechanisms include fluid transfer across the placenta and secretions from the fetal oro-nasal cavities.

Clinical assessment of AFV is unreliable, and objective definitions of abnormalities in AVF depend essentially on non-invasive methods such as ultrasound. These include the deepest vertical pool (DVP) or the amniotic fluid index (AFI), which is the total of the DVPs in each of the four quadrants and a more sensitive indicator of AFV throughout gestation.[1,2] In general terms, the DVP is easier to perform and has been demonstrated to be a sensitive ultrasound measure of fetal well-being.[3,4] There is some evidence that AFI is a more sensitive measure of fetal well-being [II].

OLIGOHYDRAMNIOS

Oligohydramnios defined by a DVP <2 cm complicates approximately 3.9 per cent of pregnancies.[3] When oligohydramnios occurs later in pregnancy, the perinatal outcome is poor, with perinatal mortality rates approaching 90 per cent.[4-6] This increased perinatal mortality is mainly related to the underlying aetiology and gestation from which oligohydramnios occurs. The common causes of oligohydramnios are shown in Table 16.1.

Perhaps the most common cause of oligohydramnios is preterm premature rupture of membranes (PPROM), which occurs in approximately 3–17 per cent of all pregnancies. Although clinical evidence for membrane rupture is obvious in the majority of cases, ultrasonic evidence of decreased liquor is present in only 5–44 per cent.[7,8]

Oligohydramnios may be associated with intrauterine growth restriction, when it is often associated with a fetal abdominal circumference (AC) measurement (using ultrasound) below the 10th centile for gestation, poor fetal growth velocity (ΔAC of >1 S.D. over 14 days) and abnormal umbilical artery waveform velocimetry. Such findings are

Table 16.1 Causes of oligohydramnios

Preterm premature rupture of membranes
Placental insufficiency (intrauterine growth restriction)
Congenital fetal anomalies
Renal agenesis
Urethral obstruction (atresia or posterior urethral valves)
Renal dysplasia

associated with increased perinatal risk, as is oligohydramnios in isolation.[9] In cases of early-onset intrauterine growth restriction (<24 weeks), there is a strong association with abnormal maternal uterine artery Doppler waveforms (indicating malplacentation), but if these waveform velocities are normal, the association with aneuploidy and structural anomalies is as high as 25 per cent.

Renal anomalies account for up to 57 per cent[10] of cases, with severe oligohydramnios presenting in the mid-second trimester of pregnancy. Such anomalies are severe and include bilateral renal agenesis, multicystic or dysplastic kidneys or bladder outlet obstruction, resulting in impaired urine production that is primary or secondary to urinary tract obstruction.

Fetal and maternal risks

The main fetal risks relate primarily to pulmonary hypoplasia, chorioamnionitis subsequent to PPROM, and prematurity. Perinatal mortality is increased largely due to prematurity and the association with congenital malformations. Approximately 7 per cent of pregnancies complicated by oligohydramnios are associated with congenital malformations. This incidence rises to almost 35 per cent when amniorrhexis occurs in the second trimester.[10,11] The sequelae of oligohydramnios, flattened facies, postural deformities and pulmonary hypoplasia, are referred to as the Potter syndrome, first reported in association with bilateral renal agenesis. The main risk associated with severe oligohydramnios is pulmonary hypoplasia, which depends critically on the gestation at which it occurs and, to a slightly lesser extent, on its duration and severity. At gestations less than 22 weeks, the perinatal mortality is extremely high. The true incidence of pulmonary hypoplasia is probably underestimated at between 9 and 11/10 000 live births. PPROM before 25 weeks where the DVP is <1 cm has a predicted mortality rate of more than 90 per cent.[12,13]

There are very few maternal risks, unless fetal therapy is considered (i.e. the placement of an vesicoamniotic shunt or amniodrainage). These procedures carry the risk of abruptio placentae and chorioamnionitis.

Management

The main management objective is to confirm the aetiology of the oligohydramnios and therefore to define prognosis. PPROM is often apparent from the history and clinical examination (the diagnosis and management of PPROM are discussed in Chapter 22). The earlier the amniorrhexis occurs, the higher the incidence of subsequent pulmonary hypoplasia [II].[12]

In general terms, there is a strong association with severe oligohydramnios/anhydramnios and perinatal mortality associated with pulmonary hypoplasia [II]. Small series of treatment with amnioinfusion have been attempted in the past,

but with no reduction in perinatal mortality [III]. Consequently, severe oligohydramnios prior to 24 weeks carries a poor prognosis.[12]

Clinical examination may reveal the presence of chronic hypertension or pre-eclampsia and/or a symphysiofundal height that is small for gestation. Subsequent ultrasound biometry may reveal intrauterine growth restriction[9] or the presence of structural anomalies. A combination of biophysical studies and Doppler waveform analyses (of both uterine and umbilical circulations) may be used to assess fetal well-being and as indirect measures of placental function [Ia].[14]

The exclusion of congenital anomalies in combination with aneuploidy or isolated is mandatory. Renal agenesis may be difficult to confirm because of the large size of the fetal adrenal glands. However, the inability to visualize a fetal bladder on serial ultrasound examinations and bilateral absence of renal arteries using colour/power Doppler increase the sensitivity of this diagnosis. In cases of urinary outflow tract obstruction, vesicoamniotic shunting in selected cases may significantly increase fetal survival [Ia].[15]

- The aetiology of oligohydramnios has a large impact on subsequent perinatal mortality [II]. This group is heterogenous in terms of fetal survival.
- There is a strong association between early-onset oligohydramnios and perinatal mortality, because of an association with preterm labour in amniorrhexis and developmental pulmonary hypoplasia [II].

POLYHYDRAMNIOS

Polyhydramnios is usually defined as a DVP ≥ 8 cm or an AFI above the 95th centile for the gestational age. It complicates between 1 per cent and 3.5 per cent of all pregnancies,[4,16,17] and has been shown to be an independent risk factor for perinatal mortality and intrapartum complications among preterm births.[17] In general, polyhydramnios may be caused by increased production of urine from the renal system or by impaired swallowing and intestinal reabsorption of amniotic fluid. The mechanism of polyhydramnios in maternal diabetes mellitus is thought to be secondary to osmotic diuresis in the fetus. However, a large proportion of cases are idiopathic as no obvious cause can be ascertained. The common causes of polyhydramnios are summarized in Table 16.2.

Fetal and maternal risks

Maternal complications of polyhydramnios mainly relate to distension of the uterus and include preterm labour,

Table 16.2   Causes of polyhydramnios

Idiopathic
Diabetes mellitus
Intestinal obstruction (oesophageal or duodenal atresia)
Impaired fetal swallowing (anencephaly, aneuploidy, muscular dystrophy)
Fetal polyuria (twin–twin transfusion syndrome, Barter syndrome)
Cardiac failure secondary to significantly lowered fetal vascular resistance (i.e. sacrococcygeal teratoma, vein of Galen aneurysm) or fetal anaemia (i.e. maternal alloimmunization or parvovirus B19 infection)
Fetal infections

abdominal discomfort and uterine atony postpartum. Unstable lie, placental abruption and an increased incidence of caesarean section also result from severe polyhydramnios.

Perinatal mortality in cases of polyhydramnios is increased 10–30 per cent[14,18] and is secondary to the presence of congenital malformations and preterm delivery.

Management

It is important to evaluate each case thoroughly in a systematic manner. A careful history, with attention to maternal symptoms, diseases such as diabetes mellitus or red cell alloimmunization or recent viral infections, is important.

High-resolution ultrasound should be performed to assess the degree of polyhydramnios, identify multiple pregnancies, and target assessment of fetal anomalies. Fetal assessment should include examination of the fetal thorax, central nervous system and gastrointestinal and renal systems. Karyotyping should be offered, particularly in association with structural anomalies. If a viral infection is suspected, appropriate fetal and maternal samples should be obtained (see Chapters 7.4 and 13). If the excess liquor is associated with anaemia, the fetus is almost always hydropic. Correction of the underlying condition with serial in-utero fetal transfusions frequently results in amelioration of the polyhydramnios [II].

A major management aim is to reduce maternal discomfort and prolong the pregnancy. Treatment is only indicated when there is severe polyhydramnios (AFI ≥ 40 cm; DVP ≥ 12 cm), as this is associated with increases in intra-amniotic pressure [II].[19]

Treatment options include pharmacological management with cyclo-oxygenase inhibitors (i.e. indomethacin and sulindac). Prostaglandin synthase inhibitors and, more recently, selective cyclo-oxygenase-2 (COX-2) inhibitors may also be used to decrease fetal urine output and hence reduce the polyhydramnios. Prostaglandin synthase inhibitors such as indomethacin are associated with renal failure in neonates and premature closure of the ductus arteriosus, resulting in perinatal mortality [IV]. There are also reports of necrotizing enterocolitis and intracranial haemorrhage in infants treated with indomethacin in utero [IV]. Serial amnioreduction in singleton pregnancies has been advocated but carries the risk of precipitating preterm labour and leads to rapid re-accumulation of liquor.

Polyhydramnios associated with twin–twin transfusion syndrome (stage II or above) is often treated with serial amnioreduction. Alternatively, disruption of the communicating placental vessels with laser therapy may correct the haemodynamic imbalances causing the disease and result in resolution of the polyhydramnios (see Chapter 12).

- Polyhydramnios is associated with increased perinatal morbidity and mortality [II].
- A careful search for the underlying cause is mandatory.
- In cases in which no secondary cause is identifiable, the gestational age of delivery may be prolonged by the use of cyclo-oxygenase inhibitors [III]. However, this form of pharmacotherapy is not without risk.

KEY REFERENCES

1. Moore TR, Cayle JE. The amniotic fluid index in normal human pregnancy. *Am J Obstet Gynecol* 1990; **162**(5):1168–73.
2. Moore TR. Superiority of the four-quadrant sum over the single-deepest-pocket technique in ultrasonographic identification of abnormal amniotic fluid volumes. *Am J Obstet Gynecol* 1990; **163**(3):762–7.
3. Philipson EH, Sokol RJ, Williams T. Oligohydramnios: clinical associations and predictive value for intrauterine growth retardation. *Am J Obstet Gynecol* 1983; **146**(3):271–8.
4. Chamberlain PF, Manning FA, Morrison I, Harman CR, Lange IR. Ultrasound evaluation of amniotic fluid volume. II. The relationship of increased amniotic fluid volume to perinatal outcome. *Am J Obstet Gynecol* 1984; **150**(3):250–4.
5. Barss VA, Benacerraf BR, Frigoletto FD Jr. Second trimester oligohydramnios, a predictor of poor fetal outcome. *Obstet Gynecol* 1984; **64**(5):608–10.
6. Mercer LJ, Brown LG. Fetal outcome with oligohydramnios in the second trimester. *Obstet Gynecol* 1986; **67**(6):840–2.
7. Gonik B, Bottoms SF, Cotton DB. Amniotic fluid volume as a risk factor in preterm premature rupture of the membranes. *Obstet Gynecol* 1985; **65**(4):456–9.
8. Robson MS, Turner MJ, Stronge JM, O'Herlihy C. Is amniotic fluid quantitation of value in the diagnosis and conservative management of prelabour membrane rupture at term? *Br J Obstet Gynaecol* 1990; **97**(4):324–8.
9. Chang TC, Robson SC, Boys RJ, Spencer JA. Prediction of the small for gestational age infant: which ultrasonic measurement is best? *Obstet Gynecol* 1992; **80**:1030–8.

10. Moore TR, Longo J, Leopold GR, Casola G, Gosink BB. The reliability and predictive value of an amniotic fluid scoring system in severe second-trimester oligo-hydramnios. *Obstet Gynecol* 1989; **73**(5 Pt 1):739–42.

11. Mercer LJ, Brown LG, Petres RE, Messer RH. A survey of pregnancies complicated by decreased amniotic fluid. *Am J Obstet Gynecol* 1984; **149**(3):355–61.

12. Kilbride HW, Yeast J, Thibeault DW. Defining limits of survival: lethal pulmonary hypoplasia after midtrimester premature rupture of membranes. *Am J Obstet Gynecol* 1996; **175**(3 Pt 1):675–81.

13. Kilbride HW, Thibeault DW. Neonatal complications of preterm premature rupture of membranes. Pathophysiology and management. *Clin Perinatol* 2001; **28**(4):761–85.

14. Alfirevic Z, Neilson JP. Doppler ultrasonography in high-risk pregnancies: systematic review with meta-analysis. *Am J Obstet Gynecol* 1995; **172**:1379–87.

15. Clark TJ, Martin WL, Divakaran TG, Whittle MJ, Kilby MD, Khan KS. Prenatal bladder drainage in the management of the fetal lower urinary tract obstruction: a systematic review and meta-analysis. *Obstet Gynecol* 2003.

16. Hill LM, Breckle R, Thomas ML, Fries JK. Polyhydramnios: ultrasonically detected prevalence and neonatal outcome. *Obstet Gynecol* 1987; **69**(1):21–5.

17. Mazor M, Ghezzi F, Maymon E et al. Polyhydramnios is an independent risk factor for perinatal mortality and intrapartum morbidity in preterm delivery. *Eur J Obstet Gynecol Reprod Biol* 1996; **70**(1):41–7.

18. Carlson DE, Platt LD, Medearis AL, Horenstein J. Quantifiable polyhydramnios: diagnosis and management. *Obstet Gynecol* 1990; **75**(6):989–93.

19. Fisk NM, Tannirandorn Y, Nicolini U, Talbert DG, Rodeck CH. Amniotic pressure in disorders of amniotic fluid volume. *Obstet Gynecol* 1990; **76**(2):210–14.

Chapter 17

Fetal Hydrops

Sailesh Kumar

MRCOG standards

- Know the pathophysiology of fetal hydrops.
- Understand the various causes of fetal hydrops (particularly non-immune hydrops).
- Appreciate the non-Rh causes of immune fetal hydrops.
- Know the relevant maternal and fetal investigations.

INTRODUCTION

Hydrops is defined as the accumulation of fluid in the interstitial tissue (skin) and two serous cavities.[1,2] It is further subdivided into 'immune' (IH) or 'non-immune' (NIH), a distinction made on the presence of maternal alloimmunization (i.e. blood group incompatibility). Table 17.1 indicates the distribution of aetiologies of hydrops fetalis in a contemporary published series. In general terms, it carries a high perinatal mortality (in some series up to 80 per cent) but the variability of outcome is reflected in its many possible underlying aetiologies.[1,2]

INCIDENCE

Historically, Rhesus (Rh) alloimmunization accounted for the majority of cases of fetal hydrops. However, with the advent of large-scale antenatal anti-D prophylaxis, NIH now represents the major challenge facing obstetricians and most contemporaneous studies indicate that NIH is more common.[1,2] The true incidence of NIH is population variable and probably also subject to seasonal variation. For example, homozygous alpha-thalassaemia is the commonest cause of

Table 17.1 Number of cases of hydrops by aetiology ($n = 63$)[2]

Aetiology	Number	Percentage
A – Immune hydrops	**8/63**	**12.7**
Anti-D antibodies[a]	5/8	62.5
Anti-Kell antibodies	2/8	25
Anti-c	1/8	12.5
B – Non-immune hydrops	**55/63**	**87.3**
HPVB19	8/55	14.5
Thoracic/pulmonary causes	6/55	10.9
Chylothorax	4/6	66.7
Cystic adenomatoid malformation	1/6	16.7
Diaphragmatic hernia	1/6	16.7
Chromosomal abnormality	14/55	25.5
Trisomy 21	6/14	42.9
Trisomy 13	1/14	7.1
Turner's syndrome	5/14	35.7
Others[b]	2/14	14.2
Feto-maternal haemorrhage	1/55	1.8
Cardiac causes	5/55	9.1
SVT	3/5	60
CCHB	1/5	20
Congenital heart defects	1/5	20
Cystic hygroma	6/55	10.9
Fetal akinesia	1/55	1.8
Congenital myotonic dystrophy	1/55	1.8
TTTs	2/55	3.6
Idiopathic	8/55	14.5
Unclassified	3/55	5.5

[a]Anti-C antibodies were found in the maternal serum of four patients, and anti-E + Fya antibodies in the fifth.

[b]The karyotypes were 46XY add10,q24 (de novo) and 46XX, t(1;4) (q42;q32) (de novo).

HPVB19, human parvovirus B19; SVT, supraventricular tachycardia; CCHB, complete congenital heart block; TTTs, twin-to-twin transfusion syndrome.

Reproduced from reference 2 with permission from Parthenon Publishing.

fetal hydrops in South East Asia and arguably the leading cause of NIH worldwide. However, this is an uncommon cause of the condition in the UK, aneuploidy, structural anomalies and human parvovirus being more commonly noted associations.[2,3]

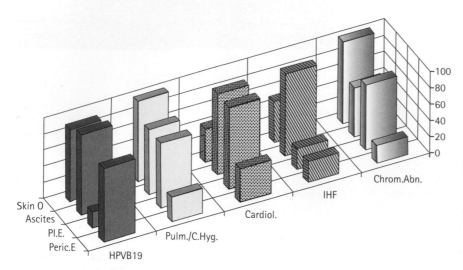

Figure 17.1   The alterations in fluid distribution by body cavity for different aetiologies.[2] Cardiol., cardiac anomaly; Chrom. Abn., chromosomal abnormalities; HPVB 19, human parvovirus B19; IHF, immune hydrops fetalis; Peric. E., pericardial effusion; Pl. E., pleural effusions; Palm./C. Hyg., pulmonary anomaly and cystic hygoma; Skin O., skin oedema. Reproduced from reference 2 with permission from Parthenon Publishing.

DIAGNOSIS

The diagnosis of fetal hydrops is made most commonly on ultrasound examination of the fetus, although it can be made pathologically. The condition is characterized by skin oedema and serous effusion in two or more body cavities (pleural or pericardial effusions and ascites).[3] There is some evidence that the distribution of serous effusion relates to the underlying aetiologies (Figure 17.1) [III]. The umbilical cord and placenta are frequently affected and are often oedematous. Polyhydramnios is also a common association (see Chapter 16).

PATHOPHYSIOLOGY OF FETAL HYDROPS

The exact pathophysiological process is not defined, but the microvascular fluid exchange system is defined by Starling's law controlling intravascular–interstitial fluid exchange. This is believed to be associated with changes in the movement of fluid across transmembranous pathways associated with a combination of reduced lymphatic drainage, raised intravascular hydrostatic pressure, decreased intravascular oncotic pressure or raised interstitial oncotic pressure [IV]. A disturbance of one or a combination of such factors may lead to the development of fetal hydrops.

Commonly, anaemia, hypoproteinaemia, cardiac dysfunction and obstruction to lymphatic flow are the principal clinical associations with fetal hydrops. Each of these is discussed briefly. Fetal anaemia is associated with reduced vascular 'afterload' with a compensatory increase in cardiac output. If associated with heterotopic erythropoiesis, particularly in the liver and spleen, there may be an end-stage rise in portal and finally central venous pressure. Secondary liver dysfunction causes severe hypoproteinaemia, and poor perfusion leads to

tissue hypoxia (especially on the myocardium), heart failure and, ultimately, widespread endothelial dysfunction and increased capillary permeability.[4]

COMMON CONDITIONS CAUSING FETAL HYDROPS (TABLE 17.2)[2,3]

Cardiac abnormalities

Cardiac malformations account for the majority of cases of hydrops. These include hypoplastic left or right heart syndrome, atrioventricular canal abnormalities and valvular lesions. The likely mechanism leading to fetal hydrops is raised central venous pressure secondary to increased right heart pressure or juxtaposition of systemic arterial pressure onto the right heart causing myocardial failure.

Cardiac dysrhythmia is associated with fetal hydrops, with both tachyarrhythmia and bradyarrhythmia being implicated. Atrial flutter, supraventricular tachycardia (SVT) and complete heart block can all cause hydrops secondary to abnormalities of diastole and direct hypoxia upon myocardial function. As a result, the central venous pressure may rise, causing transudation of fluid into the interstitial space and a consequent inability of the lymphatic system to return the excess fluid into the vascular compartment.

Sacrococcygeal teratomas, placental chorioangioma and vein of Galen aneurysms can all cause hydrops by acting as a large peripheral arteriovenous shunt (decreasing peripheral vascular resistance and afterload). Finally, 'high output' heart failure occurs in utero.

Aneuploidy

Chromosome abnormalities are commonly associated with fetal hydrops in association with or independent of congenital structural anomalies. Turner's syndrome and trisomy 21

Table 17.2   Conditions associated with non-immune hydrops

Cardiovascular	Twin pregnancy
Hypoplastic left heart	Twin–twin transfusion syndrome
Hypoplastic right heart	Acardiac twin
A-V canal defects	
Premature closure of foramen ovale	
Transposition of the great vessels	
Ebstein's anomaly	
Atrial flutter	
Supraventricular tachycardia	
Complete heart block	
Placental chorioangioma	
Sacrococcygeal teratoma	
Umbilical cord haemangioma	
Cardiomyopathy	
Chromosomal	
45X	
Trisomy 13, 18, 21	
Triploidy	
Thoracic	
Congenital cystic adenomatoid malformation of the lung	
Diaphragmatic hernia	
Pulmonary sequestration	
Primary hydrothorax	
Bronchogenic cyst	
Intrathoracic mass	
Haematologic	
Alpha-thalassaemia	
Feto-maternal haemorrhage	
Red cell enzyme deficiencies	
Infections	
Parvovirus B19	
Cytomegalovirus	
Syphilis	
Herpes	
Rubella	
Genetic syndromes	
Arthrogryposis	
Lethal multiple pterygium syndrome	
Pena-Shokeir syndrome	
Myotonic dystrophy	
Metabolic disorders	
Gangliosidosis	
Galactosialidosis	
Gaucher's disease	

together account for the majority of cases and are commonly associated with septate or non-septated cystic hygromata.[2,3] Karyotyping is therefore always indicated as one of the primary investigations in these fetuses.

Thoracic anomalies

Diaphragmatic hernia, congenital cystic adenomatoid malformation of the lung and pulmonary sequestration cause hydrops by significantly raising intrathoracic pressure and impairing venous return. Compression of the oesophagus may also obstruct fetal swallowing and cause polyhydramnios. Longstanding compression of the fetal lung, either by effusions or by herniated abdominal contents, can cause pulmonary hypoplasia, with accordingly increased perinatal mortality.

Fetal infections

Parvovirus B19 (erythema infectiosum, Fifth disease) is a significant cause of fetal hydrops; the infection commonly results in an erythematous rash and has high infectivity amongst young children.[5] The transplacental infection rate is approximately 33 per cent, with 9 per cent fetal loss rate. This virus has also been implicated in unexpected stillbirths at term and late miscarriages.[5,6] Parvovirus causes anaemia by destroying cells of the erythroid series, although neutrophils and platelets may also decrease.[6,7] Parvovirus can also directly infect cardiomyocytes and cause myocarditis and cardiac dysfunction, thereby further aggravating the hydrops.[7] The diagnosis of human parvovirus B19 in a hydropic fetus is difficult and requires the isolation of either the viral DNA using polymerase chain reaction (PCR) or parvovirus-specific immunoglobulin M (IgM) from fetal samples.[8] Hydrops tends to occur 2–4 weeks after fetal infection and, as this virus is not known to be associated with congenital malformations or long-term sequelae, fetal therapy in the form of intrauterine, intravascular transfusion(s) may be of benefit. Typically, transfusion of red cells can be of considerable benefit in salvaging some anaemic hydropic fetuses [IV].[9,10] However, there has been a report of congenital red cell aplasia in infants who underwent in-utero transfusions following parvovirus infection, and hence fetuses treated antenatally should be followed up to detect this potential complication.

A multitude of other viruses (cytomegalovirus, rubella, herpes simplex, coxsackie), bacteria (streptococci), spirochaete (syphilis) and parasites (*Toxoplasma*) can cause fetal infection and occasionally hydrops (see Chapter 13). However, the effects are variable and no organism consistently or predictably results in either congenital infection or fetal hydrops. Although it is believed that the most common mechanism for the development of hydrops is anaemia, myocarditis and/or hepatitis, other pathways that have yet to be identified may also be responsible. These other viral agents are often associated with high perinatal morbidity and mortality.

Other causes of fetal hydrops

Structural anomalies of the urinary tract (i.e. urethral atresia) may cause isolated ascites but rarely true hydrops. Urinary ascites occurs when there is rupture of the bladder or renal pelvis secondary to over-distension in lower urinary tract obstruction (posterior urethral valves or urethral atresia). In such cases, both renal dysplasia and severe oligohydramnios are usually present.

Genetic conditions, metabolic disorders and skeletal dysplasias can all cause hydrops by different means. The diagnosis should be considered when a pregnant woman has a positive family history. It is important to try to make as accurate a diagnosis as possible, as many of these conditions carry significant recurrence risks, and these patients should receive genetic counselling. In the absence of a family history or definitive diagnosis, most genetic disorders will be undiagnosed and the cause of the hydrops will remain speculative and unexplained. In twin–twin transfusion syndrome complicating monochorionic twins (stage IV or above), the recipient fetus may show signs of hydrops associated with high-output cardiac failure (see Chapter 12).

Maternal risks and complications

The maternal 'mirror' syndrome can be associated with fetal hydrops. This is characterized by an unusual type of pre-eclampsia, which has an extremely rapid onset and deterioration. This appears to occur when the placenta is severely oedematous. An increased risk of postpartum haemorrhage and amniotic fluid embolism has also been reported [III].[2]

KEY POINTS

- There are no EBM guidelines for the treatment of non-immune fetal hydrops; most evidence is in the form of small series from specialist centres [II].
- It is extremely important to exclude aneuploidy and structural malformations using ultrasound.
- Anaemia caused by parvovirus infection is potentially the most treatable condition [IV].
- Management should be in a tertiary referral fetal medicine centre [IV].

IMMUNE HYDROPS

The Rh blood group system consists of five major antigens, D, C, c, E and e, all of which can produce erythrocyte alloimmunization.[11] The erythrocyte D antigen is strongly immunogenic and therefore both more important and more common than the other Rh antigens.[11] In classical Rh disease, the mother is RhD negative and the fetus RhD positive. Fetal red cells can enter the maternal circulation at any time during pregnancy through occult fetomaternal haemorrhage. The risk of fetomaternal haemorrhage antenatally increases with gestation from 3 per cent in the first trimester to approximately 65 per cent in the last.

Once maternal sensitization occurs, IgG crosses the placenta and may have very serious effects on the fetus.[11] The concentration of antibody appears to be the most important factor in determining the severity of the disease. The fetus may develop anaemia due to anti-D antibody binding to fetal RhD-positive red blood cells, which are then sequestered in

the fetal spleen and undergo haemolysis. Erythropoiesis is stimulated in the fetal liver, which enlarges but is eventually unable to meet the increased demand. Large numbers of erythroblasts are found in the fetal circulation (hence the historical term erythroblastosis fetalis). Severe anaemia develops with cardiac failure, skin oedema, hepatosplenomegaly, ascites and pericardial and pleural effusions. Untreated, these fetuses die or are delivered with hydrops. Less severely anaemic fetuses may be delivered before hydrops occurs but will experience increasingly severe hyperbilirubinaemia (icterus gravis neonatorum), which may proceed to kernicterus due to deposition of unconjugated bilirubin in the grey matter nuclei of the central nervous system.

The frequency and pattern of this condition has changed considerably over the last half-century following the introduction of effective prophylaxis using anti-D immunoglobulin administered to the mother after delivery or after any sensitizing events that occur antenatally. Deaths attributable to RhD alloimmunization fell from 46/100 000 births in 1969 to 1.6/100 000 in 1990 in the UK. Similar decreases in prevalence have also been seen worldwide.

The list of antigens other than the Rh system that may cause haemolytic disease is extensive. In practice, atypical antibodies most likely to cause problems include anti-c, anti-kell and anti-E. Haemolytic disease of the ABO system is frequently mild, tends to occur in the first pregnancy and rarely causes severe anaemia or hydrops, causing neonatal jaundice. In contrast to Rh disease, antibodies produced in maternal Kell alloimmunization may cause unpredictably severe and early-onset fetal anaemia [II]. This is secondary to both reticulo-endothelial erythrocyte destruction and suppression of erythropoiesis.[11] The severity and outcome of this form of alloimmunization appear equally unpredictable, whether caused by fetomaternal haemorrhage or exogenous antigen presentation (i.e. transfusion). From 1996, many regions in the UK use Kell-type packed red cells for transfusion in women of reproductive age.

KEY POINTS

- The incidence of Rh disease has decreased dramatically due to the implementation of effective anti-D prophylaxis programmes [Ia].
- Management of Rhesus disease should be based on:
  - the maternal antibody titres,
  - the paternal genotype,
  - the past obstetric history,
  - specific screening tests of fetal anaemia.
  These factors are designed to detect fetal anaemia prior to the onset of hydrops [II].
- Kell alloimmunization may produce severe early-onset fetal anaemia out of proportion to the antibody titres [II].
- Management should be co-ordinated in fetal medicine centres [IV].

MANAGEMENT OF THE FETUS WITH HYDROPS

Patients whose fetuses are affected with hydrops should be referred to a fetal medicine centre where the necessary expertise and experience are available [IV]. A detailed ultrasound scan, including Doppler insonation of the fetal cerebral vasculature and liquor volume, is mandatory [II]. The ultrasound scan must also include careful evaluation of the fetal anatomy and, particularly if skeletal dysplasia is suspected, all the long bones, hands, feet, skull shape and thoracic circumference must be examined.[3]

The placenta and umbilical cord should be carefully examined to exclude a chorioangioma or other vascular abnormalities. This should also include fetal echocardiography, excluding cardiac malformations and noting normal atrial and ventricular rate and rhythm. Some indication of the cause of hydrops may be obtained from the sites of fluid collection. More recently, the finding that fetal anaemia can be predicted with up to 100 per cent sensitivity using the peak systolic velocity in the middle cerebral artery[12] has significantly improved the assessment of these fetuses. This non-invasive method of monitoring fetuses at risk of fetal anaemia may be used as an adjunct to traditional methods of screening such as amniocentesis for the measurement of optical density or fetal blood sampling [II].

Invasive fetal assessment in hydrops almost always involves fetal blood sampling [II]. This enables fetal blood to be obtained for a variety of investigations (full blood count, karyotype, virology, enzyme studies, liver function tests, acid–base status and protein concentrations). The volume of blood required for these tests is small and should not compromise the fetus. Some of the investigations, such as karyotype or viral studies, can also be done on amniotic fluid or chorionic villi; however, fetal blood is preferable for complete haematological, biochemical and metabolic information. The risks of fetal blood sampling in a hydropic fetus are significantly greater than in the non-hydropic state. However, when balanced against the high mortality in such situations, the risk becomes more acceptable [IV].

Maternal blood should also be checked for atypical antibodies (indirect Coombs test), full blood count and haemoglobin electrophoresis, viral serology (TORCH titres) and, in selected cases, G6PD and pyruvate kinase carrier status. A Kleihauer–Betke test should be performed to exclude a fetomaternal haemorrhage.[13] Other tests, such as for the presence of anti-Ro and anti-La antibodies, should be performed if the hydropic fetus is severely bradycardic. It must be emphasized that many of the tests are selected according to the clinical picture and family history. If more evidence emerges of unusual viral infections causing hydrops, specific tests to detect these agents will be necessary.

TREATMENT

Fetal anaemia is treated by in-utero intravascular transfusions in hydrops.[13,14] This is the treatment of choice for fetuses affected by red cell alloimmunization, and in experienced hands carries a risk of perinatal death of <10 per cent, with perinatal loss in the hydropic cohort being higher, at 12–15 per cent [II]. Arrhythmias of the fetal heart can be treated either indirectly by administering specific cardiotrophic drugs to the mother or directly to the fetus [II, IV]. Although the transfer of drugs through an oedematous placenta is believed to be impaired, cardioversion is certainly possible in many instances.[15]

Pleural effusions can be treated by pleuroamniotic shunting [II],[16,17] and large fetal tumours can be treated either in utero or occasionally by open surgery [II, IV]. Hydrops in the recipient fetus in twin–twin transfusion syndrome may be treated by either serial amnioreduction or direct fetoscopic laser ablation of communicating placental vessels (see Chapter 12) [II]. In severe cases where the recipient fetus is hydropic and pre-terminal, selective fetocide using cord occlusion may be the only option if its co-twin is to survive [II].

OUTCOME

Overall, perinatal mortality in cases of NIH is high (>85 per cent).[2,18,19] This is because of the high incidence of aneuploidy, structural and non-treatable infectious causes responsible for fetal hydrops. In this cohort, termination of pregnancy is a common outcome. The outcome in cases of IH treated by serial intrauterine transfusions is much better (85–88 per cent survival).[20] In severe twin–twin transfusion syndrome, the outcome is poor, especially in stage IV disease when the recipient is hydropic.[21]

CONCLUSION

Although the aetiology in many cases of NIH is now clearer, fetal NIH remains a difficult clinical problem. Recent advances in fetal therapy have increased the number of treatable conditions, but the overall perinatal morbidity and mortality rates remain high.

KEY REFERENCES

1. Warsof SL, Nicolaides KH, Rodeck C. Immune and non-immune hydrops. *Clin Obstet Gynecol* 1986; 29(3):533–42.

2. Ismail KMK, Martin WL, Ghosh S, Whittle MJ, Kilby MD. Etiology and outcome of hydrops fetalis. *J Maternal–Fetal Med* 2001; **10**:1–7.

3. Saltzman DH, Frigoletto FD, Harlow BL, Barss VA, Benacerraf BR. Sonographic evaluation of hydrops fetalis. *Obstet Gynecol* 1989; **74**(1):106–11.

4. Poeschmann RP, Verheijen RH, Van Dongen PW. Differential diagnosis and causes of nonimmunological hydrops fetalis: a review. *Obstet Gynecol Surv* 1991; **46**(4):223–31.

5. Tolfvenstam T, Papadogiannakis N, Norbeck O, Petersson K, Broliden K. Frequency of human parvovirus B19 infection in intrauterine fetal death. *Lancet* 2001; **357**(9267):1494–7.

6. Potter CG, Potter AC, Hatton CS et al. Variation of erythroid and myeloid precursors in the marrow and peripheral blood of volunteer subjects infected with human parvovirus (B19). *J Clin Invest* 1987; **79**(5):1486–92.

7. Naides SJ, Weiner CP. Antenatal diagnosis and palliative treatment of non-immune hydrops fetalis secondary to fetal parvovirus B19 infection. *Prenat Diagn* 1989; **9**(2):105–14.

8. Smoleniec JS, Pillai M. Management of fetal hydrops associated with parvovirus B19 infection. *Br J Obstet Gynaecol* 1994; **101**(12):1079–81.

9. Brown KE, Green SW, Antunez de Mayolo J et al. Congenital anaemia after transplacental B19 parvovirus infection. *Lancet* 1994; **343**(8902):895–6.

10. Ismail KMK, Kilby MD. Human parvovirus B19 infection and pregnancy. *Obstet Gynecol* 2003; **5**:4–9.

11. Moise KJ, Schumacher B. Anaemia. In: Fisk NM, Moise KJ (eds). *Fetal Therapy: Invasive and Transplacental.* Cambridge: Cambridge University Press, 1995, 141–63.

12. Mari G, Deter RL, Carpenter RL et al. Noninvasive diagnosis by Doppler ultrasonography of fetal anaemia due to maternal red-cell alloimmunization.

Collaborative Group for Doppler Assessment of the Blood Velocity in Anemic Fetuses. *N Engl J Med* 2000; **342**(1):9–14.

13. Montgomery LD, Belfort MA, Adam K. Massive fetomaternal hemorrhage treated with serial combined intravascular and intraperitoneal fetal transfusions. *Am J Obstet Gynecol* 1995; **173**(1):234–5.

14. Fairley CK, Smoleniec JS, Caul OE, Miller E. Observational study of effect of intrauterine transfusions on outcome of fetal hydrops after parvovirus B19 infection. *Lancet* 1995; **346**(8986):1335–7.

15. van Engelen AD, Weijtens O, Brenner JI et al. Management outcome and follow-up of fetal tachycardia. *J Am Coll Cardiol* 1994; **24**(5):1371–5.

16. Rodeck CH, Fisk NM, Fraser DI, Nicolini U. Long-term in utero drainage of fetal hydrothorax. *N Engl J Med* 1988; **319**(17):1135–8.

17. Chan V, Greenough A, Nicolaides KN. Antenatal and postnatal treatment of pleural effusion and extra-lobar pulmonary sequestration. *J Perinat Med* 1996; **24**(4):335–8.

18. McCoy MC, Katz VL, Gould N, Kuller JA. Non-immune hydrops after 20 weeks' gestation: review of 10 years' experience with suggestions for management. *Obstet Gynecol* 1995; **85**(4):578–82.

19. Iskaros J, Jauniaux E, Rodeck C. Outcome of nonimmune hydrops fetalis diagnosed during the first half of pregnancy. *Obstet Gynecol* 1997; **90**(3):321–5.

20. Harman CR, Bowman JM, Manning FA, Menticoglou SM. Intrauterine transfusion–intraperitoneal versus intravascular approach: a case-control comparison. *Am J Obstet Gynecol* 1990; **162**(4):1053–9.

21. Mari G, Roberts A, Detti L et al. Perinatal morbidity and mortality rates in severe twin–twin transfusion syndrome: results of the International Amnioreduction Registry. *Am J Obstet Gynecol* 2001; **185**(3):708–15.

Chapter 18

Malpresentation

David Somerset

INTRODUCTION

Presentation refers to the lowermost part of the fetus presenting to the maternal pelvis and lower uterine segment. At term, approximately 96–97 per cent of fetuses have a cephalic presentation.[1] For the purpose of this chapter, *malpresentation* includes all presentations other than cephalic and also brow and face presentations, but not mal*positions* of the occiput. Malpresentation is historically associated with increased maternal and neonatal morbidity and mortality.[2] Maternal morbidity and mortality are related to obstructed labour and the surgical and anaesthetic risks associated with emergency operative delivery. In regions with poor access to medical care, failure to intervene in obstructed labour can be associated with tissue necrosis and subsequent fistula formation, or uterine rupture, sepsis and death. Fetal morbidity and mortality are associated antenatally with congenital malformations, prematurity and intrauterine death. Intrapartum risks to the fetus include hypoxia from prolonged labour or cord prolapse, and traumatic delivery.

BREECH PRESENTATION

Incidence and aetiology

The incidence of breech presentation at term is quoted as between 3 and 4 per cent, but it is commoner preterm – 15 per cent at 32 weeks and 20 per cent at 28 weeks.[3] Not surprisingly given these figures, prematurity is the commonest association, with a quarter of breech deliveries occurring preterm.[2,4] Maternal factors associated with breech presentation include nulliparity, older age, uterine abnormalities (e.g. bicornuate uterus), abnormal placental site (e.g. placenta praevia or cornual implantation), diabetes, smoking, late/no antenatal care and white ethnicity.[4] Fetal factors include fetal abnormalities (e.g. hydrocephalus or neuromuscular dysfunction causing abnormal posture or dyskinesia), intrauterine growth restriction (IUGR), polyhydramnios, short umbilical cord, extended legs and multiple pregnancy.[5]

Clinical findings

Classically, the term mother may complain of subcostal discomfort, particularly on the right side. Abdominal palpation should reveal the hard, round, ballotable head at the uterine fundus. Vaginal examination (depending on cervical dilatation) should reveal an unusually soft presenting part with the only bony landmarks being the ischial tuberosities. The anus and genitalia may also be palpable. Clinical confusion with face presentation (see below) is reported. Over 30 per cent of breech presentations are not diagnosed until labour, and ultrasound examination to confirm presentation and exclude fetal and maternal anomalies that may influence management is mandatory. Breech presentation is subdivided into three categories: extended or frank, with hips flexed and knees extended (≈70 per cent); flexed or complete, with hips and knees flexed, and buttocks presenting; footling or incomplete, with hips and knees flexed, and feet presenting.

Fetuses presenting by the breech have an increased rate of perinatal morbidity and mortality.[5] Separating out the individual risks ascribed to the breech position itself, the mode of delivery and underlying fetal abnormalities has proved difficult. Perinatal mortality remains increased even when delivery is by elective caesarean section, despite correction for gestational age, birth weight and congenital abnormality.[6] Furthermore, whereas breech presentation is a risk factor for the development of cerebral palsy, mode of delivery is not.[7]

Clinical trials

Mode of delivery at term

In 2000, the Term Breech Trial Collaborative Group led by Mary Hannah published the results of a large, multicentre, randomized trial of planned vaginal versus caesarean delivery for breech presentation at term.[8] This trial involved 2088 women at 121 centres in 26 countries. The results showed that 90 per cent of the planned caesarean section group delivered by caesarean section, versus 43 per cent of the planned vaginal delivery group. There was no significant difference in maternal morbidity or mortality between the two groups other than a slight decrease in urinary incontinence at 3 months in the caesarean section group.[9] However, there was a significant decrease in fetal morbidity – 1.4 per cent versus 3.8 per cent, relative risk (RR) 0.36 (0.19–0.65) – and mortality – 0.3 per cent versus 1.3 per cent, RR 0.23 (0.07–0.81) – in the planned caesarean section group.[8] When the analysis was restricted to countries with a low perinatal mortality rate ($<20/1000$), the difference in mortality between the two groups was no longer significant, but the protective effect of planned caesarean section on neonatal morbidity was increased – 0.4 per cent versus 5.1 per cent, RR 0.08 (0.02–0.32).

The latest Cochrane Review[10] includes two older trials (1980 and 1983) but only 302 extra women. The results are therefore dominated by the Term Breech Trial. Neonatal mortality (Figure 18.1a), and combined neonatal morbidity and mortality were significantly reduced by intention to deliver by caesarean section. Interestingly, short-term maternal morbidity was slightly increased in the intention to deliver by caesarean section group (Figure 18.1b). As the Term Breech Trial did not show this, it may reflect an improvement in the safety of caesarean section over the last 20 years. In his discussion, Hofmeyr[10] makes two interesting points. First, none of the trials assessed future maternal morbidity due to the effects of a uterine scar in subsequent pregnancies, which may therefore be much higher in the intended caesarean section group. Second, within the high perinatal mortality countries in the Term Breech Trial, there was a tendency for very early neonatal discharge with reduced follow-up, so that some short-term neonatal morbidity may have been missed relative to those in the low perinatal mortality countries, thereby possibly hiding a further protective effect of intended caesarean section.

Mode of delivery preterm

The effect of mode of delivery on perinatal morbidity/mortality associated with breech presentation in preterm labour has not been so well addressed. Numerous retrospective studies have suggested that caesarean section improves outcomes, but it is generally acknowledged that all these studies are subject to bias.[1,5] There are concerns that the preterm fetus may be more vulnerable to hypoxic injury than the term fetus, and also that since the fetal head is relatively larger than the body preterm (biparietal diameter >bi-trochanteric diameter), there is a greater risk of entrapment of the after-coming head. However, elective caesarean delivery is complicated by the fact that 80 per cent of women in threatened preterm labour will deliver at term (see Chapter 21). Hence there is a significant risk of iatrogenic prematurity if babies are delivered by caesarean section before labour is established. Furthermore, elective preterm caesarean section does not escape the risk of head entrapment, and midline uterine incisions or inverted 'T' incisions carry increased risks of scar rupture in the future. Although attempts have been made, no satisfactory randomized trial has been able to recruit sufficient numbers of patients to provide an answer as to how best to deliver the preterm breech. Furthermore, it is generally accepted that for the fetus prior to 34 weeks, the risks associated with prematurity and congenital anomalies far outweigh those associated with mode of delivery.[1]

External cephalic version

In an attempt to reduce the number of breech presentations at term, the Royal College of Obstetricians and Gynaecologists (RCOG) recommends offering external cephalic version (ECV) to all women found to have an uncomplicated breech presentation at >37 completed weeks.[1] A Cochrane Review[11] of six randomized trials involving 612 women showed a significant reduction in caesarean sections (Figure 18.2a) and a significant reduction in non-cephalic births (Figure 18.2b), without any change in perinatal mortality or morbidity documented (Figure 18.2c). However, the numbers involved were probably too small to have demonstrated any change in perinatal morbidity/mortality. In a Cochrane Review[12] of three trials involving 889 preterm patients, ECV was not shown to be effective in reducing the incidence of either breech presentation at term or caesarean section. However, the role of ECV in breech *preterm labour* has not been assessed, and a randomized trial is currently underway in Toronto (the Early ECV Trial).

Management

External cephalic version

RCOG Guideline No. 20[1] was updated following publication of the Term Breech Trial.[8] ECV should be offered to all women with an uncomplicated breech presentation at term [Ia]. Table 18.1 lists absolute and relative contraindications to ECV. There is good evidence that ECV is more successful if used in combination with tocolysis, either selectively or routinely [Ia] (e.g. terbutaline 0.25 mg subcutaneously 15–30 minutes prior to ECV[13]); however, the RCOG does not at

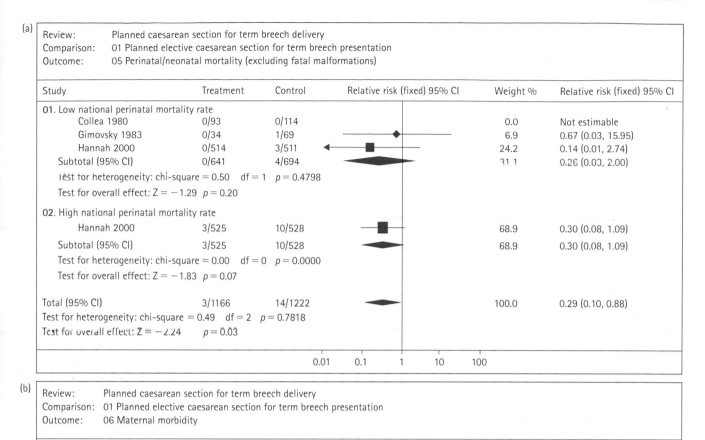

Figure 18.1   (a) Reduced perinatal mortality associated with intention to deliver by caesarian section.[10] (b) Increased maternal morbidity associated with intention to deliver by caesarian section[10]

present recommend any specific tocolytic regimen. ECV should be carried out following ultrasound assessment of the fetus to exclude contraindications [IV] and with informed consent from the patient. Cardiotocography (CTG) should be performed prior to and following attempted ECV [IV], and facilities for emergency delivery should be available [IV]. Transient fetal heart rate abnormalities (typically baseline bradycardias) are seen following up to 10 per cent of ECV attempts and usually resolve within 5 minutes.[14] The need for emergency delivery is usually given as <1 per cent, but no good data exist to quantify this more accurately. Real-time ultrasound may be of use during an attempted ECV for defining fetal position. The incidence of feto-maternal haemorrhage following attempted ECV has been reported to be as high as 18 per cent;[13] a maternal Kleihauer test to quantify the transfusion and anti-D administration is therefore mandatory for any Rhesus-negative mother [IV]. Compound

presentation and cord presentation have also been reported as rare complications of ECV. Successful ECV has been described during the first stage of labour with intact membranes and following a previous caesarean section, although no trials have been published.

Persistent breech presentation at term

If ECV fails, is declined or is contraindicated, elective caesarean section at 39 weeks' gestation is now the recommended mode of delivery [Ia].[1] The risks and benefits of this procedure should be explained to the mother, together with the implications for her future obstetric performance. Owing to the small chance of spontaneous version prior to an elective section, ultrasound examination immediately prior to surgery to confirm the lie is vital [IV].

If the mother declines an elective caesarean section, advice should be given to maximize the success and safety

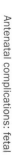

(a)
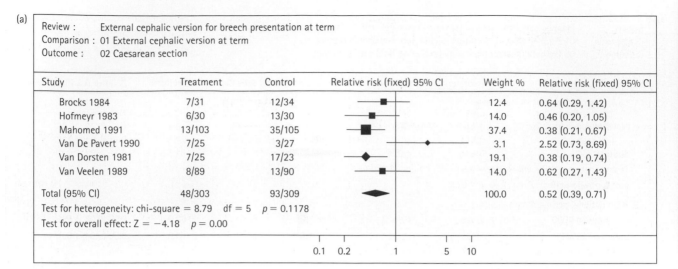

(b)
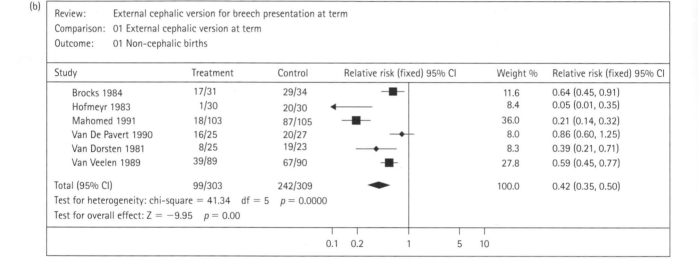

(c)
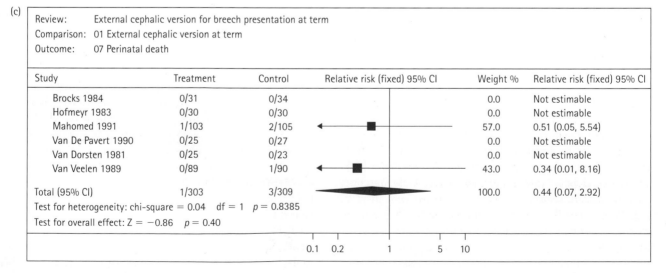

Figure 18.2   (a) Reduction in caesarian sections following attempted external cephalic version (ECV).[11] (b) Reduction in non-cephalic births following attempted ECV.[11] (c) Relative risk of perinatal death following attempted ECV[11]

Table 18.1 Contraindications to external cephalic version [IV]

Absolute	Relative
Multiple pregnancy	Uterine scar
Significant antepartum haemorrhage	Moderate/severe hypertension
Placenta praevia	Nuchal cord
Severe fetal abnormality	Intrauterine growth restriction
Hyper-extended head	Oligohydramnios
Ruptured membranes	Maternal obesity
Other indication for caesarean section	

of the attempt. Contraindications to vaginal delivery should be excluded (e.g. placenta praevia). Ultrasound assessment should be used to exclude an overly large fetus (>4000 g),[5,14] hyperextension of the fetal neck and a cord presentation or footling breech (which carries a high risk of cord prolapse) [IV]. There is no evidence to support X-ray or computerized tomography (CT) pelvimetry, but clinical assessment of the pelvis is recommended [IV].[1] The importance of careful intrapartum monitoring of both fetal well-being and progress in labour should be emphasized [IV].[1] The Seventh Annual Confidential Enquiry into Stillbirths and Deaths in Infancy (CESDI) Report highlights failure to act on suspicious fetal heart rate recordings or failure to monitor adequately as one of the most important deficiencies of care during the management of breech deliveries.[15] Fetal blood sampling from the buttocks should be used to investigate suspect CTG traces. Induction of labour and augmentation may be justified in selected cases [IV].[1] Although there is no evidence to support the routine use of epidural anaesthesia [IV], the possibility of fetal manipulation in the second stage and instrumental delivery should be discussed. Labour should be supervised by a senior obstetrician experienced in breech delivery [IV]. Progress should be similar to cephalic presentation, and any delay in cervical dilatation or descent should prompt careful consideration of whether caesarean section is advisable.[5]

The active second stage begins with the appearance of the breech at the introitus. The accoucher must be familiar with the management of the second stage, including the techniques of assisted delivery.[2,5] From delivery to the level of the umbilicus to delivery of the head should take no more than three contractions and 5–10 minutes [IV]. A paediatrician and anaesthetist should be in attendance [IV]. Although much emphasis is placed on careful case selection prior to labour, the RCOG advises that 'assessment of the undiagnosed breech in labour by experienced medical staff can allow safe vaginal delivery' [III].[1]

Preterm labour

As discussed above, there is no evidence to support routine caesarean section for preterm breech presentation [III]. Decisions about the mode of delivery in such cases should therefore be individualized and take into account the views

of the parents as well as the attending obstetric and paediatric staff.[1] If delivery is by caesarean section, the use of a tocolytic to reduce the risk of entrapment of the after-coming head is advised [IV].

Twin pregnancy

With regard to breech presentation in twin pregnancies, the RCOG guideline states that 'there is insufficient evidence to support Caesarean section for the delivery of the first or second twin' [III].[1] It is argued that the Term Breech Trial included only singleton pregnancies and twins are 'different', in that they are smaller and continuous electronic fetal monitoring is standard practice. The risk of 'locked twins' (where the presenting twin is breech, the second twin is cephalic and their heads lock above the pelvic inlet preventing delivery of the first twin) is thought to be rare (1/817). Other evidence cited includes an observational study of 82 twin pregnancies from a single centre in Israel, which showed no fetal benefit from an increase in caesarean section rate from 21 per cent to 95 per cent over time, despite an increase in maternal febrile morbidity; and a randomized study of 60 twin gestations in which the second twin was non-cephalic, which showed no fetal benefit from elective caesarean section but an increase in maternal febrile morbidity. Nevertheless, it should be remembered that lack of evidence for a benefit does not imply evidence for a lack of benefit. None of the studies referred to above and in the RCOG guideline with regard to twin delivery was powered to detect a difference in fetal morbidity or mortality.[1] Most obstetricians in the UK would recommend elective caesarean section where the presenting twin is breech [IV].[14]

KEY POINTS

- ECV after 37 weeks' gestation is effective at reducing the incidence of non-cephalic births and caesarean sections [Ia].
- Elective caesarean section for persistent breech presentation at term reduces perinatal morbidity and mortality [Ia].
- There is no evidence to support a policy of elective caesarean section for breech presentation in preterm labour [III].

FACE PRESENTATION

Incidence and aetiology

Historically, the incidence of face presentation has been reported as around 1/500. However, in modern obstetric practice, the incidence is likely to be lower, as few cases of undiagnosed anencephaly (previously a common cause of face presentation) should occur.[2] Prematurity was associated with between 25 per cent and 34 per cent of cases, and most mothers (70 per cent) were multiparous.[16] Multiple pregnancy is cited as a 'frequent' cause; however, whether this is independent of the effects of prematurity and/or polyhydramnios is unclear.[2,16] Less common associated factors include fetal problems such as thyroid goitres and uterine abnormalities such as pelvic tumours, bicornuate uterus, placenta praevia and polyhydramnios.

Clinical findings

Seventy-seven per cent of cases are reported to be mento-anterior, with 50 per cent of cases remaining undiagnosed until delivery is imminent.[16] Ritchie reports: 'Between the anterior shoulder and the head prominence there is a characteristic deep depression in which no fetal part can be felt',[2] but in truth the diagnosis is made on vaginal examination. The 'landmarks' include the mandible, mouth, nose, malar and orbital ridges. Care should be taken to avoid damaging the eyes. Historically, in obstructed labour with oedema, differentiating between a face and frank breech presentation could be difficult;[2] in modern practice, ultrasound examination should resolve any doubt.

During labour, delay in the second stage is common. Abdominal palpation is important, as the widest part of the fetal head is some 7 cm behind the face; thus vaginal examination can be misleading with regard to descent. As long as the position is mento-anterior, once the face is seen at the introitus, the head may be born by flexion, assisted by forceps if required. Because the head is presenting a very wide diameter, considerable perineal trauma is likely and a generous episiotomy is traditionally advised.[2] Mento-posterior position is incompatible with vaginal delivery unless rotation occurs or the fetus is small enough for the shoulders to enter the pelvis at the same time as the head. Following delivery, the fetal face is usually very oedematous and may be bruised. This usually persists for several days and may cause feeding difficulties.

Clinical trials

There are no clinical trials involving face presentation, and management is therefore based on expert opinion [IV].[2,16,17]

Management

The correct management of face presentation involves ultrasound examination (if not already done) to exclude fetal or pelvic abnormality that may preclude vaginal delivery. In modern obstetric practice, if the diagnosis is made during the first stage of labour, a candid discussion with the mother about the risks to both her and her fetus of both vaginal and caesarean delivery is advised. The risks from vaginal delivery include soft tissue trauma to the fetal face, perineal damage including anal sphincter injury to the mother, and second-stage emergency caesarean section. It should be remembered that by the time the diagnosis is made, considerable soft tissue trauma to the fetal face may already have occurred, which will not be prevented by abdominal delivery. Furthermore, around half the cases of mento-posterior position will rotate during the second stage to mento-anterior.[2] Frequently, the diagnosis will be made in conjunction with failure to progress, and caesarean section is usually indicated. The use of oxytocic augmentation in these circumstances is controversial, and abdominal delivery should certainly be advised if there is no progress within 2 hours.[17] In the second stage of labour, given a mento-anterior position and good progress, a vaginal delivery can be expected; however, senior obstetric assistance should be readily available.

KEY POINTS

- Face presentation may precede vaginal delivery if the position is mento-anterior.
- Caesarean section may avoid maternal perineal trauma and reduce fetal facial oedema and bruising [IV].

BROW PRESENTATION

Incidence and aetiology

Historically, the incidence of brow presentation is reported as around 1/1000 deliveries.[2] Many brow presentations in early labour are transient and either flex into a vertex presentation or further extend into a face presentation. The aetiology is the same as for face presentation, with prematurity associated with 20 per cent.

Clinical findings

Abdominal findings typically include a large, high head, as the mento-vertical diameter (≈ 13 cm at term) is unlikely to engage. Vaginally, the brow (bregma) is felt as a hard, rounded structure in the centre of the cervix with the anterior fontanelle to one side and the orbital ridges (and occasionally nose) opposite. The face is more commonly anterior than posterior; however, the diagnosis is often made late in labour because the cervix needs to be considerably dilated to feel the landmarks. In the presence of a large caput secundum, it may be impossible to make the diagnosis with confidence.[2]

Vaginal delivery is possible if the vertex is small and the pelvis 'capacious'. With the face anterior, once the brow appears at the introitus, the head initially flexes to yield the occiput before extension to deliver the face.

Clinical trials

There are no clinical trials involving brow presentation, and management is therefore based on expert opinion [IV].[2,16,17]

Management

Ultrasound assessment to exclude fetal or pelvic abnormalities is essential (unless already performed). Given the difficulty in diagnosis, most cases will present late in the first stage with failure to progress. If augmentation with syntocinon has not been attempted, this could be considered, although there is no evidence of its efficacy in this situation. Furthermore, extreme caution is advised in multipara and grand-multipara due to the risk of uterine rupture.[17] If the diagnosis is made early in the first stage, it would seem prudent to await events, as the majority will either resolve to vertex or progress to face, and management can be tailored appropriately. However, in all cases, if the head remains high and the brow presentation persists, delivery by caesarean section is required.

KEY POINTS

- Brow presentation in early labour may convert into vertex or face presentation.
- If the brow persists and the head remains high, delivery by caesarean section is required [IV].

UNSTABLE LIE/TRANSVERSE LIE/OBLIQUE LIE

Incidence and aetiology

Historical studies suggest an incidence of around 1/320; unstable/transverse/oblique lies are much more common in multiparae than nulliparae.[2] Aetiological factors involve abnormalities of the uterus, pelvis or fetus. The effect of parity is likely to reflect increasing laxity in the abdominal wall musculature failing to orientate and hold the fetus in a longitudinal lie. There is no evidence to support the commonly held view regarding increasing laxity of uterine tone.

Predispositions include polyhydramnios, which allows the fetus greater freedom of movement. Uterine septae are rarely associated with unstable lie, but more commonly associated with breech presentation, especially in their more severe forms (e.g. uterine didelphus). Placenta praevia and, less commonly, cornual placenta discourage pelvic engagement of a fetal pole and thereby predispose to unstable lie. Pelvic anomalies may also prevent engagement of a fetal pole. These include transient factors such as a full urinary bladder, and fixed obstructions such as pelvic tumours (including fibroids and ovarian cysts) and deformity or contracture of the bony pelvis. Fetal factors include multiple pregnancy, macrosomia, hydrocephaly, tumours of the neck or sacrum, fetal abdominal distension or neuromuscular dysfunction (abnormal posture/dyskinesia).

Clinical findings

Inability to locate a fetal pole in the pelvis on either abdominal or vaginal examination should suggest an unstable or non-longitudinal lie, whether in the antenatal period or during labour.

Clinical trials

There are no randomized trials on which to base the management of these problems, which is therefore based on expert opinion [IV].[2,18]

Management

Ultrasound examination should be used to confirm the lie, exclude fetal anomaly and pelvic tumours, and localize the placenta. However, it is not usually possible to diagnose congenital uterine anomalies using ultrasound during late pregnancy. Clinical examination of the pelvis following exclusion of placenta praevia is considered sufficient to exclude significant pelvic deformity or space-occupying tumour. These investigations may reveal an indication for delivery by caesarean section, which can then be arranged at the appropriate gestation. Owing to the risk of cord prolapse, all women with unstable/non-longitudinal lies should be instructed to attend for assessment if they begin to contract or suspect loss of liquor.

Given that thorough assessment has not revealed an indication for delivery by caesarean section, management may be planned as an outpatient or inpatient, and may be expectant or active. Spontaneous version to longitudinal lie will occur in 80–85 per cent of women prior to labour or membrane rupture. However, due to the risk of cord prolapse where labour occurs prior to version, inpatient management is suggested after 37 weeks' gestation. This allows for rapid intervention/delivery should this occur. Expectant inpatient management involves daily assessment and discharge home once the lie has stabilized longitudinally for 48 hours. Active management involves attempting ECV, either alone, with discharge home if successful, or in conjunction with induction of labour – 'stabilizing induction'. A 'stabilizing induction' requires a favourable cervix and the use of an oxytocic infusion to procure regular uterine contractions, prior to a controlled amniotomy once cephalic presentation has been established. The risk of cord prolapse should be explained to the mother, and preparations made for an emergency caesarean section should this occur.

If the fetal lie remains non-longitudinal post-term $(41^{+3}-42^{+0}$ weeks), elective caesarean section should be offered. Should the patient present in labour or with ruptured membranes, the choice lies between an emergency caesarean section and ECV. There is no place for attempting internal podalic version, except on occasion for the second twin. Delivery at caesarean section may be complicated by both lack of liquor and an inability to manoeuvre the fetus into a longitudinal lie. Consideration should therefore be given to a vertical uterine incision.

KEY POINTS

- 80–85 per cent of unstable lies will resolve spontaneously.
- Inpatient management from 37 weeks until resolution is advised, due to the risk of cord prolapse if labour intervenes [IV].
- Delivery by caesarean section may be difficult following rupture of the membranes.

SHOULDER PRESENTATION/COMPOUND PRESENTATION/CORD PRESENTATION

Incidence and aetiology

Historically, the incidence of cord presentation or prolapse is given as 1/200–300 deliveries.[2] Cord presentation is defined as the umbilical cord lying below the fetus, but the membranes remaining intact. Cord prolapse occurs when the membranes rupture and the cord descends through the cervix into the vagina. Compound presentation occurs when more than one fetal part presents simultaneously, most commonly a head with an arm. All are complications of labour superimposed on an unstable lie, although cord prolapse can also complicate breech presentation (especially footling breech). As with all other malpresentations, including shoulder presentation, prematurity and prior intrauterine death are common associations.

Clinical findings

In early labour, and especially when the membranes are intact and the presenting part is high, ultrasound assessment can be invaluable to detect cord presentation. In advanced labour the findings are self-explanatory.

Clinical trials

There are no clinical trials on which to base management, which is therefore based on expert opinion [IV].[2]

Management

Cord prolapse represents a clinical emergency. Direct pressure on the umbilical cord from the presenting part against the bony pelvis may occlude the fetal placental circulation, leading to acute fetal hypoxia. The drop in ambient temperature if the cord prolapses beyond the introitus may cause premature umbilical artery spasm, again precipitating acute fetal hypoxia. Immediate management therefore involves replacing prolapsed cord in the vagina and elevating the presenting part to reduce cord compression against the pelvic wall. Acceptable techniques involve placing a hand inside the vagina to displace the head manually, using an acute head-down tilt in the bed, or turning the mother onto her hands and knees, with her head resting on the bed such that her pelvis is higher than her head. Delivery should then be expedited by the most expedient route, which will usually be via caesarean section. Rarely, a cord prolapse will occur following membrane rupture at full dilatation (typically in a multiparous patient or with the second twin). Given good descent of the head into the pelvis, an instrumental delivery may then be feasible.

Compound presentation of a limb alongside the fetal head may be managed expectantly, as long as progress is satisfactory and fetal distress does not intervene.[2] The limb will often retract as the head descends, and a normal delivery can be anticipated. Shoulder presentations and other compound presentations necessitate delivery by caesarean section before significant maternal (ruptured uterus) or fetal trauma occurs. Delivery at caesarean section may be complicated by both lack of liquor and an inability to manoeuvre the fetus into a longitudinal lie. Consideration should therefore be given to a vertical uterine incision.

KEY POINTS

- Cord prolapse is managed by replacement of cord into the vagina, elevation of the presenting part and immediate delivery (usually by caesarean section) [IV].
- Compound presentation involving a limb alongside the vertex often resolves and may lead to vaginal delivery if progress is satisfactory [IV].
- All other compound presentations/shoulder presentation necessitate delivery by caesarean section if the fetus is still alive [IV].
- Delivery at caesarean section may be extremely difficult.

CONCLUSION

Malpresentation may occur by chance, but is often associated with abnormalities of the fetus, uterus or pelvis. It is associated with increased perinatal morbidity and mortality due to both antenatal and intrapartum factors. Where possible, detailed ultrasound assessment is advised to guide management. Caesarean section may be the safest option for both the mother and fetus in many cases, and is now recommended by the RCOG for singleton breech presentation at term where ECV has failed, was not indicated or was declined. Given the mass of trial data and meta-analysis in the Cochrane Database, the management of breech presentation is a likely topic for the MRCOG Part 2 examination.

KEY REFERENCES

1. RCOG. *The Management of Breech Presentation.* RCOG Guideline No. 20. London: RCOG Press, 2001.
2. Ritchie JWK. Malpositions of the occiput and malpresentations. In: Whitfield CR (ed.). *Dewhurst's Textbook of Obstetrics and Gynaecology for Postgraduates.* Oxford: Blackwell Science, 1995, 346–420.
3. Hickok DE, Gordon DC, Milberg JA, Williams MA, Daling JR. The frequency of breech presentation by gestational age at birth: a large population-based study. *Am J Obstet Gynecol* 1992; **166**(3):851–2.
4. Rayl J, Gibson PJ, Hickok DE. A population-based case-control study of risk factors for breech presentation. *Am J Obstet Gynecol* 1996; **174**(1 Pt 1):28–32.
5. Penn ZJ. Breech presentation. In: James DK, Steer PJ, Weiner CP, Gonik B (eds). *High Risk Pregnancy Management Options.* London: WB Saunders, 1999, 1025–50.
6. Schutte MF, van Hemel OJ, van de Berg C, van de Pol A. Perinatal mortality in breech presentations as compared to vertex presentations in singleton pregnancies: an analysis based upon 57819 computer-registered pregnancies in The Netherlands. *Eur J Obstet Gynecol Reprod Biol* 1985; **19**(6):391–400.
7. Nelson KB, Ellenberg JH. Antecedents of cerebral palsy. Multivariate analysis of risk. *N Engl J Med* 1986; **315**(2):81–6.
8. Hannah ME, Hannah WJ, Hewson SA, Hodnett ED, Saigal S, Willan AR. Planned caesarean section versus planned vaginal birth for breech presentation at term: a randomised multicentre trial. Term Breech Trial Collaborative Group. *Lancet* 2000; **356**(9239):1375–83.
9. Hannah ME, Hannah WJ, Hodnett ED et al. Outcomes at 3 months after planned cesarean vs planned vaginal delivery for breech presentation at term: the international andomized Term Breech Trial. *J Am Med Assoc* 2002; **287**(14):1822–31.
10. Hofmeyr GJ, Hannah ME. Planned Caesarean section for term breech delivery (Cochrane Review). In: *The Cochrane Library*, Issue 2. Oxford: Update Software, 2002.
11. Hofmeyr GJ. External cephalic version facilitation for breech presentation at term (Cochrane Review). In: *The Cochrane Library*, Issue 2. Oxford: Update Software, 2002.
12. Hofmeyr GJ. External cephalic version for breech presentation before term (Cochrane Review). In: *The Cochrane Library*, Issue 2. Oxford: Update Software, 2002.
13. Fernandez CO, Bloom SL, Smulian JC, Ananth CV, Wendel GD Jr. A randomized placebo-controlled evaluation of terbutaline for external cephalic version. *Obstet Gynecol* 1997; **90**(5):775–9.
14. Green PM, Wilkinshaw S. Management of breech deliveries. *Obstet Gynecol* 2002; **4**(2):87–91.
15. *Confidential Enquiry into Stillbirths and Deaths in Infancy.* 7th Annual Report. London: Maternal and Child Health Research Consortium, 2000.
16. Posner LB, Rubin EJ, Posner AC. Face and brow presentation: a continuing study. *Obstet Gynecol* 1963; **21**:745–9.
17. Chua S, Arulkumaran S. Poor progress in labor including augmentaion, malpositions and malpresentations. In: James DK, Steer PJ, Weiner CP, Gonik B (eds). *High Risk Pregnancy Management Options.* London: WB Saunders, 1999, 1103–20.
18. MacKenzie IZ. Unstable lie. In: James DK, Steer PJ, Weiner CP, Gonik B (eds). *High Risk Pregnancy Management Options.* London: WB Saunders, 1999, 1051–6.

Chapter 19

Prolonged Pregnancy

Murray Luckas

MRCOG standards

There are no established standards for this topic, but we would suggest the following points for guidance.

- Understand the definition of prolonged pregnancy and be able to distinguish it from post-maturity.
- Understand the controversies in the management of prolonged pregnancy.
- Be able to counsel a woman about the risks of prolonged pregnancy.

INTRODUCTION

Prolonged pregnancy is a cause of anxiety for both women and obstetricians. It is a common situation and is perceived as being a cause of increased risk to the fetus. In addition, many women find the physical burden of pregnancy at or near term to be intolerable and the concept of having to go past their estimated date of confinement unbearable. Nevertheless, debate continues over the merits of a policy of routine induction of labour at a set gestation to avoid the risks compared with a conservative wait-and-see approach.

Fetal and neonatal risks of post-term pregnancies

Post-term pregnancy per se is not a pathological condition and should not be confused with the post-maturity syndrome described by Clifford in 1954.[1] This syndrome closely resembles intrauterine growth restriction, with associations with meconium-stained amniotic fluid, oligohydramnios and fetal distress and evidence of loss of subcutaneous fat and dry, cracked skin reflecting placental insufficiency. It is apparent that not every post-term pregnancy is complicated by the post-maturity syndrome, but it is likely that the majority of

morbidity and mortality associated with post-term pregnancies arises because of post-maturity.

It has long been recognized that post-term pregnancies are associated with excess perinatal mortality and morbidity. It would appear that, unlike the 37–42-week period in which antepartum deaths contribute about two-thirds of the total, in prolonged pregnancies antepartum deaths are similar in frequency to intrapartum and neonatal deaths.[2] However, the exact risks of fetal death are a matter of ongoing debate. In the older data sets, about 25 per cent of the excess mortality risk in post-term pregnancy can be accounted for by lethal congenital abnormalities, mainly due to cranial neural tube defects, which, by their very nature, are more likely to result in post-term pregnancy. Butler and Bonham showed that delivery at 42 weeks of gestation was associated with a doubling of the perinatal mortality rate compared with delivery at 39–41 weeks; however, congenital abnormalities were not excluded.[3] Nevertheless, the doubling in the induction rates between 1958 and 1970 was partly attributable to an attempt to reduce the numbers of post-term pregnancies.

Analysis of post-term pregnancy in Dublin[2] demonstrated that total stillbirth rates were not significantly different in term and post-term pregnancies. A different picture emerges, however, when the data are analysed in a gestation-specific manner, and the risk of fetal demise is expressed in terms of ongoing pregnancies at that gestation. A retrospective analysis of 171 527 notified births in the UK revealed a rate of 2.3 stillbirths/1000 total births at term (37–41 weeks) and 1.9/1000 post-term. When calculated per 1000 ongoing pregnancies, however, the rate of stillbirth increased from 0.86/1000 at 40 weeks to 2.12/1000 at 43 weeks – almost a three-fold increase.[4] The same study demonstrated that the neonatal and post-neonatal mortality rates double from 1.57/1000 at 40 weeks to 3.71/1000 at 43 weeks.

Where lethal congenital abnormalities were excluded, intrapartum fetal death was four times more common and neonatal death was three times more common in infants born after 42 weeks' gestation. In addition, meconium staining of the amniotic fluid and the need for intrapartum fetal blood sampling were much more common in post-term pregnancies compared to those delivered at 40 weeks.[2]

Prolonged pregnancy is thus associated with an increased risk not only of meconium staining of the liquor, but also of intrapartum fetal hypoxia, which may result in fetal acidosis, neonatal seizures and perinatal death.[5] Post-term pregnancy is also a risk factor for birth trauma and shoulder dystocia.

Maternal risks of post-term pregnancy

Maternal risks of post-term pregnancies include increased operative delivery, haemorrhage and maternal infection. In addition, post-term pregnancies are associated with considerable psychological morbidity.[6] The pregnancy is perceived by many women as becoming high risk once the estimated date of confinement is passed; this leads to increased maternal anxiety.

DEFINITIONS

The definition of post-term pregnancy varies. However, the standard international definition accepted by both the World Health Organization (WHO) and the International Federation of Gynecology and Obstetrics (FIGO) is 42 completed weeks or more (294 days or more).

INCIDENCE

Using the definition of 294 days, the incidence of post-term pregnancy lies between 4 and 14 per cent; the average incidence is 10 per cent.[7] It is recognized that women who attend late for antenatal care may be of uncertain gestation and may be over-represented in populations of post-term pregnancies. Dating by the last menstrual period (LMP) alone has a tendency to overestimate the gestational age. Gardosi et al. have argued that most pregnancies that are induced for post-term are not, in fact, post-term when assessed by ultrasound dates. The use of early ultrasound alone to calculate the rate of post-term pregnancy in women who laboured spontaneously significantly reduced the post-term rate from 9.5 per cent to 1.5 per cent.[8]

Meta-analysis of four randomized, controlled trials (RCTs) included in a Cochrane Review has demonstrated that the routine use of early ultrasound to calculate gestational age significantly reduces the incidence of post-term pregnancy.[9] It is therefore apparent that accurate calculation of the estimated date of confinement using ultrasound will have a significant effect in reducing the incidence of post-term pregnancy [Ia].

AETIOLOGY

The cause of prolonged pregnancy is not clear and it may represent simple biological variation. Post-term pregnancy is more common in primigravid women, and those with a single previous post-term pregnancy have a 30 per cent chance of recurrence.

Infants who suffer fetal distress at term have elevated cortisol levels, whereas those with fetal distress post-term have reduced cortisol levels. A relative adrenocortical insufficiency may contribute to a delay in the onset of labour and an increased risk of intrapartum hypoxia or even death in post-term pregnancy. Further support for the theory that some infants born post-term may have an inherent biological defect comes from the fact that infants delivered following a post-term pregnancy are at increased risk of demise up to 2 years of age. Sudden infant death syndrome is also more common in infants born after 41 completed weeks of gestation. However, the hypothesis that post-term fetuses are fundamentally different from term fetuses remains unproven.

Amniotic fluid volumes fall in otherwise normal post-term pregnancies.[10] However, there appears to be no deterioration in cardiac output in post-term fetuses in otherwise uncomplicated pregnancies, compared to term fetuses. Doppler velocimetry in uterine, umbilical, middle cerebral, thoracic descending aorta and renal arteries in uncomplicated post-term pregnancies is no different from that in term pregnancies. Long-term pulse interval measured by computerized evaluation of the fetal heart rate correlates with fetal oxygenation and seems to fall progressively from 41 weeks.[11]

MANAGEMENT

The data from 19 RCTs comparing elective induction of labour have been included in a systematic review, which now governs policy for many units.[9] The conclusions of the analysis favour a policy of induction of labour at 41+ weeks because of reduced perinatal mortality, decreased meconium staining of the amniotic fluid and a small decrease in caesarean section, compared to conservative management [Ia]. However, the extent to which generalizations may be made from the meta-analysis has been questioned because of the high caesarean section rate and the low number of perinatal deaths in the conservatively managed groups in the trials (2.3/1000). Analysis of perinatal death rates in both groups reveals that 460 women will have to be induced at 41+ weeks to potentially prevent one perinatal death.[12]

Further criticism comes from the fact that the largest included trial[13] prohibited the use of prostaglandin in the induction process of conservatively managed women, whereas it was used in women undergoing routine induction, a bias which may have accounted for the significant reduction in caesarean delivery seen in this trial. Proponents of conservative management claim that sophisticated fetal monitoring can reduce this excess perinatal mortality, but there are no trial data to support this.

Other interventions designed to reduce the incidence of post-term pregnancy include nipple stimulation, but have not been shown to be of benefit [Ia].[9] However, sweeping the membranes at or beyond 40 weeks does appear to significantly reduce the incidence of post-term pregnancy[14] and should be offered to women [II].

MONITORING POST-TERM PREGNANCY
(see Chapter 14)

There is no consensus about what constitutes appropriate surveillance for post-term pregnancy.[15] The perinatal mortality rate does not significantly rise until 42 weeks' gestation and it is thus illogical to offer fetal monitoring prior to this gestation if it is not offered at term [IV].

Stemming from the work of Crowley et al.,[16] some form of measurement of the amniotic fluid volume usually forms part of the assessment [II]. It has been suggested that amniotic fluid index (AFI) is preferable to maximum pool depth (MPD) liquor volume assessment in these pregnancies. However, there is still debate about what constitutes the best cut-off values for both measurements, as liquor volumes fall after term. (For example, values of 4.2 cm, 3 cm and 2.1 cm for MVPD have all been advocated.) There is only one RCT of the two methodologies for liquor assessment; use of the AFI did not improve perinatal outcomes but was associated with an increase in the intervention rate.[5] Thus MPD is probably the tool of choice for assessing liquor in these post-term pregnancies [Ib]. More complex fetal monitoring with a formal biophysical scoring system has been suggested, but an RCT shows that it holds no advantage over simple monitoring with non-stress test (NST) cardiotocography (CTG) and liquor assessment [Ib].[15]

On the basis of observational data,[17] the NST CTG is usually applied, although it is of no proven benefit [III]. It has been suggested that computerized CTG may be superior to conventional CTG, but this has yet to be tested in clinical trials. The use of Doppler analysis of various fetal arterial systems has also been advocated in the assessment of post-term pregnancies, but again this has not been evaluated by RCT. In addition, complex arterial Doppler assessment is not suitable as a screening tool in standard practice. The use of umbilical artery Doppler is claimed to be of benefit; however, the alterations in the waveforms are subtle.[18]

Patient preference is also given as a reason for conservative management; however, in the largest study to date, only 31 per cent of women at 41 weeks' gestation were agreeable to conservative management despite this being the unit's policy.[6] Despite this, many women will see induction as interference with a natural process, and loss of maternal choice is a major determinant of maternal dissatisfaction with the

management of pregnancy and labour. It is therefore vital that each woman is treated on an individual basis and counselled regarding the risks of post-term pregnancy, to allow her to make her own decision about induction.

- Systematic review of four RCTs indicates that the use of early ultrasound dating reduces the incidence of post-term pregnancy.
- Systematic review of 19 RCTs indicates that induction of labour after 41+ weeks reduces perinatal mortality rates and may also reduce caesarean section rates.
- One RCT demonstrates that sweeping the membranes significantly reduces the incidence of post-term pregnancy.
- No clear evidence exists to support the hypothesis that fetal monitoring can reduce the perinatal mortality in post-term pregnancy.
- Uncontrolled studies support the use of NST CTG and liquor assessment in monitoring post-term pregnancy.
- MPD is the tool of choice for monitoring liquor in post-term pregnancy.

KEY POINTS

- Post-term pregnancy is a condition that continues to evoke anxiety in clinicians and women alike.
- Assessing the perinatal mortality rate underestimates the risk; it is appropriate to calculate the risk of stillbirth in terms of ongoing pregnancies at a particular gestation, and this gives a six-fold increase in risk from 37 to 43 weeks' gestation.
- Induction of labour at 41+ weeks significantly reduces the perinatal mortality rate and possibly the caesarean section rate. Nevertheless, some women will opt for conservative management with fetal surveillance.
- Available data suggest that the simplest monitoring is as effective as more sophisticated testing. Amniotic fluid volume assessment by MVPD is the test of choice. The role of CTG, or indeed the type of CTG, remains to be determined.

KEY REFERENCES

1. Clifford S. Postmaturity with placental dysfunction. *J Pediatr* 1954; **44**:1–13.
2. Crowley P. Post-term pregnancy: induction or surveillance? In: Chalmers I, Enkin M, Kierse M (eds).

Effective Care in Pregnancy and Childbirth. Oxford: Oxford University Press, 1989, 776–91.

3. Butler N, Bonham D. *Perinatal Mortality.* Edinburgh: Churchill Livingstone, 1963.

4. Hilder L, Costeloe K, Thilaganathan B. Prolonged pregnancy: evaluating gestation-specific risks of fetal and infant mortality. *Br J Obstet Gynaecol* 1998; 105:169–73.

5. Alfirevic Z, Luckas M, Walkinshaw SA, McFarlane M, Curran R. A randomised comparison between amniotic fluid index and maximum pool depth in the monitoring of post-term pregnancy. *Br J Obstet Gynaecol* 1997; 104:207–11.

6. Roberts LJ, Young KR. The management of prolonged pregnancy – an analysis of women's attitudes before and after term. *Br J Obstet Gynaecol* 1991; 98:1102–6.

7. Bakketeig LS, Bergsjo P. Post-term pregnancy: magnitude of the problem. In; Chalmers I, Enkin M, Kierse M (eds). *Evidence-based Care in Pregnancy.* Oxford: Oxford University Press, 1989, 765–75.

8. Gardosi J, Vanner T, Francis A. Gestational age and induction of labour for prolonged pregnancy. *Br J Obstet Gynaecol* 1997; 104:792–7.

9. Crowley P. Interventions for preventing or improving the outcome of delivery at or beyond term. *Cochrane Database Syst Rev* 2000, CD000170.

10. Nwosu EC, Welch CR, Manasse PR, Walkinshaw SA. Longitudinal assessment of amniotic-fluid index. *Br J Obstet Gynaecol* 1993; 100:816–19.

11. Mandruzzato G, Meir YJ, Dottavio G, Conoscenti G, Dawes GS. Computerised evaluation of fetal heart rate in post-term fetuses: long term variation. *Br J Obstet Gynaecol* 1998; 105:356–9.

12. Grant JM. Induction of labour confers benefit in prolonged pregnancy. *Br J Obstet Gynaecol* 1994; 101:99–102.

13. Hannah ME, Hannah WJ, Hellmann J, Hewson S, Milner R, Willan A. Induction of labor as compared with serial antenatal monitoring in post-term pregnancy. A randomized controlled trial. The Canadian Multicenter Post-term Pregnancy Trial Group. *N Engl J Med* 1992; 326:1587–92. [Published erratum appears in *N Engl J Med* 1992; 327(5):368.]

14. Allott HA, Palmer CR. Sweeping the membranes: a valid procedure in stimulating the onset of labour? [see Comments]. *Br J Obstet Gynaecol* 1993; 100:898–903.

15. Alfirevic Z, Walkinshaw SA. A randomised controlled trial of simple compared with complex antenatal fetal monitoring after 42 weeks of gestation. *Br J Obstet Gynaecol* 1995; 102:638–43.

16. Crowley P, O'Herlihy C, Boylan P. The value of ultrasound measurement of amniotic fluid volume in the management of prolonged pregnancies. *Br J Obstet Gynaecol* 1984; 91:444–8.

17. Fleischer A, Schulman H, Farmakides G, Perrotta LA, McGovern G, Katz N. Antepartum nonstress test and the postmature pregnancy. *Obstet Gynecol* 1985; 66:80–3.

18. Fischer RL, Kuhlman KA, Depp R, Wapner RJ. Doppler evaluation of umbilical and uterine-arcuate arteries in the postdates pregnancy. *Obstet Gynecol* 1991; 78:363–8.

Antenatal complications: fetal

Routine Intrapartum Care: An Overview

Harold Gee

MRCOG standards

Theoretic skills
- Revise anatomy of uterus (corpus and cervix) and birth canal.
- Understand the endocrinology and pharmacology governing labour.
- Understand the biochemistry controlling corpus and cervix in labour.
- Know the stages of labour.
- Know the definitions of labour descriptors.
- Understand fetal response in labour.

Practical skills
- Be able to interpret routine data collected in labour.
- Be able to define normal and abnormal progress in labour.
- Know how to manage delay in labour.
- Be able to interpret fetal monitoring and act appropriately.
- Be confident in operative skills: caesarean section and instrumental vaginal delivery.

Definitions

- *Presentation*: that anatomical part of the fetus which presents itself first through the birth canal.
- *Denominator*: an arbitrary point on the presenting part, chosen by convention, to describe the relationship of the presenting part to the birth canal.
- *Position*: the relationship between the denominator and the birth canal for any given presentation.
- *Lie*: the relationship between the long axis of the fetus and the long axis of the uterus.
- *Attitude*: whether the presenting part is flexed or de-flexed.
- *Engagement*: when the widest part of the presenting part has passed through the brim of the true pelvis.
- *Station*: the relationship between the lowest point of the presenting part and the ischial spines.

Stages of labour:

First: from the onset of labour to full dilatation of the cervix.
Process: cervical effacement and dilatation.

Second: from full dilatation of the cervix to delivery of the baby.
Process: descent of the fetus through the birth canal.

Third: from delivery of the baby to delivery of placenta and membranes.
Process: delivery of placenta and membranes.

INTRODUCTION

Our current concepts of labour management began during the 1960s and 1970s.

The association between prolonged labour and increased morbidity and mortality was recognized. It was reasonable to assume that correction of delay would avoid the sequelae.

Friedman's documentation and graphical representation of cervical dilatation and descent of the presenting part offered the prospect of early detection of aberrant progress.

In the equation governing progress, only the powers were considered open to manipulation. The other two variables, the passages and passenger, could only be influenced indirectly via the powers. Oxytocin provided the means. A pragmatic step was taken to use intravenous oxytocin on a 'try and see' basis to augment the powers, correct delay and resolve the problems of prolonged labour.[1] The enthusiasm for the perceived benefits overtook scientific evaluation. Problems with poor progress remained, and still do. Not until the 1990s was practice questioned. Since that time, randomized, controlled clinical trials and meta-analyses have shown that although rule-of-thumb interventions such as oxytocin augmentation to correct poor progress and routine amniotomy may speed up labour, they do not improve clinical outcomes [Ia].[2-6] This is not to say that management strategies that include these have no merit, but the effective items in the packages, for example the correct diagnosis of labour, psychological support of the woman in labour and one-to-one midwifery care, have been overlooked.[7]

THE ONSET OF LABOUR

Labour is physiological but, despite its frequency and the apparent simplicity of the uterus, its essential features remain poorly understood. The myometrium changes from quiescence in pregnancy to rhythmic, forceful activity in labour, while, simultaneously, the cervix loses its rigidity to become compliant. There are common mediators for these changes but they have different effects on myometrium and cervix, for example oestrogens and prostaglandins. Furthermore, and this makes investigation more difficult, these agents are often paracrine in their activity, i.e. they have their effects over short distances. For example, the decidua and membranes, which produce prostaglandins, are in direct contact with the myometrium and cervix on which they act.

Progesterone inhibits labour. Oestrogens and prostaglandins are facilitatory, and oxytocin maintains labour once the process has begun. Though there are changes in the balance of these hormones, no single 'trigger' for labour has been defined in the human. Evidence indicates that the fetus has a part to play (Figure 20.1). Placental corticotrophin-releasing hormone (PCRH) acts on the fetal pituitary to stimulate adrenal corticosteroid production via adrenocorticotrophic hormone (ACTH). Dehydroepiandrostenedione (DHEA) from the adrenal is metabolized by the placenta, producing a rise in maternal oestriol. Progesterone down-regulates the PCRH gene, while adrenal steroids up-regulate it. The sensitivity of the gene is greater to adrenal steroids than to progesterone. Thus, during most of pregnancy, progesterone is dominant, but small increments in DHEA will up-regulate the gene and at some point 'switch' it over to large output of PCRH through stimulation of a positive feedback loop in the fetus.

In the mother, rising oestriol has many effects. It changes smooth muscle cell membrane potentials towards their firing threshold, thereby increasing spontaneous activity. It induces prostaglandin synthesis in the decidua and promotes cervical ripening.

No sudden fall in peripheral serum progesterone has been demonstrated in the human, though it has in other mammals. However, there is a relative reduction in its effect as oestrogen levels rise. Furthermore, as the uterus grows, the placental implantation site, relative to the total internal uterine surface, decreases. Thus, more of the myometrium escapes the paracrine suppressive effect of progesterone from the placenta. Uterine distension itself increases spontaneous activity of the myometrium.

No sudden change in circulating oxytocin levels has been detected at the onset of labour but prostaglandins from the decidua potentiate oxytocin, that is to say the activity produced by the action of oxytocin plus prostaglandin is more than the sum of their individual effects alone. Oxytocin binds to specific receptors, opening calcium-activated channels and depolarizing the cell membrane. This depolarization, in turn, opens voltage-dependent calcium channels, resulting in an influx of calcium ions, action potentials and contractions. Thus, spontaneous smooth muscle activity increases. However, propagation across the myometrium is slowed, ensuring more muscle fibres are active for any single source. This source can be effective from anywhere in the myometrium – not, as was once thought, only in the cornua. The result is a more rhythmic, co-ordinated myometrium. Release of prostaglandins with contractions further stimulates this positive feedback system in the mother.

Positive feedback loops carry potential dangers. They have no built-in safety mechanism, as do negative feedbacks. Care has to be exercised when stimulating these systems, for example when augmenting uterine activity in an attempt to correct delay.

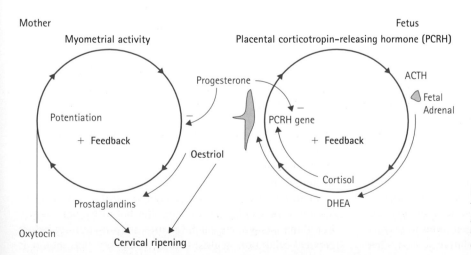

Figure 20.1 Maternal and fetal positive feedback systems in the initiation of labour. ACTH, adrenocorticotrophic hormone; DHEA, dehydroepiandrostenedione; PCRH, placental corticotrophin-releasing hormone

UTERINE PHYSIOLOGY IN LABOUR

Myometrium

Smooth muscle cells are spontaneously active. Contractions occur in the myometrium throughout pregnancy. However, pregnancy activity is decremental, i.e. activity arising in one cell is unlikely to activate many of its neighbours. Oestrogens and prostaglandins develop specialized gap junctions between muscle cells that preferentially conduct electrical potentials. Thus, under their influence at the time of labour, spontaneous activity becomes propagated.

The myometrium develops tension. In the first stage of labour, contractions are virtually isometric, i.e. tension is developed without significant change in length. This results in a rise in intrauterine pressure (IUP). IUP can be measured with catheters and intrauterine transducers, but because repetition frequency, amplitude and duration are physiologically linked, albeit non-linearly, semi-objective assessment by timing of repetition frequency and duration is adequate for clinical needs [Ia].[8]

In the second stage, contractions become isotonic, i.e. there is shortening of the muscle fibres as the uterine contents are expelled, with little change in tension. Permanent shortening is known as retraction. Retraction of the fibres compresses blood vessels as they traverse the myometrium to the placenta, and at the same time a shrinking placental implantation site shears off the placenta. Separation of the placenta and control of blood supply to the placenta are crucial to the prevention of haemorrhage in the third stage, although the process begins at some point in the second. These physiological changes may account for some of the fetal heart rate irregularities seen at full dilatation and into the second stage.

The cervix and cervical ripening

The cervix consists primarily of connective tissue in which collagen fibres are embedded in ground substance. Collagen is inelastic and highly tensile (strong). Ground substance is a gel. Its physical properties can be changed rapidly depending on its chemical composition and physical attributes, for example degree of hydration. Gelatin, which constitutes the jelly that we eat, is the most familiar example of a ground substance. In its concentrated form it is hard and rubbery, but when treated with water and/or heated, it softens and flows.

During cervical ripening, structural glycoproteins (dermatin sulphate and chondroitin sulphate) that bind collagen are reduced in concentration, while 'packing' glycoproteins without such affinity (heparan sulphate) increase. Hyaluronic acid, which carries with it water, also increases, thereby increasing hydration of the connective tissue. These changes in the ground substance allow the collagen fibres to become more loosely packed and able to move relative to each other.

Thus, the cervix changes from its pregnancy state – a rigid, tubular structure, whose canal is held closed by tightly wound, circumferential, collagen fibres bonded together by a firm ground substance – to one in which the ground substance becomes fluid, permitting change in the whole form of the cervix, with the effect that its resistance to delivery is reduced. The process by which tissue is redistributed from the cervix is recognized as *effacement* and the reduction in resistance it produces facilitates subsequent dilatation. The redistributed connective tissue helps to form the lower segment (with which every obstetrician is familiar), despite the fact that the processes and anatomical changes are more conceptual than precisely known.

EFFECTS OF LABOUR ON THE FETUS

Contractions affect placental blood flow. Observations in vivo suggest that significant impairment takes place when the intrauterine pressure rises above 35 mmHg (about half to two-thirds maximum IUP) during physiological contractions. During this time, the fetus may experience transient hypoxaemia. The response of a healthy fetus to this may be bradycardia. Bradycardia may also be caused by the response of baroreceptors in the circulatory system to external IUP. Head compression during contractions may also produce the same response. Thus, decelerations on cardiotocography may arise from physiological changes in the fetal environment, none of which is going to harm the fetus. Even the hypoxaemia is only transient, providing there is adequate recovery time between contractions. However, if hyperstimulation is induced, this may not be the case; poor utero-placental function may impair recovery, and growth-restricted fetuses may not have the energy reserves to maintain anaerobic metabolism during periods of hypoxia. In these instances, labour itself may pose a threat to the fetus.

CLINICAL DIAGNOSIS OF LABOUR

This is perhaps the single most crucial point in labour management.

Labour is recognized by the combination of two features:

- regular, purposeful uterine activity (contractions),
- cervical change,

but there are many vagaries here. Is there a threshold to define labour's uterine activity? No. Does cervical change mean effacement or has there to be evidence of dilatation? Opinions differ.

Friedman defined labour as regular painful contractions. Most women would identify with this, but often, particularly in nulliparous women, such features are present long before cervical dilatation begins. Others would say that labour is established only when there is progressive cervical dilatation and anything prior to this is 'pre-labour'. This may appear merely to be a matter of semantics, but *when applying limits to progress it is essential they are applied only to that part of labour for which they were designed.*

In practice, cervicograms describe cervical dilatation in the active phase of labour. Thus, for practical purposes, it is better to diagnose 'labour' only when there is evidence of progressive cervical dilatation to indicate entry into the active phase, i.e. cervical dilatation at, or beyond, 3 cm. There is another reason for this. Oxytocin augmentation for poor progress (slow cervical dilatation) is relatively ineffective in the latent phase. Thus, when women present in early labour (<3 cm), particularly if they are nulliparous, check that all is well with mother and baby, explain that preparation is under way for progressive labour, be patient and buy time. Once 3 cm has been reached and there is evidence of progressive cervical change, diagnose that active labour is established and start cervicograph monitoring.

PROGRESS IN LABOUR

Classically, progress is defined in terms of:

- powers
- passenger
- passages.

Powers

Efficient contractions impart tension to the cervix and produce dilatation in the first stage and, coupled with maternal effort, rotation and descent in the second. Flexion and rotation of the presenting part depend on good expulsive forces. There is no doubt that efficient powers are at the centre of efficient labour, and in any labour showing poor progress, poor uterine activity should be excluded first and treated.

Measurement of IUP appears a precise and objective way to quantify the forces, and there are several indices of uterine activity derived from the pressure measurement. However, the interpretation is not simple, and observation of contraction rate, duration and subjective assessment by an experienced attendant have been found to be adequate for clinical practice, with no advantage from invasive monitoring.[8] IUP is used mainly as a research tool but may be indicated when contractions are difficult to palpate, for example in obese patients.

Paradoxes

There are everyday paradoxes that indicate power/force and progress are not always in a simple, direct relationship.

- Multiparous women have faster labours than nulliparous and expend less uterine activity and power. Thus, less force can result in better progress.

- Precipitate spontaneous labour may be associated with low levels of uterine activity. Any reported morbidity associated with such deliveries usually results from delivery in unprepared settings rather than from the labour itself.
- Many premature deliveries take place with minimal uterine activity.

These paradoxes can be explained if resistance, for example from the cervix, is taken into account. Reduction of resistance may prove more physiological than increasing force, especially if uterine activity already appears to be adequate. The problem remains that the means to these ends are not currently available – only the powers are easily manipulated.

Passages

These have usually been considered in terms only of the bony pelvis, with the soft tissues taking second place. However, the cervix offers resistance to delivery in the first stage (that has been its prime function for the whole of pregnancy) and the perineum does so in the later part of the second stage. Poor ripening and abnormal glycoprotein balance in the cervix have been associated with poor progress. Perhaps the soft tissues should be considered more in future.

Passenger

There is statistical evidence for slight increases in birth weight over time, but these are unlikely to be clinically significant. The presenting part offers complex geometry to the birth canal. Flexion and rotation are all-important for an efficient mechanism.

FRIEDMAN'S DIVISION OF LABOUR AND GRAPHIC REPRESENTATION OF PROGRESS (Figure 20.2)

The first stage of labour was subdivided by Friedman into two main phases: latent and active. The latent phase is very variable because its onset is not precise. Friedman's data show that the latent phase in nulliparous women could last up to 20 hours (mean 8.6 hours), and 14 hours (mean 5.3 hours) in multiparae. During the latent phase there is relatively little dilatation, but effacement is taking place. Effacement and dilatation tend to be more discrete in first labours than in subsequent ones.

The active phase of dilatation is characterized by rapid, progressive dilatation of the cervix. Friedman divided the active phase further into three parts: phases of acceleration and deceleration on either side of the most important part, that of maximum slope. The phases of acceleration and deceleration have been questioned, but most cervicograms

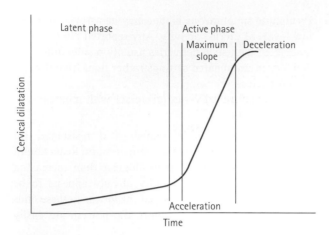

Figure 20.2   Friedman's division of labour

depict an accelerating rate of dilatation at the entry to the active phase and then an approximately linear section corresponding to Friedman's maximum slope.

Friedman identified 200 primigravidae retrospectively from a larger heterogeneous group of patients (a second paper follows the same practice for multigravidae) to identify 'ideal' labour, i.e. no iatrogenic interventions (apart from 'prophylactic low forceps'), vaginal deliveries and average-sized, healthy neonates. These patients' labour curves were analysed to identify statistical limits. Means and standard deviations were calculated.

From these data the lower limit of maximum slope dilatation of 1 cm/hour was produced. This value has now become almost universally accepted for clinical practice, but it may be an overestimate for the following two reasons.

1   The data are not normally distributed, with a tail skewed towards higher rates of dilatation. *No upper limit was set.*
2   Most clinicians use an average minimum of 1 cm/hour for the whole of the active phase, including the slower phases of acceleration and deceleration and not just the phase of maximum slope.

Progress in the second stage of labour is judged by descent and rotation of the presenting part. This can be done in two ways: by the amount of the presenting part palpable per abdomen or by the station of the presenting part on vaginal examination. The former is practical only with cephalic presentations. The latter can be performed with malpresentations and allows determination of position as well.

MONITORING

Partogram

The partogram (Figure 20.3) is a composite, graphical record of key data entered against time as labour progresses. Both maternal and fetal data are represented.

Maternal

- Vital signs (blood pressure, pulse rate, temperature, urinalysis).
- Uterine activity.
- Cervimetric progress.
- Drugs given.
- Analgesia.
- Fluid balance.

Fetal

- Heart rate.
- Descent/station.
- Presentation.
- Position.
- Liquor – membranes intact or not and presence of meconium.

The use of partograms with definitions of established labour and agreed policies for intervention has been shown to reduce the use of oxytocin, and to have small but significant benefits in terms of outcome [II].[9]

Cervicogram

An essential part of the partogram is the cervicogram. Vaginal examination to assess cervical dilatation may be performed 2, 3 or 4 hourly. The interval does not affect clinical outcome.

It is common practice to set an alert line at 1 cm/hour for the active phase dilatation and then an action line 2 hours later. The rationale for this is unclear. Philpott and Castle[10,11] were the first to use these terms, but their action line was 4 hours after the alert. Studd[12] set a 2-hour action line but, using his data, transgression of this limit gives only a 50:50 chance of accurately predicting the need for surgical intervention. It must be remembered that alert and action lines were not originally devised to indicate surgical intervention, but to enable attendants to make appropriate arrangements for surgical delivery should it be necessary. Today, in UK practice, where the vast majority of deliveries take place in fully equipped obstetric units, the use has changed without scientific verification.

Cervicograms should be aids to the management of labour. Aberrant progress and patterns thereof do not constitute a diagnosis in themselves. They are signs for which underlying diagnoses should be sought. This may not always be successful.

Uterine activity

Contractions are most commonly assessed by palpation and recorded as frequency per 10 minutes. Duration may also be timed. Uterine activity normally increases as the first stage progresses towards full dilatation. There is no fixed frequency or level of uterine activity for spontaneous, progressing

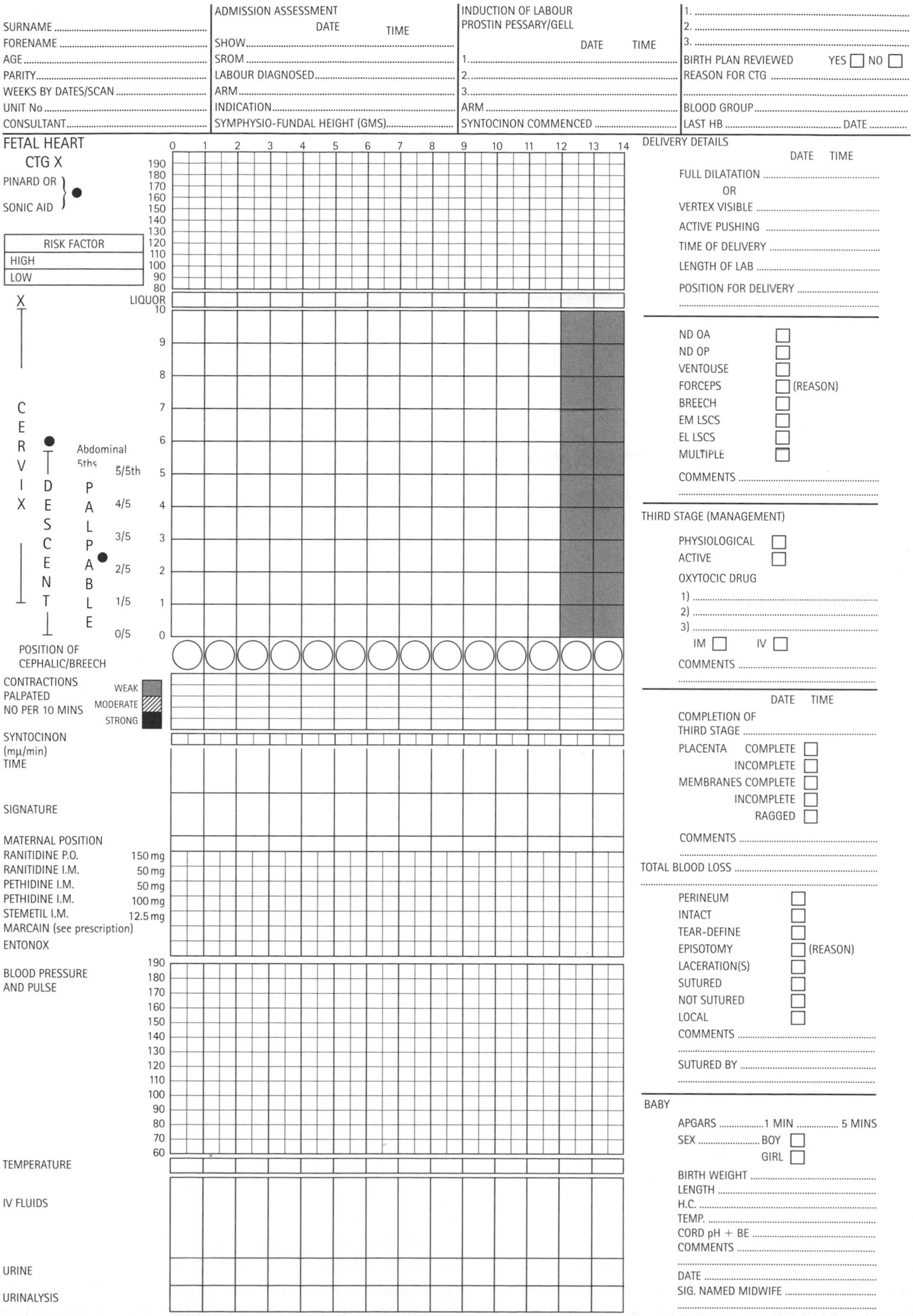

SURNAME ....

FORENAME ....

AGE ....

PARITY ....

WEEKS BY DATES/SCAN ....

UNIT No ....

CONSULTANT ....

ADMISSION ASSESSMENT

DATE   TIME

SHOW ....

SROM ....

LABOUR DIAGNOSED ....

ARM ....

INDICATION ....

SYMPHYSIO-FUNDAL HEIGHT (GMS) ....

INDUCTION OF LABOUR
PROSTIN PESSARY/GELL

DATE   TIME

1. ....

2. ....

3. ....

ARM ....

SYNTOCINON COMMENCED ....

1. ....

2. ....

3. ....

BIRTH PLAN REVIEWED   YES ☐ NO ☐

REASON FOR CTG ....

BLOOD GROUP ....

LAST HB .... DATE ....

FETAL HEART

CTG X

PINARD OR }
SONIC AID }   ●

RISK FACTOR
HIGH
LOW

X

C
E
R
V
I
X

D
E
S
C
E
N
T

P
A
L
P
A
B
L
E

Abdominal
5ths

5/5th
4/5
3/5
2/5
1/5
0/5

POSITION OF
CEPHALIC/BREECH

CONTRACTIONS
PALPATED
NO PER 10 MINS

WEAK
MODERATE
STRONG

SYNTOCINON
(mµ/min)
TIME

SIGNATURE

MATERNAL POSITION

RANITIDINE P.O.   150 mg
RANITIDINE I.M.   50 mg
PETHIDINE I.M.   50 mg
PETHIDINE I.M.   100 mg
STEMETIL I.M.   12.5 mg
MARCAIN (see prescription)
ENTONOX

BLOOD PRESSURE
AND PULSE

TEMPERATURE

IV FLUIDS

URINE

URINALYSIS

DELIVERY DETAILS

DATE   TIME

FULL DILATATION ....

OR

VERTEX VISIBLE ....

ACTIVE PUSHING ....

TIME OF DELIVERY ....

LENGTH OF LAB ....

POSITION FOR DELIVERY ....

....

ND OA   ☐
ND OP   ☐
VENTOUSE   ☐
FORCEPS   ☐ (REASON)
BREECH   ☐
EM LSCS   ☐
EL LSCS   ☐
MULTIPLE   ☐

COMMENTS ....
....

THIRD STAGE (MANAGEMENT)

PHYSIOLOGICAL ☐
ACTIVE   ☐

OXYTOCIC DRUG

1) ....
2) ....
3) ....

IM ☐   IV ☐

COMMENTS ....
....

DATE   TIME

COMPLETION OF
THIRD STAGE ....

PLACENTA   COMPLETE   ☐
            INCOMPLETE ☐
MEMBRANES COMPLETE   ☐
            INCOMPLETE ☐
            RAGGED   ☐

COMMENTS ....

TOTAL BLOOD LOSS ....

PERINEUM   ☐
INTACT   ☐
TEAR-DEFINE   ☐
EPISOTOMY   ☐ (REASON)
LACERATION(S) ☐
SUTURED   ☐
NOT SUTURED   ☐
LOCAL   ☐
COMMENTS ....
....

SUTURED BY ....

BABY

APGARS .... 1 MIN .... 5 MINS

SEX .... BOY ☐
            GIRL ☐

BIRTH WEIGHT ....

LENGTH ....

H.C. ....

TEMP. ....

CORD pH + BE ....

COMMENTS ....
....

DATE ....

SIG. NAMED MIDWIFE ....
....

Figure 20.3 A typical partogram

Obstetrics: intrapartum

labour. When augmentation is performed, three to four contractions per 10 minutes is taken as the upper limit.

External guard-ring tocodynamometers, as part of continuous electronic fetal heart rate monitoring, give no indication of amplitude. They will record repetition frequency but not necessarily the true duration, as positioning on the abdomen affects sensitivity.

Fetal monitoring

Fetal monitoring is performed in all labours. Low-risk labours should be monitored by intermittent auscultation by ear or by using hand-held Doppler devices. High-risk labours employ continuous electronic fetal heart rate monitoring. Either way, the rate is entered on the partogram every 15 minutes.

Posture

It has become customary in Western society for women to labour on beds in a recumbent position. Pregnant women should not lie supine, as this can produce vena caval compression and compromise the placental circulation. Conventional epidural analgesia limits mobility and may have contributed to current trends. If all is well, the labouring woman can adopt whatever position she finds most comfortable. Kneeling on all fours is commonly chosen. Maternal position has not been shown to affect fetal position or the mechanics of labour.

An upright posture for the second stage has been shown to increase spontaneous vaginal delivery, but perineal trauma and blood loss may be greater [Ia],[13] although there are few good-quality clinical trials.

Water births have been fashionable. Immersion in warm water plus buoyancy offers a soothing environment, which may relax the mother and reduce her requirement for analgesia. Delivery of the baby into water is more controversial and there are risks associated with the water temperature, infection and clearing the baby's oropharynx.

PROFESSIONAL ROLES

In the UK, the role of the midwife has been highly developed. The midwife is the expert in normal childbirth and will be in contact with the woman more than any other professional. (S)he should prepare the mother-to-be for labour, give her confidence and offer support, advice and encouragement during labour. This is crucial [Ia].[14] Ideally, there should be continuity of care so that the mother is familiar with her midwife. Even if this is not possible, there should be one-to-one midwifery care in labour. Midwives are independent practitioners and can thus offer total care to low-risk cases.

When complications are found, the midwife should liaise with the medical team to ensure continuity. The roles of midwife and obstetrician are complimentary. Even with medical need, the midwife will continue to collect and record data and support the woman through the rest of labour and delivery.

PSYCHOLOGICAL SUPPORT

Childbirth is a highly emotive event that engenders anxiety and apprehension for all concerned, but not least the mother. Such feelings can be ameliorated by surroundings familiar to the mother and by supportive companions, whether professional or otherwise. These are reasons why some women opt for home delivery. There has been, and still is, a long-running debate about the safety of home delivery. With careful selection and proper attention to contingencies, home delivery can be rewarding.

If the woman understands what is happening and is well prepared, she feels more in control. All too often, the delivery environment has focused on perceived medical need, and economies have eaten away at professional input to the preparation for labour. Management decisions may not be explained, thereby disempowering the woman. The result is apprehension and anxiety. These feelings may impact negatively on the labour in a number of ways, for example reduced pain threshold, need for more analgesia, increased stress hormones and muscular tension.

These 'soft' issues were once ignored, but of all the ploys in labour management, preparation and support of the woman have the strongest impact on clinical outcome [Ia].[14] Doulas (non-professional patient supporters) have been shown to be highly effective [Ia][15] and may have advantages over midwives in that they are not distracted from their prime purpose – supporting the labouring woman – by routine monitoring duties.

KEY POINTS FOR GOOD LABOUR MANAGEMENT

- Understand the physiology.
- Do not diagnose 'labour' until clearly established – evidence of progressive cervical dilatation ($\geqslant 3$ cm dilatation).
- Understand the monitoring and what it tells us.
- When there is aberrance, try to identify a diagnosis (though this may not always be possible).
- Understand interventions and identify what you want from them.
- Establish guidelines and practice on best available evidence.
- Agree guidelines across professional groups so that practice is consistent.
- Audit against these standards.
- **Prepare women for their labour and support and encourage them during it.**

KEY REFERENCES

1. O'Driscoll K, Jackson JA, Gallagher JT. Prevention of prolonged labour. *BMJ* 1969; **2**:447–80.

2. Thornton JG, Lilford RJ. Active management of labour: current knowledge and research issues. *BMJ* 1994; **309**:366–9.

3. Lopez-Zeno JA, Peaceman AM, Adashek JA et al. A controlled trial of a program for the active management of labor. *N Engl J Med* 1992; **326**:450–4.

4. Frigoletto FDJ, Lieberman E, Lang JM. A clinical trial of active management of labor. *N Engl J Med* 1995; **333**:745–50.

5. Cammu H, Van Eeckhout E. A randomised controlled trial of early versus delayed use of amniotomy and oxytocin infusion in nulliparous labour. *Br J Obstet Gynaecol* 1996; **103**:313–8.

6. Glantz JC, McNanley TJ. Active management of labor: a meta-analysis of cesarean delivery rates for dystocia in nulliparas. *Obstet Gynecol Surv* 1997; **52**:497–505.

7. Olah KS, Gee H. The active mismanagement of labour. *Br J Obstet Gynaecol* 1996; **103**(8):729–31.

8. Chua S, Kurup A, Aralkumaran et al. Augmentation of labour: does internal tocography result in better obstetric outcome. *Obstet Gynecol* 1990; **76**:164–7.

9. Anonymous. World Health Organization partograph in management of. *Lancet* 1994; **343**:1399–404.

10. Philpott RH, Castle WM. Cervicographs in the management of labour in primigravidae. I. The alert line for detecting abnormal labour. *J Obstet Gynaecol Br Commonwealth* 1972; **79**:592–8.

11. Philpott RH, Castle WM. Cervicographs in the management of labour in primigravidae. II. The action line and treatment of abnormal labour. *J Obstet Gynaecol Br Commonwealth* 1972; **79**:599–602.

12. Studd J. Partograms and nomograms of cervical dilatation in management of primigravid labour. *BMJ* 1973; **4**:451–5.

13. Gupta JK, Nikodem VC. Woman's position during seconds stage of labour. *Cochrane Syst Rev* 2000(4).

14. Scott KD, Berkowitz G, Klaus M. A comparison of intermittent and continuous support during labor: a meta-analysis. *Am J Obstet Gynecol* 1999; **180**:1054–9.

15. Klaus MH, Kennell JH. The doula: an essential ingredient of childbirth rediscovered. *Acta Paediat* 1997; **86**:1034–6.

SECTION C

Late pregnancy/intrapartum events

SECTION C

Preterm Labour

Griff Jones

INTRODUCTION

There are two major clinical subtypes of preterm births. Indicated preterm deliveries, undertaken for maternal or fetal reasons, make up approximately one-third of all such births. The remaining two-thirds are classified as spontaneous preterm births and have two subdivisions: (1) spontaneous preterm labour and (2) preterm pre-labour rupture of the membranes (PPROM).

DEFINITION

In the UK, preterm birth traditionally includes all deliveries between 24^{+0} and 36^{+6} weeks. Many developed countries now officially register all deliveries with a birth weight above 500 g.

In 1994–95, 6.6 per cent of all UK births were preterm, amounting to approximately 40 000 per annum. For reasons related to aetiology, outcome and recurrence risk, preterm deliveries should be divided into three gestational epochs: mildly preterm births at 32^{+0} to 36^{+6} weeks (incidence 5.5 per cent), moderately preterm births at 28^{+0} to 31^{+6} weeks (incidence 0.7 per cent) and extremely preterm births at 24^{+0} to 27^{+6} weeks (incidence 0.4 per cent).

Significantly higher rates of preterm birth of up to 12 per cent are reported from the USA. Conversely, many Nordic countries quote rates below 5 per cent. This must reflect differing aetiological, socio-economic and cultural factors.

NEONATAL OUTCOMES

Survival

When counselling parents, doctors must use perinatal statistics that are up to date and, where possible, reflect local outcomes. Figures from a total population within a UK Health Region have been published (Figure 21.1).[1] Predicted survival

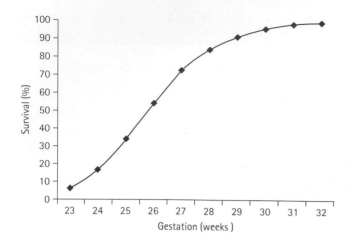

Figure 21.1   Median survival of European infants alive at the onset of labour in the Trent Health Region for 1994–97

can be modified by accurate estimates of fetal weight or antenatal assessments of fetal well-being.

Morbidity

The risks of later neurodevelopmental impairment, disability and handicap are especially significant within the 24–26-week gestational window. The recent UK-based EPIcure Study reported that 50 per cent of the survivors at 23–25 weeks' gestation were impaired, half with severe disability.[2] In another study, up to 40 per cent of survivors born before 26 weeks' gestation were found to have a head circumference below the 3rd centile at 2 years of age, after which little 'catch-up' growth is possible.[3] Follow-up of very low birth weight children to school age has also shown later educational difficulties. Additional concerns relate to social behaviour and criminality, as well as subsequent influences on adult health.

AETIOLOGY

Infection

Subclinical infection of the choriodecidual space and amniotic fluid is the most widely studied aetiological factor underlying spontaneous prematurity. Many indirect lines of evidence support the role of subclinical infection in human preterm labour, including the following.

- Vaginal colonization with a variety of micro-organisms has been associated with an increased risk of spontaneous prematurity. However, it is plausible that the presence of such pathogens may simply be markers for other socio-economic, sexual or behavioural factors that ultimately lead to preterm labour.

- If an amniocentesis is performed in preterm labour with intact membranes, 10–15 per cent of amniotic fluid samples result in positive cultures.[4]

- Histological chorioamnionitis is much commoner after spontaneous preterm birth.[5] Of note, most cases are subclinical, with only 10 per cent of histologically proven cases of chorioamnionitis having overt clinical signs of infection.

Vascular

Spontaneous prematurity has been associated with an increase in membrane haemosiderin deposits, thought to reflect decidual haemorrhages. The link between placental abruption and either uterine activity or PPROM is well recognized.

Uterine over-distension

Multiple pregnancy
In 1999, 1.44 per cent of all maternities in the UK involved multiple pregnancies. The vast majority were twin gestations. The median gestation at delivery for twins is approximately 35 weeks and for triplets 33 weeks. Presently, assisted reproduction techniques are responsible for 35 per cent of twin pregnancies and 77 per cent of triplets, leading to an increasing burden of preterm births. Multi-fetal reduction has been shown to reduce risk in higher order pregnancies and should always be considered.

Polyhydramnios
Fetal anomalies, such as atresias of the gastrointestinal tract, are the most common cause of polyhydramnios leading to preterm delivery.

Cervical weakness

This remains a notoriously difficult diagnosis to make either within or outside of pregnancy. Even a careful review of the clinical events leading up to preterm labour and delivery does not necessarily show correlation with the aetiology.

Intercurrent illness

Serious infective illnesses such as pyelonephritis, appendicitis and pneumonia are associated with preterm labour. This association is presumed to be due either to direct blood-borne spread of infection to the uterine cavity or indirectly to chemical triggers, such as endotoxins or cytokines. Many other medical complications, such as cholestasis of pregnancy, and any surgical procedures are associated with preterm labour, although the mechanisms remain obscure.

Relationship between gestation and aetiology

Studies involving the use of amniocentesis in threatened preterm labour found most positive amniotic fluid cultures to be from pregnancies presenting before 30 weeks' gestation. The incidence and severity of histological chorioamnionitis also show an inverse relationship with gestational age. Clearly, the earliest births carry the highest risk of an infectious aetiology.

Intrauterine infection has also been associated with an increased risk of various neonatal morbidities, independent of gestation at birth. These include:

- periventricular leukomalacia
- cerebral palsy
- bronchopulmonary dysplasia.

These pathologies are presumed to be secondary to high circulating levels of inflammatory cytokines. This leads to the paradox of prematurity, in that when there may be the most to gain by delaying delivery, leaving the fetus in utero may carry the greatest risk.

RISK GROUPS

Owing to limited resources and a paucity of beneficial interventions in low-risk women, most aspects of prematurity prevention should be targeted at women with major risk factors for preterm birth. These major risk factors include the following.

- *Previous preterm birth*. After one preterm birth, the risk in the next pregnancy is approximately 20 per cent. After two preterm deliveries, this risk increases to 35–40 per cent. Where the most recent birth was at term but the penultimate delivery was preterm, recurrence risks are intermediate. As well as a tendency for preterm births to recur in the same gestational age group, the earliest births have the highest recurrence risks.[6] This presumably reflects differing aetiologies predominating at different gestations.
- *Uterine over-distension*. Multiple pregnancies or pregnancies known to be at risk of polyhydramnios require careful monitoring.
- *Uterine abnormalities*. Cervical surgery such as cone biopsy remains a classic risk factor. Also, epidemiological evidence from Australia casts doubt on the benign nature of surgical cervical dilatation, the risk of subsequent preterm delivery increasing with the number of previous cervical dilatations.[7]
  Although there is little evidence upon which to estimate either individual risk or the total contribution to preterm births, the malformed uterus has long been associated with spontaneous prematurity. This may be mediated by cervical weakness, although recent evidence suggests that abnormalities of uterine vascularity may also play a role.

Maternal diethylstilboestrol (DES) exposure in the 1960s led to a cohort of female offspring with congenital uterine and cervical anomalies. The women in this cohort are now approaching the end of their reproductive years. The role of fibroids in preterm delivery remains controversial; considering their frequency, their influence is probably minimal in the absence of cervical involvement.

- *Factors in current pregnancy*. Examples include:
  - intercurrent illness
  - surgery
  - recurrent vaginal bleeding.

There is also a variety of minor risk factors for spontaneous preterm birth that carry importance in epidemiological terms. The relative risk attributable to each factor is small. Attempts have been made to develop scoring systems (such as the Creasy Score) but these have not proved helpful.

Some minor risk factors, such as:

- smoking
- low body mass index (BMI)
- interpregnancy interval of less than 1 year,

carry importance because they are potentially modifiable.

Others risk factors that are not amenable to influence include:

- maternal age (teenage multiparae)
- parity (primiparous or grandmultiparous)
- ethnicity (black women)
- socio-economic deprivation
- unemployment
- low levels of education.

MANAGEMENT OF ASYMPTOMATIC HIGH-RISK WOMEN

A careful analysis of events surrounding last birth must be undertaken. The risk of recurrence may be adjusted if there were non-recurring phenomena such as fetal anomaly or intercurrent illness.

Investigation and treatment outside of pregnancy

Ideally, women should be seen postnatally and the events leading to their preterm birth reviewed. The benefit of specialized tests of cervical and uterine anatomy such as hysterosalpingography is unproven. The most important thing to come from a postnatal visit is a clear management plan for any subsequent pregnancy [IV]. The importance of smoking cessation should be stressed [II] and the potential benefit of

Late pregnancy/intrapartum events

leaving 12 months between pregnancies should be discussed [II]. Dietician referral may be appropriate for women with a low BMI.

Investigation and treatment during pregnancy

Early dating scan

A first trimester dating scan is essential to time subsequent investigations. It also ensures precise gestational age assessment should preterm labour recur near the limits of neonatal viability [IV].

Bacterial vaginosis

Bacterial vaginosis (BV) has been associated with an increased risk of preterm birth in many observational studies. The detection of BV does not involve conventional culture techniques. A vaginal swab is rolled onto a glass slide in a similar fashion to a cervical smear test. Gram staining and microscopy are then used to diagnose BV, using the Nugent scoring system. Randomized studies, such as that of Hauth et al.,[8] have demonstrated that oral metronidazole significantly lowers the risk of preterm birth, by 60 per cent in high-risk women positive for BV [Ia].

As there is concern that BV may reflect chronic intrauterine infection, 5–7 days of oral therapy at standard doses seems appropriate. A large trial using briefer therapy has not shown benefit. Several randomized, placebo-controlled studies have suggested an increase in moderately preterm birth (<32–34 weeks) in BV-positive women randomized to vaginal clindamycin cream. One hypothesis is that topical therapy adequately treats vaginosis but fails to affect pre-existing intrauterine infection.

Asymptomatic bacteriuria

This carries an increased risk of preterm birth. Although it may simply be a marker for heavy vaginal microbial colonization, a meta-analysis of many trials confirms that risk is reduced by appropriate antibiotic treatment [Ia]. An alternative explanation for the association with preterm birth may be an increased risk of pyelonephritis in women presenting with asymptomatic bacteriuria.

Group B streptococcal colonization

Group B streptococcal (GBS) colonization has been linked to prematurity. Preterm infants are certainly more susceptible to early-onset GBS infection, acquired during passage through the birth canal. However, evidence that it is one of the major causal organisms behind spontaneous prematurity remains weak. In women known to be at increased risk of preterm delivery, testing for GBS antenatally allows appropriate intrapartum prophylaxis to be planned. Optimal screening involves the use of a combined low vaginal/rectal swab. As maternal carriage can change during pregnancy, later repeat screening should be considered. *Only intrapartum treatment should be given* [Ia], as antenatal antibiotics have not been shown to lower perinatal transmission.

It is, of course, very common for women who know they are colonized to request antenatal treatment. Women should be advised that several studies from North America have reported that over-aggressive prophylactic treatment of GBS has led to an increase in neonatal infections with penicillin-resistant *Escherichia coli*. In pregnancy, as elsewhere, antibiotics have the potential for harm.

Other organisms

Organisms such as *Chlamydia trachomatis*, *Neisseria gonococcus* and *Trichomonas vaginalis* have been associated with preterm delivery, but again, a causal link has not been established. Antenatal treatment of chlamydia has not been shown to lower prematurity rates, although it may prevent perinatal transmission. Treatment of chlamydia and gonococcus must always include contact tracing and treatment of the partner. These are best accomplished in conjunction with the department of genitourinary medicine. A test of cure should always be performed.

Cervical ultrasound

Cervical length can be accurately and repeatedly measured by ultrasound. The risk of prematurity is inversely related to cervical length [II].[9] These measurements should only be made by transvaginal scanning, as the full bladder necessary for visualization transabdominally leads to false lengthening and can obliterate gross funnelling. Transvaginal ultrasound has been shown to be more accurate than digital measurements for assessing cervical length. The test has predictive ability in all groups of women (low risk, high risk, twins, symptomatic etc.).

In asymptomatic women with a short cervix, the risk of moderately preterm delivery rises only slightly, to 4 per cent with lengths of 11–20 mm. At 10 mm, the risk is 15 per cent and it increases dramatically as length decreases further. The technique is certainly able to identify a group of women at risk of cervical weakness. The exact cut-off point for intervention remains unknown but is currently under investigation.

Cervical cerclage

After documentation of a shortened cervix on ultrasound, randomized trials of cerclage versus observation are currently giving contradictory results. Perhaps more importantly, cervical ultrasound is able to exclude weakness – if the cervix is long, surgical intervention can be avoided. The Medical Research Council Randomised Trial of Cervical Cerclage highlighted over-intervention based on simple clinical assessment, suggesting benefit in only 4 per cent of cases.[10] In a more detailed analysis, cerclage led to improved outcomes only after three or more previous very early deliveries [Ib]. The relative merits of McDonald versus Shirodkar cerclage have long been debated and remain unresolved. Certainly a

Shirodkar cerclage is located much closer to the internal os. Whether this translates into better outcomes is unknown.

Some authors have advocated transabdominal sutures. These are placed at the level of the internal os via a Pfannenstiel incision. They are permanent and necessitate caesarean section for delivery. Their use has not been subjected to rigorous testing. They have a number of theoretical disadvantages, including the need for abdominal delivery if preterm labour occurs regardless of gestation, and they are associated with the operative morbidity of any abdominal procedure. They are probably only rarely required and their use should be restricted to trials only at this stage in development.

Cervico-vaginal fibronectin testing/IGFBP1

This is undertaken after 23 weeks, as levels are often high prior to this gestation. Fetal fibronectin (fFN) is a 'glue-like' protein binding the choriodecidual membranes. It is rarely present in vaginal secretions between 23 and 34 weeks. Any disruption at the choriodecidual interface results in fFN release and possible detection in the cervico-vaginal secretions. Two tests are available.

- A quantitative laboratory-based assay gives absolute values.
- A rapid qualitative bedside test is available that gives a positive/negative result.

Technique is important in performing the bedside test.

1 The swab must be that supplied with the testing kit (Dacron).
2 The swab should be rotated in the posterior fornix for 15–20 seconds to ensure the tip is saturated.
3 Endocervical swabbing should not be undertaken.
4 The test result should be read within 15 minutes if using the bedside kit.

False-positive results can occur if:

- there has been sexual intercourse within 24 hours;
- there is vaginal bleeding;
- the filter becomes blocked and a result cannot be obtained – this occasionally occurs when there are large amounts of cervical mucus.

For high-risk asymptomatic women with a positive fibronectin test at 24 weeks' gestation, 46 per cent will deliver before 30 weeks' gestation.[11] Conversely, the chance of such an early birth is less than 1 per cent with a negative test.

There is no proven treatment for a positive fFN test, although several groups are studying the potential role of antibiotics. Presently, clinicians can use the high negative predictive value to either withhold treatments or optimize their timing.

A new test utilizing insulin-like growth factor binding protein 1 (IGFBP1) (Actin Partus™) has similar sensitivity and specificity and is less prone to false positives when blood or semen is present.

Salivary oestriol

A salivary oestriol surge has been reported up to 3 weeks before onset of labour. Its usefulness in predicting preterm birth has not been proven.

Home uterine activity monitors

An increase in painless uterine activity may precede the onset of labour. However, the early detection of this increased activity has not been found to reduce the incidence of prematurity. This is not surprising, as no effective prophylactic treatment has yet been found that suppresses contractions. Many studies, meta-analyses and reviews have shown no evidence of benefit from oral ritodrine. At present, the conclusions for other maintenance tocolytics such as nifedipine or glyceryl trinitrate (GTN) patches must be similar, given the paucity of well-controlled studies supporting their use.

Lifestyle modification

Women at high risk should be counselled about smoking [II].

Work from France suggested that increased social and economic support for women believed to be at risk of preterm delivery led to a reduction in early births. Such results have not been replicated elsewhere. Randomized trials of social support in the UK failed to improve pregnancy outcomes [Ib]. In some situations, hospitalization for bed rest led to an increase in preterm births [Ia]. The roles of sexual abstinence and/or psychological support are no clearer and should not be recommended as a universal or general measure in high-risk women.

MANAGEMENT OF SYMPTOMATIC WOMEN

History

The diagnosis of preterm labour remains notoriously difficult in the absence of advanced dilatation or ruptured membranes. Pre-assessment odds of spontaneous preterm delivery based on historical risk factors are a useful starting point, analogous to the diagnostic approach for thromboembolism or screening for Down's syndrome.

A detailed review of current symptoms is necessary. Symptoms such as low backache or cramping are often cyclical. Vague complaints, such as pelvic pressure or increased discharge, are usually common. The co-existence of vaginal bleeding should always be taken seriously. In a women presenting with contractions, the risk of delivery within 7 days if she has vaginal bleeding and a closed cervix is actually greater than if she presented with no bleeding but 2 cm of cervical dilatation. Too much emphasis is also placed on the contraction frequency; in isolation, it correlates poorly with the risk of preterm birth. Markers of contraction intensity, such as analgesic requirements or simple bedside clinical impression, may add far greater refinement.

Examination

Abdominal examination may reveal the presence of uterine tenderness, suggesting abruption or chorioamnionitis. A careful speculum examination by an experienced clinician can yield valuable information. Pooling of amniotic fluid, blood and/or abnormal discharge should all be commented on. A visual assessment of cervical dilatation is usually possible and has been shown to be as accurate as digital examination findings. Medical staff should try to limit digital examinations to cases in which speculum assessment is inconclusive, as they are known to stimulate prostaglandin production and may introduce organisms into the cervical canal. When undertaken in cases of PPROM, digital examinations are associated with a significant reduction in the latent interval before labour.

Further investigation

Repeat vaginal examination

Repeat vaginal examination in 1–4 hours should be considered essential in the absence of secondary tests. The interval between assessments should be guided by the severity of the symptoms.

Post-assessment risk

This should be based on the complete picture. A realistic endpoint should be the chance of delivery within the next 7 days. If this risk is judged to be low, serial observation and review are appropriate. If the risk is high, treatment strategies to optimize perinatal outcome should be implemented.

Bedside fibronectin testing/IGFBP1

This offers a rapid assessment of risk in symptomatic women who do not have advanced dilatation. If done correctly, these tests have a greater predictive value than digital examination. In one study, 30 per cent of women with a positive fibronectin test delivered within 7 days, compared with only 10 per cent of women who were 2–3 cm dilated.[12]

Cervical length measurement

Cervical length measurement by transvaginal ultrasound in symptomatic women has also been shown to improve diagnostic accuracy. Although measurements can be repeated frequently and with little expense, skilled ultrasonographers and suitable machines with transvaginal probes are required.

In symptomatic women, a positive fibronectin test carries a risk of delivery within 28 days of up to 70 per cent, regardless of initial cervical length. Combination testing refines the prediction of deliveries in the next 7 days. In the group with a positive fibronectin test but a normal cervical length, only 5 per cent will deliver within 1 week.[13] However, if the cervix is also short when tested, the risk of delivery within 7 days climbs to 50 per cent. This is particularly useful, as many interventions (tocolytics, steroids and in-utero transfer) should be based on this end-point.

Transplacental therapy

Steroids

Current evidence shows that a single course of maternal steroids given between 28 and 34 weeks' gestation and received within 7 days of delivery results in markedly improved neonatal outcomes [Ia], with a significant reduction in rates of:

- respiratory distress syndrome
- neonatal death
- intraventricular haemorrhage.

Maximum benefit from the injection is seen after 48 hours. In the Cochrane Database, treatment before 28 weeks did not result in statistical benefit. However, courses received less than 48 hours or more than 7 days before delivery still led to a significant reduction in respiratory distress syndrome.

In general, no convincing difference is seen between betamethasone and dexamethasone, although a recent study hinted at improved neurological outcomes with betamethasone.

There is considerable reassuring evidence about the long-term safety of **single courses** of maternal steroids from paediatric follow-up into the teenage years. However, clinicians should only cautiously employ repeat courses, as there is growing concern about adverse consequences and little evidence of improved outcome.[14]

Published examples of potentially harmful effects of **repeated doses** include:

- increased sepsis in PPROM,
- restricted fetal body and brain growth,
- adrenal suppression.

Most worrying is the increased risk of neonatal death seen when three or more courses of antenatal steroids were given in the American Thyrotropin Releasing Hormone (TRH) Study.[15]

Any extensions to the accepted gestational window should also be made cautiously. There may be a limited steroid responsiveness in fetuses at or below 25 weeks' gestation. As there is little proof that steroids are beneficial, their use may lead to over-optimism. Although the Royal College of Obstetricians and Gynaecologists guideline *Antenatal Corticosteroids to Prevent Respiratory Distress Syndrome* recommends steroids from 24 weeks' gestation, this recommendation is not based on evidence from randomized trials. More worryingly, using steroids when inappropriate may hinder later use, particularly when clinicians are wary of multiple courses. The upper gestation at which steroids should be used is also controversial. In comparison to PPROM and pretem labour (PTL), elective non-labour deliveries after

33 weeks are at increased risk of respiratory difficulties and may benefit from prophylactic steroids.

Although there is a paucity of proof that steroids are beneficial in multiple pregnancy, most expert opinion supports their use. Even more caution should be used before embarking on repeat courses in this situation.

Corticosteroids can cause significant glycaemic disruption in diabetic women. They should be used in conjunction with increased glucose monitoring and adjusted insulin doses. The effects can last up to 24 hours after the second dose of steroids.

Thyrotrophin releasing hormone, vitamin K or phenobarbitone

The use of TRH, vitamin K and phenobarbitone to improve neonatal outcome has been studied in randomized trials but has not been shown to be beneficial [Ib].

Tocolytics

The Canadian trial remains the most influential tocolytic trial to date.[16] This trial concluded that ritodrine had no significant benefit on perinatal mortality or the prolongation of pregnancy to term, although it was able to reduce the number of women delivering within 48 hours by 40 per cent [Ia]. This window of opportunity is the sole rationale for using tocolytics. The use of tocolytics is usually inappropriate if steroids have been given and intensive care cots are available.

BETA-AGONISTS

These drugs have significant maternal side effects, including hypotension, tachycardia, anxiety and palpitations. Maternal deaths from acute cardiopulmonary compromise are described, with greatest risks:

- if beta-agonists are given in large fluid volumes,
- in multiple pregnancy,
- in women with cardiac disease.

In women with diabetes, significant extra glycaemic disruption additional to that caused by steroids occurs with beta-agonists.

OXYTOCIN ANTAGONIST

The oxytocin antagonist atosiban now has a UK product licence. Although side effects are less frequent, its clinical effectiveness is no greater than that of the beta-agonists and the cost is much higher [Ib].

OTHER AGENTS

Other smooth muscle relaxants used to treat preterm labour include magnesium sulphate, nifedipine and GTN. There is little evidence to suggest increased efficacy or improved outcomes [Ib] and none has a license for use in pregnancy.

As prostaglandins appear to be one of the pivotal chemicals involved in parturition, non-steroidal anti-inflammatory drugs (NSAIDs) such as indomethacin have attracted considerable interest as tocolytics. There are potential fetal side effects, but these can be limited by restricting their use to less than 72 hours and only below 30 weeks' gestation.

Clinical effort must focus on diagnostic accuracy and appropriate use of tocolytics.

Antibiotics

The UK Oracle Study found no evidence of benefit for the use of antibiotics in uncomplicated preterm labour [Ia].[17]

Most North American centres routinely give intrapartum antibiotics to women in preterm labour unless GBS status is known to be negative. This is not yet recommended within the UK.

Emergency cervical cerclage

Occasionally, women present in the mid-trimester with relatively minor symptoms (pelvic pressure, watery discharge, etc.) and, when examined, are found to have membranes bulging into the upper vagina. If considering emergency cerclage, clinicians need to be aware that there is no randomized evidence for guidance and few reports of the outcome after expectant management. Two clinical issues must be considered.

First, is this a reflection of marked cervical weakness or is the cervix responding to uterine activity? A history of significant cervical surgery may be helpful. If symptomatic contractions are present, the answer is clear. Otherwise, all clinicians can do is reassess the cervical dilatation after several hours. This can be precisely and repeatedly measured non-invasively using transperineal ultrasound.

Second, is there any evidence of intrauterine infection? Only 10 per cent of cases of chorioamnionitis are clinically obvious but, if present, cerclage is doomed to fail. The optimal way to assess this is by amniocentesis. Combining it with a prophylactic amnioreduction may also assist in later membrane reduction. Although full culture results take several days, a rapid Gram stain should be available within a few hours. If ascending infection is not present at presentation, the chances of it occurring will increase as the duration of membrane exposure increases. Therefore, once the amniocentesis is performed, broad-spectrum intravenous antibiotics should be commenced. NSAIDs may be useful to reduce intrauterine pressure, reduce fetal urine production and limit the release of prostaglandins at any subsequent cerclage. If the Gram stain comes back as negative and there is no evidence of uterine activity or progressive cervical change, it may be reasonable to attempt emergency or rescue cerclage [IV]. The practice of observing events for several days simply allows infection to occur and the membranes to weaken further. Even sterile amniotic fluid does not guarantee that the membranes themselves are not already infected.

Membrane reduction can be achieved using a combination of the following:

- cervical traction and head-down tilt,
- mounted swab,

- amnioreduction,
- bladder distension,
- transcervical inflation of a 30 mL Foley catheter balloon.

There is a significant risk of intraoperative membrane rupture. Even if the procedure is successful, many patients will develop membrane rupture or overt infection over the next few days or weeks. The chances of reaching term are slim.

In-utero transfer

In-utero transfer to a unit with adequate neonatal facilities is recommended where these are not available in the admitting unit [III]. It would seem logical that this will improve outcome for babies. It should certainly be considered where neonatal stabilization would be difficult or impossible. It may also help to keep mother and baby together where transfer of the mother after delivery is likely to be difficult. All units should have guidelines for referral and communication.

FETAL ASSESSMENT

Maternal steroid therapy can suppress both fetal activity and heart rate variability. However, umbilical artery Doppler studies are not influenced.

When labour has started or is thought to be imminent:

- whenever possible, the presentation in preterm labour should be confirmed by ultrasound, as clinical palpation is notoriously unreliable;
- an accurate estimated fetal weight, particularly below 28 weeks, can aid parental counselling.

There are considerable difficulties surrounding the interpretation of the fetal heart rate in preterm infants, particularly at extremely early gestations. Simply applying the criteria used at term is inappropriate. Some work has suggested that the baseline rate is more important than either decelerations or variability. Of note, randomized, controlled trials have failed to show any benefit from continuous as opposed to intermittent monitoring in moderately preterm births [Ib].[18] Decisions regarding monitoring in labour at very preterm gestations must be discussed with parents. Intervention on the basis of fetal heart rate monitoring may not be justifiable near the limits of viability.

MODE OF DELIVERY

Many clinicians feel that fetal morbidity and mortality, the difficulty in diagnosing intrapartum hypoxia/acidosis and the maternal risk do not justify caesarean section for fetal indications below 26 weeks. At this early gestation, intrapartum caesarean section has not been shown to improve neonatal outcomes.

As gestation advances, both neonatal outcomes and the ability to diagnose fetal compromise improve, and intervention for fetal reasons becomes universally appropriate. The safety of breech vaginal delivery is often questioned, based on observational data suggesting an increased mortality and morbidity to the preterm breech born vaginally (see Chapter 35). However, there are recent similar studies that conclude the opposite.[19] Although the obstetric community agreed on the need for a well-conducted randomized trial to answer this question, this was not translated into recruitment when trials were attempted. A careful attempt at vaginal breech delivery, preferably under epidural analgesia, is not absolutely contraindicated [II].

Type of caesarean section

At the earliest gestations, the lower segment is poorly formed, often leading to vertical uterine incisions. A classical uterine incision carries up to a 5 per cent risk of uterine rupture in subsequent pregnancies, some of which will occur antenatally. The modified DeLee vertical lower segment incision does not appear to carry any greater risk than a conventional transverse incision and should be used in preference [III]. Alternatively, it is often possible to perform an en-caul delivery through a transverse incision if the membranes are left intact.

ANALGESIA

In terms of intrapartum analgesia, the use of epidural anaesthesia is frequently advocated. There has been little research on the subject. Postulated benefits include avoiding expulsive efforts before full dilatation or a precipitous delivery, a relaxed pelvic floor and perineum, and the ability to proceed quickly to abdominal delivery. Concerns are often expressed about the prolonged effects of narcotic analgesia on a preterm infant with limited metabolic capacity.

COMMUNICATION

There are two vital areas of communication in the management of women with threatened preterm labour:

- communication with the woman and her family *and*
- communication with the neonatal paediatricians.

Where possible, a clear management plan should be discussed with the parents. This should include monitoring in labour, potential interventions, and what will happen to the baby afterwards. Involvement of the neonatal paediatricians is helpful; especially where there are difficult issues to cover, such as the management of an extremely preterm infant. Even when resuscitation would not be appropriate, parents often appreciate the opportunity to have discussed the care of their baby with the paediatricians.

When labour does occur, it is vital to alert the neonatologists. Outcomes in very preterm infants have been shown to be improved if there is a senior paediatrician present at delivery. This can usually only be accomplished with some advanced warning.

- Oral metronidazole significantly lowers the risk of preterm birth, by 60 per cent in high-risk women positive for bacterial vaginosis.
- Asymptomatic bacteriuria carries an increased risk of preterm birth; the risk is reduced by appropriate antibiotic treatment.
- Mothers at risk of preterm delivery should be screened for GBS colonization. If positive, intrapartum antibiotics should be offered.
- When based on historical factors alone, cervical cerclage improves outcomes only in women with three or more previous very early deliveries.
- Hospitalization for bed rest leads to an increase in preterm births.
- Tocolytics have no significant benefit on perinatal mortality or the prolongation of pregnancy to term, but do reduce the number of women delivering within 48 hours by 40 per cent.
- A single course of maternal steroids given between 28 and 34 weeks' gestation and received within 7 days of delivery results in markedly improved neonatal outcomes.
- There is no evidence of benefit for the use of antibiotics in uncomplicated preterm labour.

KEY POINTS

- Beneficial antenatal treatments for high-risk women include metronidazole for bacterial vaginosis, antibiotics for asymptomatic bacteriuria and cerclage for three or more second trimester losses or very preterm births.
- In symptomatic women, the following factors are associated with a high risk of delivery within 7 days: cervical dilatation ≥ 3 cm, ruptured membranes or any vaginal bleeding.
- A single course of corticosteroids should be given when delivery before 34 weeks is likely within the next 7 days. In general, repeat courses should be avoided, as they may carry risk without conferring benefit.
- After the diagnosis of preterm labour is confirmed, consideration should be given to the issues of neonatology consultation, fetal monitoring, mode of delivery and intrapartum antibiotics if a known GBS carrier.

PUBLISHED GUIDELINES

American College of Obstetricians and Gynaecologists Practice Bulletin. Assessment of risk factors for preterm birth. *Obstet Gynecol* 2001; **98**:709–16.

Australian National Health and Medical Research Council Clinical Practice Guideline. *Care around Preterm Birth.* <www.health.gov.au/hfs/nhmrc>.

Joint Statement of the Fetus and Newborn Committee, Canadian Paediatric Society and Maternal–Fetal Medicine Committee, Society of Obstetricians and Gynaecologists of Canada. *Management of the Woman with Threatened Birth of an Infant of Extremely Low Gestational Age.* <www.cps.ca/english/statements>.

Royal College of Obstetricians and Gynaecologists. Clinical Guideline. *Tocolytic Drugs for Women in Preterm Labour.* London: RCOG Press, Oct. 2002. <www.rcog.org.uk>.

Royal College of Obstetricians and Gynaecologists. Clinical Guideline. *Antenatal Corticosteroids to Prevent Respiratory Distress Syndrome.* London: RCOG Press, Dec. 1999. <www.rcog.org.uk>.

Scottish Obstetric Guidelines and Audit Project. *Preparation of the Fetus for Preterm Delivery.* <www.show.scot.nhs.uk/SIGN/sogap3.htm>.

KEY REFERENCES

1. Draper ES, Manktelow B, Field DJ, James D. Prediction of survival for preterm births by weight and gestational age: retrospective population based study. *BMJ* 1999; **319**:1093–7.
2. Wood NS, Marlow N, Costeloe K, Gibson AT, Wilkinson AR. Neurologic and developmental disability after extremely preterm birth. EPIcure Study Group. *N Engl J Med* 2000; **343**: 378–84.
3. Bohin S, Draper ES, Field DJ. Health status of a population of infants born before 26 weeks gestation derived from routine data collected between 21 and 27 months post-delivery. *Early Hum Dev* 1999; **55**:9–18.
4. Tsatsaris V, Carbonne B, Cabrol D. Place of amniocentesis in the assessment of preterm labour. *Eur J Obstet Gynaecol Reprod Biol* 2000; **93**:19–25.
5. Mueller-Heubach E, Rubinstein DN, Schwarz SS. Histologic chorioamnionitis and preterm delivery in different patient populations. *Obstet Gynecol* 1990; **75**:622–6.
6. Mercer BM, Goldenberg RL, Moawad AH, et al. for the National Institute for Child Health and Human Development Maternal–Fetal Medicine Network. The Preterm Prediction Study: Effect of gestational age and cause of preterm birth on subsequent obstetric outcome. *Am J Obstet Gynecol* 1999; **181**:1216–21.
7. Lumley J. The epidemiology of preterm birth. *Ballière's Clin Obstet Gynecol* 1993; **7**:477–98.

Late pregnancy/intrapartum events

8. Hauth JC, Goldenberg RL, Andrews WW, DuBard MB, Copper RL. Reduced incidence of preterm delivery with metronidazole and erythromycin in women with bacterial vaginosis. *N Engl J Med* 1995; **333**:1732–6.

9. Heath VCF, Southall TR, Souka AP, Elisseou A, Nicolaides KH. Cervical length at 23 weeks gestation: prediction of spontaneous preterm delivery. *Ultrasound Obstet Gynecol* 1998; **12**:312–17.

10. MRC/MRCOG Working Party on Cervical Cerclage. Final report of the Medical Research Council/Royal College of Obstetricians and Gynaecologists Multicentre Randomised Trial of Cervical Cerclage. *Br J Obstet Gynaecol* 1993; **100**:516–23.

11. Goldenberg RL, Iams JD, Merer BM et al. for the National Institute for Child Health and Human Development Maternal–Fetal Medicine Network. The Preterm Prediction Study: The value of new versus standard risk factors in predicting early and all spontaneous preterm births. *Am J Pub Health* 1998; **88**:233–8.

12. Iams JD, Casal D, McGregor JA et al. Fetal fibronectin improves the diagnosis of preterm labor. *Am J Obstet Gynecol* 1995; **173**:141–5.

13. Rizzo G, Capponi A, Arduini D, Lorido C, Romanini C. The value of fetal fibronectin in cervical and vaginal secretions and of ultrasonographic examination of the uterine cervix in predicting premature delivery for patients with preterm labor and intact membranes. *Am J Obstet Gynecol* 1996; **175**:1146–51.

14. National Institutes of Health Consensus Development Panel. Antenatal corticosteroids re-visited: repeat courses – National Institutes of Health Consensus Development Conference Statement. *Obstet Gynecol* 2001; **98**:144–50.

15. Banks BA, Cnaan A, Morgan MA et al. and the North American Thyrotropin-Releasing Hormone Study Group. Multiple courses of antenatal corticosteroids and outcome of premature neonates. *Am J Obstet Gynecol* 1999; **181**:709–17.

16. Canadian Preterm Labour Investigators Group. Treatment of preterm labour with the beta-adrenergic agonist ritodrine. *N Engl J Med* 1992; **327**:308–12.

17. Kenyon SL, Taylor DJ, Tarnow-Mordi W et al. for the ORACLE Collaborative Group. Broad-spectrum antibiotics for spontaneous preterm labour: the ORACLE II randomised trial. *Lancet* 2001; **357**:989–94.

18. Shy KK, Luthy DA, Bennett FC et al. Effects of electronic fetal heart rate monitoring, as compared with periodic auscultation, on the neurologic development of premature infants. *N Engl J Med* 1990; **322**:588–93.

19. Wolf H, Schaap AHP, Bruinse HW, Smolders-de Hass H, van Ertbruggen I, Treffers PE. Vaginal delivery compared with caesarean section in early preterm breech delivery: a comparison of long-term outcome. *Br J Obstet Gynaecol* 1999; **106**:486–91.

Chapter 22

Pre-Labour Rupture of the Membranes

Griff Jones

MRCOG standards

- Candidates should be able to diagnose and manage rupture of the membranes in term and preterm pregnancies.

  In addition, we would suggest the following.

Theoretical skills
- Understand the changes in amniotic fluid volume at different gestational ages.
- Understand the physical and biochemical properties of amniotic fluid that can be used diagnostically.
- Be aware of the risks associated with pre-labour rupture of the membranes (PROM), both at term and preterm.
- Have a thorough knowledge of the management options for PROM at term.
- Know the organisms likely to cause chorioamnionitis along with their appropriate antibiotic therapies.

Practical skills
- Be able to confirm membrane rupture using clinical history, examination and specialized tests.
- Assess amniotic fluid volume using ultrasound.
- Be able to diagnose clinical chorioamnionitis by examination and additional testing.

INTRODUCTION

Pre-labour rupture of the membranes is a common clinical problem, and the assessment of women with possible membrane rupture is a management issue faced in everyday practice. When PROM occurs, the fetus loses the relative isolation and protection afforded within the amniotic cavity.

DEFINITION

In general, PROM refers to rupture of the membranes with leakage of amniotic fluid in the absence of uterine activity. The interval between membrane rupture and the onset of contractions is referred to as the latency. Some authorities advocate there must be a minimum latency (such as 1 hour or 4 hours) for the diagnosis of PROM to stand. In the active management of labour, as practised in Dublin, PROM at term plus uterine contractions equals labour, regardless of cervical findings.

At term, approximately 75 per cent of women will labour within 24 hours of membrane rupture. The latency period tends to be longer with decreasing gestational age: at 26 weeks, only half of women are in labour within 1 week; at 32 weeks, half will labour within 24–48 hours.

INCIDENCE

Pre-labour rupture of the membranes occurs in approximately 8 per cent of term pregnancies. It also complicates 2–3 per cent of pregnancies that have not reached 37 weeks' gestation, when it is referred to as preterm PROM or PPROM. Preterm PROM is associated with approximately one-third of all deliveries before 37 weeks' gestation. It is important to make a distinction between term PROM and preterm PROM, as the conditions have different aetiologies, risks and recommended management plans.

AETIOLOGY

An extensive review of the physiology and pathophysiology underlying membrane rupture has been undertaken by French and McGregor.[1]

Term PROM

Rupture of the membranes at term usually reflects physiological (as opposed to pathophysiological) processes. Apoptosis (programmed cell death) refers to the natural deterioration and breakdown of cells and cellular structure over time. The role of apoptosis in PROM has attracted considerable research interest.

As term approaches, uterine activity is known to increase and Braxton–Hicks contractions are prominent. Such repetitive stretching of the membranes may lead to weakening via several mechanisms. First, it induces focal thinning of the membranes. Second, it leads to strain hardening, a biomechanical phenomenon associated with materials becoming less elastic and less able to withstand stress. Such stretch-induced weakening will be most likely at the internal cervical os, where physiological ripening of the cervix will allow a degree of membrane prolapse.

Preterm PROM

In contrast to the 'natural' phenomenon occurring at term, PPROM usually has pathological origins. Ascending infection appears to be one of the major causes and, indeed, appears to be a more frequent aetiology than in preterm labour with intact membranes. That chorioamnionitis can be associated with membrane weakening is easily understood. As with preterm labour, the majority of these infections are subclinical and give few signs or symptoms until fluid loss has occurred.

Another factor strongly linked with PPROM is antepartum haemorrhage, particularly when it occurs recurrently. A weak cervix can also predispose to early membrane rupture. It will fail as a barrier to ascending infection and, by allowing membrane prolapse, will allow localized biomechanical weakening, as described for term PROM.

There is a strong epidemiological link between maternal smoking and PPROM, which is dose dependent. As smoking is a modifiable behaviour and a reduction in smoking has been shown to reduce risk, this should be pointed out to women, particularly those with a history of PPROM in a previous pregnancy.

CLINICAL ASSESSMENT

The correct diagnosis of PROM, either preterm or at term, is crucial – many interventions will be based upon the diagnosis. If undertaken unnecessarily, these interventions will undoubtedly increase maternal and fetal morbidity.

History

A history from the mother of 'a gush of fluid' followed by recurrent dampness will correctly identify over 90 per cent of cases of pre-labour membrane rupture.[2]

Examination

Pre-labour rupture of membranes should be confirmed by a sterile speculum examination, performed after the mother has rested supine for 20–30 minutes. Amniotic fluid should be seen pooling in the posterior fornix, either spontaneously or after fundal pressure. The presence of meconium is always concerning. At preterm gestations, meconium is suggestive but not diagnostic of intra-amniotic infection; at term, it is a relative contraindication to expectant management. The absence of any pooling is an equally important finding. The cervix can usually also be seen, allowing assessment of length and dilatation.

A digital examination must be avoided unless the patient is thought to be in established labour, as it is known to increase the incidence of:

- chorioamnionitis
- postpartum endometritis
- neonatal infection.

A digital examination also decreases the length of the latent period before the onset of labour, with the greatest decreases seen at the earliest gestations.[3]

Basic bedside tests

Concern about the consequences of misdiagnosing true PROM has led investigators to seek secondary tests that can be used at presentation. The two commonest tests use either nitrazine sticks (relying on the higher alkaline pH of amniotic fluid) or the ferning pattern seen when amniotic fluid is dried onto a glass slide and then viewed under a microscope. Importantly, neither of these tests has been shown to be more reliable than a basic history and examination.[2] Both have appreciable false-positive and false-negative rates, which appear to be further increased in women with prior negative speculum examinations.

Misdiagnosed PROM

Ladfors et al.[4] have studied the outcome of women presenting with possible PROM after 34 weeks' gestation in whom amniotic fluid could not be seen on speculum examination. Vaginal samples were taken and blindly analysed later for diamine oxidase, an enzyme that is absent from urine or vaginal secretions but present in large amounts in amniotic fluid. Of the women with negative speculum examinations, 12 per cent tested positive for diamine oxidase. Nearly 90 per cent of these diamine oxidase-positive women went into labour within 48 hours, compared to only 45 per cent of the diamine oxidase-negative women. Crucially, no difference in maternal or neonatal outcome was seen between the two groups. This suggests that a delay in the diagnosis of PROM in women with an initially negative speculum examination is of no clinical consequence [II].

Specialized tests

Vaginal swabs

Many more technologically advanced and expensive tests have been proposed to confirm or refute the diagnosis of PROM in women with negative speculum examinations. Three strong contenders are fetal fibronectin, insulin-like growth factor binding protein 1 (IGFBP1) and beta-human chorionic gonadotrophin (β-hCG). All are present in high concentration in amniotic fluid and all have commercially available rapid bedside tests. Actin PROM™ utilizes a monoclonal antibody to test for a form of IGFBP1 that is predominantly found in liquor. The form found in liquor is less phosphorylated and can be distinguished from the tissue-produced form if tested with Actin Partus™. It has a sensitivity of 94–99 per cent and a specificity of 98–100 per cent. Unfortunately, there is no rapid and simple test for diamine oxidase.

Ultrasound

Amniotic fluid volume can be assessed by ultrasound. Even at term, the normal variation in directly measured amniotic fluid volume is considerable, ranging from 250 to 1200 mL. This limits the usefulness of ultrasound as a primary diagnostic tool. However, ultrasound may be a useful additional investigation in those women with a strong history of PROM but a negative speculum examination, particularly if their symptoms persist for 48 hours or more. As the variation in amniotic fluid volume can be much greater in preterm gestations, the diagnostic role of ultrasound in PPROM is very limited. Despite this, the ultrasound assessment of amniotic fluid volume has been reported to correlate with latency in PPROM and with neonatal mortality and morbidity in mid-trimester PROM.

CLINICAL MANAGEMENT

Term PROM

The predominant risk to the fetus after PROM at term is ascending infection. The risks to the mother are of uterine infection, via either chorioamnionitis or postpartum endometritis. The risks of a policy of induction of labour must also be considered. These include intrapartum complications, operative delivery and postnatal morbidity.

The Canadian TERMPROM Study[5] and subsequent secondary analyses[6–10] have provided considerable evidence to share with prospective parents. The trial compared four management policies, namely immediate induction with intravenous oxytocin, immediate induction with vaginal prostaglandins, expectant management for up to 4 days followed by induction

Table 22.1 Delivery outcomes after membrane rupture at term, TERMPROM Study[5]

	Immediate induction		Expectant management	
	Oxytocin (%)	Prostaglandin (%)	Oxytocin (%)	Prostaglandin (%)
C-sect (overall)	10.1	9.6	9.7	10.9
C-sect (multiparous)	4.3	3.5	3.9	4.6
C-sect (nulliparous)	14.1	13.7	13.7	15.2
C-sect (nulliparous, unfavourable cervix)	14.8	14.1	15.0	14.9
SVD, nulliparous	60.8	60.8	58.0	58.9
Use of oxytocin	91.9	43.1	49.9	43.8
PROM-delivery interval	17.2 hours	23.0 hours	33.3 hours	32.6 hours

C-sect, caesarean section; SVD, spontaneous vaginal delivery; PROM, pre-labour rupture of membranes.

Table 22.2 Perinatal infectious morbidity after membrane rupture at term, TERMPROM Study[5]

	Immediate induction		Expectant management	
	Oxytocin (%)	Prostaglandin (%)	Oxytocin (%)	Prostaglandin (%)
Fever before or during labour	3.8	5.8	8.7	6.7
Antibiotics before or during labour	7.5	9.0	11.9	11.6
Postpartum fever	1.9	3.1	3.6	3.0
Neonatal infection	2.0	3.0	2.8	2.7
Neonatal antibiotics	7.5	10.9	13.7	12.2
NICU stay >24 hours	6.6	9.2	11.6	10.2

NICU, neonatal intensive care unit.

with oxytocin, or expectant management followed by induction with vaginal prostaglandins. As the absolute risks associated with any policy were found to be small, personal preference should be allowed considerable influence [Ia]. Table 22.1 outlines the differences in labour outcome among the four management policies. *None reached statistical significance.* In Table 22.2, the risks of maternal and neonatal infection are reviewed. Although clear trends are obvious in these tables, readers are referred to the original publication for tests of significance.

Four points from the original trial are worthy of separate mention.

1 The use of prostaglandins did not reduce the subsequent need for oxytocin; this was no different between the two groups randomized to prostaglandins and the expectantly managed group randomized to induction with oxytocin.
2 Only a minority of women (approximately 18 per cent) randomized to expectant management waited 4 days before induction.
3 The four babies that unexpectedly died in the trial were all in the expectant management arms. Two were antepartum stillbirths and two were related to fetal distress in advanced labour, both of which started spontaneously.
4 The views of the women participating in the trial showed a preference for immediate induction, as opposed to expectant management.

Later publications from the same investigators showed that the least expensive policy was immediate induction of labour using oxytocin.[10] In terms of where to undertake expectant management, the evidence suggested an increased risk of infection and caesarean section when women were allowed home. If this was translated into clinical practice, and women needed to remain in hospital, it would clearly increase the cost of expectant management further. In contrast, maternal satisfaction, particularly amongst multiparous women, was greater with management at home.[8]

Regardless of whether a policy of immediate induction or expectant management is pursued, factors linked with perinatal infection include an increasing number of vaginal examinations after membrane rupture, an increasing interval between membrane rupture and labour onset, and an increasing duration of active labour.[6,7] There is also clear evidence that immediate induction of labour using oxytocin should be recommended for women known to be colonized with group B *Streptococcus* [Ib].[9] Expectant management in this situation was associated with a three – four-fold increase in risk of neonatal infection, and even immediate induction with prostaglandins failed to lower this.

In general, the evidence suggests that immediate induction is associated with less maternal and neonatal infection and a shorter interval from membrane rupture to delivery [Ia]. There is no evidence that mode of delivery is influenced. When oxytocin is used initially, healthcare costs are lower and the interval to delivery is shortest. However, meta-analysis has suggested that the use of epidural analgesia is increased [Ia]. When prostaglandins are used initially, infection risks may be marginally greater, the interval to delivery slightly increased, and oxytocin required subsequently in nearly half of the women [Ia].

Recent work is investigating the role of misoprostol in this situation. The cost of misoprostol is dramatically lower than that of the other agents, and the ability to use it orally may lower the risk of infection. Large studies are awaited.

Preterm PROM

The major risks in preterm PROM are:

- chorioamnionitis
- abruption
- preterm delivery.

Other risks include cord prolapse and operative delivery. Many tests have been used to predict chorioamnionitis, which is usually subclinical. Serum markers, such as white cell count and C-reactive protein, have a poor predictive ability and should principally be used to support a clinical diagnosis. Oligohydramnios, as assessed by ultrasound, can select a group at higher risk of infection and/or earlier delivery, but again is not diagnostic. Amniocentesis can give the most valuable information but remains technically difficult when little amniotic fluid remains. In contrast to preterm labour with intact membranes, transvaginal ultrasound measurements of cervical length are not predictive of early delivery. As well as PPROM being a common sequela of antepartum haemorrhage, early membrane rupture carries a 5 per cent risk of subsequent abruption. However, this risk varies inversely with gestational age and is reportedly as high as 50 per cent below 24 weeks.[11]

Although neonates born after PPROM are reported to have lower incidences of respiratory distress syndrome when compared to preterm labour, maternal steroids still appear to reduce the risk further [Ia]. There does not appear to be any significant increase in maternal sepsis after **single** steroid courses. Tocolytics are relatively contraindicated in this situation and are known to be less effective.

The recent ORACLE Trial suggests a role for oral erythromycin in PPROM.[12] In this study, women with PPROM were randomized to one of four oral regimes:

- erythromycin (250 mg qds)
- co-amoxiclav (325 mg qds)
- both erythromycin (250 mg qds) and co-amoxiclav (325 mg qds)
- placebo.

The antibiotics were taken for 10 days. In singleton pregnancies, erythromycin alone was associated with a significant reduction (from 14.4 per cent to 11.2 per cent) in the composite primary outcome, a measure of neonatal mortality and major morbidity [Ia]. The reductions with either co-amoxiclav or both antibiotics failed to reach significance. Unfortunately, the 10-day course of co-amoxiclav led to a significant increase in proven neonatal necrotizing enterocolitis, from 0.5 per cent to 1.9 per cent. Once again, antibiotics have been demonstrated to have the potential for harm.

Chorioamnionitis remains a notoriously difficult diagnosis. For research purposes, it requires:

- a maternal pyrexia (>38°C)

and at least two of either:
- maternal tachycardia >100 bpm,
- fetal tachycardia >160 bpm,

- uterine tenderness,
- raised C-reactive protein,
- offensive vaginal discharge.

When clinically suspected, delivery is almost always appropriate, as antibiotic therapy is rarely curative. Based on the culture results after amniocentesis in PPROM, anaerobes are the commonest isolate, followed by group B *Streptococcus* and then other streptococci.

Novel management strategies have included serial transabdominal amnio-infusion, which has been suggested to increase latency and reduce perinatal mortality. When PPROM occurs in the presence of cervical cerclage, suture removal should be considered [IV]. The care of women known to be group B *Streptococcus* carriers has been simplified by the ORACLE Trial, as the organism is usually sensitive to erythromycin. After completion of a 10-day course, further antibiotics should probably be withheld until labour starts.

There are two gestational age epochs that require special consideration.

Previable PROM below 23–24 weeks' gestation

Lung development has reached a critical stage and appears to be at least partly reliant on normal amniotic fluid volumes. There are significant risks of lethal pulmonary hypoplasia, a condition that cannot be reliably predicted on prenatal ultrasound. These risks are highest early in the mid-trimester and when severe oligohydramnios is found on serial ultrasound monitoring.

As there are additional risks of:

- chronic pulmonary morbidity
- fetal limb contractures
- extremely preterm birth with consequent co-existent morbidity and mortality,

many parents will opt for termination of pregnancy. Current research is investigating the role of minimally invasive surgery and membrane sealants in this situation, as the prognosis is otherwise very poor.

PPROM at 34–37 weeks' gestation

This is another controversial area. Randomized trials have suggested that a policy of induction, as opposed to expectant management, may lead to less hospitalization, less perinatal infection and less neonatal morbidity [Ib].[13,14]

- At term, the outcomes for women with PROM are as good in women induced immediately as in those managed conservatively. Where possible, women should be offered the choice.
- At term, women known to be colonized with group B *Streptococcus* should be encouraged to allow immediate induction of labour using oxytocin after PROM.

- Immediate induction is associated with increased use of epidural analgesia.
- Maternal steroid use in PPROM reduces the risk of respiratory distress syndrome.
- Erythromycin used for 10 days after PPROM is associated with a significant reduction (from 14.4 per cent to 11.2 per cent) in neonatal mortality and major morbidity.
- Co-amoxiclav when used for PPROM leads to a significant increase in proven neonatal necrotizing enterocolitis, from 0.5 per cent to 1.9 per cent.

KEY POINTS

- Term PROM is usually a reflection of normal physiology, whereas pathological processes, such as infection and antepartum haemorrhage, often underlie PPROM.
- Accurate diagnosis of membrane rupture is essential and can usually be achieved by simple history and speculum examination alone.
- A digital vaginal examination should always be avoided after (P)PROM unless advanced labour is suspected.
- At term, early induction using oxytocin appears to reduce perinatal infection and shorten hospital stay without increasing operative intervention. It should be strongly recommended to women known to be group B *Streptococcus* positive.
- After PPROM, optimal management includes maternal steroids and oral erythromycin.

PUBLISHED GUIDELINES

Royal College of Obstetricians and Gynaecologists Evidence-based Clinical Guideline Number 9. *Induction of Labour*. London: RCOG, June 2001.

KEY REFERENCES

1. French JI, McGregor JA. The pathobiology of premature rupture of membranes. *Semin Perinatol* 1996; 20:344–68.
2. Friedman ML, McElin TW. Diagnosis of ruptured fetal membranes. Clinical study and review of the literature. *Am J Obstet Gynecol* 1969; 104:544–50.
3. Lewis DF, Major CA, Towers CV, Asrat T, Harding JA, Garite TJ. Effects of digital vaginal examination on the

latency period in preterm premature rupture of the membranes. *Obstet Gynecol* 1992; **80**:630–4.

4. Ladfors L, Matsson L-A, Eriksson M, Fall O. Is speculum examination sufficient for excluding the diagnosis of ruptured fetal membranes? *Acta Obstet Gynecol Scand* 1997; **76**:739–42.

5. Hannah ME, Ohlsson A, Farine D et al. Induction of labor compared with expectant management for prelabor rupture of the membranes at term. *N Engl J Med* 1996; **334**:1005–10.

6. Seaward PG, Hannah ME, Myhr TL et al. International Multicentre Term Prelabor Rupture of Membranes Study: evaluation of predictors of clinical chorioamnionitis and postpartum fever in patients with prelabor rupture of membranes at term. *Am J Obstet Gynecol* 1997; **177**:1024–9.

7. Seaward PG, Hannah ME, Myhr TL et al. International Multicentre Term PROM Study: evaluation of predictors of neonatal infection in infants born to patients with prelabor rupture of membranes at term. *Am J Obstet Gynecol* 1998; **179**:635–9.

8. Hannah ME, Hodnett ED, Willan A, Foster GA, DiCecco R, Helewa M. Prelabor rupture of the membranes at term: expectant management at home or in hospital? *Obstet Gynecol* 2000; **96**:533–8.

9. Hannah ME, Ohlsson A, Wang EE et al. Maternal colonization with group B *Streptococcus* and prelabor rupture of membranes at term: the role of induction of labor. *Am J Obstet Gynecol* 1997; **177**:780–5.

10. Gafni A, Goeree R, Myhr TL et al. Induction of labor versus expectant management for prelabor rupture of the membranes at term: an economic evaluation. *CMAJ* 1997; **157**:1519–25.

11. Holmgren PA, Olofsson JI. Preterm premature rupture of membranes and the associated risk for placental abruption. Inverse correlation to gestational length. *Acta Obstet Gynecol Scand* 1997; **76**:743–7.

12. Kenyon SL, Taylor DJ, Tarnow-Mordi W. Broad-spectrum antibiotics for preterm, prelabour rupture of fetal membranes: the ORACLE I randomised trial. *Lancet* 2001; **357**:979–88.

13. Mercer BM, Crocker LG, Boe NM, Sibai BM. Induction versus expectant management in premature rupture of the membranes with mature amniotic fluid at 32 to 36 weeks: a randomized trial. *Am J Obstet Gynecol* 1993; **169**:775–82.

14. Naef RW, Allbert JR, Ross EL, Weber M, Martin RW, Morrison JC. Premature rupture of membranes at 34 to 37 weeks gestation: aggressive versus conservative management. *Am J Obstet Gynecol* 1998; **178**:126–30.

Chapter 23

Antepartum Haemorrhage

Lucy Kean

INTRODUCTION

Definitions

Antepartum haemorrhage (APH) is variously described as bleeding from the genital tract in pregnancy before the onset of labour at gestations from 20 to 24 weeks. For the purposes of this chapter, the threshold of 20 weeks will be used, as this is often the gestation at which women will be admitted to the labour suite rather than the gynaecology ward.

Antepartum haemorrhage is one of the commonest reasons for admission in pregnancy. It affects approximately 4 per cent of all pregnancies and is associated with increased rates of fetal and maternal morbidity and mortality.

Aetiology

The causes of APH can be divided into three main groups:

- placenta praevia
- placental abruption
- others:
  - marginal placental bleeding
  - show
  - friable cervical ectropion/cervical trauma
  - local infection of the cervix/vagina
  - genital tract tumours
  - varicosities
  - vasa praevia.

Placenta praevia and abruption together account for 50 per cent of bleeding and represent the greatest threat to the fetus and mother. Despite the other causes appearing to be more minor (vasa praevia when a fetal vessel ruptures being the exception), these carry an increased perinatal mortality of at least 3 per cent, and must therefore represent a group of pathological conditions. Thus all APH must be taken seriously.

PLACENTA PRAEVIA

The incidence of placenta praevia is variable depending on the population and background caesarean section rate, with rates from 0.4 to 0.8 per cent reported.

Definitions

Placenta praevia is defined as a placenta partially or wholly situated in the lower uterine segment. It is graded in two ways, as either grades 1–4 or minor/major.

- Grade 1: the placental edge is in the lower segment but does not reach the internal os.
- Grade 2: the placental edge reaches but does not cover the internal os.

Table 23.1 The relationship between placenta praevia and caesarean section

Number of previous caesarean sections	Incidence of placenta praevia (%) [total 0.3%]	Incidence of placenta accreta in those with placenta praevia (%)	Overall risk of placenta accreta (%)
0	0.26	5	0.01
1	0.65	24	0.16
2	1.8	47	0.85
3	3	40	1.2
4	10	67	6.7

These grades represent a minor degree of placenta praevia.

- Grade 3: the placenta covers the internal os and is asymmetrically situated.
- Grade 4: the placenta covers the internal os and is centrally situated.

These grades represent a major placenta praevia.

Aetiology and associations

Uterine surgery

Placenta praevia is strongly associated with previous uterine surgery. Its incidence increases with the number of procedures performed (Table 23.1) [II].[1]

Women with two or more previous abortions have a 2.1 (95 per cent CI 1.2–3.5) times increased risk of subsequently developing placenta praevia. Other procedures such as curettage and myomectomy also increase the risks of praevia.

Maternal age

Placenta praevia increases dramatically with advancing maternal age, with women older than 40 years having a nearly nine-fold greater risk than women under the age of 20, after adjustment for potential confounders, including parity [II].[1]

Smoking

The relationship between smoking and placenta praevia is not clear but there does appear to be a small but significant increase in risk in smokers.

Associations

- Fetal abnormality: the rate of fetal abnormality is approximately doubled in women with placenta praevia [II].[1]
- Intrauterine growth restriction is common in women with multiple bleeds from a placenta praevia. The overall rate is 15 per cent [II].
- Ten per cent of women with a bleeding placenta praevia will have a co-existent abruption [II].

Diagnosis

- Placenta praevia usually presents with painless bleeding (though 10 per cent will have concurrent abruption).
- Often a small bleed will precede a much larger one (though this is not always the case).
- The presenting part is usually high, being prevented from engaging by the placenta lying in the lower segment.
- The fetal condition generally remains good until the maternal blood loss causes compromise.

It is difficult to diagnose a placenta praevia until the lower segment begins to form at about 28 weeks; however, a low-lying placenta can cause bleeding from the second trimester onwards.

Many cases are now detected on routine ultrasound at 18–23 weeks. Five per cent of women have ultrasound evidence of a low placenta at 16 to 18 weeks, but only 0.5 per cent have a placenta praevia at delivery. In many units a repeat ultrasound is only performed in women who have had symptoms or signs of a persistently low placenta, as the second trimester findings carry such a low sensitivity.

Transabdominal ultrasound is usually the test first performed, although it can be very difficult to determine the placental edge with a posterior placenta. Using transvaginal imaging is better and the woman does not need a full bladder, thus avoiding maternal discomfort. Also there is less distortion of the anatomy of the lower uterine segment and cervix. Transvaginal ultrasound does not appear to provoke vaginal bleeding [Ib].[2]

Magnetic resonance imaging has also been used to identify placenta praevia, though it is expensive and probably not superior to TV scanning performed by an experienced person.

The following factors on second trimester ultrasound are associated with the persistence of a placenta praevia in the third trimester:

- The placenta covers the internal os with an overlap of greater than 2.5 cm [III].[3]
- The leading edge of the placenta is thick [III].[4]

Morbidly adherent placenta

Morbidly adherent placentae occur in approximately 1 in 200–400 deliveries in the USA and 1 in 800 deliveries in the UK. The major risk factor is uterine scarring, and thus the incidence is increasing with the increasing caesarean section rate. However, prior manual removal or uterine curettage may also cause scarring and an increase in risk.

Three degrees of adherence have been described, accreta, increta and percreta, where the placenta adheres to or invades into or through the uterine wall because of abnormal development of the decidua basalis.

Accreta is the most common, comprising 80 per cent. Postpartum haemorrhage will occur in most cases, particularly if the accreta is partial, where non-contracted portions of myometrium are adjacent to adherent placenta. Though the diagnosis has been made in a small number of cases antenatally, most cases are diagnosed in the third stage. Antenatal diagnosis using ultrasound and magnetic resonance imaging has been described. It is worthwhile trying to determine whether an accreta is present in women at most risk (repeated caesarean sections with an anterior placenta praevia), as it can be helpful in forward planning and discussion of options with the woman.

MANAGEMENT OF PLACENTA PRAEVIA

Management of the woman who does not bleed or in whom bleeding is minor and settled

Maternal risks

BLEEDING

Antepartum haemorrhage is the cardinal sign of placenta praevia and it is unusual for a woman to reach the late third trimester without vaginal bleeding. Bleeding becomes more likely as the frequency and strength of contractions increase, causing shearing of the placenta at the level of the internal os. The bleeding is said to be painless, though a considerable number (10 per cent) of women who bleed from a placenta praevia will have a co-existent abruption. It is also reported that most women experience a minor bleed before any major bleeding. Whilst this is true for many women, some will have a significant haemorrhage as their first event.

HOSPITALIZATION

There are few data on which to base the management of placenta praevia. The only randomized study performed examined hospital versus home care for *symptomatic women*, i.e. women who had already experienced bleeding.[5] This study included only 47 women and concluded that there was no advantage in hospitalizing women with symptomatic praevia. However, one of the women with haemorrhage enough to require immediate delivery was in the home care arm.

Management decisions regarding women who have not bled are difficult and must be individually made. Important factors may include:

- whether the placenta praevia is major or minor;
- where the woman lives in relationship to the hospital and whether she has an adult with her at home;
- the gestation;
- other factors that may make a placenta praevia more difficult to manage, such as a scarred uterus.

Because there have been no trials on this aspect of management, the decision to manage as an outpatient must be made at a senior level and fully discussed with the woman and

her partner. It is important to remember that long-term hospitalization carries significant financial and psychological implications for women and their families and may not be justified for women who have never bled.

For women who have had bleeding, most obstetricians would recommend inpatient management. However, there may be exceptions, such as a placenta that migrates enough for vaginal delivery to become an option, or women with very early bleeding only and a minor degree of placenta praevia. Women who are managed as inpatients show a trend towards later delivery. The Royal College of Obstetricians and Gynaecologists recommends inpatient management, although this is not based on any good evidence [IV].[6]

Surveillance

The rate of fetal abnormality is approximately double the background rate in women with placenta praevia. When a diagnosis is made, a careful reassessment of the fetal anatomy must be undertaken.

In women who have not bled, the assessment of the placental edge will be of significance in the group in which placental migration is a possibility. A full assessment should take place at approximately 36 weeks. A major praevia is unlikely to move after that time but a minor praevia may still migrate and a further assessment may be required.

Tocolysis

Tocolysis for the treatment of uterine activity has been used to good effect in some studies [III].[7] It appears to be safe to use, gaining on average 13 days when compared to women in whom it was not used. It must be used judiciously to settle uterine activity that is causing bleeding. It must never be considered in women who show signs of cardiovascular instability or where there is evidence of fetal compromise. Agents other than beta-agonists should be considered first. Given the lack of cardiovascular side effects, an oxytocic antagonist would probably be the first choice.

Planning for delivery

In the woman who has not bled or in whom bleeding has been minor there are a number of factors that need to be taken into account. These include:

- making a final decision about how to deliver for women with minor praevia;
- timing in relationship to the gestation of the pregnancy;
- ensuring a fully experienced and prepared team is assembled for delivery.

Deciding when to attempt a vaginal delivery

There has been much debate about when a vaginal delivery can be expected and when it is unlikely to occur. One large observational study has shown that if the placenta is within 2 cm of the internal os, the vast majority of women will require caesarean section [III].[8] This is therefore accepted as a reasonable cut-off for expecting to need to perform a caesarean section. However, where the leading edge of the placenta is thick, the placenta may still have an impact at this distance.[4] Once the placenta is more than 4.5 cm from the internal os it is unlikely to be problematic. The grey area of 2–4.5 cm must be managed clinically and will depend on features such as the station of the fetal head and the position of the placenta (anterior or posterior, anterior being slightly less problematic as the anterior lower segment tends to retract more in labour).

Occasionally an examination in theatre may be required to determine the true relationship between the placental edge and cervix. This may be needed when:

- facilities are not available for ultrasound assessment and delivery needs to be considered;
- despite ultrasound assessment, a clear diagnosis cannot be reached;
- there is a suspicion of a low accessory lobe where the main body of the placenta is normally sited;
- the placenta is said to be a minor praevia, the clinical picture suggests a vaginal delivery may be feasible, and bleeding or labour requires a decision regarding delivery to be made.

Procedure for examination in theatre

This should only be undertaken when a decision has been made that delivery should be expedited and that a vaginal delivery is considered a safe and valid option if feasible (i.e. the mother and fetus are well and a major placenta praevia is not suspected).

The team should be assembled so that if a placenta praevia is confirmed a caesarean section can be performed.

A full assessment is much easier with some form of anaesthesia. Given that regional anaesthesia is now becoming more widespread (see below) for delivery in the presence of a praevia, an epidural or combined spinal/epidural is probably appropriate. This can then provide analgesia for labour if required.

Blood must be cross-matched in advance.

The woman should be placed in the lithotomy position and draped. The bladder should be empty to allow full descent of the head. Initially, a vaginal examination is performed to palpate in each fornix. The placenta can be felt as sponginess between the fetal head and the fornix. The whole 360 degrees of the cervix should be palpated against the fetal head. If, on working round the cervix, no placenta is felt, an index finger should be passed through the cervix and a gentle examination performed to feel for the edge of the placenta. This is the most difficult part in practice, but if placenta is felt it usually precipitates bleeding, making the diagnosis. If the fetal head is felt with no apparent placenta and no bleeding, the membranes should be ruptured and Syntocinon started if the labour has not already begun.

If the cervix is so unfavourable as not to allow a rupture of the membranes, delivery by caesarean section is probably the safest option.

PLANNED CAESAREAN SECTION FOR PLACENTA PRAEVIA

Timing of caesarean section

Pre-labour caesarean section carries an increased risk of respiratory complications in the newborn. Occasionally these are severe enough to require intensive intervention. Table 23.2 shows the incidence of respiratory morbidity for each week of gestation in babies delivered prior to labour from 37 to 41 weeks [III].[9]

It has also been noted that the incidence of respiratory distress syndrome is higher amongst infants born to mothers delivered by elective caesarean section for placenta praevia that relates to lower cortisol levels in these infants [II].[10] This suggests that the maturing processes in these infants are not accelerated. These data suggest that when bleeding has not occurred, caesarean section should be planned no earlier than 38 weeks, and if a planned caesarean section is to be performed before this time for placenta praevia, it may be worthwhile administering corticosteroids 48 hours prior to delivery.

When bleeding is occurring, the risks and benefits of delivery versus conservative management can only be assessed on an individual basis. However, there is often pressure to deliver earlier because of hospital inpatient management. If there are no compelling medical reasons for delivery before 38 weeks, the risks to the fetus must be fully discussed with the mother before delivery.

Planning the caesarean section

The degree of technical difficulty of caesarean section for placenta praevia will be related to:

- gestation,
- the degree of praevia,
- whether the praevia is anterior,
- the presence of other risk factors making a morbidly adherent placenta more likely,
- multiple previous abdominal procedures, which may make the access to the uterus more difficult,
- morbid obesity.

Table 23.2   Respiratory morbidity amongst infants delivered by elective caesarean section

Gestation	Respiratory morbidity/ 1000 (95% CI)	Odds ratio compared to vaginal delivery at term (95% CI)
37 + 0–37 + 6	73.8 (49.1–106.1)	14.3 (8.9–23.1)
38 + 0–38 + 6	42.3 (31.1–56.2)	8.2 (5.5–12.3)
39 + 0–39 + 6	17.8 (8.0–33.5)	3.5 (1.7–7.1)

It is useful to have as much idea as possible prior to the procedure about the likelihood of placenta accreta. This will enable the mobilization of appropriate personnel and resources (blood etc.).

Autologous blood transfusion is not recommended in the management of placenta praevia, as when blood is needed it is often required in very large amounts.[6] Haemoglobin should be optimized before delivery.

Consent

It is important that the potential outcomes are discussed with the mother before delivery. This must include a discussion of management in the presence of continued or heavy bleeding and the possibility of the need for hysterectomy or other techniques.

A planned caesarean section must enlist the help of all those thought to be necessary. This will include at the very least:

- senior obstetrician,
- senior anaesthetist,
- experienced midwives, anaesthetic assistants and theatre staff.

Where a morbidly adherent placenta is a strong possibility, discussion with a surgical/urological team may be necessary as bladder involvement is not uncommon.

When a caesarean section is likely to involve significant haemorrhage, the haematology staff (medical and laboratory) should be alerted. The appropriate amount of blood should be cross-matched in advance. The laboratory should be warned if there is likely to be a need for more blood or blood products.

Type of anaesthetic

The type of anaesthesia used is the ultimate responsibility of the anaesthetist. The final decision can only be made when the anaesthetist has all the facts at his or her disposal. Good communication before the delivery is vital.

There is increasing evidence that blood loss at caesarean section for placenta praevia is less when regional anaesthesia is used and that this does not compromise mothers [II].[11] (Elective delivery is different from delivery of the cardio-vascularly unstable woman with acute bleeding, as discussed below.) When procedures are likely to take slightly longer, a combined spinal–epidural approach may be enlisted.

Surgery

The surgery must be performed or supervised by an experienced obstetrician. The Confidential Enquiry into Maternal Deaths in the United Kingdom 1994–1996 recommended that a consultant be present during surgery for a placenta praevia.

The main reason for this recommendation is that a decision to proceed to life-saving hysterectomy is likely to be made earlier by a senior person. Despite this recommendation, there were four deaths due to placenta praevia in the last enquiry, even though a consultant obstetrician was present in three of the four cases.

The surgeon must avail him/herself of all the available information before commencing the caesarean section. It is prudent to try to plan how the uterine incision will relate to the placenta before starting. Careful ultrasound mapping of the placental site prior to operation may help the surgeon to know in which direction the nearest edge of a placenta-overlying uterine incision will be located.

It is also the responsibility of the surgeon to ensure that appropriate consent has been gained, that all the team members are aware the procedure is about to commence, and that the blood is available in theatre. These vital steps should not be delegated to anyone else in an elective situation.

Technique

Uterine incision
Caesarean section is usually performed through a transverse skin incision and through the lower segment of the uterus, but if there is an anterior placenta praevia, the vessels may cover the entire anterior lower segment and the placenta will be encountered underneath the uterine incision. Some authors have recommended a classical caesarean section in this situation, but this may make any repeat caesarean section even more hazardous, and lower segment bleeding can be difficult to see and secure in this case.

Delivery
The baby may be delivered by the obstetrician passing a hand round the margins of the placenta, or by incising the placenta. It is often easier to bring down one of the baby's feet and perform breech extraction than to try to deliver a very high head past the placenta that occupies the uterine incision. Prolonged delay in delivery can lead to fetal exsanguination if the placenta has been cut. Some authors have recommended clamping the cord as soon as the uterine incision is made, to prevent fetal bleeding if the placenta is cut [IV]. However, in many cases this is not easy and often adds unnecessary delay.

Third stage
Oxytocics should be administered (5 units Syntocinon i.v.) as soon as the baby is delivered. An oxytocin infusion may then be commenced to continue uterine contraction. The uterine angles should be secured with Green–Armytage clamps before delivery of the placenta, and any large bleeding venous sinuses in the incision can also be secured.

The placenta should be delivered by controlled cord traction. If at this point a placenta accreta is diagnosed (and it is usually obvious, as no plane of cleavage can be found where the placenta adheres to old scar), a decision to proceed to hysterectomy should be made. It is an advantage if regional anaesthesia is being used, as this can be explained to the mother.

Once the placenta is delivered, the lower segment can be examined. Delivery of the uterus may improve visualization. Bleeding with a placenta praevia at this stage is most troublesome from the lower segment as this contracts poorly. Various strategies have been employed to improve haemostasis. These include:

- over-sewing individual bleeding sinuses;
- packing the uterine cavity;
- siting a balloon device, which can be inflated to provide uterine compression and removed later per vaginum;
- extra oxytocics, including prostaglandin $F_{2\alpha}$, intramyometrial vasopressin;
- radiographic embolization techniques;
- uterine or internal iliac artery ligation.

What is most important is that if haemorrhage is continuing and excessive, early recourse to hysterectomy is the safest strategy and the abdomen should not be closed until haemostasis is assured.

Post-delivery monitoring

Women delivered with a major placenta praevia or who have had significant intraoperative haemorrhage must be carefully monitored in a high-dependency setting until continuing loss has been excluded.

The management of major postpartum haemorrhage is discussed in Chapter 42. Again it is vital that if haemorrhage is continuing, early recourse to hysterectomy is undertaken.

Postnatal counselling

When haemorrhage has been severe, women will need the opportunity to go through events with the senior member of the team. The anaesthetist may wish to be involved. It is important that women understand what implications there may be for future deliveries, especially where there has been particularly difficult surgery.

The management of women with severe antepartum bleeding with placenta praevia utilizes the steps above. Further management of the woman with severe bleeding is discussed below.

PLACENTAL ABRUPTION

Definition

Abruption is defined as bleeding following premature separation of a normally sited placenta.

It occurs in as many as 5 per cent of pregnancies, though the majority of these are small and only visible on placental examination after delivery. It can most easily be graded as follows.

- An asymptomatic retroplacental clot seen after placental delivery.
- Vaginal bleeding and uterine tenderness; visible retroplacental clot after delivery.
- Revealed bleeding may or may not be present but placental separation is significant enough to produce evidence of fetal compromise and retroplacental clot visible after delivery.
- Revealed bleeding may or may not be seen but there are significant maternal signs (uterine tetany, hypovolaemia, abdominal pain), with late stage fetal compromise or fetal death. Thirty per cent of these women will develop disseminated intravascular coagulopathy (DIC).

Abruption has historically been associated with very poor fetal and maternal outcomes. Perinatal mortality rates vary widely as the diagnostic criteria are generally clinical and broad. The minimal perinatal mortality rate is at least 4 per 1000. In the last Confidential Enquiry into Maternal Deaths, three deaths were due to abruption, though these were not thought to have been preventable.

Aetiology and associations

The aetiology of placental abruption is unclear, but there are a number of recognized associations.

The risk factors for abruption include:

- previous abruption
- fetal abnormality
- rapid uterine decompression (rupture of membranes with polyhydramnios)
- trauma
- chronic chorioamnionitis
- smoking
- abnormal placentation (circumvallate placenta etc.)
- pre-eclampsia
- underlying thrombophilias.

It is clear that abnormal placentation in its widest context predisposes to abruption. This probably encompasses the last four associations, all of which may represent disturbances in placentation. Abruption is increased in the majority of thrombophilias, including factor V Leiden and prothrombin gene heterozygotes and homozygotes, protein C and S deficiency, antiphospholipid syndromes and homocysteinaemia [II].[12] It is possible that the association with homocysteinaemia may underlie the association suggested with folate deficiency as long ago as 1966, although the failure to demonstrate any improvement in supplementation may have been because only a very small number of women would have benefited. What is as yet unproven is whether there are any effective interventions to prevent abruption in women with underlying thrombophilias. Women who have previously had an abruption are approximately six times more likely to do so again than women who have never abrupted.

Given that placental abruption is associated with disturbed placentation, any factor also seen in these cases will be associated with an increased risk of abruption. These include growth restriction, oligohydramnios, fetal abnormality (especially aneuploidy) and abnormal umbilical artery Doppler velocities.

Diagnosis

The diagnosis of placental abruption is primarily a clinical one. There may or may not be revealed bleeding. The woman may have had pain preceding or during the bleed and the uterus may be irritable; alternatively, if a large abruption is present, the uterus may be hard and tetanic.

In grades 2 and 3, the clinical picture is usually clear and the management will be dictated by the fetal and maternal condition. Grades 0 and 1 may be much more difficult to diagnose. There will be much overlap between women with marginal bleeding and bleeding due to other causes. This is largely irrelevant clinically, as all women with APH represent a high-risk group for whom surveillance in pregnancy needs to be increased.

Ultrasonography is not a good method of diagnosing placental abruption. Small areas are difficult to visualize and, in the acute phase, large abruptions can be isoechoic and look like placenta. When an abruption is clinically suspected, it is prudent to manage with that as the diagnosis. Ultrasound should be used to:

- confirm fetal viability
- assess fetal growth
- measure liquor volume
- perform umbilical artery Doppler velocities
- confirm fetal normality as far as possible
- exclude placenta praevia.

Management specific to abruption

When to deliver

The main management decision to be made with abruption is whether to deliver the fetus. Approximately 50 per cent of women who abrupt will present in labour, and the decision then must be how to deliver the fetus.

When fetal compromise is confirmed, the aim should be to deliver the fetus. Studies comparing neonatal outcomes at gestations of viability suggest that caesarean section is a better choice for the fetus; however, even when caesarean section is performed, perinatal mortality rates of 15–20 per cent are reported in this group. At very low gestations, a vaginal delivery should be the aim. Labour is often quick and although prostaglandins can be used, they are rarely needed.

It is important when performing a caesarean section to alert the haematology laboratory and to arrange to have blood cross-matched as soon as possible (see below). Whether there is time to delay to await the results of clotting screens and cross-matching will depend on the degree of maternal bleeding and the condition of the fetus.

It is important to:

- remember that there may already be considerable unrevealed bleeding which may increase the blood loss well above that which has been revealed;
- be as prepared as possible;
- seek senior help if this is thought likely to be necessary;
- expect heavy postpartum bleeding.

If the fetus is already dead, a vaginal delivery should be the expectation. At least 30 per cent of women will develop DIC and delivery should be expedited. The management is discussed further below.

The time taken to achieve delivery will depend entirely on the rate of bleeding, the rate of change in the clotting studies and the clinical condition of the mother. Fortunately, delivery is usually rapid and after delivery the DIC will usually begin to resolve.

If the abruption is small, the fetus uncompromised and the mother well, a conservative approach may be utilized. There can only be gains for the mother and fetus if there are benefits in terms of maturity and the option to give steroids. If abruption is thought to be the diagnosis and the fetus is mature, delivery in a controlled manner is probably the best management plan. After 38 weeks in most cases of suspected abruption, delivery should be considered. Between 34 and 38 weeks, cases must be managed on an individual basis. When a conservative approach is undertaken, increased surveillance is essential. In the acute phase, a period of inpatient management with twice-daily cardiotocography until stability is confirmed is warranted. Fetal growth must be serially assessed, and umbilical artery Doppler waveform analysis is also helpful.[13]

Bleeding of other causes

The group of other causes comprises a wide range of conditions. As a group, these causes carry an increased risk of perinatal mortality of approximately five-fold and therefore warrant careful consideration.

Management will depend on the individual cause, but there are some general principles.

- It is preferable to err on the side of caution, and safer to increase surveillance rather than to assume that the cause must be benign.
- There is no evidence to support a policy of delivery at term in the well fetus, but steps to ensure fetal well-being must be continued if a conservative approach is adopted.

MANAGEMENT OF THE WOMAN PRESENTING WITH ANTEPARTUM HAEMORRHAGE

Management at initial presentation

A rapid assessment of the condition of both the mother and the fetus is a vital first step.

A clinical history can be quickly taken in an acute situation. A more detailed history can be taken once the immediate clinical picture is established. When taking the initial history, questions should be asked regarding:

- dates by menses and previous scan,
- amount of bleeding,
- associated or initiating factors,
- abdominal pain,
- coitus,
- trauma,
- leakage of fluid,
- previous episodes of bleeding,
- previous uterine surgery (including induced abortions and surgically managed miscarriages),
- smoking and use of illegal drugs (especially cocaine),
- fetal movements,
- blood group,
- position of the placenta, if known from a previous scan.

Smoking increases the risk of placenta praevia, placental abruption and marginal bleeding. This is a dose-dependent effect. Fetal growth restriction is associated with both marginal placental bleeding and placental abruption. The mother may have noticed a reduction in fetal movements. The use of cocaine and crack cocaine is strongly associated with placental abruption.

Maternal assessment

In the initial stages, this should include:

- pulse,
- blood pressure,
- uterine palpation for size, tenderness, presenting part.

A vaginal examination must not be performed until a placenta praevia has been excluded.

Fetal assessment

It should be established whether a fetal heart can be heard, making sure it is fetal not maternal (the mother may be very tachycardic). If a fetal heart is heard and the gestation is estimated to be 26 weeks or more, fetal heart rate monitoring should be commenced.

These initial steps take very little time. Following this initial assessment, women will fall into one of two categories.

1 The bleeding is minor or settling and neither the mother nor fetus is compromised.
2 The bleeding is heavy and continuing and the mother or fetus is or soon will be compromised.

Group 1: bleeding is minor or settling and neither the mother nor fetus is compromised

This is the most common group. It is usually clearly apparent that neither mother nor fetus is in danger on admission. Time can then be taken to conduct a full and thorough history and examination.

Once it is clear that the placenta is not low, a vaginal examination can be undertaken with the following aims:

- to assess the degree of bleeding;
- to ascertain cervical changes, which may be indicative of labour;
- to assess local causes of bleeding (trauma, polyps etc.);
- to take bacteriological samples if infection is suspected (high vaginal and endocervical swabs, urine polymerase chain reaction (PCR) or endocervical swabs for chlamydia, plus viral swabs if herpes is suspected).

After a careful history and examination, is should be possible to use selected investigations to help establish a diagnosis.

Further investigations
- Full blood count.
- Kleihauer testing in women known to be Rhesus negative or in women with unknown blood group.
- Grouping and saving of serum, with blood cross-matched if there is continuing or severe bleeding.
- Clotting screen in cases of suspected abruption or heavy bleeding.

Ultrasound is useful for:

- measurement of fetal size,
- assessment of liquor volume,
- location of the placenta in relation to the internal cervical os,
- establishment of fetal well-being:
  - biophysical profile (see Chapter 14)
  - umbilical artery Doppler velocimetry.

Ultrasound is not generally helpful in diagnosing abruption. Acute abruptions can be difficult to see as they may have the same echogenicity as placenta. It should be made clear that the ultrasound examination is primarily to assess the position of the placenta and the well-being of the fetus. Women are often disappointed if they have been led to believe the ultrasound will identify the cause of the bleeding.

If the source of bleeding is fetal, the fetus is usually quickly compromised. This may present with a fetal tachycardia progressing rapidly to a sinusoidal cardiotocography and finally a terminal bradycardia. Very rarely, an Apt's test (which relies on the resistance of fetal haemoglobin to denaturization by acid) can help if fetal blood loss is suspected.

A Kleihauer test is mandatory for all Rhesus-negative women. All RhD-negative women will require 500 IU anti-D (unless they are already sensitized). The Kleihauer test must be done to determine whether there has been a large fetomaternal haemorrhage, in which case more anti-D will be needed.

The Kleihauer is not a useful test to differentiate small abruptions from bleeding of other causes [II].[14] Fetal cells may appear in the maternal circulation in as many as 15 per cent of women at some time in pregnancy, and a lack of fetal cells in the maternal circulation does not preclude an abruption.

Surveillance after a limited antepartum haemorrhage

Although most units admit women who have had APH for 24 hours, there is no evidence to suggest that this improves outcome once fetal and maternal well-being has been established. Management must be individualized, taking into account the suspected cause of bleeding, gestation, fetal assessment and continuing maternal risk factors.

The following must be borne in mind.

- No bleeding, however light, should be dismissed without full investigation.
- Once APH has occurred, the pregnancy becomes high risk, and a management plan for ongoing fetal surveillance must be formulated and discussed with the mother.
- Women must be advised to watch for warning signs such as a decrease in the frequency of fetal movements, further bleeding or pain, and should be assessed again should any of these occur.

Planning for the rest of pregnancy

If bleeding settles and the mother is discharged, a clear plan for the remainder of the pregnancy should be made. Even if the cause is thought to be minor, extra fetal surveillance is needed as a higher fetal mortality rate is seen compared with background. Fetal surveillance for growth and well-being should be instituted, as guided by the clinical picture. If all remains well, induction of labour at term is not needed, but the degree of surveillance after the due date may need to be increased.

Group 2: severe ongoing bleeding, compromised mother and/or fetus

Delivery must be expedited if the mother is compromised. If the fetus is compromised, the decision to deliver will be based on the gestational age. In most cases, delivery will be indicated.

The method of delivery will be determined by the cause and severity of the bleeding, the fetal gestation and status. Women with major haemorrhage from a placenta praevia will need delivery by caesarean section.

Placental abruption causing maternal or fetal compromise necessitates delivery. If the fetus is already dead, vaginal delivery after stabilization of the mother is usually the safest option. However, if the bleeding continues, and the mother's condition cannot be stabilized, delivery should be achieved by the quickest method, which may be caesarean section. Coagulopathy will only begin to resolve once the placenta is delivered, and may be severe enough to warrant replacement with fresh frozen plasma (FFP), cryoprecipitate and platelets. These women usually labour very quickly. Epidural or spinal anaesthesia must not be used if the clotting studies are abnormal or not available. Central venous pressure (CVP) lines can be useful, but should be sited through an antecubital long line, and not sited or removed until clotting is normal.

It can be difficult to measure obstetric blood loss accurately, as the loss may be concealed (placental abruption) or diluted by amniotic fluid.

Major haemorrhage can be defined by blood loss and/or vital signs:

- disturbance of conscious state,
- systolic pressure <100 mmHg,
- blood pulse >120 beats per minute (bpm),
- blood loss >1500 mL,
- reduced peripheral perfusion.

Disturbances of coagulation due to loss or consumption of platelets and clotting factors may occur during haemorrhage. DIC is the coagulation problem most often encountered in obstetric patients. This and the other complications – fetal or maternal death, adult respiratory distress syndrome, renal and hepatic failure – are more likely to occur if adequate replacement of blood volume is not instigated rapidly.

> **Aims of treatment of major haemorrhage**
>
> - Rapid restoration of the circulation blood volume and oxygen-carrying capacity.
> - Cessation of further blood loss.
> - Restoration/maintenance of normal blood coagulation.
> - Delivery of the live fetus (where appropriate).

Resuscitation should aim to keep the haemoglobin concentration above 10 g/dL, the pulse rate below 100 bpm, and the systolic blood pressure above 100 mmHg. Four units of cross-matched blood should be available at all times.

The success of treatment is dependent on careful organization as well as prompt treatment and the use of appropriate blood products and non-blood volume expanders. The patient, her partner and relatives must be kept fully informed.

When major haemorrhage is identified

1 Call for help. The immediate team will consist of:
- the obstetric specialist registrar
- the obstetric senior house officer
- the anaesthetic registrar
- the senior midwife.

A member of staff should be nominated to run samples and record events.

2 Start facial oxygen 8 L/min (hypoxia will reduce uterine contractions).

3 Insert two intravenous cannulae (14 gauge-brown) one into each antecubital fossa.

4 Take 30 mL of blood for:
- full blood count (FBC)
- clotting screen (including fibrinogen and fibrin – degradation products or D-dimers if DIC is suspected)
- cross-match 6 units
- urea and electrolytes.

5 Commence the following infusions:
- up to 2 L normal saline/Hartmann's solution
- colloid (up to 1.5 L – remember risk of anaphylaxis)
- uncross-matched Rh-negative blood or group-specific blood (if clinical condition is critical)
- cross-matched blood as soon as available.

Cross-matched blood is the ideal but crystalloid first and colloid second should be used until blood is available. Group O RhD-negative blood should only be used as a last resort, but can be life saving when haemorrhage is severe. Group O RhD-negative blood **must not** be given to patients known to have anti-c antibodies from their antenatal records.

6 One member of staff should be assigned to record the following:
- pulse
- blood pressure
- CVP (half-hourly) if a line is present (see below)
- continuous fetal heart rate (where appropriate)
- fundal height (abruption/postpartum haemorrhage)
- urine output (catheterize and aim to keep output <30 mL/h)
- fluid input (type, volume and i.v. site)
- any drug administration (time, type, dose)
- measured blood loss.

7 Site an indwelling catheter to monitor urine output and aim to keep output above 30 mL/h.

8 The senior obstetrician present should co-ordinate and manage the clinical situation, i.e. prompt treatment of the cause of haemorrhage, adequate fluid replacement and regular checking of FBC and clotting status in order to prevent and treat DIC.

A major haemorrhage box is an asset on any acute unit. It should contain everything needed for the initial resuscitation (fluids, cannulae, tourniquet, blood bottles and forms, oxytocics etc., Figure 23.1).

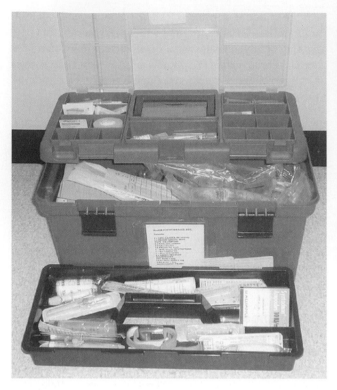

Figure 23.1   A major haemorrhage box

BLOOD TRANSFUSION CONSIDERATIONS

Packed cells and stored blood lack platelets and clotting factors. Fresh whole blood is not available because of potential hazards of viral transmission. FFP and sometimes cryoprecipitate are usually necessary to compensate after transfusion of 6 units. Stored blood also is a source of thromboplastins and can lead to or exacerbate DIC when large amounts are transfused. In most units, up to 4 units of FFP may be issued before the coagulation screen result is known for a patient in critical condition (usually 6 units already transfused and blood loss continuing), provided that coagulation studies are being processed.

Thrombocytopenia can also occur during massive transfusion, but in DIC a platelet transfusion is rarely required unless the platelet count falls below 50×10^9 and there is continued blood loss.

Blood should be administered through blood-warming equipment and rapid administration of fluid should be achieved by the use of a compression cuff on the infusion bag. The use of a blood filter is not necessary. Cold injury increases the risk of DIC.

Extra blood and products should be ordered early – the amount of each will depend on the clinical situation and FBC and coagulation screen results. In established DIC, extra FFP or cryoprecipitate and platelets may be needed, according to instructions from the haematologist.

Once bleeding has been stopped, the patient should be managed in an obstetric high-dependency setting or adult intensive therapy unit.

Central venous pressure monitoring

Central venous pressure monitoring can be helpful where there has been massive haemorrhage, concealed blood loss or when blood loss is continuing.

A long line should be used if there are concerns regarding clotting.

A pressure between 3 and 7 cmH$_2$O, using the angle of Louis as the reference zero, should be established.

- Ensure that the rate of transfusion at least equals the rate of continuing blood loss and is, in addition, adequate to replace the loss already measured.
- Do not over-transfuse the patient with cell free colloid as this will result in a severely anaemic patient, with a high CVP, preventing further blood transfusion.
- Do not exceed a CVP of 7 cmH$_2$O (this leads to a high risk of pulmonary oedema due to low colloid oncotic pressure).
- Do not use or rely on increasing the CVP excessively to correct oliguria.
- Consider using a fluid challenge test if you are unsure of the adequacy of fluid replacement:

Infuse 250 mL Hartmann's or normal saline rapidly (<2 minutes). Observe the CVP changes over the following 5–10 minutes.

- *Hypovolaemia*: rapid rise and fall back to previous CVP level.
- *Isovolaemia*: rise and fall back to slightly higher CVP level.
- *Hypervolaemia*: rise to higher CVP level sustained for more than 10 minutes.

MAJOR HAEMORRHAGE AND SPECIFIC ANTEPARTUM CONDITIONS

Placenta praevia

It is unusual for the placental site to be unknown, as most women have a detailed fetal anomaly scan. Bleeding significant enough to cause maternal hypotension requires delivery.

If the placenta is known to be praevia, delivery by caesarean section is needed. If the placental site is unknown, the following strategy is helpful.

- Is the presenting part engaged? If so, a placenta praevia is less likely.

- Ultrasound scan can be performed to confirm the leading edge of the placenta, but only if the practitioner is trained to do so.
- If the presenting part is high and delivery is needed, an examination in theatre should be considered if the diagnosis is still unclear.
- The consultant must be informed prior to delivery and should be present for delivery or as soon as possible.

MAJOR ABRUPTION

Large abruptions can lead on to DIC in 30 per cent of women. Management must be directed at ensuring the safety of the mother and fetus. Abruption is associated with a high risk for postpartum haemorrhage.

- Usually presents with pain and vaginal bleeding with a woody, hard, tender uterus.
- If fetal heart is present, continuous monitoring is needed.
- Vaginal examination should be performed with due caution.
- Follow the guidelines for massive obstetrics haemorrhage above.
- Prevent postpartum haemorrhage and monitor for renal failure.
- Discuss with consultant haematologist.
- If no fetal heart is detected, ultrasound confirmation should be performed, membranes should be ruptured and Syntocinon commenced to empty the uterus.
- FBC and clotting must be monitored at least 4-hourly as these can deteriorate quickly.

DISSEMINATED INTRAVASCULAR COAGULATION

This is defined as inappropriate activation of the clotting cascade, leading to widespread coagulation, increased fibrinolysis and end organ failure.

The obstetric causes can be divided into three areas.

1 Injury to vascular endothelium:
   - pre-eclampsia
   - hypovolaemic shock
   - septicaemia
   - cold injury (large amounts of cold fluid).
2 Release of thrombogenic tissue factors:
   - placental abruption
   - amniotic fluid embolism
   - prolonged intrauterine fetal death.

Late pregnancy/intrapartum events

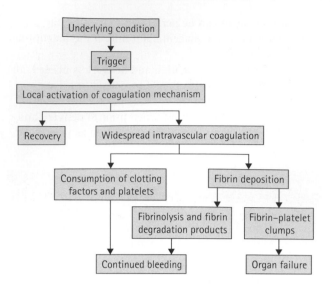

Figure 23.2 Evolution of disseminated intravascular coagulation

3 Production of procoagulant phospholipids:
 – incompatible blood transfusion
 – septicaemia.

Disseminated intravascular coagulation represents a cascade of events which can vary in severity, and range from a compensated state with only laboratory evidence of increased coagulation and fibrinolytic factor turnover, through to massive uncontrollable haemorrhage with very low concentrations of plasma fibrinogen, raised fibrin degradation products (FDPs) and thrombocytopenia. The evolution of events leading to DIC is shown in Figure 23.2. End organ damage is caused by hypotension, fibrin–platelet clump deposition in small vessels, and persisting endothelial damage leading to increased vascular permeability.

The following organs are most susceptible to damage.

- Kidneys:
 – acute tubular necrosis
 – glomerular damage.
- Lungs:
 – pulmonary oedema
 – adult respiratory distress syndrome/systemic inflammatory response syndrome.
- Central nervous system:
 – infarcts
 – cerebral oedema.

The principles of management are:

- maternal resuscitation
- treatment of the cause
- replacement of blood and clotting factors
- intensive monitoring until resolution.

Prompt and aggressive fluid replacement will limit damage to the endothelium and allow rapid clearance of fibrin–platelet clumps.

A full coagulation screen should be obtained for any patient at risk of DIC (this should include FPDs or D-dimers and fibrinogen; a thrombin time is useful if fibrinogen testing cannot be done). In DIC, all aspects of the routine clotting study are deranged (activated partial thromboplastin time, partial thromboplastin time and thrombin time). In pregnancy, the normal range for fibrinogen is increased, with the lower limit of normal being 4 g/dL. In any woman in whom the fibrinogen falls to 1 g/dL, a cryoprecipitate infusion (which is rich in fibrinogen) should be considered. Measurement of fibrin degradation products can be useful; D-dimers that are more specific may also be measured when other indices of coagulation are abnormal.

Management of disseminated intravascular coagulation

Senior haematological advice should always be sought if DIC is suspected. The mainstay of the management of massive haemorrhage treatment is to stop further loss of blood and resuscitate with appropriate blood products. Mild DIC may be controlled by adequate transfusion with stored blood and FFP. More FFP will be required in severe cases. FFP provides factors V and VIII, other labile coagulation factors and some antithrombin IIIa and fibrinogen. Cryoprecipitate (with a higher concentration of fibrinogen) and platelets may also be needed. After initial resuscitation, management will be dependent on repeated checks of the haemoglobin, platelet count and coagulation status.

- Remember that stored blood contains thromboplastins and can exacerbate DIC once 6 units have been given.
- Remember fibrinogen reference range in pregnancy is >4 g/dL. Any woman with a fibrinogen of <1 g/dL requires cryoprecipitate if there is active bleeding.

Treatment of the cause

Disseminated intravascular coagulation will not settle until the cause resolves. The urgency of treatment will be determined by the severity of the DIC and other factors such as maternal and fetal condition.

In general, following abruption and intrauterine fetal death, vaginal delivery should be the aim. Usually this will be accomplished within 4–6 hours. If DIC becomes uncontrollable during this time, more rapid delivery will be needed. Although it is considered that transfusion of replacement clotting factors may add fuel to the fire of DIC, it is recommended that replacement is aggressively pursued whilst delivery is being accomplished.

After delivery, steps to avoid postpartum haemorrhage should be instituted.

Post-delivery surveillance

The aims are to:

- ensure adequate blood and clotting factor replacement,
- prevent further bleeding,
- monitor renal function and urine output until resolution,
- be vigilant for signs of impending lung involvement.

Fortunately, most women make a rapid recovery following delivery. It is important to ensure that the patient and her partner have the opportunity for a full debriefing.

SUMMARY

Antepartum haemorrhage increases the risk of perinatal death regardless of the cause. All women with APH therefore warrant careful fetal and maternal evaluation. In many cases a cause cannot be found, but the increase in perinatal mortality requires careful fetal surveillance for the remainder of all such pregnancies. Abruption carries the largest fetal and maternal risk. Women with underlying placental disease carry the highest risk for abruption.

Placenta praevia is becoming increasingly prevalent. As repeated caesarean sections are performed, the risk of a placenta praevia with a morbidly adherent placenta increases. A multidisciplinary approach is needed to ensure good maternal outcomes in the most difficult cases.

- Transvaginal ultrasound provides the most information and is safe in the diagnosis of placenta praevia.
- The risk of placenta praevia and accreta increases with each subsequent caesarean section.
- Regional anaesthesia for elective caesarean section for placenta praevia is safe and is associated with less maternal bleeding than general anaesthesia.

KEY POINTS

- The major causes of APH abruption, placenta praevia and a mixed category of other causes.
- APH of any cause carries an increase in the risk of perinatal death for that pregnancy.
- Maternal deaths related to abruption and placenta praevia continue to be reported. Senior involvement is needed in the delivery of women with placenta praevia.

- Placenta praevia and accreta are likely to become more common as the caesarean section rate rises.
- Increased surveillance is required for all ongoing pregnancies complicated by APH.
- Large abruptions carry a high risk of DIC and require a multidisciplinary approach to optimize care.

KEY REFERENCES

1. Sheiner E, Shoham-Vardi I, Hallak M, Hershkowitz R, Katz M, Mazor M. Placenta previa: obstetric risk factors and pregnancy outcome. *J Matern Fetal Med* 2001; **10**:414–19.
2. Sherman SJ, Carlson DE, Platt LD, Medearis AL. Transvaginal ultrasound: does it help in the diagnosis of placenta praevia? *Ultrasound Obstet Gynecol* 1992; **2**:256–60.
3. Becker RH, Vonk R, Mende BC, Ragosch V, Entezami M. The relevance of placental location at 20–23 gestational weeks for prediction of placenta previa at delivery: evaluation of 8650 cases. *Ultrasound Obstet Gynecol* 2001; **17**:496–501.
4. Ghourab S. Third-trimester transvaginal ultrasonography in placenta previa: does the shape of the lower placental edge predict clinical outcome? *Ultrasound Obstet Gynecol* 2001; **18**:103–8.
5. Wing DA, Paul RH, Millar LK. Management of the symptomatic placenta praevia: a randomized, controlled trial of inpatient versus outpatient expectant management. *Am J Obstet Gynecol* 1996; **175**:806–11.
6. Royal College of Obstetricians and Gynaecologists. *Placenta Praevia: Diagnosis and Management.* Green Top Guideline No. 27. London: RCOG, 2001.
7. Besinger RE, Moniak CW, Paskiewicz LS, Fishes SG, Tomich PG. The effect of tocolytic use in the management of symptomatic placenta praevia. *Am J Obstet Gynecol* 1995; **172**:1770–8.
8. Oppemheimer LW, Farine D, Knox Ritchie JW, Lewinsky RM, Telford J, Fairbanks LA. What is a low-lying placenta? *Am J Obstet Gynecol* 1991; **165**:1036–8.
9. Morrison JJ, Rennie JM, Milton PJ. Neonatal respiratory morbidity and mode of delivery at term: influence of timing of elective caesarean section. *Br J Obstet Gynaecol* 1995; **102**:101–6.
10. Bekku S, Mitsuda N, Ogita K, Suehara N, Fujimura M, Aono T. High incidence of respiratory distress syndrome (RDS) in infants born to mothers with placenta previa. *J Matern Fetal Med* 2000; **9**:110–13.

11. Parekh N, Husaini SWU, Russell IF. Caesarean section for placenta praevia: a retrospective study of anaesthetic management. *Br J Anaesth* 2000; **84**:725–30.

12. Alfirevic Z, Roberts D, Martlew V. How strong is the association between maternal thrombophilia and adverse pregnancy outcome? A systematic review. *Eur J Obstet Gynecol Reprod Biol* 2002; **101**:6–14.

13. Neilson JP, Alfirevic Z. Doppler ultrasound for fetal assessment in high risk pregnancies (Cochrane Review). In: *The Cochrane Library*, Issue 2. Oxford: Update Software, 2002.

14. Emery CL, Morway LF, Chung-Park M, Wyatt-Ashmead J, Sawady J, Beddow TD. The Kleihauer–Betke test. Clinical utility, indication, and correlation in patients with placental abruption and cocaine use. *Arch Pathol Lab Med* 1995; **119**:1032–7.

Chapter 24

Intrauterine Fetal Death

Lucy Kean

INTRODUCTION

Intrauterine fetal death (IUFD) or stillbirth is variously defined in different countries, by gestation or birth weight (usually 500 g). The variety of definitions makes comparisons of stillbirth rates difficult. However, for the purposes of this chapter fetal death after 20 weeks' gestation is taken as the focus, as these women are generally managed on the labour ward.

The stillbirth rate in England and Wales is approximately 5.5/1000 births.[1] In the UK, a stillbirth is defined as the delivery of a baby with no signs of life after 24 weeks of pregnancy.

AETIOLOGY

The ability to determine the cause of an IUFD will be related to the rate of uptake of post-mortem examination, the quality of the examination and the experience of the examiner. It is hoped that the recognition of the need for specialized paediatric pathology services will reduce the number of IUFDs categorized as unexplained. In large recent studies, the fetal deaths stated as unexplained have been reduced to 10 per cent from previously quoted rates of 40 per cent.

It has also been reported that amongst the group of unexplained IUFD there is a large proportion of fetuses for which poor growth is suspected, if maternal characteristics are included when calculating birth-weight centiles.[2] The implication of this finding is that fetal undergrowth is associated with many unexplained losses, although the pathological mechanism remains unclear [II].

The causes of fetal death are many (Table 24.1); however, an understanding of these can better direct investigations.

Table 24.1 Causes of intrauterine fetal death

Fetal
- Cord accidents
- Feto-fetal transfusion
- Feto-maternal haemorrhage
- Chromosomal and genetic disease
- Structural abnormality
- Infection
- Anaemias of fetal origin e.g. alpha-thalassaemia

Direct maternal effects
- Obstetric cholestasis
- Metabolic disturbance e.g. diabetic ketoacidosis
- Reduced oxygen states e.g. cystic fibrosis, obstructive sleep apnoea
- Uterine abnormalities e.g. Ashermann's syndrome
- Antibody production e.g. Rhesus disease, platelet alloimmunization, congenital heart block

Maternal placental effects
- Pre-eclampsia
- Renal disease
- Antiphospholipid syndromes
- Thrombophilia
- Smoking
- Drug abuse e.g. cocaine

ASSOCIATIONS

It is recognized that IUFD is more common amongst certain groups, though the exact aetiology for the increase in risk is uncertain. Advanced maternal age, obesity, advanced gestation and social deprivation are all associated with increased risk [II].[3]

The contribution of each of the above factors to fetal death may be variable. Many of these diseases or conditions are common and yet fetal death is uncommon. It is vitally important not to ascribe causation, as this may lead to important further information being missed. Although abruption may lead to fetal demise, it may not be the whole story, as abruption is commoner in fetal abnormality, thrombophilias, growth restriction, smoking and drug use. Equally, thrombophilias are common (affecting more than 5 per cent of the population), and whilst they have been shown to contribute to fetal death in some women, they may also be an incidental finding after a fetal death of another cause.

Obstetric cholestasis is discussed further in Chapter 6.8. It is strongly associated with fetal death as gestation increases. It is an important diagnosis to make, as it may recur in up to 80 per cent of subsequent pregnancies. It is a difficult diagnosis to make at post mortem, as the features are very non-specific in the fetus (generally just an anoxic mode of death). Direct questioning about itching may point to the diagnosis, which can be confirmed by measurement of maternal bile acids.[4]

DIAGNOSIS OF THE DEATH

Intrauterine fetal death presents with decreased fetal movement in as many as 50 per cent of cases. Others present with an unexpected finding at a routine ultrasound or antenatal visit or with signs of an acute event such as abruption, ruptured membranes or the onset of labour. When an IUFD is suspected, it is vitally important to establish the diagnosis as soon as possible. It is natural for parents to cling on to every shred of hope for as long as possible, and delay in diagnosis can lead to a false elevation of hope.

Fetal death must be diagnosed by ultrasound. Cardiotocography can be very misleading, as the heart rate tracing of an anxious mother is usually identical to that of a fetus. Even heart rate tracings achieved by scalp electrode can record the maternal heart rate when the fetus is dead.

The ultrasound must be performed by someone trained to do it. Colour-flow mapping can be very useful, especially in the obese woman. It is sometimes, but not always, helpful to the parents to be shown the still fetal heart.

Ultrasound can also confirm features that may be helpful in further investigation. There may be:

- Spalding's sign (overlapping of the fetal skull bones when the fetus has been dead for some time),
- oligohydramnios,
- signs of fetal hydrops.

Once the ultrasound has confirmed fetal death, it is very important that the news is given to the parents in an unambiguous and sensitive way. Phases such as 'I cannot see a fetal heart beat' can be taken by parents to mean that the operator cannot be sure or is not sufficiently trained. It is much better to explain that the baby has died and to express your sorrow.

The initial reaction of parents will vary according to their prior suspicions, and many parents will initially feel anger. It is helpful for parents to be able to express their distress freely and without interruption. Do not try to challenge anger expressed against medical or midwifery staff at this time. If the pregnant woman has family with her, they should be allowed time together to come to terms with the findings.

All units should have a clear protocol for the management and investigation of women with fetal death. It should encompass lines of responsibility so that steps are not inadvertently omitted or repeated.

It is important to establish the events leading up to the fetal death, as there may be factors that will impact on the next pregnancy. It does not take long to take a history of events, and mothers may forget important factors later. It is an important process for the mother; she may feel the need to go through events preceding the admission. Although some of the information that parents volunteer is not relevant, it should be listened to sympathetically and never dismissed as irrelevant.

PROVIDING CHOICE AND ESTABLISHING THE SAFETY OF THE MOTHER

At this point it is important to accede to mothers' choices in regard to management as long as these do not compromise safety.

Measurement of blood pressure and urinalysis should be undertaken to rule out significant pre-eclampsia. Where the fetal death is due to an abruption, clinical signs are usually apparent from the outset. If it is felt that the fetus has been dead for some time, a clotting screen should be performed to ensure that there is no coagulopathy.

PREVENTION OF RHESUS (D) ISOIMMUNIZATION

Massive feto-maternal haemorrhage is one cause of fetal death and may have occurred hours or even days before clinical presentation. If the woman is Rhesus (D) negative, blood for Kleihauer testing should be taken soon after the diagnosis for an estimation of the volume of fetal – maternal transfusion. Anti-Rh (D) immunoglobulin should be given as soon as possible after presentation and not delayed. Delivery may not occur until after the 72-hour watershed beyond which immunoprophylaxis is less effective, A further dose of anti-Rh (D) immunoglobulin might be necessary once the Kleihauer result is known.

HOW TO DELIVER

If the mother is well, the next step is to decide how and when to deliver her. Many women are horrified that a vaginal delivery is recommended. This must be approached in a sympathetic manner. Most women will understand that a straightforward vaginal delivery will minimize the length of postnatal inpatient time and speed their general recovery. There may be circumstances in which caesarean section has to be considered. These will include women for whom this management was previously planned, women with a major placenta praevia and women who simply cannot bear the concept of a vaginal delivery. There can be no hard and fast rules and each case must be individually managed. There have been no studies that have assessed the psychological impact of different delivery strategies in this context.

DELIVERY

Women should be offered the choice of when they would like to deliver. Some women will want to spend a short time at home before commencing induction and others will want to start the process as soon as possible.

Women should be cared for within the delivery suite in order that maternal safety is not compromised. In many units, a dedicated room is set aside for their management. It is good practice to allow partners and other family members to stay.

Women should have full access to analgesia as required. Diamorphine or morphine is a better option in this setting (as compared to pethidine) as both have a longer half-life. Epidural analgesia should be available for women with normal clotting, and patient-controlled analgesia may be useful for those who cannot receive epidural analgesia.

INDUCTION OF LABOUR

There are various strategies that have been used for induction of labour after fetal death. Whichever method is used, it is important to remember that complications such as uterine rupture and shoulder dystocia can occur and management must be safe. Until relatively recently, third trimester induction was generally achieved with standard prostaglandin E2 preparations. This was because of their safety profile in relation to uterine rupture. More recently, the combination of the antiprogesterone mifepristone and the prostaglandin analogue misoprostol has been used to good effect with low complication rates. The advantage of this protocol is that the induction to delivery time is shorter (median 8.5 hours). However, in order for the process to work efficiently, the mifepristone needs to be given 24–48 hours before starting misoprostol. Although this time can be spent at home, many women do not wish to delay starting, and in these women misoprostol alone or prostaglandin E2 may be used. There is usually a longer time from induction to delivery in these cases [II].[5,6]

A standard protocol for mifepristone/misoprostol induction is shown below.

- Mifepristone: 200 mg 24–48 hours before induction.
- Misoprostol: 200 μg p.v. then 200 μg orally every 3–4 hours.

In gestations of 34 weeks or more, doses of 100 μg of misoprostol appear to be effective.

Extra-amniotic infusions are rarely used now, even in economically deprived areas, as misoprostol is safe and cheap. However, extra-amniotic saline has been shown to be reasonably effective as an alternative [Ib].[7]

Where possible, membranes should be left intact for as long as possible, as ascending infection can rapidly occur.

Postpartum haemorrhage is not uncommon; especially where there is pre-eclampsia, abruption, prolonged fetal death or infection. Prolonged chorioamnionitis and repeated small abruptions predispose to retained placenta. When this occurs it should be dealt with quickly and antibiotic prophylaxis given.

INVESTIGATIONS

It is important not to make assumptions about the cause of the IUFD that may deny parents full investigations. This is particularly so when a true knot or placental abruption is seen. Parents may wish to have a clear cause quickly identified, but it is the role of the medical and midwifery team to explain that only complete information can provide real answers.

The fetus should be carefully examined after birth. The birth weight should be recorded and the placenta weighed.

Any dysmorphic signs should be noted and if there is a suspected abnormality at this stage, an examination by a clinical geneticist or interested paediatrician can be helpful (this is particularly important if post mortem is declined).

Sexing the baby is essential for identity and naming, but may be very difficult in early fetal deaths. Also, where there are dysmorphic features, there may be ambiguity. There must be no attempt to guess the sex by obstetricians or midwives, as this may prove very damaging if the assessment is wrong. If necessary, it may be better to await the result of the initial post-mortem findings or karyotype.

No samples of any kind should be taken from the fetus without the consent of the parents (see below). When consent is obtained, the following should be considered:

- fetal blood for karyotyping
- fetal skin for karyotyping
- fetal blood for infection screening
- full fetal X-ray.

Investigation of the mother should include the following.

- Maternal blood for:
  - infection screen
  - lupus anticoagulant
  - anticardiolipin antibodies
  - possibly thrombophilia screening (see below)
  - HbA1c
  - bile salts
  - Kleihauer (regardless of blood group)
  - anti-Ro antibodies if the fetus is hydropic.
- Maternal genital swabs should be taken if infection is suspected.
- Maternal urine can be sent for urine drug screening with permission.
- Placenta:
  - swabs for infection should be taken; ideally, the membranes should be separated and a swab taken from between the two,
  - a small sample for karyotype should be sent in saline (with consent),
  - the whole placenta should be sent for pathology if the parents consent.

Other information may become available later, which may require further investigations. These would include parental karyotype if a fetal translocation were found or antiplatelet antibodies if intracranial haemorrhage is seen.

Karyotype analysis often fails. Where there are specific concerns, the genetic laboratory may be able to help with specific diagnoses by utilizing other techniques such as fluorescent in-situ hybridization or polymerase chain reaction. Fetal chondrocytes provide the most prolonged cell viability, and a small sample from the iliac crest can sometimes provide a diagnosis. Some have recommended performing a fetal karyotype by transabdominal chorionic villus sampling to avoid problems associated with delay and infection of the placenta during delivery. Whereas this may be ideal, it will be unacceptable to many mothers at this time.

The Kleihauer test will become negative very quickly if there is ABO incompatibility. This test must therefore be performed as soon after confirmation of fetal death as possible and should not be delayed until after delivery. Mothers who have experienced huge feto-maternal transfusion may describe an episode of shivering, feeling unwell or rigors that may pinpoint the event; transfusion reactions have been described in this context.

Maternal glucose metabolism returns to normal almost as soon as the fetus dies. Blood sugar estimation is therefore generally unhelpful. Also, as the derangement is generally mild, HbA1c measurements are usually normal. A suspicion of disordered glucose metabolism may arise if the fetal weight is excessive and islet cell hyperplasia is confirmed (though other diagnoses such as Beckwith syndrome can also present in this manner). Women with unexplained stillbirth have a four-fold increase in glucose abnormalities in subsequent pregnancies. Therefore, if this diagnosis is suspected, formal glucose testing should be undertaken in the next pregnancy [II].[8]

It is established that antiphospholipid syndrome can lead to IUFD, and there is evidence that low-dose aspirin and low-molecular-weight heparin improve pregnancy outcome amongst those women who present with recurrent miscarriage (see Chapter 6.8). When compared with controls, women with unexplained stillbirth are more likely to be heterozygous for factor V Leiden mutation, protein S deficient or protein C deficient. Interestingly, these fetuses may not be growth restricted, although there may be placental features that point to an underlying thrombophilia.[9] Although there is increasing evidence of the association between thrombophilia and fetal death, there are no studies to guide management in the subsequent pregnancy.

Obstetric cholestasis has been suggested as being implicated in as many as 40 per cent of fully investigated unexplained stillbirths. The diagnosis can be made by serum bile acid estimation. Measurement of liver function alone may miss the diagnosis in many cases. It is unclear how quickly the bile acids return to normal after fetal death, but given the high recurrence risk, it is worth performing this test as soon as possible.[4]

It is possible to screen maternal urine for the presence of illegal drugs. This should only be done with the consent of the mother and, in this author's experience, is unhelpful. Most mothers feel guilty enough if they think they have contributed to the death of their baby without needing concrete evidence. Those who divulge information about illicit drug use do not need the additional burden of proof. Those who do not provide this information are unlikely to consent to urine testing.

POST MORTEM

The uptake of post mortem has declined recently following adverse publicity concerning organ retention. Many parents are unclear as to what a post mortem entails and may have quite unjustified fears about the process.

Of all the investigations offered to parents, this is the most important. New information becomes available in as many as 40 per cent of cases, and even when an ultrasound diagnosis has been made, 25 per cent will have new or different findings. For many parents this will be their best or only chance of finding out what happened [II].[10]

The issues to be discussed with parents must include the following.

What the procedure is designed to do and how it is performed

Parents need to know that the person performing the examination is a dedicated perinatal pathologist. Unfortunately, and particularly recently, this may not be the case. Some regions perform their perinatal pathology in a main centre. When this is the case, parents should be told that the baby will need to be transferred and will be rapidly and safely returned. Babies classified as stillborn under UK law must be transferred by the undertaker.

The baby is always treated with dignity and respect. The incisions are closed and do not involve the face or limbs. In most cases the baby when dressed will look no different from the way it did before the post mortem. The exception may be the very small macerated fetus whose skin is so thin that suturing is not possible. In these cases, the baby is wrapped.

What tissues are kept

In general, the pathologist will not need to keep any organs. Samples for histology may be retained, but even these can be returned should the parents wish. Where a post mortem is performed in the first trimester, organs are so small that occasionally whole organs need to be retained to make microscope slides. Again, these can be returned if wished.

Where there is a suspected central nervous system abnormality, the brain should be fixed before examination. This can take many days, especially in a large term fetus. If this is an important aspect of the post mortem (usually if there has been antenatal suspicion of abnormality), parents have three options:

1 to forego this extra information,
2 to delay funeral arrangements until this process is complete,
3 to allow the pathologist to retain the fetal brain and to proceed with funeral arrangements without the brain being returned.

Most parents who have given consent for post mortem will want to wait, and to delay arrangements until the baby can be returned intact.

Can anything else be offered to parents who do not want a post mortem?

Placental pathology should be offered regardless of whether a full post mortem is to be performed. Parents can be offered a limited post mortem that examines specific areas. X-rays of the baby are useful, especially if there are dysmorphic features. Magnetic resonance imaging has been used to examine fetal morphology post mortem, and may have some advantages, especially with central nervous system lesions; however, it cannot replace a complete post-mortem examination.

Parents need careful counselling by someone who is experienced in dealing with this situation and who understands the processes involved. There has been much debate about whether the pathologist should obtain consent. The difficult logistics involved in this and the fact that most perinatal pathologists are currently only just coping with their workload are likely to preclude this. However, it is important that obstetricians are trained to seek consent in these cases and understand fully the issues involved. An excellent leaflet explaining post mortem to parents is published by the Confidential Enquiry into Stillbirths and Deaths in Infancy.

The final facet of obtaining good information at post mortem is to give the pathologist all the relevant information. Where there are specific suspicions, the pathologist should be informed of these. It is usually helpful to speak directly with the pathologist about the case. This will also enable the doctor responsible for the case to attend the post mortem if possible.

AFTER DELIVERY

After delivery there are many processes that need to be completed before discharge. The first and most important is to allow the parents as much (or as little) time with the baby as they need. It has previously been believed that parents should be encouraged to see and hold the baby. However, recent interesting evidence from a case-controlled study showed that behaviours that promote contact with the stillborn infant were associated with worse outcome.[11] Women who had held their stillborn infant were more depressed than those who only saw the infant, while those who did not see the infant were least likely to be depressed – 13 of 33 (39 per cent), versus 3 of 14 (21 per cent), versus 1 of 17 (6 per cent) ($p = 0.03$). Women who had seen their stillborn infant had greater anxiety ($p = 0.02$) and higher symptoms of post-traumatic stress disorder than those who had not ($p = 0.02$). Women who had seen their infant were also more likely to show disorganized attachment behaviour towards their next infant – 18 of 43 (42 per cent), versus 1 of 12 (8 per cent) ($p = 0.04$). As these data were acquired from a case-controlled study, there may be many variables that are having an impact. Women who did not wish to see or hold their stillborn baby may have very different coping mechanisms from those who held the baby. Mothers who hold or see the baby may be a self-selected group who form attachments differently. However, these data do show that professionals should not unduly encourage women who do not wish to see or hold the baby to do so, as they may not benefit from this [II].

Parents should be offered the opportunity to have photographs taken and, if these are not wanted at the time, they can be kept, as many parents request them later (sometimes a long time later). The parents may want footprints or handprints of the baby to be taken.

Importantly, the above study indicated that having a funeral and keeping mementoes were not associated with further adverse outcomes, but the small numbers involved limited interpretation. Photographs should only be taken after seeking the parents' wishes, as in some cultures taking photographs of the dead is unacceptable.[12]

Most units have a bereavement team to take on the funeral arrangements with the parents. These teams are usually acutely aware of cultural requirements and may provide an important liaison between the family and the pathologist, especially where there is a need for funeral arrangements to proceed without delay. Unfortunately, it is often those who have the most to gain from post mortem who feel the most cultural pressure not to delay. Sympathetic discussion can often provide a way forward, and many pathologists will provide an out-of-hours service so that delays can be minimized.

Parents should be provided with the telephone numbers of organizations that may also offer support, such as the Stillbirth and Neonatal Death Society (SANDS), as they sometimes need to talk to people unconnected with the hospital. The bereavement team will also provide a contact number.

LEGAL ISSUES

It is necessary for parents to register the birth of any baby born after 24 weeks' gestation. This is often a traumatic time for parents and the bereavement team can be helpful in assisting with this. The parents need the stillbirth certificate in order to register the baby. When the certificate is completed, it is important not to use abbreviations, and not to attempt to guess the cause of death. It is extremely difficult to have death certificates changed and parents can be deeply upset to find that a baby has a registered cause of death that is not accurate. The Registrar's office may need to contact the doctor signing the death certificate, so it is always important to sign and print the name, and important information such as recognized General Medical Council qualifications must not be omitted. The less well the form is completed, the more time the bereaved parents will have to spend at the Registrar's office while he or she tries to contact the doctor involved.

It is the law that no matter when the fetus was known to die, it is the expulsion from the mother that dates the birth. Therefore, any fetus expelled from the mother after 24 weeks' gestation must be registered. This means that where there has been a co-twin death or selective termination, if the fetus is recognizable, it must be registered if delivery occurred after 24 weeks.

The law does not recognize fetal deaths before 24 weeks. The lack of legal recognition means that parents will not have a death certificate for these early fetal losses. It does not mean that they cannot arrange a funeral or cremation if they wish.

The Coroner does not have any legal jurisdiction in cases of stillbirth (even intrapartum), and cases should not need to become the remit of the Coroner.

SUPPRESSION OF LACTATION

The onset of lactation often catches women by surprise and is a source of considerable distress when it starts in earnest at about 48 hours. Although not all women need or want lactation suppression, discussion should take place so that advice can be given about how to cope. For most women, simply a good supportive bra, non-steroidal anti-inflammatory agents if there is discomfort, and time will be enough. However, for some women pharmacological measures are needed and a single dose of cabergoline, a long-acting dopamine agonist, is highly effective. Dopamine agonists for the inhibition of lactation should not be used in women with pre-eclampsia or a personal or strong family history of thromboembolic disease.

CONTRACEPTION

This subject is best covered by the general practitioner or consultant later, but women do need to know that they can conceive before their first period. A pregnancy conceived quickly may delay the grieving process and, before women go home, it does no harm to include a leaflet on contraception that will meet their needs.

GOING HOME

Although every effort is made to ensure women go home quickly, premature discharge must be avoided. It is undoubtedly more painful for women to have to return with problems, and safety is paramount. Many units have a bereavement suite or family room so that other family members can stay for support until discharge can safely be achieved.

Contact telephone numbers should be given to the woman or a companion, and there should be a contact who knows what has happened and who is easily available should problems occur. The community team will play a central role in the care of the family, and detailed communication with the general practitioner and community midwife is of paramount importance. They must be informed by telephone on the day of the woman's return to the community, and all antenatal appointments must be cancelled.

BEREAVEMENT CARE

As perinatal death becomes less common, couples can feel increasingly isolated in their grief. The bereavement team and the community midwife and general practitioner need to be aware of the situation and to react quickly when problems appear to be mounting. It is particularly those couples with high expectations and little family or social support who can be most vulnerable at this time. It is helpful to ensure before discharge that provision is made for the partner to have some time off work, as he will often be forgotten at this time. Also, if the fetal loss has occurred early (20–24 weeks), the patient will need a sick note, as maternity leave will not be applicable.

Parents who have other children often wish to receive guidance about explaining the death of the baby to them. Children's books about death are available. Self-help groups (such as SANDS) also offer support that may sometimes be lacking from professionals. The couple's response to bereavement cannot be predicted by whether they already have children, or the gestation of the fetal loss. Couples respond in different ways and take different amounts of time to heal. The loss of a baby with a severe malformation should not be interpreted as a blessing; it may leave parents with significant fears for the future.

The death of one twin with the survival of the other is especially distressing for parents, who are faced with contradictory psychological processes. It is very difficult to celebrate the birth of one healthy baby and to grieve the death of the other. In this situation, mourning may get postponed or give rise to symptoms of failed grieving, which include the inability to care for and relate to the surviving child appropriately and may contribute to postnatal depression.

FOLLOW-UP

The obstetrician involved in the antenatal care is the usual choice to conduct the follow-up. However, there may be occasions when the woman requests follow-up by a different practitioner, and when this occurs it should not be questioned. It has traditionally been arranged for follow-up to take place at around the time of the usual postnatal visit. This may mean that important information is kept until this visit that may provide some solace to the grieving family. A provisional post mortem is often reported by 2 weeks, and a subsequent visit can always be scheduled.

Women often experience extreme anxiety coming back to the hospital where they have had such a devastating experience. If possible, a neutral venue should be chosen. In every case, there should be enough time to discuss events.

Ideally, the name of the baby should be ascertained before the interview. The bereavement team should be able to supply this. Not all parents will have named the baby.

Generally, parents need to have time to go through events as they recall them, to ask questions that are important to them, and to receive and understand the results of any tests that have been performed.

Often the issues that are most troubling parents are not those that the medical team see as important, so it is vital to keep an open mind, to encourage parents to talk spontaneously and to be honest in replies. Parents may want to apportion blame to individuals or actions. When this occurs, it is important to be honest and to offer apology where this is deemed necessary. Where there has been a failure of care, parents need to receive sincere apologies and reassurance that action to prevent a similar occurrence will take place. Being half-truthful or dishonest will not prevent or reduce litigation. However, where there has been no failure of care, it is important to support other colleagues' management in discussion with parents.

When an underlying cause for the fetal death has been identified, this must be clearly explained. There may be the need to involve other professionals, such as clinical geneticists, at a later date.

When no cause has been found, parents are often very frustrated. This is always difficult for professionals, as the wish to provide answers is one of our most ingrained rationales. It is important not to try to provide unfounded reassurance, but in all cases a clear plan of management for the next pregnancy should be outlined.

Parents often ask when they can try for another pregnancy. It must not be assumed that all couples will wish to do so, and this issue must be covered sensitively. In general, there are few sound medical reasons why couples should delay conception. However, it is important that the grieving process is complete (as much as can ever be so) before the next child. Mothers who conceive very quickly may have more problems with depression, post-traumatic stress disorder and disordered bonding after the next birth, although the evidence is very tenuous.[13]

It is helpful for parents if the issues discussed can be provided for them in a letter. Many women will not wish to book their next pregnancy at the same hospital, and a clear letter will help the future team to understand events. It is also helpful for parents as an aide memoire, as they may not clearly remember some of the points covered. Finally, parents must be given the opportunity to come back if they are unclear about certain aspects and, for some, a preconceptual visit is helpful.

MANAGEMENT OF THE NEXT PREGNANCY

The most important facet of management is to try to adhere to the plans that were formulated after the loss of the baby. It is unusual for professionals to disagree to such an extent that a previously agreed plan has to be changed. There may be minor differences of opinion, but it is better to put these aside in the interests of maintaining the faith of the patient in their care when at all possible. When the plan needs to be changed (such as may occur when new information comes to light), it is important to explain clearly why the changes need to be made and how this will improve the prospects of a healthy pregnancy.

After the birth of the next child, parents may require much reassurance that the baby is healthy. An examination by a senior paediatrician can do much to allay fears.

SUMMARY

The management of women with fetal loss is an integral and important aspect of good obstetric care. If done well, it can help the grieving process.

- There is little that can be cited as evidence in this field. Most of the suggested management is based on the experience of various professionals and support groups.
- Regimens utilizing mefipristone/misoprostol in the third trimester appear safe and achieve shorter induction to delivery times but require pre-priming before induction, which adds to the total time before delivery [III].

KEY POINTS

- Confirm fetal death quickly by ultrasound.
- Offer parents choice wherever possible.
- The support of a bereavement team is an integral part of care.
- Do not discharge the mother home until it is safe to do so.
- Information should be provided at all stages in a form that parents can understand.
- Management of the next pregnancy should try to follow previously set plans.

KEY REFERENCES

1. Confidential Enquiry into Stillbirths and Deaths in Infancy. 8th Annual Report. London: Maternal and Child Health Consortium, 1999.
2. Gardosi J, Mul T, Mongelli M, Fagan D. Analysis of birthweight and gestational age in antepartum stillbirths. *Br J Obstet Gynaecol* 1998; **105**:524–30.
3. Froen JF, Arnestad M, Frey K, Vege A, Saugstad OD, Stray-Pedersen B. Risk factors for sudden intrauterine unexplained death: epidemiologic characteristics of singleton cases in Oslo, Norway, 1986–1995. *Am J Obstet Gynecol* 2001; **184**:694–702.
4. Milkiewicz P, Elias E, Williamson C, Weaver J. Obstetric cholestasis. *BMJ* 2002; **324**:123–4.
5. El-Refaey H, Hinshaw K, Templeton A. The abortifacient effect of misoprostol in the second trimester. A randomised comparison with gemeprost in patients pre-treated with mifepristone (RU486). *Hum Reprod* 1993; **8**:1744–6.
6. Wagaarachchi PT, Ashok PW, Narvekar NN, Smith NC, Templeton A. Medical management of late intrauterine death using a combination of mifepristone and misoprostol. *Br J Obstet Gynaecol* 2002; **109**:443–7.
7. Mahomed K, Jayaguru AS. Extra-amniotic saline infusion for induction of labour in antepartum fetal death: a cost effective method worthy of wider use. *Br J Obstet Gynaecol* 1997; **104**:1058–61.
8. Robson S, Chan A, Keane RJ, Luke CG. Subsequent birth outcomes after an unexplained stillbirth: preliminary population-based retrospective cohort study. *Aust NZ J Obstet Gynaecol* 2001; **41**:29–35.
9. Alfirevic Z, Roberts D, Martlew V. How strong is the association between maternal thrombophilia and adverse pregnancy outcome? A systematic review. *Eur J Obstet Gynecol Reprod Biol* 2002; **101**:6–14.
10. Weston MJ, Porter HJ, Andrews HS, Berry PJ. Correlation of antenatal ultrasonography and pathological examination in 153 malformed fetuses. *J Clin Ultrasound* 1993; **21**:387–92.
11. Hughes P, Turton P, Hopper E, Evans CDH. Assessment of guidelines for good practice in psychosocial care of mothers after stillbirth: a cohort study. *Lancet* 2002; **360**:114–18.
12. Gatrad AR, Sheikh A. Muslim birth customs. *Arch Dis Child Fetal Neonatal Ed* 2001; **84**:F6–8.
13. Turton P, Hughes P, Evans CDH, Fainman D. Incidence, correlates and predictors of post-traumatic stress disorder in the pregnancy after stillbirth. *Br J Psychiatry* 2001; **178**:556–60.

SECTION D

First stage of labour

Chapter 25

Induction of Labour

Richard Hayman

DEFINITION

An induction of labour refers to the process of artificially initiating uterine contractions, prior to their spontaneous onset, with the intention to effect progressive effacement and dilatation of the cervix and, ultimately, the delivery of a baby. The term 'induction of labour' generally refers to procedures performed in the third trimester, but occasionally may be applied to pregnancies at gestations greater than the legal definition of fetal viability (24 weeks in the UK) when fetal survival is an anticipated outcome. Any procedure performed prior to this gestation may be classified as a termination of pregnancy, and will not be considered here further.

The management of labour induction remains a difficult problem for today's obstetrician. As a result of audit, clinical experience and evidence-based research, the National Institute for Clinical Excellence (NICE) has issued formal guidelines based on those published by the Royal College of Obstetricians and Gynaecologists (RCOG) for the management of induction of labour, which should be read by all undertaking such interventions.

INCIDENCE

Induction of labour is a common procedure and although it is currently employed in 15–20 per cent of all term pregnancies in the UK, this represents a fall from the peak levels of 40 per cent in the 1970s. These figures are not constant and have a wide variation, within and between regions which reflects differences in opinion and practice. The 'correct' level of intervention remains a matter of debate.

INDICATIONS FOR INDUCTION OF LABOUR

The purpose of an induction is to achieve benefit to the health of the mother and/or baby, which must exceed that to be gained by continuing the pregnancy, excluding those situations for which delivery by planned caesarean section is prudent.

There are many reasons for induction of labour. The commonly cited indications are detailed below. It is not the purpose of this chapter to outline all the possible reasons for induction, and many are not included here.

- Pregnancy passing 41 weeks.
- Pre-labour spontaneous rupture of membranes.
- Maternal request.
- Maternal disease, e.g.:
  - diabetes
  - hypertensive/renal disease
  - autoimmune disease, e.g. systemic lupus erythematosus.
- Pregnancy-related conditions:
  - pre-eclampsia
  - intrahepatic cholestasis of pregnancy
  - recurrent antepartum haemorrhage (APH)
  - APH at term
  - placental abruption.

- Fetal:
  - intrauterine growth restriction
  - oligohydramnios
  - isoimmunization
  - intrauterine fetal demise.

It is also common to find that an induction of labour is performed for cumulative reasons which, when considered in isolation, would not constitute a sufficient indication. It is vitally important that whatever the indication for induction, the gestational age must be calculated accurately so that appropriate resources and staff can be provided (dexamethasone to promote fetal lung maturation, in-utero transfer to a suitable unit etc.).

Pre-labour rupture of membranes is covered extensively in Chapter 22 and will therefore not be dealt with further here.

INDUCTION OF LABOUR FOR POST-MATURITY

In the UK, the commonest indication for labour induction is prolonged pregnancy. This accounts for approximately 70 per cent of all inductions.

When the expected date of confinement is unknown, because the patient is uncertain of the date of her last menstrual period or has an erratic menstrual cycle, confirmation of the gestation at an early booking scan will reduce the incidence of iatrogenic prematurity. This will also have the benefit of allowing the definition of the maximum period of gestation and will thus reduce the maternal anxiety associated with the passing of the expected date of delivery with no sign of labour. Where routine dating is performed, less than 5 per cent of women will reach 42 weeks. However, women who have already experienced a prolonged pregnancy have a 30–40 per cent chance of doing so again.

The recommended clinical practice in this area has recently been modified as a result of a large multicentre, randomized, controlled trial comparing the induction of labour at 41 weeks with a policy of ongoing fetal surveillance whilst awaiting spontaneous onset of labour.[1] This Canadian trial showed benefit of induction of labour at 41–42 weeks of pregnancy, with a reduction in caesarean section rates (21.2 vs 24.5 per cent), operative vaginal delivery rates, fetal distress (5.7 vs 8.3 per cent), meconium staining of the liquor and perinatal mortality [Ib].[1]

Critics of this study and of the meta-analysis of all the available data raise the following issues.

- The effect on perinatal mortality may be overestimated, as only two of the seven deaths in the meta-analysis were related to post-maturity in monitored pregnancies.
- Induction of labour in the conservatively managed group in the Canadian study was by oxytocin alone,

a method with a higher incidence of caesarean section than when combined with prostaglandin (see below).
- The trials could not possibly be blinded and clinicians may have had different thresholds for recommending operative delivery in the conservative group.

At 41 weeks' gestation, approximately 19 per cent of women remain undelivered. This drops to 3.5 per cent at 42 weeks. The timing of induction will thus have critical workload implications. The NICE and RCOG guidelines recommend offering induction beyond 41 weeks, but commencing further fetal surveillance at 42 weeks for women who do not wish induction. The later the induction is performed in the 41–42-week period, the fewer inductions will be needed [Ia].

It is important to remember that approximately 1000 women will need to be induced to prevent stillbirth during this period of gestation. Induction of labour prior to 41 completed weeks will generate an increase in the workload without reducing perinatal mortality, and may have substantial effects on the incidence of caesarean section amongst nulliparae, with a potential doubling in rates.

Assessment of the post-dates pregnancy

Many different tests of fetal well-being are performed for the assessment of the post-term fetus. These include:

- cardiotocography (CTG)
- ultrasonographic testing
- amniotic fluid index
- biophysical profiles
- umbilical artery Doppler waveform analyses.

An amniotic fluid index <5 cm or maximum pool depth <2 cm is associated with higher rates of fetal heart rate decelerations and meconium staining of amniotic fluid in labour and both are indications for delivery. Equally, a biophysical score of 6/10 or less or abnormal umbilical artery Dopplers would also constitute a reason for delivery. However, the mechanism of fetal death in the late term pregnancy is poorly understood. The above assessments of fetal well-being are likely to identify those fetuses that are compromised for reasons such as placental infarction/insufficiency, but this is probably a different mechanism from that occurring in the death of many post-term fetuses. Consequently, obstetricians are unable to offer complete reassurance to the expectant mother who continues to await spontaneous onset of her labour. However, some form of monitoring additional to CTG must be offered, if only to detect fetuses compromised in assessable ways. The guidelines recommend at least twice-weekly CTG and ultrasound for amniotic fluid volume.

INDUCTION OF LABOUR FOR MATERNAL REQUEST

Induction of labour is sometimes performed for the convenience of the mother in the absence of any definite medical indication or clear health benefit (often described as social induction). Such inductions must be justified according to the particular circumstances involved, and any decision should be taken on an individual basis after fully informing the woman of any potential disadvantages. However, as with any intervention in pregnancy, induction of labour is not free from unwanted side effects and should not be undertaken lightly.

The personal characteristics of women requesting elective, rather than selective, induction of labour have been extensively studied. Such patients often experience more problems in the antenatal period and appear to be more anxious with regard to labour and delivery than their counterparts. However, as advocated in *Changing Childbirth*,[2] women should be allowed reasonable choices in their obstetric and midwifery care. If pregnancy has reached term and the cervix is favourable, there are no clear benefits for the fetus in delaying the onset of labour.

In multiparae with a favourable cervix, the risks are few; however, there is an increase in the incidence of instrumental deliveries and caesarean sections in nulliparae undergoing elective induction after 39 weeks [II].[3]

Consequently, it should be explained that if an induction fails, the risks of delivery by caesarean section might outweigh any possible social benefits that may be gained. Patients can only make an informed decision after careful consultation, with the risks and benefits clearly and appropriately presented.

A final comment is that a request for early induction of labour will sometimes present logistical problems to busy labour wards and the needs of women who require induction of labour for medical reasons must always be of paramount importance. Occasionally this needs to be explained when a request for induction cannot be met.

MECHANISMS OF PARTURITION

Although many theories have been postulated, the exact mechanisms underlying the onset of parturition in humans are not fully understood. However, the initiation of human labour must involve a constellation of changes that leads to a swing in the balance between quiescence and activity within the uterus.

Some clues may be gleaned from animal models. In the sheep, the production of fetal cortisol causes an increase in the production of placental oestrogens and prostaglandins, which sensitize the myometrium to circulating oxytocics,

Table 25.1   Factors involved in the onset of labour

Rise	Fall	Other
Endogenous prostaglandins	Prostaglandin dehydrogenase	Fetal ACTH
Serum oestrogens	Serum progesterone	Cervical remodelling
Oxytocin release	Cervical remodelling	Increase in number and sensitivity of uterine stretch receptors
Dihydroepiandrostenedione	Increase in uterine stretch receptors	
Basal cortisol	Fetal ACTH	
Interleukin-8 activity	Up-regulation of oxytocin receptors	

ACTH, adrenocorticotrophic hormone.

and in turn initiate labour. These changes are mediated by the hypothalamic–pituitary axis. However, this situation appears dissimilar to that in humans, in whom anencephalic fetuses demonstrate no tendency to prolonged gestations.

This suggests that other processes are responsible, and although many mechanisms have been postulated, the exact role played by each of the suggested agents has not been clearly elucidated (Table 25.1).

INDUCTION OF LABOUR

The methods currently employed in labour induction modulate only a limited part of the labour processes. Induction does not usually involve just a single intervention, but a complex set of interventions that present challenges for clinicians and women. Therefore it should not be surprising that induction of labour sometimes fails.

The methods currently employed include the following.

- Those employed by women that do not require formal medical prescription or involvement – ingestion of castor oil, acupuncture, herbal remedies, breast and nipple stimulation, and sexual intercourse.
- Those that rely on mechanical forces to promote cervical effacement and dilatation and the initiation of uterine contractions – membrane sweeping, hygroscopic and mechanical dilators, extra-amniotic infusion of saline, and amniotomy.
- Those that employ pharmacological agents to alter the cervical state, initiate uterine activity, or act by a combination of methods – prostaglandins, oxytocin, oestrogens, relaxin, antiprogestogens (mifepristone).

As a general rule, the more remote from term, the more difficult induction of labour will be, frequently requiring more than one technique over a period of a few days. There are fewer complications with methods employed closer to term, as they precede the probable onset of spontaneous labour by only a few hours or days, some of the receptor and biochemical changes are already established.

First stage of labour

Assessment before induction commences

As with any intervention, before the attendant physician proceeds with an induction, it is important to ensure that the indication for induction still exists, and that any specific labour management issues that may occur as a consequence of the intervention are highlighted. The clinician must confirm the fetal lie and presentation by abdominal palpation, and assess the well-being of the fetus (commonly by electronic monitoring of the fetal heart rate).

The likelihood of either successful induction or its failure may be most specifically ascertained by assessing the condition of the cervix. A variety of clinical scoring techniques have been reported for the assessment of the cervix prior to induction; the most commonly employed is the Bishop's Score, or a modification of this (Table 25.2). The most predictive elements in this system are the station of the presenting part, the length and dilatation of the cervix; as could be predicted, the shorter and more dilated the cervix, the shorter the intervention-to-delivery interval.

Fetal fibronectin

Fetal fibronectin is released from the amniotic membranes into the cervical transudate, and concentrations >50 g/mL are associated with a favourable cervix and a decrease in intrapartum morbidity. The fibronectin concentration has also been shown to correlate more favourably with the outcome of labour induction, with a shorter induction-to-delivery interval and length of labour than may be predicted by clinical assessment of the cervical state alone.[4] Measurement of this glycoprotein may help tune the timing of labour induction by allowing a more accurate correlation between the state of the cervix, changes in uterine activity and the responsivity to prostaglandins. In general, however, as induction should always be clinically indicated, this test has limited additional benefit. Perhaps it has a role in dissuading women requesting induction early, when a negative fetal fibronectin may indicate a higher chance of failure.

Table 25.2   Modified Bishop's Score

Factor	Score			
	0	1	2	3
Cervical dilatation (cm)	<1	1–2	3–4	>4
Cervical length (cm)	>4	2–4	1–2	<1
Station of the head	−3	−2	−1	0
Consistency	Firm	Average	Soft	
Position of the os	Posterior	Medium	Anterior	

The modified Bishop's Score is the summation of the individual scores for each of the observations.

Induction methods traditionally utilized by women

Castor oil

This medication, when taken orally, stimulates contractions of the large and small intestine via an effect on the smooth muscle within the viscera. Accompanying this unpleasant 'side effect' is a stimulation of uterine activity, but much more common are profuse diarrhoea and abdominal cramps. Its safety profile for mothers and babies has never been fully investigated and its use must be discouraged. It may potentially increase the incidence of meconium staining of liquor, as it has an effect on a term fetus similar to that on the mother [III].

Acupuncture

The use of acupuncture for labour induction is based on the traditions of Chinese medicine that date back at least 30 centuries. The published data from Western literature are too small to address the issues of efficacy or safety, and its use outside the remits of clinical studies cannot be recommended.

Herbal remedies

Traditional remedies employed to stimulate the onset of labour rely on products that contain ergot derivatives in various strengths that consequently exhibit a weak uterine stimulant effect. The dose and purity of these compounds are often variable, and there is not sufficient evidence to support their use. The efficacy of raspberry leaf tea, whose potential for labour induction stems from observations on brood mares, is equally dubious.

Breast and nipple stimulation

Breast stimulation is thought to work by stimulating the release of oxytocin from the posterior pituitary. Although many different studies have attempted to standardize the 'treatment' provided (either through mechanical pumps or electrical stimulation), none has been shown to produce consistent and reproducible results.

There are case reports of nipple stimulation being associated with uterine hypertonus and fetal bradycardia. These same studies suggest that if nipple stimulation is to be advocated as a method of labour induction, continuous fetal monitoring should be employed at the same time. The studies that look at larger groups employing such techniques are fraught with technical difficulties and at best are difficult to interpret and at worst, meaningless.

Sexual intercourse

Semen is rich in naturally occurring prostaglandins; however, there is little evidence to support the belief that sexual intercourse enhances cervical ripening.

Medical interventions

Mechanical

MEMBRANE SWEEPING

The practice of sweeping the membranes during vaginal examination has long been advocated as a method for stimulating the onset of labour. This procedure involves passing a finger through the cervical os, sweeping it around the internal surface of the cervix and gently pushing the membrane surface away.

It is recommended that all women be offered membrane sweeping prior to induction of labour (see 'Further reading'), as it is associated with:

- increased likelihood of spontaneous labour within 48 hours (63.8 vs 83 per cent, relative risk (RR) 0.77, 95 per cent confidence interval (CI) 0.7–0.84, number needed to treat (NNT) 5);
- decreased incidence of prolonged pregnancy of 41 weeks or more (18.6 vs 29.9 per cent, RR 0.62, 95 per cent CI 0.49–0.79, NNT 8).

On a population basis, this may result in a decrease in the induction rate of 15 per cent, with no differences in maternal or fetal outcome [Ia].

However, it is important that before this is undertaken, women understand:

- the procedure is designed to impact as above,
- it may be a little uncomfortable,
- they may experience frequent contractions following the procedure,
- there may be a little vaginal bleeding following the procedure.

If the woman gives her consent for a membrane sweep, the procedure should be performed with gentleness and consideration. If consent is not given, membranes should not be swept under any circumstances.

HYGROSCOPIC AND MECHANICAL DILATORS

When compared with their frequent use in the process of procuring a first or early second trimester abortion, cervical dilators have been employed with relative infrequency for the induction of labour.

Hygroscopic dilators work by absorbing water by osmosis, with a resulting change in their size and shape. When placed into the cervical canal over a period of hours (>12 hours – often overnight), they produce a mechanical dilatation, which then permits an amniotomy to be performed. These agents may also stimulate the local release of prostaglandins, which may have additional benefits on cervical ripening.

Balloon devices and Foley catheters placed within the cervical canal in an attempt to dilate the cervix mechanically have also been investigated. As with the hygroscopic devices, they have been shown to be effective in facilitating cervical dilatation, but overall have not improved the number of successful labour inductions.

With all these devices, insertion is best performed with the patient in the lithotomy position, using an aseptic technique to visualize the cervix, which must be exposed with a Cusco's speculum. One or more hygroscopic agents are then inserted into the cervical canal as judged appropriate by the cervical state, and left in situ for the period of time necessary to provide the required improvement in the cervical condition. Synthetic polyvinyl alcohol polymer sponges impregnated with magnesium sulphate (Lamicel) and the polyacrylonitrite tents are more rapidly effective than their naturally occurring counterpart (Laminaria Tent) [Ib].

Once the cervix has reached the required dilatation, the induction may be advanced by amniotomy ± administration of oxytocin. However, with any intracervical device, concerns regarding the introduction of iatrogenic infection have been raised. This risk probably increases in proportion to the duration of retention of any mechanical device, and consequently careful monitoring of the maternal pulse and temperature and the fetal heart rate must be undertaken.

Currently, there appear to be few indications for such interventions, as the efficacy, and safety, of prostaglandins make them almost redundant.

EXTRA-AMNIOTIC INFUSION OF SALINE

The infusion of 0.9 per cent saline solution into the extra-amniotic space via a Foley catheter has been used as a method of inducing labour. This technique appears to be equally effective at inducing labour as topical prostaglandins, with no difference in the incidence of maternal or neonatal infectious morbidity between the groups. There may be a trend towards an increase in the rate of caesarean section with the infusion intervention, although the studies to date have been too small to assess the clinical significance of this. Further studies are recommended.

AMNIOTOMY

Traditionally, amniotomy (rupturing of the amniotic membrane) has been either hindwater (performed with a Drew–Smythe catheter) or forewater (a procedure performed with an amniotomy hook – 'Amnihook' – or toothed forcep). The risks inherent with the hindwater approach – namely, uterine, placental and fetal trauma – make this intervention difficult to justify in modern obstetric practice. By comparison, the forewater procedure is safe, but still carries the risks of cord prolapse, placental abruption and the introduction of infection into the uterine cavity.

Prior to any amniotomy, an abdominal palpation must be performed to confirm the fetal lie and presentation as well as to allow auscultation of the fetal heart. Following this, the cervix is examined to confirm that the forewaters are intact. The station of the presenting part is noted and the membranes ruptured. This releases amniotic fluid, the quantity and colour of which should be noted (absence or presence of meconium). A check is made to ensure that the presentation/station and position of the presenting part remain unchanged and that there is no prolapse of the umbilical cord. If required, a fetal scalp electrode may be sited.

The success of amniotomy is dependent upon the state of the cervix (dilatation and effacement), the parity of the woman and the station of the presenting part at the time of intervention. Up to 88 per cent of women with a favourable cervix will labour within 24 hours after amniotomy alone.[5] Amniotomy with the commencement of an early oxytocin infusion (commonly within 2–6 hours if prostaglandins have been used for cervical ripening) produces a significant reduction in the number of women remaining undelivered at 24 hours compared with those managed expectantly [Ib].[6]

Biochemical

PROSTAGLANDINS

Prostaglandins are long-chain fatty acids derived from arachadonic acid via the cyclo-oxygenase pathway, and exert a powerful effect on the cervix and myometrium at all stages of gestation. Not only do they modify the ground substance within the cervix, increasing its compliance, they also stimulate the onset of uterine contractions, and thus induce labour. They are therefore particularly useful for labour induction where the cervix is unfavourable.

Prostaglandins of the E_2 and $F_{2\alpha}$ class have been used to initiate labour, although there are few studies employing the latter in preference to the former. More recently, prostaglandin E_1 analogues (e.g. misoprostol) have received attention.

Prostaglandins may be given via the oral, intravaginal, intracervical or intravenous routes to good effect (Table 25.3). However, intracervical gel and intravaginal preparations have fewer systemic side effects compared with the other routes of administration. Meta-analyses have shown that there are advantages to the use of prostaglandins for ripening the cervix and for induction of labour, compared with oxytocin alone. These are:

- increased successful vaginal delivery within 24 hours,
- decreased incidence of caesarean section,

- decreased risk of the cervix remaining unfavourable at 48 hours,
- reduced epidural usage.

This is at the expense of increased gastrointestinal side effects and uterine hypertonus, which occur in approximately 1 per cent of pregnant women receiving no more than two 2 mg intravaginal gels.[7]

Even in women with a favourable cervix, prostaglandins are associated with increased rates of successful vaginal delivery at 24 hours, though there are no differences in caesarean section or epidural rates [Ia]. It is recommended that prostaglandins are the first-line method for all women regardless of cervical score. Interestingly though, in the group with a favourable cervix, prostaglandins were associated with reduced levels of maternal satisfaction.

Intravaginal prostaglandin E_2 (either gel or tablets) appears to be marginally superior to intracervical preparations, with an increase in the success of induction and a decreased need for oxytocin. Failure rates of 10 per cent for the intracervical route versus <3 per cent for the intravaginal route have been quoted, although several studies have not demonstrated any difference.[7]

There are theoretical advantages to the use of the gel over tablets; namely, that plasma levels are higher with the gel. Some studies suggested higher rates of instrumental vaginal delivery with gel in comparison to tablets, but this is not a universal finding. At present, given the lack of evidence for different clinical effects, the differential cost implications have led to the recommendation that tablets should be used (NICE Guideline, induction of labour).

There are many randomized trials of prostaglandins, but as the populations, protocols, routes, dosages and dosage intervals are so heterogeneous, providing firm management conclusions is very difficult. Some protocols use repeated prostaglandin treatments at 6-hourly intervals for three doses, whereas others prescribe amniotomy and infusion of oxytocin 15 hours after a single prostaglandin treatment,

Table 25.3   Route of administration for prostaglandins in induction of labour

Route of administration	Prostaglandin type/dose and frequency	Benefits	Problems
Oral	E_2 tablets 0.5 mg hourly every 2 hours to a max. of 2 mg	Avoids potential iatrogenic introduction of infection	Gastrointestinal side effects
Intravenous	E_2 infusions at 0.1 μg/min to a max of 4 μg/min $F_{2\alpha}$ 3 μg/min to a max. of 30 μg/min	Enables titration against effect to be closely monitored	Gastrointestinal side effects Local tissue reactions (erythema) at infusion site
Intracervical	E_2 tablets	Reduced incidence of systemic side effects when compared with other routes of administration	Higher failure rate (10% vs 3%), more difficult to administer and less efficient at ripening the cervix than intravaginal preparations Potential iatrogenic introduction of infection
Intravaginal	E_2 tablets, viscous gel, wax pessary 2–5 mg in biodegradable form – latent period of 12 hours Sustained release preparations 5–10 mg in non-biodegradable form	Reduced incidence of systemic side effects when compared with other routes of administration	Potential iatrogenic introduction of infection

Table 25.4   Recommended regimens for prostaglandin E$_2$ administration

Type	Interval	Total dose
Tablets	6 hourly	3 mg, 3 mg all women
Gel	6 hours	2 mg, 1 mg, 1 mg in nulliparae
		1 mg, 1 mg, 1 mg in multiparae

unless labour is already established. There is only a marginal benefit in using more than three or four doses. Similarly, dosage intervals of <6 hours or doses of >4 mg do not appear to be advantageous (Table 25.4).[7]

Prostaglandin E$_2$ is also available as a sustained release preparation (Propess, Ferring AB, Malmo, Sweden). This polymer-based vaginal insert contains 10 mg of prostaglandin E$_2$ that is released continuously over a 12-hour period, producing metabolite levels within the circulation that are similar to those found with 1 mg of intravaginal prostaglandin E$_2$ gel. A potential benefit of this preparation is that the insert can be removed from the vagina if uterine hypertonus or fetal distress develops. Although comparison with placebo indicates that it is probably a safe and effective induction agent, the preparation is expensive and its efficacy may be affected by the pH of the vagina. Further clinical trials are therefore necessary.

In summary, intravaginal prostaglandin E$_2$ is currently the agent of choice [Ia].

There is often debate about whether further doses can be given when women are experiencing mild tightenings in response to a gel given 6 hours previously. This is always a difficult area, and there are no studies on which to base practice. The manufacturer's leaflet suggests that uterine activity contraindicates a repeat dose, but this has to be a clinical decision. Where there is doubt, it is best to delay giving another dose if the cervix is unfavourable (if favourable, an amniotomy can be performed or the establishment of labour awaited). It may be best not to delay too long (especially not to leave women unassessed overnight), as this can lead to a very protracted and exhausting induction process. Usually it is apparent by 8–10 hours that labour is commencing or contractions are settling.

MISOPROSTOL

This prostaglandin E$_1$ analogue was initially developed for the treatment and prevention of peptic ulcer disease. It was subsequently noted to produce uterine contractions and has recently been utilized as an abortifacient with marked success. In addition, misoprostol is cheaper and more easily stored than the other prostaglandins.

Several studies have shown that misoprostol appears to be as effective an induction agent as the currently available prostaglandin preparations in inducing labour in the third trimester, but the safest and most effective administration protocols have yet to be established. It has been used in doses ranging from 50 μg (administered 4 hourly per vaginum to a maximum of five doses) to 100 μg (as single or repeat doses), and although the induction-to-delivery interval is reduced with increasing doses, this is often at the increased risk of uterine hypertonus [Ib].

There are considerable concerns regarding the rates of postpartum haemorrhage when misoprostol is used for induction, and of uterine dehiscence in women who have a previous caesarean section scar. Consequently, further work needs to be performed to establish a safe dosing regimen that carries a low risk of hypertonus and uterine dehiscence whilst maintaining an effect as a labour inductificant. Misoprostol remains unlicensed for labour induction and until the best dose regimen is determined, its use in labour induction should be confined to clinical trials.

OXYTOCIN

Oxytocin is an octapeptide hormone secreted from the supraoptic and paraventricular nuclei of the hypothalamus. It is transported to the posterior pituitary along the axons of these neurons, where it is stored and then released in a pulsatile manner. Despite its short half-life in the circulation, oxytocin stimulates uterine activity, with the frequency and force of contractions being proportional to the oxytocin concentration in the plasma. Oxytocin also exhibits antidiuretic properties, a consequence of a structural similarity with vasopressin. Therefore, the possibility of fluid overload must always be borne in mind during administration in labour.

Although many different infusion regimens exist, it is generally recommended that oxytocin should be given via an infusion pump or syringe driver with a 'non-return valve', and the fluid load minimized. Most infusion regimens commence at low rates (1–2 mU/minute) and increase variably (titrated against contractions), arithmetically or logarithmically at intervals of between 10 and 30 minutes up to a maximum of approximately 32 mU/minute. The aim is to attain contractions at a frequency of 3–4 per 10 minutes, and in some cases this may be established with 12 mU/minute or less.

There is no evidence of benefit in using intervals of less than 30 minutes to increase the dose, as most, but not all, of the reports indicate that the use of longer intervals reduced uterine hypertonus, decreased maximum and total dose of oxytocin, and decreased the rate of caesarean section for fetal heart rate abnormalities. This seems to be a logical approach as it takes 30–45 minutes for the plasma levels of oxytocin to reach a 'steady state'. Such a regimen also appears to have no adverse effects on induction–delivery intervals.[8]

Pulsatile infusion regimens, in which boluses of oxytocin are given at 20–30-minute intervals, have been suggested to be more physiological, and more logical in view of the half-life of oxytocin and its receptor occupancy in labour. It is possible that such regimens require less oxytocin overall, with reduced risk of hyperstimulation, but so far there is little evidence to suggest they have any great advantage over those currently used.

First stage of labour

The pregnant uterus is relatively insensitive to oxytocin and first requires priming with either endogenous or exogenous prostaglandins for oxytocin to have any substantial effect on uterine contractility. Consequently, medical priming with prostaglandin E_2 followed by an amniotomy (mechanical induction) and oxytocin infusion is the common sequence of interventions in an induction of labour. If oxytocin infusion is commenced at the time of amniotomy rather than delayed, there are advantages of a significantly shorter induction–delivery interval, reduced operative delivery rates and a reduction in postpartum haemorrhage. However, it is recommended that oxytocin should not be prescribed within 6 hours following the administration of vaginal prostaglandins. Whether these benefits outweigh the disadvantages of intravenous cannulation with consequent restricted mobility should be left to individual patients who, after appropriate counselling, can then make an informed choice.

Agents currently being researched

NITRIC OXIDE DONORS

Nitric oxide donors stimulate cyclo-oygenase activity. When administered per vaginum, they are believed to increase the production of prostaglandins within the cervix, and cause cervical remodelling and effacement. However, they may also exert a tocolytic effect on the term uterus, and may be associated with an increase in the induction-to-delivery interval and in the rates of caesarean section and postpartum haemorrhage. Further studies are required.

RELAXIN

In a few small clinical trials, this agent has been administered as a vaginal gel in an attempt to induce cervical ripening. At a dose of between 1 and 4 mg, the recombinant product of synthetic manufacture has been singularly unsuccessful in inducing labour when compared with placebo. It is possible that an increase in the prescribed dose or route of administration may provide different results.

ANTIPROGESTOGENS (MIFEPRISTONE – RU486)

As an agent for ripening the cervix, this class of drugs exhibits great potential. In a prospective, randomized, controlled trial involving 120 women of mixed parity, 56 per cent of those given mifepristone commenced labour, compared with 22 per cent of the placebo group. However, other outcomes between the two groups were no different; the incidence of delivery by caesarean section was equal in both groups.[9] As mifepristone also crosses the placenta, and has the potential to cause disturbances in aldosterone and glucocorticoid metabolism, there exists the possibility of fetal or neonatal side effects, although none has so far been observed.

INTERLEUKIN-8

Interleukin-8 is a pro-inflammatory cytokine, produced in vivo by choriodecidual cells and implicated in the onset of spontaneous labour. Interleukin-8 production is stimulated

by mifepristone and it has synergistic actions to the prostaglandins. This agent has good theoretical potential as a cervical collagenolytic and uterine stimulant, although its clinical application has yet to be investigated, as research is currently limited to rabbits.

PRACTICAL CONSIDERATIONS CONCERNING INDUCTION OF LABOUR

Where should induction of labour take place?

The main proviso for safe induction of labour is that it should be conducted in a setting in which there are adequate staffing levels to monitor both the fetus and mother where necessary. For prostaglandin administration, it may be that a ward area provides the necessary levels of surveillance. However, when induction is performed with a potentially compromised fetus or increased risks in the mother (prior caesarean section, high parity etc.), the extra level of surveillance provided by a labour ward should be the norm.

Once labour is established or oxytocin commenced, the labour ward is the appropriate setting, and women should be cared for on a one-to-one basis.

The 4th Annual Report of the Confidential Enquiry into Stillbirth and Deaths in Infancy (CESDI) cited an induction of labour as a contributory cause in 54 cases. The main problems identified were:

- inadequate monitoring and supervision in high-risk cases,
- lack of monitoring after prostaglandin induction,
- the use of prostaglandins in higher than recommended doses and for too long,
- repeated doses of prostaglandins (often without examination) causing hypertonus,
- use of oxytocin for too long despite lack of progress in labour,
- use of oxytocin despite evidence of good progress in labour,
- use of oxytocin despite clear signs of cephalo-pelvic disproportion or fetal compromise.

The report also highlighted the special care required when induction of labour is undertaken in a woman with a previous caesarean section, especially if the cervix is unfavourable and prostaglandin or oxytocin is employed.

When to perform induction

Uterine contractility has a natural circadian rhythm, with the period of maximal activity occurring between 2200 and 2400 hours. The inference from this observation is that inductions of labour performed at this time would stand a greater chance of being successful than those commenced at other times. However, there are no data to support this hypothesis.

Many units have moved to a first dose of prostaglandin being inserted in the evening, with the aim of reducing the number of deliveries in the early hours. There are anecdotal reports that this is effective, but randomized trials have not been performed [III].

FETAL SURVEILLANCE FOLLOWING INDUCTION OF LABOUR

There are no trials that indicate the level of fetal surveillance required during an induction; however, as induction is a process most commonly undertaken when there are minimal risks to the fetus or mother, it would seem prudent to ascertain, as far as is possible, that the fetus is in good health before it is submitted to any stressful intervention. Therefore, when prostaglandins are used for cervical ripening, CTG should be performed for 20 minutes before its administration and for 60 minutes thereafter and should be recommenced when contractions ensue. Continuous CTG is also recommended throughout the induction process whenever an oxytocin infusion is used and if there are other risk factors, for example fetal growth restriction, diabetes or pre-eclampsia. If fetal status is reassuring, pregnancy has been uncomplicated and labour ensues with prostaglandin alone, intermittent monitoring may be employed [IV].

COMPLICATIONS OF INDUCTION OF LABOUR

Failed induction of labour

It has been estimated that a 'failed induction' occurs in up to 35 per cent of cases induced with oxytocin alone and in 3–5 per cent of cases in which prostaglandins have been used. However, making a formal diagnosis of induction failure is frequently difficult, as many different definitions exist and a consensus has yet to be reached. It may be applied to:

- cases in which the cervix remains unfavourable and amniotomy is not possible 6 hours after 4 mg of prostaglandin has been administered in nulliparae and 3 mg in multiparae;
- cases in which the cervix fails to dilate beyond 3 cm during a period of appropriate stimulation with oxytocin – this is commonly quoted as 6 hours after the maximal infusion rate of syntocinon has been attained (a level determined by local protocols).

These clinical scenarios present different dilemmas to the attendant obstetrician. Where the induction has involved the administration of prostaglandins alone, there is often little immediate risk to the mother or baby. The next stage of management must therefore be to question the indication for delivery and review the clinical scenario in this light. If the indication is weak, such as social convenience, a delay of a few days while awaiting the onset of spontaneous labour or a further attempt at induction may be indicated. In the interim, a suitable level of maternal and fetal surveillance must be undertaken, perhaps incorporating daily CTGs and twice-weekly biophysical scores. If the indication remains strong, however, there is little else to do but persist with the induction or deliver by caesarean section. This decision must be made at a senior level and in conjunction with the woman.

Where oxytocin has been employed, the risks to both mother and baby are greatly increased. Not only are there risks of infection with prolonged rupture of the membranes, but also of:

- continued uterine stimulation and the effect on the fetal acid–base status;
- the antidiuretic effect of oxytocin on maternal and fetal electrolyte balance (especially if the indication for induction is pre-eclampsia);
- maternal, and paternal, exhaustion;
- rarely, uterine rupture.

The attendant physician may choose to resort to delivery by caesarean section (by far the easiest and perhaps safest option), but careful assessment (including confirming that the forewaters are indeed absent) may determine that a further period of observation should be employed. If no further change occurs after this time (e.g. 2 hours), delivery by caesarean section must be offered.

Cord prolapse

An amniotomy performed without the presenting part located within or 'over' the pelvis runs the risk of cord prolapse. However, the occurrence of such a problem during labour induction is fortunately rare. Should the cord present during such a procedure, pressure on the cord should be reduced by placing the patient in the knee/chest position and a doctor/midwife should displace the presenting part by the introduction of their hand within the vagina. Inserting a Foley catheter per urethram and filling the bladder with 400 mL normal saline may achieve a similar effect. Delivery must then be effected as quickly as possible to reduce the risks of hypoxia to the fetus.

Abruption

A placental abruption may occur if rapid uterine decompression complicates an amniotomy. Care should therefore be taken if polyhydramnios is suspected and, if so, adequate precautions (e.g. intravenous access, theatre team aware etc.) must be in place before the procedure is performed.

First stage of labour

Maternal

Hyponatraemia

This avoidable complication often occurs as a consequence of prolonged intravenous oxytocin infusions. The fluid retention, electrolyte disturbance, coma, convulsions and death that may follow can be avoided by careful fluid balance management and by administering the oxytocin in an appropriate concentration (e.g. 40 IU in 500 mL normal saline). Similar electrolyte disturbances can occur in the neonate and lead to neonatal seizures in extreme cases.

Uterine hyperstimulation

Any technique used to stimulate labour carries the potential risk of inducing uterine hyperstimulation – an inappropriate reaction of the myometrium to exogenous oxytocics, as a result of either drug hypersensitivity or drug overdose. The resultant uterine hypertonus is associated with an elevation in the resting intrauterine pressure, which in turn causes fetal hypoxia. The incidence of hyperstimulation appears to be related to the efficiency of the technique employed to stimulate labour. Misoprostol carries the greatest risk; whereas both prostaglandins and oxytocin appear to be less troublesome (each carrying a risk of hyperstimulation of approximately 1:500 inductions).[10]

The potential management options include the following.

- In cases associated with oxytocin stimulation, the infusion should be decreased or discontinued.
- Administration of an intravenous bolus dose of a suitable tocolytic to reduce the hypertonus and allow the fetal heart to recover: e.g. terbutaline 250 µg subcutaneously (NB. inhaled medication is of questionable benefit).
- Expedition of delivery (assisted vaginal delivery if fully dilated or delivery by caesarean section) within 30 minutes.

There is no research evidence evaluating the benefits and risk associated with the short-term use of facial oxygen therapy in cases of suspected fetal compromise. Prolonged use of maternal facial oxygen therapy may be harmful to the fetus and should therefore be avoided (see Chapter 29).

Postpartum haemorrhage

Women delivered following labour induction have a higher incidence of postpartum haemorrhage than those delivering after a spontaneous onset of labour. This problem should therefore be anticipated and managed accordingly.

Fetal

Prematurity

Situations in which an infant is born prematurely may be the consequence of a deliberate preterm induction, where the maternal or fetal condition merits intervention for example pre-eclampsia. However, erroneous iatrogenic prematurity should not occur in modern obstetric practice, as ultrasound confirmation of the gestation will invariably have been performed, and all dates should be confirmed before an induction is undertaken. Where dates are uncertain, usually because of late presentation for antenatal care or missing early scans, fetal well-being should be established by ultrasound. Once it is established that the fetus is healthy, a policy of watchful waiting can be adopted. There may be a need to repeat tests of well-being. Induction can be planned once the cervix is favourable or if concerns arise regarding the mother or fetus.

Hyperbilirubinaemia

Neonatal jaundice has been reported following the use of oxytocin, but not prostaglandin, during labour induction. In most cases this jaundice is mild, short lived and does not require treatment.

SPECIAL CASES

Induction following caesarean section

This subject is covered extensively in Chapter 26. Decisions regarding induction should be made at a senior level.

Grand multiparae

Induction of labour in the grand multipara is associated with an increased incidence of precipitate labour, uterine rupture and postpartum haemorrhage. In this group of women, it is reasonable to increase syntocinon more slowly, with 45-minute increments at the most. This appears to be safe in the majority of women.[8]

SUMMARY

A summary of the points covered in this chapter is shown in Table 25.5.

- An ultrasound to confirm gestation should be offered before 20 weeks' gestation, as this reduces the need for induction for perceived post-term pregnancy.
- Women with uncomplicated pregnancies should be offered an induction of labour beyond 41 weeks.
- Prostaglandin should be used in preference to oxytocin when induction is undertaken in either nulliparous women or multiparous women with intact membranes, regardless of their cervical favourability.

Table 25.5   Suggested methods for labour induction as guided by cervical status

Bishop's Score	Method of induction	Proven efficacy	Mechanism of action	Followed by
<5	*Mechanical*		Mechanical cervical dilatation	Amniotomy ± oxytocin
	Catheters	X		
	Balloons	X		
	Hygroscopic dilators	X		
	Medical		Cervical modification and myometrial stimulation	Repeated doses if required – then amniotomy ± oxytocin
	Prostaglandins	√		
	Anti-progestogens	√		
	Oestrogens	X		
	DHEAS	X		
	Relaxin	X		
5–8	*Mechanical*		Cervical modification and myometrial stimulation	Oxytocin infusion immediately or after a short delay
	Amniotomy	√		
	Medical			Repeated doses if required – then amniotomy ± oxytocin infusion
	Prostaglandins (oral or vaginal)	√		
>8	*Mechanical*		Cervical modification and myometrial stimulation	Oxytocin infusion immediately or after a short delay 6 hours before oxytocin if prostaglandins
	Amniotomy	√		
	Medical			
	Prostaglandins			

DHEAS, dihydroepiandrostenedione.

- Either prostaglandins or oxytocin may be used when induction is undertaken in nulliparous or multiparous women who have ruptured membranes, regardless of cervical status, as they are equally effective.
- When induction is undertaken with prostaglandins, intravaginal prostaglandin E_2 tablets should be considered in preference to gel formulations or intracervical administration.
- In the presence of abnormal fetal heart rate patterns and uterine hypercontractility (not secondary to oxytocin infusion), tocolysis should be considered. A suggested regimen is subcutaneous terbutaline 250 μg.

- The accurate assessment of each patient and her suitability for induction may help to increase the success rate of each intervention whilst decreasing the iatrogenic problems that currently do not occur infrequently.

KEY REFERENCES

1. Hannah ME, Hannah WJ, Hellman J, Hewson S, Milner R, Willan A. Canadian Multicenter Post-Term Pregnancy Trial Group. Induction of labour as compared with serial antenatal monitoring in post-term pregnancy. A randomized controlled trial. *N Engl J Med* 1992; **326**:1587–92.
2. Department of Health. *Changing Childbirth*, Part 1. Report of the Expert Maternity Group. London: HMSO, 1993.
3. Smith LP, Nagourney BA, McLean FH, Usher RH. Hazards and benefits of elective induction of labour. *Am J Obstet Gynecol* 1984; **148**(5):579–85.
4. Garite TJ, Casal D, Garcia-Alonso A. Fetal fibronectin: a new tool for the prediction of successful induction of labour. *Am J Obstet Gynecol* 1996; **175**:1516–21.
5. Booth JH, Kurdizak VB. Elective induction of labour: a controlled study. *Can Med Assoc J* 1970; **103**:245–8.
6. Keirse MJNC. Amniotomy plus early vs. late oxytocin infusion for induction of labour. In: Ankin MW, Keirse MJNC, Renfrew MJ, Neilson JP, Crowther C

KEY POINTS

- Induction of labour is a common procedure and is now performed in 15–20 per cent of all term pregnancies in the UK.
- Induction seldom involves a single intervention, but rather a complex set of interventions that can present challenges for both clinicians and mothers to be.
- Many agents have had their role in the process of labour induction, established by carefully controlled trials, whereas others have been less formally assessed.

(eds). *The Cochrane Pregnancy and Childbirth Database*. Oxford: The Cochrane Collaboration, 1995, 262–8.

7. Keirse MJNC. Any prostaglandin (by any route) vs oxytocin (any route) for induction of labour. In: Enkin MW, Keirse MJNC, Renfrew MJ, Neilson JP, Crowther C (eds). *The Cochrane Pregnancy and Childbirth Database*. Oxford: The Cochrane Collaboration, 1995, 308–13.

8. Orhue AA. A randomized trial of 30-min and 15-min oxytocin infusion regimen for induction of labour at term in women of low parity. *Int J Gynaecol Obstet* 1993; **40**:219–25.

9. Frydman R, Lelaidier C, Barton-Saint-Mleux C. Labour induction in women at term with mifepristone (RU486): a double-blind, randomized, placebo-controlled study. *Obstet Gynecol* 1992; **80**:972–5.

10. MacKenzie Z, Burns E. Randomised trial of one versus two doses of prostaglandin E2 for induction of labour. 1. Clinical outcome. *Br J Obstet Gynaecol* 1997; **104**:1062–7.

Chapter 26

Management after Previous Caesarean Section

Lucy Kean

MRCOG standards

- Candidates are expected to be able to manage the labour of a woman with a previous caesarean section.

In addition, we would suggest the following.

Theoretical skills
- Be able to counsel a woman regarding planning for subsequent delivery after a single caesarean section.
- Know the rates of vaginal delivery in women undergoing labour after prior caesarean section in your unit.
- Revise the signs and symptoms of scar dehiscence.

Practical skills
- Be able to recognize a morbidly adherent placenta at manual removal and manage with senior assistance.

INTRODUCTION

Delivery by caesarean section accounts for 21.3 per cent of deliveries in England. In many units, caesarean section rates for primigravidae of 24 per cent are seen.[1] Consequently, the problem of management of women with a scarred uterus in subsequent pregnancies is one of the most common reasons for hospital referral in multigravidae. It is a vital part of antenatal care that women are given a clear understanding of the plan of management from early in pregnancy, with the caveat that this may need to be adapted if the pregnancy presents unexpected problems.

UNDERSTANDING THE RISKS

Relative maternal morbidity and mortality

It is almost impossible to assess the relative mortality from caesarean section, as the indication for the caesarean section will undoubtedly impact on the outcome. There are no trials to instruct us in this, and adapting information from published reports such as the Confidential Enquiry into Maternal Deaths is fraught with difficulty.

The most recent Confidential Enquiry quotes the figures in Table 26.1.

The relative risks of mortality for indirect deaths are also similar, 4.5 (2.85–7.06) for all caesarean sections.

Of the three reported deaths from placenta praevia, all were women with previous uterine surgery, two of whom had had previous caesarean section. It is also commented upon that in several cases placenta accreta attributable to previous caesarean section contributed to the maternal death. In addition, seven deaths from thromboembolism after caesarean section were reported.

Table 26.1 Estimated case fatality rates per million maternities and relative risk by type of delivery for direct deaths, UK 1997–99

Type of delivery	Total	Delivered direct deaths	Death rate/ million	Relative risk (95% CI)
All maternities	2124	63		
Vaginal deliveries	1710	29	16.9	1.0
All caesarean section	413	34	82.3	4.9 (2.96–7.97)
Emergency	69	14	202.9	12.0 (6.32–22.65)
Urgent	137	14	102.2	6.0 (3.18–11.4)
Scheduled	78	1	12.8	0.8 (0.1–5.55)
Elective	130	5	38.5	2.3 (0.88–5.86)

CI, confidence interval.

This knowledge is vital in counselling women with regard to subsequent delivery. However, it must be balanced against the risks of trial of vaginal delivery after caesarean section.

The risks of both placenta praevia and placenta accreta increase exponentially with each repeat caesarean section, from a baseline risk of 0.26 per cent and 0.01 per cent respectively in an unscarred uterus to 10 per cent and 6.7 per cent after a fourth caesarean section (see Chapter 31).

When discussing management with a patient, the individual risks and benefits must be considered.

Repeat elective caesarean section: risks and benefits

Maternal benefits

Caesarean section avoids labour with its risks of:

- perineal trauma (urinary and faecal problems),
- the need for emergency caesarean section,
- scar dehiscence or rupture with subsequent morbidity and mortality.

It also has the advantage of allowing a planned delivery.

Maternal risks

- Increased bleeding.
- Thromboembolism.
- Febrile morbidity.
- Prolonged recovery.
- Bladder dysfunction long term.
- Increased risks of placenta praevia and accreta in subsequent pregnancies.

Fetal benefit

- No risk from intrapartum scar rupture.

Fetal risk

- Increased risk of transient tachypnoea/respiratory distress syndrome.

The aim of this chapter is to attempt to quantify these risks, in order that, for each individual, appropriate counselling can be undertaken in planning the next delivery.

It is important to realize that women make decisions for a variety of reasons and that their choices may not always be those that we would make ourselves. The debate about choice with regard to delivery is not one that can be fully covered here, but it is apparent from the *Sentinel Caesarean Section Audit* that women are given far greater choice in planning their next delivery if their previous delivery was by caesarean section.

There is remarkably little evidence to inform practice with regard to the management of previous caesarean section. There are no randomized trials comparing trial of labour with elective caesarean section, and most of the available data relate to observational studies.

It is important to recognize that small asymptomatic scar dehiscences occur in women delivered both vaginally and by elective caesarean section. Most published studies do not differentiate between scar dehiscence and rupture. A meta-analysis of observational and comparative studies examining maternal and fetal morbidity and mortality following trial of labour compared with women undergoing repeat elective caesarean section showed the combined scar dehiscence and rupture rates for lower segment scars were 1.8 per cent for all trials of labour, 1.9 per cent for women undergoing repeat caesarean section without labour (no difference), and 3.3 per cent for women who underwent emergency caesarean section during a trial of labour [III]. Maternal febrile morbidity was significantly lower after a trial of labour than after an elective repeat caesarean section (9.6 vs 17.4 per cent, $p < 0.001$).

Table 26.2 shows the odds ratios for scar dehiscence/ rupture from the meta-analysis by Rosen et al.[2] The rate of scar problems in the successful VBAC group will be very low, as the majority of these women will not have undergone examination of the scar and small asymptomatic dehiscences will therefore not be noted.

Fetal morbidity was also assessed in the meta-analysis of trial of labour compared with repeat elective caesarean section by Rosen et al. After excluding antepartum deaths, fetuses weighing $<750\,$g, and congenital anomalies incompatible with life, there were no differences in perinatal death rates. If the scar truly ruptures, the perinatal mortality rate is 2.5 per cent. The proportion of 5-minute Apgar scores of $\leqslant6$ was higher after a trial of labour (2.4 vs 1.6 per cent, $p < 0.01$), but it was not possible to exclude very low birth weight fetuses or those with congenital anomalies from this analysis.[2]

Table 26.3 shows the odds ratio for a low Apgar score at 5 minutes from Rosen et al.[2]

The risks of maternal death were very low, with most studies reporting no or one death. Deaths were predominantly related to placenta accreta, though rupture-related

Table 26.2 Rate of uterine dehiscence or rupture by type of delivery

Type of delivery	Patients (n)	No. dehiscence/ 1000	OR rupture/ 1000
Elective CS	3611	19	1.0
All TOL	2771	18	0.8
Failed TOL	584	33	2.8
Successful VBAC	1613	12	0.7

OR, odds ratio; CS, caesarean section; TOL, trials of labour; VBAC, vaginal birth after caesarean section.

Table 26.3   Neonatal morbidity and mortality by type of delivery

Type of delivery	Patients n	No. Apgar ≤ 6/1000	Odds ratio
All TOL	1444	24	2.1
Failed TOL	286	38	2.6
VBAC	584	17	1.8
Elective repeat CS	1955	16	1.0

TOL, trials of labour; VBAC, vaginal birth after caesarean section; CS, caesarean section.

Table 26.4   Successful vaginal delivery in subsequent labour by reason for previous caesarean section (CS)

Indication for previous CS	Success rate (%)
Malpresentation	85
Any reason + previous vaginal delivery	84
Fetal distress	75
Dystocia	67
Oxytocin in this labour	63

deaths were reported. The absolute risk of maternal hysterectomy was about 0.05 per cent.

CHOOSING WHO SHOULD UNDERGO A SUBSEQUENT LABOUR

It is generally agreed that the expectation should be for a straightforward labour before advising a trial of labour. Women with multiple pregnancies have usually been advised against trial of labour, although the evidence that this is necessary is lacking. Only one study addressed this issue, and found no increase in perinatal or maternal morbidity in those women who laboured.

When advising on management, as much information about the previous caesarean section as possible should be sought. It is good practice to ask for a copy of the case notes of the previous surgery before making a final decision, as occasionally features may be seen that will alter management, such as extensions of the uterine incision that the woman may be unaware of. It is also important to gain any available information about the circumstances leading to the caesarean section.

Type of scar

It is recognized that vertical upper segment uterine scars have a high risk of rupture, often with catastrophic results. Therefore, it is usual to recommend repeat pre-labour caesarean section for women who are known to have undergone previous classical caesarean section. However, despite this, some women will arrive in labour. A scar rupture rate of 12 per cent has been seen in this group.[2] Lower segment vertical scars are associated with lower rates of uterine rupture, but it is often very difficult to be sure that the scar did not encroach into the upper segment, and, in general, women with a vertical uterine incision should be advised against trial of labour. It should not be assumed that a vertical abdominal incision means that the uterine incision will also be vertical; indeed, in most cases a vertical abdominal incision is associated with a transverse uterine incision. Given the extremely high rates of uterine rupture with vertical upper segment incisions, it is best to err on the side of caution whenever there is doubt.

Indication for previous caesarean section

The extent to which the reason for previous caesarean section impacts on subsequent successful trial of labour has been evaluated in a meta-analysis of observational studies [III].[3] The results are shown in Table 26.4.

DOES CERVICAL DILATATION AT TIME OF PREVIOUS CAESAREAN SECTION IMPACT ON DELIVERY?

This question has been addressed through observational studies. Only women whose prior caesarean section was for 'failure to progress' were included (Table 26.5).[4]

These data accord with an overall rate of vaginal delivery for dystocia in the previous labour of 69 per cent, which compares well with the data from Rosen et al.,[3] and show that dilatation at arrest does not signify who will achieve successful delivery next time [III].

Table 26.5   Successful vaginal delivery related to dilatation at arrest of the previous labour

Dilatation at arrest (cm)	Vaginal delivery (%)
0-5	61
6-9	80
10	69

TRIAL OF LABOUR IN WOMEN WITH MORE THAN ONE PRIOR CAESAREAN SECTION

An observational study examined outcomes for women undergoing trial of labour at Los Angeles County and University of Southern California Women's Hospital over a 10-year period (1983–92). Trial of labour was used in 80 per cent of women with one previous caesarean section, in 54 per cent with two, and in 30 per cent with three or more. The success rate was significantly higher in women

First stage of labour

with only one previous caesarean section (83 per cent) than in those with two or more (75.3 per cent). Uterine rupture was three times more common with two or more previous caesarean sections. Among women undergoing a trial of labour, there were three rupture-related perinatal deaths and a single rupture-related maternal death.[5]

A further prospective comparative study, comparing women undergoing trial of labour with two prior caesarean sections with those delivering by planned repeat caesarean section, did not show higher rates of uterine dehiscence associated with labour than in women who did not labour. However, the rates of uterine dehiscence in both groups were twice as high as those in women who had only one previous section.[6] It is likely, therefore, that the rate of uterine dehiscence/rupture is two to three times that for women having only one section previously [III]. Whereas the majority of these may be asymptomatic, on rare occasions there are catastrophic consequences for the mother or baby. Patients who wish to consider a trial of labour after two caesarean sections should therefore be counselled that the chance of successful vaginal delivery is lower than after only one caesarean section, but remains reasonable (this will vary from unit to unit). The absolute risk of scar dehiscence is about 2 per cent; if this does occur, the baby will die in about 1 in 40 cases, and in the same number a hysterectomy will be required.

TRIAL OF LABOUR IN WOMEN WITH MORBID OBESITY

In the case of women with a scarred uterus and obesity, decision-making is often difficult. It is recognized that fetal birth weight is usually larger than average, and the prior caesarean section will often have been performed for poor progress in labour. The wish to avoid a further abdominal delivery must be balanced against the increased morbidity that occurs if an emergency caesarean section is required. Observational data suggest that for women weighing in excess of 135 kg, the chance of vaginal delivery is very low (13 per cent) and elective caesarean section may be a better option in this very obese group.[7]

ANTENATAL MANAGEMENT

Counselling and documentation

Wherever possible, the records of the delivery leading to caesarean section should be reviewed [IV]. Occasionally, facts that the patient may be unaware of may come to light. It is especially important to review records where there is any doubt about the type of uterine scar used. Counselling the patient with regard to the likelihood of success is also important, and review of the previous labour is a necessary part of this counselling.

It is very important to document the discussion of the risks and benefits of both vaginal delivery and caesarean section with the patient carefully.

Planning the delivery

Value of pelvimetry

Pelvimetry performed either clinically or radiographically does not provide any useful information [Ia]. Four trials of more than 1000 women were included in the most recent Cochrane Review. The trials were generally not of good quality. Women undergoing pelvimetry were more likely to be delivered by caesarean section (odds ratio 2.17, 95 per cent confidence interval 1.63–2.88). No impact on perinatal outcome was detected.[8]

Value of ultrasound for scar thickness

Ultrasound evaluation of the scar antenatally has been investigated as a method of determining women at higher risk of scar rupture during labour. Unfortunately, results do not give a high enough sensitivity for this modality to be used in everyday clinical practice.

Documenting the plan and setting limits

Women are generally keen to avoid a repeat of the previous labour, and so it may be reasonable to avoid the circumstances that led to problems in the previous labour, such as avoiding induction if the caesarean section was for failed induction. Women who underwent caesarean section for poor progress usually need reassurance that limits will be placed on their next labour so that they do not undergo a prolonged labour. Women are significantly more likely to request a repeat caesarean section if they had their initial surgery because of failure to progress in labour than if their initial caesarean section was because of suspected fetal compromise.

It is important when discussing delivery in the antenatal period to agree a clear plan of management with the patient and for this to be carefully documented and easily available to carers in labour. If the agreed plan is for delivery by elective caesarean section, it is good practice to give the patient a date for this assuming an uncomplicated pregnancy. This can be made with the proviso that if circumstances change, it can be amended, but it does allow women to plan in advance and minimizes requests for early delivery later in pregnancy that can compromise neonatal well-being. In general, an elective caesarean section should be performed in the 39th week of pregnancy. It is possible to apply a little common sense where women have persistently laboured at 38 weeks before, but it must be remembered that if women have a tendency to go well past their dates, even 39 weeks may be early for some babies.

MANAGEMENT OF LABOUR

All carers on labour wards must be trained in the identification of the signs and symptoms of scar rupture. This is a requirement in the UK for accreditation at Level 2 for the Clinical Negligence Scheme for Trusts (CNST). Dehiscence is usually asymptomatic and may only be apparent at the time of caesarean section.

Signs and symptoms of scar rupture

The cardinal signs of imminent uterine rupture are:

- worsening cardiotocography (CTG) changes (especially prolonged variable or late decelerations),
- haematuria,
- secondary arrest,
- small amounts of vaginal bleeding.

Signs of uterine rupture are:

- fetal bradycardia,
- upward displacement of the presenting part,
- sudden loss of contractions,
- maternal hypotension,
- heavy vaginal bleeding.

If the fetus or placenta is extruded into the abdomen, there is very little time to salvage the fetus. Delivery needs to be accomplished within 10 minutes. Most fetuses in this situation are profoundly acidotic at the time of delivery.

Conduct of the labour

General management

Some general steps can be taken on admission in labour to minimize the risks to the mother and fetus. These include:

- read the plan for labour in the notes and note any discussion points,
- site intravenous access (though this can be capped and flushed),
- group and save blood,
- discuss active management of the third stage,
- perform continuous electronic fetal monitoring once labour is established.

The use of electronic fetal monitoring

There are no trials assessing the various modalities of monitoring of the fetus in labour. It is widely recognized that in most cases changes in the CTG precede uterine rupture; therefore the consensus opinion of the Expert Committee recommends continuous fetal monitoring in labour for women with a uterine scar [IV].[9]

The use of oxytocin

The use of oxytocin in labour in women with previous caesarean section is contentious. There are no randomized studies to help and only observational data are available [III]. A comparative study across eight hospitals is the largest to address this issue.[10]

Women undergoing vaginal birth after caesarean section (VBAC) needing oxytocin in labour were compared with those who did not receive oxytocin (Table 26.6). More than one prior caesarean section was not a contraindication to oxytocin, and induction of labour with oxytocin was included. Breech presentations and twin pregnancies were excluded. Women whose prior caesarean section was for suspected cephalopelvic disproportion were not excluded. A total of 1776 women were studied, of whom 485 (27 per cent) were treated with oxytocin.

Lower rates of vaginal delivery with oxytocin were seen only in the group whose prior caesarean section was for failure to progress. Oxytocin corrected labour patterns in all other groups, and vaginal delivery rates were similar to those of women not requiring oxytocin. However, just as for women with an unscarred uterus, trials of the use of Syntocinon or waiting have not been performed, and therefore the outcomes for a conservative approach are unknown. It is of concern that the rates of uterine rupture/dehiscence are two to three times higher amongst women receiving oxytocin. A larger study may have reached statistical significance. Results from the meta-analysis by Rosen et al.[2] also suggested a rate of dehiscence of 2.3 per cent in women needing oxytocin, compared with 1.5 per cent in the no-oxytocin trial of labour group.

It is vital that before considering Syntocinon, all steps are taken to optimize labour progress. With the advent of small fetal monitors and more mobility with epidural analgesia, it should be possible to allow women the opportunity to mobilize without compromising fetal surveillance. Forty per cent of women will respond to simple measures such as rehydration (see Chapter 27). A more flexible approach should be adopted in women with a uterine scar, and allowance should be made for lower rates of progress before resorting to Syntocinon. When Syntocinon is thought to be necessary, the decision should be made at consultant level and the risks and benefits should be discussed with the mother [IV].

Table 26.6 Outcomes for trial of labour for women needing oxytocin compared with women not needing oxytocin

	Oxytocin (%)	No oxytocin (%)	p
Vaginal delivery (total)	64	78	<0.001
Vaginal delivery if prior CS for poor progress	54	70	<0.001
Uterine rupture/dehiscence	1.4	0.54	0.07
True uterine rupture	0.41	0.08	0.18

CS, caesarean section.

INDUCTION OF LABOUR

There have been many concerns voiced about induction of labour in women with a scarred uterus. Only four small, randomized trials assessing the method of induction have been performed, and none has assessed induction against a conservative approach. These were too small to provide any meaningful data. Several observational studies have been performed, but it is likely that these are biased, in that women with a softer more favourable cervix are more likely to be induced by amniotomy and oxytocin, with a higher success rate than for those women receiving prostaglandin.

Artificial rupture of membranes (ARM) and oxytocin

Women who were induced with oxytocin were included in the study mentioned above;[10] vaginal delivery rates of 56 per cent were seen if the cervix was 0–2 cm dilated at the start of oxytocin, and 72 per cent if the cervix was 3–4 cm dilated. Uterine dehiscence/rupture rates from other studies appear to be in keeping with the figures presented above.

Prostaglandin induction of labour

There are eight observational studies that have focused on the use of prostaglandin for induction of labour. The composite vaginal delivery rate is 63 per cent, with a uterine rupture rate of 0.6 per cent and a uterine dehiscence rate of 0.58 per cent (total 1.2 per cent). These figures are very similar to those seen with oxytocin in labour [III].

Very recently, a further observational study has been published which has suggested a much higher rate of uterine rupture following prostaglandin induction of labour.[11] This population-based retrospective cohort study assessed data from 1987 to 1996 from 20 095 women delivering in a single area. The data were collected from discharge data by discharge codes ICD-9-CM – codes 665.0, rupture of uterus before onset of labour, and 665.1, rupture of uterus during labour. There is no distinction between rupture and dehiscence in the coding.

The study suggests that in women with a prior caesarean section, the risk of rupture or dehiscence is 0.16 per cent in non-labouring women. The relative risk (RR) for uterine rupture/dehiscence for spontaneous labour is 3.3 (a rate of 0.52 per cent), for induction with oxytocin RR = 4.9 (0.77 per cent), and for induction with prostaglandin RR = 15.6 (2.45 per cent). This represents a doubled rate for prostaglandin induction compared with the rates previously quoted. It must be recognized that the codes used for this study do not differentiate asymptomatic dehiscence from true rupture. It is suspicious that the rates for elective caesarean section are much lower than reported by Rosen et al.,[2]

suggesting that, when found at elective caesarean section, a dehiscence is much less likely to be reported or coded as it is clinically insignificant.

The codes used for this study have been examined in a previously published study by the Massachusetts Department of Public Health, the Massachusetts Maternal Mortality Review Committee and the Centers for Disease Control (CDC) in 2000. This study showed an overall positive predictive value for any degree of uterine rupture of only 39.8 per cent using ICD-9 codes, and concluded that ICD-9 codes related to uterine rupture lack adequate specificity for surveillance.

It has also been suggested that the high rates of uterine rupture/dehiscence suggested may relate to the change in practice in the USA over the last few years. A single uterine closure has become the norm (compared to the UK, where a two-layer closure is commonly practised). Only one small observational study exists, which suggests a doubling in the rates of uterine rupture in women whose previous uterine incision was closed in a single layer.[12] This study is very small and does not provide enough data to answer the question.

The reality remains that only good-quality, randomized, prospective studies will provide the answers to these questions. Until these are performed, it is vital that every possible step is taken to ensure as safe practice as possible.

Indications for induction

The indications for induction must be weighed against the risks of adopting a conservative approach and awaiting spontaneous labour. Where delivery is deemed necessary, a full discussion with the patient must take place, with the risks and benefits being carefully discussed.

Post-maturity as an indication for induction of labour *must not* be considered in the same light as induction for this indication in a woman with an unscarred uterus. In the largest randomized, controlled trial assessing this indication for induction, previous caesarean section was an exclusion factor. This trial suggested that 476 women need to be induced to prevent one stillbirth. Induction of labour in 476 women with a scarred uterus is likely to cause at least three uterine ruptures. A conservative approach with fetal surveillance is therefore safer than induction of labour in this group. Elective caesarean section should be considered in women with an unfavourable cervix who do not wish to await spontaneous labour. If induction occurs, women should be counselled about the increased risk of scar rupture, and a true rupture risk of 0.2–0.6 per cent quoted.[13]

Several recommendations have been made by the Confidential Enquiry into Stillbirths and Deaths in Infancy (CESDI) aimed at reducing risk. The following should be taken as good practice.

- The involvement of a senior obstetrician in decisions regarding mode of delivery, the need for induction and intrapartum care.

- Management plans should be fully documented.
- There should be a high level of intrapartum surveillance.
- Local guidelines should be developed.
- There should be adequate education of all staff, ensuring awareness of risk factors.

MANAGEMENT OF THE THIRD STAGE

Postpartum haemorrhage is commoner in women who have a scarred uterus, probably because of the inability of the scar tissue to contract and increased placental adherence. Therefore, a low threshold for very active management of the third stage should be implemented.

This should include:

- oxytocics at delivery of the shoulders,
- prompt delivery of the placenta after separation,
- consideration of continued Syntocinon infusion for 4 hours after delivery.

If the placenta is retained, the possibility of a placenta accreta must be borne in mind. Therefore, before proceeding to a manual removal, important steps must be taken.

1 Establish the probable placental site from the previous scan reports. Accreta is much more likely if the placenta was noted to be anterior.
2 Cross-match 4 units of blood.
3 Obtain the patients' consent and note that the possibility of accreta has been discussed, with its potential problems and management options.
4 Ensure that senior staff are aware and, if you are inexperienced, ask for help *before* you go to theatre.

If at the time of manual removal a clear plane of cleavage cannot be defined, placenta accreta is likely. Different management options have been tried with variable success.

Hysterectomy

Two large studies have shown that maternal mortality is lower if an aggressive operative approach, i.e. hysterectomy, is instituted, and this must be considered as the *safest approach* where haemorrhage is severe.[14,15] However, because there are cases in which preservation of fertility is of over-riding importance to the woman, several conservative measures have been reported.

Leaving the entire placenta in place

This has been described where no plane of cleavage can be identified. Bleeding becomes much more likely once the placenta has been partially removed. Some units have used just expectant management or with additional methotrexate. Haemorrhage, sepsis and persistent placental retention are recognized complications, but successful pregnancies have been reported subsequently.

Blunt dissection and curettage

This technique entails attempting to remove as much placenta as possible, utilizing oxytocin to help control bleeding and considering later curettage once bleeding is controlled. This approach has been successful in a few cases, but may lead to intractable haemorrhage and the need for hysterectomy.

Conservative surgery

This encompasses local oversewing of bleeding areas or defects and uterine and internal iliac artery ligation. The degree of blood loss is likely to be great, and early recourse to hysterectomy should be instituted when blood loss is continuing.

Subendometrial vasopressin has been reported to be effective in one case in which all other measures had failed, and uterine artery embolization under radiographic control has also reportedly been effective in individual cases.

If a conservative option is chosen, meticulous observation must be instituted, and recourse to hysterectomy considered if haemorrhage persists.

CONCLUSIONS

The current rates of caesarean section of 24 per cent in primiparae will inevitably lead to large numbers of women needing to choose the best method for delivery next time. Vaginal delivery after caesarean section is a safe option if precautions are taken. Induction of labour and augmentation lead to increased rates of scar rupture and must only be undertaken with caution. However, the risks of repeated caesarean section must also be considered, as it is recognized that placenta accreta increases in incidence exponentially with each repeat caesarean section (see Chapter 31). Keeping primary caesarean section rates to a minimum will help to prevent the morbidity associated with both VBAC and repeated caesarean section.

> There is a huge paucity of evidence on this subject. The only evidence relates to pelvimetry and suggests that it is unhelpful.

First stage of labour

KEY POINTS

- A thorough history and examination of the notes should be made when booking a patient who has undergone a previous caesarean section.
- Where information is lacking, it should be sought.
- Vaginal delivery is a valid option after almost any prior lower segment caesarean section.
- After classical caesarean section, vaginal delivery should be avoided.
- Repeated caesarean sections carry exponentially increasing risks of placenta praevia and accreta, with significant maternal morbidity.
- The risk of scar dehiscence or rupture in labour after a single caesarean section is approximately 1.8 per cent, but most of this is asymptomatic dehiscence. This rate is the same as that found in elective caesarean section.
- Oxytocin use in labour probably increases this risk by two to three times.
- Induction of labour may lead to at least a doubling in risk of scar problems but it is possible that the magnitude of increase is higher if prostaglandins are needed. Induction of labour for post-maturity should not be embarked upon without a detailed discussion with the patient, as the risks of induction probably outweigh the benefits.
- The risk of scar rupture is two to three times higher after more than one caesarean section. Therefore, repeat caesarean section should be offered and, if declined, carers must maintain high levels of vigilance for scar rupture.
- Vigilance for scar rupture in labour is of paramount importance.
- Active management of the third stage should be standard.
- Placenta accreta must be considered if an anteriorly placed placenta is retained.

KEY REFERENCES

1. Thomas J, Paranjothy S, Royal College of Obstetricians and Gynaecologists Clinical Effectiveness Support Unit. *National Sentinel Caesarean Section Audit.* London: RCOG Press, 2001.

2. Rosen MG, Dickinson JC, Westhoff CL. Vaginal birth after caesarean: a meta-analysis of morbidity and mortality. *Obstet Gynecol* 1991; **77**:465–70.

3. Rosen MG, Dickinson JC. Vaginal birth after caesarean: a meta-analysis of indicators for success. *Obstet Gynecol* 1994; **84**:255–8.

4. Ollendorff D, Goldberg JM, Minogue JP, Socol ML. Vaginal birth after Caesarean section for arrest of labour: is success determined by maximum cervical dilatation during the prior labour? *Am J Obstet Gynecol* 1988; **159**:636–9.

5. Miller DA, Diaz FG, Paul RH. Vaginal birth after Caesarean section; a 10 year experience. *Am J Obstet Gynecol* 1996; **175**:194–8.

6. Phelan JP, Ahn MO, Diaz F, Brar HS, Rodriguez MH. Twice a caesarean, always a caesarean? *J Reprod Med* 1993; **38**:289–92.

7. Chauhan SP, Magann EF, Carroll CS, Barrilleaux PS, Scardo JA, Martin JN. Mode of delivery for the morbidly obese with prior Caesarean delivery: vaginal versus repeat Caesarean. *Am J Obstet Gynecol* 2001; **185**:349–54.

8. Pattinson RC. Pelvimetry for fetal cephalic presentations at term (Cochrane Review). In: *The Cochrane Library*, Issue 2. Oxford: Update Software, 2002.

9. Royal College of Obstetricians and Gynaecologists. *The Use of Electronic Fetal Monitoring.* Evidence-based Clinical Guideline No. 8. London: RCOG Press, 2001.

10. Flamm BL, Goings JR, Fuelberth N, Fischermann E, Jones C, Hersh E. Oxytocin during labour after previous Caesarean section: results of a multicenter study. *Obstet Gynecol* 1987; **70**:709–12.

11. Lydon-Rochelle M, Holt V, Easterling T, Martin D. Risk of uterine rupture during labour among women with a prior caesarean delivery. *N Engl J Med* 2001; **345**:3–8.

12. Bujold E, Bujold C, Gauthier R. Uterine rupture during a trial of labour after a one-versus two-layer closure of a low transverse caesarean. *Am J Obstet Gynecol* 2001; **184**:S18.

13. Vause S, Macintosh M. Use of prostaglandins to induce labour in a woman with a previous Caesarean section scar. *BMJ* 1999; **318**:1056–8.

14. Fox H. Placenta accreta, 1945–1969. *Obstet Gynecol Surv* 1972; **27**:475–89.

15. Read JA, Cotton DB, Miller FC. Placenta accreta: changing clinical aspects and outcome. *Obstet Gynecol* 1980; **56**:31–4.

Chapter 27

Poor Progress in Labour

Richard Hayman

INTRODUCTION

The management of labour and its complications is an issue of great importance worldwide. In low-income countries, prolonged labour is commonly associated with high levels of fetal and maternal morbidity and mortality as a consequence of inadequate levels of healthcare, obstructed labour, sepsis, uterine rupture and postpartum haemorrhage. Many of these problems might be overcome by the timely use of antibiotics and delivery by caesarean section, but unfortunately these are often unavailable. In the 'developed' world, deliveries are not problem free, although the consequences are of a lesser magnitude to society as a whole. In both settings, however, a careful and methodical approach to the management of labour and its abnormalities will be of benefit to the individual mother and her baby.

Augmentation of labour for poor progress is now such a common event on labour wards in the UK that as many as 50 per cent of nulliparae may receive oxytocin in labour.

Policies incorporating such interventions in labour are not without consequences, and in the UK more than 20 per cent of all deliveries are by caesarean section. Although there is a multitude of indications for such interventions, many are performed for 'dystocia' or 'abnormal' patterns of labour. Many authorities argue that this level of intervention is too high. UNICEF, WHO and UNFPA guidelines recommend that, as a general rule, a minimum of 5 per cent of deliveries are likely to require a caesarean section in order to preserve the life and health of the mother or infant, and rates higher than 15 per cent indicate inappropriate use of the procedure.[1] However, it is uncertain as to how these rates have been determined and consequently as to what the 'appropriate' rate should be. Whilst it is irrefutably the case that caesarean section will contribute to the overall levels of maternal morbidity and mortality, especially when performed in an emergency situation, there is undoubtedly a place for caesarean sections in modern obstetric practice, albeit at a lower rate than that currently observed.

Good communication is of paramount importance on any labour ward. It is therefore particularly important that all practitioners use standard definitions, especially when different staff members perform serial examinations on the same patient – an inevitable consequence of the frequent shift changes that now occur.

DEFINITIONS

Effacement relates to the length of the cervix. Recording effacement may be useful during the latent phase, during induction of labour and in threatened preterm labour. It reflects cervical remodelling and is usually defined either as cervical length in centimetres or as no/partial/full effacement.

Dilatation, the single feature on which most management decisions in labour are made, is defined in centimetres. By convention, full dilatation, where no cervix is palpable, is taken as 10 cm. Of course, this will be a variable dependent on fetal head size, and consequently there may be large interobserver differences amongst examinations in labour. When management decisions need to be made, repeat examinations by the same individual are important.

Presentation is the part of the fetus within the pelvis adjacent to the cervix. Presentations that can be delivered vaginally at term are:

- vertex
- face (mento-anterior)
- breech.

Malpresentations are defined as anything other than a vertex. (Note that cephalic presentations will include face and brow, which are malpresentations.) Presentations that are not deliverable vaginally at term will include:

- mento-posterior face
- brow
- shoulder.

A cord presentation may be delivered vaginally when diagnosed late in the second stage, and where it is anticipated that a quick vaginal delivery can be safely accomplished.

All presentations may deliver vaginally if the fetus is very preterm.

Position is defined as the relationship of the denominator of the presenting part of the fetus to fixed points of the maternal pelvis.

The denominator is the most definable point of the presenting part:

- occiput for vertex presentations
- sacrum for breech presentations
- mentum for face presentations.

The fixed points on the maternal pelvis are:

- the symphysis pubis anteriorly
- the sacrum posteriorly.

Station of the presenting part relates to descent within the pelvis. It should be first defined by abdominal palpation as number of fifths palpable. This is particularly important when there is moulding, as this may exaggerate the fetal head shape, with seemingly better descent on vaginal examination.

Only after abdominal palpation should the station be defined vaginally. This is notoriously prone to interobserver difference. By convention, station is defined in relationship to the ischial spines in centimetres above or below this landmark.

Moulding is an important part of a vaginal examination as it relates to the fit of the fetal head through the pelvis. Various different methods have been used to define moulding. The

easiest is to palpate the sagital suture and note the following:

- no moulding: sutures a little apart
- 1+: sutures together with no gap
- 2+: sutures overlap but reduce with gentle pressure
- 3+: sutures overlap and do not reduce with gentle pressure.

Caput is a reflection of scalp oedema. Although it may be seen in prolonged labour, it may be present in normal labour and is not helpful in management planning.

The above features should be represented graphically on a partogram where possible and carefully documented at every vaginal examination.

NORMAL LABOUR: STANDARDS FOR DEFINITION OF PROGRESS

The start of a normal labour is difficult to define precisely, although it is often cited as being from the onset of painful uterine contractions that are associated with effacement and dilatation of the cervix beyond 3 cm with descent of the head in a vertex presentation. This process culminates in the birth of a baby and is followed shortly afterwards by the delivery of a placenta.

Such a complex process has many interacting components, and the safe passage of the fetus through the pelvis is dependent less upon absolutes and more upon a series of unknown variables that include:

- cervical remodelling,
- the efficiency of uterine contraction,
- the flexibility of the bony and ligamentous pelvis,
- the moulding of the fetal head,
- the adaptability of the fetus' physiology.

Many observers have attempted to provide a simple and logical approach to analysing each of these areas and thus to untangle the intricate pathways involved.

Friedman's meticulous examination of patterns of progress in labour in the 1950s enabled clinicians to monitor each labour with reference to a 'known standard'.[2,3] He noted that the first stage of parturition was usually a continuous process, extending from the time of admission to the labour ward to the full dilatation of the cervix. This period could also be divided into latent and active phases (Figure 27.1).

During the latent phase, the cervical canal shortens from 3 cm in length to <0.5 cm, whilst dilating to 3 cm. This process encompasses little cervical dilatation in comparison to the changes within the cervical collagen content, ground substance and alignment with the birth canal. In any individual, comparing progress in labour with time is fraught with difficulties. Labour is only an accentuation of uterine activity that is present throughout pregnancy. Defining the onset of labour is therefore problematic; during the latent phase, cervical change may be subtle and difficult to assess accurately.

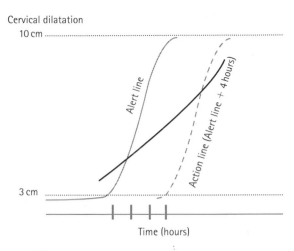

Figure 27.1

By comparison, the active phase is associated with changes in cervical dilatation, from 3 cm to 10 cm, and may be divided into:

- acceleration: between the latent phase and maximum slope,
- maximum slope: linear dilatation with time,
- deceleration phase: at the end of the active phase and prior to full dilatation.

Friedman's examination of such 'labour curves' in both multiparae and nulliparae suggested that a maximum slope dilatation of 1 cm/hour should be the minimum rate of progression.[2,3] Although this value is often quoted, there are several problems with the universal acceptance of this figure as the 'gold standard', namely:

- the original data were not normally distributed, but skewed towards higher rates of dilatation;
- the lower limit of 1 cm/hour refers to the maximum slope phase, and not to the whole of the active phase of labour.

These figures were never intended as a method of choosing which labours needed augmentation, although they have been used for this purpose.

Several researchers have subsequently aimed to modify the original data to make them suitable for application to different demographic groups.[4] Although such analyses allowed the detection of labours with 'sub-optimal' progress at an early stage, the claims that the instigation of appropriate management strategies would result in an improved outcome in the active management arm in comparison to the control population have not been met. In fact, many of these methods result in an increase in operative intervention when arbitrary delays in cervical dilatation are observed, without any improvement in the overall labour outcome.

Many of the perceived problems may actually be a result of:

- artefact inherent upon the misdiagnosis of the onset of labour;

- confounding variables, e.g. the Hawthorne effect (merely performing research may improve the outcome for reasons other than those under scrutiny);
- methodological flaws (rendering many of the findings unsuitable for application to the general population);
- failure to establish, test and substantiate 'norms and limits of biological variation' and not actual problems with labour itself.

THE PASSAGES, THE PASSENGER AND THE POWERS

An improved understanding of the physiology of labour has enabled a more scientific approach to the management of the commonly encountered problems. Whereas specific patterns of deviation from the normal may be linked with possible pathologies, labour is still evaluated in the traditional terms of the passages, the passenger and the powers.

The *passages* relate to the bony components of the pelvis and the soft tissues within this semi-rigid structure. In developed countries where nutritional status in childhood is generally good, significant bony pelvic pathology is rare. However, the influence of the soft tissues on the outcome of labour is often ignored. Abnormalities of remodelling of the cervix and space-occupying viscera within the pelvis such as impacted rectum, full bladder, cervical fibroids and ovarian cysts may all lead to delay in the active phase. An impacted rectum and full bladder are problems easily remedied without resorting to surgical interventions, unlike the other scenarios for which delivery by caesarean section may be the safer of the options.

The *passenger* refers to the fetus. Although there is evidence to suggest that birth weights are rising in developed countries, the amount (30 g over 12 years) is unlikely to be of any biological significance. Whilst induction of labour at term may seem reasonable to reduce the potential for macrosomia and its complications, positive benefits for either the mother or fetus have not been observed in the trials performed to date. The fetal head is designed to mould during labour to fit through the pelvis. Its smallest diameter (suboccipito-bregmatic) is that found with an occipito-anterior position in second stage. Larger diameters present when a fetal head does not rotate correctly during labour. Dystocia caused by malposition or malpresentation is discussed later in this chapter.

The *powers*, i.e. uterine contractions, are the only component that can truly be manipulated. The forces that expel the baby and its placenta originate in the upper uterine segment, propagating through the myometrium towards the lower segment. This wave of activity is associated with the myometrial fibres located in this area contracting, relaxing and retracting, i.e. after relaxation they retain a length that is not as great as before the onset of the contraction. At the same time, the fibres of the lower uterine segment become

First stage of labour

elongated, thinned and incorporated into the supravaginal portions of the cervical canal. These factors interact to cause descent of the presenting part, and expulsion of the fetus.

Through the use of oxytocin, the frequency, intensity and duration of the contractions can be augmented. However, there are limits to the maximum effect that may be achieved, especially when the potential for inducing iatrogenic fetal compromise is taken into consideration. There is also little evidence to show that the outcome of labour, in terms of successful vaginal delivery, can be improved when the uterine activity is normal.

PATTERNS OF CERVICAL DILATATION

Graphical representation of cervical change over time may be charted on a partogram, along with other maternal and fetal observations. Data presented in this way allow a rapid analysis of many inter-related facts, and although this may have many advantages, incorrect inclusion of the latent phase, inaccurate data recording and subjective assessment of the visual data may give an erroneous impression of suboptimal progress and, in turn, increase the likelihood of operative intervention.[5]

DISORDERS OF LABOUR

Three major disorders of labour are characterized and, once diagnosed, details concerning the aetiological factors, efficacy of modalities of treatment and prognostic outlook can be determined (Figure 27.2).

Prolonged latent phase

During the latent phase, changes occur in the ground substance glycoprotein, collagen content and hydration state of the cervix, which result in the remodelling and effacement

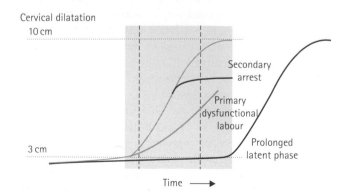

Cervical dilatation
10 cm

Secondary arrest

Primary dysfunctional labour

Prolonged latent phase

3 cm

Time ⟶

Figure 27.2

that may be observed during this period. Friedman described the latent phase as lasting up to 20 hours in nulliparae (median 8.6 hours) and 14 hours in multiparae (median 5.3 hours), although the absolute duration is dependent upon the definition of the onset of labour.[2,3]

During the latent phase, women may experience painful contractions and need a lot of support. However, it is important that unnecessary interventions to accelerate labour are not implemented at this point, as clinical studies have demonstrated that oxytocin augmentation during this phase does not result in an increase in the vaginal delivery rate, but rather a ten-fold increase in the incidence of caesarean delivery and a three-fold increase in low Apgar scores [Ib].[6,7]

In place of active intervention, careful explanation and the provision of adequate analgesia may be all that is required before the cervical changes complete and the active phase of labour is entered. Any decision to augment in the latent phase should be based on medical or obstetric indications. In such an event, management along the lines consistent with an induction of labour may be the most appropriate, although the risks of uterine hyperstimulation may be increased.

Primary dysfunctional labour

Primary dysfunctional labour (PDL) is defined as poor progress during the active phase of labour. This affects up to 26 per cent of nulliparae and 8 per cent of multiparae and, whereas no single aetiology is responsible for all cases, 70 per cent of nulliparae and 80 per cent of multiparae will respond to oxytocin.[6] This observation suggests that poor/inco-ordinate uterine activity is a significant factor, although an improvement in the rate of cervical dilatation does not correlate with improved outcomes in terms of vaginal delivery. PDL may culminate in an obstructed labour and is associated with higher rates of maternal infection, uterine rupture and postpartum haemorrhage [II].[6]

Interventions will include:

- optimization of maternal well-being (hydration, pain relief etc.);
- the provision of one-to one care or a professional maternal companion if this is not already provided;
- a longer period of time to allow labour to progress;
- mobilization;
- augmentation with oxytocin;
- delivery by caesarean section.

The relative risks and benefits of these are discussed below.

Secondary arrest

Secondary arrest affects approximately 6 per cent of nulliparae and 2 per cent of multiparae, and may be defined as a cessation of cervical dilatation following a normal period of active-phase dilatation.[6] Whereas any of the factors implicated in PDL may contribute to this abnormal labour pattern, secondary arrest is more likely to be associated with a significant underlying pathological process, with cephalo-pelvic disproportion (CPD), both relative and absolute, occasionally being encountered.

It should also be acknowledged that, up to the stage of arrest, the uterine activity has been sufficient to produce a normal response in terms of cervical effacement and dilatation. Thus, although augmentation may be considered, a diagnosis must be sought before such an intervention is commenced in order to reduce the complications associated with cases of absolute CPD. Nevertheless, in one series of patients with secondary arrest, 60 per cent of nulliparae and 70 per cent of multiparae demonstrated an improvement in progress with oxytocin.[6] However, the caesarean section rate was ten times greater in the treatment arm than in the uncomplicated cohort. CPD cannot usually be properly diagnosed until the latter stages of labour, and it is in these cases that particular care must be taken.

Secondary arrest in the decelerative phase

Friedman observed that delay during the decelerative phase on a partogram, between cervical dilatations of 7 and 10 cm, was associated with an increased risk of failure to respond to oxytocin augmentation and difficulty in procuring a successful instrumental vaginal delivery. Before any intervention is considered, a careful clinical assessment must be performed, noting:

- an estimate of fetal size (a fetus measuring >40 cm on symphysis–fundal height measurement at this stage of labour is likely to be large);
- the degree of engagement (fifths palpable per abdomen);
- position of the presenting part;
- signs of obstruction (moulding);
- presence of pelvic masses;
- descent of the presenting part with contractions;
- contraction frequency;
- fetal well-being.

Variable decelerations and a rising baseline are common in obstructed labour. Where fetal scalp sampling reveals a normal pH, the suspicion must be that the CTG changes could represent obstruction rather than fetal intolerance to labour.

Options at this stage are much as defined for PDL and are discussed below.

Secondary arrest in the second stage of labour

The second stage of labour is the period from full cervical dilatation to delivery of the fetus, a continuum in the process of labour and not a static phase. It may also be divided into pelvic and perineal stages, representing the differences between full dilatation with the head high and the over-whelming sensation a patient feels when the presenting part is deep in the pelvis and exerting pressure on the rectum.

In the presence of a malposition, the second stage may become lengthened. The second stage may also lengthen when an epidural is present, an effect contributed to by relaxation of the pelvic floor and failure of the Ferguson reflex. As long as the fetal condition remains satisfactory, oxytocin infusion in combination with the provision of additional time for the co-ordination of maternal efforts with uterine activity can reduce the incidence of instrumental vaginal deliveries.

INTERVENTIONS IN LABOUR

Maternal hydration and pain relief

Data demonstrating that in primary dysfunctional labour approximately 40 per cent of nulliparae will respond to normal saline infusions (either before oxytocin is considered or after it has failed) highlight the fact that factors such as maternal hydration are vitally important in labour.

Pain relief and consequent effects on labour are discussed in Chapter 30. It is important that before augmentation is considered, pain relief is discussed with the patient. Although there is a transient reduction in contraction frequency after epidural analgesia is commenced, this usually resolves and with careful management should not impact on the first stage of labour [1a]. It is important to recognize that although epidural analgesia is associated with an increase in the rate of instrumental vaginal delivery, this is not the case with delivery by caesarean section.

The provision of one-to-one care

If there is any evidence for any intervention in the management of labour that improves outcomes it is for this one. The carer does not have to be a midwife, but should not be the husband/partner (though of course his presence may be welcomed). Meta-analysis of randomized, controlled trials (RCTs) shows that the continuous presence of a caregiver reduces the likelihood of medication for pain relief, instrumental vaginal delivery, caesarean section and a 5-minute Apgar score <7.[8] Continuous support is also associated with a slight reduction in the length of labour [Ia].

Mobilization

Much has been made of the contribution of mobility in the progress of labour, but in fact there is a remarkable paucity of good data. Only one good RCT is available, which compares two types of epidural analgesia (mobile vs conventional). In the mobile epidural group, women were encouraged to walk. There was no difference in the length of labour, need for augmentation or type of delivery between the two groups [Ib].

Amniotomy

Amniotomy has traditionally been practised to shorten the length of labour. Recent meta-analysis of the trials incorporating routine early amniotomy into the management of spontaneous labour shows that amniotomy is associated with a reduction in labour duration of between 60 and 120 minutes [Ia].[9]

However, with early amniotomy there was:

- a marked trend towards an increase in the risk of caesarean delivery (odds ratio (OR) 1.26; 95 per cent confidence interval (CI) 0.96–1.66);
- a decrease in the likelihood of a 5-minute Apgar score <7 (OR 0.54; 95 per cent CI 0.30–0.96);
- a decrease in the use of oxytocin (OR 0.79; 95 per cent CI 0.67–0.92).[8]

Other markers of neonatal well-being are similar between the two groups (arterial cord pH, neonatal intensive care unit admissions).

Given that the reduction in length of labour is not large and that there is a potential for increase in the need for urgent delivery for suspected fetal compromise, it has been suggested that amniotomy should be reserved for women with abnormal labour progress.

OXYTOCIN FOR LABOUR AUGMENTATION

- Inco-ordinate uterine activity is a descriptive term for the observations from a tocographic recording.
- Inefficient uterine activity is a failure of the uterus to function in a way that results in normal progression of labour.
- Inco-ordinate uterine activity does not need to be addressed if progress in labour is normal.

Despite widespread use in clinical practice, there is a huge paucity of evidence to demonstrate that the use of oxytocin to augment labour improves either the maternal or fetal outcomes. There have been few RCTs, and those that have been performed are generally small. This is in part due to ethical committees not giving permission for a placebo arm, or poor trial recruitment in the presence of a placebo arm. In one small recent RCT assessing the use of oxytocin for PDL, improvement in progress of labour was seen, but this was not reflected in improved outcomes for mothers or babies. Although this trial did show that mothers randomized to oxytocin had higher satisfaction scores than those in the control arm, the numbers were too small to draw decisive conclusions [Ib].[10]

Comparative studies and one RCT demonstrate that 60–80 per cent of women will respond to Syntocinon in terms of improved rates of cervical dilatation but not other outcomes of labour.[6,11]

In order to answer the real questions about outcome, larger trials are needed. A multicentre RCT is currently being run in the north east of England, with the major outcome measure being the rate of caesarean section and psychological morbidity. It is hoped that this trial will provide a major body of much-needed evidence.

Any decision to augment should be based on the clinical findings, and a full clinical assessment as described above must be made. *This is mandatory when augmentation is to be considered in multiparous women.* If CPD is thought to be present, caesarean section should be performed.

Augmentation of labour in multiparae is one of the greatest contributing factors to uterine rupture. A decision to augment a multipara who presented in spontaneous labour must be made by an experienced person and only after a complete clinical re-evaluation of the case.

WHEN TO AUGMENT LABOUR

Augmentation with oxytocin has been advocated when the progress of labour falls behind that which would be considered optimal. This vague definition reflects the wide variations in clinical practice currently in operation. O'Driscoll et al. advocated augmentation when labour was noted to be progressing at a rate of <1 cm/hour when reassessed 1 hour later.[12] Others have employed 'action lines' – markers on the partogram drawn parallel but 2–4 hours behind the alert line. By allowing a delay before commencement of augmentation, the number of patients requiring oxytocin will be significantly reduced, with no increase in the incidence of complications, at the expense of a slight increase in the duration of labour (Figure 27.3).[7]

Debate therefore exists about not only when oxytocin should be started, but also whether it should be used at all, especially where labour is progressing, albeit slowly.

The Royal College of Obstetricians and Gynaecologists (RCOG) audit standards suggest that caesarean section should

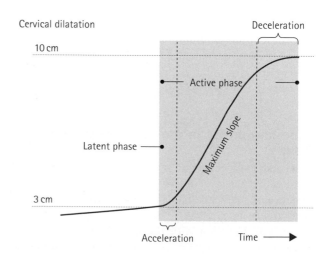

Figure 27.3

not be performed for poor progress in nulliparae before a trial of oxytocin. It must be realized that this recommendation is not based on any evidence from randomized trials.

Once commenced, oxytocin should be titrated to provide a contraction frequency of four in 10 minutes, with each contraction lasting approximately 40 seconds. Such a regimen has been shown to be compatible with normal progress in labour (≥ 1 cm/hour) with minimal adverse sequelae, as long as the appropriate action is taken if signs of maternal or fetal compromise develop. The frequency and duration of contractions may be assessed by either internal or external tocography; uterine tone and quantification of uterine activity can only be measured by internal tocography.

Advocates of invasive monitoring claim that uterine hyperstimulation can be identified earlier and, in patients with a previous caesarean section scar, that dehiscence can be diagnosed more promptly with a consequent improvement in neonatal outcome. However, a prospective randomized study failed to show an improvement in the obstetric outcome when an intrauterine pressure catheter was employed in an augmented labour when compared with an external tocograph [Ib].[13] In clinical practice, it is undoubtedly easier, cheaper and less invasive to monitor uterine activity using an external monitor.

Oxytocin given intravenously takes 30–45 minutes to reach steady-state levels. Increments for increase should not be performed more frequently than half-hourly. Many units use similar concentrations and maximum doses as for induction of labour (RCOG Guideline on Induction of Labour, 2001) (see Chapter 25).

HOW LONG TO AUGMENT

Debate continues about how long unsuccessful augmentation should continue before it can be confidently established that vaginal delivery will not be achieved. The data currently available suggest that a period of augmentation exceeding 8 hours' duration is unlikely to result in a successful vaginal delivery in the presence of persistent poor progress. However, it will not be appropriate to leave all women this long, and decisions must be taken in the context of full clinical assessment. Between 8 per cent of multiparae and 22 per cent of nulliparae will fail to respond to oxytocin and require delivery by caesarean section, although the majority of patients will deliver vaginally within this time with few risks of intrapartum injury [II].[6] It is important to recognize that as fetal compromise may result from augmentation of the forces, continuous monitoring of the fetus should be employed.

ACTIVE MANAGEMENT OF LABOUR

In order to reduce the incidence of complications related to long labour, and to manage a clinical workload effectively,

the concept of 'active management' of labour was formulated by O'Driscoll et al.[12] They adopted a pragmatic approach in which delay *in nulliparae*, whether due to inadequate uterine activity, relative CPD or other aberrant mechanisms, was treated by manipulation of the powers, as this was the only variable open to alteration. They observed that an oxytocin infusion in conjunction with a strict diagnosis of labour, early amniotomy and one-to-one care resulted in a marked reduction in the rate of interventional deliveries.

The Dublin team makes every effort to ensure that it is understood that this strategy is **not applicable** to multiparae, though this message is often forgotten in other units.

The low rates of caesarean section achieved in Dublin have not been matched in other units. Furthermore, the meta-analysis of the studies employing 'the complete' active management protocols fails to show an effective reduction in the rates of caesarean section and other operative vaginal deliveries.[14] By contrast, the provision of continuous professional support in labour has been found to reduce both types of operative interventions, although the effect on the incidence of caesarean section was confined to those settings in which partners were excluded from the delivery room [Ib].

OTHER CONTRIBUTORS TO POOR PROGRESS

Relative cephalo-pelvic disproportion in cases of malposition

If the progress of labour remains unsatisfactory despite adequate augmentation of contractions, mechanical factors such as malposition or deflexion of the head may be found to contribute to the observed delay.

Rather than the presentation of the optimal suboccipito-bregmatic diameter (9.5 cm in an 'average' term fetus) in a well-flexed occipito-anterior position, the larger occipito-frontal diameter (11 cm) or other positions will result in relative CPD. However, the dynamic nature of labour will continuously alter the dimensions of the presenting part through flexion, rotation and moulding in relation to the pelvis. Likewise the shape of the pelvis undergoes subtle changes and is not simply a static bony conduit. The relative combinations of the passenger and the passages to the delay may therefore be difficult to evaluate.

In cases of malposition, it is important to assess progress not only in terms of dilatation, but also in terms of rotation and descent. Therefore, accurate definition of position is very important when labour is not progressing (Table 27.1).

Face presentation

A face presentation may be diagnosed by palpation of the chin, mouth, nose and orbital ridges per vaginam. The

Table 27.1 Definitions and potential causes

Diagnosis	Fetal
Malposition	Occipito-posterior
	Occipito-lateral
	Deflexion
Malpresentation	Face (if mento-posterior)
	Diabetes
Macrosomia	Congenital abnormality
	Post-dates

Table 27.2 Contributory factors in absolute CPD

Diagnosis	Maternal	Fetal
Bony abnormalities	Severe kyphosis	
	Severe scoliosis	
	Poliomyelitis	
	Maternal dwarfism	
	Rickets	
	Pelvic fracture	
Soft tissue abnormalities	Cervical fibroids	Hydrocephalus
	Ovarian tumour	Iniencephaly
	Pelvic kidney	Anencephaly
	Excessive fat	Conjoined twins
	Cervical cancer	
	Vaginal\vulval atresia	
	Vaginal septum	
	Gartner's duct cysts	
Malpresentation		*Incidence at term*
	Face (if mento-posterior) – brow	1:500
	Shoulder	1:1500
	Compound presentations	3:10 000

presenting diameters are those of the transverse biparietal (9.5 cm) and the saggital submento-bregmatic (9.5 cm). When the chin (mentum) is anterior, a face presentation may deliver spontaneously or following assistance with forceps, as a consequence of a presentation with 'favourable diameters' and the ability of the head to flex beneath the symphysis pubis while 'crowning'. In face presentations, a lower threshold for delivery by caesarean section is usually adopted, as avoidance of a difficult vaginal delivery is important.

When the chin is posterior, the head is almost fully extended and unable to flex due to the sacral 'obstruction'. Although vaginal delivery may be possible if the head rotates during labour or with rotational forceps, in all but the most experienced hands, intervention by caesarean section is usually warranted.

Contributory factors in absolute cephalo-pelvic disproportion (Table 27.2)

Maternal causes
PELVIC ABNORMALITIES
Congenital
These are rare and include the following.

- Incorporation of the sacrum into the fifth lumbar vertebrae: this results in the sacral promontory being higher than usual, with an apparent lengthening of the sacrum and an increase in the angle of inclination. Although women with sacralization of the fifth lumbar vertebra may successfully deliver vaginally, it contributes to CPD in a number of women.
- Protrusio acetabulae (the Otto pelvis): the acetabular heads protrude medially to distort the pelvic cavity and obstruct labour.

Acquired
These are more common and include the following.

- Kyphoscoliosis: kyphosis of the thoracic spine promotes a compensatory lumbar lordosis, with consequent contractions in the pelvic anterior–posterior diameters. Scoliosis produces deformities of the pelvic inlet. Kyphoscoliosis combines these problems, and there may be additional maternal respiratory embarrassment.

- Pelvic fractures and disuse atrophy: direct pelvic trauma may result in a pelvis of any shape, which may or may not accommodate the passage of a fetus during childbirth. Rickets (vitamin D deficiency) may affect pelvic development in childhood, with a resultant narrowing of the pelvic inlet (sacral promontory pushed forward). This results in marked asynclitism of the presenting part and a significant risk of shoulder dystocia if the head is successfully delivered. Disuse atrophy may be the consequence of any primary pathology (poliomyelitis, spina bifida, tuberculosis, suppurative arthritis etc.) and may result in a pelvis of any shape.

SOFT TISSUE ABNORMALITIES
- Congenital abnormalities of the vagina are rarely a problem, as the soft tissues will distort in the face of fetal descent, and can often be pushed to one side, for example vaginal septum. Congenital or acquired strictures, on the other hand, may significantly impede descent and, because of the close proximity of the bladder anteriorly and the rectum posteriorly, delivery by caesarean section should be the treatment of choice.

Fetal causes
BROW PRESENTATION
A brow presentation is due to a deflexed head. The presenting diameters are those of the transverse biparietal (9.5 cm) and the saggital mento-verticular (13 cm). The mid-cavity of the pelvis measures only 12 × 12 cm in the average woman, and a brow is unlikely to negotiate its way through this passage unless it undergoes flexion to a vertex or extension to a face.

Diagnosis is usually made by a combination of:

- poor progress in labour (often apparent at early stages),
- at least two to three fifths of the head palpable per abdomen,
- vaginal station of $-2 - -3$ cm,
- orbital ridges palpable on vaginal examination.

If a brow is diagnosed early in labour, two courses of action are acceptable.

1 Conservative: a short time (2–3 hours) may be allowed without oxytocin augmentation to see whether spontaneous flexion or extension occurs. This is the best strategy if uterine contractions are good and in multiparae.

2 Active: a short period of oxytocin augmentation may be allowed (1 hour) to see whether additional 'power' will resolve the problem. Caution must be taken with this line of management, especially in multiparae, and it should *never* be initiated in grande multiparae.

In either case, if no change in the presentation occurs over the time allotted, delivery should be by caesarean section.

The accoucheur should be aware that all malpresentations are more common preterm than at term. Therefore, they may not pose the same problems, as the diameters of the fetal head are comparatively small. However, the same principles of management apply, and failure to progress should be dealt with in the safest manner (often caesarean section).

Problems with:

- fetal abnormalities (e.g. brow presentations: thyroid goitre, anencephaly – see list above),
- maternal abnormalities (see list above),

must always be considered when a malpresentation is identified.

- A latent phase of up to 20 hours in nulliparae (median 8.6 hours) and 14 hours in multiparae (median 5.3 hours) is normal, although absolute duration is dependent upon when the definition of the onset of labour is made. Oxytocin augmentation during this phase does not result in an increase in the vaginal delivery rate, but rather a ten-fold increase in the incidence of caesarean delivery and a three-fold increase in low Apgar scores.
- PDL affects up to 26 per cent of nulliparae and 8 per cent of multiparae. While no single aetiology is responsible for all cases, 70 per cent of nulliparae and 80 per cent of multiparae will respond to oxytocin in terms of improvement in the rate of cervical dilatation.
- Secondary arrest affects approximately 6 per cent of nulliparae and 2 per cent of multiparae, and

may be defined as a cessation of cervical dilatation following a normal period of active-phase dilatation. Sixty per cent of nulliparae and 70 per cent of multiparae demonstrated an improvement in progress with oxytocin.

- Improved rates of cervical dilatation with oxytocin do not necessarily lead to improved outcomes for mothers and babies.
- Meta-analysis of the studies employing the 'complete' active management protocols failed to show an effective reduction in the rates of caesarean section and other operative vaginal deliveries. By contrast, the provision of continuous professional support in labour reduces operative interventions and the need for pain relief, shortens labour and leads to infants being delivered in better condition.

KEY POINTS

- Abnormalities of the progression of labour are common problems on the modern labour ward, due in part to classification systems that may overdiagnose these complications.
- Prolonged labour is not a diagnosis; it is an abnormality that may be detected during parturition, and for which a cause must be identified before treatment is instigated.
- Although the majority of cases of 'delay' will respond to uterine stimulation with oxytocin, this may not improve outcomes and should not cloud a clinician's objectivity. Cases of absolute CPD should be identified and managed accordingly.
- Delivery by caesarean section should not be regarded as a failure, but rather as an appropriate intervention after a full assessment.
- It is recommended that caesarean section should not be performed in nulliparae for delay in labour before oxytocin has been tried (RCOG audit standards).
- Instrumental delivery may be challenging after correction of poor progress in labour and should only be performed by experienced practitioners.

KEY REFERENCES

1. AbouZahr C, Wardlaw T. Maternal mortality at the end of a decade: signs of progress? *Bull WHO* 2001; 79:561–8.
2. Friedman EA. Primigravid labor. *Obstet Gynecol* 1955; 6:567–89.

3. Friedman EA. Labor in multiparae. *Obstet Gynecol* 1956; **8**:691–703.

4. Studd J. Partograms and nomograms of cervical dilatation in management of primigravid labour. *BMJ* 1973; **4**:451–5.

5. Cartmill RS, Thornton JG. Effect of presentation of partogram information on obstetric decision-making. *Lancet* 1992; **339**:1520–2.

6. Cardozo LD, Gibb DM, Studd JW, Vassant RV, Cooper DJ. Predictive value of cervicometric labour patterns in primigravidae. *Br J Obstet Gynaecol* 1982; **89**(1):33–8.

7. World Health Organization. Maternal health and safe motherhood programme. World Health Organization partograph on management of labor. *Lancet* 1994; **343**:1399–404.

8. Hodnett ED. Caregiver support for women during childbirth (Cochrane Review). In: *The Cochrane Library*, Issue 2. Oxford: Update Software, 2002.

9. Fraser WD, Turcot L, Krauss I, Brisson-Carrol G. Amniotomy for shortening spontaneous labour (Cochrane Review). In: *The Cochrane Library*, Issue 3. Oxford: Update Software, 2002.

10. Blanch G, Lavender T, Walkinshaw S, Alfirevic Z. Dysfunctional labour: a randomised trial. *Br J Obstet Gynaecol* 1998; **105**:117–20.

11. Bidgood KA, Steer PJ. A randomized control study of oxytocin augmentation of labour 1. Obstetric outcome. *Br J Obstet Gynaecol* 1987; **94**:512–17.

12. O'Driscoll K, Stronge JM, Minogue M. Active management of labour. *BMJ* 1973; **31**(5872):135–7.

13. Chua S, Kurup A, Arulkumaran S, Ratnam SS. Augmentation of labor: does internal tocography result in better obstetric outcome than external tocography? *Obstet Gynecol* 1990; **76**(2):164–7.

14. Frigoletto FDJ, Lieberman E, Lang JM. A clinical trial of active management of labour. *N Engl J Med* 1995; **333**:745–50.

Chapter 28

Meconium

Sandie Bohin

INTRODUCTION

The detection of meconium-stained amniotic fluid during labour often causes anxiety in the delivery room because of its association with increased perinatal mortality and morbidity.

Meconium is composed of swallowed amniotic fluid debris, bile pigment and the residue from intestinal secretions. It is a sterile, durable compound made up primarily of water (75 per cent), with mucous glycoproteins, lipids and proteases. Although meconium is sterile, its passage into amniotic fluid is important because of the risk of meconium aspiration syndrome (MAS) and its sequelae. Infants delivered through meconium-stained amniotic fluid are more likely to be depressed at birth and to require resuscitation and neonatal intensive care.[1]

INCIDENCE

The passage of meconium in utero occurs in approximately 12–15 per cent of all fetuses, with the highest rates reported from North America.[2] Meconium-stained liquor is rare in premature infants (<5 per cent of preterm pregnancies); if it does occur, there is an association with infection and chorioamnionitis. Passage of meconium is increasingly common in infants >37 weeks' gestation and occurs in up to 50 per cent of post-mature infants (>42 weeks).[2]

The incidence of MAS varies between 1 and 5 per cent of all deliveries where there has been meconium-stained liquor, with higher rates reported from North America compared to Europe. There are a number of factors associated with an increased risk of developing MAS; these include a lack of antenatal care, black race, male fetus, abnormal fetal heart rate monitoring, thick meconium, oligohydramnios, operative delivery, poor Apgar scores, no oropharyngeal suctioning and the presence of meconium in the trachea.[2]

AETIOLOGY

Many theories have been proposed to explain the passage of meconium in utero; however, the precise mechanisms remain unclear. The fetal bowel has little peristaltic action and the anal sphincter is contracted. It is thought that hypoxia and acidaemia cause the anal sphincter to relax, whilst at the same time increasing the production of motilin, which promotes peristalsis.[3]

PATHOPHYSIOLOGY

Meconium aspiration syndrome is a disease of term and post-term infants and its severity is inextricably linked to co-existing fetal asphyxia. Aspiration of meconium into the distal airways can occur either antenatally or postnatally, but in the majority of affected infants the exact timing is not clear.

Production of fetal lung fluid is a continuous process, with a net movement of fluid out of the lung. During normal fetal breathing, lung fluid is not usually drawn into the distal airway. It is suggested that prolonged fetal hypoxia stimulates fetal gasping and that the consequent acidaemia stimulates deep breathing – resulting in meconium being drawn into the distal airway of the fetus via the oropharynx and nasopharynx.

Aspiration is known to occur prior to delivery, as meconium has been found in the lungs of stillbirths and in infants delivered pre-labour by caesarean section without evidence of fetal distress. Postnatal inhalation can occur late in the second stage or immediately after delivery if the infant gasps or makes breathing movements while the oropharynx, nasopharynx or trachea contains meconium-stained liquor.

Meconium has a number of adverse effects on the neonatal lung, which may ultimately lead to the respiratory failure (and hypoxaemia) which characterizes MAS.[4] First, it causes mechanical blockage of the airway, creating a ball-valve effect, so that gas can pass over the meconium plug into the lung but cannot be exhaled. This causes air trapping, hyperinflation and an increased risk of pneumothorax. Second, it acts as a chemical irritant causing pneumonitis, alveolar collapse and cell necrosis. The presence of organic material in the airway, although initially sterile, predisposes to secondary bacterial infection. Finally, meconium is known to inhibit the surface tension properties of surfactant at alveolar level, thus further increasing airway resistance.

PREVENTION OF MECONIUM ASPIRATION SYNDROME

Given the potential morbidity and mortality from MAS, prevention would clearly be beneficial. This has led to a number of antenatal, intrapartum and postnatal preventative therapies being explored, with a varying degree of success. Many of these remain controversial and have not been subjected to the scrutiny of randomized, controlled trials.

Antenatal therapies

Amnioinfusion

This potential therapy is used in North America but remains controversial. The rationale behind amnioinfusion is that by increasing the liquor volume, meconium will be diluted. In addition, in cases of oligohydramnios, the increased volume will prevent cord compression, subsequent hypoxia, fetal gasping and passage of meconium. A meta-analysis of amnioinfusion trials showed that this therapy has a role in the prevention of MAS [Ia].[5] However, the use of amnioinfusion requires further evaluation, as the therapy is associated with a number of complications, including a higher incidence of instrumental delivery and endometritis.

Delivery by caesarean section

Although most studies suggest that infants with MAS are more likely to be delivered by caesarean section than by vaginal delivery, this is largely due to the suspicion or confirmation of fetal compromise. There is currently no evidence to suggest that MAS would be prevented by elective delivery by caesarean section of infants with meconium-stained

liquor; perhaps this is not surprising, as neither the conditions for nor the timing of aspiration can be predicted.

Maternal sedation

It has been suggested that the administration of narcotics to labouring women will prevent fetal gasping in utero by suppressing fetal breathing. Although there has been success in the prevention of MAS in animal models, there are no data to support this therapy in humans. Moreover, the likely maternal and neonatal complications would preclude its use [IV].

Intrapartum/postpartum management

Oropharyngeal suctioning

Suction of the oropharynx and nasopharynx before delivery of the shoulders and trunk is a well-established practice that has been used since the 1970s [II]. It seems reasonable that suctioning in this way would minimize the amount of meconium in the upper airway and thus reduce the amount aspirated during the onset of respiration. This intervention is based on a non-randomized cohort study using historical controls and very small numbers. Subsequent studies using a similar suctioning approach have been unable to match the low incidence of MAS observed in the original study.

The evidence for oropharyngeal suction prior to the delivery of the body in the prevention of MAS is therefore conflicting. What is clear, however, is that meticulous cleaning of the upper airway after delivery is beneficial in reducing MAS [Ia].[6]

Physical manoeuvres

It has been suggested that MAS may be prevented if the infant is prevented from breathing after delivery. Methods advocated include thoracic compression, in which the thoracic cage of the infant is compressed by a healthcare professional in order to prevent respiration and subsequent aspiration of the contents of the upper airway, and cricoid pressure, in which external pressure is applied to the cricoid, thus preventing aspiration. It is suggested that if used, these interventions be continued until a second resuscitator undertakes oral and/or endotracheal suctioning. There is no evidence supporting the use of either of these methods in preventing MAS. In fact, both are potentially dangerous and cannot be recommended [IV].

Postnatal intervention

Intratracheal suctioning

Until relatively recently, *all* infants with meconium-stained amniotic fluid underwent endotracheal intubation and suction, as this was known to reduce the incidence of MAS. More recently, evidence has suggested a change in practice depending on whether or not an infant is deemed *vigorous*. A recent meta-analysis suggests that routine intubation of vigorous term infants in order to aspirate the lungs should be abandoned [Ia]. Suctioning of the oropharynx may be beneficial, but endotracheal suctioning should be reserved for depressed or non-vigorous infants or those who deteriorate following initial assessment.[6]

Aspiration of gastric contents to remove swallowed meconium is still practised in many centres. However, this practice has never been evaluated. The passage of an orogastric tube is likely to cause apnoea and/or bradycardia and is potentially harmful. This practice should be abandoned [IV].

Saline lavage and physiotherapy are used in order to loosen meconium. No randomized studies have shown physiotherapy in infants with MAS to be beneficial. Saline lavage is potentially harmful, as saline will displace endogenous surfactant, which could in turn worsen the respiratory illness. In cases where saline lavage has been used, infants developed respiratory distress secondary to 'wet lung'.

DELIVERY ROOM MANAGEMENT OF INFANTS BORN WITH MECONIUM-STAINED LIQUOR

It is important that a person experienced in neonatal resuscitation attends the delivery of all infants in whom *thick* meconium-stained liquor is noted, particularly if accompanied by suspected fetal compromise, as it is in these cases that MAS is likely to be a problem.

The Neonatal Resuscitation Program of the American Academy of Pediatrics incorporates guidelines for the management of these infants (Figure 28.1).[7]

If an infant is *vigorous* after delivery:

- no tracheal suctioning should be undertaken,
- secretions should be cleared from the mouth and nose using a wide-bore suction catheter,
- routine care should be given.

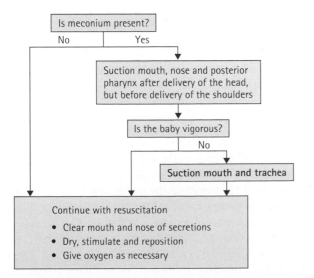

Figure 28.1   Guidelines for the initial management of infants born in meconium-stained liquor[7]

However, if an infant is *not vigorous* after birth (defined as depressed respirations, decreased muscle tone and/or heart rate <100 beats per minute):

- direct endotracheal suctioning should be undertaken as soon as possible,
- suction should be applied for no more than 5 seconds and the tube withdrawn,
- if meconium is aspirated from below the cords, the infant should be re-intubated and the process repeated, unless the infant has a profound bradycardia, in which case:
  - resuscitation should proceed with intermittent positive pressure ventilation (IPPV) without suctioning,
  - further suctioning can be attempted at a later stage.

If after the first suctioning no meconium is aspirated, no further suctioning should be attempted and the infant should be resuscitated using IPPV via an endotracheal tube.

CLINICAL MANIFESTATIONS OF MECONIUM ASPIRATION SYNDROME

Infants usually have signs of post-maturity, with dry, flaking skin that is often stained green/yellow by meconium. The most obvious feature of MAS is respiratory distress, characterized by tachypnoea with respiratory rates up to 100/minute, subcostal recession, nasal flaring and an expiratory grunt. As air trapping is a feature of this condition, hyperinflation of the chest is common. Meconium causes widespread crepitations throughout the chest on auscultation. Asphyxiated infants may be apnoeic, but exhibit identical physical signs once ventilated. The respiratory course varies depending on the severity of the MAS; however, the respiratory symptoms in most infants will have resolved by 14 days, and in some by 48 hours. Up to 60 per cent of infants with severe MAS will require mechanical ventilation[1,2] and many will have concomitant pulmonary hypertension of the newborn.[8] Infants with MAS may show signs of neonatal encephalopathy, depending on the degree of asphyxial insult. Jitteriness and irritability are common features and may last for several days. An early chest X-ray will show widespread patchy infiltrates with areas of hyperinflation. In mild cases the X-ray may return to normal by 72 hours. In severe cases the X-ray will show diffuse homogeneous opacification of the lung fields, reflecting the pneumonitis and interstitial oedema. Such changes may remain for up to 14 days or more.

TREATMENT

No specific treatments are available for MAS. Infants should receive appropriate neonatal intensive care support until the meconium is cleared and respiratory function returns to normal. Special attention should be paid to the treatment of respiratory failure, acid–base status and secondary infection. Unless affected by co-existing asphyxia, many infants can be initially managed by administering humidified oxygen therapy via a headbox.

Continuous positive airway pressure (CPAP) is not indicated in these infants, as it increases the risk of pneumothorax and causes abdominal distension, which may lead to splinting of the diaphragm and exacerbate the respiratory symptoms [IV].

Mechanical ventilation is often required.[2]

Intubation and ventilation are indicated if:

- the infant is asphyxiated and apnoeic,
- the infant is tiring,
- despite FiO_2 concentrations of 80 per cent, the infant remains hypoxic,
- the $PaCO_2$ increases above 8–9 kPa (60–67 mmHg).

Sedation with an opiate infusion is routinely used in neonates who require ventilation for any reason. However, in infants with MAS, in whom peak inspiratory pressures are often high, the additional use of a muscle relaxant makes ventilatory management easier and reduces the risk of pneumothorax.

For infants who remain hypoxic on conventional ventilation, high-frequency oscillatory ventilation may be used. If despite good ventilatory management there is continuing hypoxia and co-existing pulmonary hypertension of the newborn, the use of inhaled nitric oxide or extracorporeal membrane oxygenation (ECMO) is recommended. ECMO has been shown to improve the survival of infants with severe MAS [Ib].[9]

Surfactant has been used in a number of ways in MAS. First, surfactant replacement therapy has been shown to reduce the need for ECMO in infants with MAS [Ia].[10] Second, airway lavage with diluted surfactant has been used in an attempt to wash residual meconium from the airway [III]. Initial results are promising, but further work is needed.

COMPLICATIONS, MORBIDITY AND MORTALITY

It is difficult to give precise details of morbidity in MAS, as complications and outcome are linked to concomitant neonatal encephalopathy and persistent pulmonary hypertension of the newborn.

Pneumothoraces are the most common complication of MAS and occur in up to 20 per cent of non-ventilated infants and up to 50 per cent of ventilated infants. Chronic lung disease is relatively uncommon, occurring in only 5 per cent of ventilated infants,[1] whereas up to 40 per cent of children who previously had MAS have asthma and about 50 per cent have abnormal lung function lasting many years.[11]

Persistent pulmonary hypertension of the newborn is a common complication, particularly in fatal cases.[9] Treatment includes ventilation plus the use of inhaled nitric oxide or ECMO.

Neurological morbidity is usually attributable to any co-existing neonatal encephalopathy, although damage may result from severe hypoxia secondary to the disease itself or to pulmonary air leaks. The neurological outcome for infants without neonatal encephalopathy is very good.

With improvements in neonatal care, the widespread availability of inhaled nitric oxide therapy and ECMO, deaths from MAS should now be rare. The mortality appears to have fallen from around 35 per cent in the 1970s to less than 5 per cent currently.[2] Most deaths are due to respiratory failure, but some are due to the renal or neurological sequelae of severe asphyxia.[9]

- There is no evidence supporting the use of saline lavage, chest physiotherapy, gastric aspiration or thoracic compression in the prevention of MAS.
- The evidence relating to routine suctioning of the oropharynx as a preventative measure is conflicting.
- Intratracheal suctioning should be reserved for the non-vigorous baby.
- The administration of surfactant in severe MAS reduces the need for ECMO.

KEY POINTS

- Meconium-stained liquor is associated with increased morbidity and mortality in babies.
- MAS is linked to perinatal asphyxia.
- Good neonatal resuscitation skills reduce the incidence of MAS.

KEY REFERENCES

1. Cleary GM, Wisewell TE. Meconium stained amniotic fluid and the meconium aspiration syndrome: an update. *Pediatr Clin North Am* 1998; **45**:511–29.
2. Wisewell TE. Handling the meconium-stained infant. *Semin Neonatol* 2001; **6**:225–31.
3. Lucas A, Christophides ND, Adrian TE, Bloom SR, Aynsley-Green A. Fetal distress, meconium and motilin. *Lancet* 1979; i:718.
4. Tyler DC, Murphy J, Cheney FW. Mechanical and chemical damage to lung tissue caused by meconium aspiration. *Pediatrics* 1978; **62**:454–9.

5. Hofmeyr GJ. Amnioinfusion for meconium-stained liquor. *Curr Opin Obstet Gynecol* 2000; 12:129–32.

6. Halliday HL, Sweet D. Endotracheal intubation at birth for preventing morbidity and mortality in vigorous, meconium-stained infants born at term (Cochrane Review). In: *The Cochrane Library*, Issue 3. Oxford: Update Software, 2003.

7. Kattwinkel J, Niermeyer S, Carlo W et al. *Textbook of Neonatal Resuscitation*, 4th edn. Elk Grove Village, IL: American Academy of Pediatrics, 2000.

8. Wisewell TE, Tuggle JM, Turner BS. Meconium aspiration syndrome: have we made a difference? *Pediatrics* 1990; 85:715–21.

9. UK Collaborative ECMO Trial Group. UK collaborative randomised trial of neonatal extracorporeal membrane oxygenation. *Lancet* 1996; 348:75–82.

10. Soll RF, Dargavile P. Surfactant for meconium aspiration syndrome in full term infants (Cochrane Review). In: *The Cochrane Library*, Issue 3. Oxford: Update Software, 2003.

11. Swaminathan S, Quinn J, Stabile MW et al. Long-term pulmonary sequelae of meconium aspiration syndrome. *J Pediatr* 1989; 114:356–60.

Chapter 29

Fetal Compromise in the First Stage of Labour

Griff Jones

MRCOG standards

- The ability to recognize, classify and act appropriately on cardiotocograph patterns.
- The ability to perform fetal blood sampling and to be able to interpret the results.

In addition, we would suggest the following.

Theoretical skills
- Know the risk factors for fetal compromise and how they can be recognized either antenatally or in early labour.
- Understand the alterations in placental blood flow during contractions.
- Know the acute intrapartum complications that can lead to fetal compromise.
- Be aware of the different techniques available for assessing fetal well-being in labour as well as their individual indications and limitations.
- Be able to quote the risk of serious neonatal morbidity and mortality.

Practical skills
- Be confident in your ability to interpret a cardiotocograph, particularly with regard to recognizing those babies requiring immediate delivery.
- Be able to perform and interpret additional tests of fetal well-being for non-reassuring cardiotocographs that do not necessitate immediate delivery.
- Be able to apply a scalp electrode or perform a real-time ultrasound scan when it is not possible to obtain an adequate fetal heart rate trace using conventional Doppler techniques.
- Be familiar with intrauterine resuscitation techniques.

INTRODUCTION

Members of the public (and indeed the legal profession) commonly relate childhood handicap to a 'difficult' labour and delivery. However, the Consensus Statement of the International Cerebral Palsy Task Force reported that intrapartum hypoxia could at most be responsible for only one in ten cases of cerebral palsy.[1] Nevertheless, as labour represents about 0.4 per cent (1/280) of the total duration of pregnancy, a 10 per cent contribution to sub-optimal neonatal outcomes reminds us that it is a relatively 'high-risk' period. The fact that uterine perfusion is dramatically reduced during each contraction emphasizes the additional stress that labour places on fetuses.

DEFINITIONS

The aim of monitoring fetal well-being during labour is to prevent birth asphyxia and so reduce perinatal mortality, morbidity and long-term handicap. Although all three of these outcomes are uncommon, the use of operative delivery for 'non-reassuring fetal status' remains an everyday occurrence on delivery suites in the UK. This is in part because of a wish to deliver on the downwards slope towards a 'poor outcome', before it actually occurs. But what are the 'poor outcomes' that we are trying to prevent? Current recommendations suggest focusing on long-term 'absolute outcomes' (death and handicap) in combination with 'intermediate measures' that reflect neonatal condition at birth (Royal College of Obstetricians and Gynaecologists (RCOG) Guidelines, *The Use of Electronic Fetal Monitoring*) (Table 29.1).

ABSOLUTE OUTCOMES

Perinatal mortality

This remains a widely accepted measure of maternity care, but such crude figures provide little help in assessing

Table 29.1 Statistics for outcomes in labour

Caesarean section for suspected fetal compromise (Sentinel Study, RCOG 2001)	5%
NICU admissions at term	4%
Umbilical artery acidosis (pH <7.20)	15%
Umbilical artery metabolic acidosis (pH <7.20, Base deficit >12 mmol/L)	2.5%
5-minute Apgar <7 at term	2%
Neonatal encephalopathy at term	0.5%
Cerebral palsy	0.2%

RCOG, Royal College of Obstetricians and Gynaecologists; NICU, neonatal intensive care unit.

intrapartum monitoring. First, they are heavily distorted by very preterm births, in which fetal condition at birth is only one of many factors influencing outcome. Second, perinatal mortality rates also include stillbirths. It is self-evident that fetal monitoring can only be of use when the baby is alive at the onset of labour. Intrapartum term stillbirths may be a more appropriate mortality figure, as they are often related to events occurring during parturition. The intrapartum stillbirth rate in term singleton pregnancies is reported as only 0.3 per 1000.[2] The influence of fetal monitoring on such a rare event will remain difficult to study.

Handicap

The achievement of normal long-term neurodevelopment is another major aim of intrapartum fetal assessment. The incidence of cerebral palsy is widely quoted as 2 per 1000. However, as mentioned previously, only in 10 per cent of cases (or 1 in 5000 births) are intrapartum events thought to have been of influence. Once again, the ability of fetal monitoring to impact on such a rarity is difficult to prove or disprove.

All obstetricians should therefore appreciate that intrapartum operative interventions carried out at term because of 'non-reassuring fetal status' are trying to prevent suboptimal outcomes seen in approximately 1 in 2000 births. It is necessary not only for obstetricians to react appropriately but also to avoid over-reaction.

INTERMEDIATE MEASURES

Apgar scores

To improve the recognition of intrapartum factors contributing to the absolute outcomes referred to above, markers of potential long-term morbidity have been used.

The influence of the condition of the baby at birth using Apgar scores taken at 1 and 5 minutes has been widely investigated, particularly in the earliest studies. All now agree that the 1-minute Apgar score purely reflects the need for neonatal resuscitation, regardless of aetiology. Unfortunately, the

5-minute Apgar score also appears to provide little predictive ability for long-term complications unless very low (<4) or moderately low (<7) and remaining so beyond 10 minutes of age.

There is not yet enough evidence to support the use of other similar markers, such as the need for intubation or ventilation.

Arterial or capillary pH

Hypoxaemia will result when gas exchange across the placenta is impaired, with a gradual fetal accumulation of CO_2. This eventually leads to fetal acidaemia, which can be detected by analysing fetal capillary or neonatal arterial pH. The widely accepted lower limit of normal for fetal or neonatal pH is 7.20. This represents two standard deviations below the mean fetal pH seen from intrapartum studies. It must be stressed that this value was chosen for statistical reasons, not primarily because of an association with neonatal morbidity. Clinical studies suggest that an umbilical arterial pH below 7.00 may be a more reliable marker of potential long-term problems; the figure of 7.20 remains in everyday use to provide a wide margin of safety. The type of acidosis is also important. In a respiratory acidosis, the PCO_2 is elevated but the base excess is normal, a condition that will be easily resolved with the onset of neonatal respiration and gas exchange. Metabolic acidosis is associated with a transition to anaerobic metabolism and an accumulation of acids such as lactate. It is defined by a base deficit >12 mmol/L and is a marker of moderate to severe neonatal morbidity in its own right. More recently, an umbilical arterio-venous PCO_2 difference of >25 mmHg or 3.33 kPa has been suggested as the most sensitive and specific marker of significant infant morbidity, including long-term neurodevelopmental problems.[3]

Neonatal encephalopathy

Neonatal behaviour and early-onset medical complications also provide some prognostic information. Neonatal encephalopathy refers to disturbed neurological function in the first week of life. Signs include difficulty maintaining respiration, depressed tone and reflexes, altered level of consciousness and seizures. Moderate to severe neonatal encephalopathy will be seen in most cases of brain damage secondary to intrapartum complications. However, neonatal encephalopathy has poor sensitivity; 75 per cent of cases having no clinical signs of intrapartum hypoxia.

Criteria for intrapartum hypoxic events

No individual intermediate measure can precisely link intrapartum complications to absolute outcomes. Several groups have proposed pathways by which combinations of intermediate measures can help to define a causal intrapartum hypoxic event. The International Cerebral Palsy Task Force has listed criteria essential to link brain injury to an earlier intrapartum hypoxic event.[1] They include:

- evidence of a metabolic acidosis at birth (pH <7.00 and base deficit ≥12 mmol/L,
- early-onset moderate or severe encephalopathy,
- cerebral palsy of the spastic quadriplegic or dyskinetic type.

Other features that support an intrapartum hypoxic event include:

- a sentinel hypoxic event around the time of labour,
- a deterioration in the fetal heart rate pattern around the time of the sentinel event after a previously normal pattern,
- Apgar scores of <7 for longer than 5 minutes,
- early-onset multi-organ dysfunction,
- early imaging evidence of an acute cerebral abnormality.

WHAT TYPE OF FETAL MONITORING IS BEST?

The Dublin Trial of Intermittent versus Continuous Monitoring remains the classic study in this field.[4] Despite subsequent studies, the conclusions are largely unchallenged. In low-risk pregnancies, electronic continuous monitoring was better at detecting fetal acidosis and led to a reduced incidence of neonatal seizures. However, it did not appear to have any influence on the absolute outcomes of mortality and long-term handicap. Meta-analysis seems to support these conclusions, although it is recognized that the data are insufficient to detect a true difference in the rare absolute outcomes of death and handicap [Ia]. Most authorities agree that continuous monitoring leads to an increase in operative intervention, although this can be at least partially mitigated by the use of secondary tests of fetal well-being.

WHAT IS A LOW-RISK PREGNANCY?

Although the entry criteria to the Dublin trial included preterm births from 28 weeks onwards and multiple gestations, most units would now classify such pregnancies as high risk.

Meconium staining of the amniotic fluid remains a marker of risk and is covered in more detail in Chapter 28. In the Dublin trial, artificial rupture of the membranes was performed on admission, and the 5 per cent of women with either no fluid or significant meconium were excluded from

the trial. Despite continuous monitoring and fetal blood sampling, the perinatal mortality rate in this group was 11 per 1000, compared to 2.1 per 1000 in the remaining trial participants. The significance of meconium in low-risk term pregnancies has been re-iterated more recently in a contemporary Israeli study.[5] The 16.6 per cent of uncomplicated term pregnancies with any degree of meconium staining of the amniotic fluid had a perinatal mortality rate of 1.7 per 1000, compared to only 0.3 per 1000 when the amniotic fluid was clear.

The presence of any of the following risk factors at the onset of labour would label a fetus as being at 'high risk' of intrapartum hypoxia, for which the consensus is that continuous fetal monitoring should be offered [IV].

- Hypertension/pre-eclampsia
- Diabetes
- Antepartum haemorrhage (APH)
- Significant maternal medical disease
- Intrauterine growth restriction (IUGR)
- Preterm gestation
- Isoimmunization
- Multiple pregnancy
- Breech presentation
- Previous caesarean section
- Significant meconium staining of the amniotic fluid
- Post-term pregnancy
- Epidural analgesia
- Induced or augmented labour

It is attractive to base intrapartum monitoring plans on a pre-labour assessment of risk. However, risk can change as labour progresses, with examples including the onset of vaginal bleeding, the development of meconium staining of the amniotic fluid or slow progress. Ongoing risk appraisal can assist the clinician in deciding how long to tolerate a non-reassuring (but not pathological) cardiotocograph (CTG) before employing secondary tests. It must be remembered that at least 40 per cent of cases of moderate to severe birth asphyxia in term pregnancies will occur to women in whom no antepartum risk factors were identified.[6]

ADMISSION TESTS

Equally attractive to the pre-labour assignment of risk is an early labour re-assessment in low-risk pregnancies. In this situation, a screening test is applied to try to identify those fetuses that are more likely to develop intrapartum complications. Tools that have been used in this situation include CTGs, ultrasound assessment of amniotic fluid volume and umbilical artery Doppler. Research suggests that an abnormal admission test is associated with increased levels of obstetric intervention but no significant reduction in adverse perinatal outcomes [Ib].[7,8] The RCOG Guideline on Monitoring in Labour now recommends that an admission test is not necessary in women with uncomplicated pregnancies labouring at term.

INTERMITTENT AUSCULTATION

In the low-risk situation, intermittent auscultation, either by Pinnard stethoscope or by hand-held Doppler, is often advocated. Conventional guidelines, such as those issued by the RCOG and the Society of Obstetricians and Gynaecologists of Canada, suggest auscultating the fetal heart rate every 15 minutes in the active phase of the first stage of labour. This should be for 60 seconds following a contraction, in order to detect significant decelerations.

The main criticisms of intermittent monitoring are that:

- the above standards are often not achievable on busy delivery suites;
- gradual changes such as an increasing baseline or falling variability will be missed;
- there is no certification process for practitioners using intermittent monitoring;
- no hard record from the monitoring is generated and therefore it is impossible to audit any guidelines related to performing the technique.

CONTINUOUS ELECTRONIC FETAL MONITORING

The mainstay of 'high-risk' fetal assessment, electronic fetal monitoring (EFM), relies on several assumptions:

- that abnormal patterns in the fetal heart rate will be seen in the presence of compromise;
- that sufficient warning will be given to allow potentially beneficial interventions to be undertaken;
- that caregivers will recognize the abnormality and take appropriate action.

Many events, such as cord prolapse or abruption, may be so acute as to have no preceding period of deterioration in fetal well-being. Fetal monitoring may allow recognition of the problem but no advance warning. A similar rapid deterioration may be seen in fetuses with diminished reserves at the onset of labour, such as those babies with IUGR. Alternatively, it has been suggested that a chronically compromised baby may not exhibit the same type of fetal heart rate changes when acute compromise is superimposed. CTG abnormalities in this situation may be subtle or even atypical. Low et al. found that only 80 per cent of term births with metabolic acidosis exhibited a predictive fetal heart rate pattern.[6] In other words, in one-fifth of cases, the obstetrician

would have found the CTG acceptable. The pathophysiology behind other causes of neonatal harm, such as infection, may not be associated with severe or typical 'non-reassuring' fetal heart rate abnormalities until almost pre-terminal. Finally, events related to the actual delivery (trauma, shoulder dystocia, problems during resuscitation) contribute to morbidity and mortality but cannot be predicted by intrapartum monitoring.

Some cases of abnormal intrapartum monitoring may have their roots in fetal development. Fetal cardiac anomalies are frequently undiagnosed antenatally and carry considerable morbidity and mortality. It is logical to assume that an abnormal heart will respond to the haemodynamic changes of labour atypically. Similarly, it can be difficult to disentangle prenatal neurological damage, occurring before the onset of labour, from that arising during labour. As the control of fetal heart rate involves higher centres, damage to them will lead to abnormal cardiovascular responses in labour. The common assumption is that a stressful labour, reflected by the abnormal CTG, led to the neurological damage. The alternative possibility is that the pre-existing neurological damage led to the abnormal cardiovascular response to labour.

WHAT IS A NORMAL CARDIOTOCOGRAPH?

A useful approach that helps to avoid over-reaction is initially to extract those features of a CTG that are normal by systematically reviewing baseline rate, heart rate variability and accelerations.

- *Baseline.* The normal fetal baseline heart rate is 110–160 beats per minute (bpm). There is a small fall in baseline rate as gestation advances. A stable baseline over time is also important. With a lengthy trace, this can be assessed by folding the CTG up and viewing the lateral side edge-on (Figure 29.1). Many women will also have had recent admissions, generating earlier CTGs for comparison.
- *Variability.* Fetal heart rate variability appears to result from a balance between sympathetic and parasympathetic influences. Therefore, a well-oxygenated nervous system is required for its full expression. Normal variability is >5 bpm. Short periods of reduced variability (particularly when associated with an inactive baby) can be entirely physiological, but in most cases variability will have recovered within 45 minutes.
- *Accelerations.* Fetal heart rate accelerations represent a response to many minor stresses. Commonly, this is fetal movement, but it also includes palpation or noise. It implies a fetus responsive to external stimuli and, therefore, intact neurocardiac pathways. Most authorities report 'accelerations to be the hallmark of fetal well-being'.

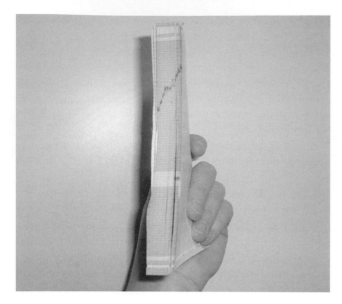

Figure 29.1   Rising baseline

WHAT IS AN ABNORMAL CARDIOTOCOGRAPH?

- *Baseline.* The only fetal heart rate pattern that indicates fetal hypoxaemia is a continuous and progressive bradycardia. Fetal bradycardia can arise with any acute reduction in fetal oxygenation, such as cord compression, abruption or uterine hyperstimulation. If the bradycardia is moderate to severe or associated with other CTG abnormalities and the cause cannot be corrected promptly, abdominal delivery will be necessary. An isolated tachycardia is rarely, if ever, associated with fetal compromise. Such a tachycardia may be appropriate in some situations. If the baby is very active, the mother will know and the variability will usually be excellent. A fetal tachycardia may arise secondary to a maternal tachycardia, often in response to pain. Clinicians must always be wary of an underlying diagnosis of chorioamnionitis as the fetus is in a hazardous environment that will not be reflected by scalp pH.
- *Variability.* A prolonged period of reduced variability, lasting >90 minutes, is clearly abnormal. The most concerning cause of decreased variability is fetal hypoxaemia, usually chronic, that has globally depressed central nervous system function. Other aetiologies include pre-existing neurological problems, maternal drugs and congenital heart block.
- *Accelerations.* These will rarely be seen in the presence of a compromised fetus.
- *Decelerations.* Decelerations arouse instant concern in many observers, particularly the less experienced. However, they should never be viewed in isolation, only as a part of the whole picture. Decelerations are usually divided into one of three types, but this can

only be determined after observing a pattern repeating over time.

- *Early decelerations.* These decelerations begin with the onset of a contraction and mirror the shape of the contraction trace. They are usually thought to arise from vagal nerve stimulation secondary to cord compression. They are seen in 1 in 20 first-stage CTGs and, in isolation, are rarely associated with fetal compromise (Figure 29.2).
- *Variable decelerations.* Variable decelerations are just that – variable. Each deceleration has a different shape and their timing with regard to contractions is unpredictable. They are the most common type of deceleration and are seen in up to 1 in 8 first-stage traces (Figure 29.3). They are classically thought to arise from chemoreceptor stimulation secondary to cord compression. They may also result from head compression. Isolated mild to moderate variable decelerations are rarely associated with fetal compromise. However, severe variable decelerations (rate drops by >60 bpm or to <60 bpm or deceleration lasts longer than 60 seconds) can be associated with fetal acidosis.
- *Late decelerations.* Late decelerations begin 20–30 seconds after the contraction, the nadir occurs after the contraction apex and the baseline does not return to normal until after the contraction has finished (Figure 29.4). Only 1–2 per cent of labours demonstrate late decelerations in the first stage of labour. Late decelerations have been postulated to result from direct fetal myocardial depression secondary to hypoxaemia. There may be an additional contribution from chemoreceptor stimulation. Although isolated late decelerations with no other fetal heart rate abnormality are rarely associated with fetal compromise, the presence of any other co-existing abnormalities justifies secondary testing.

No one element of the CTG should be interpreted in isolation. Regardless of how much intellectual activity is put into the interpretation of the CTG, it remains a screening test only. Even the most worrying pattern (late decelerations with reduced variability) is only associated with acidosis in 50 per cent of cases. Diagnostic or secondary tests are necessary to avoid unnecessary obstetric intervention.

SECONDARY TESTS OF FETAL WELL-BEING

Vibroacoustic stimulation

The use of vibroacoustic stimulation applied to the maternal abdomen in the presence of a non-reactive antenatal CTG is

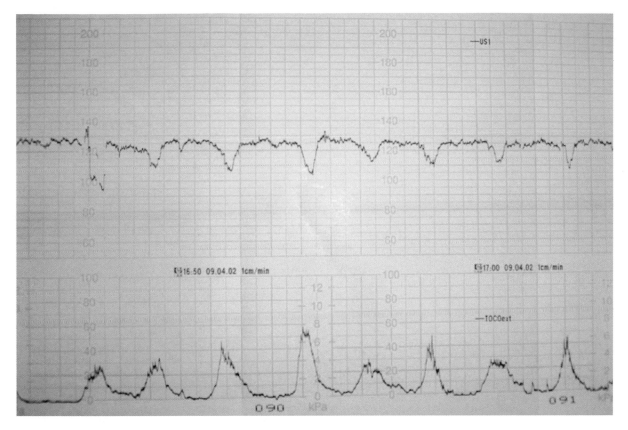

Figure 29.2   Early decelerations

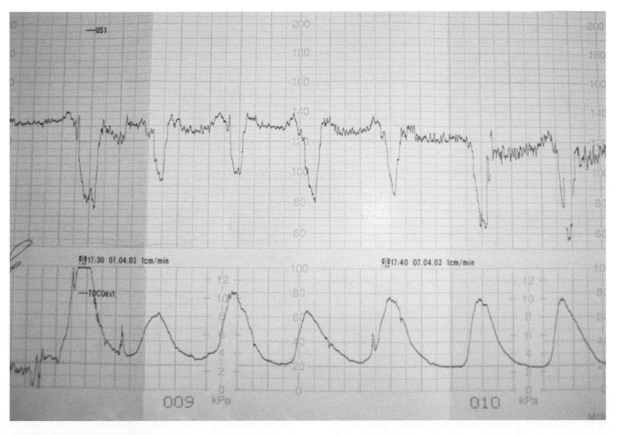

Figure 29.3   Variable decelerations

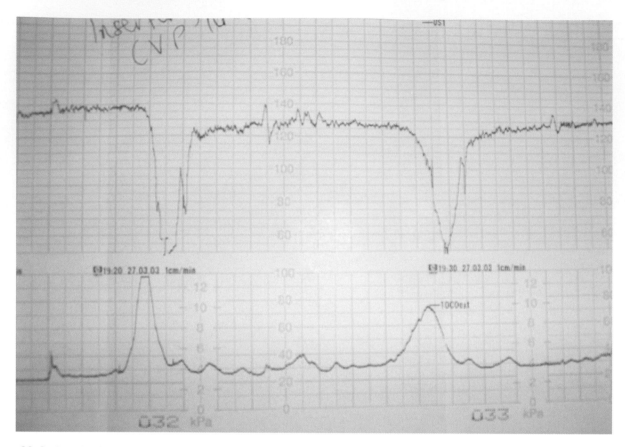

Figure 29.4 Late decelerations

well documented.[9] The healthy fetus responds with an acceleration in fetal heart rate. The same technique has been applied in the intrapartum period. An acceleration evoked by vibroacoustic stimulation immediately prior to scalp sampling was never associated with a pH of <7.25. Vibroacoustic stimulation cannot completely eliminate the need for scalp sampling, as only 30 per cent of non-responders will be found to be acidotic. However, it can reduce the need for scalp sampling by up to 50 per cent [II].

Fetal blood sampling

Fetal scalp pH studies remain the principal secondary test of intrapartum fetal well-being. It is recommended that all units offering continuous EFM have facilities for fetal blood sampling. The scalp pH lies somewhere between the arterial and venous pH but it cannot be determined to which it is closer in advance. As mentioned previously, the lower limit of normal is accepted as a pH of 7.20 in order to allow a wide margin of error. Ideally, the base excess should also be measured to distinguish metabolic from respiratory acidosis. There is interest in simply measuring the capillary lactate levels, which provide similar information. Testing systems have now been developed that require smaller volumes of fetal blood than conventional pH studies. This, in conjunction with the ability to sample at lesser dilatations, has led to a lower 'failure-to-sample' rate.

Scalp stimulation

Most clinicians will have noted that fetuses that respond to scalp sampling with an acceleration almost always have a normal pH. This has been confirmed in formal studies, which showed 93 per cent of fetuses with a scalp pH >7.20 respond with an acceleration, compared to none of those that are acidotic.[10] This can be useful information when technical difficulties preclude sample collection. However, clinicians should always be wary of scalps that do not bleed, as this may reflect peripheral vasoconstriction in a compromised fetus.

Fetal electrocardiogram

Recent work using the fetal electrocardiogram (ECG) PR interval in addition to the CTG failed to show any improvement in the detection of acidaemia or any reduction in operative intervention. In contrast, the use of fetal ECG ST-wave analysis plus conventional CTG resulted in less metabolic acidosis (0.7 per cent vs 2.0 per cent) and a small reduction in operative delivery for fetal distress [Ib].[11] Fetal monitors are now being marketed that incorporate this technology.

Fetal pulse oximetry

The largest trial to date of fetal pulse oximetry failed to show any overall reduction in operative delivery with the use of this technology, although it was suggested that the detection of acidosis was improved [Ib].[12]

THE MANAGEMENT OF SUSPECTED FETAL COMPROMISE

- Improve placental blood supply.
  1 Correct maternal hypovolaemia and/or hypotension.
    - Maternal positioning to avoid aorto-caval compression.
    - Intravenous fluids when appropriate.
    - Vasoconstrictors such as ephedrine for lower limb vasodilatation secondary to epidural analgesia. Remember, arm blood pressure may be normal in this situation.
  2 Diminish uterine activity, particularly if excessive.
    - Decrease or stop any oxytocin infusion.
    - Remove vaginal prostaglandins if given recently. This may require vaginal lavage if gels have been used.
    - Use bolus tocolytics (e.g. terbutaline 0.25 mg) [II]. It is illogical to use beat-agonist inhalers in this situation. Even women with chronic asthma often have poor inhaler technique and the whole point of inhaled therapy is to limit systemic effects.
- Improve maternal oxygenation.
  1 Maternal oxygen therapy should not be used for more than a short period of time unless there is documented low maternal oxygen saturation. There is no evidence of benefit and a suggestion of possible detrimental effect when applied for more than a few minutes [Ia].
- Improve umbilical blood flow.
  1 Increase amniotic fluid volume. Transcervical amnioinfusion may reduce cord compression and frequently leads to an improvement in the fetal heart rate. One randomized trial showed a significant reduction in operative intervention and an improvement in cord pH at delivery [Ia].[13] Common protocols include infusing 500 mL of Hartmann's solution over 20–30 minutes followed by up to 250 mL/hour. To minimize the risk of amniotic fluid embolus and over-distension, the infusion should be gravity fed. It has also been suggested to improve fetal outcome by diluting meconium.
- Decide if delivery is indicated, based upon:
  1 clinical tests – such as the CTG and secondary tests of fetal well-being;

2 the whole picture – including obstetric risk factors and progress in labour;

3 untreatable fetal complications – such as abruption, cord prolapse and chorioamnionitis, scar dehiscence.

A clinical approach to reviewing intrapartum CTGs in the first stage of labour

Does the abnormality require immediate delivery if it continues?
Yes (Think little, do lots)
1 Is there a possible precipitant?
  - cord prolapse/recent epidural/excessive uterine activity/bleeding/scar dehiscence etc.
  - If possible, rapidly take steps to correct any precipitants identified.
  - If no corrective steps are possible or there is no response, deliver by caesarean section.
No (Do little, think lots)
1 For comparison, has there been a 'normal' CTG:
  - earlier in labour?
  - within a few weeks of admission?
2 On the current CTG, what normal features are present?
  - Stable baseline with normal rate
  - Good variability
  - Accelerations.
3 On the current CTG, what abnormal features are present?
Compare 1 and 2 with 3 to decide on the 'severity' of any CTG abnormality.
4 Is there a possible precipitant?
  - Cord prolapse/cord compression/recent epidural/excessive uterine activity/bleeding/scar dehiscence etc.
If possible, take steps to correct any precipitants identified in 4.
5 What risk factors were present in the antenatal period?
6 Were there any recent changes immediately prior to labour?
  - Maternal illness/reduced fetal activity etc.
7 Have any risk factors developed during labour?
  - Meconium/bleeding/poor progress/fever etc.
Then use 5, 6 and 7 to decide:
  - if and for how long this abnormality can be tolerated before delivering or employing secondary tests of fetal well-being, *and*
  - when to next review the CTG – a deliberate plan is the best approach.
Always try to answer 'What is causing this CTG abnormality?'.
Do not forget 'benign' causes, such as recent narcotic analgesia or a rapidly progressing labour.

- Maternal oxygen therapy does not improve fetal outcomes in the acutely compromised fetus.
- Intermittent monitoring in problem-free pregnancies is associated with long-term outcomes as good as those in labours monitored continuously.
- Admissions testing is not necessary in problem-free pregnancies and leads to increased intervention without improved outcomes.

PUBLISHED GUIDELINES

Royal College of Obstetricians and Gynaecologists Evidence-based Clinical Guideline No. 8. *The Use of Electronic Fetal Monitoring.* London: RCOG, May 2001.

Society of Obstetricians and Gynaecologists of Canada Clinical Practice Guideline. *Fetal Health Surveillance in Labour: Executive Summary. J Obstet Gynaecol Can* 2002; 24:250–62.

KEY POINTS

- Intrapartum events rarely lead to perinatal mortality or neurodevelopmental handicap after uncomplicated term pregnancies.
- Electronic fetal monitoring is a crude screening test with a poor predictive value for acidosis.
- Always review electronic fetal monitoring in the context of the whole pregnancy.
- Secondary tests of fetal well-being after non-reassuring CTGs are necessary to avoid over-intervention.
- Intrauterine therapy can improve non-reassuring CTGs and reduce operative delivery.

KEY REFERENCES

1. MacLennan A, for the International Cerebral Palsy Task Force. A template for defining a causal relationship between acute intrapartum events and cerebral palsy: international consensus statement. *BMJ* 1999; 319:1054–60.

2. Smith GCS. Life-table analysis of the risk of perinatal death at term and post term in singleton pregnancies. *Am J Obstet Gynecol* 2001; 184:489–95.

3. Belai Y, Goodwin T, Durand M, Greenspoon J, Paul R, Walther F. Umbilical arteriovenous PO_2 and PCO_2 differences and neonatal morbidity in term infants with severe acidosis. *Am J Obstet Gynecol* 1998; 178:13–17.

4. MacDonald D, Grant A, Sheridan-Pereira M, Boylan P, Chalmers I. The Dublin randomized controlled trial of intrapartum fetal heart rate monitoring. *Am J Obstet Gynecol* 1985; 152:524–9.

5. Maymon E, Chaim W, Furman B, Ghezzi F, Shoham Vardi I, Mazor M. Meconium stained amniotic fluid in very low risk pregnancies at term gestation. *Eur J Obstet Gynaecol Reprod Biol* 1998; 80:169–73.

6. Low JA, Pickersgill H, Killen H, Derrick EJ. The prediction and prevention of intrapartum fetal asphyxia in term pregnancies. *Am J Obstet Gynecol* 2001; 184:724–9.

7. Mires G, Williams F, Howie P. Randomised controlled trial of cardiotocography versus Doppler auscultation of fetal heart at admission in labour in low risk obstetric population. *BMJ* 2001; 322:1457–61.

8. Chauhan SP, Washburne JF, Magan EF, Perry KG, Martin JN, Morrison JC. A randomised study to assess the efficacy of the amniotic fluid index as a fetal admission test. *Obstet Gynecol* 1995; 86:9–13.

9. Polzin GB, Blakemore KJ, Petrie RH, Amon E. Fetal vibro-acoustic stimulation: magnitude and duration of fetal heart rate accelerations as a marker of fetal health. *Obstet Gynecol* 1988; 72:621–5.

10. Clark SL, Gimovsky ML, Miller FC. Fetal heart rate response to scalp blood sampling. *Am J Obstet Gynecol* 1982; 144:706–9.

11. Amer-Wahlin I, Hellsten C, Noren H et al. Cardiotocography only versus cardiotocography plus ST analysis of fetal electrocardiogram for intrapartum fetal monitoring: a Swedish randomised controlled trial. *Lancet* 2001; 358:534–9.

12. Garite TJ, Dildy GA, McNamara H et al. A multicenter controlled trial of fetal pulse oximetry in the intrapartum management of non-reassuring fetal heart rate patterns. *Am J Obstet Gynecol* 2000; 183:1049–53.

13. Schrimmer DB, Macri CJ, Paul RH. Prophylactic amnioinfusion as a treatment for oligohydramnios in laboring patients: a prospective, randomized trial. *Am J Obstet Gynecol* 1991; 165:972–8.

Chapter 30

Obstetric Anaesthesia and Analgesia

David M. Levy

MRCOG standards

Candidates are expected to:

- understand and be able to counsel women about the options for pain relief in labour, including their risks;
- understand the impact of various complications of pregnancy and labour (e.g. pre-eclampsia, coagulopathy and major haemorrhage) on the different modes of anaesthesia.

INTRODUCTION

Obstetric *analgesia* is pain relief in labour; *anaesthesia* is the abolition of sufficient sensation to allow operative delivery.

Analgesia is one of the most important aspects of the modern management of labour. Women receive education antenatally about the options for analgesia in labour and often have very high expectations on admission to the delivery suite.

Regional (spinal, epidural or combined spinal–epidural) anaesthesia is now used for the vast majority of caesarean sections.

ANALGESIA FOR LABOUR

Methods of analgesia include:

- relaxation therapy
- immersion in warm water
- aromatherapy
- transcutaneous electrical nerve stimulation (TENS)
- nitrous oxide/oxygen inhalation
- parenteral opioids
- regional analgesia.

In units providing an 'on-request' regional analgesia service, it is not uncommon for as many as 70 per cent of nulliparous women to request this intervention. The role of the caregiver in labour must not be overlooked. The requirement for pharmacological pain relief in labour is reduced when a known practitioner provides continuous support [Ia].[1]

Transcutaneous electrical nerve stimulation

Electrical impulses applied to the skin via flexible carbon electrodes from a battery-powered stimulator modulate the transmission of pain by closing a 'gate' in the dorsal horn of the spinal cord. The effect is similar to massage of the lower back by a birthing partner.

- TENS is used in about 1 in 20 labours in the UK. The technique is completely free from adverse effects, and can diminish the need for other analgesic interventions.
- A study comparing TENS and 'sham' TENS (TENS devices which appeared to be working but had been disabled) failed to demonstrate reduced pain scores in labour. After delivery, however, those women who had had working TENS retrospectively rated their analgesia more highly. More women from this group stated they would choose TENS again in a future labour [Ib].[2]

Opioid analgesia

Clinical studies of pain scores have cast doubt on the analgesic efficacy of opioids in labour. The drugs are undoubtedly sedative, and induce a feeling of disorientation, thereby making pain more tolerable.[3]

- Maternal gastric emptying is inhibited, and the incidence of nausea and vomiting increased.
- All opioids can induce maternal and neonatal respiratory depression (decreased Apgar and neurobehavioural scores).

- A reduction in baseline variability on the cardiotocograph (CTG) can make interpretation difficult.
- Midwives can prescribe and administer controlled drugs in accordance with locally agreed policies and procedures. In the UK, pethidine is the most widely used intramuscular (i.m.) opioid. A usual dose of 100 mg lasts around 3 hours.
- Plasma pethidine concentrations are maximal in the neonate when the mother has received the drug about 3 hours before delivery. It is therefore illogical to withhold the drug at any particular juncture for fear of causing neonatal respiratory depression.
- Neonatal respiratory depression is readily reversible with naloxone, a specific opioid antagonist. The neonatal dose is 10 μg/kg i.m., repeated if necessary.
- Comparisons of pethidine 100 mg with diamorphine 5 mg, meptazinol 100 mg and tramadol 100 mg have failed to demonstrate any convincing benefits.
- An anti-emetic (e.g. cyclizine 50 mg or prochlorperazine 12.5 mg) should be given i.m. with the chosen opioid.
- Because of the additive risk of respiratory depression, i.m. opioids should never be given in the event of inadequate regional analgesia without prior reassessment of the woman by an anaesthetist.

Patient-controlled analgesia

Remifentanil is an opioid with a fast onset time and short duration of action. It has been evaluated for intravenous patient-controlled analgesia (PCA) in labour. Bolus doses of 0.5 μg/kg with a 2-minute lockout setting provided demonstrable analgesia (reduced visual analogue pain scores) without neonatal depression. Remifentanil by PCA is potentially useful in women with thrombocytopenia or other haematological reason for avoiding regional analgesia or i.m. injections.

Nitrous oxide

Sixty to 70 per cent of labouring women in the UK seek to achieve analgesia by inhalation of a 50:50 mixture of nitrous oxide and oxygen (N_2O/O_2). Marketed as Entonox® and Equanox®, the gas mixture is supplied in cylinders with a blue body and blue/white shoulders and is piped to delivery rooms in many hospitals.

- The gas is self-administered by inspiration through a facemask or mouthpiece, which opens a demand valve. Diffusion from alveoli to pulmonary capillaries and delivery to the brain by the cardiac output are not instantaneous. Inhalation should therefore start as soon as a contraction begins, in order that maximum effect is achieved at its peak.
- The drug is non-cumulative, and does not affect the fetus. N_2O/O_2 causes sedation, which is highly variable

amongst patients. Some appear to be dreaming or drunk; others become somnolent or even briefly unrousable.

- Hyperventilation with N_2O/O_2 can be followed by a short period of apnoea; therefore, the woman should always hold the mouthpiece or mask herself. If she loses consciousness, she will let go. A few breaths of air eliminate the N_2O and consciousness is invariably soon regained.
- A number of studies have questioned the analgesic effect of N_2O/O_2. Pain is often still perceived under the influence of the drug – it is merely rendered more bearable by the intoxicated state. Thirty to 40 per cent of women in labour derive no benefit.[4]
- The risk of cross-contamination between patients sharing breathing systems dictates that mouthpieces and masks should be disposable, or sterilized between patients. Either a new disposable breathing system should be used for each patient, or a disposable breathing system filter interposed between the tubing and mouthpiece/mask [IV].

Regional analgesia for labour

Regional analgesia is the provision of pain relief by blockade of the sensory nerves as they enter the spinal cord. Local anaesthetic can be introduced into epidural or subarachnoid (intrathecal) spaces, or both. Compared with every other analgesic modality, pain relief from regional blockade is undoubtedly superior. Ninety per cent of consultant obstetric units in the UK provide a 24-hour epidural service; the average epidural rate is 24 per cent. Contraindications to regional blockade are outlined in Table 30.1. Subcutaneous low-molecular-weight heparin (LMWH) within the previous 8 hours is a relative contraindication. Previous spinal surgery might make identification of the epidural space difficult, and spread of local anaesthetic solution may be impeded by scar

Table 30.1 Contraindications to regional analgesia, with associated risks

Contraindication	Risk
Uncorrected anticoagulation or coagulopathy	Vertebral canal haematoma
Local or systemic sepsis (pyrexia >38°C not treated with antibiotics)	Vertebral canal abscess
Hypovolaemia or active haemorrhage	Cardiovascular collapse secondary to sympathetic blockade
Patient refusal	Legal action
Lack of sufficient trained midwives for continuous care and monitoring of mother and fetus for the duration of epidural blockade	Maternal collapse, convulsion, respiratory arrest; fetal compromise

tissue. However, regional blockade might nevertheless be feasible – early referral (ideally with the postoperative radiographs) should be made to an obstetric anaesthetist.

Epidurals and spinals

The epidural space is identified by the loss of resistance to depression of a syringe plunger as a Tuohy needle is advanced (Figure 30.1) through the ligamentum flavum. A catheter is then threaded through the Tuohy needle (Figure 30.2) to facilitate bolus top-ups or a continuous infusion. The subarachnoid space, which contains cerebrospinal fluid (CSF), is a few millimetres deeper, inside the meninges. Needles used for deliberate spinal injection are much finer than Tuohy

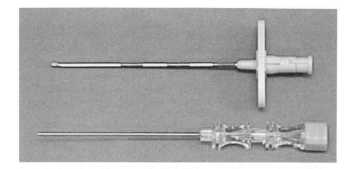

Figure 30.3 Epidural Tuohy (above) and spinal needles

needles (Figure 30.3). Intermittent epidural boluses, continuous epidural infusions and patient-controlled epidural analgesia all provide comparable pain relief and maternal satisfaction. Unlike local anaesthetics, which prevent the conduction of nerve impulses, opioids act on specific receptors in the spinal cord. Synergistic mixtures of local anaesthetic and opioids (usually fentanyl) have permitted significant reductions in the amount of local anaesthetic used. Side effects specific to the use of opioids are respiratory depression (in the most unlikely event that opioid spreads cephalad to reach the brainstem) and pruritus.

Dural tap

Inadvertent meningeal puncture with a Tuohy needle is called a dural tap. Eighty-five per cent of women who have a dural tap will develop a severe postural headache, caused by leakage of CSF. Only the presence of headache during labour is an indication for elective forceps or vacuum extraction at full dilatation. The definitive treatment is epidural injection of 20 mL of autologous blood – a 'blood patch', best undertaken at 24–48 hours post-delivery.

Total spinal

Five to ten times the dose of local anaesthetic is required for an equivalent effect after epidural as opposed to subarachnoid injection. Any communication between the epidural and subarachnoid spaces introduces the risk of local anaesthetic intended for the epidural space reaching the subarachnoid space and causing a block high enough to cause respiratory arrest – known as a total spinal. A total spinal should be a survivable event for mother and fetus. The mother will undergo emergency tracheal intubation and treatment of hypotension. The urgency of caesarean section will be dictated by the fetal heart trace. Tracheal extubation should be feasible within 2–3 hours once the high block has regressed.

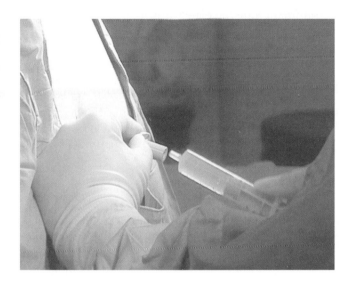

Figure 30.1 Tuohy needle with loss-of-resistance syringe

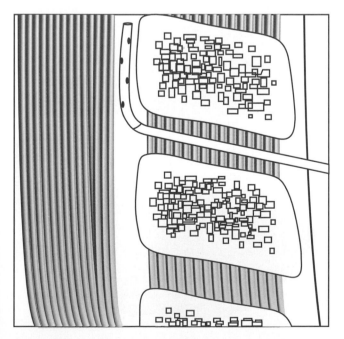

Figure 30.2 Tuohy needle advanced through the ligamentum flavum, with the catheter in the epidural space

Local anaesthetic toxicity

If local anaesthetic is injected inadvertently into an epidural vein, symptoms and signs of local anaesthetic toxicity (Table 30.2) can arise from the effect of high concentrations of local anaesthetic in the central nervous system (CNS). Initial treatment follows the 'ABC' principle: airway, breathing and circulation (with relief of aorto-caval compression).

Table 30.2   Symptoms and signs of local anaesthetic toxicity

Symptoms	Signs
Numbness of tongue or lips	Slurring of speech
Tinnitus	Drowsiness
Light-headedness	Convulsions
Anxiety	Cardiorespiratory arrest

Table 30.3   COMET: analgesic regimen and mode of delivery

Delivery	'Traditional' epidural ($n = 353$)	Combined spinal epidural ($n = 351$)	Low-dose infusion epidural ($n = 350$)
Normal vaginal	124 (35%)	150 (43%)	150 (43%)
Instrumental vaginal	131 (37%)	102 (29%)	98 (28%)
Caesarean section	98 (28%)	99 (28%)	102 (29%)

$p = 0.04$, 1DF (degree of freedom) for normal vs other deliveries.

Combined spinal–epidural techniques

Combined spinal–epidural analgesia entails an initial subarachnoid injection of fentanyl mixed with a tiny amount of local anaesthetic. The spinal injection makes the onset of analgesia considerably faster (5 minutes, as opposed to at least 20 minutes with an epidural). The resulting motor block is sufficiently minimal for women to retain sufficient muscle power to walk in labour. However, proprioception (information from joint receptors to maintain balance) can be impaired. The Comparative Obstetric Mobile Epidural Trial (COMET) found that both low-dose infusion epidurals and combined spinal–epidural analgesia resulted in a lower incidence of instrumental vaginal deliveries compared to traditional intermittent bolus epidurals (Table 30.3).[5] It is presumed that this finding is attributable to the preservation of motor tone and the bearing-down reflex, as mode of delivery was not influenced by whether or not women walked in labour.

Regional analgesia and progress of labour

Regional analgesia has been shown to improve uteroplacental blood flow in labour. However, a fall in blood pressure after a bolus dose of local anaesthetic can precipitate a fetal bradycardia. This will usually be resolved by treatment of the hypotension: if the CTG returns to normal, no further action is necessary.

There has been much debate about the effects of regional analgesia on labour. Since blockade of motor fibres causes relaxation of pelvic floor muscles and impairs expulsive efforts, provision of adequate maternal analgesia with as little motor block as possible has emerged as a goal common to all regional analgesia regimens.

A Cochrane Review has found that epidural analgesia was associated with better pain relief than other methods of analgesia, but with longer first and second stages and an increased incidence of fetal malposition. There was greater

use of Syntocinon and an increased vaginal instrumental delivery rate, although no effect on the caesarean section rate [Ia].[6] The link between epidural analgesia and backache has been thoroughly investigated and no evidence of a causative effect found [Ia].

ANAESTHESIA FOR CAESAREAN SECTION

A UK-wide survey of more than 60 000 caesarean sections in 1997 revealed that 78 per cent were completed under regional anaesthesia (Figure 30.4), although the proportion varied from centre to centre.[7] It is likely, however, that the increasing caesarean section rate has kept the overall number of general anaesthetics broadly the same as when regional techniques were in the minority. Across the 14 hospitals of the South Thames (West) region, the caesarean section rate increased by 10 per cent from 1993 to 1998. Although the proportion of caesarean sections performed under general anaesthesia fell by two-thirds, the actual number decreased by only one-third.

Categorization of urgency

Good communication between the obstetric and anaesthetic staff is a vital part of the organization for a caesarean section. A four-point classification of urgency of caesarean section (Table 30.4), similar to that used by the National Confidential Enquiry into Perioperative Deaths, has been validated by close

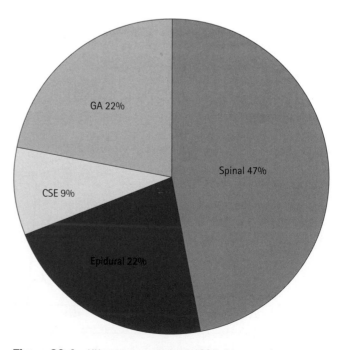

Figure 30.4   UK caesarean sections, 1997. GA, general anaesthesia; CSE, combined spinal–epidural

Table 30.4   Classification of urgency for caesarean section

Category	Definition (at time of decision to operate)
Emergency	Immediate threat to life of woman or fetus
Urgent	Maternal or fetal compromise that is not immediately life threatening
Scheduled	Needing early delivery but no maternal or fetal compromise
Elective	At a time to suit the woman and maternity team

agreement between anaesthetists' and obstetricians' gradings of more than 400 cases.[8] Mutual adoption of this classification should aid decisions about which mode of anaesthesia is appropriate in non-elective cases. A decision-to-delivery interval of 30 minutes has become widely adopted as an audit standard, despite lack of any evidence that 30 minutes is a critical threshold in the development of intrapartum hypoxia. Spinal anaesthesia is often appropriate for urgent (Table 30.4) caesarean section, although a recent Confidential Enquiry into Stillbirths and Deaths in Infancy (CESDI) has deemed repeated attempts at regional anaesthesia to be inadvisable in the absence of significant risk factors for general anaesthesia.[9]

Mortality

Maternal mortality attributed to anaesthesia has fallen considerably over the last 30 years (Figure 30.5). In the Report on Confidential Enquiries into Maternal Deaths (CEMD) in the UK for 1994–96, there were no deaths from general anaesthesia: the solitary anaesthetic death followed combined spinal–epidural anaesthesia.

CESDI highlighted four cases from the same period in which general anaesthesia was associated with life-threatening hazards (two cases of anaphylaxis, two airway crises). In the 1997–99 CEMD there were three deaths:

- cardiac arrest after an excessively high spinal compounded by obstetric haemorrhage,
- aspiration pneumonitis,

- fatal airway obstruction in a woman who had undergone tracheostomy in an intensive care unit (ICU) after obstetric haemorrhage.

Antacid prophylaxis

Fasting intervals of 6 hours for food and 2 hours for fluids (tea/coffee with semi-skimmed milk, or fruit squash) are appropriate for women scheduled for elective caesarean section. Ranitidine 150 mg should be prescribed 2 hours before an elective operation and administered 8-hourly to women in labour with risk factors for caesarean section to reduce gastric acid secretion. The administration of a measure of sodium citrate 0.3 M immediately before every caesarean section is almost universal practice. The risk of aspiration is not confined to general anaesthesia: protective reflexes may be obtunded in the event of an excessively high regional block.

Regional anaesthesia

Single-shot spinal anaesthesia
Single-shot spinal anaesthesia has become the most popular anaesthetic technique for caesarean section (Figure 30.4), largely as a consequence of the widespread adoption of pencil-point-tip needles (Figure 30.6). Compared to standard cutting bevel or Quincke needle tips, there is less leakage of CSF and a lower incidence of headache requiring epidural blood patch.

Preload
A crystalloid fluid preload has become recognized as an ineffective means of preventing hypotension after spinal injection. In contrast to colloid, its short intravascular half-life prevents the necessary sustained increase in cardiac output before sympathetic blockade. In one study, 1 L of hydroxyethyl starch produced a mean increase in cardiac output of more than 40 per cent, and prevented hypotension

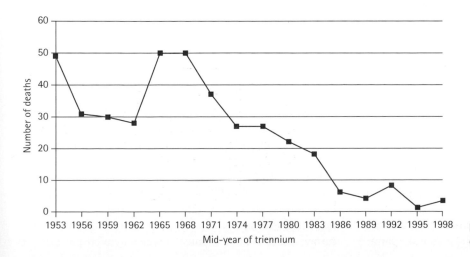

Figure 30.5   Maternal mortality (number of deaths) from anaesthesia 1952-99

First stage of labour

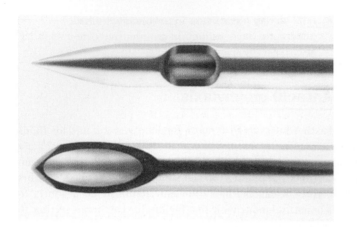

Figure 30.6   Pencil-point (above) and cutting bevel-tip spinal needles

in more than 80 per cent of women. However, all colloids incur a risk of anaphylaxis, and concern has been raised that the further increase in cardiac output from autotransfusion of blood as the uterus contracts after delivery might precipitate circulatory overload.

Hypotension is best managed by:

- strict avoidance of aorto-caval compression,
- prompt boluses of vasopressor,
- infusion of crystalloid immediately *after* intrathecal injection.

Level of injection

Magnetic resonance imaging has shown that the conus medullaris of the spinal cord extends below the level of the body of L1 in 20 per cent of patients. Moreover, anaesthetists commonly underestimate the height of their approach. A series of case reports describing damage to the conus medullaris has led to an authoritative recommendation that spinal needles should not be inserted higher than the L3/4 interspinous space [IV] – practically, the space at or immediately above a line joining the highest points of the iliac crests.

Dose of local anaesthetic

Virtually all UK obstetric anaesthetists use hyperbaric bupivacaine 0.5 per cent. Gestation is important when deciding upon the dose for a single-shot spinal. In one study, loss of cold sensation to T4 was achieved with 2.25 mL in all of a group of women at term but only 16 per cent of women at 28–35 weeks' gestation. The progressively gravid uterus causes increasing vena caval compression, epidural venous engorgement and consequent displacement of the dura and reduced subarachnoid space volume. Postural manoeuvres after intrathecal injection, such as moving from right to left lateral or flexing the knees and thighs, promote cephalad spread of the injectate by influencing vertebral canal blood volume.

Most UK anaesthetists ascertain block height by defining loss of temperature sensation with ethyl chloride spray.

However, there is evidence that loss of light touch sensation to T5 is a better predictor of pain-free caesarean section under (opioid-free) spinal bupivacaine anaesthesia. Light touch can be tested by gently dabbing the skin with cotton wool. The extent of the block and modality of testing should be recorded routinely, in case a subsequent claim of intra-operative pain has to be defended. The obstetrician must clarify with the anaesthetist that it is appropriate to start surgery.

Opioids

The addition of intrathecal fentanyl, diamorphine or morphine can reduce the incidence of intraoperative visceral pain, although fentanyl does not contribute significantly to postoperative analgesia. Over 70 per cent of respondents to a survey of UK obstetric anaesthetists added an opioid, most often fentanyl. Diamorphine was used by less than a quarter of those using an opioid, morphine by less than 10 per cent. Reports of respiratory depression after intrathecal doses of opioids in obstetric practice are conspicuous by their absence. Intraoperative pain should be treated promptly by intravenous alfentanil (0.5 mg increments) or inhaled isoflurane 0.25 per cent in an N_2O/O_2 50:50 mixture, or conversion to general anaesthesia.

Vasopressors

Ephedrine (alpha and beta sympathomimetic) has generally been regarded as the vasopressor of choice in obstetrics. Persist-ing reservations about the effects of alpha-agonists on utero-placental blood flow have been founded on a 30-year-old study of Columbian ewes – which did not undergo regional anaesthesia. A randomized comparison of i.v. boluses of ephedrine and phenylephrine in women undergoing caesarean section found similar changes in maternal systolic pressure and cardiac output, and no changes in umbilical artery (UA) Doppler waveforms. Mean UA pH was significantly *lower* in neonates whose mothers had received ephedrine. Increased fetal metabolic rate secondary to ephedrine-induced beta-adrenergic stimulation may be the explanation. However, if phenylephrine is used indiscriminately to treat hypotension, it is liable to cause maternal bradycardia, necessitating i.v. atropine or glycopyrrolate. Phenylephrine is most useful in 50–100 μg increments for the treatment of hypotension in the presence of tachycardia. Doses of this magnitude offset the haemodynamic effects of bolus doses of Syntocinon given after delivery.

Spinal anaesthesia and pre-eclampsia

Over the last few years, it has become accepted by many that pre-eclampsia is not necessarily a contraindication to single-shot spinal anaesthesia; if the abnormal vasoconstriction is of humoral rather than neural aetiology, sympathetic blockade should not cause precipitous hypotension. Prior vasodilatation by effective anti-hypertensive treatment (e.g. oral methyldopa or i.v. hydralazine) with limited intravascular volume expansion seems to avert problematic hypotension. Judicious increments of either ephedrine or phenylephrine do not cause arterial pressure overshoot.

Postoperative analgesia

Supplementation of intrathecal diamorphine or morphine by regular oral or rectal paracetamol (1 g 6-hourly) *and* diclofenac (50 mg 8-hourly, 12 hours after an initial 100 mg postoperative dose), with oral dihydrocodeine if required (60 mg 4-hourly), makes patient-controlled i.v. morphine unnecessary for most women. Non-steroidal anti-inflammatory drugs (NSAIDs) are contraindicated in the initial postoperative period if caesarean section has been complicated by excessive bleeding or there is concern about the adequacy of haemostasis (e.g. uterine atony).

Epidural anaesthesia

Few elective caesarean sections are now performed under epidural anaesthesia, because the quality of anaesthesia is generally poorer than that afforded by subarachnoid block. In the 1997 survey, the rate of conversion to general anaesthesia for epidurals (6 per cent) was three times greater than that for spinals. Epidural anaesthesia is still favoured by many when gradual establishment of block is desired to minimize hypotension, although combined spinal–epidural techniques are gaining in popularity. In severe pre-eclampsia, postoperative infusion of epidural bupivacaine/fentanyl in a high-dependency area will confer optimal analgesia and contribute to blood pressure control. A South African study demonstrated that women who were fully conscious and co-operative after an eclamptic seizure could safely undergo caesarean section under epidural anaesthesia. All women had platelet counts $>100 \times 10^9$/L and had been treated with magnesium sulphate.[10]

Conversion of labour analgesia

In women in labour deemed high risk for caesarean section – and those with potentially difficult airways – consideration should be given to instituting epidural analgesia early. It should be established that the block is working well, without missed segments. If analgesia in labour has been poor, it is unlikely that anaesthesia for caesarean section will be satisfactory. Conversion of analgesia for labour to surgical anaesthesia for caesarean section is not the same as establishing epidural anaesthesia de novo. Plain bupivacaine 0.5 per cent alone has been shown to convert low-dose bupivacaine/fentanyl labour epidural analgesia to surgical anaesthesia for caesarean section as swiftly and effectively as lidocaine 2 per cent with adrenaline, or a 50:50 mixture of the two solutions. The impact of adding bicarbonate has not been studied in this situation. Use of bupivacaine 0.5 per cent alone circumvents the time spent and risks inherent in the hurried preparation of alkalinized drug mixtures. Good communication among midwives, obstetricians and anaesthetists should make general anaesthesia for the woman with a working epidural a rarity. Even in the event of cord prolapse, traditionally managed without question by

general anaesthesia, there might be time for an epidural top-up, provided upward pressure on the presenting part is effective in avoiding cord compression.

Combined spinal–epidural anaesthesia

Studies over the last 15 years have confirmed the superior quality of combined spinal–epidural anaesthesia compared to that of epidural anaesthesia alone for caesarean section. Many units have adopted combined spinal–epidural anaesthesia as their standard technique for caesarean section, despite lack of evidence of overall superiority compared with single-shot spinals in respect of the following variables:

- speed of establishment of surgical anaesthesia;
- incidence of hypotension;
- incidences of nausea/vomiting and shivering;
- requirement for i.v./inhalational supplementation and conversion to general anaesthesia;
- quality of muscle relaxation;
- incidence of dangerously high block requiring emergency airway management;
- incidence of postoperative headache, neuropathy and CNS infection.

Use of a Tuohy needle inevitably incurs a risk of accidental dural puncture and its consequences. In a needle-through-needle technique, the spinal needle is typically advanced up to 15 mm beyond the tip of the Tuohy needle. Unlike a single-shot spinal, the needle is not gripped by successive tissue layers during its passage. Moreover, the tip of a pencil-point needle is 1 mm or so distal to the aperture. Compared to a bevel-tipped needle, unrestrained deeper insertion before flashback of CSF might predispose to the alleged greater incidence of paraesthesiae and possible increased risk of neural damage. The risk of meningitis is theoretically greater for combined spinal–epidural anaesthetics compared to single-shot spinals because of the proximity of a catheter to a dural hole.

Placenta praevia

Combined spinal–epidural anaesthesia is useful when surgery is predicted to outlast a single-shot spinal block. In the event of protracted surgery (e.g. caesarean hysterectomy in a woman with placenta praevia), an epidural catheter will allow extension of the block, typically around 90 minutes after a standard intrathecal dose. Recent UK and American retrospective studies have compared regional and general anaesthesia for caesarean section with placenta praevia. Regional anaesthesia was associated with reduced estimated blood loss and transfusion requirements. The commonly held obstetric view that placenta praevia dictates general anaesthesia was not supported. However, anterior placenta praevia in a woman over 35 who has undergone previous caesarean sections suggests a particularly high risk of placenta accreta and massive haemorrhage. General anaesthesia with provision for postoperative ICU admission might be considered prudent [IV].

First stage of labour

General anaesthesia

General anesthesia may be indicated for 'emergency' caesarean sections (Table 30.4) and for other cases for which a regional block is absolutely contraindicated, or has failed.

Good communication between the anaesthetist and obstetrician is vital in these cases, and the safety of the mother must always remain of paramount importance.

If the history or evaluation of the airway suggests that tracheal intubation might be difficult, awake fibre-optic intubation should be considered. The principal risks of general anaesthesia are:

- airway problems (e.g. failed tracheal intubation),
- aspiration of gastric contents,
- anaphylaxis (principally to succinylcholine).

In the event of anaphylaxis, adrenaline (epinephrine) is likely to improve rather than reduce utero-placental blood flow. Rapid operative delivery while the anaesthetist administers pharmacological treatment should aid maternal resuscitation.

Depth of anaesthesia

The regimen of thiopental, succinylcholine and intubation has remained standard and largely unchanged since it superseded mask and ether 40 years ago, and permitted a lighter plane of inhalational general anaesthesia. Although babies born to mothers anaesthetized with ether were undoubtedly sleepier than those whose mothers who had light anaesthesia facilitated by neuromuscular block, they were not necessarily compromised. General anaesthesia is 'innocuous and reversible' for the baby, provided maternal oxygenation and normocarbia are maintained, aorto-caval compression is avoided, and a paediatrician is present to support ventilation. Fetal compromise to which uterine hyperstimulation has been contributory might actually be relieved by uterine relaxation conferred by a volatile agent. In contrast, a maternal stress response to excessively *light* general anaesthesia will be to the detriment of utero-placental blood flow. With inhalational agent monitoring now universally available, the risk of awareness in obstetric anaesthesia should have been consigned to history.

Special considerations in pre-eclampsia

Uncorrected coagulopathy is an indication for general anaesthesia. Prior communication with a paediatrician is essential in order for preparation to be made for antagonism of opioid and provision of ventilatory support for the neonate.

Any dubious notion of light general anaesthesia for the baby's benefit should be over-ridden by efforts to protect the mother's cerebral circulation.

The onset and duration of succinylcholine are unaffected by therapeutic serum magnesium concentrations. However, the durations of action of all non-depolarizing drugs are potentiated, and the use of a peripheral nerve stimulator is essential to ensure adequate reversal at the end of surgery.

There should be a low threshold for blood pressure monitoring by radial arterial line, both in theatre and postoperatively in the high-dependency unit.

Any patient whose larynx was noted to be swollen at laryngoscopy or in whom intubation was traumatic is at particular risk of laryngeal oedema. Postoperative care must be undertaken in an ICU or high-dependency area with an anaesthetist immediately available. The ominous significance of stridor (impending airway obstruction) must be understood, and vigilance maintained. Should stridor develop, an anaesthetist must be called immediately.

PRE-ASSESSMENT AND THE ROLE OF THE ANAESTHETIST

All units should have a referral system between obstetricians and obstetric anaesthetists. Trainees providing out-of-hours cover should never be presented with complex cases 'out of the blue'. Obstetric referrals to a specialist physician's clinic (e.g. cardiology) should be notified to a consultant obstetric anaesthetist.

Anaesthetists' principal concerns are:

- the feasibility of regional block – which depends on flexion of the lumbar spine and normal blood coagulation;
- whether tracheal intubation at emergency caesarean section might be hazardous, e.g. because of limited neck flexion/mouth opening;
- the influence of medical conditions and their treatment on the safe conduct of regional or general anaesthesia.

The presence of morbidly obese women admitted in labour or to the antenatal ward should be brought to the attention of the duty obstetric anaesthetist. Regional blockade will almost certainly be a challenge, and general anaesthesia hazardous.

The criteria for referral are listed in Table 30.5.

- The need for analgesia in labour is reduced by the continuous presence of a professional carer.
- Regional analgesia produces the most satisfactory pain relief for labour.
- Regional analgesia does not increase the incidence of postnatal backache.
- Epidural analgesia is associated with an increase in the requirement for instrumental vaginal delivery, but not caesarean section.
- Continuous low-dose epidural infusions and CSEs are associated with a lower risk of instrumental vaginal delivery than conventional top-up epidural analgesia.

Table 30.5 Criteria for antenatal anaesthetic referral

Cardiovascular problems
Congenital heart disease
Valvular heart disease
Arrhythmias
Cardiomyopathy
Poorly controlled hypertension

Respiratory problems
Severe asthma (requiring steroids or hospital admission)
Breathlessness which limits daily activity
Cystic fibrosis, or any other chronic chest disease

Neurological/musculoskeletal problems
Any back surgery, e.g. laminectomy, surgery for scoliosis
Congenital conditions, e.g. spina bifida
Muscular dystrophy, myotonia
Myasthenia gravis
Demyelinating disease (multiple sclerosis)
Spinal cord injury
Rheumatoid arthritis or any condition affecting neck/jaw
Cerebrovascular disease, e.g. aneurysm, arteriovenous malformation

Haematological problems
Anticoagulation
Blood clotting/platelet disorders
Patients who have been treated for malignancy, e.g. lymphoma, leukaemia

Airway problems
Previous difficulty with intubation
Inability to open mouth or move jaw or head normally

Drug-related problems
Cholinesterase abnormalities - succinylcholine (Scoline) apnoea
Allergy or adverse reaction to anaesthetic drugs
Malignant hyperthermia
Drug abuse

Other problems
Morbid obesity - body mass index (weight ÷ height squared) >40 kg/m^2
Needle phobia
Panic attacks
Any obscure eponymous syndrome that no one seems to have heard of ...
which may pose problems if emergency anaesthesia is needed
Any patients with concerns regarding analgesia or anaesthesia,
e.g. previous problems with inadequate epidural for labour, or
pain/awareness during caesarean section

KEY POINTS

- Compared to intermittent bolus epidurals, low-dose epidural infusions and combined spinal–epidural analgesia result in a lower incidence of instrumental vaginal deliveries.
- In 1997, 78 per cent of caesarean sections in the UK were performed under regional anaesthesia.
- Single-shot spinals are the commonest regional technique for caesarean section. The addition of opioid to the local anaesthetic can reduce the incidence of intraoperative pain and provide postoperative analgesia.
- Epidural anaesthesia is generally of poorer quality than spinal anaesthesia. A combined

spinal–epidural technique is useful when it is anticipated that surgery might be protracted.

- General anaesthesia is indicated for the majority of emergency caesarean sections (i.e. when there is immediate threat to the life of the mother or fetus) and when a regional technique is absolutely contraindicated or has failed.
- The principal risks of general anaesthesia are airway problems, aspiration of gastric contents and anaphylaxis (principally to succinylcholine).
- The risk of aspiration is not confined to general anaesthesia: protective reflexes may be obtunded in the event of an excessively high regional block. Ranitidine should be prescribed for women in labour with risk factors for caesarean section.
- Placenta praevia does not necessarily dictate general anaesthesia for caesarean section. Risk factors for placenta *accreta* are predictive of massive haemorrhage.
- All units should have a referral system between obstetricians and anaesthetists. Morbid obesity should ring as many alarm bells as does severe pre-eclampsia.

KEY REFERENCES

1. Hodnett ED. Caregiver support for women during childbirth (Cochrane Review). In: *The Cochrane Library*, Issue 2. Oxford: Update Software, 2002.
2. Harrison RF, Woods T, Shore M et al. Pain relief in labour using transcutaneous electrical nerve stimulation (TENS). A TENS/TENS placebo controlled study in two parity groups. *Br J Obstet Gynaecol* 1986; 93:739–46.
3. Elbourne D, Wiseman RA. Types of intra-muscular opioids for maternal pain relief in labour (Cochrane Review). In: *The Cochrane Library*, Issue 2. Oxford: Update Software, 2002.
4. Yentis SM, Clyburn P. The use of Entonox® for labour pain should be abandoned. *Int J Obstet Anesth* 2001; 10:25–9.
5. Comparative Obstetric Mobile Epidural Trial (COMET) Study Group UK. Effect of low-dose versus traditional epidural techniques on mode of delivery: a randomised controlled trial. *Lancet* 2001; 358: 19–23.
6. Howell CJ. Epidural versus non-epidural analgesia for pain relief in labour (Cochrane Review). In: *The Cochrane Library*, Issue 2. Oxford: Update Software, 2002.

First stage of labour

7. Shibli KU, Russell IF. A survey of anaesthetic techniques used for caesarean section in the UK in 1997. *Int J Obstet Anesth* 2000; **9**:160–7.

8. Lucas DN, Yentis SM, Kinsella SM et al. Urgency of caesarean section: a new classification. *J R Soc Med* 2000; **93**:346–50.

9. Focus Group. Obstetric anaesthesia delays and complications. In: *Confidential Enquiry into Stillbirths and Deaths in Infancy, 7th Annual Report.* London: Maternal and Child Health Research Consortium, 2000, 41–52.

10. Moodley J, Jjuuko G, Rout C. Epidural compared with general anaesthesia for caesarean delivery in conscious women with eclampsia. *Br J Obstet Gynaecol* 2001; **108**:378–82.

Chapter 31

Caesarean Section

Richard Hayman

MRCOG standards

Candidates are expected to:

- be able to perform a caesarean section and an uncomplicated surgical repeat caesarean section;
- have attended a basic surgical skills course.

Theoretical skills
- Have a thorough knowledge of abdominal and pelvic anatomy.
- Understand the setting of caesarean section in the context of abnormal labour and its management.
- Be able to counsel a woman in a subsequent pregnancy concerning a trial of vaginal delivery.

Practical skills
- Be confident to effect delivery by caesarean section in a wide range of clinical scenarios.
- Where possible, have seen a classical caesarean section and have witnessed a caesarean hysterectomy.

INTRODUCTION

Birth by caesarean section has become a commonplace intervention on the modern labour ward. According to some, the caesarean section rate has reached epidemic proportions and requires a dramatic rethink of obstetric management.

Delivery by caesarean section has been part of human culture since ancient times, but despite rare references to operations on living women, the initial purpose was essentially to retrieve the infant from a dead or dying mother as a measure of last resort. It was not until much later that intervention with a good outcome for both mother and baby became possible.

Today's clinical setting

Currently in the UK, slightly more than one in seven women experiences complications during labour that provide an indication for surgical delivery. These problems can be life threatening for the mother and/or baby (e.g. eclampsia, abruptio placenta) and, in approximately 40 per cent of such cases, caesarean section provides the safest solution. In the UK, more than 21 per cent of all babies are now delivered by caesarean section – approximately 120 000 babies in the year 2000. The principal aims must be to ensure that those women and babies who need delivery by caesarean section are so delivered, and that those who do not are saved from unnecessary intervention. In 1985, concern regarding the increasing frequency of caesarean section led the World Health Organization (WHO) to hold a Consensus Conference. This conference concluded that there were no health benefits above a caesarean section rate of 10–15 per cent. The Scandinavian countries managed to hold caesarean section rates at this level during the 1990s, with outcomes comparable to or better than those of countries with higher caesarean section rates.

Although many factors have been associated with an increase in the caesarean section rate, not all have been to the detriment of the mother or baby. Interestingly, whilst the caesarean section rate has risen over the two preceding decades, the instrumental vaginal delivery rate has remained relatively constant, at approximately 10 per cent.

FACTORS THAT MAY CONTRIBUTE TO AN INCREASE IN THE RATES OF CAESAREAN SECTION

Dating the pregnancy

Many practitioners combine the information obtained from a carefully taken history with that from a dating ultrasound scan, particularly when the date of the last menstrual period is uncertain. This approach enables the expected period of confinement (37–42 weeks) to be calculated and the maximum limit of the pregnancy discussed at an early stage. Such management helps to reduce the anxiety experienced by many women when they pass their 'expected date of delivery' and also reduces the requests for 'early' induction of labour.

In units that do not routinely date the pregnancy by ultrasound scanning before 20 weeks, an opportunity for accurate dating may be missed. This may be of particular importance in units that have a policy of offering routine induction of labour to women who are 41 weeks' gestation or more. By decreasing the rate of inappropriate interventions, the complications of caesarean delivery when an induction 'fails' may be avoided.

Fetal monitoring

Following its introduction in the 1970s, electronic fetal monitoring (EFM) was universally implemented without the appropriate trials. This resulted in an increase in the incidence of caesarean section without a demonstrable improvement in perinatal outcome. Undoubtedly inappropriate monitoring increases the rate of interventions and current recommendations are for intermittent auscultation to be performed in all 'low-risk pregnancies', with continuous EFM in those pregnancies deemed to be 'high risk' or 'low risk with additional risk factors' (see Chapter 29).

Analgesia in labour

Epidural analgesia has become increasing available and utilized on labour wards in the UK.

Several studies have reported an increase in the incidence of instrumental vaginal deliveries when epidural analgesia is provided to more than 50 per cent of parturients. However, epidural analgesia has not been associated with a higher rate of caesarean section (9.6 per cent in the epidural cohort vs 13.6 per cent in the opioid group – relative risk (RR) 0.70; 95 per cent confidence interval (CI) 0.38–1.31) [Ia].[1]

Macrosomia

Maternal concern about fetal size is a common problem that frequently engenders anxiety amongst obstetricians and midwives. Although there is evidence to suggest that birth weights are rising in developed countries, the amount (30 g over 12 years) is unlikely to be of any biological significance. Unfortunately, both clinical and ultrasonographic estimations of fetal size are prone to inaccuracy (especially in large term infants), and many unnecessary inductions of labour and caesarean deliveries are performed as a consequence (see Chapter 25).

Maternal request

Traditionally, caesarean sections have been reserved for situations guided by standard clinical indications. However, requests for delivery by an elective caesarean section where there is not a compelling obstetric indication are becoming more common.

Maternal request was given as the primary reason for 7 per cent of caesarean deliveries in the UK in 2001.[2] There is, however, huge heterogeneity in studies examining the effect of maternal request on caesarean section rates. Study results range from 1.5 to 28 per cent in the contribution of request as the primary reason for section, and this is due, in major part, to the differing definitions of 'request'.[2] The arguments surrounding this area are complex, and combine ethical dilemmas, the fetal and maternal risks of vaginal and surgical deliveries and the financial consequences of permitting such a preference.

During the antenatal period, the dialogue between patients and their doctors has increased over recent years. *Changing Childbirth*[3] enshrined in practice the principle of total involvement of the pregnant woman in her own care. Implicit in this is the consideration of her wishes relating to delivery. Therefore, discussions must be accompanied by the careful imparting of information, counselling and advice, but should the patient's opinions differ from those of her healthcare providers, these cannot simply be ignored. The risks of caesarean section and labour are different, and the risks of recurrent caesarean deliveries are additive (increasing risk of placenta praevia, accreta, operative complications etc.). However, if these risks are fully explained to the woman, she should be allowed to accept one set of risks over the other. Consequently for a fully informed patient, an elective caesarean section should not be viewed as bad practice, but rather as an appropriate management plan.

A woman's request for caesarean section appears to be treated more favourably if she has previously undergone caesarean section, though this may not necessarily be a valid approach.[2]

INDICATIONS

There are many different reasons for performing a delivery by caesarean section. The four major indications accounting for more than 70 per cent of operations are: previous caesarean section, dystocia, malpresentation and suspected acute fetal compromise. Other indications, such as multi-fetal pregnancy, abruptio placenta, placenta praevia, fetal disease and maternal disease, are less common.[2] No list can be truly comprehensive and, whatever the indication, the over-riding principle is that whenever the risk to the mother and/or the fetus from vaginal delivery *exceeds* that from operative intervention, a caesarean section should be undertaken.

Absolute indications for recommending delivery by cae-sarean section are few; almost all indications are relative and there will be circumstances in which caesarean section may be best for one woman but not another. Lack of consent by a woman with the capacity to give consent will prohibit caesarean section regardless of the clinical need, as dis-cussed below.

The indications may be divided into groups as follows:

Indications for which elective caesarean section would be the strongly recommended means of delivery

- Past obstetric history:
  - previous classical caesarean section,
  - interval pelvic floor or anal sphincter repair,
  - previous severe shoulder dystocia with significant neonatal injury.
- Current pregnancy events:
  - significant fetal disease likely to lead to poor tolerance of labour,
  - monoamniotic twins,
  - placenta praevia,
  - obstructing pelvic mass,
  - active primary herpes at onset of labour.
- Intrapartum events:
  - acute fetal compromise in the first stage,
  - maternal disease for which delay in delivery may compromise the safety of the mother,
  - absolute cephalo-pelvic disproportion (brow presentations etc.).

There are many other reasons why a caesarean section may be recommended that are too numerous to list; in almost every case there will be practitioners who believe that vaginal delivery is feasible or a better option, and therefore each woman deserves a personal evaluation of her individual needs.

MORBIDITY AND MORTALITY

Although caesarean section is becoming increasingly safe and evidence is mounting regarding the risks of labour and vaginal delivery, pregnant women, their midwives and doc-tors need to understand and appreciate the maternal risks associated with the different modes of delivery. Some mater-nal deaths following caesarean section are not attributable to the procedure itself, but rather to medical or obstetric dis-orders that lead to the decision to deliver using this approach. Many women who deliver vaginally encounter the same problems.

The Confidential Enquiries enable the risks associated with each method of delivery to be analysed.[4] A comparison

Table 31.1 Direct death rates per million maternities by mode of delivery in UK, 1997–99[4]

Mode of delivery	Calculated maternities (×1000)	Direct deaths	Death rate per million maternities	Relative risk (95% CI)
Vaginal	1710	29	16.9	1.0
Caesarean section	413	34	82.3	4.9 (2.96–7.97)
Elective	130	5	38.5	2.3 (0.88–5.86)
Emergency	69	14	202.9	12 (6.32–22.65)
Urgent	137	14	102.2	6.0 (3.18–11.4)
Scheduled	78	1	12.8	0.8 (0.1–5.55)
All maternities	2123	63	29.7	

of fatality rates can be useful, but it is preferable to restrict the analysis to direct deaths, as many women whose deaths were classified as indirect had pre-existing illness. Direct deaths are specifically those that result from obstetric com-plications of the pregnant state, from interventions, omis-sions or incorrect treatment, or from a chain of events that occur after any of the above.

Using hospital episode statistics data, it is possible to esti-mate the overall number of caesarean sections that took place in the UK between 1997 and 1999. Estimated case fatality rates can thus be calculated and are shown in Table 31.1.

It can be seen that the case fatality rate for all caesarean sections is five times that for vaginal delivery, and for emer-gency caesarean delivery this may be 12 times greater. These differences are highly significant. Even for elective cae-sarean section, the rate is more than twice as great, although this does not reach statistical significance. In the absence of other evidence (e.g. from randomized, controlled trials of different modes of delivery), it is not appropriate to be dog-matic about best practice. Consequently, any decision to undertake major surgery with an associated mortality should be taken very seriously by all concerned. The Confidential Enquiry emphasizes that a caesarean section constitutes major surgery.

REPEAT CAESAREAN SECTION

Providing the first operation was carried out for a non-recurrent cause, and providing the obstetric situation close to term in the succeeding pregnancy is favourable, a trial of vaginal delivery is appropriate. The factors to be weighed when determining the recommended mode of delivery depend on the balance between the desires of the mother, the risks of a repeat operation, the risks to her child of labour, and the risk of labour on the strength of the old scar (see Chapter 26).

First stage of labour

PROCEDURE

Informed consent

Full informed consent must always be obtained prior to operation. The level of information discussed must be commensurate with the urgency of the procedure, and a commonsense approach is needed. Although it is often difficult to impart complete and thorough information when caesarean sections are performed as emergency procedures, mothers must understand what is being planned and why. Where possible, all women must be educated in pregnancy about caesarean section and the circumstances in which it may be urgently needed. It is important to remember that no adult may give consent for another (although it is good practice to keep relatives fully informed). Where there is incapacity to consent (as may occur with conditions such as eclampsia), the doctor is expected to act in the patient's best interests.

Resistance to a recommended emergency caesarean section is rare, as long as the indications for delivery are discussed in an appropriate and considerate manner. When it occurs, it is often the consequence of a failure in communication. Full documentation of the recommendation and its refusal is mandatory, but no healthcare provider can force a competent adult to undergo surgery against her will. One must always respect the wishes of the patient and her cultural and religious beliefs, no matter how challenging the consequences appear. In an elective or unhurried atmosphere, where there is significant doubt about capacity to consent, two medical opinions are required to over-ride patient wishes. It is advised, though not mandatory, that one of these should be obtained from a psychiatrist.

The national consent forms require both the risks and benefits to be discussed with patients and recorded on the consent form. Common medical practice is to highlight risks but not benefits. It is important to remember that the operation is being offered because of perceived benefits, both maternal and fetal in many cases. It is suggested that the top copy of the form should be offered to the patient, although in extreme emergencies this may not be appropriate.

Surgical basics

Following on from Munro Kerr's description of the lower segment procedure in the early twentieth century, more than 90 per cent of caesarean sections are performed using adaptations of this technique.[2]

Routine preoperative preparation with suprapubic shaving should be undertaken. The bladder should be emptied before the procedure. It is the policy in many units for a catheter to remain in situ perioperatively and for a defined period thereafter (commonly 24 hours or until the patient is mobile). Although this approach may improve patient comfort postoperatively and reduce the incidence of over-distension of the bladder (a complication of regional anaesthesia), there is a risk of iatrogenic urinary tract infection.

A left lateral tilt minimizes compression of the maternal inferior vena cava and reduces the incidence of hypotension (with its consequent reductions in placental perfusion). The patient should then be draped in the standard manner, although more recent advances with plastic adhesive drapes may prove more effective than standard drapes in the prevention of wound infections.

The choice of incision and closure should be individualized to the characteristics of the woman and the circumstances demanding operative intervention.

Skin incisions

Two basic skin incisions are used – suprapubic and midline vertical.

The transverse incision has the advantages of improved cosmetic results, decreased analgesic requirements and thus less postoperative pulmonary compromise and superior wound strength.

The vertical incision, on the other hand, provides greater ease of access to the pelvic and intra-abdominal organs and may be enlarged more easily. Haeri demonstrated no difference between the two incisions when comparing overall operative time, postoperative haemoglobins of <10 g/dL, or postoperative febrile morbidity [III].[5] However, Mowatt and Bonnar reported an eight-fold increase in the incidence of wound dehiscence with the midline incision when compared to a transverse abdominal approach (this difference may be reduced by mass closure techniques) [III].[6]

The Pfannenstiel incision

The skin and subcutaneous tissues are incised using a transverse curvilinear incision at a level of two fingerbreadths above the symphysis pubis, extending from and to points lateral to the lateral margins of the abdominal rectus muscles. The subcutaneous tissues are separated by blunt dissection and the rectus sheath is incised transversely along the middle 2 cm. This incision is then extended with scissors before the fascial sheath is separated from the underlying muscle by further blunt dissection. Separation is performed cephalad to permit adequate exposure of the peritoneum in a longitudinal plane. Perforating blood vessels must be cauterized to minimize the risks of development of subrectus haematomas. The recti are separated from each other, the peritoneum incised and the abdominal cavity entered.

The Cohen incision

This incision is similar to the Pfannenstiel incision, but permits a more rapid and bloodless entry into the peritoneal cavity. A straight transverse incision is made between two points inferior and medial to the anterior superior iliac spine, the subcutaneous tissues are divided in the midline for 3 cm and the central rectus sheath is similarly divided. By blunt dissection and vertical traction, the subfascial space is opened, the peritoneum exposed and the abdominal cavity entered high above the bladder. Entry with this technique into the abdominal cavity is often not suitable for repeat caesarean sections, where scarring may distort the underlying fascial planes.

The infra-umbilical incision

The vertical skin incision is specifically indicated in cases of extreme maternal obesity, if the need for caesarean section is coupled with the suspicion of other intra-abdominal pathology necessitating surgical intervention, or where access to the uterine fundus may be required (classical caesarean section).

The lower midline incision is made from the lower boarder of the umbilicus to the symphysis pubis, and may be extended caudally towards the xiphisternum if required. Sharp dissection to the level of the anterior rectus sheath is performed, which is then freed of subcutaneous fat in the midline. The rectus sheath is then incised, taking care to avoid damage to any underlying bowel, and extended inferiorly to the vesical peritoneal reflection and superiorly to the upper limit of the abdominal incision.

Uterine incisions

As with the skin incision, the nature of the uterine incision is determined by the clinical situation. The lower uterine incision is used in more than 95 per cent of caesarean deliveries due to ease of repair, reduced blood loss and lower incidence of dehiscence or rupture in subsequent pregnancies when compared with the alternative incisions.

There are relatively few absolute indications for classical section. However, these include a lower uterine segment containing fibroids or a lower segment covered with dense adhesions, both of which may make entry difficult. Such obstruction may be associated with heavy bleeding or may distort the anatomy to such an extent that the lower segment approach is not safe. Other indications include placenta praevia, transverse lie with the back down and especially when associated with prolapse of a fetal arm (a more satisfactory delivery will be achieved through a lower segment incision after correction of the lie), fetal abnormality (e.g. conjoined twins), or caesarean section in the presence of a carcinoma of the cervix (so as to avoid damage to the cervix and its vascular and lymphatic supplies).

The uterus is palpated to identify the size and presenting part of the fetus and to determine the direction and degree of rotation of the uterus. A Doynes or similar retractor blade is inserted inferiorly and the loose reflection of vesico-uterine serosa overlying the uterus picked up with toothed forceps, opened with scissors and divided laterally. The underlying lower uterine segment is reflected with blunt dissection, and the developed bladder flap held rostrally with the retractor. The uterus is then opened in a transverse plane for a distance of 1–2 cm; the incision may be extended laterally with either blunt dissection (lateral and upward pressure with the index fingers) or scissors. Such an incision should be adequate to allow delivery of the fetus without extension into the broad ligament or uterine vessels. If necessary, cutting the incision upward unilaterally (J-incision) or bilaterally (U-shape) will avoid such an extension and provide extra room. Damage to the uterine vessels or broad ligament, when it occurs, is associated with an increase in maternal morbidity (especially blood loss) and prolonged hospitalization. If a midline extension is required, the T-incision, in future pregnancies vaginal delivery will be contraindicated because of an increased risk of uterine rupture [III].

A modified classical or De Lee incision should also be in the surgeon's repertoire. This entry is vertical on the uterus in the sagittal plane, is extended to the level of entry of the round ligaments, but is not taken onto the fundus (unlike a true classical section). Although delivery through this incision decreases the risk of rupture in subsequent pregnancies compared with a classical incision, most would recommend future deliveries by elective caesarean section.

The fetal lie is then stabilized, the membranes are ruptured if still intact, and the accoucheur's hand is positioned below the presenting part. If cephalic, the head is flexed and delivered by elevation though the uterine incision, either manually or with forceps. Fundal pressure is then applied to aid the delivery. However, this should not be commenced until the presenting part is located within the incision – for fear of converting the lie from longitudinal to transverse.

Specific manoeuvres must be employed at caesarean section, prior to membrane rupture for stabilization of transverse or oblique lies, and for delivery of the breech.

Once the fetus is delivered, an oxytocic (5 IU Syntocinon i.v.) is administered to aid uterine contraction and placental separation. Prophylactic antibiotics should be administered to reduce the incidence of postoperative endometritis, and although no one regimen has been shown to have a clear advantage over any other, a single dose of either a first-generation or second-generation cephalosporin ± metronidazole, or ampicillin with clavulanic acid would be suitable [Ia]. There is no evidence to suggest that a prolonged course of antibiotics is more beneficial than a single dose when used for prophylaxis [Ia].

The placenta should be delivered by combined cord traction; manual removal significantly increases the intraoperative blood loss and postoperative infectious morbidity [Ia].[7] The uterus should then be inspected to ensure complete removal of the placenta and membranes. Some authors advise confirmation of a patent cervical canal to ensure a patent passage for the drainage of lochia, although this is not necessary in labouring women.

Repair of the incision may be performed with the uterus in situ or following exteriorization. Exteriorization is not routinely necessary, but enhances visualization of the lower segment and thus facilitates surgical repair; especially when there have been lateral extensions to the incision margins.

First stage of labour

Evidence comparing blood loss between the two techniques is contradictory. One trial reported a decrease in the haematocrit fall with exteriorization compared with intraperitoneal procedures (6.2 ± 0.35 vs 7.0 ± 0.43, $p < 0.01$), whereas another did not. The main problems with exteriorization are increases in maternal pain, vagal-induced vomiting and the incidence of venous air emboli, although the incidence of infectious morbidity is not altered. There is currently not enough information to evaluate adequately the routine use of exteriorization of the uterus for repair of the uterine incision.

Uterine closure

Placement of Green–Armytage forceps on the inferior uterine edge in addition to each angle improves visualization and reduces blood loss further, especially in the presence of bleeding venous sinuses. Closure should be performed in either single or double layers with continuous or interrupted sutures. The initial suture should be placed just lateral to the incision angle, and the closure continued to a point just lateral to the angle on the opposite side. A running stitch is often employed and this may be locked to improve haemostasis. If a second layer is used, an inverting suture or horizontal suture should overlap the myometrium. There are only two reported randomized, controlled trials comparing single-layer versus two-layer closure. A single-layer closure is associated with reduced operating time, with no statistically significant differences in the use of extra haemostatic sutures, incidence of endometritis, decrease in postoperative haematocrit or use of blood transfusion [Ib]. There have recently been some concerns regarding single-layer closure, as one widely reported observational study of scar dehiscence in subsequent labours showed a higher incidence than previously reported. One possible aetiological factor that has been suggested is the move to single-layer closure during the time period studied.[8]

In cases associated with extended 'tears', once the uterine angles are secure, the defect should be repaired as a primary procedure prior to uterine closure. Lacerations involving uterine tissue are usually repaired without difficulty. However, vertical lacerations into the vagina or lateral extensions into the broad ligament may be associated with substantial blood loss and the potential for ureteric damage. To minimize bleeding from the perforated myometrial vessels in such cases, the needle must be positioned just distal to the apex of the laceration and, once inserted, should not be withdrawn.

Once repaired, the incision is assessed for haemostasis and 'figure-of-eight' sutures can be employed to control bleeding. The uterus, tubes and ovaries are inspected, elective or emergency adnexal procedures performed (e.g. tubal ligation ovarian cystectomy for dermoid cyst), and the paracolic gutters cleaned. Peritoneal closure is unnecessary and may result in a higher incidence of adhesion formation than would otherwise occur [Ia]. Many surgeons routinely place drains in the subfascial space to reduce haematoma formation, but such management is most appropriate in the presence of infection or in the obese, where a large 'space' is potentially left. In all cases, attention to haemostasis is the key.

Abdominal closure

Closure is performed in the anatomical planes with high-strength, low-reactivity materials such as polyglycolic acid or polyglactin (Dexon® and Vicryl®). Interlocking of the sutures should be avoided, as this can devascularize the tissues and delay the healing process. Closure of a midline incision differs at the level of the rectus sheath. Here, repair should be effected with a running continuous suture of polyglycolic acid, large-bore monofilament polypropylene or nylon, which have delayed/prolonged absorption characteristics.

In any patient with an increased risk of haematoma formation, such as severe pre-eclampsia, HELLP syndrome or morbid obesity, a closed drainage system located anterior to the rectus sheath may be required. Subcutaneous sutures to approximate Camper's fascia should be used in women with more than 2 cm of subcutaneous fat, as they have been shown to reduce the incidence of wound disruption and seroma formation, and potentially may lower the overt infection rate [II]. The skin may be closed using any number of techniques. The most common involve surgical staples, subcuticular stitches or tension sutures (interrupted or continuous/polyglycolic acid, large-bore monofilament polypropylene or nylon). However, lower transverse abdominal skin incisions closed with a subcuticular stitch result in less postoperative discomfort and are more cosmetically appealing at the 6-week postoperative visit when compared to incisions closed with staples [Ib].

COMPLICATIONS

It must never be forgotten that caesarean section is a major abdominal surgical procedure and carries with it all the risks inherent in such an approach.

Intraoperative complications

Bowel damage
Bowel damage is rare at caesarean section, but may occur during a repeat procedure or if adhesions are present from previous surgery. Damage is often recognized by smell or the observation of faecal soiling. The management is dependent on the site of the injury, and is best conducted in conjunction with a general surgeon. Small bowel damage is repaired using a two-layer closure with 2-0 Vicryl® or equivalent. Large bowel damage is managed likewise, but in addition a temporary defunctioning colostomy may be required. Post-repair peritoneal lavage is mandatory, as is a treatment course with broad-spectrum antibiotics, for example a cephalosporin and metronidazole.

Haemorrhage

Haemorrhage accounts for 6 per cent of deaths associated with caesarean section and an unknown proportion of operative morbidity. This complication may be due to the operative procedure as a consequence of damage to the uterine vessels, or may be incidental as a consequence of uterine atony or placenta praevia. There are many manoeuvres that may be employed to manage such cases, which range from bimanual compression, infusions of oxytocin and administration of 15-methyl prostaglandin $F_{2\alpha}$ to conservative surgical procedures such as uterine compression sutures, to the more radical, but life-saving, hysterectomy.

Placenta praevia

The proportion of patients with a placenta praevia is increasing as a consequence of caesarean section. The incidence increases almost linearly after each previous caesarean section (Table 31.2), and as the risks of such a complication increase with increasing parity, future reproductive intentions are very relevant to any individual decision for operative delivery.

Clark et al.[9] also reported that 25 per cent of women undergoing caesarean delivery for placenta praevia in the presence of one or more uterine scars subsequently underwent caesarean hysterectomy for placenta accreta.

In patients with an anticipated high risk of haemorrhage, for example known cases of placenta praevia, 4 units of blood should be routinely cross-matched, and must be available in theatre before the procedure is commenced. A combined approach to the management of such patients, with the anaesthetists, haematologists and obstetricians working together, will result in the best standard of care.

Urinary tract damage

Direct injury to the bladder is not uncommon during caesarean section. The transverse lower abdominal incision carries the risk of cystotomy, especially after prolonged labours where the bladder is displaced caudally, after previous caesarean section where scarring obliterates the vesico-uterine space, or where a vertical extension to the uterine incision has occurred. Preoperative catheterization in association with careful operative technique should reduce the likelihood of damage occurring. If damage to the bladder is

suspected, transurethral instillation of methylene blue-coloured saline will help to delineate the extent of the defect. When such an injury is observed, a repair with 2-0 Vicryl® as a single continuous or interrupted layer is appropriate. The urinary catheter will need to remain in situ for 7–10 days and prophylactic antibiotics prescribed.

Damage to the ureters is uncommon, as reflection of the bladder displaces them rostrally, but if suspected, the ureters should be investigated and repaired in conjunction with a urological surgeon.

Caesarean hysterectomy

The most common indication for caesarean hysterectomy is uncontrollable maternal haemorrhage, a situation not infrequently associated with a morbidly adherent placenta. This operation, whilst a major undertaking, should not be left too late, as the risk of operative complications, maternal morbidity and mortality increase with increasing haemorrhage.

Although postpartum haemorrhage is relatively common (occurring after about 1 per cent of deliveries), life-threatening haemorrhage requiring immediate treatment affects only 1 in 1000 deliveries.[4] There is no 'clinical standard' at which intervention by hysterectomy is recommended, so local protocols must be formulated to address this specific issue and to guide the individual clinician to intevene if the loss remains uncontrollable after, for example, 2.5 L. It is important to note that the Confidential Enquiries continue to cite delays in performing definitive surgery, for example a hysterectomy, as an avoidable cause of maternal mortality.[4]

The most important risk factor for emergency postpartum hysterectomy is a previous caesarean section, especially when the placenta overlies the old scar and increases the risks of placenta accreta. This complication alone accounts for 30 per cent of emergency caesarean hysterectomies.

From the early stages, such cases should be managed by an experienced obstetrician and anaesthetist.[4] It is also important to counsel such patients accordingly, and to gain consent preoperatively for caesarean hysterectomy when appropriate.

Other common indications for hysterectomy are:

- atony (43 per cent),
- uterine rupture (13 per cent),
- extension of a low transverse incision (10 per cent),
- leiomyomata preventing uterine closure and haemostasis (4 per cent).

Hysterectomies performed for atony are significantly associated with the following factors when compared to hysterectomies performed for other indications:

- amnionitis,
- caesarean section for labour arrest,

Table 31.2 Risk of placenta praevia and accreta with repeat caesarean sections

Number of previous caesarean sections	Incidence of placenta praevia (%) [total 0.3%]	Incidence of placenta accreta in those with placenta praevia (%)	Overall risk of placenta accreta (%)
0	0.26	5	0.01
1	0.65	24	0.16
2	1.8	47	0.85
3	3	40	1.2
4	10	67	6.7

First stage of labour

- oxytocin augmentation of labour,
- magnesium sulphate infusion,
- excessive fetal weight.

It should be remembered that the pelvic tissues in the pregnant woman are lax, with increased vascularity. They are therefore prone to bleed more freely than in the non-pregnant state, and extra care must be taken to ensure the pedicles are correctly ligated. Identification of the lower margin of the cervix may be exceedingly difficult, and a subtotal procedure may need to be considered.

Postoperative complications

Infection and endometritis

The single most important risk factor for postpartum maternal infection is caesarean delivery, and women undergoing caesarean section have a 5–20-fold greater risk of an infectious complication when compared with a vaginal delivery [III]. These complications include fever, wound infection, endometritis, bacteraemia, other serious infection (including pelvic abscess, septic shock, necrotizing fasciitis and septic pelvic vein thrombophlebitis) and urinary tract infection. Such sequelae are an important and substantial cause of maternal morbidity and are often associated with a significant increase in the length of the hospital stay. It should be remembered that fever can occur after any operative procedure, and a low-grade fever following a caesarean delivery may not necessarily be a marker of infection. Other common causes that enter the differential diagnosis include haematoma, atelectasis and deep vein thrombosis.

The incidence of postoperative wound infection has been quoted to be between 1 and 9 per cent. The following factors are associated with an increased risk of postoperative infection:

- preterm labour
- ruptured membranes
- prolonged labour
- delivery by an inexperienced surgeon
- the number of vaginal examinations
- internal fetal monitoring
- urinary tract infection
- anaemia, blood loss
- diabetes
- general anaesthesia
- obesity
- low socio-economic status.

Labour, its duration and the presence of ruptured membranes appear to be the most important factors, with obesity playing a particularly important role in the occurrence of wound infections.

The most important source of micro-organisms responsible for post-caesarean section infection is the genital tract, particularly if the membranes are ruptured preoperatively.

Even in the presence of intact membranes, microbial invasion of the intrauterine cavity is common, especially with preterm labour. Infections are commonly polymicrobial.

The pathogens isolated from infected wounds and the endometrium include:

- *Escherichia coli*
- other aerobic Gram-negative rods
- group B *Streptococcus*
- other *Streptococcus* species
- *Enterococcus faecalis*
- *Staphylococcus aureus*
- coagulase-negative staphylococci
- anaerobes (including *Peptostreptococcus* species and *Bacteroides* species)
- *Gardnerella vaginalis* and genital mycoplasmas.

Although *Ureaplasma urealyticum* is commonly isolated from the upper genital tract and infected wounds, it is unclear whether it is a pathogen in this setting. Wound infections caused by *Staphylococcus aureus* and coagulase-negative staphylococci arise from contamination of the wound with the endogenous flora of the skin at the time of surgery.

The general principles for the prevention of any surgical infection include careful surgical technique, skin antisepsis and antimicrobial prophylaxis. Without prophylaxis, the incidence of endometritis is reported to range from 20 to 85 per cent and the rates of wound infection and serious infectious complications may be as high as 25 per cent. The reduction in the risk of endometritis with antibiotics appears to be similar across a spectrum of patient groups:

- elective caesarean section: RR = 0.24
  (95 per cent CI = 0.11–0.48)
- emergency caesarean section: RR = 0.30
  (95 per cent CI = 0.25–0.35)
- undefined or all patients: RR = 0.29
  (95 per cent CI = 0.26–0.33) [Ia].[10]

Overall, the use of prophylactic antibiotics at caesarean section results in a major, clinically important and statistically significant reduction in the incidence of episodes of fever, endometritis, wound infection, urinary tract infection and serious infections.

The common regimens have been subjected to a number of trials and have been summarized by meta-analysis [Ia].[10] Almost all trials included endometritis, febrile morbidity, wound infection and urinary tract infection as outcome measures. In only three trials were antibiotics given preoperatively, making comparison of the timing of the first dose impossible.

The analysis examined types of antibiotic prophylaxis, single-dose versus multiple-dose regimens and method of administration (systemic vs peritoneal lavage).

The drug regimens compared included comparisons of different types of cephalosporins, extended spectrum penicillins, ampicillin and ampicillin plus gentamicin.

No drug regimen was superior to any other, with the exception that second-generation or third-generation cephalosporins were associated with fewer urinary tract infections than extended spectrum penicillins (odds ratio (OR) 0.38, 95 per cent CI 0.17–0.83). Multiple-dose regimens did not reduce the rates of febrile morbidity (OR 1.32, 95 per cent CI 0.95–1.84), endometritis (OR 0.92, 95 per cent CI 0.7–1.23) or wound infection (OR 0.91, 95 per cent CI 0.58–1.43). However, fewer urinary tract infections were seen in the multiple-dose group (OR 0.6, 95 per cent CI 0.43–0.83).

There continues to be some debate about the necessity of antibiotics in women at very low risk undergoing elective caesarean section. The most recent large randomized, controlled trail (not included in the meta-analysis) suggested again that prophylactic antibiotics might be unnecessary [Ib].[11] Four hundred and eighty women undergoing elective caesarean section had cefoxitin or placebo. Wound infection occurred in 13.3 per cent and 12.5 per cent of women in the placebo and cefoxitin groups, respectively. Prophylactic antibiotics did not decrease febrile morbidity, wound infection, endometritis, urinary tract infection and pneumonia. Hospital stay was on average a day less than for those who received placebo. Putting the data from this trial into the meta-analysis gives a relative risk for endometritis in the treatment group of 0.4 (95 per cent CI 0.2–0.79), suggesting that prophylactic antibiotics do reduce the risk of endometritis after elective caesarean section, but do not reduce the incidence the of other infective morbidity.

The best guidance is that, at the very least, antibiotics should be used whenever there are risk factors in women undergoing caesarean section.

Pulmonary emboli and deep vein thrombosis (venous thromboembolism)

Pulmonary embolism (PE) remains the leading direct cause of maternal death. However, there has been a dramatic fall in deaths from PE after caesarean section following criticism made in the 1994–97 Confidential Enquiry into Maternal Deaths and the subsequent Royal College of Obstetricians and Gynaecologists (RCOG) recommendations for thromboprophylaxis. It is also likely that the inclusion of thromboembolism prophylaxis guidelines as part of the Clinical Negligence Scheme for Trusts standards has contributed to the widespread application of these guidelines. In the last reported triennium, 31 deaths from PE were reported and only seven were after caesarean section.[4] The major areas for attention now encompass recognition of thromboembolism in women presenting to general practitioners or in accident and emergency departments.

It is difficult to be specific about the incidence of non-fatal PEs post-caesarean section, as these are notoriously difficult to record, due to presentation at different times and to many different professionals. Everyone dealing with pregnant or recently pregnant women needs to be aware of the following symptoms.

- Deep vein thromboembolism (DVT): leg pain or discomfort (especially in the left leg), complaints of pulled muscles or muscle strain, swelling, tenderness, increased temperature and oedema, lower abdominal pain and elevated white cell count. One or many of these symptoms may present.
- PE: dyspnoea, collapse, chest pain, haemoptysis, faintness, raised jugular venous pressure, focal signs in chest, and symptoms and signs associated with DVT. Remember that pelvic veins account for most post-caesarean section PEs and leg signs may not be present.

The subjective, clinical assessment of DVT and PE is unreliable, and less than half of the women with clinically suspected venous thromboembolism have the diagnosis confirmed when objective testing is employed. However, the index of suspicion must be high, and consequently treatment should be commenced whilst awaiting diagnostic confirmation.

The incidence of such complications can undoubtedly be reduced by the perioperative administration of prophylactic heparin and the prompt initiation of treatment, when required, in accordance with the guidelines issued by the RCOG (see Chapter 6.5).

Psychological

The spontaneous birth of a live infant can convey a huge degree of both satisfaction and achievement for both the mother and her partner. Although all women entering labour face the risks of an emergency delivery, the majority will achieve a normal vaginal delivery without complications. Whatever the outcome, pain, exhaustion and the demands of a newborn baby can complicate the recovery and, when combined with fear of the unknown and a sense of 'loss of control', may have dramatic effects on the woman both in the long and the short term. The recovery period after labour thus depends on a large number of interacting factors.

It is commonly believed that the general recovery after caesarean section is more prolonged than after vaginal delivery. It is recognized that all difficult deliveries carry increased maternal psychological and physical morbidity. Recent evidence suggests that the compromised postpartum psychological functioning in women delivered by caesarean section may be secondary to delayed contact with the baby. This is important, as it is a factor that in most cases should be amenable to remedy.

- Effective thromboembolism prophylaxis has reduced the number of deaths from pulmonary embolism after caesarean section and should be a routine part of caesarean section management.
- Repeat caesarean sections increase the risks of placenta praevia and accreta.

First stage of labour

- There is a significant reduction in the risk of endometritis with antibiotics across a spectrum of patient groups:
  - elective caesarean section: RR = 0.24 (95 per cent CI = 0.11–0.48)
  - emergency caesarean section: RR = 0.30 (95 per cent CI = 0.25–0.35)
  - undefined or all patients: RR = 0.29 (95 per cent CI = 0.26–0.33).
- Repeated courses of antibiotics for routine prophylaxis are not necessary.
- Antibiotic drug regimens covering the common organisms are equally as effective as prophylaxis.
- Manual removal of the placenta at caesarean section increases the risk of endometritis.
- Single-layer closure of the uterus is as effective as a two-layer closure but the trial numbers are relatively small and the question of uterine dehiscence has not been addressed in relationship to this technique.
- Peritoneal closure is not necessary routinely.

KEY POINTS

- The rate of delivery by caesarean section continues to be an issue of great concern to many midwives, obstetricians, politicians and society as a whole, but should not be considered in isolation from other changes taking place in society.
- Maternal satisfaction is an important part of childbirth and must be taken into consideration when implementing any changes in childbirth policy. There is no evidence that there will be a widespread increase in maternal requests for caesarean section.
- There is a real need for national debate about whether maternal choice is a valid indication and, if agreed, this should be fully funded.
- Placenta praevia, particularly in patients with a previous uterine scar, may be associated with uncontrollable uterine haemorrhage at delivery, and caesarean hysterectomy may be necessary. A very experienced operator is essential and a consultant must be readily available.
- Every unit must have a protocol for the management of massive haemorrhage.

KEY REFERENCES

1. Thomas J, Paranjothy S, Royal College of Obstetricians and Gynaecologists Clinical Effectiveness Support Unit. *National Sentinel Caesarean Section Audit*. London: RCOG Press, 2001.
2. Howell CJ. Epidural versus non-epidural analgesia for pain relief in labour. Cochrane Review. In: *The Cochrane Library*, Issue 3. Oxford: Update Software, 2002.
3. *Changing Childbirth*. Report of the Expert Maternity Group. London: HMSO, 1993.
4. The Confidential Enquiries into Maternal Deaths in the United Kingdom. *Why Mothers Die 1997–1999*. London: RCOG Press, 2001.
5. Haeri AD. Comparison of transverse and vertical skin incisions for Caesarean section. *South African Med J* 1976; 52:33–4.
6. Mowatt J, Bonnar J. Abdominal wound dehiscence after Caesarean section. *BMJ* 1971; 2:256–7.
7. Wilkinson C, Enkin MW. Manual removal of placenta at caesarean section. In: *The Cochrane Library,*Issue 3. Oxford: Update Software, 2002.
8. Enkin MW, Wilkinson C. Single versus two layer suturing for closing the uterine incision at Caesarean section. In: *The Cochrane Library*, Issue 2. Oxford: Update Software, 2002.
9. Clark SL, Yeh SY, Phelan J, Samuel B, Paul RH. Emergency hysterectomy for obstetric haemorrhage. *Obstet Gynecol* 1984; 64(3):376–80.
10. Hofmeyr GJ, Smaill F. Antibiotic prophylaxis regimens and drugs for cesarean section. In: *The Cochrane Library*, Issue 2. Oxford: Update Software, 2002.
11. Bagratee JS, Moodley J, Kleinschmidt I, Zawilski W. A randomised controlled trial of antibiotic prophylaxis in elective Caesarean delivery. *Br J Obstet Gynaecol* 2001; 108:143–8.

SECTION E

Second stage of labour

Chapter 32

Fetal Compromise in the Second Stage of Labour

Griff Jones

INTRODUCTION

The management of suspected fetal compromise in the second stage of labour demands considerable skill, in terms of both decision-making and practical ability. Uterine contractions have peaked in terms of strength and frequency, and the resulting intrauterine and uterine wall pressures are further increased by maternal pushing. These pressures will frequently be greater than maternal arterial blood pressure, temporarily abolishing placental perfusion. Compression of the fetal head and umbilical cord is at its greatest, as the amniotic fluid volume has reached a nadir and passage through the rigid bony pelvis has begun. After many hours of stressful labour, fetal reserves may also be reduced or depleted. All these factors combine to make fetal heart rate abnormalities particularly common, although many of these abnormalities will be entirely benign. Having reached full dilatation, there is also an expectation that vaginal birth will be achieved.

Despite the factors detailed above, clinicians must remain wary of undertaking difficult assisted vaginal deliveries in the presence of fetal compromise. For this reason, secondary tests of fetal well-being still have a place in the second stage of labour. Such tests can give reassurance that further time for head descent and/or rotation can be allowed, converting a difficult delivery into an easier one or even a spontaneous birth.

DEFINITIONS

See Chapter 29.

WHAT TYPE OF FETAL MONITORING IS BEST IN THE SECOND STAGE?

There is no evidence to support different conclusions regarding fetal monitoring in low-risk pregnancies in the second stage of labour compared to the first stage. However, with intermittent monitoring, it will be difficult for the obstetrician called to undertake an assisted delivery to confirm fetal well-being. Any concern regarding a difficult delivery should be met with either a short period of electronic fetal monitoring or fetal scalp blood sampling.

Intermittent auscultation

In the low-risk situation, intermittent auscultation, either by Pinnard stethoscope or by hand-held Doppler, remains popular. Conventional guidelines, such as those issued by the Royal College of Obstetricians and Gynaecologists (RCOG) and the Society of Obstetricians and Gynaecologists of Canada, suggest auscultating the fetal heart rate every 5 minutes in the second stage. Usually this is for 60 seconds following a contraction, in order to detect significant decelerations [IV].

WHAT IS A NORMAL SECOND STAGE CARDIOTOCOGRAPH?

In an early large study of 1755 second stage heart rate traces, 75 per cent maintained a normal baseline rate, with about 5 per cent becoming tachycardic.[1] The remaining 20 per cent of traces developed a baseline bradycardia that was transient in one-third, persistent in one-third and progressive in the remaining third.

Overall, a normal baseline in combination with an absence of decelerations was seen in only one-quarter of second stage heart rate tracings. However, 60 per cent of these 'normal' traces either exhibited no accelerations or poor variability, resulting in 90 per cent of all second stage cardiotocographs (CTGs) showing some degree of abnormality.

Therefore, the definition of a normal second stage CTG is difficult. Using standards applied for antenatal or even first stage CTGs, a normal CTG would appear to be rare in the second stage of labour.

Early studies of second stage CTG abnormalities related neonatal outcome to Apgar scores rather than cord pH. Provided the baseline heart rate remained normal, only 2 per cent of neonates ended up with a 5-minute Apgar score <7 [II].[1] Later studies found a similar risk of metabolic acidosis in this situation.[2–5]

WHAT IS AN ABNORMAL SECOND STAGE CARDIOTOCOGRAPH?

- *Baseline.* Apart from late decelerations, the only fetal heart rate patterns that are strongly suggestive of fetal hypoxaemia are a continuous or progressive bradycardia.

    Approximately 10 per cent of persistent or progressive bradycardias in the second stage will lead to 5-minute Apgar scores <7.[1] Neither superimposed early nor variable decelerations influence these figures. In later studies, fetal bradycardia was linked with neonatal acidosis.[3–5] Both Piquard et al.[6] and Cordoso et al.[3] found the mean umbilical artery pH to be lower in the presence of a fetal bradycardia. The severity of the bradycardia also correlates with perinatal risk. Acidosis was found in 30–40 per cent of moderate to severely bradycardic fetuses;[4,5] in more than half of the cases there was a metabolic acidosis. One study found that a fetal heart rate of <70 beats per minute (bpm) increased the risk

of acidosis 26-fold and the risk of metabolic acidosis five-fold.[2]

A baseline tachycardia is reportedly associated with low 5-minute Apgar scores in 6 per cent of cases[1] and with neonatal acidaemia in up to 20 per cent.[4,5] However, it is rarely linked with a base excess >12.[5]

- *Variability.* The work of Gilstrap et al.[4] suggested that absent variability dramatically increased the risk of neonatal acidosis, even in the presence of an otherwise normal CTG. A cord pH <7.20 was seen in 24 per cent of cases with isolated absent variability, compared to 3 per cent of completely normal second stage traces. Gull et al.[7] investigated the inter-relationship between baseline bradycardias and variability. In the presence of a baseline heart rate <100 bpm, the risk of neonatal metabolic acidaemia increased as the interval before loss of variability shortened and as the duration of loss of variability increased. This suggests that loss of variability corresponds to fetal decompensation.
- *Accelerations.* These are not commonly present in the second stage.
- *Decelerations.* Decelerations are remarkably common, and are seen in more than 70 per cent of second stage heart rate traces.
  - *Early decelerations* occur in 14 per cent of second stage traces. They never appear to increase the risk of a low 5-minute Apgar score,[1] and should be viewed as benign – regardless of baseline rate.
  - *Variable decelerations* are much commoner, being seen in approximately half of second stage CTGs. After taking into account the baseline heart rate, mild variable decelerations have little influence on the incidence of low Apgar scores.[1] However, deep variable decelerations, with a drop in fetal heart rate of >70 bpm, are associated with ten-fold increase in the risk of metabolic acidosis [II].[2]
  - *Late decelerations* are relatively uncommon in the second stage, being seen in only 5 per cent of traces. However, their presence dramatically increases the chances of a low 5-minute Apgar score, regardless of baseline rate.[1] If the baseline rate is normal, a 5-minute Apgar score <7 is seen in 10 per cent of cases. This increases to 20–25 per cent when superimposed on a persistent or progressive baseline bradycardia. The combination of a baseline tachycardia and late decelerations is associated with a 14 per cent risk of low Apgar scores. The presence of late decelerations increases the risk of metabolic acidosis 17-fold.[2]

ACTIVE VERSUS PASSIVE SECOND STAGE

Many clinicians now divide the second stage of labour into a passive and an active phase. During the former, continued descent of the fetal head occurs with neither maternal effort nor urge to push. The risks of acidosis in this passive phase are probably similar to those of the active first stage. Certainly, Nordstrom et al. showed fetal scalp lactate to increase in parallel with the length of *active* pushing in the second stage [II].[8]

SECONDARY TESTS OF FETAL WELL-BEING

Fetal blood sampling

Fetal scalp pH studies remain the principal secondary test of fetal well-being in the second stage of labour. There is no evidence that their accuracy falls, and they are usually technically very easy.

Other secondary tests

There has been little investigation into the prognostic ability of other secondary tests of fetal well-being, such as vibro-acoustic stimulation, scalp stimulation, fetal electrocardiogram (ECG) or pulse oximetry in the second stage of labour.

THE MANAGEMENT OF SUSPECTED FETAL COMPROMISE IN THE SECOND STAGE OF LABOUR

- Improve placental blood supply.
  - Maternal positioning to avoid aorto-caval compression.
  - Intravenous fluids when appropriate.
  - Vasoconstrictors such as ephedrine for lower limb vasodilatation secondary to epidural analgesia. Remember, arm blood pressure may be normal in this situation.
- Improve maternal oxygenation.
  - Maternal oxygen therapy may be helpful if used for a short period while other measures are instituted. However, the routine use of oxygen therapy in the second stage was found to lead to an increase in newborn acidosis [Ia].[9]
- Diminish uterine activity if excessive.
  - Decrease or stop any oxytocin infusion. In the second stage, bolus intravenous tocolytics have been associated with an increase in instrumental delivery but no improvement in fetal outcome [Ia].[10] Their use in this situation should be restricted to cases in which a short delay is expected before operative delivery can be undertaken.

- Decide if delivery is indicated, based upon:
  - the severity of the CTG abnormality and results of any secondary tests of fetal well-being;
  - response to the above interventions to improve the situation;
  - the 'whole picture', including obstetric risk factors, progress in labour and potential difficulty of an assisted delivery;
  - untreatable fetal complications such as abruption, cord prolapse and chorioamnionitis, and scar dehiscence.

There is little evidence to support the use of amnioinfusion in the second stage of labour to reduce cord compression and improve umbilical blood flow.

A clinical approach to reviewing abnormal second stage CTGs

Always ask yourself: What factors are present that increase the neonatal risk of instrumental delivery? – meconium/macrosomia/malposition/mid-cavity arrest/diabetes/previous shoulder dystocia.

Does the abnormality require immediate delivery? Yes

Is an assisted delivery likely to be easy?
- Yes – occiput anterior (OA)/low station/little caput or moulding
  - Deliver in room
- No – malposition/mid-cavity arrest/major moulding or caput
  - Undertake delivery in theatre either as trial or directly by caesarean section
  - Strongly consider fetal blood sampling before trial of instrumental delivery

No

Is an assisted delivery likely to be easy?
- Yes – OA/low station/little caput or moulding
  - Has progress been steady in active second stage?
  - Yes: offer mother choice of continued pushing for set time before recommending assisted delivery
  - No: consider oxytocin (±fetal blood sampling beforehand) if mother wishes to avoid assisted delivery
  - If no intervention possible to improve situation, recommend assisted delivery in room
- No – malposition/mid-cavity arrest/major moulding or caput)
  - Has progress been steady in active second stage?

– Yes: consider fetal blood sampling to allow more time and convert to an easier delivery
– No: consider fetal blood sampling and then oxytocin
– If inappropriate to intervene to improve progress, recommend delivery
– In theatre either as a trial or directly by caesarean section, strongly consider fetal blood sampling before trial of instrumental delivery

- Routine use of oxygen therapy in the second stage leads to an increase in newborn acidosis.
- In the second stage, bolus intravenous tocolytics are associated with an increase in instrumental delivery but no improvement in fetal outcome.

KEY POINTS

- CTG abnormalities are very common in the second stage but many are benign.
- Particular attention should be paid to marked bradycardias, any bradycardia with reduced variability and late or severe variable decelerations.
- Use fetal scalp sampling to avoid potentially difficult instrumental deliveries in the presence of pre-existing fetal compromise.

PUBLISHED GUIDELINES

Royal College of Obstetricians and Gynaecologists Evidence-based Clinical Guideline No. 8. *The Use of Electronic Fetal Monitoring.* London: RCOG Press, May 2001.

Society of Obstetricians and Gynaecologists of Canada Clinical Practice Guideline. *Fetal Health Surveillance in Labour*: Executive Summary. *J Obstet Gynaecol Can* 2002; **24**(3):250–62.

KEY REFERENCES

1. Krebs HB, Petres RE, Dunn LJ. Intrapartum fetal heart rate monitoring. V. Fetal heart rate patterns in the second stage of labor. *Am J Obstet Gynecol* 1981; **140**:435–9.
2. Sheiner E, Hadar A, Hallak M, Katz M, Mazor M, Shoham-Vardi I. Clinical significance of fetal heart rate tracings during the second stage of labor. *Obstet Gynecol* 2001; **97**:747–52.
3. Cardoso CG, Graca LM, Clode N. A study on second stage cardiotocographic patterns and umbilical acid–base balance in cases with first stage normal fetal heart rates. *J Matern Fetal Invest* 1995; **5**:144–9.
4. Gilstrap LC, Hauth JC, Toussaint S. Second stage fetal heart rate abnormalities and neonatal acidosis. *Obstet Gynecol* 1984; **63**:209–13.
5. Gilstrap LC, Hauth JC, Hankins GD, Beck AW. Second stage fetal heart rate abnormalities and type of neonatal acidemia. *Obstet Gynecol* 1987; **70**:191–5.
6. Piquard F, Hsiung R, Mettauer M, Schaefer A, Haberey P, Dellenbach P. The validity of fetal heart rate monitoring during the second stage of labor. *Obstet Gynecol* 1988; **72**:746–51.
7. Gull I, Jaffa AJ, Oren M, Grisaru D, Peyser MR, Lessing JB. Acid accumulation during end-stage bradycardia in term fetuses: how long is too long? *Br J Obstet Gynaecol* 1996; **103**:1096–101.
8. Nordstrom L, Achanna S, Naka K, Arulkumaran S. Fetal and maternal lactate increase during active second stage of labour. *Br J Obstet Gynaecol* 2001; **108**:263–8.
9. Thorp JA, Trobough T, Evans R, Hendrick J, Yeast JD. The effect of maternal oxygen administration during the second stage of labor on umbilical cord blood gas values – a randomized controlled trial. *Am J Obstet Gynecol* 1995; **172**:465–74.
10. Campbell J, Anderson I, Chang A, Wood C. The use of ritodrine in the management of the fetus during the second stage of labour. *Aus N Z J Obstet Gynecol* 1978; **18**:110–16.

Chapter 33

Shoulder Dystocia

Griff Jones

INTRODUCTION

Shoulder dystocia is an acute obstetric emergency requiring rapid intervention to prevent neonatal morbidity and mortality. The relative infrequency of shoulder dystocia means that few obstetricians are truly experienced in the management of this complication. However, its unpredictability means that all labour ward practitioners must possess a detailed knowledge of the condition and how to overcome it.

DEFINITION

Classically, shoulder dystocia is recognized when the fetal chin retracts firmly back onto the perineum immediately after delivery of the head, the so-called 'turtle-neck' sign. However, there is no universally accepted definition of shoulder dystocia. Labelling a delivery as complicated by shoulder dystocia is often a subjective opinion influenced by relative experience.

A logical approach to the assessment of severity of an earlier shoulder dystocia is essential. Events surrounding the delivery should be considered under three headings.

1 Additional manoeuvres.
   - What steps were required to effect delivery? See 'simple', 'advanced' and 'heroic' under 'Management' below.
2 Fetal complications.
   - Apgar scores and degree of resuscitation required.
   - Neonatal unit admission.
   - Direct fetal trauma (Erb's palsy, fractures).
   - Long-term handicap (neurodevelopmental, palsy).
3 Maternal complications.
   - Perineal trauma (extended episiotomy or tear, third degree tear).
   - Postpartum haemorrhage.

INCIDENCE

The lack of a universally agreed definition for shoulder dystocia hampers any estimate of incidence. As a rough guide, approximately 1 per cent of deliveries are complicated by shoulder dystocia.

CONSEQUENCES

Fetal

Short-term complications such as fractures of the humerus or clavicle are not uncommon. However, these heal well and have an excellent prognosis. Transient brachial plexus injury, such as Erb's palsy, is also relatively common. Fortunately, with early recognition, prompt physiotherapy and even neurosurgical treatment, most improve over time, leaving only 1–2 per cent of shoulder dystocia cases with long-term dysfunction. Hypoxic–ischaemic encephalopathy may develop after severe cases and carries a risk of later neurodevelopmental handicap. Perinatal mortality secondary to shoulder dystocia was reported in 56 cases in the UK in 1994–95, an incidence of approximately 1 in 25 000 births.[1]

Maternal

Excessive blood loss from extensive perineal, vaginal and even cervical lacerations is possible. Extension of perineal trauma into third or fourth degree tears is also recognized.

AETIOLOGY

The mechanics underlying shoulder dystocia have been reviewed by Johnstone and Myerscough.[2] Although the bisacromial diameter is larger than the biparietal diameter, the shoulders have the advantage of inherent mobility. As the fetal head passes through the pelvic outlet, the shoulders simultaneously enter the pelvic inlet. Ideally, the shoulders should enter the pelvis transversely, although they are usually oblique, with the posterior shoulder moving towards the sacrosciatic notch. As restitution of the fetal head occurs, the shoulders rotate through the pelvis and the anterior shoulder presents under the symphysis pubis.

In true cases of shoulder dystocia, either the anterior shoulder or, in severe forms, both the anterior and posterior shoulders are arrested at the pelvic inlet. It is a common misconception that the pelvic outlet and perineum contribute to shoulder dystocia. This is in part fuelled by the advice to perform an extended episiotomy in this situation. It must be understood that in this situation the episiotomy is to create the space necessary for vaginal manipulations.

PREDISPOSING FACTORS

Excessive fetal size

The incidence of shoulder dystocia is known to increase in line with birth weight. Below 3.5 kg, the reported incidence is 0.2–0.8 per cent, rising to 5–23 per cent with birth weights above 4.5 kg.[3,4]

Despite this relationship, half of all shoulder dystocia cases occur with babies of normal birth weight. This may be because some babies that fail to meet an absolute criterion for macrosomia (such as a birth weight >4.0 kg) are actually relatively 'large for gestation' for that particular woman. Unfortunately, it is difficult to know in advance the 'intended' birth weight for any individual woman's offspring. However, customized fetal growth charts are increasingly available; these use maternal ethnic origin, build and parity to individualize predicted fetal weight at any gestation.

Clinicians must remain wary of any clinical situation or condition that is likely to increase fetal weight beyond Mother Nature's original intention. **Maternal diabetes**, long known to be associated with a risk of excessive fetal growth, is a major risk factor [Ib].[5] Other causes of fetal macrosomia, either relative or absolute, include **maternal obesity, multiparity** and **post-dates pregnancies** (ACOG Practice Bulletin 22 Guideline).

Intrapartum events

Relative disproportion is often suggested by **poor progress** in labour, but this is a poor predictor of subsequent shoulder dystocia.[4,6] Shoulder dystocia has been associated with **mid-cavity instrumental deliveries**,[6] but since this reflects a significant failure of descent, it is again highlighting poor progress in labour.

Parturition has long been linked with the three Ps – the passages, the passenger and the powers. It may be that inefficient uterine contractile activity underlies some cases of shoulder dystocia. Recent reports have suggested that the endogenous powers pushing the shoulders through the birth canal in cases of shoulder dystocia are actually more important than the traction forces generated by the obstetrician.[7] An aetiological role for the 'powers' is also suggested by the increased incidence of shoulder dystocia found in induced labours, long associated with an increased risk of dysfunctional labour and operative delivery.[4,6,8]

MANAGEMENT

Antenatal assessment

Recurrence risks

Overall recurrence risks for shoulder dystocia are approximately 10–15 per cent.[9,10] These low estimates of recurrence are further evidence of both imprecision in diagnosis and the potential importance of contraction strength and maternal effort. The above studies suggest increased risks in overweight women or with large or 'larger' babies in the subsequent pregnancy.

Review of previous delivery

A careful review of the events surrounding an earlier delivery is essential, using the system outlined under 'Incidence'. This must include a review of the previous maternity notes, which may necessitate correspondence with other units.

Screening for gestation diabetes

If there is any suspicion of excessive fetal growth in a previous pregnancy (regardless of birth weight), a glucose tolerance test should be arranged for 28 weeks' gestation. If impaired glucose tolerance is found, measures should be implemented to minimize any fetal effects [II].

Pelvimetry

There is no evidence to support the routine use of pelvimetry in this situation. Its use should be highly selective. Examples of situations in which it might be considered include marked shoulder dystocia with a small baby or a predisposing factor for pelvic contraction, such as a previous significant fracture.

Antenatal intervention

Identification of fetal macrosomia

The prediction of fetal weight, either clinically or by ultrasound, is notoriously inaccurate (ACOG Practice Bulletin 22 Guideline). Precision also falls with increasing fetal size. The information gained from prenatal assessment of size can only be used as one risk factor to be applied to the overall picture. It facilitates advance planning and preparation but, in isolation, should not dictate any particular management. The recognition of significant macrosomia in association with other risk factors, particularly diabetes or a previous birth with shoulder dystocia, requires careful assessment.

Early induction

Evidence from observational and randomized trials does not support the use of induction to prevent shoulder dystocia in suspected macrosomia (ACOG Practice Bulletin 22 Guideline) [Ib].[8,11,12] As mentioned previously, induced labours are reported to have a higher incidence of shoulder dystocia.

Elective caesarean section

The American College of Obstetricians and Gynecologists recommends considering elective caesarean section when the birth weight is predicted to be greater than 5 kg in non-diabetics or 4.5 kg in diabetics (ACOG Practice Bulletin 22 Guideline) [IV]. Despite this, it acknowledges that such a policy would result in 443 caesarean sections in diabetic women to prevent a single permanent newborn injury. These calculations are strongly influenced by our inability to reliably predict macrosomia antenatally. At present, there are few grounds on which to recommend elective caesarean section on the basis of fetal size alone. Decisions should be individualized, based on an appreciation of all risk factors present.

Diabetic control

It is logical to suppose that tight diabetic control may reduce the incidence of fetal macrosomia. At present, there is a small body of evidence to support this assumption [II].

Intrapartum management

Advance planning

Antenatal risk factors for shoulder dystocia should be noted.

- **Reassessment of risk** should be carried out if there is poor progress in labour. In women believed to be at significant risk, advance preparation is essential.
- Midwifery and medical staff should establish a **contingency plan** involving:
  - who needs to be aware of the potential problem,
  - who will be present at the delivery, and
  - what steps will be taken should difficulties arise.

In mothers who have failure of descent in the second stage, the presence of other risk factors for shoulder dystocia will influence not only if but also where and by whom an instrumental delivery is attempted (ACOG Practice Bulletin 22 Guideline). Although a trial of instrumental delivery in theatre does not reduce the risk of shoulder dystocia, it ensures the presence of adequate staffing to deal with it efficiently.

An **epidural** should always be considered in situations in which there is judged to be a considerable risk of shoulder dystocia, particularly if it is felt that maternal distress may interfere with co-operation.

Early diagnosis allows prompt intervention. The 'turtle sign' is usually obvious, but if there is delay in delivery of the shoulders, examination to define the location of the anterior shoulder (above or below the symphysis) can be helpful.

Treatment

There are no randomized trials to provide guidance for the management of this obstetric emergency. In women judged to be at particularly high risk, obstetricians should consider the prophylactic use of some of the simple measures described below in order to avoid delay in delivery of the shoulders. In this situation, it is probably still worth waiting for the next contraction before completing the delivery. Help should always be summoned as soon as a problem is recognized. As well as additional midwives, neonatology and anaesthetic staff should be called. Manipulations to overcome shoulder dystocia cannot be learnt from a book. Practical training in obstetric emergencies must be undertaken, as offered on an ALSO© Course or similar. Manipulations should be considered under three headings.

SIMPLE MEASURES

These measures should always be tried first and will be successful in 90 per cent of cases. Remember to maintain the head in a neutral position, avoiding excessive lateral traction. In the absence of medical staff, midwives will have often already tried placing the mother in a lateral position, which is reported to have some benefit.

- *McRoberts manoeuvre* involves hyperflexion of the maternal thighs onto the maternal abdomen, either by the mother herself or by a pair of assistants. It has been shown radiographically to flatten the lumbosacral curve and lessen any obstruction from the sacral promontory.
- *Suprapubic pressure* is often used simultaneously. Using a stance similar to that of cardiopulmonary resuscitation (CPR), pressure is exerted obliquely on the posterior aspect of the anterior shoulder. The aim is to move the shoulders into the wider oblique diameter of the pelvis and force the anterior shoulder under the symphysis pubis.

ADVANCED MEASURES

Failing correction of the problem with simple measures, more aggressive manipulations will be required. These may involve considerable discomfort to the mother (and distress to her partner) and warning should be given. In order that a hand can be introduced into the vagina, a generous episiotomy is required.

- Initially, attempts should be made to *rotate the shoulders into the oblique diameter* of the pelvis, using a finger hooked into one axilla. Ideally, one should attempt to move the fetus in a direction that allows the shoulder to move inwards towards the chest, which will decrease the dimensions of the shoulders. Once disimpacted, traction can again be tried.
- If simple rotation fails and the posterior shoulder is below the sacral promontory, *Wood's screw manoeuvre* should be attempted. This involves rotating the posterior shoulder through 180° so that it becomes the anterior shoulder. By simultaneously combining this with a degree of downward traction, the rotated shoulder remains within the pelvis and appears under the symphysis.

If all the above fail or both shoulders are above the pelvic inlet, two choices remain.

- One is to advance your hand into the uterus posteriorly and, after finding the fetal hand, deliver the posterior arm by sweeping it across the fetal chest. Although this may sound easy on paper, by definition space is extremely restricted.
- An alternative choice is deliberately to fracture the fetal clavicle(s).

HEROIC MEASURES

If all the above measures have been tried and retried and the baby is still alive, heroic measures could be considered.

However, the likelihood of any individual obstetrician gaining experience of these techniques within the UK is remote. Furthermore, publication bias means that clinicians often only report their successes. It is likely that heroic measures have, on many occasions, been followed by stillbirth, neonatal death or profound handicap, at a cost of considerable maternal morbidity.

- In the *Zavenelli manoeuvre*, the fetal head is replaced into the uterus by reversing the steps of parturition. This may require additional uterine relaxation, using either bolus tocolytics or general anaesthesia. Abdominal rescue describes intrauterine manipulation through a transabdominal hysterotomy to facilitate vaginal delivery.
- *Symphysiotomy* can lead to a 2–3 cm increase in the bony pelvic diameters. However, there is a significant risk of long-term maternal morbidity. Special skills and equipment are required, including a solid-bladed scalpel. The urethra must be catheterized and displaced laterally. In the absence of an epidural, local anaesthesia is needed. It is likely that the fetus will have been severely compromised by the time a symphysiotomy could be safely performed on most UK labour wards.

DOCUMENTATION

After a delivery complicated by shoulder dystocia, it is important that the details surrounding the delivery are accurately recorded. This is important not only for medico-legal reasons, but also for helping form a plan in any subsequent pregnancy. The information discussed under 'Diagnosis' should all be recorded, together with the interval between delivery of the head and shoulders. In the heat of the moment, this is often not recorded, although neonatologists often note this using the resuscitaire clock.

In terms of psychological benefit, the role of maternal de-briefing remains controversial. However, mothers must understand what went wrong, both to minimize inappropriate blame of themselves or others and so that they may alert their caregivers in their next pregnancy.

- Evidence from observational and randomized trials does not support the use of induction to prevent shoulder dystocia in suspected macrosomia.
- There is a need to address the issue of induction of labour for the prevention of shoulder dystocia by large randomized, controlled trials.

KEY POINTS

- Neither fetal macrosomia nor shoulder dystocia can be reliably predicted.
- Most strategies to prevent shoulder dystocia are either ineffective (early induction) or lead to excessive intervention (elective caesarean section).
- The presence of known risk factors, particularly two or more, should trigger advance preparations to deal with or avoid the situation, before it actually arises.
- Since shoulder dystocia will often occur without warning, obstetricians must have well-rehearsed strategies to overcome it.

PUBLISHED GUIDELINES

American College of Obstetricians and Gynecologists. ACOG Practice Bulletin Number 22. *Fetal Macrosomia.* Clinical Management Guidelines for Obstetricians/ Gynecologists. November 2000.

Focus Group – Shoulder dystocia. In: *Confidential Enquiry into Stillbirths and Deaths in Infancy*, 5th Annual Report, Section 8, Focus Group – Shoulder Dystocia. London: HMSO, 1996.

KEY REFERENCES

1. Hope P, Breslin S, Lamont L et al. Fatal shoulder dystocia: a review of 56 cases reported to the Confidential Enquiry into Stillbirths and Deaths in Infancy. *Br J Obstet Gynaecol* 1998; **105**:1256.

2. Johnstone FD, Myerscough PR. Shoulder dystocia. *Br J Obstet Gynaecol* 1998; **105**:811–15.

3. Mocanu EV, Greene RA, Byrne BM, Turner MJ. Obstetric and neonatal outcome of babies weighing more than 4.5 kg: an analysis by parity. *Eur J Obstet Gynecol Reprod Biol* 2000; **92**:229–33.

4. Acker DB, Sachs BP, Friedman EA. Risk factors for shoulder dystocia in the average-weight infant. *Obstet Gynecol* 1986; **67**:614–18.

5. Acker DB, Sachs BP, Friedman EA. Risk factors for shoulder dystocia. *Obstet Gynecol* 1985; **66**:762–8.

6. McFarland M, Hod M, Piper JM, Xenakis EM-J, Langer O. Are labor abnormalities more common in shoulder dystocia? *Am J Obstet Gynecol* 1995; **173**:1211–14.

7. Gonik B, Walker A, Grimm M. Mathematical modelling of forces associated with shoulder dystocia: a comparison of endogenous and exogenous forces. *Am J Obstet Gynecol* 2000; **182**:689–91.

8. Dublin S, Lydon-Rochelle M, Kaplan RC, Watts DH, Critchlow CW. Maternal and neonatal outcomes after induction of labour without an identified indication. *Am J Obstet Gynecol* 2000; **183**:986–94.

9. Smith RB, Lane C, Pearson JF. Shoulder dystocia: what happens at the next delivery? *Br J Obstet Gynaecol* 1994; **101**:713–15.

10. Lewis DF, Raymond RC, Perkins MB, Brooks GG, Heymann AR. Recurrence rate of shoulder dystocia. *Am J Obstet Gynecol* 1995; **172**:1369–71.

11. Combs CA, Singh NB, Khoury JC. Elective induction versus spontaneous labor after sonographic diagnosis of fetal macrosomia. *Obstet Gynecol* 1993; **81**:492–6.

12. Gonen O, Rosen DJD, Dolfin Z, Tepper R, Markov S, Fejgin MD. Induction of labour versus expectant management in macrosomia: a randomized study. *Obstet Gynecol* 1997; **89**:913–17.

Chapter 34

Instrumental Vaginal Delivery

Richard Hayman

MRCOG standards

Candidates are expected to:

- have a thorough knowledge of abdominal and pelvic anatomy;
- understand the setting of instrumental vaginal delivery in the context of labour and its management;
- be confident to effect delivery by ventouse and/or obstetric forceps in a wide range of clinical scenarios, including rotational deliveries.

INTRODUCTION

Although the use of instruments to facilitate a birth was initially reserved for the extraction of dead infants via destructive techniques, there exist reports from as early as 1500 BC of successful deliveries of live infants in obstructed labours. Chamberlen's development of the modern obstetric forceps in the late sixteenth century dramatically changed the aim of intrapartum intervention in favour of delivery of a live infant, and following from William Smellie's description of the use of forceps in midwifery, instrumental intervention in the process of labour has become a more widely accepted practice.

Between 1st April 1998 and 31st March 1999, of the 661 934 births recorded in the UK, 74 824 (11.3 per cent) were assisted with forceps/ventouse. However, the incidence of instrumental intervention varies widely both within and between countries and may be performed as infrequently as 1.5 per cent or as often as 26 per cent of cases.[1] Such differences may often be related to variations in the management of patients on the labour ward.

STRATEGIES FOR REDUCING THE NEED FOR INSTRUMENTAL VAGINAL DELIVERY

Many different strategies have been suggested and employed to help lower the rates of assisted delivery. However, only a few of these are evidence based.

- Provision of a caregiver in labour.[2] This is associated with a reduction in the need for operative vaginal delivery (odds ratio (OR) 0.77). The effect is seen in women who are both accompanied and unaccompanied by a family member.
- Active management of the second stage with Syntocinon in nulliparous women with epidural analgesia.
- Delayed pushing in nulliparous women with epidural analgesia.[3]

The incidence of difficult delivery is reduced with delayed pushing (relative risk (RR) 0.79) with a reduction in mid-pelvic procedures being especially noted (RR 0.72). It is also important to recognize that the chance of a spontaneous delivery is slightly more common among women who delay pushing, the practice of fetal blood sampling in the second stage providing the confidence to delay the onset of 'active parturition'.

Other techniques that are commonly used but have no evidence to support their usage are upright positions in labour[4] and allowing epidural anaesthesia/analgesia to wear off before expulsive efforts are commenced [II]. Indeed, allowing a previously effective epidural to wear off to the point that the mother has considerable pain is likely to be detrimental to a successful second stage rather than helpful, and seems unnecessarily cruel.

Operative vaginal delivery has been clearly identified as a major risk factor for fetal morbidity and mortality as well as for early and late maternal morbidity (including faecal incontinence). The Royal College of Obstetricians and Gynaecologists (RCOG) has issued clinical guidelines regarding the use of instruments to aid vaginal delivery, stating that, 'Obstetricians should be competent and confident in the use of both instruments [forceps and ventouse]'. The emphasis of the guideline is on the relative merits of the two instruments, the indications for their use and their associated complications. It also states that, 'practitioners should use the most appropriate instrument for individual circumstances'.[5]

INDICATIONS FOR ASSISTED VAGINAL DELIVERY

There are two basic categories into which the indications for assisted vaginal delivery may be placed.

Fetal

The most common fetal indications are those concerning malpositions of the fetal head (occipito-transverse and occipito-posterior). Such positions occur more frequently with regional anaesthesia, as a consequence of alterations in the tone of the pelvic floor that impede spontaneous rotation to the optimal occipito-anterior position. Epidural analgesia has been shown to be associated with longer first and second stages of labour, increased incidence of fetal malposition, increased use of oxytocin and increased incidence of instrumental vaginal deliveries.[6] It is possible that the increasing incidence of instrumental deliveries may reflect the rising demand for regional anaesthesia.

Fetal distress is a commonly cited indication for instrumental intervention, although it is infrequently the fetus that is actually distressed. Presumed fetal compromise is a more comprehensive term, especially when employed in conjunction with a precise description of the situation surrounding the intervention in order to validate the decision.

The use of *elective* instrumental intervention for infants of reduced weight is more controversial. In infants of less than 1.5 kg, delivery with forceps offers no advantage over spontaneous delivery and may, in fact, increase the incidence of intracranial haemorrhage [II]. Ventouse carries the same risks, but in addition should be avoided in infants of less than 35 completed weeks of gestation.

Maternal

The most common maternal indications for intervention are those of maternal distress, exhaustion or undue prolongation of the second stage of labour. Labour may be deemed to be prolonged if the second stage lasts >2 hours in a primigravida (3 hours if an epidural is in situ) or >1 hour in a multipara (2 hours if an epidural is in situ).

Less common indications include medically significant conditions such as aortic valve disease with significant outflow obstruction or myasthenia gravis.

The reasons cited for intervention are often imprecise, as one or more factors may interact, for example delay in the second stage as a consequence of poor maternal effort and transitional malposition. Determining which is the more important may be a case of semantics. Independently or conjointly, they are an indication for delivery. However, they are not necessarily an indication for delivery by a specific instrument.

Delivery options in the second stage include caesarean section and this should particularly be considered if there is a high 'index of suspicion' of delivery failure. It is therefore suggested that most mid-cavity procedures, which by their nature have a higher rate of complications than outlet or low deliveries,[7] should be performed in theatre. However, the psychological consequences of transferring a patient to an operating theatre in the second stage should not be underestimated.

INSTRUMENT CHOICE AND MANAGEMENT OPTIONS

The choice of instrument employed by the accoucheur should be based on a combination of indication, experience and training, and it is the last two of these issues that must be formally addressed in light of today's changes in junior 'doctor's hours' and working practices. It is certainly the case that only adequately trained or supervised practitioners should undertake any vacuum or forceps delivery.

Systematic review[8] has shown the vacuum extractor, when compared to the forceps, to be:

- significantly *more* likely to [Ia]:
  - fail at achieving a vaginal delivery (OR 1.7; 95 per cent confidence interval (CI) 1.3–2.2; NNH 20),
  - be associated with a cephalohaematoma (OR 2.4; 95 per cent CI 1.7–3.4; NNH 17),
  - be associated with retinal haemorrhage (OR 2.0; 95 per cent CI 1.3–3.0; NNH 50),
  - be associated with maternal worries about the baby (OR 2.2; 95 per cent CI 1.2–3.9; NNH 17),
  (NNH = number needed to harm, i.e. for every 20 vacuum deliveries there is one 'extra' failure cf. forceps)
- significantly *less* likely to be associated with [Ia]:
  - use of maternal regional/general anaesthesia (OR 0.6; 95 per cent CI 0.5–0.7; NNT 12),
  - significant maternal perineal and vaginal trauma (OR 0.4; 95 per cent CI 0.3–0.5; NNT 10),
  - severe perineal pain at 24 hours (OR 0.54; 95 per cent CI 0.31–0.93; NNT 17),
  (NNT = number needed to treat, i.e. for every ten ventouse deliveries one less case of significant maternal perineal trauma will occur)

Second stage of labour

- *equally* likely to be associated with [Ia]:
  - delivery by caesarean section (OR 0.6; 95 per cent CI 0.3–1.02),
  - low 5-minute Apgar scores (OR 1.7; 95 per cent CI 0.99–2.8),
  - the need for phototherapy (OR 1.08; 95 per cent CI 0.7–1.8).

The incidence of maternal injuries in deliveries performed with the vacuum is significantly reduced when compared with forceps; anal sphincter injury in particular is twice as common with forceps delivery.

Unfortunately, there is a paucity of long-term follow-up data for both the mother and the baby. However, one of the largest randomized, controlled trials showed no difference in the groups delivered by forceps or ventouse when the women were assessed at approximately 5 years. Bowel urgency was commoner in the ventouse group (26 vs 15 per cent, $p =$ 0.06), but this just failed to reach statistical significance. This study also demonstrated no differences in the infants at this age.[9]

Although the degree of rotation required is a significant indicator of a potentially difficult delivery, the data currently available from the published trials cannot be analysed separately to compare the use of ventouse and forceps (e.g. Kiellands) for rotational deliveries.

ROTATIONAL INSTRUMENTAL VAGINAL DELIVERY VERSUS CAESAREAN SECTION

Often the decision facing the obstetrician is whether to perform a rotational vaginal delivery or caesarean section. Caesarean section has often been viewed as the less harmful of the two interventions; however, there are limited data comparing the morbidity of second stage caesarean section with instrumental vaginal delivery. One prospective cohort study of 393 women with term, singleton, liveborn, cephalic pregnancies requiring operative delivery in theatre at full dilatation showed that factors increasing the likelihood of caesarean section included:[10]

- maternal body mass index (BMI) >30
- neonatal birth weight >4.0 kg
- occipito-posterior position.

Women who were delivered by caesarean section were more likely to have a major haemorrhage of more than 1 L and to need a hospital stay of >5 days. On the other hand, babies delivered by caesarean section were less likely to have trauma than babies delivered by forceps but more likely to require admission for intensive care. It is important to note that serious trauma was not limited to the vaginally delivered group, and that the experience of the operator was directly related to the chance of major haemorrhage whatever the

mode of delivery. It should therefore be the aim at this stage in labour to deliver women vaginally, unless there are clear signs of cephalo-pelvic disproportion. It is undoubtedly the case that skilled obstetricians should supervise complex operative deliveries, whatever time of day they occur [II].

Pre-requisites for *any* instrumental delivery

- Confirmed rupture of the membranes.
- The cervix must be fully dilated (except second twin and rare other situations – see below).
- Vertex presentation with identification of the position.
- For occipito-anterior and transverse positions, no part of the fetal head should be palpable abdominally. For occipito-posterior positions, it is acceptable that one-fifth of the head may be palpable. The presenting part should be at +1 or more below the ischial spines.
- Adequate analgesia/anaesthesia.
- Empty bladder/no obstruction below the fetal head (contracted pelvis/pelvic kidney/ovarian cyst etc.).
- A knowledgeable and experienced operator with adequate preparation to proceed with an alternative approach if necessary.
- An adequately informed and consented patient (consent must be obtained though not necessarily sought in writing).

For forceps, all the pre-requisites above apply, but in addition:

- it is essential that the operator checks the pair of forceps to ensure that a matching pair has been provided and that the blades lock with ease (both before and after application).

Basic rules

It has been suggested that failure rates of less than 1 per cent should be achieved with well-maintained apparatus and the use of the correct technique. However, many feel that this is an unrealistic target, an observation illustrated by the study of Johanson et al., who achieved a vaginal delivery with the first instrument in only 86 per cent of cases.[11] They cited the following as factors contributing to delivery failure.

- Failure to select the correct cup type: inappropriate use of the silastic cup, especially in the presence of deflexion of the fetal head, excess caput, a macrosomic infant or prolonged second stage of labour.
- Inadequate initial case assessment: high head, misdiagnosis of the position and attitude of the head.
- Incorrect cup placement: positioning either too anterior or lateral.

- Failure due to traction in the wrong plane.
- Poor maternal effort, with inadequate use of Syntocinon to aid expulsive efforts in the second stage.

Patient evaluation

A careful pelvic examination is essential to determine whether there are any 'architectural' contraindications to performing an instrumental vaginal delivery. If, for example, a contracted pelvis is the cause of failure to progress in the second stage, due consideration must be paid to determining the type of instrument to be employed, or whether it may be more prudent to perform a caesarean section. The shape of the subpubic arch, the curve of the sacral hollow, the presence of flat or prominent ischial spines all contribute to the decision as to whether a vaginal delivery may be safely performed. Anthropoid (narrow), android (male/funnel-shaped), or platypelloid (squashed) pelvises all make instrumental deliveries more difficult and may preclude the use of rotational forceps.

With any difficult instrumental delivery, the risk of shoulder dystocia occurring after successful delivery of the fetal head should always be remembered, as should the subsequent and probable postpartum haemorrhage. As a consequence, the accoucheur must be able to develop the skills necessary to anticipate such events and to manage the consequences in a logical and calm manner.

CONTRAINDICATIONS

The ventouse should not be used:

- in gestations of <35 completed weeks because of the risk of cephalohaematoma and intracranial haemorrhage,[12]
- in cases of face presentation.

There is minimal risk of fetal haemorrhage if the vacuum extractor is employed following fetal blood sampling or application of a spiral scalp electrode, and no excess bleeding was reported in two randomized trials comparing deliveries performed with forceps or ventouse.[8]

Forceps and vacuum extractor deliveries before full dilatation of the cervix are contraindicated, although possible exceptions occur with the vacuum delivery of a second twin where the cervix has contracted or with a prolapsed cord at 9 cm if rapid delivery is anticipated [IV].

ANALGESIA

Analgesic requirements are greater for forceps than for ventouse delivery. Where rotational forceps are needed, regional analgesia is preferred. For a rigid cup ventouse delivery, a pudendal block with perineal infiltration may be all that is needed and, if a soft cup is used, analgesic requirements may be minimal. A requirement for haste should not preclude the use of analgesia. No operator would consider performing a caesarean section without the appropriate anaesthesia, and the same should be true for a vaginal delivery.

POSITIONING

Instrumental deliveries are traditionally performed with the patient in the lithotomy position and using as aseptic a technique as is possible. The angle of traction needed requires that the foot of the bed be removed. For patients with limited movements, such as those with symphysis dysfunction, it may be necessary to limit abduction of the thighs to a minimum. It is the accoucheur's duty to ensure that the bladder is emptied.

INSTRUMENT TYPES

Ventouse/vacuum extractors

The basic premise of such instruments is that a suction cup, of a silastic or rigid construction, is connected, via tubing, to a vacuum source. Either directly through the tubing or via a connecting 'chain', direct traction can then be applied to the presenting part to expedite delivery. Recent developments have removed the need for cumbersome external suction generators and have incorporated the vacuum mechanism into 'hand-held' pumps, for example OmniCup™ (Figure 34.1). Such devices appear to be more acceptable to patients than standard equipment and have no obvious effects on instrumental delivery success or on the incidence of maternal or fetal complications, but large trials have yet to be performed.

Choosing the type of cup

Soft cups are significantly more likely to fail to achieve vaginal delivery than rigid cups; however, they are associated with less scalp injury (OR 1.65) [Ia]. There appears to be no difference in terms of maternal injury between the groups. Metal cups appear to be more suitable for 'occipito-posterior', transverse and difficult 'occipito-anterior' position deliveries where the infant is larger or there is a marked caput. The soft cups are appropriate for straightforward deliveries with an occipito-anterior position as they produce less scalp trauma (OR 0.45).[13]

The vacuum extractor can be used during the delivery of a second twin (this also being the only routine situation where application of an instrument with the cervix less than fully dilated is permitted), but should never be used with a breech presentation.

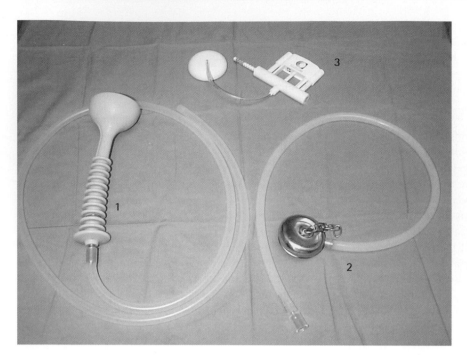

Figure 34.1   Three different types of ventouse. (1) A siliastic cup ventouse, and (2) a metal cup ventouse for posterior application – the 'Bird cup'. Both of these require external vacuum generators. (3) A hand-held ventouse (with a pump incorporated in the handle)

Technique

For successful use of the ventouse, determination of the flexion point is vital. This is located at the vertex, which, in an average term infant, is on the saggital suture 3 cm anterior to the posterior fontanelle and thus 6 cm posterior to the anterior fontanelle. The centre of the cup should be positioned directly over this, as failure to do so will lead to a progressive deflexion of the fetal head during traction, and an inability to deliver the baby [Ib].

The operating vacuum pressure for nearly all ventouse is between −0.6 and −0.8 kg/cm² (−60 to −80 kPa/−500 to −800 cmH₂0). No evidence exists that incremental 'stepwise' increases in pressure improve the rate of success of delivery when compared with a linear increase. Using the latter technique with a silastic cup, a caput secundum is formed instantly, and with the metal cup, an adequate chignon is produced in less than 2 minutes. The standard teaching has been that the largest cup that can be placed should be; however, in practice a 5 cm cup is suitable for nearly all deliveries. It is prudent to increase the suction to 0.2 kg/cm² first and then to recheck that no maternal tissue is caught under the cup edge. When this is confirmed, the suction can then be increased.

Traction must occur in the plane of least resistance along the axis of the pelvis – the traction plane. This will usually be at exactly 90 degrees to the cup, and the operator should keep a thumb and forefinger on the cup at the traction insertion to ensure that the traction direction is correct and to feel for slippage. Safe and gentle traction is then applied in concert with uterine contractions and voluntary expulsive efforts. This minimizes undue traction and the risk of trauma to the fetus. With the ventouse, the operator should allow no more than two episodes of breaking the suction in any vacuum delivery, and the maximum time from application to delivery should ideally be less than 15 minutes. If there is no evidence of descent with the first pull, the patient should be reassessed to ascertain the reason for failure to progress (Figure 34.2). This may simply be a failure of the equipment to provide adequate traction as a consequence of a leakage of the vacuum or the presence of a large caput. Inclusion of maternal soft tissues within the cup, traction along the incorrect plane, misdiagnosis of the position of the fetal head with incorrect equipment placement, choice of the wrong instrument, and cephalopelvic disproportion are other reasons for failure of delivery.

Rotation is achieved by the natural progression of the head through the pelvis. The operator must **never** try to assist rotation by turning the cup manually, as this is unhelpful and can lead to **severe** scalp lacerations [IV].

It is not acceptable to use a ventouse when:

- the position of the fetal head is unknown;
- there is a significant degree of caput that may either preclude correct placement of the cup or, more sinisterly, indicate a substantial degree of cephalopelvic disproportion;
- the operator is inexperienced in the use of the instrument.

Forceps

Types of forceps

The basic forceps design has not radically changed over many years and all types in use today consist of two blades with shanks, joined together at a lock, with handles to provide a point for traction. However, the specific details of construction vary between the instruments. The blades may

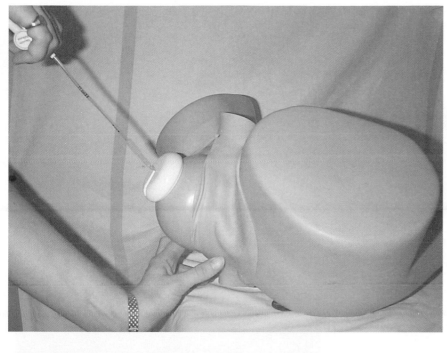

Figure 34.2 Application of a hand-held ventouse (Kiwi OmniCup™). The cup should be positioned over the flexion point to ensure optimal delivery technique. Manipulation of the cup during crowning of a fetus in an occipito-anterior position is shown

be fenestrated (open), pseudofenestrated (open with a protruding ridge), or solid. Likewise, the length of the shanks, the design of the lock (convergent, divergent or sliding) and the fashioning of the handles are instrument specific (Figure 34.3).

Technique

Once the patient has been optimally positioned, the pelvis must be examined to establish the positions and station of the vertex and the contours of the pelvis. At this stage, the accoucheur should always be prepared to abandon the vaginal route of delivery if a safer alternative is more appropriate. The forceps should then be held in front of the patient so as to visualize how they will be inserted per vaginum and placed around the fetal head.

It is appropriate to use non-rotational forceps when the head is occipito-anterior ±15°. Where the head is positioned >15° from the vertical, rotation must be accomplished before traction (which for minor degrees may often be accomplished by manual rotation).

By convention, the left blade is inserted before the right with the accoucheurs hand protecting the vaginal wall from direct trauma. With proper placement of the forceps blades, they come to lie parallel to the axis of the fetal head and between the fetal head and the pelvic wall. The operator then articulates and locks the blades, checking their application before applying traction. If the application is not correct, the blades *must* be repositioned.

Traction should be applied intermittently in concert with uterine contractions and maternal expulsive efforts. The axis of traction changes during the delivery and is guided along the J-shaped curve of the pelvis. As the head begins to crown, the blades are directed to the vertical, a Ritgen manoeuvre is performed or an episiotomy fashioned (Figure 34.4). Once the

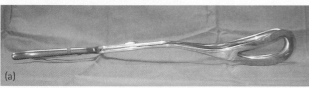

(a)

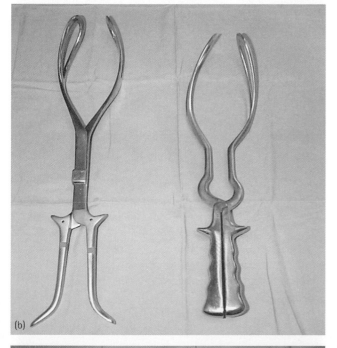

(b)

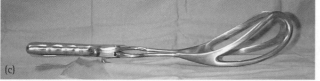

(c)

Figure 34.3 Rotational and non-rotational obstetric forceps

Second stage of labour

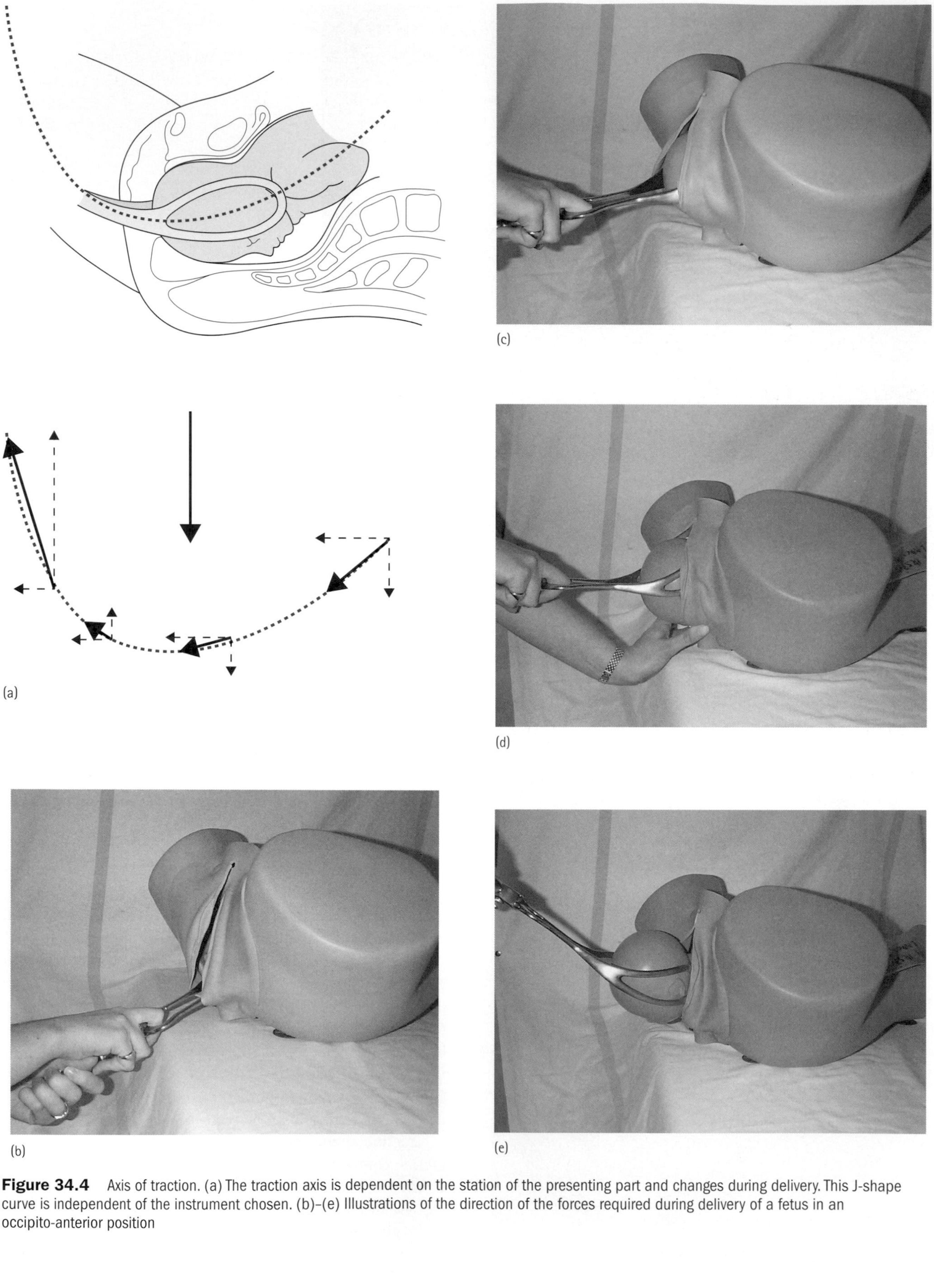

Figure 34.4   Axis of traction. (a) The traction axis is dependent on the station of the presenting part and changes during delivery. This J-shape curve is independent of the instrument chosen. (b)–(e) Illustrations of the direction of the forces required during delivery of a fetus in an occipito-anterior position

head is delivered, the forceps are removed in the reverse order to which they were inserted, and the delivery is completed in the normal fashion.

Kiellands forceps are the most commonly utilized instrument for rotational forceps deliveries and, as specific techniques are required, only those who have been properly trained in their use should employ them. These forceps are unique in their design, having a minimal pelvic curve to allow rotation around a fixed axis, and a sliding lock to enable correction of asynclitism.

The method of application of the Kiellands blades differs from the standard forceps technique. It is commonly described as the 'wandering method', a specific application to a head in the transverse position, which need not be employed for direct occipito-posterior positions. As with the standard technique, the forceps are assembled and held in position to enable visualization of their final position prior to application. The anterior blade is chosen, introduced in the standard manner, but subsequently manoeuvred over the fetal face until it comes to lie over the parietal bone. The internal hand is used for guidance and protects the maternal soft tissues from trauma. The posterior blade, which occupies the sacral hollow, can be directly inserted in most instances, but if this proves not to be possible, application in the manner of the anterior blade should be performed, but in reverse. Rotation should be performed between contractions and may be accomplished by pushing the head 'up' to the level of the pelvic mid-cavity, or by gentle traction at the level at which the head has reached.

The axis of traction is more in the vertical in the first instance and then proceeds as previously described, but extra care must be taken towards the end of the delivery as the lack of the forceps pelvic curve makes perineal damage more likely. Rotational forceps deliveries have been abandoned in many institutions, as they have been associated with spiral tears of the vagina and other soft tissue injuries, and in some cases uterine rupture. However, for those experienced in their use, they still have a role, as the ventouse is associated with a higher incidence of failure of delivery in occipito-posterior and occipito-transverse positions.

Episiotomy

It has been recommended that an episiotomy be cut whenever an instrumental vaginal delivery is performed [IV]. This is not based on any robust evidence. It is recognized in spontaneous vaginal delivery that episiotomy does not protect against third-degree and fourth-degree tears, but does reduce the incidence of anterior vaginal trauma. Perineal trauma will occur in most nulliparous women undergoing instrumental vaginal delivery, and episiotomy should be considered in these women in order to limit multiple lacerations. In multiparae, particularly those requiring only a simple ventouse, an episiotomy may not be needed.

Special considerations

Failure of the chosen instrument

Failures can occur when the choice of instrument is wrong (e.g. a silastic cup ventouse for a rotational delivery), when the positioning of the ventouse cup is wrong or when the position has been wrongly defined, leading to larger diameters presenting to the pelvis in occipito-posterior positions. Failure is also more common if the fetus is large or maternal effort poor. Fourteen to 27 per cent of deliveries will not be accomplished when the ventouse is the instrument of first choice. The lower figures are achieved when a rigid posterior cup is used for rotational deliveries. If forceps are chosen first, up to 10 per cent of deliveries may not be accomplished.[8]

In many circumstances, the head may then have descended to a point at which caesarean section becomes even more hazardous. The art of obstetrics is not to find oneself in this position to start with, by choosing a correct instrument and using it properly.

There have been no randomized studies assessing the best approach in this circumstance. Observational studies show that the outcomes for babies are worse than if the instrument of first choice is successful, but this is hardly surprising. In addition, the rates of third-degree and fourth-degree tears are higher when a second instrument is used.[14]

Unfortunately, there are no easy answers. A policy of delivering all such women by caesarean section will undoubtedly also lead to an increase in maternal morbidity and perhaps mortality.

Where the first instrument fails, the following scenarios may pertain.

- The reason for cup failure was detachment (the reason for failure in 40 per cent of ventouse deliveries attempted), but the head is occipito-anterior and on the perineum. A full reassessment should be made. If it is confirmed that this is still the case (i.e. occipito-anterior, head on the perineum), a simple lift-out forceps is acceptable. If there are any concerns, senior help *must* be sought before using a second instrument.
- The instrument failed because there was little or no descent with the first pull. Where there has been *little or no* descent, delivery must be by caesarean section.
- The instrument failed because the position was wrongly defined. In this case, the next option will be either a rotational forceps or caesarean section. Already the fetus will have been subjected to traction, probably with minimal descent. Only after a full assessment by a senior person in theatre could a further instrumentation be considered. In many cases, delivery by caesarean section may be the safer option for the fetus.

ROTATIONAL DELIVERIES IN CASES OF SUSPECTED FETAL COMPROMISE

Concern has been expressed that the risk incumbent with rotational delivery for fetal compromise, especially with Kiellands forceps, should persuade the accoucheur to opt for delivery by caesarean section instead. Such advice is based on little evidence, and mainly reflects the views of one study in which there was observed to be a significant difference in base deficit in cord venous blood, but no difference in pH, in infants delivered by rotational when compared to non-rotational deliveries.[15] The main factor to consider must be the ease with which delivery will be accomplished. This will relate to the fetal position, station and size, the progress of the labour, the degree of analgesia and the experience of the operator. Each case must be judged on an individual basis. An easy forceps will be preferable to a difficult caesarean section, and vice versa.

Complications

Assisted deliveries with both vacuum and forceps can be associated with significant maternal and fetal complications.

There have been maternal deaths associated with cervical tears in women delivered by ventouse before full cervical dilatation was attained. In the most recent report of the Confidential Enquiries into Maternal Deaths, the only death directly attributable to instrumental delivery was secondary to a traumatic uterine rupture following a forceps delivery.

Traumatic vaginal delivery is considered the most important risk factor for faecal incontinence in women and may occur not only after recognized third-degree perineal tears, but also after apparently non-traumatic vaginal delivery [Ib].[16] The incidence of such damage is increased by intervention with any instrument, rising from an approximate baseline incidence of 10 per cent to 25 per cent following ventouse and 40 per cent following forceps.[16] Studies using endo-anal ultrasonography have shown that persisting sphincter defects are the main cause of faecal incontinence and not, as was previously believed, neurological damage. However, at 5-year follow-up there are no discernible differences in symptoms between women delivered by forceps and those delivered by ventouse.[9] Successful delivery by the instrument of first choice will limit damage. Good technique and adequate training are also imperative.

Postpartum haemorrhage is commoner in women needing instrumental vaginal delivery compared to women who deliver spontaneously, but less common than in women delivered by caesarean section in the second stage. Measures to limit this include:

- prophylactic Syntocinon infusion post-delivery,
- prompt suturing,
- careful identification of high tears.

Underestimation of blood loss at instrumental vaginal delivery is common. Where possible, loss should be measured through the weighing of swabs and towels.

Fetal complications are no less important; however, combined evidence from all available controlled trials (1175 babies in the vacuum extractor groups and 1155 babies in the forceps groups) allows conclusions to be drawn only about the relatively common neonatal outcomes. Although concerns about risks of intracranial and subgaleal haemorrhage remain, in a recent review of 583 340 live-born singleton infants born to nulliparous women, the rate of subdural or cerebral haemorrhage in vacuum deliveries did not differ significantly from that associated with forceps use or caesarean section during labour.[17] Overall, the risks of perinatal trauma using the vacuum extractor correlate with [Ia]:

- the duration of application,
- the station of the fetal head at the commencement of the delivery,
- the difficulty of the delivery,
- the condition of the baby at the time of commencement of the procedure.[12]

It is important to remember that the risks of such damage significantly increase amongst babies who are exposed to multiple attempts at both vacuum and forceps delivery.[14,17]

CLINICAL RISK MANAGEMENT IN OBSTETRICS

Instrumental vaginal delivery has never been free from criticism, and is certainly not without risks, although most instrumental deliveries have normal outcomes and give no reason for complaint. However, in today's litigious society, the risks of litigation against accoucheurs or the hospital in which they practice are increased by a bad outcome.

Common allegations against practitioners that are cited in lawsuits include (amongst others): inadequate indication; failure to exclude cephalo-pelvic disproportion; improper use of instruments with excessive use of force resulting in fetal or maternal injury; lack of informed consent (although this may not be fully possible in an emergency situation); and inadequate supervision.[18]

The basis of any defence following an adverse outcome will rely upon the quality of the record keeping. Proper documentation is a critical part of the surgeon's responsibility in performing any operative delivery, and should include, as a basic minimum, a statement of the indication for the procedure, the anaesthesia used, the personnel involved and an outline of the procedure performed. Additional comments about the difficulty of the extraction, the performance of rotation, fetal injuries, maternal soft-tissue trauma and their repair, and an estimate of the blood loss should be included.

The fear of litigation *must not* dictate good medical practice, and assisted vaginal deliveries remain an appropriate intervention when practised with the appropriate safeguards. It should be remembered that although both intrapartum asphyxia and, to a lesser degree, intrapartum trauma contribute to neonatal morbidity, abnormal fetal growth, prematurity, chromosomal abnormalities, intrauterine infection and other non-genetic chromosomal disorders contribute more significantly to permanent neonatal complications.

TRAINING OBSTETRICIANS IN PRACTICAL SKILLS

Good outcomes are achieved if training is thorough and supervision is requested when any delivery is thought to be potentially more difficult than the operator is used to.

Accurate application of the forceps or the vacuum extractor and close adherence to standard techniques are essential in the safe performance of all instrumental deliveries. Practical procedures can be learnt only in action, and descriptions are a poor substitute for seeing and doing them. However, comprehensive descriptions of the techniques of forceps and ventouse deliveries are accessible and should be read.

With many of the 'more difficult' vaginal deliveries being abandoned in many institutions, and a generalized de-skilling in their use, training in some centres may be deemed to be less than comprehensive. As a profession, we are in danger of abandoning methods of procuring a successful vaginal delivery because of the perceived danger of specific instruments, when the danger lies, not with the instrument, but in the inadequate training and competence of the accoucheur.

CONCLUSIONS

Despite the known risks, instrumental vaginal delivery undoubtedly continues to have a role in the management of the second stage of labour. Caesarean sections performed at this stage are not infrequently traumatic for both patients and staff, and are themselves associated with a significant morbidity and mortality.

> - Failure rates are higher with soft than with rigid cups and with ventouse than with forceps.
> - Soft cups should not be used for rotational deliveries.
> - Use of a second instrument increases the risks of fetal and maternal damage.
> - Caesarean section in the second stage is associated with higher rates of haemorrhage than instrumental delivery.

KEY POINTS

- Careful assessment of each patient, combining history and examination, must be performed before any intervention is undertaken.
- 'Sang froid' should be the motto of choice, and the accoucheur should always consider the available alternative.
- Instruments should only be used by those trained to do so.

KEY REFERENCES

1. Stephenson PA. *International Differences in the Use of Obstetrical Interventions.* Copenhagen: WHO (EUR/ICP/MCH), 1992.
2. Hodnett ED. Caregiver support for women during childbirth (Cochrane Review). In: *The Cochrane Library*, Issue 2. Oxford: Update Software, 2002.
3. Fraser WD, Marcoux S, Krauss I, Douglas J, Goulet C, Boulvain M. Multicenter, randomized, controlled trial of delayed pushing for nulliparous women in the second stage of labor with continuous epidural analgesia. The PEOPLE (Pushing Early or Pushing Late with Epidural) Study Group. *Am J Obstet Gynecol* 2000; **182**:1165–72.
4. Gupta JK, Nikodem VC. Position for women during second stage of labour (Cochrane Review). In: *The Cochrane Library*, Issue 2. Oxford: Update Software, 2002.
5. Johanson RB. *Instrumental Vaginal Delivery.* Clinical Green Top Guidelines No. 26. London: RCOG Press, 1999.
6. Howell CJ. Epidural versus non-epidural analgesia for pain relief in labour. (Cochrane Review). In: *The Cochrane Library*, Issue 2. Oxford: Update Software, 2002.
7. American College of Obstetricians and Gynecologists. *Operative Vaginal Delivery.* Technical Bulletin No. 196. Washington: American College of Obstetricians and Gynecologists, 1994.
8. Johanson RB, Heycock E, Carter J, Sultan AH, Walklate K, Jones PW. Maternal and child health after assisted vaginal delivery: five year follow-up of a randomised controlled study comparing forceps and ventouse. *Br J Obstet Gynaecol* 1999; **106**:544–9.
9. Johanson RB, Menon BKV. Vacuum extraction vs. forceps delivery (Cochrane Review). In: *The Cochrane Library*, Issue 2. Oxford: Update Software, 2002.
10. Murphy DJ, Liebling RE, Verity L, Swingler R, Patel R. Early maternal and neonatal morbidity associated with

operative delivery in second stage of labour: a cohort study. *Lancet* 2001; **358**:1203–7.

11. Johanson RB, Rice C, Doyle M et al. A randomised prospective study comparing the new vacuum extractor policy with forceps delivery. *Br J Obstet Gynaecol* 1993; **100**:524–30.

12. Vacca A. The trouble with vacuum extraction. *Curr Obstet Gynaecol* 1999; **9**:41–55.

13. Johanson R, Menon V. Soft versus rigid vacuum extractor cups for assisted vaginal delivery (Cochrane Review). In: *The Cochrane Library*, Issue 2. Oxford: Update Software, 2002.

14. Gardella C, Taylor M, Benedetti T, Hitti J, Critchlow C. The effect of sequential use of vacuum and forceps for assisted vaginal delivery on neonatal and maternal outcomes. *Am J Obstet Gynecol* 2001; **185**:896–902.

15. Baker PN, Johnson IR. A study of the effect of rotational forceps delivery on fetal acid–base balance. *Acta Obstet Gynecol Scand* 1994; **73**: 787–9.

16. Sultan AH, Kamm MA, Hudson CN. Anal sphincter disruption during vaginal delivery. *N Eng J Med* 1993; **329**:1905–11.

17. Towner D, Castro MA, Eby-Wilkens E, Gilbert WM. Effect of mode of delivery in nulliparous women on neonatal intracranial injury. *N Engl J Med* 1999; **341**:1709–14.

Chapter 35

Breech Presentation

Richard Hayman

INTRODUCTION

The management of a fetus presenting by the breech has been an area of great controversy and changing practice. From a situation in which the breech was considered advantageous, presumably because the midwife could pull on the legs to expedite delivery, to 'once a breech, always a caesarean section', changes in observed practice have frequently reflected the attitudes of the attendant birth professionals rather than following principles determined by suitable randomized, controlled trials.

Although the Term Breech Study has done much to clarify thinking around delivery of the breech infant at term, some management issues still remain areas of intense controversy.

AETIOLOGY

The incidence of breech presentation varies with gestational age, and is between 14 and 20 per cent at 28 weeks and 2.2 and 3.7 per cent at term. Thus a major reason for breech presentation in labour is preterm delivery, as most fetuses will turn spontaneously towards term. Although these babies tend to be structurally normal, there are unfortunately higher perinatal mortality and morbidity with breech presentation when compared with cephalic-presenting contemporaries. This is due principally to the increased risks from birth asphyxia or trauma.[1]

Another important cause for breech is maternal or fetal abnormality, with up to 18 per cent of preterm and 5 per cent of term breeches having congenital abnormalities, compared with 2.5 per cent of term cephalic babies.

Maternal abnormalities associated with breech presentation

- Uterine abnormality, e.g. bicornuate uterus.
- Pelvic abnormality.
- Pelvic mass (cervical fibromyomata, ovarian cyst).
- Drug and alcohol abuse.
- Anticonvulsant therapy.

Fetal abnormalities associated with breech presentation

- Intrauterine growth restriction.
- Abnormality, especially central nervous system (CNS):
  - hydrocephalus
  - myelomeningocele
  - Prader–Willi syndrome
  - aneuploidy/trisomy.

Feto-maternal abnormalities associated with breech presentation

- Preterm.
- Placenta praevia.

- Previous pregnancy complicated by a breech presentation at term.
- Multiple pregnancy.
- Oligohydramnios or polyhydramnios.

Breech presentation, whatever the mode of delivery, is a signal for potential fetal handicap and this should inform antenatal, intrapartum and neonatal management. It is important to remember that the perinatal mortality remains increased even when the delivery is by caesarean section and corrected for gestation, congenital defects and birth weight.[1]

Caesarean section for breech presentation has been suggested as a way of reducing the associated fetal problems, and in many countries in northern Europe and North America, caesarean section has become the normal mode of delivery in this situation.

DIAGNOSIS

Three clinical breech presentations are recognized.

- Extended (frank): the legs of the fetus are flexed at the hip and extended at the knee. Such a presentation occurs in 60–70 per cent of all breech presentations at term, and carries the lowest risks of cord prolapse and feto-pelvic disproportion.
- Flexed (complete): the hips and knees are flexed so the feet present to the pelvis. (Feeling a foot at the cervix does not constitute a footling; most are flexed breeches.)
- Footling (incomplete): at least one leg extended at the hip and knee, the buttocks therefore not being within the pelvis at all. This presentation carries the highest risks of cord prolapse and feto-pelvic disproportion.

Clinical diagnosis of the breech presentation may be difficult by palpation alone. Suggestive features are:

- a history of subcostal discomfort, with the palpation of a 'solid' fetal pole at the uterine fundus;
- auscultation of the fetal heart sounds above the umbilicus;
- palpation of the fetal ischial tuberosities, sacrum and anus during vaginal examination. (Differentiation from a face presentation may be difficult, but in a face presentation careful palpation will frequently distinguish the bony landmarks of the malar eminences, mentum and mouth with its obvious bony margin.)

Such observations are frequently imprecise, and it is estimated that 30 per cent of breech presentations are not diagnosed until the onset of labour. As abdominal palpation has been shown to have a sensitivity of 28 per cent and specificity of 94 per cent, confirmation by ultrasound scan must therefore be regarded as the 'gold standard'.

MANAGEMENT OPTIONS FOR BREECH PRESENTATION

When determining the mode of delivery that is most suitable, many factors must be taken into consideration. The main comparison must be between maternal and fetal risks and benefits, a difficult equation to calculate, even at the best of times.

In all studies of breech presentation, maternal morbidity is increased in women delivered by caesarean section when compared to those having a vaginal delivery. Such morbidity includes haemorrhage, hysterectomy, uterine and wound haematomas and infections, urinary tract infection and deep vein thrombosis and pulmonary embolism.[1] The risks associated with future deliveries are also not inconsiderable, especially with preterm breech deliveries through a vertical uterine incision, and should feature in any risk versus benefits equation.[2,3]

However, it is inappropriate to compare maternal risks and fetal/neonatal risks directly, as the potential adverse consequences of each complication affect the recipient in vastly different ways. Only the mother can determine where the balance lies, and it should be the role of the attendant clinician to empower her to reach a carefully formulated and clinically sound decision.

Preterm: 26–36 completed weeks

- This encompasses approximately 2 per cent of all pregnancies with viable fetuses.
- Approximately 25 per cent of all babies delivered at these gestations will be by the breech.
- The overall incidence of breech presentation between these gestations is 0.5 per cent.

When compared with vertex-presenting counterparts, the premature breech often:

- is small for gestational age,
- has a higher head to body circumference ratio,
- has a higher association with antepartum stillbirth and neonatal demise.

Caesarean delivery is not always an atraumatic option for the fetus, and a preterm breech infant faces some formidable difficulties whatever the mode of delivery. During a vaginal breech delivery, the occipital bone of the fetus is particularly exposed to damage due to its impact upon the maternal pubis during decent of the fetal head in the second stage of labour. Such forces may act to separate the central portion of the occipital bone from the lateral part (occipital diastasis), with potential damage to the cerebellum and herniation of brain tissue through the foramen magnum. If this does not result in stillbirth or early neonatal death, the diagnosis may be delayed until the child is older, when signs of ataxic cerebral palsy may be displayed. Fortunately, this is a rare occurrence.

More frequently, problems of intraventricular and periventricular damage due to hypoxia or haemorrhage during the antenatal, peripartum, intrapartum and postpartum courses may be inflicted on the fetus. Although these injuries may be related to the mechanics of vaginal delivery, avoiding such circumstances may not prevent them occurring.

Other common problems faced by the breech fetus include the following.

- Damage to the internal organs, transection of the spinal cord, nerve palsies and fractures of the long bones – these frequently result from the injudicious use of traction on the presenting parts [III].[4]
- Entrapment of the after-coming head. The risk of such a problem increases when the active second stage is begun *before* full cervical dilatation is achieved (more common with footling than with other presentations). Although prevention is preferable to intervention, should this problem occur, incising the cervix at 4 and 8 o'clock with a pair of scissors may result in its resolution. A complete examination must be performed following delivery, the haemorrhage must be arrested and the defect repaired.

The preterm breech usually presents in labour. Although *routine* external cephalic version (ECV) before term has not been shown to confer any advantages in such a case, ECV could be considered if the membranes are intact.

Evidence from the Term Breech Trial *cannot* be directly extrapolated to preterm breech delivery, which remains an area of clinical controversy.

There is insufficient evidence to support routine caesarean section for preterm breech delivery [II].

Although the majority of obstetricians use delivery by caesarean section for the uncomplicated preterm breech, only a minority believe that there is sufficient evidence to justify this policy. There is general acknowledgement (including in some reports) that the numerous retrospective studies that suggest that caesarean section confers a better outcome in this situation have been subject to bias. The poor outcome for very low birth weight infants is mainly related to complications of prematurity and *not* to the mode of delivery.[2] Grant reviewed the controlled trials assessing the value of elective versus selective caesarean delivery of the 'small baby'.[5] He concluded that the data 'are not sufficient to justify a policy of elective Caesarean section', and, in the absence of good evidence that a preterm baby needs to be delivered by caesarean section, the decision about the mode of delivery should be made after close consultation with the labouring woman and her partner. Attempts have been made to answer the questions concerning preterm breech delivery, but clinicians were unwilling to randomize women, leading to the abandonment of the trial.

Management of the preterm breech in labour

When a woman is not in labour and an indication exists for expediting delivery, the preferred route should be by caesarean section. When time permits, such an intervention should always be preceded by the mother being given a course of antenatal steroids.

In labour the management depends on:

- an accurate diagnosis of labour (50 per cent of cases of presumed preterm labours settle spontaneously);
- tocolysis to delay labour whilst steroids are administered or transfer to another unit is arranged;
- confirmation of the presentation;
- exclusion of a fetal abnormality (a detailed ultrasound scan should be performed if time and labour permit).

As with all preterm labours, many will be precipitate and several will be associated with antecedents that are often pathological. The decision regarding the best method of delivery must take into account the following.

- Gestation: the very preterm infant is unlikely to benefit from caesarean section and maternal risks will be higher.
- Fetal abnormality.
- The progress of labour: this is often very quick, and caesarean section may not be realistic.
- Fetal status: at gestations with expected good outcomes, non-reassuring fetal status may indicate caesarean section.

Full discussion with the parents, with realistic evaluation of the fetal and maternal risks, should take place.

Procedure: preterm breech delivery

An experienced obstetrician should supervise vaginal delivery of the breech. An epidural should be sited and effective, to prevent pushing prior to full cervical dilatation. This will also enable intradelivery manipulations, the painless application of forceps to the after-coming head, or rapid recourse to operative delivery. As with all preterm deliveries, a paediatrician should be present and an anaesthetist available. Delivery with the membranes intact has been shown to confer some advantage to the fetus [III].[3]

Should the cervix clamp down around the fetal head following delivery of the body, gentle flexion by insertion of the index finger into the fetal mouth may be advantageous. If this does not succeed, incision of the cervix should be performed as previously described.

Caesarean delivery can nearly always be performed through a transverse lower abdominal incision. The nature of the most beneficial uterine incision is less certain, although from a maternal viewpoint, a J-shaped extension to the lower uterine incision has many advantages over a classical/De Lee or inverted-T approach. However, with a fetal mortality of up to 80 per cent with breech presentations below 28 weeks, it may not be in the mother's best interests to compromise her future childbearing by employing a classical approach.

Second stage of labour

Presentation at term

The decline in the incidence of breech presentations towards term suggests that spontaneous version is a common occurrence, with approximately 57 per cent turning between 32 and 36 weeks and 25 per cent thereafter. Even if a primigravid patient with a fetus in an extended breech presentation (one of the least favourable for spontaneous version) is to be delivered by caesarean section, the presentation should be confirmed by ultrasound scan, as the chance of spontaneous version at this stage is not insignificant. This is even more important in multiparous patients offered this management.

Reducing the incidence of breech presentation at term

POSTURE

Four randomized trials have been undertaken to establish whether or not postural management (knee–chest position for up to 10 minutes a day) is effective in converting breech to cephalic presentations. No significant benefits were found in these studies,[6] and there is no evidence to support routine recommendation of the knee–chest position [Ia].

EXTERNAL CEPHALIC VERSION

External cephalic version has been practised since the time of Hippocrates and has been demonstrated to be associated with a significant reduction in the risk of caesarean section (odds ratio (OR) 0.4; 95% confidence interval (CI) 0.3–0.6) without any increased risk to the baby. It is current best practice that all women with an *uncomplicated* breech pregnancy at term (37–42 weeks) should be offered ECV [Ia]. However, as with all procedures, ECV should only be undertaken by appropriately trained professionals in an appropriate setting.[7] It should not be offered routinely before term, as it does not improve outcomes.[7,8]

Although several studies have reported significant benefits from routine tocolysis in facilitating the procedure of EVC, with success rates ranging from 3 per cent to 40 per cent in these trials, there remains insufficient evidence upon which to base the routine use of tocolysis. Because of the recognized adverse effects of beta-sympathomimetics, there is considerable interest in the evaluation of the benefits and risks of alternative agents.[7]

Despite this, ECV has been successfully introduced into routine practice in many units in the UK. Although the success rates (conversion to cephalic presentation) are less than those quoted in some countries (e.g. 40 per cent in the UK, >80 per cent in Africa), a more comprehensive nationwide implementation would result in a significant reduction in the numbers of caesarean sections performed for breech presentation. It is possible to achieve higher success rates with case selection, and it is undoubtedly the case that operators improve with experience. Patients can be informed that, following successful ECV, 97.5 per cent of fetuses remain cephalic.

A number of factors have been found to increase the likelihood of successful ECV. These include:

- multiparity,
- adequate liquor volume,
- breech above the pelvic brim,
- fetal head easy to feel.

Although primarily intended for the management of the uncomplicated breech pregnancy at term, ECV has also been carried out successfully during early labour. It can be performed in women who have had a prior caesarean section and appears to be safe, though trials are not randomized and are only small. This may be acceptable to some women as, if the fetus stays breech, many will decide on elective caesarean section for delivery, which makes the choices much more limited should they have future pregnancies.

Although various interventions for improving the success rate of ECV have been suggested, neither vibroacoustic stimulation nor amnio-infusion has been proven to be effective in controlled trials and each requires further evaluation.

A few small randomized, controlled studies have shown that regional epidural anaesthesia improves version success without any increase in fetal or maternal morbidity. However, a more recent study of spinal anaesthesia has been published that does not support improved outcome with regional anaesthesia. Once again, no adverse effects on the mother or fetus were reported. In addition, an economic analysis has suggested that with epidural use in institutions where caesarean sections are systematically performed for breech presentations, substantial cost savings are possible. However, no studies have reported any outcomes related to maternal satisfaction or quality of life. Further research in this area is recommended.

It must be remembered that following EVC, whether successful or not, anti-D should be administered to all women who are Rhesus negative.

Benefits to the fetus of external cephalic version

External cephalic version reduces the incidence of breech presentation at term. However, it should be noted that the rate of delivery by caesarean section may be higher than average for those babies successfully turned when compared to 'genuine' cephalic presentations. It should also be remembered that even when EVC has been successful, these now cephalic-presenting fetuses, when subject to the stress of labour, are more likely to display signs of fetal compromise, and thus should still be regarded as a high-risk group requiring continuous monitoring in labour.

Risks to the fetus of external cephalic version

Transient bradycardia occurs in up to 8 per cent of cases. Abruption or direct effects on the placenta or cord (prolapse or direct trauma) occur far less frequently.[7] Feto-maternal haemorrhage has an occurrence rate of between 5 and 28 per cent, although this is often minor and of little clinical significance as long as anti-D is administered appropriately.

It is important that such risks are always compared with those incurred during vaginal *or* abdominal breech delivery, procedures that are not risk free themselves.

Benefits to the mother of external cephalic version

Implementing the practice of ECV has been shown to result in a decrease in the number of vaginal breech deliveries and deliveries by caesarean section. Such practice invariably reduces maternal morbidity and mortality (both of which are increased by caesarean section and vaginal breech delivery).

Procedure of external cephalic version

Such procedures are best managed by following an agreed protocol (Figure 35.1).

Indications for external cephalic version
- Any breech presentation after 37 completed weeks in an otherwise uncomplicated pregnancy.
- Maternal request.

Absolute contraindications for external cephalic version
- Multiple pregnancy.
- Antepartum haemorrhage (after 20 weeks).
- Need for caesarean section regardless of presentation (e.g. placenta praevia).
- Ruptured membranes.
- Fetal abnormality.
- Need for urgent delivery to ensure fetal well-being – any suspected fetal compromise.
- Cord completely encircling fetal neck on ultrasound.
- Declined consent.

Relative contraindications
- Previous LSCS.
- Maternal disease, e.g. hypertension, diabetes.
- Fetal growth restriction or oligohydramnios.
- Maternal obesity: if the maternal body mass index (BMI) is >20 per cent of ideal, the procedure is less likely to succeed.

Although there is no evidence that reduced fetal growth makes ECV any more difficult to perform, it may be a marker for the existence of some fetal compromise already, and it is for the protection of the operator that it is advised not to turn these fetuses.

Before attending for ECV, women should be asked to drink plenty of fluid, as this has been shown to optimize liquor volume [Ia].[9] There should be no need to starve women before the procedure, as the chance of emergency caesarean section being required is very small.

Ultrasound is useful before ECV to:
- confirm the breech,
- confirm the presence of a normal fetus,
- ensure an adequate liquor volume,
- confirm the placental position,
- observe for the presence of a nuchal cord,
- detail the fetal attitude and position of the fetal legs.

It should be routine practice to:
- perform a cardiotocogram (CTG) to confirm a normal reactive pattern,
- obtain informed consent, specifically detailing the risks (failure, caesarean delivery, need for anti-D if Rhesus negative),
- ensure that facilities for delivery by immediate caesarean section are present.

External cephalic version should be performed in a facility with rapid access for operative delivery if required.[10] Once the prerequisites have been completed, the woman is positioned supine with slight lateral tilt. Tocolysis may be given (e.g. 250 μg terbutaline i.v./s.c.) and a short time allowed for the drug to exert its effect.

The operator should perform the ECV in one manoeuvre and uterine manipulation should be limited to a total of 10 minutes' duration (the vast majority will turn within 5 minutes). A variety of techniques may be employed, but essentially:
- the breech is manipulated out of the pelvis by steady and continuous abdominal pressure (the patient having a full bladder may aid this manoeuvre, although this often increases the abdominal discomfort experienced);
- a forward or backward roll/somersault of the fetus can then be performed; pressure should be maximally aimed at moving the breech upward; one hand can be used to maintain the head in flexion – a rocking manoeuvre is sometimes helpful;
- if this sequence should prove unsuccessful, rotation in the opposite direction may be tried; a fetus will often rotate easily one way but not the other; it is not always easy to predict which way will be more successful.

If successful, the attitude of the fetus should be maintained manually for a couple of minutes, during which time fetal monitoring can be commenced. Fetal monitoring should also be commenced if the procedure is unsuccessful. The CTG should be continued until a normal and reassuring pattern can be observed and, once this has been obtained, the patient should be allowed home with an appointment after a few days to confirm the persistence of the cephalic presentation.

Mothers should be told that:
- the procedure does not normally precipitate labour,
- only 2 per cent of babies will revert to a breech,
- the fetus should continue to be active and that a reduction in fetal movements must be reported,
- any vaginal loss (blood or fluid) must be reported.

If reversion to breech occurs, a repeat ECV may be attempted or delivery by caesarean section may be offered. If the ECV is unsuccessful, a full discussion should take

Date ....

Identification label

Exclude the following (tick)

☐   Multiple pregnancy

☐   Previous Caesarean section

☐   Antepartum haemorrhage after 20 weeks'

☐   Need for caesarean section regardless of presentation

☐   Ruptured membranes

☐   IUGR/oligohydramnios

☐   Fetal abnormality

Parity [   ]   Gestation by scan [   ]

Explain the procedure and the following risks

• Need for immediate caesarean section if signs of fetal distress on CTG following procedure

• Small risk of feto-maternal haemorrhage therefore anti-D needed if rh negative.

• Need to return for check of presentation next week.

• Very small risk that the baby can turn back (no documented cases in our experience to date)

Procedure

Ultrasound scan
Presentation   Breech extended [ ]   Flexed [ ]   Footling [ ]   Cephalic [ ]

Nuchal cord   No [ ]

Liquor volume   Normal [ ]   Increased [ ]

Placental site   Anterior [ ]   Posterior [ ]

Pre ECV CTG satisfactory   Yes [ ]

Fetal head easy to feel   Yes [ ]   No [ ]

Breech deep in pelvis   Yes [ ]   No [ ]

Ritodrine dose .... (see protocol)

Procedure

Signed ....

Successful   Yes [ ]   No [ ]

Post ECV CTG satisfactory   Yes [ ]   No [ ]

Blood group .... Kleihauer .... Anti-D given .... date

Outcome   Home (without ECV) [ ]   Home after ECV [ ]

                Immediate delivery [ ]

Figure 35.1   Proforma, external cephalic version

place regarding delivery. It should be remembered that ECV can be offered in early labour if the membranes are intact.

As mentioned previously, if the patient is Rhesus negative, anti-D may be administered prophylactically once maternal blood has been obtained for Kleihauer estimation of feto-maternal transfusion.

External cephalic version: summary

- Tocolysis is effective, both when used routinely and when used selectively.
- ECV should be done near to facilities for emergency delivery.
- CTG is necessary before and after ECV.
- Ultrasound is helpful.

Elective caesarean section versus planned vaginal breech delivery at term

At term, the first question that must be addressed when confronted by a breech presentation is 'Where is the placenta?'. Once this question has been successfully answered, a rational approach may be applied to further management.

For the fetus, the best method of delivering a term frank or complete breech singleton is by planned caesarean section [Ia].[9,10]

Before 2001, much of the evidence supporting elective caesarean section in preference to vaginal breech delivery was obtained from two small randomized trials and data from hospital audit. These studies, which revealed outcomes for vaginal delivery and delivery by caesarean section rather than comparing a policy of intended caesarean section with a policy of intended vaginal birth, showed no differences in mortality between the groups. However, an increase in short-term morbidity was noted amongst those babies delivered vaginally.[12]

The Canadian Medical Research Council (MRC) funded an international multicentre randomized, controlled trial of planned vaginal delivery versus planned elective caesarean section for the uncomplicated term breech.[12]

Sub-analysis was undertaken after excluding deliveries that occurred:

- after a prolonged labour,
- after labours induced or augmented with oxytocin or prostaglandins,
- in cases where there was a footling or uncertain type of breech presentation at delivery,
- in cases for which there was no skilled or experienced clinician present at the birth.

In this sub-analysis, the risk of the *combined outcome* of perinatal mortality, neonatal mortality or serious neonatal morbidity with planned caesarean section compared with planned vaginal birth was 16/1006 (1.6 per cent), compared with 23/704 (3.3 per cent) (relative risk (RR) 0.49; 95 per cent CI 0.26–0.91; $p = 0.02$).

In a further sub-analysis, results were separated into those obtained from countries with higher perinatal mortality ($>20/1000$) and those from countries with a lower perinatal mortality ($<20/1000$). The findings suggested that the benefits of delivery by caesarean section became even more significant in countries with a low perinatal mortality rate, but were not as significant in countries with a higher perinatal mortality rate. There were no differences between any of the groups in terms of maternal mortality or serious *early* maternal morbidity.

However, this study did not evaluate long-term outcomes for child or mother, and many have raised serious questions about the study design.[13] Although it is possible that careful exclusion of growth-restricted infants, better intrapartum monitoring and full pelvimetry and umbilical cord assessment might have improved the prospects for a vaginal breech delivery, the results of the Term Breech Trial led the Royal College of Obstetricians and Gynaecologists (RCOG) to the recommendation that 'the best method of delivering a singleton fetus at term with an extended or flexed breech presentation is by planned LSCS'. This information should be disseminated to pregnant women, their families and all clinicians involved in maternity care.[10]

It remains likely that some women will choose to deliver vaginally and that some women for whom a caesarean section is planned will labour too quickly for the operation to be undertaken (nearly 10 per cent of women assigned to deliver by caesarean section in the Term Breech Trial delivered vaginally). It therefore remains important that clinicians and hospitals are prepared for vaginal breech delivery.

Criteria for the selection of patients in whom a trial of vaginal delivery may be appropriate

Issues to be considered when counselling a woman planning a vaginal birth are:

- the careful selection of patients,
- appropriate intrapartum management,
- the skill, experience and judgement of the intrapartum attendant.

It is undisputed that a trial of labour should be precluded in the presence of medical or obstetric complications that are likely to be associated with mechanical difficulties at delivery. Likewise, a trial of vaginal breech delivery is more likely to be successful if both mother and baby are of 'normal' proportions.[14]

When contemplating a trial of vaginal breech delivery, the fetal presentation should be either extended (frank) or flexed (complete), with no evidence of feto-pelvic disproportion and a clinically 'adequate' pelvis. Although clinical judgement is subjective, no other form of pelvimetry has been proven to be of increased benefit and not need to be used routinely. X-ray pelvimetry has figured prominently in protocols for planned vaginal birth, but none of these studies was able to confirm the value of this examination in selecting women who were

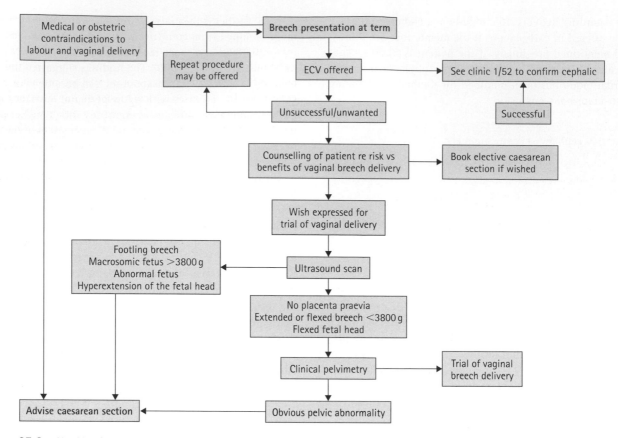

Figure 35.2   Algorithm for the management of breech presentation at term. ECV, external cephalic version

more likely to succeed in a trial of labour or in having any effect on perinatal outcome. In another sub-analysis of the Term Breech Trial, the use of radiological pelvimetry was not linked to improved outcome [Ib].[12]

Ultrasonographic estimation of the fetal weight should be undertaken, with macrosomic infants >3800 g being excluded. By performing such a scan, fetuses with severe abnormalities, hyperextension of the fetal neck or presenting with a footling breech may be excluded.

A management algorithm is shown in Figure 35.2.

INTRAPARTUM MANAGEMENT

Should the patient choose to opt for a trial of vaginal delivery, careful monitoring of fetal well-being must be ensured. In the 7th Annual Confidential Enquiry into Stillbirth and Deaths in Infancy (CESDI) report, the single and most avoidable factor associated with breech stillbirths and deaths among breech babies was suboptimal care in labour. It is important to remember that an accurate assessment of the fetal acid–base status may be obtained by sampling blood from the fetal buttocks when the fetal heart rate trace is suspect.[15] However, many clinicians will advise that, should fetal blood sampling be required to facilitate the management during a breech delivery, intervention by caesarean section should be the management course of choice.

It is important to note that despite the 'rigid' entry criteria of the Term Breech Trial, there were still frequent incidents of

suboptimal care, including the misinterpretation of suspicious or pathological CTGs, delays in asking for senior help and clinical inexperience at the time of delivery that may well have exacerbated the risks for an already hypoxic baby.[11]

Procedure: vaginal term breech delivery

Ultrasonographic examination of the fetus is essential in determining those infants suitable for trial of vaginal delivery.

- An estimation of the fetal weight, within its limitations of ±15 per cent at term, may exclude those macrosomic fetuses for whom a vaginal delivery would be somewhat more hazardous. A cut-off of 3.8 kg has been suggested (a figure not based on any specific scientific evaluation), but it should be remembered that the error of ultrasound estimation of fetal weight is greater in the breech than in the vertex-presenting fetus.
- The presence of a 'star gazing' or hyperextended fetal neck is an important finding associated with spinal cord and brain injuries during birth. Although the aetiology is not known, proposed causative factors include a nuchal cord (cord around the fetal neck), fundal placenta, spasm of the fetal neck musculature and uterine abnormalities. Extension >90° is associated with a particularly poor prognosis, and delivery by caesarean section is to be recommended with such findings.

Table 35.1 Fetal and maternal morbidity as a result of breech delivery

Fetal	Low Apgar scores at birth reflecting poor 'overall' condition
	Intracranial haemorrhage
	Medullary coning
	Occipital diastasis
	Severance of the spinal cord
	Hypopituitarism
	Brachial plexus injury
	Long-term neurological damage
	Fracture of the fetal long bones and epiphyseal separation
	Rupture of the internal organs
	Genital damage in the male
	Damage to the mouth and pharynx
Maternal	Soft tissue injuries to genital tract with increased morbidity

It is probably wise to perform a clinical examination of the pelvis to exclude the obvious deformities associated with a contracted pelvis, but more formal estimation of the pelvic structures is of limited value.

Close consultation with the mother and her partner and counselling about the implications of the choice of vaginal breech delivery versus delivery by caesarean section are some of the most important issues to be addressed.

Risks of vaginal breech delivery

All risks to both the mother and fetus must be by comparison with the alternative method of delivery available, specifically caesarean section. Whereas short-term problems are often obvious, many of the more subtle long-term problems encountered may actually be due to the fact that breech presentation itself may be a bad prognostic variable, and that being born by breech is risky regardless of the route of delivery (Table 35.1).

In the Term Breech Trial, the excess neonatal morbidity was approximately 1 per cent and the neonatal morbidity 15 per cent.

Procedure: breech delivery

The principle of vaginal breech delivery is to allow the spontaneous delivery of the fetus through the combination of uterine activity and maternal expulsive efforts. Operator intervention should be limited to a few well-timed manoeuvres, with injudicious traction on the fetal body or limbs avoided at all costs. Not only can traction lead to direct injury, such interventions may also increase displacement of the fetal limbs from their normal attitude, increasing the relative disproportion between fetus and pelvis that may already exist.

The mechanism of delivery is divided into three stages: delivery of the fetal hips (bitrochanteric diameter), delivery of the shoulders (bi-acromial diameter), and delivery of the head (biparietal diameter).

With a breech, the presenting part usually engages with the bitrochanteric diameter occupying the oblique or transverse plane at the pelvic inlet. With the sacrum anterior, the

anterior hip leads and, on meeting the pelvic floor, is rotated anteriorly beneath the pubic arch. Should the posterior hip reach the pelvic floor first, it undergoes long anterior rotation. The breech is then held up behind the pubic arch, lateral flexion allowing the posterior hip to be born first. The fetus then straightens as the anterior hip is delivered, the legs and feet following. As the shoulders enter the brim in the oblique or transverse diameters, the trunk undergoes external rotation. The shoulders then descend and undergo internal rotation, which brings them into the antero-posterior diameter of the pelvic outlet. The third and final part to enter the pelvis is the fetal head. This rotates until the posterior part of the neck becomes fixed under the subpubic arch and the head is born by flexion.

MANAGEMENT DURING THE FIRST STAGE

Labour should be conducted within a setting that allows rapid intervention by caesarean section should the clinical situation demand it (in the Term Breech Trial, 50 per cent of emergency caesarean deliveries were for failure to progress and 29 per cent for fetal distress).[11] On arrival in the labour ward, the diagnosis of labour and presentation of the fetus by the breech should be confirmed, intravenous access established and fetal monitoring commenced.

An epidural anaesthetic *may* be recommended in order to prevent involuntary expulsive efforts prior to full cervical dilatation, and to permit emergency delivery by caesarean section should the clinical situation demand it. However, **epidural anaesthesia is not essential**, and in fact there may be a higher chance of obtaining a successful vaginal delivery without it [III].[16] The use of oxytocin to stimulate uterine contractions should be discouraged in the light of the Term Breech Trial findings, and any failure to make the expected progress in cervical dilatation or for the breech to descend appropriately in the first stage of labour should prompt careful consideration of whether caesarean section is advisable. However, augmentation of uterine activity may still have a place in the management of a few select cases, but only after careful review of the facts, senior obstetric advice and, most importantly, discussion with the mother and her partner concerning their wishes.

MANAGEMENT DURING THE SECOND STAGE

The active second stage of labour only begins with full cervical dilatation and visualization of the fetal anus at the perineum, and *must* be managed by an operator trained in the delivery of the breech. There are different opinions about the best way to manage a breech delivery and there is no evidence to support one method above the other. In some countries (such as The Netherlands), spontaneous breech delivery is the norm. In the UK assisted delivery is taught, and in some parts of the USA the Bracht manoeuvre is popular.

In an assisted breech delivery the lithotomy position should be adopted, supine hypotension being avoided by lateral tilt by insertion of a wedge. A pudendal block can be provided if an epidural is not in situ. An episiotomy may be

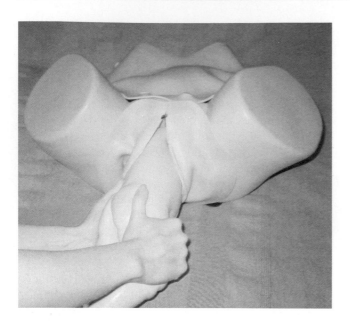

Figure 35.3   Breech delivery (see text for details)

performed at this stage as it will facilitate the manual and forceps manipulation of the after-coming head and may be exceedingly difficult to perform at a later stage of the delivery process.

The breech should be allowed to deliver spontaneously to the level of the umbilicus, rotation of the fetus to sacro-anterior being the only correction permitted if it is not in this position already (Figure 35.3). Flexion of the fetal knee by pressure in the popliteal fossa associated with abduction of the thigh will aid delivery of the legs, which should then be supported. A loop of cord is then 'brought down' to minimize traction and the risks of traumatic cord injury. Ideally, the remainder of the delivery from this stage should be achieved with the minimum of interference, but this is seldom the case.

Once the legs and abdomen have emerged, the fetus should be allowed to hang from the perineum until the wings of the posterior scapula are seen. The arms are frequently folded across the fetal chest, and require no particular manoeuvres to expedite their delivery. No attempt should be made to deliver an arm until the scapula and one axilla are visible. If injudicious traction is employed, extension of the arms above the fetal head may require Lovset's manoeuvre to free them. In this case, the fetus is grasped over the bony pelvis, with the accoucheur's thumbs along the sacrum, and turned so as to bring the posterior arm anterior (Figure 35.4) The elbow will appear below the symphysis pubis and that arm is subsequently delivered by sweeping it across the fetal body (Figure 35.5). This manoeuvre should then be repeated with the other arm.

A nuchal arm – the arm lying above and behind the fetal head (flexed at the elbow and extended at the shoulder) – is often the consequence of inappropriate traction on the breech. It is best dealt with in one of the following ways.

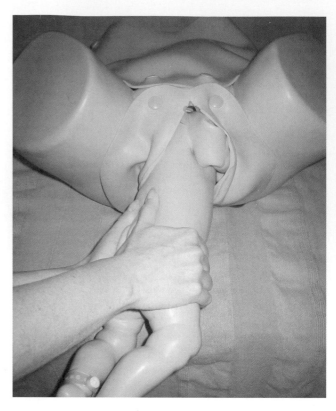

Figure 35.4   Lovset's manoeuvre. The fetus is grasped over the bony pelvis with the accoucheur's thumbs along the sacrum. The fetus is the turned so as to bring the posterior arm anterior

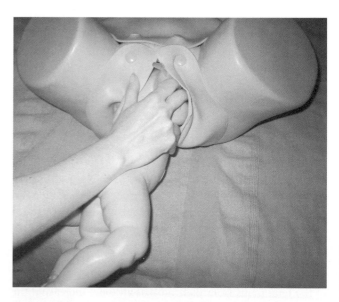

Figure 35.5   Lovset's manoeuvre. The elbow will appear below the symphysis pubis and that arm is subsequently delivered by sweeping it across the fetal body

- A modified Lovset's manoeuvre – rotating the fetal back in the direction of the trapped arm, thus forcing the elbow towards the fetal face and over the fetal head. Once 'free', a more traditional Lovset's intervention may then be performed.

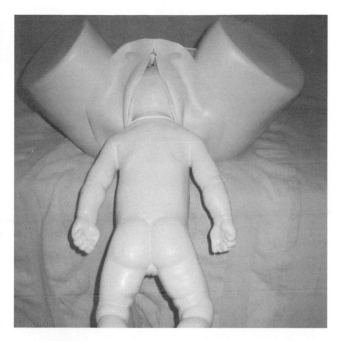

Figure 35.6 Once the legs and abdomen have emerged, the fetus should be allowed to hang from the perineum until the wings of the posterior scapula are seen

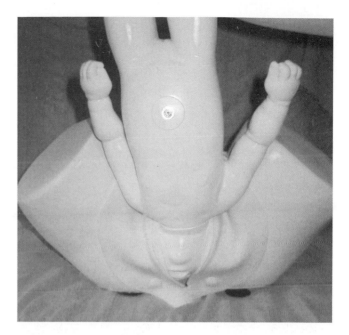

Figure 35.7 The Burns-Marshall technique (see text for details)

- If this technique fails, grasping the arm by hooking a finger over it may result in its delivery – but is also likely to result in a humeral fracture.
- If this does not work, as a last resort, general anaesthesia should be induced, the body of the fetus 'pushed up' the hand passed along the ventral surface and the most accessible arm brought down.

The fetus should then be allowed to hang from the vulva for a few seconds – 'as long as it takes the accoucheur to wash their hands' (Figure 35.6) – until the nape of the neck is visible at the anterior vulva. This allows the head to descend into the pelvis and avoid the complications of hyperextension that can occur with traction at this stage. The duration of time that should be allowed to lapse from the visualization of the umbilicus to the fetal mouth clearing the perineum is 10–15 minutes.

Delivery of the fetal head
THE BURNS-MARSHALL TECHNIQUE (Figure 35.7)
The operator's assistant should grasp the ankles of the fetus and raise the body vertically above the mother's abdomen. This promotes flexion of the fetal head and encourages it into the anterior–posterior diameter of the pelvic outlet. This often allows spontaneous delivery of the fetal head without further intervention, and it is therefore advisable to protect the perineum, by covering it with a hand, to prevent precipitate delivery and severe perineal trauma. Forceps may be applied in the usual fashion to facilitate and slow delivery of the fetal head. Too rapid an extraction may result in decompression forces on the fetal skull inducing intracranial bleeding or tentorial tears.

MAURICEAU–SMELLIE–VEIT MANOEUVRE
(Figure 35.8)
With the fetus supported on the right forearm of the accoucheur, the middle finger is placed into the fetal throat and the forefinger and ring finger are placed either on the malar eminences. Pressure is applied to the fetal tongue to encourage flexion of the head and thus present the favourable suboccipito-bregmatic diameters to the pelvis. The accoucheur's left hand is then employed to exert pressure on the fetal occiput to encourage further flexion.

FORCEPS APPLICATION (Figure 35.9)
The application of forceps may be required to aid delivery of the head. Straight forceps, such as Kielland' forceps, are often easier to apply than Neville–Barnes or Andersons. (Piper's forceps are specifically designed for this task but are unavailable in most obstetric units in the UK.) These should be applied in the usual fashion but must be placed below the fetal body. As the smallest part of the fetal head is lowest in the vagina, the accoucheur must ensure that the forceps blades accommodate the occiput. Premature straightening of the blades may not only result in undue pressures on the fetal head, but may also expose the maternal soft tissues to the perils of instrumental trauma.

Whatever technique is employed, the fetal head should be delivered slowly to reduce the chances of decompression injuries occurring to the fetal skull and brain.

Should the head fail to descend into the pelvis following delivery of the shoulders:

- the body of the fetus should be turned sideways and suprapubic pressure applied to increase flexion and encourage entry through the pelvic inlet in the

Second stage of labour

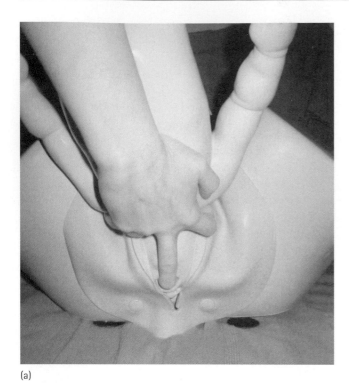

(a)

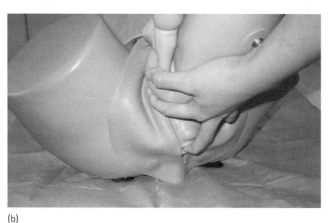

(b)

Figure 35.8   The Mauriceau–Smellie–Veit manoeuvre (see text for details)

occipito-lateral position; a McRobert's manoeuvre may help;

- consideration must be given to incising the cervix (preferably at 4 and 8 o'clock) should descent have begun before full cervical dilatation is achieved;
- consideration must be given to the possibility of fetal abnormalities such as hydrocephalus – ultrasound confirmation may be helpful; vaginal delivery may only be possible in cases of hydrocephalus by drainage of cerebrospinal fluid aspiration through the foramen magnum.

It is important to note that a paediatrician should always be present at delivery.

Although these manoeuvres have been practised for many years, they actually bear little resemblance to what happens

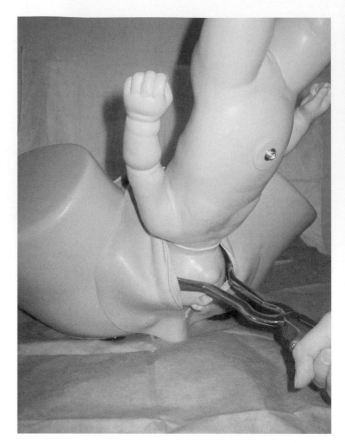

Figure 35.9   The application of forceps (see text for details)

during a spontaneous breech delivery. Bracht has described an alternative set of manoeuvres, which not only appear to be safe for the mother and baby, but are also less complicated for the accoucheur to perform.[17]

Breech extraction

With breech extraction, the obstetrician delivers the infant with little or no assistance from the mother. The only indication for performing a breech extraction is to deliver a second twin. Before starting, the accoucheur must ensure that the cervix is fully dilated and that there are no mechanical obstacles to delivery. A footling presentation is frequently easier to extract than a flexed or extended breech, and in such a case Pinard's manoeuvre should be employed to deliver the foot. Groin traction is performed to draw the breech over the perineum, Lovset's manoeuvre to facilitate delivery of the arm, and downward traction to bring the fetal head into the pelvis.

Caesarean section (see Chapter 31)

Both elective and emergency caesarean delivery for the term breech should present few problems for the obstetrician, although extension of the uterine incision into a J shape may be required to facilitate access. However, performance of a caesarean section does not prevent the possibility of birth injury, especially with injuries concerning the fetal abdominal organs, spine and head, and precautions similar to those undertaken with a vaginal breech delivery should be observed.

Training

There have been major changes in the organization of junior doctors' work patterns over the last few years and coincidentally in the management of breech pregnancies. Over a 10-year period it appears that there has been a ten-fold reduction in vaginal breech delivery experience for UK registrars. As this number can be expected to fall further following the conclusions of the Term Breech Trial, alternative methods of training urgently need to be introduced (e.g. videos, models and scenario teaching) and regular updates performed.

Any woman who gives birth to a breech vaginally should be cared for by an attendant(s) with suitable experience.

Management of the twin breech

In the majority of studies to date, the major problems associated with vaginal breech delivery relate to fetal distress in labour and difficult delivery. However, these trials only include singleton pregnancies and do not specifically address the problems for twins. Nevertheless, the plan for delivery will need careful consideration and full discussion with the parents, preferably before the onset of labour.

Although many clinicians choose caesarean section when the first twin presents as a breech because of concern about 'interlocking', this complication is extremely rare. It is equally as important to realize that no changes in neonatal morbidity or mortality in breech-presenting twins (first and second) were noted in one study over a time period during which the caesarean section rate increased dramatically (21 per cent to almost 95 per cent) [III].[18] There was, however an increase in maternal mortality in association with caesarean delivery during the same interval.

Where the second twin is non-vertex (about 40 per cent of twins), it is the consensus opinion that vaginal delivery is safe [IV]; studies show no difference in 5-minute Apgar scores or in any other indices of neonatal morbidity or mortality between the two groups.

There is insufficient evidence to support caesarean section for the delivery of the first or second twin.

Documentation

It is essential that all details of care be clearly documented, including:

- the risks and benefits to both the mother and baby of each management plan discussed,
- the agreed management plan for labour,
- clear contemporaneous documentation of the events of labour,
- the identity of all those involved in the procedures,
- postnatal cord blood pH records.

- Thirty per cent of breech presentations are not diagnosed until the onset of labour. Abdominal palpation has been shown to have a sensitivity of 28 per cent and specificity of 94 per cent. Confirmation of the presentation by ultrasound scan should be regarded as the 'gold standard'.
- ECV has been demonstrated to be associated with a significant reduction in the risk of caesarean section (OR 0.4; 95 per cent CI 0.3–0.6).
- The Term Breech Trial confirmed that vaginal delivery is more hazardous than elective caesarean section, with the overall risk of perinatal death for the term frank/complete breech fetus when delivered by planned caesarean birth being reduced by 75 per cent (RR 0.23; 95 per cent CI 0.07–0.8).
- In a sub-analysis of the Term Breech Trial, the risk of the *combined outcome* of perinatal mortality, neonatal mortality or serious neonatal morbidity with planned caesarean section compared with planned vaginal birth was 16/1006 (1.6 per cent) compared with 23/704 (3.3 per cent) (RR 0.49; 95 per cent CI 0.26–0.91; $p = 0.02$).

KEY POINTS

- Breech presentation, whatever the mode of delivery, is a signal for potential fetal handicap and this should inform antenatal, intrapartum and neonatal management. Each patient requires individualized attention and evaluation.
- At term, the first question that must be addressed when confronted by a breech presentation is 'Where is the placenta?'; the second is 'Is the fetus normal?'.
- All women with an uncomplicated breech pregnancy at term (37–42 weeks) should be offered ECV.
- Planned caesarean section greatly reduces both perinatal/neonatal mortality and neonatal morbidity, at the expense of somewhat increased maternal morbidity. The questions of long-term morbidity and the cost implications of implementing a policy of caesarean section for all breech deliveries have not been addressed.
- Evidence from the Term Breech Trial *cannot* be directly extrapolated to preterm breech delivery. As a consequence, the management of the preterm breech remains an area of clinical controversy. ECV before term has not been shown to offer any benefits.

- The most experienced obstetrician available should manage labour, with continuous fetal monitoring as standard. Epidural anaesthesia may be provided if the mother so wishes, but is not compulsory. Premature expulsive efforts must be discouraged, as these can lead to head entrapment, nuchal arms and hyperextension of the fetal head.

KEY REFERENCES

1. Cheng MH. Breech delivery at term: a critical review of the literature. *Obstet Gynecol* 1993; **82**:605–18.
2. Danielian PJ, Wang J, Hall MH. Long-term outcome by method of delivery of fetuses in breech presentation at term: population-based follow up. *BMJ* 1996; **312**:1451–3.
3. Penn ZJ. Breech presentation. In: James DK, Steer PJ, Weiner CP, Gonik B (eds). *High Risk Pregnancy, Management Options.* London: WB Saunders, 1999, 1025–50.
4. Mazor M, Hagay ZJ, Leiberman J, Biale Y, Insler V. Fetal abnormalities associated with breech delivery. *J Reprod Med* 1985; **30**:884–6.
5. Grant A. Elective vs. selective caesarean for delivery of the small baby (Cochrane Review). In: *The Cochrane Library*, Issue 2. Oxford: Update Software, 2002.
6. Hofmeyr GJ, Kulier R. Cephalic version by postural management for breech presentation. In: *The Cochrane Library*, Issue 2. Oxford: Update Software, 2002.
7. Hofmeyr GJ, Kulier R. External cephalic version for breech presentation at term. *In: The Cochrane Library*, Issue 2. Oxford: Update Software, 2002.
8. Hofmeyr GJ. External cephalic version for breech presentation before term (Cochrane Review). In: *The Cochrane Library*, Issue 2. Oxford: Update Software, 2002.
9. Hofmeyr GJ, Gülmezoglu AM. Maternal hydration for increasing amniotic fluid volume in oligohydramnios and normal amniotic fluid volume (Cochrane Review). In: *The Cochrane Library*, Issue 2. Oxford: Update Software, 2002.
10. Royal College of Obstetricians and Gynaecologists. *The Management of Breech Presentation*, Guideline No. 20. London: RCOG Press, 2001.
11. Tatum RK, Orr JW, Soong S, Huddleston JF. Vaginal breech delivery of selected infants weighing more than 2000 g. A retrospective analysis of 7 years of experience. *Am J Obstet Gynecol* 1985; **152**:145–55.
12. Hannah ME, Hannah WJ, Hewson SA, Hodnett ED, Saigal S, Willan AR. Term Breech Trial Collaborative Group. Planned caesarean section versus planned vaginal birth for breech presentation at term: a randomised multicentre trial. *Lancet* 2000; **356**:1375–83.
13. Lumley J. Any room left for disagreement about assisting breech births at term? [Commentary] *Lancet* 2000; **356**:1368–9.
14. Recommendations of the FIGO Committee on Perinatal Health on Guidelines for the Management of Breech Delivery. *Eur J Obstet Gynecol Reprod Biol* 1995; **58**:89–92.
15. Brady K, Duff P, Read JA, Harlass FE. Reliability of fetal buttock sampling in assessing the acid–base balance of the breech fetus. *Obstet Gynecol* 1989; **74**:886–8.
16. Chadha YC, Mahmood TA, Dick MJ, Smith NC, Campbell DM, Templeton AA. Breech delivery and epidural analgesia. *Br J Obstet Gynaecol* 1992; **99**:96–100.
17. Edelstone DI. Breech presentation. In: Kean LH, Baker PN, Edelstone DI (eds). *Best Practice in Labor Ward Management.* Edinburgh: WB Saunders, 2000, 141–65.
18. Oettinger M, Ophir E, Markovitz J, Stolero E, Odeh M. Is caesarean section necessary for delivery of a breech first twin? *Gynecol Obstet Invest* 1993; **35**:38–43.

Chapter 36

Perineal Trauma

Lucy Kean

INTRODUCTION

Perineal trauma is a common event in first labours, affecting up to 90 per cent of first-time mothers. It is a cause for concern for many women and in some countries has led to a large increase in the numbers of women requesting elective caesarean section. Considerable postnatal morbidity and occasionally mortality can be attributed to this, and therefore a clear understanding of the best management of perineal trauma is mandatory for every clinician working in obstetrics.

ANATOMY OF THE PELVIC FLOOR AND DEFINITIONS OF TRAUMA

In order to understand the pathophysiology of perineal trauma, an understanding of the anatomy of the pelvic floor is required.

First-degree and second-degree trauma corresponds to lacerations of the vaginal epithelium alone or including the perineal body, transverse perineal and bulbocavernosus muscles. Larger incisions or tears may include the pubococcygeous and extend into the ischiorectal fossa. Figure 36.1 shows the muscles of the perineum and the usual extensions of mediolateral and midline episiotomy.

Third-degree extensions involve any part of the anal sphincter complex (external and internal sphincters) and fourth-degree encompasses extension into the rectal mucosa.

The Royal College of Obstetricians and Gynaecologists (RCOG) of the UK recommends classifying anal sphincter damage as follows.[1]

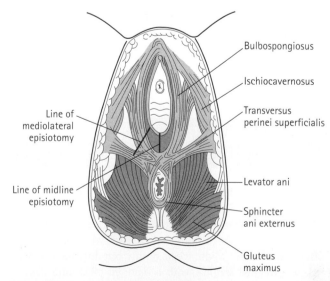

Figure 36.1 Muscles of the perineum

Bulbospongiosus

Ischiocavernosus

Transversus perinei superficialis

Line of mediolateral episiotomy

Line of midline episiotomy

Levator ani

Sphincter ani externus

Gluteus maximus

– 3a: less than 50 per cent of the external anal sphincter is torn.
– 3b: more than 50 per cent of the external anal sphincter is torn.
– 3c: tear involving the internal anal sphincter (almost always involves complete disruption of the external sphincter).
– Fourth degree: injury to the anal sphincter complex extending into the rectal mucosa.

The college acknowledge that identification of trauma to the internal sphincter is very difficult in the acute setting, therefore the simpler definition of third-degree and fourth-degree trauma is likely to be more applicable in practice.

SECOND-DEGREE PERINEAL TRAUMA

In a first pregnancy, second-degree trauma affects up to 90 per cent of women, with episiotomy rates of 40–60 per cent being common in many large hospitals. The perineum following delivery is often the source of much discomfort and pain for many women. Morbidity to the perineum may persist for weeks to years post-delivery. This can result in a cascade of events such as dyspareunia, psychosexual dysfunction, maladjustment to motherhood and relationship breakdown. Minimizing the risk of perineal trauma should therefore be at the forefront of care during labour.

RISK FACTORS FOR PERINEAL TRAUMA

It is recognized that perineal trauma is associated with:

- larger infants,
- prolonged labour,
- instrumental delivery.

Instrumental delivery and forceps delivery carry a particularly large increase in the risk of extended trauma, with as many as 60 per cent of women experiencing ultrasonographically visible anal sphincter defects in research studies. Long second stage also appears to contribute to perineal damage.

REDUCING THE RISK OF PERINEAL TRAUMA

The role of episiotomy

Liberal use of mediolateral episiotomy does not appear to reduce the incidence of third-degree tears, with the exception of two small trials. Midline episiotomy certainly increases the risk of extended trauma, with a reported odds ratio (OR) of 4.5–6 for third-degree or fourth-degree tears. It is important to recognize that there are significant differences in extension rates for mediolateral and midline episiotomies. Meta-analyses that do not make this distinction are unlikely adequately to assess the effect of episiotomy. Where episiotomy is restricted, an increase in anterior vaginal trauma is seen, but this does not necessarily equate to an increase in urinary problems. Thus there is now good evidence to support a restrictive policy for episiotomy (absolute risk difference −0.23, 95 per cent confidence interval [CI] −0.35, −0.11 [Ib].[2]

Perineal massage

In nulliparae during the weeks before giving birth, perineal massage appears to protect against perineal trauma (risk difference −0.08, 95 per cent CI −0.12, −0.04) [Ia].[3]

The conduct of delivery has also been examined in the 'Hands on or Hands Poised' study, in which the standard delivery technique of controlled delivery of the head was compared with a more spontaneous delivery. Changing established practice is obviously difficult, as there was only 73 per cent compliance in the 'hands poised' group (vs 95 per cent in 'hands on'). The rates of perineal trauma were similar in both groups: 29 per cent first-degree trauma and 37 per cent second-degree trauma. There were slightly fewer episiotomies in the 'hands poised' group (10 vs 13 per cent) and very slightly less pain at 10 days in the 'hands on' group (34 vs 31 per cent). Thus, conduct of the delivery in this setting showed no advantage of one method over the other [Ib].[4]

Mode of delivery

Mode of delivery has a large impact on rates of perineal trauma. Of course, elective caesarean section prevents damage to the perineum from labour-related events, and reducing the rates of instrumental vaginal delivery will reduce the incidence of perineal trauma.

Ventouse delivery appears to be associated with less perineal trauma (see Chapter 34). Ventouse delivery (risk difference −0.06, 95 per cent CI −0.10, −0.02) and spontaneous birth (−0.11, 95 per cent CI −0.18, −0.04) causes less anal sphincter trauma than forceps delivery.[3] However, at 5-year follow-up there is no difference in reported symptoms in women delivered by either ventouse or forceps. Therefore, given that the highest rates of severe perineal damage occur in women for whom two instruments are needed to achieve delivery, the first choice must be the instrument most likely to deliver the baby safely and with which the obstetrician is experienced.[5,6]

Episiotomy has been recommended when instrumental vaginal delivery is performed. This is not based on any evidence, and a more flexible approach is needed. Ventouse delivery in a multiparous woman may not require any episiotomy, and an intact perineum may result. However, a forceps delivery in a nulliparous woman is likely to require episiotomy.

Epidural analgesia and prolonged second stage

There are two issues here. The first is that epidural analgesia has been shown to be associated with an increased risk of instrumental vaginal delivery, with the attendant perineal morbidity.[7] The second is that there is an association between long second stage and perineal trauma, with increased risk of severe trauma in women experiencing long second stages. However, it has been shown that allowing a passive second stage in nulliparae with continuous epidural analgesia reduces the incidence of difficult instrumental delivery (relative risk (RR), 0.79; 95 per cent CI, 0.66–0.95). Spontaneous delivery is also slightly more likely among women who delay pushing (RR, 1.09; 95 per cent CI, 1.00–1.18).[8] Given that instrumental delivery represents the greatest risk to the perineum, it is probably better to allow descent of the head with passive second stages, but further research is needed to evaluate the risks and benefits fully.

Position for delivery

The mother's position during the second stage has little influence on perineal trauma (supported upright vs recumbent: risk difference 0.02, 95 per cent CI, −0.05, −0.09).[3] Women should be allowed to adopt any position for delivery that they are comfortable with, provided delivery can be achieved safely.

REPAIR TECHNIQUES FOR FIRST-DEGREE AND SECOND-DEGREE TRAUMA

Adequate lighting, analgesia and any necessary assistance are mandatory before attempting to repair a tear or episiotomy. It is unacceptable to perform a perineal repair with inadequate analgesia.

Before commencing a repair, a full examination should take place. The vaginal apex must be identified and the anal sphincter inspected.

The standard technique is to close the vaginal epithelium, perineal muscles and then skin (three stage). An interlocking suture to the vaginal epithelium is often taught, to prevent foreshortening of the vagina. There is no evidence that a locking suture is necessary, and a loose unlocked suture may be less uncomfortable for the mother (see below).

Minor first-degree trauma that is not bleeding does not need closure. Some authors use a continuous suture technique to perform the entire repair, finishing with a subcuticular skin suture. It is vital to ensure that the apex of the vaginal component is secured, as paravaginal haematoma formation can occur if the apex is missed. When individual bleeding arteries are identified, they should be ligated separately. Once the repair is complete, it is important to perform the following.

1 Remove any vaginal tampon placed to aid visualization.
2 Count swabs and ensure none is retained.
3 Count and dispose carefully of any needles.
4 Inspect the repair to ensure vascular haemostasis.
5 Perform a rectal examination to ensure no sutures have breached the rectal mucosa and to palpate the anal sphincter to ensure it is intact.
6 Prescribe analgesia.

Evidence for suture technique

There has been little change to the standard method of perineal repair. However a Cochrane Review has examined the evidence for interrupted versus subcuticular skin repair and shown that subcuticular sutures are associated with less pain up to 10 days (OR 0.68; 95 per cent CI 0.53–0.86) [Ia].[9] The Ipswich Childbirth Study randomized women to either a two-stage or a three-stage repair (two stages are closure of vagina and perineal tissue but not skin, as long as the skin edges can be approximated to within 5 mm). A two-stage repair was associated with less long-term perineal dysaesthesia (30 per cent vs 40 per cent; RR 0.75, 95 per cent CI 0.61–0.91) and less discomfort when sexual intercourse resumed [Ib].[10]

Recent work shows that a continuous repair utilizing a non-locking vaginal suture is associated with less pain at 10 days than a standard interrupted repair ($p < 0.0001$, 95 per cent CI 0.38–0.58). This difference was seen regardless of the experience of the operator or the material used.[11] Also, significantly less suture material was needed with a continuous repair, with 79 per cent of repairs being completed with a single suture packet compared with 32 per cent of repairs using an interrupted technique. More women in the continuous suture group felt that they were back to normal at 3 months. However, no differences in outcomes at 12 months were seen between the groups [Ib].

Evidence for suture material

Much effort has been dedicated towards comparing different types of suture material. Catgut has been widely compared with polyglycolic acid sutures (Dexon™ and Vicryl™) and the conclusion is that catgut was associated with more short-term pain. However, in the UK the manufacturers have now withdrawn catgut. The above study assessing technique also addressed the issue of short versus medium half-life polyglactin sutures (Vicryl™ vs Vicryl Rapide™, Ethicon, UK). The primary end-point for the study of pain at 10 days showed no difference between the two suture types, though more women with standard Vicryl sutures required analgesia in the preceding 24 hours and more women experienced pain on walking. Suture material was much less likely to need removal at a later stage in the group sutured with the more rapidly absorbed polyglactin suture. At 10 days, the midwives were more likely to comment that the wound was gaping in the group sutured with the rapidly absorbed suture (6.1 per cent vs 3.4 per cent; 95 per cent CI 1.14–2.92), although at 3 months the outcomes were no different [Ib].

Braided sutures have not been compared with monofilament sutures.

Follow-up

In general, most first-degree and second-degree perineal repairs will heal without problems. Important issues relate to the failure to identify anal sphincter damage, which may only become apparent later. Women who have experienced difficult vaginal deliveries may value the opportunity to discuss their delivery at a later date.

The ideal setting for follow-up for women experiencing persistent problems after delivery is a dedicated perineal dysfunction clinic. This is not available in most units at present, but a team approach involving obstetricians and physiotherapists, with access to appropriate investigative techniques such as endoanal ultrasound and manometry, is important. Urinary problems are amenable to biofeedback techniques, and physiotherapy input is vital to ensure that these are appropriately taught and reinforced.

THIRD-DEGREE AND FOURTH-DEGREE TRAUMA

Incidence

Internal anal sphincter incompetence results in insensible faecal incontinence, whereas external anal sphincter incompetence causes faecal urgency. Third-degree tears are reported in approximately 2.8 per cent of primigravidae and 0.4 per cent of multigravidae. The reported rates will vary amongst units with different rates of instrumental delivery. New-onset symptoms of faecal incontinence are reported in 10 per cent of primigravidae undergoing instrumental vaginal delivery at 10 months, and in 3 per cent of primigravidae undergoing spontaneous vaginal delivery. Some of these new symptoms are attributable to pudendal neuropathy, as 5 per cent of women report new symptoms after emergency caesarean section, whereas new onset bowel symptoms are very uncommon after elective caesarean section. Some degree of faecal urgency probably related to occult anal sphincter damage is much more common, with 44 per cent of women reporting this at 5 years following instrumental delivery of their first baby.

Ultrasonographically visible anal sphincter defects are apparent in 82 per cent of women undergoing forceps delivery and in 48 per cent of ventouse deliveries.[12] However, most women report infrequent problems, and there is no difference in long-term follow-up between forceps and ventouse delivery.[5]

Research studies investigating anal sphincter damage have demonstrated sphincter defects visible on ultrasound in 40 per cent of women after vaginal delivery of their first baby, though two-thirds of these will be asymptomatic.[13] The much higher incidence of problems demonstrated in research studies underlines two important facts:

1 women are embarrassed about faecal problems after childbirth,
2 ultrasonographically demonstrated lesions do not translate into confirmed problems of faecal continence.

Anal sphincter damage is mainly limited to first deliveries, whereas pudendal nerve damage can be cumulative. Pudendal nerve damage occurs during labour as the nerve becomes compressed and stretched. Delivery late in first stage or second stage by caesarean section does not prevent this. It has also been shown that ultrasonographically visible anal sphincter defects can be demonstrated in women who were demonstrated to have an intact anal sphincter at the time of delivery. The mechanism for this late disruption is unclear. It may be related to infection or haematoma formation, or possibly to partial unrecognized sphincter ruptures.

Risk factors for third-degree and fourth-degree tears

The risk factors for third-degree and fourth-degree tears are shown in Table 36.1.

Shoulder dystocia is also implicated. Risk factors are cumulative, and in some cases the risks may be greater than the sum of two individual risks, for instance the risk of severe trauma when two instruments are needed is much greater than the summed risks for each individual instrument.

Table 36.1   Factors associated with increased risk of third-degree tears

	Odds ratio
Primigravida	2–7
Second stage of labour of >60 minutes (including passive second stage)	2
Instrumental vaginal delivery	1.7–7
Midline episiotomy	5–11
Macrosomia	2.9
Persistent occipito-posterior position	1.7
Epidural analgesia	1.5
Prior third-degree tear	4

Repair

Identification of extent of damage

All women sustaining perineal trauma should be carefully examined to assess the severity of damage to the perineum, vagina and rectum. All staff performing perineal repair must be confident in their ability to diagnose anal sphincter injury. It is imperative to examine carefully for rectal extension, as small buttonhole tears can be overlooked and lead to fistula formation.

When disrupted, the anal sphincter retracts, forming a dimple on either side of the anal canal. Rupture of the rectal mucosa will almost always involve damage to both the internal and external anal sphincters.

A good repair of the sphincter is imperative, as this is the factor most strongly associated with future faecal continence.

Conduct of the repair

There is no evidence to suggest that an overlap technique is better than end-to-end approximation of the muscle [Ib].[14] It is important to ensure that the muscle is correctly approximated with long-acting sutures so that it is given adequate time to heal.

The repair must be performed or directly supervised by a practitioner trained in the repair of third-degree and fourth-degree trauma. There must be adequate analgesia. In practice, this means either a regional or general anaesthetic, as local infiltration does not allow enough relaxation of the sphincter to allow a satisfactory repair. The lighting must be adequate and an assistant is usually needed.

Repair of the rectal mucosa should be performed first. 2:0 polyglycolic acid interrupted sutures with the knots placed on the mucosal side are commonly used. Next, the layers of the internal sphincter should be re-plicated across the defect. The torn external sphincter is then repaired. This should be re-approximated with either three or four figure-of-eight sutures, or an overlap technique.

A 2.0 or 3.0 polydioxanone suture (PDS) is ideal. Polyglycolic acid is also used and there is no research to establish which is superior. However, the longer tensile retention of PDS is likely to make it more suitable. Short half-life treated polyglactin sutures (Vicryl Rapide™) are not acceptable as they do not have a long enough half-life to ensure muscle healing. Also, non-absorbable sutures should not be used in the acute setting as these can form a focus for infection, requiring removal.

The remainder of the perineal repair is effected as for second-degree trauma.

Postoperative precautions

It is common practice after delayed anal sphincter repair to use a constipating regimen to allow the repair to heal before stools are passed. This is difficult in recently delivered women who have very different needs from those of the surgical patient. Constipative regimens have been compared with stool-softening regimens. It is concluded that constipative management leads to more pain and a longer postoperative stay compared to stool-softening regimens, but with no difference in repair success. Lactulose and a bulk agent such as Fybogel are recommended for 5–10 days.

It is common sense to give a broad-spectrum antibiotic. It is important to include an antibiotic that will cover possible anaerobic contamination, such as metronidazole. This should be prescribed orally rather than per rectum.

Adequate oral analgesia should be prescribed. Paracetamol, non-steroidal anti-inflammatory drugs and opioid analgesia are acceptable. However, opioids used alone can exacerbate constipation, and thus the former should be used first.

Before women go home:

- ensure that the mother has had a chance to discuss the delivery with a senior member of the team;
- prescribe necessary analgesia and stool softeners;
- advise on perineal hygiene;
- provide a contact number in case problems occur;
- make an initial plan for short-term management with a physiotherapist;
- counsel that sutures occasionally migrate and fragments may be passed per vaginum or, occasionally, per rectum; help should be sought if there are concerns;
- give an appointment for follow-up.

Follow-up

All women who have sustained a third-degree or fourth-degree tear should be offered follow-up by someone interested in this field. A team approach as outlined earlier is best. Physiotherapy should include augmented biofeedback, as this has been shown to improve continence.

At 6–12 months, a full evaluation of the degree of symptoms should take place. This must include careful questioning with regard to faecal and urinary symptoms. A standard questionnaire for women to complete before attending is helpful in precisely delineating the degree of symptoms. Symptomatic women should be offered investigation, including endoanal ultrasound and manometry. Women with demonstrable sphincter defects and continuing symptoms should be counselled regarding the pros and cons of further surgery by a colorectal surgeon. As pudendal neuropathy can take at least 6 months to improve, any further surgical intervention is best deferred until at least this time; however, in exceptional cases in which sphincter disruption is demonstrated and faecal incontinence is debilitating, surgery may be required earlier.

Counselling about subsequent delivery

Women can be divided into one of three or four groups with regard to their next delivery.

Previous third/fourth-degree tear, no ongoing symptoms

These women should be counselled that there is approximately a 4 per cent risk of further anal sphincter damage in a subsequent vaginal delivery. This recurrence is not predictable antenatally. Women who were transiently incontinent after their first delivery are particularly at risk of worsening of symptoms, and 17–24 per cent may develop worsening symptoms after subsequent delivery.[14]

When women opt for subsequent vaginal delivery, every effort should be made to avoid instrumental vaginal delivery. There is no evidence that episiotomy prevents muscle damage, and most women appreciate an intact perineum if that can be achieved. The second stage should not be prolonged. Women need careful counselling about epidural analgesia with reference to both the type of delivery and length of second stage. Where anal sphincter damage does not occur, new-onset symptoms are usually attributable to pudendal neuropathy, which usually improves with time. Transient flatus incontinence is reported by 10 per cent of women delivered without further sphincter damage.

Women who continue to be symptomatic

The majority of these women will have a demonstrable defect on ultrasound. There is a risk of worsening of symptoms, which may then make life much more difficult. Women should be carefully counselled with regard to the additional effects of worsening pudendal damage and the small risk of further muscle damage. The majority of women in this group may opt for caesarean section, but for those choosing vaginal delivery, every effort should be made to avoid operative vaginal delivery and lengthy second stage.

Women who have undergone a secondary anal sphincter repair

The consensus is that these women should be delivered by caesarean section [IV]. However, there are no data to advise women who wish to try for a vaginal delivery. Again, instrumental delivery and long second stage should be avoided where possible.

Women who are asymptomatic but have demonstrable anal sphincter defects or abnormal manometry on testing

These women have only been identified in a research setting, as in most units further investigation is limited to women with symptoms. This is a difficult group to manage, as there are few data to advise management. These women are at risk of new symptoms following subsequent delivery. Those at most risk appear to be women with a full quadrant defect, and these women may wish to choose caesarean section next time [III].[15]

The plan for delivery must be clearly documented in the case notes.

Perineal trauma and female genital mutilation (circumcision)

The practice of female circumcision is very common in parts of the Middle East and Africa. In particular women from Sudan, Somalia and Nigeria are likely to have undergone this as children. The practice involves removal of parts of the female genital organs, including the labia minora, infundibulum, clitoris and, in extreme cases, the labia majora. It is illegal in the UK and many other countries. With cultural, economic and political migration, more women are presenting in pregnancy with some form of genital mutilation.

When women who are likely to have undergone these procedures are seen in antenatal clinic it is vital that they are sensitively questioned about them and that a careful plan of management is made for delivery. It is important at this vulnerable time in a woman's life not to convey prejudice about a practice that is regarded with dismay in this country. However, it is also important that matters relating to law are clearly understood by both the woman and, particularly, her husband.

Problems arising in pregnancy as a result of circumcision include lower urinary tract infection and psychological problems (especially fear of labour).

Some bodies advocate releasing scarred areas under anaesthesia prior to delivery; however, this is unacceptable to most women, and is probably unnecessary.

Special counselling and antenatal education are important for these women. They may not realize, for instance, that vaginal examination may be needed in labour. It is also very important to counsel that it is not possible under British law to re-circumcise following delivery. The law allows the perineum to be anatomically re-sutured, but suturing together of the labia is not permitted. For many women this is culturally unacceptable. In the countries of origin, the usual practice is to perform an anterior episiotomy, releasing the fused labia, and a mediolateral episiotomy if necessary. The labia are then re-sutured in the midline anteriorly. This is illegal in the UK. Thus the edges may be oversewn but not joined. Many women will prefer to undergo mediolateral episiotomy as a first-line procedure. Unfortunately, as the perineum is often very scarred, extension of tears is not uncommon, and healing is sometimes poor and delayed.

ACUTE HAEMATOMA

Incidence

The reported incidence of puerperal haematomas varies widely, ranging from 1 in 1500 to 1 in 309. However, large and clinically significant haematomas complicate between 1 in 1000 and 1 in 4000 deliveries.

Aetiological factors

- Episiotomy (85–90 per cent of cases).
- Instrumental vaginal delivery.
- Primiparity.
- Hypertensive disorders.

Multiple pregnancy, vulval varicosities, macrosomic infants and prolonged second stage have all been implicated, but their contribution is probably small.

In two-thirds of haematomas, failure to achieve perfect haemostasis at the time of repair, particularly at the upper end of the incision, has been implicated. However, haematomas can occur without any perineal laceration.

The anatomy of the perineum and vagina plays an important part in the limitation or extension of haematoma formation. Infralevator haematomas, most commonly associated with vaginal delivery, are limited superiorly by the levator ani, medially by the perineal body and from extension onto the thigh by Colles fascia and the fascia lata. These may extend into the ischiorectal fossa. They usually arise from small vulvar or labial vessels, branches of the inferior rectal, inferior vesical or vaginal branch of the uterine arteries. They usually present as vulval pain out of proportion to that expected from an episiotomy, with an ischiorectal mass and discoloration. Continued bleeding or urinary retention may also occur.

In contrast, supralevator haematomas have no fibrous boundaries. They arise from branches of the uterine artery, the inferior vesical and pudendal artery. Bleeding can track into the broad ligament, the retroperitoneal and presacral spaces. Thus they present as rectal pain and pressure, an enlarging rectal or vaginal mass or with hypovolaemic shock.

Broad ligament haematomas will cause upward and lateral displacement of the uterus. The uterus feels well contracted and there may be little revealed vaginal bleeding. As these haematomas are above the pelvic diaphragm; they are more rarely associated with vaginal delivery, although they can occur if genital trauma extends into the fornices or if a cervical tear is sustained. They may also occur in cases of uterine rupture or scar dehiscence.

Following delivery, the vulvar and paravaginal tissues are loose and oedematous. They can accommodate large amounts of blood before a haematoma becomes obvious and gives rise to symptoms (500–1500 mL). Blood loss estimation is therefore extremely difficult and is usually grossly underestimated.

Presenting symptoms

Infralevator haematomas

- Vaginal swelling.
- Continued vaginal bleeding.
- Severe rectal/vaginal pain.
- Urinary retention.

If postpartum blood loss was moderate, bleeding into the haematoma may produce signs of shock.

Supralevator haematomas

- Cardiovascular collapse.
- Uterine displacement.
- Abdominal or rectal pain.
- Continued vaginal bleeding.

Management

Small, non-expanding haematomas of less than 3 cm can be managed conservatively. Larger or expanding haematomas require surgical management to prevent pressure necrosis, septicaemia, haemorrhage and death. Full maternal resuscitation in conjunction with anaesthetic colleagues is vital. Blood loss is likely to be significantly underestimated and early recourse to transfusion is necessary. As for repair of genital trauma, adequate analgesia, assistance and lighting are needed.

If the haematoma lies beneath a repair, this should be taken down. If no repair was made, an incision in the inferior portion of the mass near the introitus should be made. Clot is evacuated and the area involved is irrigated with saline. Individual bleeding points should be ligated, although it is more common to find diffuse ooze from very friable haemorrhagic paravaginal tissue. If the tissues allow, a layered closure or primary closure should be undertaken; however, the tissues are generally very difficult to place sutures into, as they are extremely friable. If sutures appear to be tearing out, closing the defect over a soft suction drain such as a Jackson–Pratt drain with a tight pack in the vagina for 12–24 hours may achieve the necessary reduction of dead space and control of bleeding. A urethral catheter will be needed, both to allow effective bladder emptying and to monitor urinary output. Prophylactic broad-spectrum antibiotics should be given, as the risk of subsequent infection is reasonably high and late problems are often attributable to infection. There must be a high index of suspicion if repeated symptoms occur, as the risk of recurrence in the first 12–48 hours is high (approximately 10 per cent). Special vigilance after pack removal is particularly important.

Large paravaginal haematomas can be much more complicated. Extension into the retroperitoneal space or broad ligament can be life threatening. The cervix should be carefully examined to assess cervical lacerations. This is best accomplished by grasping the cervix with a sponge holder, starting at 12 o'clock. A second sponge holder is placed at 2 o'clock and the cervix examined between the two. If intact, the first holder is moved to 4 o'clock. By working around the cervix in this way the whole circumference can be examined and tears identified. Tears must be repaired with full-thickness interrupted sutures, ensuring that the apex is identified. A combined vaginal and abdominal approach may be needed to evacuate clot, identify bleeding and secure haemostasis. An abdominal approach is always needed for tears of the cervix or upper vagina where the apex cannot be identified and bleeding is occurring. **Ureteric injury can result from blindly placed deep sutures in the fornix.**

Internal iliac artery ligation, hysterectomy and radiological embolization techniques have all been described to control intractable bleeding.

Careful observation in a high dependency area is required for 12–24 hours, as recurrence of the haematoma may occur in up to 10 per cent of cases. These women are likely to have lost very large amounts of blood and the strategy for major obstetric haemorrhage should be followed. Early recourse to surgery, antibiotics and transfusion has improved maternal mortality in this life-threatening situation.

It is important that measures to reduce thromboembolism are not ignored in these women, as they have a high risk of thrombosis. Whilst many surgeons may wish to defer heparins until the risk if recurrence is lessened, other measures such as full-length thromboembolic stockings, compression boots and leg exercises can all be safely implemented without increasing the risk of recurrence.

DOCUMENTATION

Clear written notes in black ink must be made following any perineal trauma. These must include:

- a clear record of the extent of trauma,
- type of analgesia/anaesthesia,
- comprehensive notes of the procedure undertaken and suture material used (including evidence of anal sphincter examination),
- documentation of a swab and needle count before and after the procedure,
- estimated blood loss,
- postoperative instructions covering all aspects (fluid replacement, extra monitoring, antibiotics, thromboprophylaxis, stool softeners),
- pre-discharge instructions as necessary,
- follow-up needs.

The notes must be signed, with the date and time. The operator's name should be printed and a contact or pager number given if possible.

- Episiotomy does not prevent third-degree and fourth-degree tears. Midline episiotomy increases the risk of such trauma.
- Perineal massage antepartum reduces the risk of third-degree and fourth-degree trauma in primiparae by a small amount.
- There are higher rates of ultrasonographically visible anal sphincter defects after forceps compared with ventouse, but no difference in maternal symptoms at 5 years.
- Leaving the perineal skin approximated but not closed is associated with less perineal

dysaesthesia. If the skin is sutured, a subcuticular suture causes less short-term pain.
- A loose continuous repair without locking the vaginal component is associated with less short-term pain.
- Rapidly absorbed sutures are associated with as good results as standard polyglactin sutures but require removal far less frequently.
- Overlap and end-to-end approximation of the anal sphincter produce similar results after repair of third-degree tears.

KEY POINTS

- Perineal trauma is a source of post-delivery morbidity in a large number of women, especially primiparae.
- Suture techniques can be employed that minimize pain.
- The anal sphincter must be examined whenever a perineal repair is undertaken, as many sphincter ruptures are missed.
- Third-degree and fourth-degree repairs should be performed in optimal surroundings by a suitably trained operator.
- Follow-up should be conducted by a team with an interest in the management of perineal trauma.
- Documentation should include all aspects of the repair, with clear post-repair instructions.
- Women with haematomas need vigilance for recurrence in the first 24 hours after drainage.

KEY REFERENCES

1. Royal College of Obstetricians and Gynaecologists. *Management of Third- and Fourth-Degree Perineal Tears Following Vaginal Delivery*. Clinical Green Top Guideline No. 29. London: RCOG Press, 2001.
2. Wooley R.J. Benefits and risks of episiotomy: a review of the English-language literature since 1980, Parts I and II. *Obstet Gynecol Surv* 1995; **50**:806–35.
3. Eason E, Labrecque M, Wells G, Feldman P. Preventing perineal trauma during childbirth: a systematic review. *Obstet Gynecol* 2000; **95**:464–71.
4. McCandlish R, Bowler U, Van Asten H et al. A randomised controlled trial of care of the perineum during second stage of normal labour. *Br J Obstet Gynaecol* 1998; **105**:1262–72.
5. Royal College of Obstetricians and Gynaecologists. *Instrumental Vaginal Delivery*. Clinical Green Top Guideline No. 26. London: RCOG Press, 1999.

6. Johanson RB, Heycock E, Carter J, Sultan AH, Walklate K, Jones PW. Maternal and child health after assisted vaginal delivery: five year follow-up of a randomised controlled study comparing forceps and ventouse. *Br J Obstet Gynaecol* 1999; **106**:544–9.

7. Howell CJ. Epidural versus non-epidural analgesia for pain relief in labour (Cochrane Review). In: *The Cochrane Library*, Issue 2. Oxford: Update Software, 2002.

8. Fraser WD, Marcoux S, Krauss I, Douglas J, Goulet C, Boulvain M. Multicenter, randomized, controlled trial of delayed pushing for nulliparous women in the second stage of labor with continuous epidural analgesia. The PEOPLE (Pushing Early or Pushing Late with Epidural) Study Group. *Am J Obstet Gynecol* 2000; **182**:1165–72.

9. Kettle C, Johanson RB. Continuous versus interrupted sutures for perineal repair (Cochrane Review). In: *The Cochrane Library*, Issue 2. Oxford: Update Software, 2002.

10. Gordon B, Mackrodt C, Fern E, Truesdale A, Ayers S, Grant A. The Ipswich Childbirth Study: 1. A randomised evaluation of two stage postpartum perineal repair leaving the skin unsutured. *Br J Obstet Gynaecol* 1998; **105**:435–40.

11. Kettle C, Hills RK, Jones P, Darby L, Gray R, Johanson R. Continuous versus interrupted repair with standard or rapidly absorbed sutures after spontaneous vaginal birth: a randomised controlled trial. *Lancet* 2002; **359**:2217–23.

12. Sultan AH, Johanson RB, Carter JE. Occult anal sphincter trauma following randomized forceps and vacuum delivery. *Int J Obstet Gynecol* 1998; **61**:113–19.

13. Fynes M, O'Herilhy C. The influence of mode of delivery on anal sphincter injury and faecal incontinence. *Obstet Gynecol* 2001; **3**:120–5.

14. Fitzpatrick M, Behan M, O'Connell PR, O'Herlihy C. A randomised clinical trial comparing primary overlap with approximation repair of third degree tears. *Am J Obstet Gynecol* 2000; **183**:1220–4.

15. Fynes M, Donnelly V, Behan M, O'Connell PR, O'Herlihy C. Effect of second vaginal delivery on ano-rectal physiology and fecal continence. *Lancet* 1999; **354**:983–6.

Second stage of labour

SECTION F

Postpartum complications: neonatal

Perinatal Asphyxia

Sandie Bohin

INTRODUCTION

Perinatal asphyxia is an important cause of death and disability in the term neonate. Although the pathophysiology of the asphyxial process is understood, there are currently few interventions available that preserve brain function and few treatment modalities have been subject to randomized, controlled trials. A number of clinical, biochemical and radiological markers of hypoxic–ischaemic damage are available, but their use in predicting outcome requires caution.

DEFINITION

The terms birth asphyxia and perinatal asphyxia are widely used to describe an intrapartum hypoxic–ischaemic insult in a term infant. However, the precise clinical definition varies, making interpretation of data on incidence, clinical manifestations and outcome difficult.

It is unclear if premature infants, with their immature central nervous system, exhibit the same responses to hypoxic–ischaemic insults as term infants. Preterm infants are of course at higher risk of cerebral insults outside of the intrapartum period.

INCIDENCE OF HYPOXIC–ISCHAEMIC INJURY

The incidence varies depending on the definition used and whether preterm infants are included. The incidence appears to be higher in developing countries, although preterm infants are often included in published data. With improvements in antenatal and intrapartum monitoring, the incidence appears to have fallen in some published UK studies, from 6.0 per 1000 live births in the early 1980s[1] to 1.0 per 1000 live births in the mid-1990s. However, there is a suggestion that there was a further increase in the late 1990s [III].[2]

PREVENTION

In order to prevent brain injury caused by hypoxia–ischaemia, there needs to be awareness as to when and under what conditions the injury might occur. Most available information relates to the detection of problems during the intrapartum period. However, it is clear that not all hypoxic–ischaemic insults occur intrapartum and that many occur prior to labour and delivery [II].[3] In recent years, major advances in antenatal assessment have been made and a number of tools for the antenatal assessment of fetal well-being are now widely used, including monitoring fetal movements, fetal heart rate, biophysical profiles, fetal growth and blood flow velocity in umbilical and fetal blood vessels (see Chapter 14).

The aim of intrapartum monitoring is to detect 'fetal compromise'; this is often used as a marker for hypoxia–ischaemia. Detection of fetal compromise does not help in timing the hypoxic insult, as it may reflect the infant's inability to mount a normal physiological response to an earlier hypoxic event. Intrapartum assessments of fetal well-being/fetal compromise include:

- monitoring of fetal heart rate, either intermittently or continuously,

- assessment of fetal acid–base status,
- passage of meconium in utero.

It should be noted that the detection of fetal compromise is a poor predictor of hypoxaemic–ischaemic encephalopathy (HIE) or later cerebral palsy.

Once concerns have been raised regarding the well-being of the infant, in order to ensure optimum resuscitation, it is vital that communication is made to neonatal staff prior to delivery. It is essential that staff attending the delivery are appropriately trained in neonatal resuscitation and are given any relevant details in the maternal history that may affect resuscitation, for example placental abruption, for which the infant may require blood during the resuscitation.

PATHOPHYSIOLOGY OF BRAIN INJURY

Perinatal asphyxia occurs when a lack of oxygen and acidosis cause organ impairment. Deprivation of oxygen to the brain can occur in two ways:

- hypoxaemia – a reduction in the amount of oxygen in the blood,
- ischaemia – a reduction in the amount of blood perfusing the brain.

Although brain injury occurs at the time of the hypoxic–ischaemic insult, it is now well established that neuronal damage is an ongoing process which starts at the time of the primary injury and continues, despite resuscitation, into the recovery phase (secondary injury). This is supported clinically by the delay of 24–48 hours before typical signs of encephalopathy are observed, with further delays before radiological changes are seen on either ultrasound or magnetic resonance imaging (MRI) [III].[4]

Following a hypoxic–ischaemic insult, cell death occurs in two phases. The mechanisms involved are different and are influenced by the severity and nature of the original insult. The neuronal injury resulting from hypoxic– ischaemic insult in a term infant is 'selective neuronal necrosis'. It is unaffected by resuscitation and occurs 5–30 minutes after the onset of ischaemia. *Primary* neuronal death predominantly affects the watershed areas of the cerebral cortex, is bilateral and usually symmetrical. Many neurons do not die during this primary phase; they do, however, appear vulnerable to further injury and death as a result of severe cerebrovascular dysfunction. This appears to trigger a series of biochemical events resulting in *secondary* neuronal death. There is increasing evidence that during the post-resuscitation phase, a therapeutic window exists when intervention may prevent secondary neuronal death and subsequent poor neurological outcome.[5]

AETIOLOGY

Perinatal asphyxia may be the result of an acute event or may occur as a result of chronic hypoxia (Table 37.1). It is

Table 37.1   Causes of perinatal asphyxia

Impaired maternal oxygenation
  Maternal cardiovascular disease

Impaired uterine blood flow
  Vascular disturbance – PET, diabetes
  Maternal hypotension/hypovolaemia
  Obstructed labour

Impaired placental function
  Infarction
  Abruption
  Post-maturity
  Infection

Impaired blood flow to cord
  Cord compression
  Cord prolapse

Abnormal fetal haemoglobin
  Rhesus haemolytic disease
  Twin-twin transfusion
  Feto-maternal transfusion

Maternal drugs
  Cocaine

Failure to establish adequate cardiopulmonary circulation after birth

Meconium aspiration

Congenital cardiorespiratory disease

PET, pre-eclampsia.

important to note that in many cases no single factor is identified and that asphyxia may be caused by several antenatal factors or antenatal and intrapartum factors co-existing. It is difficult accurately to quantify the timing of hypoxic-ischaemic insults, as reported studies differ widely in their definitions, methodologies and inclusion criteria. It has been estimated that approximately 20 per cent of insults occur antenatally, 35 per cent occur intrapartum, and in a further 35 per cent there are both antenatal and intrapartum factors involved.[3] It is clear that despite differences in definition, the majority of cases occur in the intrapartum period.

CLINICAL FEATURES AND MANAGEMENT OF HYPOXIC–ISCHAEMIC ENCEPHALOPATHY

Despite the subjective nature of the scoring system, the universal method employed to assess an infant's well-being at birth is the Apgar score. Infants who have been exposed to a hypoxic insult will invariably have low Apgar scores beyond 1 minute; however, other factors not associated with asphyxia can also lower the Apgar score, for example anaesthetic agents and prematurity. Despite this, there is good evidence that prolonged depression of the Apgar score is associated with death or major neurological disability [II].[6]

It is essential that personnel trained in neonatal resuscitation are present prior to the delivery of an asphyxiated infant. Resuscitation should establish a secure airway, ensure adequate oxygenation and restore circulation. Some severely affected infants will require endotracheal intubation and ventilation in the delivery room; however, others will require little in the way of initial resuscitation, but will deteriorate after the first 24 hours. Intravenous fluids, and in particular colloid, should be used with caution in restoring the circulation in severe asphyxia, the exception being where there is a clear history of antepartum haemorrhage or placental abruption; in such cases, O-negative blood should be administered in the delivery room.

If, despite appropriate resuscitation, there is no spontaneous cardiac output by 10 minutes or respiratory activity by 30 minutes, the outlook for both term and preterm infants is poor.

Post-resuscitation management

Infants who have experienced an asphyxial insult develop the clinical syndrome known as hypoxic–ischaemic encephalopathy. After resuscitation, the infant may be flaccid and unresponsive. The clinical signs progress over the first 24–48 hours before gradual improvement is seen. The severity of HIE can be graded clinically as mild, moderate or severe, as shown in Table 37.2.[1] The management after hypoxia-ischaemia is crucial, as the affected infant is still at risk of reperfusion injury.[5] Transfer to a neonatal intensive care unit with facilities for cerebral and systemic monitoring is of the utmost importance. Full supportive care is required, with great attention to detail. As well as general intensive care, specific neurological monitoring and care should also be given.

General management

During episodes of hypoxia, blood flow is distributed in order to preserve blood supplies to vital organs, namely the brain, heart and adrenals. This leaves other organs, particularly the kidney, liver and gut, prone to ischaemic damage. With this in mind, blood pressure should be continuously monitored and hypotension avoided in order to ensure cerebral perfusion and to prevent further underperfusion of other organs. Hypotension is common, but is due to myocardial dysfunction rather than hypovolaemia. It should be treated promptly with volume expansion and/or inotropes as clinically indicated. Care should be taken not to overload infants with fluid, as acute tubular necrosis and inappropriate antidiuretic hormone release are common sequelae. Fluid should

be restricted by 25 per cent for the first 48 hours or so, based on regular clinical assessment of hydration, serum and urinary electrolytes, urine output and specific gravity and the infant's weight.

Asphyxiated infants are at risk of developing necrotizing enterocolitis and therefore oral feeds should be introduced with caution. Prevention of tissue catabolism is important and thus nutritional support should be provided by parenteral nutrition until feeds are established.

Respiratory support with endotracheal intubation should only be undertaken if hypercapnia develops, if the infant has prolonged or frequent convulsions or if there is co-existing respiratory disease. Hyperventilation is not recommended, as hypocapnia reduces cerebral perfusion and may compound the ischaemic insult. Respiratory support is guided by regular arterial blood gas analysis. Hypoxia should be avoided and the PaO_2 kept between 8 and 12 kPa (60–90 mmHg).

Neonatal meningitis may present in a similar way to HIE and therefore if there is any doubt, a lumbar puncture should be performed and treatment commenced. Routine antibiotics have no part to play in the treatment of HIE.

Disseminated intravascular coagulation is not uncommon in severe cases of HIE, and therefore regular assessments of clotting status should be made. Treatment includes additional vitamin K, platelets, cryoprecipitate and/or fresh frozen plasma infusions.

Neurological management

Much of the management after hypoxic–ischaemic insults has not been subject to randomized, controlled trials.

In severe HIE, cerebral oedema and raised intracranial pressure (ICP) are commonly observed. Management strategies to lower ICP have included the administration of hyperosmolar agents and lowering $PaCO_2$. There is no evidence that hyperventilation and the ensuing hypocarbia are beneficial in reducing ICP, and therefore accepted practice is to maintain the $PaCO_2$ within the normal range [IV].

The use of hypertonic saline has been shown to be beneficial in lowering ICP in animal models and in adults. Its use has not been evaluated in the neonate and it cannot be recommended. There is no evidence for the use of mannitol, frusemide or steroids in the treatment of cerebral oedema in neonates.[7]

Seizures are a salient feature of HIE. Frequent and prolonged clinically evident seizures should be treated promptly with anticonvulsant(s). Phenobarbitone is the drug of choice, as recent evidence suggests that the use of phenytoin, diazepam or chloral hydrate confers no benefit [Ia].[7] Anticonvulsants can be stopped once seizures are controlled. The use of early prophylactic phenobarbitone as a 'neuroprotector' in HIE has been subject to a meta-analysis, which concluded that routine use is not recommended in perinatal asphyxia [Ia].[8]

Glucose metabolism in HIE has been extensively studied and yet is still not fully understood. Normoglycaemia should be maintained, as there is evidence that both hypoglycaemia and hyperglycaemia may worsen brain injury.

Table 37.2   Clinical grading for hypoxic–ischaemic encephalopathy[7]

Grade I	Grade II	Grade III
Mild	Moderate	Severe
Irritability	Lethargy	Comatose
Mild hypotonia	Marked abnormalities in tone	Severe hypotonia
Poor suck	Requires tube feeds	Failure to maintain spontaneous respiration
Hyperalert	Seizures	Prolonged seizures

New neuroprotective strategies

A number of new neuropreotective strategies have evolved in recent years.[5,7] Most have been used in animal models, with only a few trials in the human neonate. The rationale behind these interventions is in the prevention of reperfusion injury. Interventions have included magnesium sulphate, calcium channel blockers, allopurinol as a free radical scavenger, the Chinese herb *Salvia miltiorrhizae*, naloxone and hypothermia. Of these alternatives, selective hypothermia looks the most promising strategy, with a number of randomized clinical trials currently in progress.

INVESTIGATIONS

Continuous integrated single-channel electroencephalogram (EEG) monitoring is now in widespread use and may be helpful in severe cases or where muscle relaxants are in use.

The value of neuroimaging is limited in the first 24–48 hours of life. Ultrasound evidence of lesions in the thalami and basal ganglia, focal infarctions and changes in periventricular white matter are usually seen after the first 48 hours of life. Their presence before this suggests an antenatal insult.

Magnetic resonance imaging is useful in asphyxiated infants. Early scans characteristically show brain swelling and abnormal signal intensity within the basal ganglia, periventricular white matter, subcortical white matter and cortex. Late MRI findings associated with poor outcome include delayed myelination as a marker for neuronal loss and extensive white matter changes.

OUTCOME

Determining the outcome after perinatal asphyxia is difficult for a number of reasons:

- the definition of asphyxia varies,
- there is variation in the outcomes assessed – mortality, motor, behavioural etc.,
- there is varied inclusion/exclusion of preterm infants,
- the age at time of assessment varies.

What is clear, however, is that the neurological outcome depends on the severity of the insult. It is well recognized that term infants with grade I HIE (mild) have no long-term developmental problems, whereas severe HIE is associated with a poor outcome. It is more difficult to predict the outcome of moderate HIE as there are few readily available reliable markers of long-term impairment. One early predictor of adverse outcome is the severity of the neurological abnormalities found on clinical examination, particularly in association with discontinuous activity on EEG. Severe acidosis associated with poor Apgar scores, multi-organ failure and

encephalopathy immediately after birth are also markers of poor outcome [III].[9]

The major neurological sequelae in surviving infants are motor deficits and, in particular, spastic quadriplegia and dyskinetic cerebral palsy. There may also be associated visual or intellectual impairment or epilepsy. It is important to note that not all cerebral palsy is the result of perinatal asphyxia and not all asphyxiated infants develop cerebral palsy [II].[10]

- Phenobarbitone is the drug of choice for convulsions secondary to HIE.
- There is no role for routine seizure prophylaxis in infants with HIE.
- Most infants with severe HIE will develop neurological sequelae. Most infants with mild HIE will have no long-term sequelae. Infants in the moderate category remain the most difficult in whom to predict outcome.

KEY POINTS

- Most cases of HIE occur during labour. However, not all infants with HIE develop cerebral palsy, and not all children with cerebral palsy demonstrate HIE.
- Damage due to HIE occurs in two phases: the initial insult and then further reperfusion injury.
- Damage is usually symmetrical and affects watershed areas.
- A persistently depressed Apgar score is generally associated with poor outcomes.

KEY REFERENCES

1. Levene MI, Kornberg J, Williams THC. The incidence and severity of post-asphyxial encephalopathy in full term infants. *Early Hum Dev* 1985; 11:21–6.
2. *Trent Neonatal Survey Report 2000*. Trent Infant Mortality and Morbidity Studies. Leicester University, 2001.
3. Volpe JJ. Hypoxic–ischaemic encephalopathy: clinical aspects. In: *Neurology of the Newborn*, 3rd edn. Philadelphia: WB Saunders, 1995.
4. Sie LT, Van der Knapp MS, Van Wezel-Meyler G et al. Early MR features of hypoxic–ischaemic brain injury in neonates with periventricular densities on sonogram. *Am J Neuroradiol* 2000; 21:852–61.
5. Cornette L, Levene MI. Post-resuscitative management of the asphyxiated term infant. *Semin Neonatol* 2001; 6:271–82.

6. Nelson KB, Ellenberg JH. Apgar scores as predictors of chronic neurological disability. *Pediatrics* 1981; 68:36–44.

7. Whitelaw A. Systematic review of therapy after hypoxic–ischaemic brain injury in the perinatal period. *Semin Neonatol* 2000; 5:33–44.

8. Evans DJ, Levene MI. Anticonvulsants for preventing mortality and morbidity in full-term newborns with perinatal asphyxia (Cochrane Review). In: *The Cochrane Library*, Issue 3. Oxford: Update Software, 2003.

9. Yudkin PL, Johnson A, Clover LM, Murphy KW. Clustering of perinatal markers of birth asphyxia and outcome at age five years. *Br J Obstet Gynaecol* 1994; 101:774–81.

10. Blair F, Stanley FJ. Intrapartum asphyxia: a rare cause of cerebral palsy. *J Pediatrics* 1988; 112:515–19.

Chapter 38

Neonatal Resuscitation

Andrew Currie

INTRODUCTION

Health professionals involved with childbirth should be capable of providing life support to the newly born when the need arises.

To facilitate this, various professional bodies have been developed, including the UK Resuscitation Council, the European Resuscitation Council and the International Liaison Committee on Resuscitation (ILCOR).[1–3] Each professional body has produced guidelines and training programmes to improve resuscitation practices.

Much of resuscitation procedures is based on 'best practice', with very little evidence-based medicine to support it. This is hardly surprising given the ethical dilemmas that would be created by trying to perform randomized, controlled studies of resuscitation techniques.

This chapter concentrates on the essential steps required to provide safe and appropriate resuscitation to the newborn. It draws on recommendations from the above resuscitation bodies and, where possible, the evidence is reviewed.

INCIDENCE

Most studies show that approximately 90–95 per cent of all births require no resuscitation. The other 5–10 per cent need some form of respiratory support, with possibly up to 1–2 per cent requiring full cardiopulmonary resuscitation.[4]

PHYSIOLOGICAL CHANGES

Many physiological adaptations occur to the infant at birth.[5] The most important involve the cardiovascular system, respiratory system and thermoregulatory mechanisms.

Respiratory

In utero, the lungs are full of fluid (30–35 mL/kg in term infants). Pulmonary pressures are suprasystemic, thus reducing blood flow to the fetal lung. To adapt to extrauterine life, lung fluid production reduces near term. In addition, the mechanics of birth include the birth canal exerting an immense extrathoracic pressure on the infant during its descent, squeezing lung fluid from the trachea and upper airways. With delivery, a natural 'recoil' of the airways (along with the infant's first respiratory efforts) helps to inflate the lungs. Subsequent breaths become progressively easier, due to development of a functional residual capacity and improving lung compliance. Dispersal of surfactant to form a monolayer within the alveolar system further improves lung mechanics by lowering surface tension and ensuring alveoli remain open, even in expiration.

Cardiovascular

Major features of the fetal cardiovascular system include high pulmonary pressures and a series of three anatomical right-to-left shunts.

1 The ductus venosus carries blood from the placenta back to the fetus (effectively connecting the umbilical vein to the inferior vena cava).
2 The foramen ovale is important in diverting blood from the right atrium to the left, thus bypassing the lungs.
3 The ductus arteriosus diverts blood from the pulmonary artery to the aorta.

Following birth, the pulmonary pressures fall. This is as much to do with changes at a cellular level (including the effects of cytokines, prostaglandins and the influence of endogenous nitric oxide) as with the mechanics of lung infla-tion. The ductus venosus closes soon after clamping of the umbilical cord, with establishment of the normal venous cir-culation. The fall in pulmonary pressures allows greater blood flow into the pulmonary circulation. This increases the blood volume returning to the left atrium, with consequent closure of the foramen ovale and increased systemic pressures; these in turn reverse the shunting across the ductus arteriosus. The ductus arteriosus subsequently closes under the influence of increasing oxygen concentrations and prostaglandins. As a result, the normal neonatal circulation is established. The conversion of the fetal to the neonatal circulation may take several days to complete.

Thermoregulation

The infant is born naked and wet into a hostile environ-ment. Immature thermoregulatory mechanisms can lead to cold stress with serious morbidity, such as acidosis, hypo-glycaemia and respiratory distress. Equally, pyrexia may be as dangerous, studies showing that it worsens cerebral hypoxic injury.[6] Hence, an essential part of neonatal resus-citation is maintenance of a normal body temperature.

AETIOLOGY

Many causes have been associated with a potentially com-promised infant at birth. These can be divided into mater-nal, fetal and intrapartum. A list of the more common is shown in Table 38.1.

MANAGEMENT OF THE RESUSCITATION

Basic principles (fundamental to optimize patient outcome)

1 As with any resuscitation, the ABC (Airway, Breathing, Circulation) approach is the most appropriate. The vast majority of neonatal 'arrests' are primarily due to respiratory problems. Hence heavy emphasis is placed on ensuring an adequate airway and efficient ventilation delivery to the child.
2 Good preparation is essential to optimize clinical management.
3 Resuscitation of the newborn is a team approach. Clear communication is essential.
4 The ability to assess a situation and act accordingly on a regular basis is crucial. The ability to use basic knowledge in a safe, logical and adaptive manner makes resuscitation of the patient a more rewarding process.

Table 38.1 Common causes for a compromised newborn infant

Maternal
Chronic ill-health
Drug ingestion (legal and illegal)
Hypertension
Diabetes mellitus
Anatomical abnormalities
Placenta praevia

Fetal
Multiple pregnancies
Prematurity
Post-term (>42/52)
Intrauterine growth restriction
Congenital abnormalities
Liquor disturbances (oligohydramnios/polyhydramnios)
Hydrops
Isoimmunization
Intrauterine infection

Intrapartum
Fetal distress
Abnormal presentation
Prolapsed cord
Antepartum haemorrhage
Prolonged rupture of membranes
Thick meconium
Instrumental deliveries

Preparation

Good preparation is as important to a successful outcome as the actual resuscitation itself. Preparation involves more than getting equipment ready.

Keywords

– Medical history
– Personnel
– Communication
– Environment
– Equipment

Medical history

Accurate medical information is invaluable. Although a detailed medical history is ideal, time is often against this. It is vital to establish key facts quickly.

Useful questions that may influence the actual resuscita-tion process include the following.

- How many infants should we expect?
- What is the gestation?
- Are there any congenital anomalies (e.g. congenital diaphragmatic hernia)?
- Has the mother had any relevant medication in the last few hours (e.g. opiates)?
- Has there been any meconium prior to delivery?

Personnel

All workers involved in birth should be able to provide basic neonatal life support, and regular updates of skills should be undertaken. Ideally, somebody trained in advanced neonatal life support should also be readily available.

Resuscitation is a team event. Individuals should understand their roles. Ideally, two to three people make an effective team: one to look after the airway, one to look after the cardiovascular circulation and the third to assist with drugs, fluids and additional equipment. One person should take the role of leader; this ensures clarity of the roles and efficient team working.

Other important tasks that may be delegated in the acute situation include informing neonatal unit staff who will be looking after the infant following resuscitation and communicating with the parents, who need to be informed of events as early and fully as possible.

Communication and documentation

Often, the source of mishaps and complaints is poor communication. In addition, poor documentation makes post-hoc reviews very difficult. The importance of accurate information gathering, documentation and communication cannot be emphasized enough. Accurate timing must be recorded, and all records (midwifery, obstetric and neonatal) must be consistent. In the acute situation, if enough staff are available, one team member should be asked to keep a record of times and procedures.

Environment

A brightly lit, warm and draft-free room is ideal. As well as reducing morbidity due to heat loss, a good environment ensures that attendants can see and assess the infant appropriately.

The infant's temperature should be kept in the normothermic range. Hyperthermia is associated with increased neuronal damage in cases of perinatal hypoxia. Hypothermia is equally associated with increased morbidity, although it has been suggested that mild hypothermia may be neuroprotective in cases of severe perinatal hypoxia. Clinical trials are ongoing and, until this uncertainty is resolved, recommended best practice remains to aim for normothermia [IV].

Equipment

Having the right equipment, which is reliable, is paramount to a successful resuscitation. Table 38.2 shows a list of essential equipment.

Within the hospital setting, all essential equipment is found on a resuscitaire – best described as a mobile, open cot. The heat and warmth sources are located above a firm, flat surface. A clock is attached. There are usually two sources of oxygen (piped and cylinders), with two outlets. Air supplies may be available on some resuscitaires.

Suction apparatus is intrinsic in the resuscitaire. The rest of the equipment should be readily available, stored in various drawers mounted on the resuscitaire.

Table 38.2   Essential equipment for neonatal resuscitation

Light source
Source of warmth (heater and/or warmed linen)
Flat surface ($\pm$firm mattress)
Clock
Suction apparatus (able to deliver suction up to 100 mmHg)
Suction catheters
Oxygen supply
Ventilation system (either 'bag valve mask' or 'mask and T-piece', or both)
Endotracheal tubes (various sizes from 2.5 to 4.0 mm internal diameter
Introductory stylet
Fixation kit for endotracheal tube
Laryngoscopes (with straight blades and spare bulbs)
Oropharyngeal airways
Nasogastric tubes
Umbilical venous catheters
Scalpel
Intravenous cannulae
Intraosseous cannula
Syringes and needles
Fluids and medications

The resuscitaire should be situated in the delivery room.

Fluids and medications may or may not be stored with the resuscitaire. If not, they should be in a readily accessible place for emergency use.

It is the responsibility of the individuals using equipment for resuscitation to ensure that they are competent with its use and that it is working properly. All resuscitation equipment should be checked daily, as well as before and after each use.

The resuscitation process

This section assumes birth is taking place in a maternity suite with a resuscitaire; however, the principles can be applied to any setting.

Figure 38.1 shows a step-by-step approach. Each step is explained in more detail below.

Step 1

With the birth of the whole baby, the clock is started and the infant is transferred to the resuscitaire. The infant is placed with the head in the 'neutral position', towards the resuscitator. The neutral position involves the head being placed so that the eyes are looking directly upward. This position helps maintain airway patency.

The infant is dried with a warm towel to reduce heat loss. A vigorous, not aggressive, rub with the towel serves the dual purpose of drying the infant and stimulating breathing. The infant is then wrapped in a second, warm towel.

The airway must be correctly positioned and also needs to be clear. Babies have secretions in their oropharynx at birth. Assuming these are not copious and the infant is vigorous, the infant will clear them independently. **Routine oropharyngeal suctioning is to be avoided** [IV].

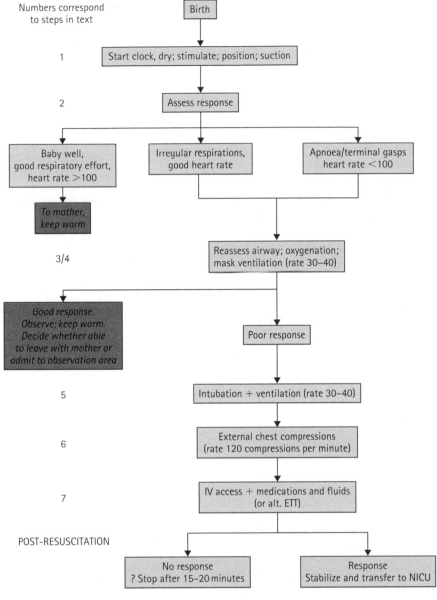

Figure 38.1   Neonatal resuscitation in the delivery room. ETT, endotracheal tube

Infants with excessive secretions, or those with thick meconium (see 'Special situations') and/or blood, need suctioning. A suction catheter can be placed in the oropharynx; care must be taken not to push the catheter too far back, and some authorities advocate not inserting it further than 5 cm. A suction pressure of 100 mmHg is appropriate. Excessive toileting of the oropharynx causes reflex bardycardia and laryngospasm.

These initial steps should take no more than 20–30 seconds.

Step 2

The infant is then assessed. Initial assessment should include heart rate, respiratory effort and colour. This should have occurred by 30 seconds of age.

Table 38.3   Apgar scoring system

Parameter	Score		
	0	**1**	**2**
Heart rate	0	<100	>100
Breathing	Apnoeic	Irregular	Good
Colour	White	Blue	Pink
Muscle tone	Floppy	Some movement	Active
Reflex response	None	Grimace	Cough, cry, sneeze

Assessment (and reassessment) is vital to a successful outcome. Many workers use the Apgar score (Table 38.3) to aid them. This was originally described by Virginia Apgar, an anaesthesiologist, in 1953. Whilst this is a useful tool, it has its limitations. Apgar scores are carried out at 1 minute and 5 minutes of life. Further scores may be done at 5-minute intervals depending on subsequent progress. It is an internationally recognized assessment tool, giving an indication of the neonate's condition after birth. However, it would be inappropriate to delay resuscitating an apnoeic infant with a profound bradycardia at birth whilst waiting for a low 1-minute Apgar score.

From the initial assessment, the infant will fall into one of three groups.

1 *Well, healthy and vigorous.* The child has a good respiratory effort, is pink centrally, and the heart rate is >100 beats per minute (bpm). This infant can be wrapped up and given to the parents.
2 *Cyanosed, poor respiratory effort, with or without a heart rate <100 bpm.* This infant needs further intervention.
3 *White, apnoeic or terminal gasps, with absent heart beat or profound bradycardia (<60 bpm).* This infant needs full intensive resuscitation.

If the child's condition is still a cause for concern, the previous interventions should be checked.

• Is the airway clear and positioned correctly?
• Has the child responded to stimulation?

Step 3

Next, facial oxygen administration should be considered. How this is delivered will depend on the state of the respiratory effort: an apnoeic infant will not respond to wafting oxygen over its face; however, it may be inappropriate to jump to mask ventilation to deliver oxygen in a child with reasonable respiratory effort who will probably respond to continued stimulation plus facial oxygen.

At present, accepted best practice is to use 100 per cent oxygen for resuscitation. There is growing evidence (from both animal work and clinical trials) to indicate that resuscitation with air in the term infant is as effective and may even be advantageous [II].[7] Concerns exist relating to the effects of oxygen on the respiratory centres as well as its direct effects on lungs by means of free radical production. Such effects are even more contentious in the preterm infant. As a result, some workers have advocated using blended oxygen mixtures to try to minimize any side effects. However, the most recent statements from the ILCOR have again advocated the use of 100 per cent oxygen [IV].[3]

Step 4

Following this intervention, the infant's response should be reassessed. If there is still concern, ventilation should be commenced.

Indications for ventilation are:

• an apnoeic infant, or one with gasping respirations despite the above interventions;
• an infant that remains cyanosed despite adequate oxygen delivery.

At this stage in the rescusitation, the infant should be no more than 1 minute of age. This is time enough to know if simple interventions are going to work, without causing further insult by undue delay.

Ventilation is performed either with a bag-valve-mask (bvm) apparatus or a face-mask plus T-piece connector.

• The *bag-valve-mask* is attached to an oxygen supply and should have a reservoir bag attached. This helps to increase the concentration of oxygen to nearer 100 per cent. (In practice it is probably nearer 60–80 per cent with a refill bag, as opposed to 30–40 per cent without; 100 per cent oxygen concentration is difficult to achieve with bvm devices due to leakage at various points.) It is recommended that 500 mL bags be used to aid efficient delivery of ventilatory breaths. These devices have a 'pop-off' valve, which is set to between 20 and 30 cmH$_2$O. (The 'pop-off' valve reduces the risk of excessive peak pressures, which could cause over-inflation.) The face-mask is applied over the nose and mouth. For neonates, a circular face-mask forms the best seal. Positive pressure is applied by squeezing the bag fully, then allowing it to re-inflate before the next breath.
• The *face-mask plus T-piece* is also attached to an oxygen supply. Again the face-mask is applied over the nose and mouth to form a seal. Above the face-mask is a hole over which the resuscitator's thumb is applied to create a positive pressure. The peak pressure can be set using a pressure gauge.

Both techniques are easily learnt, although the T-piece plus face-mask probably results in more reliable delivery of a set positive pressure compared to the bvm technique. Certain types of T-piece plus face-mask apparatus can also deliver positive end-expiratory pressure (PEEP), which is advantageous in helping to create and maintain a functional residual capacity.

When starting ventilation, five 'rescue' breaths should be administered. These are more sustained breaths, designed to overcome the high airways resistance present in the lungs of the infant who has not breathed. This is much easier to achieve using the T-piece plus face-mask technique, in which the thumb can be applied for 1–2 seconds at a set pressure. With the bvm technique, prolonged breaths are difficult to achieve, but higher pressures can be applied by locking the 'pop-off' valve.

Following these initial rescue breaths, the infant's response should be assessed. If there is still concern regarding respiration, regular ventilation should be commenced. This is delivered at a rate of 30–40 breaths per minute, with each breath lasting approximately 0.5 seconds. The peak pressure should be set to achieve adequate lung expansion without over-distension. Clinically, this can be assessed by chest movement, breath sounds, colour and heart rate, as well as improving spontaneous respiratory effort. Ventilation should be stopped once good, spontaneous, respiratory effort is achieved.

Step 5

After another 30–60 seconds of face-mask ventilation, if there is still inadequate response, endotracheal intubation for more efficient ventilation should be considered.

Indications for intubation include:

- poor respiratory effort despite appropriate interventions as above,
- thick meconium at delivery,
- anticipated need for long-term ventilatory support.

Intubation is achieved using a straight-bladed laryngoscope held in the left hand and an endotracheal tube held in the right hand. The laryngoscope blade size can be chosen to suit the infant. Thus a size 1 blade is suitable for term infants, whereas a size 0 is better suited to preterm infants. A size 00 is available for extremely premature infants with small mouths.

The blade is inserted into the mouth in the midline and the laryngoscope is pulled forward and upward, thus bringing the lower jaw and tongue up and forward until the uvula is visible. At this point it may be necessary to suction the oropharynx using a suction catheter in the right hand. The blade is then advanced over the back of the tongue into the venecular and pulled forward. This elevates the epiglottis, revealing the glottis and vocal cords. It should be remembered that the larynx in the newborn is more 'floppy' than in adults, hence to aid vision, external downward pressure over the cricoid cartilage may be needed to help bring the vocal cords into view. An alternative technique is to place the laryngoscope in the oropharynx as far as it will go, pull the lower jaw and tongue forward and upward to maximize vision and then gradually withdraw the laryngoscope until the epiglottis slips into view, with the vocal cords visible below. This is quicker, but can be more traumatic if not performed carefully.

Once the vocal cords are visualized, the endotracheal tube can be inserted. There is a choice between a straight-sided and a shouldered endotracheal tube (Coles tube). The shouldered tube is stiffer, to help intubation. An introductory stylet can be used to help stiffen whichever endotracheal tube is used.

For resuscitation purposes, oropharyngeal intubation is best practised [IV], as this is simpler and quicker than nasopharyngeal intubation – a technically more demanding skill.

Once the endotracheal tube has been positioned, the ventilatory circuit can be attached and ventilatory breaths delivered. Adequate air entry should be confirmed (equal chest movement, breath sounds, appropriate colour and heart rate). If there is any doubt about whether the tube is in the correct position, it should be removed and the infant ventilated with a face-mask system whilst the situation is reassessed.

The act of intubation should take no longer than 20–30 seconds from the time of inserting the laryngoscope blade in the mouth until the endotracheal tube is attached to the ventilatory circulation. Whilst performing this action, the infant is effectively being asphyxiated, thus undue delay is unacceptable.

Endotracheal intubation should not be attempted by inexperienced practitioners without appropriate supervision.

Ventilation breaths are delivered at a rate of 30–40/minute, the same as for mask ventilation. Slightly higher rates (up to 60 breaths/minute) may be used for premature infants.

Once intubation has been established, the practitioner must be alert to potential complications such as a blocked or displaced endotracheal tube, equipment failure and pneumothorax.

Step 6: Circulation

Once the airway and breathing have been addressed, the next step is to assess the circulation. The heart rate and pulses should be checked. Useful sites include the base of the umbilical cord or brachial pulse, as other pulses can be difficult to elicit. Infants with a heart rate <60 bpm require external chest compressions. This is performed by depressing the lower half of the sternum by one-third of the antero-posterior diameter of the chest. In practice, for most infants this equates to 1–2 cm.

Chest compressions can be performed either using both thumbs over the lower sternum, with the hands wrapped around the chest, or by placing the index and middle fingers over the lower sternum. It is more important that appropriate sternal compressions are performed, regardless of which technique is preferred. A rate of 120 chest compressions per minute (2 per second) should be attained. If ventilation is being undertaken at the same time, a ratio of three chest compressions to one breath is appropriate. Chest compressions should be stopped once the cardiac rate is >60–80 bpm.

Step 7: Vascular access, use of medication and volume expansion

- Vascular access may be needed for advanced resuscitation. Use of the umbilical vein is the quickest and most effective means of achieving access. An umbilical catheter, primed with 0.9 per cent saline, should be inserted to a depth of approximately 5 cm. Alternative forms of access include the use of peripheral intravenous cannulae (but only if a peripheral vein is readily accessible) or an intraosseous needle. The endotracheal tube can also be used for quick access for certain medications (e.g. adrenaline).
- Medication.
  - *Adrenaline* is probably the most important medication available. It can be given via any route, most commonly intravenous or endotracheal. The recommended dose is 0.1–0.3 mL/kg of 1:10 000 solution (or 10–30 µg/kg). This dose may be repeated every minute. Most recommendations incorporate a higher dose of 100–300 µg/kg (i.e. 0.1–0.3 mL/kg of 1:1000 solution) after the second dose. However, there is no evidence that this is beneficial and, indeed, some studies suggest higher doses of adrenaline may be detrimental to the infant [Ib].[3]
  - *Sodium bicarbonate* remains very controversial. It may be useful in prolonged resuscitations when sustained

cellular acidosis may affect myocardial contractility. If used, administration should be limited to a 4.2 per cent solution in aliquots of 1.0 mL/kg intravenously. The aim is to improve acidic conditions in the heart and thus improve myocardial contractility, as well as facilitating the beneficial effects of adrenaline.

– *Naloxone* may be used in the infant with respiratory depression as a result of maternal intrapartum opiate analgesia. The dose is 200 µg intramuscularly. Naloxone is not a substitute for appropriate resuscitation, which should always take precedent. Also, it should not be administered to the infants of drug-dependent mothers, as it can result in a severe withdrawal state in the infant. Finally, the caregiver should note that naloxone has a shorter half-life than most opiates and doses may need to be repeated.

– *Dextrose*. Hypoglycaemia is a major problem in prolonged resuscitations. Hence small aliquots of dextrose may be required. A dose of 2–3 mL/kg of 10 per cent dextrose should be adequate.

- Use of volume replacement.
  – Blood. If there is any suggestion of haemorrhage, O-negative blood should be used: 10–20 mL/kg can be given as a bolus and the response assessed.
  – For other causes of circulatory disturbance, volume replacement with a crystalloid or colloid can be useful in the resuscitation scenario. The dose is again 10–20 mL/kg. Following a Cochrane Review[8] that found the use of albumin to be detrimental, most authorities recommend crystalloids, such as 0.9 per cent saline [Ia]. **Glucose solutions should not be used for volume replacement.**

Post-resuscitation

Continuing care

Once the infant has been successfully resuscitated, it is essential that provision for ongoing care be provided. This may simply involve handing a well infant to the mother to keep warm and feed, with attendants available to ensure there is no deterioration, or transfer of the sick infant to a neonatal intensive care unit for ongoing intensive care.

Before any transfer, the infant should be reassessed clinically. All lines, including endotracheal tubes, intravenous cannulae, nasogastric tubes and monitoring leads, should be secured. The need for ongoing medication and fluids should be considered.

Comprehensive documentation, including interventions, responses and subsequent management plans, should be completed and signed legibly. The family should be fully informed of events.

Discontinuing care

Unfortunately, not all resuscitation attempts are successful and the decision to stop resuscitative attempts can be extremely difficult. As a guide, it is appropriate to discontinue resuscitative attempts if there is no spontaneous circulation by 15 minutes [IV].

Non-initiation of resuscitation

This can also be a contentious issue and it is important that units develop guidance in this area. Most practitioners would accept that it is inappropriate to attempt resuscitation in infants less than 23 weeks' gestation or 400 g birth weight. Equally, it is ethically acceptable not to resuscitate infants with lethal anomalies, such as anencephaly or trisomy 13 and 18.

In cases of uncertainty, an alternative approach is to commence resuscitation, and withdraw intensive care only once more information is available. However, it should be remembered that both withdrawal and withholding of intensive care are ethically equivalent.

With such decisions, the family should be fully informed and involved, as they will have to live with the consequences.

SPECIAL SITUATIONS

Extreme prematurity

These infants have much greater difficulties due to their immature physiology. Their lungs are poorly developed, lack surfactant and have poor lung compliance. They thus experience greater degrees of respiratory distress. Many infants less than 30 weeks' gestation require early ventilation, with administration of surfactant. Indeed, some practitioners advocate 'elective' intubation of all infants less than 28 weeks. This has become contentious with greater awareness of the damage caused by barotrauma and oxygen toxicity.

Premature infants have a much greater surface area to body mass ratio, and thus loose heat much more quickly than term infants. Their cardiovascular systems are also immature, with poor autoregulation of the cerebral circulation. Care should be exercised when administering volume expanders.

Meconium (see Chapter 28)

Whereas it was previously taught that all infants with meconium present prior to delivery should have their airway viewed and suctioned under direct vision, it is now accepted that this approach can be detrimental in the majority of cases [Ia].[9] As a rule, infants born in good condition with good respiratory effort do not require airway visualization or oropharyngeal suctioning. Infants that have depressed respiratory effort at birth should have their airway cleared prior to any other resuscitative efforts. The aim of this is to prevent inhalation of any meconium into the lungs of the compromised infant, as this can cause mechanical problems with breathing as well as a chemical peumonitis.

Hydrops

The main problem at birth, regardless of the cause, is the presence of large effusions (pleural, pericardial and peritoneal). These often need draining as a matter of urgency at delivery. Probably the quickest method is the use of an 18 or 20 FG cannula attached to a syringe. This can be advanced into the effusion to be drained whilst maintaining gentle negative pressure on the syringe. As soon as fluid is aspirated, the cannula should be advanced over the needle, which is removed. In this way the cannula can act as a temporary drain until a more permanent one can be inserted.

Congenital diaphragmatic hernia

At birth, the major concern is to prevent the infant swallowing air and thus inflating the stomach in the chest. The infant may be best managed with early intubation and muscle relaxation soon after birth. A large-bore nasogastric tube is inserted. Owing to lung hypoplasia, caution with positive pressure ventilation must be exercised to prevent pneumothorax.

Congenital cardiac disease

Management depends on the lesion. There are too many to discuss in this chapter, except to say that infants with duct-dependent lesions should be commenced on a prostaglandin infusion early after birth. Otherwise, for the purposes of early neonatal resuscitation, there is no need for other special measures.

Polyhydramnios

The main difference over the usual resuscitation process in this circumstance is to exclude a possible oesophageal atresia by inserting a large-bore nasogastric tube.

SUMMARY

This chapter briefly discusses the process of resuscitating the newborn infant. It emphasizes the ABC approach, with a need for continual appraisal of a situation. It should be stressed that the vast majority of infants require no, or minimal, intervention. Equally, for those that do need help, most problems are related to the respiratory system, and attention to detail with regard to the airway and ventilation will be all that is required.

- Resuscitation should initially be with 100 per cent oxygen [IV].
- In the term baby, air is as good as 100 per cent oxygen for resuscitation and may have additional benefits [Ib].
- High doses of adrenaline may be detrimental [III].

KEY POINTS

- The vast majority of infants need nothing more active than keeping warm at birth.
- Nearly all neonatal resuscitations involve respiratory failure as the primary event.
- Optimizing airway patency is the most important part of neonatal resuscitation.
- Always remember the ABC approach.
- Do not forget to keep the infant warm.

KEY REFERENCES

1. Royal College of Paediatrics and Child Health and Royal College of Obstetricians and Gynaecologists. *Resuscitation of Babies at Birth*. London: BMJ Publishing Group, 1997.
2. Phillips B, Zideman D, Wyllie J et al. European Resuscitation Council Guidelines 2000 for Newly Born Life Support. A statement from the Paediatric Life Support Working Group and approved by the Executive Committee of the European Resuscitation Council. *Resuscitation* 2001; **48**:235–9.
3. The Pediatric Working Group of the International Liaison Committee on Resuscitation (ILCOR). Part 11: Neonatal resuscitation. *Resuscitation* 2000; 46:401–16.
4. Kattwinkel J, Niermeyer S, Nadkarni V et al. Resuscitation of the newly born infant. *Circulation* 1999; **99**:1927–38.
5. Bhutani VK. Extrauterine adaptations in the newborn. *Semin Neonatol* 1997; **2**:1–12.
6. Gunn AJ, Bennet L. Is temperature important in delivery room resuscitation? *Semin Neonatol* 2001; **6**:241–9.
7. Saugstad OD. Resuscitation of newborn infants with room air or oxygen. *Semin Neonatol* 2001; **6**:233–9.
8. Alderson P, Schierhout G, Roberts I, Burn F. Colloids versus crystalloids for fluid resuscitation in critically ill patients. In: *The Cochrane Library*, Issue 2. Oxford: Update Software, 2002.
9. Halliday HL. Endotracheal intubation at birth in vigorous term meconium-stained babies. In: *The Cochrane Library*, Issue 2. Oxford: Update Software, 2002.

Chapter 39

Common Neonatal Problems

Andrew Currie

MRCOG standards

There are no defined standards relevant to this topic. However, a candidate would be expected to know the following:

- How to examine a healthy newborn infant, and thus distinguish between this and a sick infant.
- How to give simple advice regarding feeding regimens.
- What to expect from a well newborn infant in the early days of life.
- How to proceed when faced with a non life-threatening problem in the term infant.

INTRODUCTION

Most infants are born healthy and remain so throughout their lives. However, they can develop a number of common problems which, whilst not necessarily life threatening, may nonetheless cause significant morbidity and parental anxiety.

This chapter introduces the reader to the commonest problems encountered at or shortly after birth, concentrating in the main on those relating to the term infant.

At the end of this chapter there is a brief summary of the more complicated problems associated with prematurity.

INCIDENCE

There are no reliable figures relating to how often paediatricians are asked to review infants for anything other than a newborn check.

Infants requiring paediatric input fall into two main groups. The first group comprises those that require acute care. These infants are primarily seen within the delivery suite shortly after birth. Paediatricians are called either to the resuscitation or for acute problems such as 'the grunting infant'.

Table 39.1 Numbers of infants presenting with common problems on the postnatal wards over a 12-month period, in a birth populaion of 5500 per year

Clinical condition(s)	Total number
Hips	213
Jaundice	99
Cardiac murmurs	33
Antenatal anomalies	25
Birth trauma	16
Surgical	23
Hypothermia	2
Hypoglycaemia	5
Vomiting	2
Infection	23
Maternal infection	34
Other maternal conditions	23
Family history	64
Genetic	15
Skin lesions	31

The other group comprises infants seen on the postnatal wards. They are usually several hours of age, and any concern is less acute. Table 39.1 summarizes an audit of common, non-life-threatening problems seen within one unit during a 1-year period, and gives an indication of the concerns paediatricians are asked to respond to on the postnatal wards. The birth population was approximately 5500 births per year. Routine newborn examinations and acutely ill infants have been excluded.

It can be seen from this table that many common problems in the newborn period are not serious health issues, but nonetheless can cause considerable morbidity and anxiety.

COMMON NEONATAL COMPLICATIONS PRESENTING IN THE FIRST 24 HOURS

Respiratory/grunting (transient tachypnoea of the newborn)

One of the commonest problems that paediatricians review is acute respiratory embarrassment. Tachypnoea and 'grunting' are the most common concerns. 'Grunting' is the descriptive term given to the noise made by forced expiration against a closed glottis. It is essentially a sign of alveolar disease: the alveoli do not open adequately, hence the infant tries to open them by increasing his or her intrathoracic pressure. Most commonly, 'grunting' and tachypnoea are caused by excess lung fluid, which has not fully cleared following birth. These signs usually appear within the first few hours after birth and settle within 24–48 hours. The infant is otherwise well and observation is usually all that is required. This condition is often referred to as transient tachypnoea of the newborn (TTN). It must be remembered that this is a diagnosis of exclusion. More serious conditions such as sepsis, pneumothorax or respiratory distress syndrome should be excluded. The signs of acute respiratory embarrassment are the same for many aetiologies;[1] thus, such infants should be seen by a paediatrician. If the signs are not settling quickly (i.e. within a few hours), if they worsen or if there are other risk factors in the history, the infant should be admitted to a neonatal unit for further management. This complication is common amongst babies delivered by elective caesarean section, with as many as 15 per cent of neonates being affected [II].[1]

Hypoglycaemia

This subject generates much anxiety, and continues to generate much controversy.[2] It is now accepted that many newborn infants go through a period of relatively low blood glucose levels shortly after birth. Assuming they are otherwise well, they can utilize alternative fuel sources such as ketones and lactate in the short term. This means that for term infants of average birth weight, it is unnecessary to monitor blood glucose and start invasive treatments. They should be left alone to establish breast, or bottle feeding normally. The importance of hypoglycaemia is to identify and treat the 'at-risk' infant. Examples include:

- preterm infants (<36 weeks),
- growth-restricted babies,
- the infants of diabetics,
- infants with perinatal asphyxia,
- septic infants,
- infants with inborn errors of metabolism.

In these groups, a blood glucose <2.6 mmol/L is generally accepted to indicate hypoglycaemia [IV]. Any infant presenting with low blood glucose must be carefully examined for the underlying cause and treated accordingly. The treatment of hypoglycaemia involves the administration of glucose. In the well infant, feeding with milk should be the first-line treatment. If this is not successful, or if there are indicators to suggest the infant is unwell, intravenous dextrose may be needed (a 10 per cent solution should be used initially). It may be necessary to give intravenous bolus doses (small boluses of 2–3 mL/kg of 10 per cent dextrose,

followed by an infusion). All infants requiring this type of intervention should be admitted to a neonatal unit.

Hypothermia

This can be defined as a rectal temperature <36°C. It is most commonly seen in growth-restricted and preterm small infants, or as part of the clinical picture in the sick infant. Newborn infants are born exposed and wet, and can lose heat very quickly if not dried and covered adequately. Hypothermia can cause significant morbidity; infants are lethargic and feed poorly. More seriously, hypothermia is associated with hypoglycaemia, metabolic acidosis and respiratory distress.

The septic infant may also present with hypothermia rather than pyrexia. Hence, when dealing with the cold newborn, the first concern is to look for the underlying cause. Once this has been dealt with, specific measures to warm the child include a warm environment (this may seem obvious, but it is often found that delivery rooms are environmentally unfriendly for the newborn infant), drying the infant adequately and dressing him or her in warm clothes (including skin-to-skin contact with the mother and warm towels, covers), and the use of a radiant heater or warming mattresses. For extreme hypothermia, more invasive measures, such as reheating with warmed plasma expanders or exchange transfusions with warmed blood, have been used. However, it is debatable whether these convey any benefit over the use of a radiant heater and warming mattress.

Fractures

These are not common. Fracture of the clavicle is the most frequently seen, followed by the humerus, femur and skull bones. Fractures usually result from traumatic deliveries, for example in association with shoulder dystocia and difficult instrumental deliveries [III].[3]

Clavicular fractures are best treated conservatively and have an excellent prognosis. Mild analgesia may be helpful.

Fractures of long bones may require some form of simple splinting.

Skull fractures are more serious, and the possibility of underlying haemorrhage must be considered.

Cephalohaematomas

These result from bleeding between the periosteum and skull bones, and take the shape of the underlying skull bone. As they resolve, they may exacerbate jaundice, and the possibility of associated injury (such as skull fracture or intracranial bleeding) should be ruled out. Most cephalohaematomas are benign and resolve without problems. During resolution, the swelling may increase in size; this is usually due to fluid shift into the haemorrhage by osmosis as the clot breaks down. The carers should be warned of this, as it can cause concern.

Nerve palsies

Erbs palsy and facial palsy are the most common nerve palsies. Erbs palsy is due to damage to the brachial plexus (cervical roots C5, 6 and 7), and is commonly associated with traction on the neck and shoulders during difficult deliveries[3] although cases occurring in infants delivered by caesarean section have been reported. The result is usually a flaccid arm held in a pronated and internally rotated position. Recovery rates vary according to different studies. Between 49 per cent and 94 per cent make a full recovery, with most improving by 12 months of age.[4] Early physiotherapy can help, and surgical treatment techniques are now available for those cases that do not resolve spontaneously.

Facial palsies are commonly ascribed to obstetric manoeuvres such as the use of forceps causing pressure damage; however, facial palsies also occur in infants delivered normally.[3] Most are probably the result of external pressure causing a lower motor neuron injury, and the prognosis is excellent. If an upper motor neuron lesion is suspected, the infant should be investigated for possible cerebral injury or congenital disorders. There is no specific treatment required.

Sternomastoid tumours

These are the result of bleeding into the sternomastoid muscle. They are not normally recognized at birth, and do not become obvious until a few weeks of age. Physiotherapy is required to prevent contracture of the muscle.

Traumatic cyanosis

This is a petechial rash present over the face and head, and may extend to the upper body, although the rest of the child is usually spared. It is probably the result of venous congestion, resolves spontaneously and is only of importance because it has been mistaken for true cyanosis. Simple reassurance is all that is required.

Lacerations

Occasionally the infant may suffer skin lacerations during delivery, usually during caesarean section. They are usually superficial and heal without problems. Suturing or use of Steristrips may be needed for deeper wounds.

THE NEWBORN EXAMINATION

This is included in this chapter because it plays a major role in the care of the newborn. It entails a clinical examination of the infant, carried out in the first week of life. It is meant as a screening health check, although there has been much controversy concerning its usefulness. At least 80 per cent of mothers find it a useful and reassuring process.[5]

It is probably not worth performing this examination within the first 24 hours of life, as there is a high chance of both false-negative and false-positive findings. Equally, assuming the infant is well, a 24-hour interval provides a chance for the infant to recover from the stresses of birth, and allows bonding to occur.

The newborn examination should be performed in a well-lit, warm room to prevent the exposed infant getting cold.

As with all medical examinations, it helps to have a routine system. By convention, the neonatal check is performed from the head and working down. Auscultation of the heart is opportunistic, as the infant needs to be quiet. A full explanation of the examination process would be lengthy, and the reader is referred to any of the standard textbooks of neonatology for this. A few points to remember include the need for proper hand hygiene when examining infants, and that the infant should not be left exposed for prolonged periods of time. It is often best to leave the nappy area until last. As part of the newborn check, parents should be asked about the passage of urine and stool, as well as any feeding concerns. In addition, a check should be made of the weight and head circumference.

COMMON NEONATAL PROBLEMS PRESENTING ON THE POSTNATAL WARD

Feeding

This is a huge subject and is one of the commonest causes of anxiety in mothers.

There are two methods of feeding infants: breastfeeding and the use of formula milk feeds. Breastfeeding is clearly the best choice for a number of reasons, including the following:

- it adapts to the infant's nutritional needs,
- it has anti-infective properties,
- it helps with bonding,
- it helps the mother lose weight,
- it aids contraception,
- it is convenient and free.

However, there are a few problems associated with breastfeeding. Contrary to the mother's preconceptions, breastfeeding is not always established readily. This can lead to a sense of failure and to the abandonment of breastfeeding if no support is available. Ill and preterm infants do not readily feed. In this situation, facilities should be available to help with the expression of breast milk until such time as the child is ready to suckle. There are often concerns about milk volumes; these are usually helped by support and reassurance. Test weighing has been used to try to quantify the amount of milk an infant is getting; however, this may be unhelpful, and indeed can be detrimental to breastfeeding as it often instils a further sense of failure in the mother.

Other problems include concern about inverted nipples, cracked nipples, engorged breasts, overfeeding and weaning. These concerns should be easily addressed with the right support and information. Mastitis can also cause problems but is not a reason to stop breastfeeding. Antibiotics or non-steroidal anti-inflammatory agents may be indicated.

There are very few contraindications to breastfeeding. Probably the commonest are chronic ill-health in the mother (such as cystic fibrosis), potential infective risk (e.g. human immunodeficiency virus (HIV) in developed countries), acute ill-health in both the mother and infant, and certain metabolic disorders in the infant (such as phenylketonuria and galactosaemia).

Artificial feeding with formula milk is the alternative. Problems specific to this include:

- poor preparation of feeds,
- inadequate sterilization,
- cost.

Other problems common to both methods include problems with sucking and swallowing co-ordination. These may be due to anatomical factors such as cleft palates or large tongues as well as physiological factors such as immaturity of the sucking reflexes.

Vomiting can be a major problem, and is most commonly due to gastro-oesophageal reflux. Assuming that the infant is well and growing, reassurance is usually all that is needed. Examination to exclude other causes of vomiting, such as pyloric stenosis and sepsis, should be performed. Failure to thrive is often due to feeding problems, but usually presents later in life. Bilious vomiting is pathological until proven otherwise, and should always prompt the search for a cause.

Urine/stools

It is not uncommon for neonatologists to be asked to review an infant who has either not passed urine or not opened his/her bowels. Either situation is usually benign. A detailed history, including review of the antenatal progress and birth, is important. The external genitalia and anus should be examined as part of the assessment.

Most infants pass urine within the first 24 hours. This is often missed if it occurs at the time of birth. If there is any doubt but the infant otherwise appears well, it is worth placing cotton wool ball(s) in the nappy. An infant who has not passed urine within the first couple of days or in whom there is any other concern may need further investigation to exclude either obstruction (such as posterior urethral valves in males) or renal disease.

An infant who has not opened his or her bowels within the first 2–3 days should also be reviewed. Obstruction due to anal atresia should be obvious shortly after birth; however,

conditions such as anal stenosis and Hirschprung's disease are easily missed if not considered. Investigation in such situations may involve gentle rectal examination, radiological tests and possibly rectal biopsy. Advice should be sought from a neonatologist and/or paediatric surgeon.

Weight loss

It is normal for infants to lose weight in the first week of life. This is predominantly due to water loss. Breast-fed infants tend to lose slightly more weight than bottle-fed infants. By 1 week of age, infants should start putting weight on. The average weight gain is 20–30 g/day in term infants. Weight loss in excess of 10 per cent is unusual and needs further investigation. There is a long list of causes of excess weight loss, ranging from inadequate intake, through inadequate nutritional content, to feed intolerance and ill-health.

Skin lesions

Skin lesions are a common cause of concern in the otherwise well newborn infant. They include the following.

- *Birthmarks* such as the flammeus naevus (or 'stork mark') and port wine stains. It should be noted that strawberry birthmarks do not appear until a few weeks of age. Another birthmark is the Mongolian blue spot (very common in Asian and Afro-Carribean babies), which consists of blue macules found over the back and is caused by melanocytes in the deep dermal layers.
- Skin *defects* such as the aplasia cutis lesion. This is a congenital absence of the skin over the scalp. It usually has a punched-out appearance, with a healed edge, and it is important to distinguish it from trauma. These lesions usually heal spontaneously, by granulation. Plastic surgery, when older, is required for larger lesions.
- *Rashes*. Common rashes include erythema toxicum neonatorum, a red maculopapular rash, which comes and goes in the first few days and is of no clinical significance. Miliaria may also cause concern; this rash is caused by obstruction of sweat glands. Pustular rashes are common; most are sterile, but possible infection needs to be excluded. Nappy rashes include napkin dermatitis and candidiasis, both of which are very common and cause considerable anxiety.
- Skin *tags*. These can occur anywhere on the body; common sites are around the ears, anus and vagina. Pre-auricular skin tags have classically been associated with renal disorders, although the evidence is tenuous.

Facial problems

- *Clefts of the lip* are usually obvious at birth. With better antenatal screening, many are now diagnosed on antenatal ultrasonography. The possibility of an associated chromosomal disorder should be considered, although most are independent of any other disorder. Although cosmetically they may look very abnormal, the surgical results are excellent. Parents need careful counselling from an early stage, including the use of 'before and after surgery' photographs for reassurance. During the neonatal period, the main concern is one of feeding, and referral for specialist advice at an early stage is paramount.

- Isolated *clefts of the palate* are almost never detected antenatally. They may be detected at a newborn check or can present in the early neonatal period as difficulty in feeding, apnoeas, choking episodes, poor feeding and chest infection. They are often associated with syndromes, and a meticulous neonatal examination should be performed. Referral to a geneticist may be indicated if there are other dysmorphic features. The specialist cleft lip and palate centre should be involved at an early stage.

Orthopaedic

- *Talipes* ('club foot') is a common referral for paediatric assessment. It is important to differentiate between fixed talipes and positional talipes. The former needs referral to orthopaedic surgeons and physiotherapy, whereas the latter is of no consequence and the parents can be reassured.

- Examination of the *hips* is performed to detect dislocation. The hip should be held in a flexed, slightly internally rotated position, between index finger and thumb, whilst the knee is stabilized within the palm of the hand. The hip is then downwardly displaced to see if it can be dislocated. It is then externally rotated and upward pressure is exerted onto the outer trochanter of the hip with a view to reducing a dislocated hip. These are essentially the Ortolani and Barlow manoeuvres and are designed to diagnose a dislocatable or dislocated hip (in which case a 'clunk' should be felt). This is to be distinguished from a clicky hip, which is usually either due to poor examination technique or lax ligaments around the joint. Dislocated and dislocatable hips need referral to the orthopaedic team. Ultrasonography is useful to discriminate where there is uncertainty. It is also indicated in babies at greater risk of dislocated hips (breech deliveries, positive family histories). The use of double nappies is no longer recommended.

Accessory digits

It is not uncommon for infants to be born with accessory fingers and toes. Most of these are pre-axial and not associated with any other problems. The infant should be thoroughly examined for other anomalies. Most accessory digits are attached by a thread of skin, and are easily dealt with by tying off with a suture. Those with thicker bases should be referred to a plastic surgeon.

Surgical

- *Hernias.* Common hernias include umbilical and inguinal hernias.

  Umbilical hernias are easily reducible and usually resolve spontaneously. They are more common in non-white, European races.

  Inguinal hernias are more serious. They are up to six times more common in males than females and there is an increased incidence of complications in the newborn. Early referral to a paediatric surgeon for operative correction is advised. Premature infants more commonly develop inguinal hernias than term infants.

- *Bilious vomiting* always needs investigating; although it may be innocent, the risk of intestinal obstruction or other serious pathology must be considered.

- *Hydroceles* are due to fluid accumulation in the scrotum as a result of incomplete closure of the processus vaginalis. They can be differentiated from inguinal hernias because it is possible to get above them and they transilluminate. Most hydroceles resolve spontaneously.

- *Hypospadias* occurs in approximately 1 : 300 male infants. It is characterized by a congenitally short urethra that opens onto the ventral surface of the penis, an abnormally formed foreskin, and chordee of the penis. Referral to a paediatric urologist is required. The parents should be advised not to have the child circumcized, as the foreskin is vital in any reconstructive surgery. The possibility of chromosomal abnormalities (especially sex chromosome problems) needs to be considered in severe cases.

- *Undescended testes* are common in the newborn male. Most are unilateral, and reassurance that descent will occur is all that is required. If the testicle has not descended by 1 year of age, referral to a paediatric surgeon is warranted. Bilaterally undescended testicles are much more unusual and require further investigation to exclude underlying disorders such as intersex or hormonal disorders of the pituitary–adrenal–testicular axis.

Genetic

Paediatricians are commonly asked to review an infant whose appearance has given cause for concern. Most of the time, simple reassurance is all that is required. However, in all cases the child should be carefully and thoroughly examined. There are many dysmorphic features – too numerous to list here.

In cases where doubt exists, further advice should be sought from a clinical geneticist. Chromosomal tests as well as other investigations (dictated by the presenting condition) may be needed. It is important that the parents are carefully counselled. If doubt exists, this should be explained, to avoid erroneous conclusions being made.

Eyes

- The vast majority of '*sticky eyes*' are due to blocked tear ducts; simple toileting with lukewarm sterile water and cotton wool or gauze is all that is required. If the discharge persists, or is particularly copious, infections should be considered, and a swab sent for microbiological culture and sensitivity. The eyes should then be treated with topical antibiotics. Staphylococcal infections are the most common and are usually successfully treated with either topical gentamicin or neomycin. Chloramphenicol eye drops are also available and popular, but can mask chlamydial infection. Chlamydial infection should be considered if the discharge is copious or persistent; *Chlamydia* requires special culture mediums to grow, and is treated with chlortetracycline eye ointment plus systemic erythromycin.
- Congenital *cataracts* are rare. The newborn check is designed to detect them by looking for the normal red reflex with an ophthalmoscope. If a cataract is present, the red reflex will be absent, or partially obscured, depending on the size of the cataract. In this situation, urgent referral to an ophthalmologist is required. With early intervention, it is possible to improve subsequent vision.

Cardiac murmurs

Heart murmurs are a common finding in newborn infants; however, most cardiac murmurs in the newborn infant are innocent flow murmurs – these are especially audible in the first days of life. As a general rule, identification of a cardiac murmur should lead to a careful clinical examination, an electrocardiogram (ECG) and measurement of limb oxygen saturations in the right arm and lower limbs (i.e. pre-ductal and post-ductal oxygen saturations). The majority of infants will be found to have a soft systolic murmur (i.e. with a grading of 1–2/6), a normal cardiovascular examination, no significant change in pre-ductal and post-ductal oxygen saturations, and a normal ECG. These infants can be reviewed in 4–6 weeks, as the chance of a significant cardiac lesion is very small. Parents should be warned of the small risk of a cardiac defect; if they have any concerns, such as the child getting breathless, tired, not feeding or going blue, they should seek medical advice urgently.

Infants who do not meet these criteria should be referred to a paediatric cardiologist for further investigation.

Maternal group B streptococcal infection

It is generally accepted that infants of group B streptococcal (GBS) carriers are at greater risk of infection. However, quantifying that risk is difficult. Equally, given the high carriage rate amongst the normal population (estimated between 30 and 50 per cent), it is difficult to ascertain the best treatment approach.

Group B streptococcal disease is divided into early and late onset.

Early-onset disease is caused by passage of the infant through the genital tract in a carrier mother (many women are carriers and few babies are affected). It may present as:

- a clinical picture which mimics severe perinatal asphyxia,
- severe respiratory failure at birth,
- signs of early neonatal sepsis, such as temperature instability, lethargy, irritability, respiratory signs and tachycardia.

It is a neonatal emergency with potentially life-threatening consequences.

Universal pregnancy screening programmes and the use of prophylactic antibiotics are not recommended in the UK (see Chapter 22).

In an attempt to identify at-risk babies, it is recommended that infants born to mothers who are GBS carriers and have one or more of the following features deserve special attention:

- previous infant born with GBS disease,
- spontaneous onset of premature labour,
- prolonged rupture of membranes,
- evidence of invasive GBS disease in the mother.

If mothers are given sufficient antibiotics early enough in the labour, the infant should be adequately covered [Ia].[6] If this does not occur, or the infant is in any way unwell, he or she should be screened and treated with intravenous antibiotics. Subsequent management will depend on the clinical course and the results of cultures.

Late-onset GBS disease is probably related to infection after birth from a carrier mother. It can be present days or weeks later, most commonly with pneumonia or meningitis.

Renal

In addition to determining whether or not a baby has passed urine (see above), other renal problems usually relate to infants who have been found to have renal anomalies during antenatal ultrasound screening. Assuming the infant is well, repeated scanning can be performed within the first few weeks of life; many anomalies will have resolved. If there are continuing abnormalities, further investigation is required to delineate the nature of the anomaly.

Infants with significant bilateral renal anomalies on antenatal ultrasound (e.g. bilateral dysplastic, cystic kidneys or bilaterally dilated ureters) need more urgent investigation. They should also be monitored for failing renal function.

Metabolic

The Guthrie test is a screening test performed on all newborn infants within the first week of life. It involves the collection of blood drops from a heal prick, and screens for:

- hypothyroidism,
- phenylketonuria,
- cystic fibrosis (in certain parts of the UK, immunoreactive trypsin levels are measured).

The test should be performed once the infant has been established on feeds for a few days.

Sacral dimples

Sacral dimples are a common finding, usually at the base of the spinal column. It is also important to ask about bowel actions and urine excretion and to check the lower limbs for normal movements and power. Assuming the base is easily seen and there are no other abnormalities, simple reassurance is all that is required. If the base is not visualized, or if the sacral dimples are larger than 0.5 cm diameter or associated with other features such as tufts of hair, ultrasound investigation and paediatric review are indicated.

The most commonly associated problem is tethering of the spinal cord, which usually presents later in life.

Umbilical cord

The umbilical cord is a common source of concern. The cord stump usually falls off within a few days.

- The most serious problem is one of *infection*. It is common for the cord stump itself to become colonized with commensal organisms, resulting in a 'sticky' or 'smelly' cord stump. Assuming the infant is otherwise well, with no signs of ascending infection, simple toileting with sterile saline or water is all that is needed [Ia].[7] Should there be any signs of spreading infection or systemic illness, the infant must be treated immediately. Ascending infection from the cord stump is usually due to *Escherichia coli*, other Gram-negative organisms or *Staphylococcus aureus*, and is a neonatal emergency requiring intravenous antibiotics.
- Umbilical stump *granulomas* do not present until after the cord stump has separated. Most resolve, although some practitioners treat them with application of a silver nitrate stick. They must be differentiated from a patent urachus.

Jaundice

Jaundice is a common, and potentially serious, problem with numerous causes:

- physiological jaundice, due to overloading of the immature hepatic system as a result of excessive red blood cell breakdown: the infant develops an unconjugated hyperbilirubinaemia between the second and fifth days, settling by a week of age;
- sepsis;
- haemolysis due to Rhesus or ABO incompatibility.

Acute haemolytic disease usually presents within the first 24–48 hours of life, thus any baby appearing jaundiced within this time must be investigated.

Treatment may not be necessary. The most important reason for treating jaundice is to prevent kernicterus, which is associated with severe unconjugated hyperbilirubinaemia and may result in death or major neurological sequelae. Most infants can be treated with simple phototherapy, although for more serious cases exchange transfusions are needed.

Prolonged jaundice is also of concern in the neonate. As a general rule, any term infant with evidence of jaundice beyond 10–14 days of age, or a preterm infant after 3 weeks of age, should be considered as having prolonged jaundice. There are numerous causes, of which the commonest is 'breast milk jaundice' (a diagnosis of exclusion). All infants with prolonged jaundice should be investigated. It is particularly important to exclude a conjugated hyperbilirubinaemia, as this may be due to obstruction (e.g. biliary atresia), which can be treated successfully with surgical intervention if diagnosed early.[8]

PROBLEMS ASSOCIATED WITH PREMATURITY

Respiratory distress syndrome (also known as hyaline membrane disease) is due to a lack of surfactant in the lungs, leading to acute respiratory failure. The severity varies from mild respiratory symptoms, requiring minimal input, to severe respiratory failure, requiring full intensive care and complex ventilator strategies.

Respiratory distress syndrome can either recover or develop into chronic lung disease (bronchopulmonary dysplasia). Other complications include pulmonary interstitial emphysema and other airleak syndromes.

Effectively, every system in the premature infant is at greater risk of problems. Premature infants are at risk of cardiovascular instability and hypotension requiring treatment. They are susceptible to cerebral insults, especially intraventricular haemorrhage. Their immature immune systems put them at higher risk of sepsis. They easily become anaemic, due to marrow immaturity as well as the need for frequent phlebotomy. Their gastrointestinal system is vulnerable. They often show feed intolerance initially, and there is a high risk of necrotizing enterocolitis. (Necrotizing enterocolitis is a serious condition, which affects the lining of the bowel; it probably results from infection superimposed on bowel that has suffered an ischaemic insult.)

Premature infants also have a higher risk of long-term sequelae, including poor growth, neurodevelopmental disabilities and chronic lung disease.

CONCLUSION

This chapter highlights some of the more common problems faced with the newborn infant. It concentrates on common acute problems occurring in the delivery suite shortly after birth and subsequently on common concerns that subsequently present on the postnatal wards. Most of the common problems occurring after the first hours following birth are not life threatening, but do cause significant anxiety and morbidity.

KEY POINTS

- Most common neonatal problems are non-life threatening.
- Recognizing the sick infant from the well infant is vital to avoid disaster.
- The newborn examination is a clinical screening test, and as such its limitations should be borne in mind.

KEY REFERENCES

1. Dani C, Reali MF, Bertini G et al. Risk factors for the development of respiratory distress syndrome and transient tachypnoea in newborn infants. Italian Group of Neonatal Pneumology. *Eur Respir J* 1999; 14:155–9.
2. Cornblath M, Hawdon JM, Williams AF et al. Controversies regarding definition of neonatal hypoglycemia: suggested operational thresholds. *Pediatrics* 2000; 105:1141–5.
3. Perlow JH, Wigton T, Hart J, Strassner HT, Nageotte MP, Wolk BM. Birth trauma. A five-year review of incidence and associated perinatal factors. *J Reprod Med* 1996; 41:754–60.
4. Pollack RN, Buchman AS, Yaffe H, Divon MY. Obstetrical brachial palsy: pathogenesis, risk factors, and prevention. *Clin Obstet Gynecol* 2000; 43:236–46.
5. Wolke D, Dave S, Hayes J, Townsend J, Tomlin M. Routine examination of the newborn and maternal satisfaction: a randomised controlled trial. *Arch Dis Child Fetal Neonatal Ed* 2002; 86:F155–60.
6. Smaill F. Intrapartum antibiotics for Group B streptococcal colonisation (Cochrane Review). In: *The Cochrane Library*, Issue 3. Oxford: Update Software, 2002.
7. Zupan J, Garner P. Topical umbilical cord care at birth (Cochrane Review). In: *The Cochrane Library*, Issue 3. Oxford: Update Software, 2002.
8. Johnson LH, Bhutani VK, Brown AK. System-based approach to management of neonatal jaundice and prevention of kernicterus. *J Pediatr* 2002; 140:396–403.

Chapter 40

Perinatal Mortality

James Drife

MRCOG standards

Theoretical skills
- Know the definitions of the perinatal mortality rate and its subdivisions.
- Have knowledge of the way in which perinatal deaths are classified and the leading causes.
- Know how perinatal mortality rates can be kept low or reduced further.

Practical skills
- Recognize that reducing perinatal mortality requires practical obstetric skills.
- Recognize the need for attention to detail in both antenatal and intrapartum care.
- Recognize that skills in risk management are highly relevant.

INTRODUCTION

Strictly speaking, perinatal mortality is defined as stillbirths and deaths of babies in the first week of life. In all countries the perinatal mortality rate (PMR), even with this relatively limited definition, is much higher than the maternal mortality rate. In the UK in 1999 the PMR (7.9 per 1000 live and stillbirths) was around 70 times higher than the maternal mortality rate (11.4 per 100 000 maternities), though exact comparison is difficult because of the different denominators.[1]

The PMR is widely used as an indicator of the quality of obstetric care and enables comparisons to be made among nations, regions and indeed individual hospitals. Nevertheless, perinatal mortality includes a wide range of conditions – from preterm labour to sudden infant death syndrome – with a wide range of underlying causes. For useful clinical lessons to be learned, perinatal mortality must be subdivided by the time of the death and by the causes.

DEFINITIONS

The following definitions are those used in the UK and published in the annual reports of the Confidential Enquiry into Stillbirths and Deaths in Infancy (CESDI). CESDI reports are available at <www.cesdi.org.uk> and the work of CESDI is described later in this chapter.

- *Stillbirth.* The legal definition in England and Wales is 'A child which has issued forth from its mother after the 24th week of pregnancy and which did not at any time after being completely expelled from its mother breathe or show any other signs of life'.
- *Early neonatal death.* Death of a liveborn infant occurring less than 7 completed days (168 hours) from the time of birth.
- *Perinatal mortality rate.* The number of stillbirths and early neonatal deaths (those occurring in the first week of life) per 1000 live and stillbirths.

CESDI also gathers data on deaths that fall outside the strict definition of perinatal mortality. The remit of the enquiry extends from 20 weeks of pregnancy to the end of the first year of life, and this involves several other categories and definitions.

- *Late fetal loss.* Death occurring between 20 weeks + 0 days and 23 weeks + 6 days. If gestation is not known or not sure, all births of at least 300 g are reported.
- *Infant death.* Death in the first year following live birth, on or before the 365th day of life (366th in a leap year). Infant deaths therefore include early and late neonatal deaths, and post-neonatal deaths.
- *Neonatal death.* Death before the age of 28 completed days following live birth.
- *Late neonatal death.* Death from age 7 days to 27 completed days of life.
- *Post-neonatal death.* Death at age 28 days and over but under 1 year.

When infant and neonatal death rates are calculated, the denominator is 'per 1000 live births'. This is slightly different from the denominator for the late fetal loss rate, which (like that of the stillbirth rate and the PMR) is 'per 1000 live and stillbirths'.

Definitions of 'stillbirth'

Miscarriages are not included in the PMR. In the UK it is legally necessary to register stillbirths – i.e. babies born dead after 24 weeks – but registration of miscarriage is not required. The dividing line between miscarriage and stillbirth is arbitrary, however, and may vary from country to country. For example, in New York State it is 20 weeks and in Canada it is 28 weeks.

In the UK the dividing line was also 28 weeks until 1992. When it was lowered, the official stillbirth rate rose by nearly 30 per cent. The change was made because, with modern neonatal care, many fetuses born alive at under 28 weeks can now survive. Indeed, survival is possible even below 24 weeks, but this was retained as the dividing line in the UK partly because, under British law, therapeutic abortion for social reasons is allowed up to 24 weeks' gestation.

The World Health Organization (WHO) has chosen a dividing line of 22 weeks, but in many parts of the world it may be difficult to define gestation exactly and therefore fetal weight is the main basis of the WHO definition of stillbirth:

> *The death of a fetus weighing at least 500 g (or when birth weight is unavailable, after 22 completed weeks of gestation or with a crown–heel length of 25 cm or more), before the complete expulsion or extraction from its mother.*[2]

In all countries, if a baby is born alive and dies soon after delivery, this is classified as a neonatal death irrespective of the gestation. This may lead to some anomalies. For example, in the UK a baby born at 23 weeks' gestation will be included in the national statistics if death occurs after delivery but not if death occurs before delivery.

CONFIDENTIAL ENQUIRY INTO STILLBIRTHS AND DEATHS IN INFANCY

History

In England and Wales the Confidential Enquiry into Maternal Deaths (CEMD) has been running continuously since 1952. In 1992, this method of enquiry was extended to the deaths of babies with the setting up of a separate organization, CESDI. Its aim is to improve understanding of the risks of death from 20 weeks of pregnancy to 1 year after birth, and of how these might be reduced. Like CEMD, CESDI attempts to identify suboptimal care so that faults can be remedied.

However, CESDI requires a larger infrastructure than CEMD. In England, Wales and Northern Ireland there are around 10 000 deaths annually between 20 weeks' gestation and 1 year

of life, compared with only about 100 maternal deaths. CESDI was originally based on the 14 health regions of England, each of which undertook its own perinatal mortality survey and had a full-time co-ordinator with support staff. There were separate arrangements for Wales and Northern Ireland.

Since 1996, CESDI has been managed by a consortium of Royal Colleges – those of Midwives, Obstetricians and Gynaecologists, Paediatrics and Child Health, and Pathology. It is funded by the government through the National Institute of Clinical Excellence (NICE). In 2002, CEMD and CESDI joined to form the Confidential Enquiries into Maternal and Child Health (CEMACH).

Together with the Confidential Enquiry into Perioperative Deaths (CEPOD) and the Confidential Inquiry into Suicides and Homicides by People with Mental Illness (CISH), they form an important part of the work of NICE. Although these developments have produced a bewildering proliferation of acronyms, it is gratifying for obstetricians that the 'confidential enquiry' method, pioneered 50 years ago by CEMD, has been steadily extended as a way of improving care.

Methods

All deaths occurring between 20 weeks' gestation and 1 year of life are notified to the regional CESDI co-ordinator using 'Rapid Report Forms'. A full national picture of the causes of death is therefore obtained every year. In addition, a sub-set of cases is anonymized and reviewed by a specialist panel within each region. The regional data and enquiry findings are collated by a central secretariat to provide a national overview and are published in an annual report.

Each panel consists of experts from several disciplines, including as a minimum an obstetrician, paediatrician, midwife, specialist perinatal/paediatric pathologist, general practitioner and an independent chairman. Others with appropriate expertise may also be involved. Panel members are sent anonymized case notes and they summarize their cases and meet for discussion. They comment on suboptimal care, grading each case as follows.

- Grade 0 – no sub-optimal care.
- Grade 1 – sub-optimal care, but different management would have made no difference to the outcome.
- Grade 2 – sub-optimal care, different management might have made a difference to the outcome.
- Grade 3 – sub-optimal care, different management would reasonably have been expected to have made a difference to the outcome.

Recommendations are made to reduce the likelihood of sub-optimal care in future.

The work programmes of CESDI

Each CESDI report includes a detailed study of a specific subject, for example on the deaths of normal fetuses during labour. These reports have been highly influential in improving care. The programme of special studies is shown below.

- *Enquiry topic*
  - Intrapartum-related deaths >2.5 kg
  - Intrapartum-related deaths >1.5 kg
  - 'Explained' sudden deaths in infancy
  - '1 in 10' sample of all deaths >1 kg
  - All deaths 4 kg and over
- *Case-control studies*
  - Sudden unexpected deaths in infancy
  - Antepartum term stillbirths
  - Project 27/28 (deaths from 27 + 0 weeks to 28 + 6 weeks)
- *Focus groups and central reviews*
  - Should dystocia
  - Ruptured uterus
  - Planned home delivery
  - Anaesthetic complications and delays
  - Breech presentation at the onset of labour
  - Stillbirths
- *Audits and collaborative work*
  - Post-mortem reporting
  - Cardiotocography (CTG) education
  - European comparisons of perinatal care
  - Use of electronic fetal monitoring

Perinatal post-mortem examination

A particular problem in the UK in recent years has been public concern about the perinatal post mortem. This was triggered by events in Liverpool, where organs had been retained after post mortem without the permission of parents having been specifically sought. Several bodies have recently produced guidelines on post mortems and these have been summarized in the Eighth CESDI Report.[1] The key points are that parents should be better informed about the post mortem, and that those who discuss post mortems with parents must understand the process so that consent is informed. The Chief Medical Officer has recommended that all Trusts should designate a named individual to provide information to families.

INCIDENCE

Worldwide

Globally there were 132 million births in the year 2000, and 90 per cent of them took place in developing countries, where more than 80 per cent of people live.[3] Accurate data on perinatal mortality in developing countries are often lacking, but WHO estimates that there are between 7 and 8 million perinatal deaths annually. This gives a global PMR of between 50 and 60 (compared to 7.9 in the UK).

Table 40.1   Numbers of perinatal deaths in CESDI annual reports[1,9]

	1994	1999
Total births in England, Wales and Northern Ireland	677 758	644 940
Stillbirths	3 688	3 216
Neonatal deaths	2 749	2 502
Post-neonatal deaths	1 199	1 184
Total number of perinatal deaths	5 897	5 115
Perinatal mortality rate (per 1 000 live and stillbirths)	8.5	7.9
Neonatal mortality rate (per 1 000 live births)	3.4	3.3

There are wide differences among countries. Overall life expectancy in some countries is less than half that in others, and this is largely due to high death rates in small children. For example, in much of South-east Asia, 40 per cent of children die by their fourth year. The underlying reason is often malnutrition, which makes children more susceptible to infection. Malnutrition affects particularly those born into large and poorly spaced families.

There are also differences within the developed world. In Europe, the PMR in some countries is double that in others. The main reason, again, is poverty. By comparison, differences in PMRs due to minor variations in the definition of stillbirth are relatively unimportant.

The UK

Data on perinatal mortality have been collected in the UK for the last 60 years. During this time there has been a dramatic reduction in perinatal deaths. This has mainly been due to the improved health of the population, better nutrition and wider education, though the role of the healthcare services is also important, particularly in recent years.

Improvement is still continuing. In 1963 in England and Wales the stillbirth rate was >17 per 1000 total births and the neonatal death rate was >14 per 1000 live births. In 1999 these rates had fallen to 5.0 and 3.9 respectively.

During the 1990s, improvements were documented in CESDI's annual reports (Table 40.1). Perinatal deaths were first included in the report for 1994.[4] The Eighth Annual Report, published in 2002, gave the figures for 1999.[1]

This comparison shows a fall in the PMR over this 6-year period, mainly due to a reduction in the number of stillbirths. This appears to be the result of an improvement in obstetric care, which is discussed in more detail below.

AETIOLOGY

The problem in developing countries has been summed up as follows by the former Director-General of WHO:

There are between 7 and 8 million perinatal deaths, but we do not know exactly how many are stillbirths and how many are early neonatal deaths. In many cases, births of infants who die soon after birth are neither recorded nor counted. ...Although the exact medical causes in countries may differ, the problem is simple: the common denominator for these deaths is the lack of appropriate and quality services, confounded by poverty.[3]

In the developed world, by contrast, sophisticated systems have been developed not only for recording and counting perinatal deaths, but also for subdividing them according to the underlying cause.

Classification systems

CESDI uses three systems of classification: the extended Wigglesworth classification, the Obstetric (Aberdeen) classification, and the Fetal and Neonatal Factor classification. They show many similarities.

Extended Wigglesworth classification

There are nine categories in this classification. The first four categories are the main ones as far as the UK is concerned and are discussed in more detail below.

- Category 1. Congenital defect or malformation (lethal or severe).
- Category 2. Unexplained antepartum fetal death.
- Category 3. Death from intrapartum asphyxia, anoxia or trauma.
- Category 4. Immaturity.
- Category 5. Infection. This applies when there is clear microbiological evidence of infection – e.g. group B streptococci.
- Category 6. Other specific causes. Some conditions are not covered in the main four categories, e.g.
  - fetal conditions such as hydrops fetalis
  - neonatal conditions such as pulmonary hypoplasia
  - paediatric conditions such as malignancy.
- Category 7. Accident or non-intrapartum trauma. This includes confirmed non-accidental injury.
- Category 8. Sudden infant death, cause unknown. This category includes all infants in whom the cause was unknown at the time of death. Information from post mortem may be added later.
- Category 9. Unclassifiable. This category may be used, but only as a last resort.

Obstetric (Aberdeen) classification

This system includes 22 categories grouped under the following headings.

- Congenital anomaly
- Isoimmunization
- Pre-eclampsia
- Antepartum haemorrhage

- Mechanical (e.g. cord prolapse or malpresentation)
- Maternal disorder
- Miscellaneous
- Unexplained

Fetal and Neonatal Factor classification

This system includes 24 categories grouped under the following headings.

- Congenital anomaly
- Isoimmunization
- Asphyxia before birth
- Birth trauma
- Severe pulmonary immaturity
- Hyaline membrane disease
- Intracranial haemorrhage
- Infection
- Miscellaneous
- Unclassifiable or unknown

In the Fetal and Neonatal Factor classification, as in the Obstetric (Aberdeen) classification, only one category can be applied to any one death, and categories at the head of the list take priority over those lower down. For example, a baby who dies of intracranial haemorrhage (number 7 on the above list) would be categorized by the cause, such as birth trauma (number 4) or hyaline membrane disease (number 6).

Causes of perinatal mortality

The Eighth Report gave the data in Table 40.2 for England, Wales and Northern Ireland for 1999.

Table 40.2 Causes of perinatal mortality in England, Wales and Northern Ireland in 1999[1]

	Number	Percentage
Stillbirths		
Antepartum fetal death	2472	71.3
Congenital malformation	438	12.6
Intrapartum anoxia	253	7.3
Infection	83	2.4
Total	3469	
Early and late neonatal deaths		
Immaturity	1209	47.2
Congenital malformation	625	24.4
Intrapartum anoxia	233	9.1
Infection	211	8.2
Total	2559	
Post-neonatal deaths		
Congenital malformation	338	28.5
Sudden infant death	291	24.6
Infection	233	19.7
Immaturity	139	11.7
Total	1184	

Postpartum complications: neonatal

Table 40.3   Stillbirths and deaths in the first month of life

	Number	Percentage
Antepartum fetal death	2472	41
Immaturity	1209	20
Congenital malformations	1063	18
Intrapartum anoxia	486	8
Others	798	13
Total	6028	

An unfavourable outcome of obstetric care may be either a stillbirth or an early or late neonatal death, so Table 40.3 aggregates stillbirths and deaths up to the end of the first month of life, showing the four main causes in 1999.

This list slightly underestimates the importance of prematurity, which may also result in post-neonatal death, but it demonstrates the large contribution of antepartum fetal death to the overall problem of perinatal mortality. The proportion of deaths due to intrapartum anoxia has fallen to 8 per cent from 10 per cent in 1994, and the reason for this is discussed in more detail later in this chapter.

PREVENTION

Worldwide

In 2000, at the Millennium Summit in New York, world heads of state named reducing child mortality and improving maternal health as key Millennium Development Goals. Strategies for reducing perinatal mortality overlap with those for improving maternal health and reducing maternal mortality. The WHO target for 2015 is to reduce by two-thirds the under-5 mortality ratio and by three-quarters the maternal mortality ratio from their 1990 levels.

However, ambitious targets have been set before and have not been achieved. The causes of perinatal mortality in many countries are resistant to change. Poverty is a major factor, and poor women are often caught in a damaging cycle of disease and malnutrition. The WHO estimates that 15 per cent of babies weigh less than 2 500 g at birth, but in some countries one-third are below this weight, and in reality the proportion is probably much higher because only about one-third of babies are weighed at birth.

Nevertheless, improvements can be made. Family size throughout the world has been reduced by improving access to contraception, and reduced perinatal mortality can to a great extent be achieved by basic hygiene, access to trained health workers and simple, well-tried technology.[3] A randomized trial in rural Gambia showed that dietary supplementation during pregnancy in chronically undernourished women can reduce perinatal mortality.[5]

Infection is a major problem in developing countries. There is evidence that perinatal infection and mortality can

be reduced by cleansing the birth canal during labour with chlorhexidine.[6] Perinatal transmission of human immuno-deficiency virus (HIV) can be reduced by avoiding breast-feeding but this may not be widely implementable because of the lack and dangers of alternative feeding methods.[6] Promotion of breastfeeding is particularly important in developing countries. Not only does it provide appropriate nourishment for the newborn, but also it reduces the risk of infection from artificial feeding, provides passive immunity through maternal antibodies, and acts as a natural contraceptive to ensure adequate pregnancy spacing.

The UK

The potential for further reducing perinatal mortality in the UK is discussed under the headings of the four main categories of the extended Wigglesworth classification.

Category 1. Congenital malformation

Congenital abnormalities account for about 18 per cent of the perinatal deaths in the UK. Cardiovascular abnormalities constitute the largest proportion of lethal congenital anomalies at birth because of the difficulty of adequately visualizing the cardiovascular system at ultrasound screening. The fetal spine is easier to visualize, and most neural tube defects (NTDs) are identified at a gestation at which the woman can be offered termination of pregnancy. This has resulted in a decrease in perinatal mortality from this condition but an increase in therapeutic termination. Ideally, congenital malformations would be prevented altogether rather than being diagnosed early enough for termination, but this is difficult to achieve. The government has advised that all women should take periconceptual folic acid to reduce the incidence of NTDs, but only a minority do so.

Besides fetal anatomy scanning in mid-pregnancy, the other major screening programme available in the UK is biochemical screening for chromosomal abnormalities through tests such as the 'triple test'. However, the commonest chromosomal abnormality, Down's syndrome, does not usually cause neonatal death, and therefore this screening programme has little effect on perinatal mortality.

Category 2. Antepartum fetal death

Antepartum fetal death causes less soul-searching among obstetricians than intrapartum death, but it accounts for a much larger proportion of perinatal mortality. Antepartum term stillbirth was the subject of a special study in the Fifth Annual CESDI Report.[7] Cases were compared with controls and parents were interviewed in addition to the usual methods of gathering data. Of 86 cases studied, 27 were unexplained and 22 were associated with intrauterine growth restriction. Of the remainder, the two commonest conditions were placental abruption (nine cases) and abnormal glucose tolerance (nine cases). Many of the mothers had noticed a change in fetal movements or the occurrence of abdominal pain. There was an excess of mothers of non-white origin.

The Eighth CESDI Report examined 422 stillbirths in 1996–97 and found that 45 per cent of them were associated with sub-optimal care. For example, screening for intrauterine growth restriction needs to be improved – for instance by meticulous use of symphysis–fundal height measurements – and communication with mothers needs to be optimized so that those with concerns about reduced fetal movements can be seen promptly for checks on fetal well-being. A full list of the panel's comments is given below.

Nature of sub-optimal care

- Risk recognition
  - Failure to recognize high-risk woman at booking
- Growth
  - Inadequate monitoring of growth
  - Failure to recognize intrauterine growth restriction
  - Failure to act on intrauterine growth restriction
- Fetal movement
  - Failure of professional to act on decreased fetal movements
  - Importance of changes in fetal movement not explained to woman
  - Decreased fetal movements not reported by mother until after delivery
- Management
  - Failure to act on high-risk situation/history
  - Failure to act on raised blood pressure and/or proteinuria
  - No plan of care/management
  - Failure to act on suspicious antenatal CTG
  - Failure to do or repeat glucose tolerance test
  - Poor diabetic management
  - Inappropriate grade of staff involved in care
- Communication
  - Poor documentation
  - Poor communication – oral and written
- Lifestyle
  - Maternal smoking
  - Poor attendance for antenatal checks
- Post-delivery
  - Inadequate screening following stillbirth
  - Post mortems – quality issues, failure to send samples
  - Bereavement support

Particular attention needs to be focused on at-risk groups – poor women and those from ethnic minorities. In Sweden, a country with one of the lowest PMRs in the world, women who emigrated from sub-Saharan Africa have an increased perinatal mortality. A study identified sub-optimal factors in perinatal care among this group, including delay in seeking healthcare, mothers refusing caesarean sections, insufficient surveillance of intrauterine growth restriction, inadequate medication, misinterpretation of CTG and interpersonal miscommunication.[8]

Category 3. Intrapartum asphyxia

The Fourth Annual CESDI Report looked at 873 cases of death from intrapartum-related events in 1994 and 1995.[9] The risk of death in labour was 1 in 1561 births. Over 78 per cent of the cases were criticized for sub-optimal care – alternative management might (25 per cent) or 'would reasonably be expected to' (52 per cent) have made a difference to the outcome. With antepartum care, the main problem was failure to recognize risk factors. With intrapartum care, the main problem was inadequate assessment of the fetal condition by heart rate monitoring and blood sampling. In 22 per cent of cases there was also criticism of the resuscitation of the newborn.

The report's recommendations, based on these findings, were radical. Three recommendations are particularly important.

1 'The training, assessment, supervision and practice of obstetricians and midwives of all grades needs to be critically appraised by their parent bodies.'
2 Professional bodies should 'look again at how level of practical competence of professionals of all grades caring for women in labour and for babies following delivery are achieved and maintained'.
3 'A multidisciplinary initiative at national level is needed to develop guidelines covering all aspects of fetal assessment before and especially during labour.'

The Royal Colleges of Midwives and of Obstetricians and Gynaecologists responded by publishing guidelines for improved standards of care in labour, which recommended, among other things, more involvement of consultant obstetricians in the day-to-day running of delivery suites.[10] This recommendation was strongly promoted by the Royal College of Obstetricians and Gynaecologists (RCOG) and has resulted in a change in the pattern of daytime obstetric cover in Britain. National evidence-based guidelines were also produced on induction of labour and the use and interpretation of electronic fetal monitoring (EFM). A survey in the Eighth CESDI Report found that fetal blood sampling is now available as an adjuvant to EFM in most units, although the availability of EFM guidelines is still poor.

These initiatives, which involved much effort at local and national levels, have produced a gratifying improvement in this cause of perinatal mortality. The Eighth Annual CESDI Report included the following statement:

It is therefore extremely encouraging to see that intra-partum-related mortality has now decreased significantly from 0.95 (1994) to 0.62 (1999) per 1000 live births and stillbirths. Although it is not possible to

Postpartum complications: neonatal

predict if this is a continuing downward trend, it is hoped that by maintaining efforts to achieve the highest possible standard of intrapartum care this will prove to be the case.[1]

Category 4. Immaturity

Almost 50 per cent of neonatal deaths are due to prematurity, although, as mentioned above, twice as many babies are lost as antepartum stillbirths. The immediate causes of death include respiratory distress syndrome, infection, neurological causes and gastrointestinal causes. Advances in neonatal care have improved the survival of premature infants to a remarkable degree. The Eighth CESDI Report included a survey of babies born at between 27 + 0 and 28 + 6 weeks' gestation, which found that the survival rate to day 28 was 88 per cent.

The best solution to the problem of immaturity would be to prevent preterm delivery occurring, but this is an elusive goal for researchers. In the meantime, there is clear evidence that giving the mother steroids before preterm delivery will reduce the baby's risk of developing respiratory distress syndrome, and reduce perinatal mortality. Steroids must be given at least 24 hours before delivery and sometimes it is impossible to delay delivery long enough for them to work.

Clinical risk management

For many years it has been standard practice for maternity hospitals to hold perinatal mortality meetings to review cases of perinatal death. The clinical history and pathological findings are examined and the implications for the management of similar cases are discussed. This method is being extended to include 'near-miss' incidents, and hospitals are introducing 'critical incident' reporting.[11] A critical incident is any event that a member of staff feels might put patients at risk. Incidents are reported to a senior member of staff, who decides which ones should be discussed at staff meetings. It is essential that such discussions take place in a blame-free atmosphere, so that constructive suggestions can be made for improving care.

Comprehensive standards for clinical risk management have been published by the Clinical Negligence Scheme for Trusts (CNST).[12] Compliance with these standards has financial benefits for Trusts by reducing the annual premiums they pay to the CNST.

SUMMARY

Worldwide, there are between 7 and 8 million perinatal deaths annually, 90 per cent of which occur in developing countries, where the main causes are poverty, malnutrition and lack of access to healthcare. Improvements could be made by basic hygiene, access to trained healthcare workers, and promotion of breastfeeding.

In the UK, perinatal mortality is low by comparison but could be reduced still further. Intrapartum management is being improved, with better training in the interpretation of electronic monitoring and more involvement of senior staff. Congenital malformations can be detected during pregnancy, but the ideal strategy is prevention. Prevention of preterm labour remains a considerable challenge, but neonatal care has greatly improved survival rates. Antepartum fetal death is the major contributor to perinatal mortality and its reduction requires meticulous antenatal care, with better detection and management of intrauterine growth restriction. In this regard, particular attention must be paid to at-risk groups such as poor women and those from ethnic minorities.

- Maternal steroid administration before preterm delivery reduces perinatal mortality [Ia].
- The evidence does not support the routine use of EFM in low-risk labours.
- Dietary supplementation in chronically malnourished women reduces perinatal mortality [Ib].

KEY POINTS

- The perinatal mortality rate is the number of stillbirths and deaths in the first week of life per 1000 live and stillbirths.
- Globally the perinatal mortality rate is around 50–60.
- Worldwide perinatal mortality is due to poverty, malnutrition and infection and can be reduced by better hygiene and better access to healthcare.
- In the UK the perinatal mortality rate is currently 7.9.
- The causes in the UK, in round figures, are antepartum stillbirth (40 per cent), immaturity (20 per cent), congenital malformations (20 per cent), intrapartum asphyxia (10 per cent) and others (10 per cent).
- Deaths from intrapartum asphyxia have recently been reduced by implementing CESDI recommendations, particularly with regard to senior obstetric staff being present in the delivery suite.
- Antepartum stillbirths could be reduced by more focused antenatal care, concentrating on the detection of intrauterine growth restriction and on better communication with at-risk women.
- Perinatal post mortems require fully informed consent from parents, and sensitive counselling is very important.

KEY REFERENCES

1. Confidential Enquiry into Stillbirth and Deaths in Infancy. *Eighth Annual Report.* London: Maternal and Child Health Research Consortium, 2002.

2. World Health Organization. *Mother–Baby Package: Implementing Safe Motherhood in Countries.* Geneva: WHO, 1994. (Also available at <www.who.int/reproductive-health/publications>.)

3. Brundtland GH. Perinatal mortality and morbidity – a global view. Speech delivered at the XVIII European Congress of Perinatal Medicine, Oslo, 19 June 2002: <www.who.int/director-general/speeches/2002>.

4. Confidential Enquiry into Stillbirths and Deaths in Infancy. *Second Annual Report.* London: Maternal and Child Health Research Consortium, 1995.

5. Ceesay SM, Prentice AM, Cole TJ et al. Effects on birth weight and perinatal mortality of maternal dietary supplements in rural Gambia: 5 year randomised controlled trial. *BMJ* 1997; 315:786–90.

6. Hofmeyr GJ, McIntyre J. Preventing perinatal infections. *BMJ* 1997; 315:199–200.

7. Confidential Enquiry into Stillbirth and Deaths in Infancy. *Fifth Annual Report.* London: Maternal and Child Health Research Consortium, 1998.

8. Essen B, Bodker B, Sjoberg N-O et al. Are some perinatal deaths in immigrant groups linked to suboptimal perinatal care services? *Br J Obstet Gynaecol* 2002; 109:677–82.

9. Confidential Enquiry into Stillbirths and Deaths in Infancy. *Fourth Annual Report: Concentrating on Intrapartum Deaths 1994–95.* London: Maternal and Child Health Research Consortium, 1997.

10. Royal College of Obstetricians and Gynaecologists. *Report of the Working Party on Minimum Standards of Care in Labour.* London: RCOG Press, 1998.

11. Drife J. Reducing risk in obstetics. In: Vincent C (ed). *Clinical Risk Management*, 2nd edn. London: BMJ Books, 2001; 77–94.

12. NHS Litigation Authority. Risk management in practice. *NHS Litigation Authority Review*, Issue 25, Winter 2002/3 (available at <www.nhsla.com>).

SECTION G

Postpartum complications: maternal

Postpartum Collapse

Peter J. Thompson

MRCOG standards

Modules 10 and 13 cover the majority of this topic.

Theoretical knowledge
- Understand the different aetiologies and clinical presentations of postpartum collapse and to have a sufficient understanding of both the medical and surgical treatments of these patients.

Practical skills
- Recognize the cause of a postpartum collapse and be able to both initiate and co-ordinate a multidisciplinary-based plan of management, often in conjunction with senior medical staff.

INTRODUCTION

Postpartum collapse is a major cause of maternal mortality and morbidity in both the developed and developing worlds. Although the commonest causes of postpartum collapse are not confined to the immediate postpartum period, because of the rapid haemodynamic, hormonal and anatomical changes occurring at this time, there is an increased prevalence of these conditions.

Although many of these conditions require specific management plans, the generic treatment of a shocked patient, i.e. airway protection, administration of oxygen and gaining intravenous access, is common to all.

DEFINITION

Postpartum collapse is the onset of shock in the immediate period following delivery of the fetus.

INCIDENCE

There are no good denominator data available accurately to determine the incidence of this condition.

AETIOLOGY

There are many causes of postpartum collapse, with the commonest and most important being listed in Table 41.1. Many of these aetiologies have common pathways via hypovolaemia, whether it be absolute hypovolaemia, as in haemorrhage, or relative hypovolaemia secondary to changes in the autonomic nervous system, as in uterine inversion. It is noteworthy that all the main conditions that contribute to both direct and indirect maternal mortality in the UK are represented in this list.

The management of many of these conditions has been described elsewhere in this book, and will therefore not be redressed here. This chapter concentrates on the causes of postpartum collapse marked with an asterisk in Table 41.1.

Vaso-vagal attacks

Vaso-vagal attacks are relatively common occurrences and are induced by many external stimuli, which result in extreme emotions such as fright, anxiety or phobias. They are frequently preceded by a prodromal state consisting of dizziness, nausea, sweating, tinnitus and yawning. The

Table 41.1 Aetiology of postpartum collapse

Pulmonary emboli	Vaso-vagal attacks*	Uterine inversion*
Septic shock	Epileptic convulsions	Cardiac arrest*
Haemorrhage	Cerebrovascular accident	Cardiac arrhythmias
Amniotic fluid embolus*	Eclampsia	Iatrogenic*

* See text for explanation.

aetiology is one of vasodilatation, leading to a pooling of blood and therefore a relative hypovolaemia. The heart therefore begins to empty, stimulating mechanoreceptors in the wall of its left ventricle. This in turn acts centrally to initiate further vasodilatation and a bradycardia. These attacks usually resolve spontaneously, though it is advisable to position the patient flat and then elevate her legs to encourage central venous return and hence adequate filling of the heart [IV]. Similar syncopal episodes may also be present in patients with cardiac disease, specifically those women who have arrhythmias or obstructive heart disease.

Cardiac arrest

Cardiac arrest during the postnatal period is usually associated with hypovolaemia, complex congenital heart disease or obstructive heart disease. However, with increasing maternal age at the time of delivery, ischaemic heart disease is now seen. Indeed, in the last Confidential Enquiry into Maternal Mortality 1997–99,[1] five women died following myocardial infarction. Although none of these deaths was in the immediate postpartum period, three of them were in the puerperium. Other causes of reversible cardiac arrest are listed in Table 41.2.

Resuscitation of women who have had a cardiac arrest in pregnancy is usually complicated by the fact that, when supine, a gravid uterus will compress the inferior vena cava, decreasing venous return. Emptying the uterus, by delivering the fetus, will improve stroke volume by 60 per cent and is therefore mandatory if resuscitation has not been successful within 5 minutes [III]. Although this latter problem is not present in the immediate postpartum period, the uterus may still be of sufficient size to cause significant aorto-caval compression and therefore resuscitation should be conducted with the patient on a left lateral tilt [III]. This results in an increased cardiac output of 25 per cent when compared to a supine patient.[2,3] The optimum tilt is a left lateral tilt at an angle of 27°. This angle was calculated by Rees and Willis,[4] who examined all angles between 0 and 90°, comparing their efficiency for chest compression and their propensity to increase central impedance to venous return. At this angle, it is possible to exert 80 per cent of the mechanical pressure on the chest that one would if the patient were flat. As a result of this study, the Cardiff Resuscitation Wedge was designed and manufactured.

Management therefore consists of diagnosing and treating any reversible cause of the arrest whilst simultaneously following the European Resuscitation Council Guidelines 2000 for Adult Advanced Life Support;[5] these are summarized in Figure 41.1. Once a cardiac arrest has been diagnosed, a precordial thump may be administered by a trained healthcare professional, though its success rate is low if the arrest has already lasted longer than 30 seconds [III]. Basic life support should begin once the airway is secured, with ventilation at a rate of 12 breaths per minute and chest

Table 41.2   Reversible causes of cardiac arrest

Four 'H's	Four 'T's
Hypovolaemia	Tension pneumothorax
Hypoxia	Cardiac tamponade
Hyper/hypokalaemia, hypocalcaemia, acidaemia	Thromboembolic or mechanical obstruction
Hypothermia	Toxic or therapeutic substances in overdose

compression at a rate of 100 per minute. The ventilation does not need to be synchronized with chest wall compression, as substantially higher coronary artery perfusion pressures are obtained if chest wall compression is uninterrupted.

Post-resuscitation care should include transfer of the patient to a critical care unit or coronary care unit [III]. Patients who are hypothermic should not be warmed and those who are pyrexial should receive antipyretics [II].

Amniotic fluid embolus

Amniotic fluid embolism is rare, with an incidence of 1 in 80 000 pregnancies,[6,7] though good denominator data are not available. However, due to its high mortality rate of 80 per cent,[6,7] it is a relatively common cause of maternal mortality, with eight women dying from this condition in the last maternal mortality report.[1] This was a significant reduction from the previous triennial report on maternal deaths (50 per cent). The aetiology is an anaphylactic reaction to the passage of amniotic fluid and particulate matter into the lungs. This results in pulmonary hypertension and hypoxia[8] presenting as respiratory distress, central cyanosis and circulatory collapse. Approximately half of the patients who survive the initial insult develop disseminated intravascular coagulation.

Diagnosis of the condition is suspected when patients suddenly collapse either in labour or shortly after delivery with signs of central cyanosis, though confirmation of the diagnosis can be made on examination of lung tissue at post mortem, or on examination of blood films for the presence of squames or fetal hair. Management of these patients revolves around the generic treatment of shock and coagulopathies, with the former often requiring the information provided by pulmonary artery wedge pressures to guide inotropic interventions [III].

Uterine inversion

Uterine inversion is a rare condition, occurring with an incidence of 1 in 10 000 pregnancies. Although maternal death secondary to uterine inversion is well recognized, in the last Confidential Enquiry into Maternal Mortality 1997–99,[1] no such deaths were documented. The degree with which the fundus of the uterus inverts is variable, with the mildest form being dimpling of the fundus and the most severe being complete inversion, where the fundus of the uterus

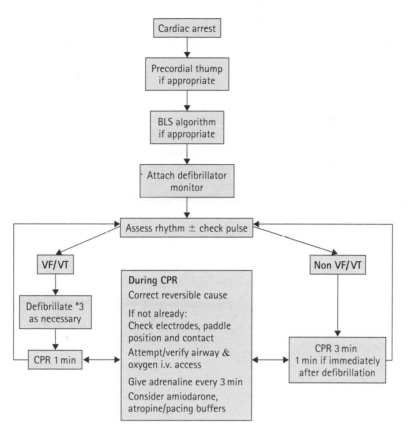

Figure 41.1   European Resuscitation Council Guidelines for Adult Advanced Life Support.[5] BLS, basic life support; VF ventricular fibrillation; VT, ventricular tachycardia; CPR, cardiopulmonary resuscitation

passes through the cervix. There is no agreement on the aetiology of this condition, though several factors appear to be associated with its occurrence. These include:

- mismanagement of the third stage of labour, either by inappropriate traction during controlled cord traction or too rapid removal of the placenta during manual removal;
- maternal age >25 years;
- a sudden rise in intra-abdominal pressure in the presence of a relaxed uterus;
- a fundally placed placenta with a short umbilical cord.

Patients present with a picture of shock in the absence of visible blood loss. This shock appears to be of neurogenic origin secondary to traction on structures adjacent to the uterus. The fundus of the uterus may be visible at the introitus; however, if not, it will be detected on vaginal examination. This latter examination is mandatory in all patients who appear to be shocked in the immediate postpartum period in the absence of visible blood loss [IV]. Not only can this lead to the exclusion of a diagnosis of an inverted uterus, but a diagnosis of a supralevator haematoma will also be excluded.

Treatment is based on the principles of managing a shocked patient and then replacing the uterus as soon as possible. If the diagnosis is made immediately, the uterus can often be replaced manually prior to the onset of shock. However, once the uterus has been inverted for only a few minutes, the tissues surrounding it constrict, preventing its replacement. In this circumstance manual replacement may be possible using general anaesthesia [III]. If this fails, O'Sullivan's hydrostatic technique may be attempted: the vagina is filled with warm saline whilst being blocked at the introitus with the attendant's fist. The hydrostatic pressure resulting from the instillation of 4–5 L of saline may be sufficient to balloon the vagina and reverse the inversion [III].

Should neither of these techniques result in replacement of the uterus, a laparotomy and Haultain's procedure should be performed before the uterus becomes ischaemic from obstruction of its blood supply. At laparotomy, traction is placed on the round ligaments and an incision is made through the muscular ring in the posterior uterine wall. Continued manual pressure on the fundus from the vagina and traction of the round ligaments will allow replacement of the uterus, and the incision is closed [III].

In all the previously described management options, once the uterus is correctly sited, a Syntocinon infusion should be commenced to encourage contraction of the uterus [IV]. It should be noted that a recurrence rate of approximately 30 per cent has been quoted in the literature, though recent figures are unavailable.

Iatrogenic causes

Iatrogenic causes of loss of consciousness in the postnatal period include inappropriate advice on positioning the woman, with a resultant syncopal episode, and reactions to the administration of drugs. Although any drugs may be administered at this time, those that are most frequently used include Syntocinon, Ergometrine and local anaesthetics.

Syntocinon may cause sudden hypotension and, in women who are supine and have recently haemorrhaged, can be sufficient to result in loss of consciousness. This situation should be managed as for any shocked patient, with the appropriate positioning of the woman, protection of the airway and the administration of intravenous fluids. In the recent Confidential Enquiry into Maternal Mortality, it was reiterated that Syntocinon should be used with care in such situations. Ergometrine, which is usually administered along with Syntocinon, is a powerful smooth muscle constrictor and is contraindicated in women with severe hypertension, as it may precipitate a hypertensive crisis and haemorrhagic cerebrovascular accident.

In women with inadequate analgesia, infiltration of the perineum with a local anaesthetic is mandatory prior to surgical repair of the perineum. Lignocaine, the most widely used local anaesthetic for this purpose, is ideally suited, with an onset and duration of action after infiltration of 5 minutes and 1 hour, respectively (maximum plasma concentrations occur at 25 minutes). Overdosage usually presents as light-headedness, sedation, paraesthesia, twitching and convulsions. However, if the drug is administered intravenously, it may result in the precipitation of cardiac arrhythmias and cardiac arrest. This is one of the reversible causes of cardiac arrest and should be managed according to the guidelines described by the European Resuscitation Council [IV].[5]

It is therefore imperative for all healthcare professionals who infiltrate with lignocaine to ensure that injections are not intravenous and to be aware of the maximum dose of lignocaine that can be administered safely. This will depend, amongst other things, upon the patient's size and the degree of vascularity of the area being infiltrated. This latter variable can be altered by the administration of vasoconstrictors to the local anaesthetic. The recommended maximum dose of lignocaine is 200 mg (500 mg if administered with adrenaline). However, this situation is complicated by the fact that most local anaesthetics are labelled in percentage solutions and hence professionals need to understand how much lignocaine there is in a specified percentage solution. This equation is shown below.

1 L of a 100 per cent solution contains 1 kg of the active ingredient. Therefore 10 mL of 0.5 per cent lignocaine contains:

$$\frac{1000\,g \times 10\,mL \times 0.5}{1000\,mL \times 100} = 0.05\,g = 50\,mg$$

- There are few randomized, controlled trials of the management of acute postpartum collapse.
- There are, however, internationally accepted evidence-based guidelines for adult resuscitation.

KEY POINTS

- All healthcare practitioners should be aware of the local guidelines to treat the shocked patient.
- European guidelines are available for resuscitation following cardiac arrest.
- Pregnant women who have had a cardiac arrest need to be placed in a left lateral tilt at an angle of 27°.
- Prompt replacement of an inverted uterus may be life saving.
- Local anaesthetic solutions are labelled in per cent and can easily be converted into milligrams.
- Local and national guidelines are essential for the management of these conditions.
- Good denominator data are not available for many of the conditions that cause postpartum collapse.

KEY REFERENCES

1. Department of Health. *Why Mothers Die:* 1997–1999. London: RCOG Press, 2001.
2. Lee RV, Rodgers LD, White LM, Harvey AC. Cardiopulmonary resuscitation of the pregnant woman. *Am J Med* 1986; 81:311–18.
3. Uckland K, Novy MJ, Peterson EN. Maternal cardiopulmonary dynamics IV. The influence of gestational age on the maternal cardiovascular response to posture and exercise. *Am J Obstet Gynecol* 1969; 104:856–64.
4. Rees GAD, Willis BA. Resuscitation in pregnancy. *Anesthesia* 1998; 43:347–9.
5. de Latorre F, Nolan J, Robertson C, Chamberlain D, Baskett P. European Resuscitation Council Guidelines 2000 for Adult Advanced Life Support. A statement from the Advanced Life Support Working Group (1) and approved by the Executive Committee of the European Resuscitation Council. *Resuscitation* 2001; 48:211–21.
6. Morgan M. Amniotic fluid embolism. *Anaesthesia* 1979; 34:20–32.
7. Mulder JI. Amniotic fluid embolism: an overview and case report. *Am J Obstet Gynecol* 1985; 152:430–5.
8. Clark SL, Colton DB, Gonik B, Greenspoon J, Phelan JP. Central dynamic alteration in amniotic fluid embolism. *Am J Obstet Gynecol* 1988; 158:1124–6.

Chapter 42

Postpartum Haemorrhage

Peter J. Thompson

INTRODUCTION

Haemorrhage is still one of the leading causes of maternal mortality in the UK with postpartum haemorrhage playing a significant role in the deaths of seven women in the last triennial report.[1] Any discussion of postpartum haemorrhage must cover both the primary and secondary conditions, although the majority of this chapter is aimed at the management of primary postpartum haemorrhage.

DEFINITIONS

The differentiation between primary and secondary postpartum haemorrhage is more than an academic discussion, as the aetiology, clinical presentation, treatment and prognosis of the two conditions are very different.

Postpartum haemorrhage is subclassified as follows:

- Primary postpartum haemorrhage is defined as the loss of 500 mL of blood from the genital tract following, but within the first 24 hours of, the delivery of the baby.

  A caveat is added in that if the blood loss is <500 mL but is sufficient to cause hypovolaemic shock in the patient, this is also classified as a primary postpartum haemorrhage. A new definition of massive postpartum haemorrhage has been introduced, being the loss of greater than 1000 mL or 1500 mL of blood. Owing to the relatively low risks of blood loss below these levels, this is thought to be of greater clinical relevance. The incidence of this complication is being used in some units as an indicator of the standard of maternity care.[2]
- Secondary postpartum haemorrhage is more of a subjective diagnosis, as its definition is blood loss from the genital tract of a volume greater than expected after the first 24 hours but within the first 6 weeks of delivery.

INCIDENCE

The incidence of primary postpartum haemorrhage in the developed world is approximately 5 per cent of all deliveries.[3] The incidence of massive postpartum haemorrhage in the UK has been reported as 6.7 per 1000.[2] This figure was obtained by analysis of a cohort of 48 865 women who delivered in a 1-year period. Although significant morbidity will be associated with this condition, other data concerning its incidence are limited. However, the risk of mortality from postpartum haemorrhage was calculated to be 0.47 per million maternities in the last triennial report on maternal mortalities in the UK.[1]

AETIOLOGY

The commonest aetiology of primary postpartum haemorrhage is uterine atony, followed by genital tract trauma.

Uterine atony may have many causes, including retained placental fragments, and is associated with prolonged labour, multiple pregnancies, polyhydramnios, instrumental deliveries and grand multiparity. Other somewhat rarer causes include coagulopathies, pathological placentation (e.g. placenta accreta) and uterine inversion. These rarer causes retain a significant level of importance because of their relative over-representation among severe cases of haemorrhage.

The major aetiological factors associated with secondary postpartum haemorrhage are retained placental fragments and endometritis.

MANAGEMENT

It is important to discuss the options for the prevention of postpartum haemorrhage with women antenatally. It has been well established that active management of the third stage of labour, with the administration of Syntometrine at the time of delivery of the infant's anterior shoulder followed by controlled cord traction, is associated with a relative risk of postpartum haemorrhage of 0.38 (95 per cent confidence interval (CI) 0.32–0.46) [Ia].[4] However, there is a substantial increase in the risk of maternal side effects such as nausea with active management of the third stage of labour when compared to physiological management.[4] Women at risk of a postpartum haemorrhage should also have an intravenous cannula inserted during labour and blood taken for estimation of the haemoglobin concentration, and serum should be grouped and saved [IV]. Such women include those in the risk categories mentioned above as well as women who have had a previous postpartum haemorrhage, who have a risk of recurrence of approximately 25 per cent. Examination of the placenta post-delivery should identify a proportion of women who have retained placental fragments and who will require manual removal of the placenta.

Significant postpartum haemorrhage is an obstetric emergency that requires a multidisciplinary team for optimum management [IV]. Initial management is dependent upon rapid diagnosis. This is difficult, as it is well recognized that both obstetricians and midwives are poor at accurately estimating blood loss at the time of delivery. This can be further confounded by the ability of fit young women to maintain their blood pressure, either with or without a tachycardia, until they have lost approximately 15 per cent of their blood volume.

Resuscitation

Immediate management will involve resuscitation of the hypovolaemic patient with the citing of two large-bore (16G) intravenous cannulae, fluid administration, the application of facial oxygen, and examination to determine the aetiology of the haemorrhage [IV]. Although for many years clinical teaching has been that fluid replacement by colloid is superior to the use of a crystalloid, examination of randomized, controlled trials in patients with hypovolaemia has failed to show any benefit with the preferential use of colloids [Ia].[5] Although these studies are in the non-pregnant population, it is reasonable to extrapolate this conclusion to fit pregnant women. In this early stage of resuscitation it is important to obtain blood for a full blood count, clotting studies and group and cross-matching.

Disseminated intravascular coagulation

Disseminated intravascular coagulation (DIC) is a life-threatening complication of massive haemorrhage. Regardless of the aetiology, the management should revolve around maintaining an adequate intravascular volume and treating the underlying cause, in this case stopping the haemorrhage. This condition is discussed in more detail in Chapter 23. However, one should aim to follow four basic principles:

1 to maintain the intravascular volume,
2 to administer fresh frozen plasma (FFP) at a rate to keep the activated partial thromboplastin:control ratio <1.5,
3 to administer packed platelets to maintain a platelet count $>50 \times 10^9$/L,
4 to administer cryoprecipitate to keep the fibrinogen level >1 g/dL.

Although administration of blood components should be guided by haematological results, as described above, this should not be delayed until the patient is moribund, as successive Confidential Enquiries into maternal mortalities have identified delay in transfusion as a significant contributor to maternal mortality [III].

Specific managements strategies

Uterine atony can be managed pharmacologically or by a combination of pharmacological and surgical intervention. If the placenta is thought to be complete, the uterus is clinically atonic and there are no significant signs of genital tract trauma, an examination in theatre may be avoided by the administration of ergometrine followed by a Syntocinon infusion. Although the former has significant side effects, including nausea, vomiting and hypertension, its tonic action on the uterine muscle is a valuable adjunct to therapy with Syntocinon alone. However, caution is necessary in patients with pre-eclampsia, who may suffer episodes of severe hypertension following the administration of ergometrine.

Should these efforts fail to control the bleeding, examination of the genital tract needs to be performed with adequate lighting and patient analgesia. This usually means examination in an operating theatre with the patient having a regional or general anaesthetic. If the bleeding is significant, this examination should not be delayed in order to

Table 42.1   Suggested dosages for uterotonics

Uterotonic	Route of administration	Dosage
Syntocinon	i.v.	Bolus dose of 5 iu, followed if necessary by an infusion of 40 iu in 40 mL of saline run at 10 mL/hour
Syntometrine	i.m.	1 mL
Ergometrine	i.v./i.m.	250–500 μg
Carboprost	i.m.	250 μg every 15–90 minutes, to a maximum of 2 mg (eight doses)
Misoprostol	p.r.	800 μg
Gemeprost	Intrauterine	1–2 mg

obtain blood results; if the anaesthetist is concerned about the risks of siting a regional anaesthetic in the presence of a possible coagulopathy, a general anaesthetic should be administered [IV].

Examination under anaesthesia should include examination of the vagina, cervix and, in the case of continued bleeding, exploration of the uterine cavity digitally to identify and remove any retained fragments of the placenta. If the uterine cavity is explored digitally, this should be covered by the administration of a broad-spectrum antibiotic. At this time, if no other cause for the haemorrhage has been identified, administration of prostaglandin analogues, either intramuscularly (if carboprost is available) or rectally (if only misoprostol or gemeprost is available), is advisable. The success of carboprost administration was as high as 88 per cent in one study.[6] Suggested dosages of these uterotonics can be seen in Table 42.1. Bimanual compression of the uterus may also need to be performed at this stage; this decreases blood loss partly because of the fact that it puts the uterine arteries under tension.

If these pharmacological and basic surgical steps have not achieved haemostasis, the uterus can be packed by either a traditional technique using gauze[7] or, as has more recently been described, balloon insufflation.[8,9] This technique can be employed regardless of whether the abdomen is open or closed, and may therefore avoid the need for open laparotomy [III]. Indeed, the provisional data on the use of balloon insufflation using a Rusch urological balloon appear very encouraging, although there are problems related to when and by how much the balloon should be deflated.

Should these steps fail, the patient will require a laparotomy. At that time either unilateral or bilateral uterine artery ligation can be performed, with success rates reported of more than 90 per cent [III].[10]

This technique involves placement of a suture through the broad ligament to include 2–3 cm of myometrium. The suture should be placed approximately 2 cm above the point where an incision for a lower segment caesarean section would be, thus ligating the ascending branch of the uterine artery and avoiding inclusion of the ureter in the suture.

Arterial ligation has been modified into a series of stepwise procedures producing uterine devascularization. This

technique, described in Egypt, involves five steps: unilateral ligation of the uterine artery at the level of the lower segment; bilateral ligation of the uterine artery at the level of the lower segment; low ligation of the uterine artery after mobilization of the bladder; unilateral ovarian vessel ligation; and bilateral ovarian vessel ligation [III].[11] The first two of these steps resulted in haemostasis in more than 80 per cent of cases in the original report. Although ligation of the internal iliac arteries has been well described in the literature, it requires a high level of surgical skill and is reported as avoiding hysterectomy in only 50 per cent of cases.[12] The surgical time and complication rate in this series were also higher than when a hysterectomy was performed. After all these levels of uterine devascularization, subsequent menstruation and successful pregnancies have been reported.

The use of compression sutures of the uterus has been reported from Switzerland and the UK,[13,14] although their exact role in the treatment of postpartum haemorrhage has yet to be established. Compression sutures are only of possible benefit if bimanual compression of the uterus results in significant decrease in blood loss. Initially, the operation described by B-Lynch involves inserting a compression suture through a lower uterine segment incision, either the caesarean section incision or making a new incision. The suture is placed 3 cm below the incision and 3 cm in from its lateral border, through the uterine wall and cavity, exiting through a similar position on the superior aspect of the incision 3 cm above and 4 cm in from the lateral border. It then passes over the uterine fundus 3–4 cm from the right cornua and passes posteriorly down the uterus to enter the posterior uterine wall at the same level as the upper anterior entry point. The suture is then placed under moderate tension whilst an assistant compresses the uterus. It is then placed back through the posterior wall on the left at a similar point as on the right. The suture is passed back over the fundus and then inserted through the upper and lower incisions on the left in a similar fashion as on the right. It is then tied. Initially, this technique was described using a 2 catgut suture on a 70 mm round-bodied hand needle. However, since the withdrawal of catgut, an alternative suture would be 1 monocryl.

A modification of the technique without opening a previously intact uterus has also been described.

Hysterectomy with ovarian conservation may be required as a life-saving procedure. It has a reported incidence of approximately 0.7 per cent following caesarean section and 0.02 per cent following vaginal delivery.[15] Experienced obstetricians need to be involved in the decision-making process during this cascade of events and, where possible, the patient and her relatives should be kept fully informed.

Selective arterial embolization has been described both prior to hysterectomy and for persistent bleeding following hysterectomy. However, at the present time its use is limited by its availability.

The postoperative management of these patients may include the use of critical care units, with careful monitoring of central venous pressure being a recommendation from consecutive maternal mortality reports [III]. In the long term, these patients may also need professional counselling, especially if they have undergone a hysterectomy, and a debriefing with the lead clinician in charge of the patient's care is likely to improve patient understanding and satisfaction [IV].

The management of secondary postpartum haemorrhage may, if severe, follow similar lines to the above. However, if milder, the management will depend upon the aetiology of the condition, with patients with suspected endometritis being treated with broad-spectrum antibiotics and those with suspected retained fragments of the placenta by uterine exploration. Because of the high incidence of infection, it is important that any uterine instrumentation is covered by administration of a broad-spectrum antibiotic [IV]. The role of ultrasound in the detection of retained products of conception is limited, because of the difficulty in distinguishing between placental tissue and an organized blood clot on ultrasonographic examination [IV].

- A systematic review of randomized, controlled trials shows that active management of the third stage of labour decreases the incidence of postpartum haemorrhage.
- A systematic review of the optimal choice of fluid for resuscitation shows no advantage in choosing a colloid before a crystalloid.
- There are few randomized, controlled trials of the management of postpartum haemorrhage.
- A series of retrospective and prospective studies has shown that even with severe haemorrhage, a combination of medical and surgical treatment should avoid the need for hysterectomy in the vast majority of cases.

KEY POINTS

- Postpartum haemorrhage is still a cause of maternal mortality in the UK.
- Active management of the third stage of labour decreases the risk of postpartum haemorrhage.
- Early identification of postpartum haemorrhage with accurate estimation of blood loss is essential.
- Acute management requires a multidisciplinary approach with the involvement of senior clinicians.
- It is important to monitor central venous pressure in severe cases.
- Early transfusion and correction of coagulopathies are fundamental.
- All units need their own detailed protocols for the management of massive postpartum haemorrhage.

KEY REFERENCES

1. Department of Health. *Why Mothers Die: 1997–1999*. London: RCOG Press, 2001, 94–103.
2. Waterstone M, Bewley S, Charles Wolfe C. Incidence and predictors of severe obstetric morbidity: case-control study. *BMJ* 2001; **322**:1089–94.
3. Annonymous. The management of postpartum haemorrhage. *Drug Ther Bull* 1992; **30**:89–92.
4. Prendiville WJ, Elbourne D, McDonald S. Active versus expectant management in the third stage of labour (Cochrane Review). In: *The Cochrane Library*, Issue 4. Oxford: Update Software, 2001.
5. Bunn F, Alderson P, Hawkins V. Colloid solutions for fluid resuscitation (Cochrane Review). In: *The Cochrane Library*, Issue 4. Oxford: Update Software, 2001.
6. Oleen MA, Mariano JP. Controlling refractory atonic postpartum hemorrhage with Hemabate sterile solution. *Am J Obstet Gynecol* 1990; **162**:205–8.
7. Maier RC. Control of postpartum hemorrhage with uterine packing. *Am J Obstet Gynecol* 1993; **169**:317–23.
8. Katesmark M, Brown R, Raju K. Successful use of a Sengstaken–Blakemore tube to control massive postpartum haemorrhage. *Br J Obstet Gynaecol* 1994; **101**:259–60.
9. Johanson R, Kumar M, Obhrai M, Young P. Management of massive postpartum haemorrhage: use of a hydrostatic balloon catheter to avoid laparotomy. *Br J Obstet Gynaecol* 2001; **108**:420–2.
10. O'Leary JA. Uterine artery ligation in the control of post cesarean hemorrhage. *J Reprod Med* 1995; **40**:189–93.
11. Abd Rabbo SA. Stepwise uterine devascularization: a novel technique for management of uncontrolled postpartum hemorrhage with preservation of the uterus. *Am J Obstet Gynecol* 1994; **171**:694–700.
12. Annonymous. Postpartum haemorrhage. *Clin Obstet Gynecol* 1994; **37**:824–30.
13. Schnarwller B, Passweg D, von Castleberg B. Erfolgreiche Behandlung einr medikamentos refraktaren Uterusatonie durch Funduskompressionsnahte. (Successful treatment of drug refractory uterine atony by fundus compression sutures.) *Geburtshilfe Frauenheilkd* 1996; **56**:151–3.
14. B-Lynch C, Coker A, Lawal AH, Abu J, Cowen MJ. The B-Lynch surgical technique for the control of massive postpartum haemorrhage: an alternative to hysterectomy? Five cases reported. *Br J Obstet Gynaecol* 1997; **104**:372–5.
15. Clark SL, Yeh S, Phelan JP, Bruce S, Paul RH. Emergency hysterectomy for obstetric hemorrhage. *Obstet Gynecol* 1984; **64**:376–80.

Postpartum Pyrexia

Peter J. Thompson

INTRODUCTION

Historically, postpartum sepsis was most commonly secondary to infection with group A *Streptococcus*, and the prognosis was poor. Although the advent of antimicrobial therapy has significantly improved the prognosis, the last triennial report demonstrates that puerperal sepsis is not a disease of the past. Indeed, in this report, maternal mortality from genital tract sepsis was identified as the cause of direct maternal deaths in 18 women.[1]

DEFINITIONS

Normal core body temperature is 37–37.5°C, with a diurnal variation of body temperature resulting in evening temperatures being 0.5–1°C higher than those in the morning. Oral and axillary temperatures are usually 0.4 and 1°C lower than core temperature respectively. Persistent elevation of body temperature above those normal levels is termed pyrexia or fever. The standard definition for puerperal fever used for reporting rates of puerperal morbidity is an oral temperature of 38.0°C or more on any two of the first 10 days postpartum, or 38.7°C or higher during the first 24 hours postpartum.

INCIDENCE

Following delivery, pyrexia is common, with fever secondary to disorders of the breast occurring in approximately 18 per cent of healthy mothers.[2,3] Benign fever with resolution in the first 24 hours occurs with an incidence of 3 per cent.[4] Fever associated with infection is more common, with urinary tract infections occurring in 2–4 per cent of women following delivery and endometritis in 1.6 per cent. Infections of the lower genital tract are uncommon and account for only approximately 1 per cent of cases of puerperal infection.[5]

AETIOLOGY

The aetiology of pyrexia following delivery can be separated into four broad categories:

- benign fever,
- breast engorgement,
- infections of the urogenital tract,
- distant infections.

The commonest infections of the urogenital tract are endometritis, urinary tract infections and infections of perineal repairs. Although not all pyrexias are of an infective origin, infection is the most important diagnosis and a thorough examination to search for a possible site of infection should be made. Rare causes of infection should be borne in mind in those patients who have recently been in tropical countries. Specific infections in the puerperium are caused by the same organisms that cause these infections at other times.

The development of endometritis is secondary to contamination of the uterine cavity with vaginal organisms during labour and delivery, with subsequent invasion of the myometrium. Endometritis is usually a polymicrobial infection associated with mixed aerobic and anaerobic flora. Bacteraemia may be present in 10–20 per cent of cases. The organisms that contribute to this condition include groups A and B beta-haemolytic *Streptococci*, aerobic Gram-negative rods, *Neisseria gonorrhoeae* and certain anaerobic bacteria.

Regardless of the aetiology of the pyrexia, the common pathway appears to be the production of endogenous pyrogens released by leucocytes in response to an antigenic stimulus. These then act on the hypothalamus, which in turn acts on the vasomotor centre, resulting in an increased production of heat and a decrease in heat loss.

MANAGEMENT

Prophylaxis

Prophylaxis against infections in the puerperium is particularly important in the case of delivery by caesarean section [Ia][6] and in women at risk of developing subacute bacterial endocarditis [III]. Although the advice contained within the *British National Formulary* only states that prophylaxis should be used in obstetric cases in which there is a history of prosthetic valves or previous endocarditis,[7] there were two indirect maternal deaths secondary to cardiac disease involving co-existent infection secondary to bacterial endocarditis reported in the last Confidential Enquiry into Maternal Deaths.[8] Therefore, although routine prophylaxis has not been recommended for all women with a heart lesion during labour, a high index of suspicion should be retained in the presence of such a lesion, and close liaison with local cardiologists should be maintained [IV].

General management

Management will depend upon the origin of the pyrexia. Because of the diverse nature of aetiologies mentioned above, a thorough history and examination need to be performed, with particular attention to examination of the breasts, chest and any wound sites. This includes an abdominal examination of the uterus for tenderness, a sign of endometritis. The endometrial cavity should be thought of as a wound site in this situation [IV]. Features that are more typical of a benign fever are the presence of early low-grade pyrexia in the absence of any other symptomatology.

Appropriate cultures should be taken and, depending on the clinical features present, these may include wound and vaginal swabs, midstream specimens of urine, sputum samples and blood cultures. Management should consist of supportive therapy to ensure hydration and, where necessary, the administration of regular paracetamol, which acts as an antipyretic and will improve patient comfort, whilst not altering the course of the disease process [Ib].[9] In cases of

severe septicaemia, transfer to a critical care unit may be required so that inotropic support can be initiated.

Specific management

This should be aimed at the administration of an appropriate antibiotic, which may need to be given intravenously in the first instance. In line with controls assurance standards, all hospitals should have an antibiotic policy determined by examination of the antibiotic sensitivities of organisms that have been detected within that unit. An example of one such policy from Birmingham Women's Hospital is included in Table 43.1.

The management of proven endometritis has been shown to be optimal if antibiotics that cover *Bacteroides fragilis* and other penicillin-resistant anaerobic bacteria are used. When uncomplicated endometritis is clinically improving on intravenous therapy, there appears to be no advantage in continuing oral therapy [Ia].[10] As no single antibiotic regimen has yet been shown to be superior to others in the treatment of urinary tract infections, therapy should be determined by policies based on the antibiotic sensitivities of bacteria isolated locally [Ia].[11]

Wound infections and endometritis may both be complicated by abscess formation. In these circumstances antibiotic therapy alone is insufficient, and surgical drainage

Table 43.1   First-line antibiotic treatment for obstetric complications at Birmingham Women's Hospital

Condition	First-line treatment	Second-line treatments
Chest infection	Amoxycillin and await cultures	Trimethoprim or clarithromycin or i.v. cefuroxime
Infective endocarditis prophylaxis	Treat relevant cardiac conditions with the policy in the BNF 'as for special risk'	
Wound infection	Flucloxacillin	Erythromycin or trimethoprim
Wound infection with cellulitis	Benzylpenicillin i.v. and flucloxacillin i.v.	Contact microbiology for advice
Septicaemia post-surgery	Cefuroxime i.v. and metronidazole p.r.	Contact microbiology for advice
Septicaemia: antenatal	Augmentin	Cefuroxime i.v. and metronidazole p.r.
Septicaemia: postnatal	Cefuroxime i.v. and metronidazole p.r.	Contact microbiology for advice
Endometritis	Augmentin oral	Trimethoprim ± metronidazole
Urinary tract infection	Await cultures unless systemically unwell, if so cefuroxime i.v.	
Prophylaxis for caesarean section	Augmentin i.v.	Cefuroxime i.v. and metronidazole p.r./i.v.

BNF, *British National Fomulary*.

will be required [IV]. The long-term complications of endometritis include subfertility [III].

The management of fever associated with breast problems is detailed elsewhere (see Chapter 45).

- Systematic reviews of randomized, controlled trials show:
  - a decrease in infective morbidity following caesarean section if prophylactic antibiotics are used;
  - in cases of endometritis, antibiotics that cover *Bacteroides fragilis* and other penicillin-resistant anaerobic bacteria should be used;
  - if the endometritis is uncomplicated, oral therapy following intravenous therapy is unnecessary.
- Randomized, controlled trials show that the administration of paracetamol to pyrexial patients increases their comfort and does not affect the progress of the disease.
- Expert opinion regarding controls assurance suggests that all hospitals should have their own antibiotic policy.

KEY POINTS

- Puerperal sepsis is still a significant cause of maternal mortality.
- A thorough examination and acquisition of appropriate cultures are mandatory.
- The National Health Service Executive have produced guidelines regarding controls assurance which suggest that all hospitals should have their own antibiotic policy.
- Paracetamol administration is safe and improves patient comfort.

KEY REFERENCES

1. Department of Health, *Why Mothers Die: 1997–1999*. London: RCOG Press, 2001.
2. Almeida OD Jr, Kitay DZ. Lactation suppression and puerperal fever. *Am J Obstet Gynecol* 1986; 154:940–1.
3. Marshall BR, Hepper JK, Zirbel CC. Sporadic puerperal mastitis. An infection that need not interrupt lactation. *J Am Med Assoc* 1975; 233:1377–9.
4. Ely JW, Dawson JD, Townsend AS, Rijhsinghani A, Bowdler NC. Benign fever following vaginal delivery. *J Fam Pract* 1996; 43:146–51.
5. Sweet RL, Ledger WJ. Puerperal infectious morbidity: a two-year review. *Am J Obstet Gynecol* 1973; 117: 1093–100.
6. Smaill F, Hofmeyr GJ. Antibiotic prophylaxis for cesarean section (Cochrane Review). In: *The Cochrane Library*, Issue 4. Oxford: Update Software, 2001.
7. Anonymous. Antibiotic prophylaxis of infective endocarditis. Recommendations from the Endocarditis Working Party of the British Society for Antimicrobial Chemotherapy. *Lancet* 1990; 335(8681):88–9.
8. Department of Health. *Why Mothers Die: 1997–1999*. London: RCOG Press, 2001.
9. Prescott LF. Paracetamol: past, present, and future. (Review.) *Am J Ther* 2000; 7:143–7.
10. French LM, Smaill FM. Antibiotic regimens for endometritis after delivery (Cochrane Review). In: *The Cochrane Library*, Issue 4. Oxford: Update Software, 2001.
11. Vazquez JC, Villar J. Treatments for symptomatic urinary tract infections during pregnancy (Cochrane Review). In: *The Cochrane Library*, Issue 4. Oxford: Update Software 2001.

Postpartum complications: maternal

Disturbed Mood

Peter J. Thompson

INTRODUCTION

There is significant morbidity and mortality associated with mood disorders in pregnancy, with the morbidity being in both social and physical terms. In the last triennial report examining maternal mortality, a new section was added: deaths from psychiatric causes. Although it seems likely that there was some under-reporting of these events, 28 cases were identified. Of these, five cases involved suicide during pregnancy and 18 in the postnatal period. Antenatal disorders of mood tend to involve the management of pre-existing psychiatric conditions, whilst postnatal disorders of mood fall into three broad categories: 'baby blues', postnatal depression and puerperal psychosis. This section aims to cover all four of these areas.

DEFINITIONS

Baby blues (or postpartum blues) is the term used to describe the transient experience of tearfulness, anxiety and irritability that frequently occurs in the first few days following delivery.

In comparison, postpartum psychosis is a disorder defined as a severe mental disorder usually occurring in the first 4 weeks of delivery, characterized by the presence of irrational ideas and unusual reactions to the baby. In addition, these patients also suffer less specific symptoms such as restlessness, irritability, insomnia and lability of mood.

The symptoms of postnatal depression do not differ from the symptoms of depression at other times of life, but a temporal association with childbirth distinguishes it from other forms of depression. There does, however, seem to be little agreement on what the limits of this temporal relationship are, which makes assessment of the literature more difficult. Most studies are limited to depression with onset within 3 months of delivery, although some studies extend this limit to 6 months.

INCIDENCE

As antenatal disorders of mood disturbance are usually due to pre-existing psychiatric conditions, the incidence is approximately the same as amongst non-gravid women of a similar age.

More than 50 per cent of women suffer from postpartum blues, usually commencing on the fourth or fifth postnatal day.[1] The incidence of postnatal depression is approximately 10–15 per cent,[2] whereas postnatal psychosis is rare, occurring in 0.1 per cent of cases.[3]

AETIOLOGY

Antenatal conditions

As already mentioned, although antenatal mood disorders are usually secondary to pre-existing conditions, they can be precipitated for the first time by a significant life event – the pregnancy. Pregnancy can place a significant strain on many relationships, not to mention the worries of future financial burdens, which may be sufficient to destabilize a susceptible individual. Therefore these conditions may be secondary to the social implications of pregnancy rather than the pregnancy itself.

Baby blues

As the immediate postnatal period is a time of significant physiological and social change, it is not surprising that a significant number of mothers suffer from disorders of mood. Baby blues is a self-limiting condition that has not been associated with any specific metabolic or endocrinological disturbance. It is commoner in women following their first delivery, and sufferers are not more likely to have a past psychiatric history than non-sufferers. Other factors such as lack of sleep, hospitalization and pain have been implicated in the aetiology of this condition.

Postnatal depression

The social and physiological changes seen at this time are also relevant to postnatal depression and puerperal psychosis. Although it is still true that no specific endocrinological change has been associated with the onset of postnatal depression, it has been hypothesized that the fall in both progesterone and oestrogen concentrations is implicated, as these hormones are known to have psychoactive properties. Indeed, it is well recognized that the peripheral blood levels of sex hormones do not accurately reflect either the concentration of the hormones within the brain or the numbers or affinity of receptors within the brain. Unlike baby blues, postnatal depression is associated with a past history of psychiatric illness. One of the problems with determining the aetiology of this condition is that not all experts even recognize it as a separate disease entity.

Puerperal psychosis

Whether puerperal psychosis is a discrete disease entity or a rapidly evolving affective psychosis is a matter of much debate. The aetiology of puerperal psychosis is poorly understood; however, it does appear to be more common following the first delivery, in patients with previous bipolar disorders and is recognized as having a 25 per cent risk of recurrence in subsequent pregnancies. Many patients also suffer from recurrent relapsing affective disorders for the remainder of their lives.[4]

MANAGEMENT

Antenatal conditions

Management of psychiatric illnesses during pregnancy is similar to that outside of pregnancy. The main concerns are the effects that psychotropic drugs may have on the fetus, due to their high transplacental transfer rates. Indeed, although these drugs are not licensed for use in pregnancy, it is well established that if medication is withdrawn for mood disorders, there are high rates of relapse during pregnancy, anxiety disorders and schizophrenia. In view of this, several reviews have been published examining the possible teratogenic effects of these drugs (see Chapter 8).[5,6]

A review of the effects of tricyclic antidepressants, fluoxetine and newer selective serotonin reuptake inhibitors attempted to determine the risk to the fetus in each of the five domains of toxic effects of fetal exposure to drugs: intrauterine death, physical malformation, growth impairment, behavioural teratogenicity and neonatal toxicity. Although there is little available information about long-term behavioural teratogenicity, there was no evidence that tricyclic antidepressants, fluoxetine or newer selective serotonin reuptake inhibitors affect the risk of intrauterine death or fetal physical malformation. Both tricyclic antidepressants and fluoxetine have been associated with neonatal withdrawal syndromes, though studies on fluoxetine have given conflicting results. Conflicting evidence is also present for the effect of these drugs on growth impairment.

Following treatment in the first trimester of pregnancy, benzodiazepines, antipsychotic medication and lithium have all been associated with small but significantly increased risks of teratogenicity in the offspring. Therefore women with a psychiatric disorder who are pregnant or who are trying to conceive should be counselled regarding the relative risks of disease relapse and fetal exposure to medication, and where appropriate an alternative, safer drug may be prescribed [II].

Women with a past history of psychiatric problems are at an increased risk of developing postnatal depression, and should therefore be identified and offered increased professional support following delivery [IV]. However, to date, antenatal screening programmes have been unsuccessful.

Baby blues

Research into the management of this condition is limited, with the only significant research being focused on an attempt to identify women who are at increased risk of developing either postnatal depression or puerperal psychosis. Management consists of providing a supportive environment for the new mother, with both professionals (particularly midwives) and the family working together [IV]. Drug therapy is not indicated, as the condition is usually self-limiting. Those women in whom the condition persists beyond 10–14 days[7] and those who have marital difficulties appear to have an increased risk of developing puerperal psychosis.

Postnatal depression

Whether or not postnatal depression is a separate disease entity from depression, there is no doubt that it can have significant long-term effects on the mother–infant relationship and the development of the infant. Therefore early detection and appropriate treatment are essential. The Edinburgh Postnatal Depression Score is a self-report scale that has ten items relating to symptoms of depression. The detection rates of postnatal depression in the community can be improved by implementation of the Edinburgh Postnatal Depression Score at a 6 weeks' postnatal check [II].[8]

The treatment of postnatal depression has mainly revolved around supportive therapy, the administration of sex hormones (oestrogen and progesterone) and the prescription of antidepressants. Early involvement of a psychiatrist with experience in this condition is essential [IV] and if the patient requires hospitalization, it is preferable to avoid separation from the baby, which will necessitate admission to a specialized mother and baby unit [III]. The three main treatments mentioned above have all been the subject of systematic reviews.

There are two randomized, controlled trials that assess the effect of increased professional input on the incidence of postnatal depression. In one of these studies the professional was a specially trained health visitor and in the other a psychologist. The meta-analysis of these studies showed an odds ratio of 0.34 (95 per cent confidence interval (CI) 0.17–0.69) for the development of postnatal depression in the treated group [Ia].[9] These studies were small, and at least one was prone to bias due to the high drop-out rate of subjects.

The role of antidepressants for the treatment of this condition has also been the subject of a systematic review; however only one randomized, controlled trial was suitable for inclusion in the analysis. This found that the administration of fluoxetine was equally as effective as cognitive–behavioural therapy [Ib].[10] However, the long-term effects of fluoxetine on the infant are less well described.

In comparison, a systematic review of studies that used oestrogen or progesterone to treat women with postnatal depression showed discouraging results. Treatment with high doses of oestrogen did appear to reduce the depression scores of women with severe postnatal depression, but the potential side effects of thromboembolic disease, endometrial hyperplasia and inhibition of lactation make this an unattractive therapy for women to take. Progesterone therapy was associated with a higher incidence of postnatal depression than placebo. This could be because the mood elevation seen with natural progesterones is not an effect of synthetic progestogens.[11] Therefore these medications cannot be recommended for women with postnatal depression [Ia].

The available evidence thus suggests that the optimum therapy for postnatal depression is increased caregiver support [Ia], with subsequent addition of fluoxetine if necessary [Ib].

Puerperal psychosis

This is a psychiatric emergency and its treatment requires hospitalization. As it is preferable to avoid separation of the mother from her infant, admission to a specialized mother and baby unit should be arranged, where antidepressant and neuroleptic medication can be initiated and supervised by psychiatrists [II]. Failure to treat the condition aggressively is associated with rates of infanticide as high as 4 per cent [II].[12] This aggressive treatment may include electroconvulsive therapy [III].

- Systematic review of two randomized, controlled trials shows progesterone therapy to be of no benefit, although oestrogen therapy may decrease the severity of depression when used as adjunctive therapy.
- A randomized, controlled trial has shown that fluoxetine is as effective as cognitive–behavioural therapy for the treatment of postnatal depression.
- Cohort studies show that the Edinburgh Postnatal Depression Score is effective in detecting women at risk of postnatal mood disorders.
- Retrospective cohort studies show that most drugs used to treat psychiatric conditions are relatively safe to use in pregnancy.

KEY POINTS

- Most drugs used to treat psychiatric disorders are relatively safe to use in pregnancy.
- Postnatal screening for postnatal depression using the Edinburgh Postnatal Depression Score is effective.
- The best treatment for postnatal depression appears to be cognitive–behavioural therapy, with the administration of antidepressants where necessary.
- Puerperal psychosis is a psychiatric emergency.

KEY REFERENCES

1. Kendell RE, McGuire RJ, Connor Y, Cox JL. Mood changes in the first three weeks after childbirth. *J Affect Disord* 1981; 3:317–26.

2. Cox JL, Murray D, Chapman G. A controlled study of the onset, duration and prevalence of postnatal depression. *Br J Psychiatry* 1993; **163**:27–31.

3. Kumar R, Robson KM. A prospective study of emotional disorders in childbearing women. *Br J Psychiatry* 1984; **144**:35–47.

4. Davidson J, Robertson E. A follow-up study of postpartum illness, 1946–1978. *Acta Psychiatr Scand* 1985; **71**(5):451–7.

5. Altshuler LL, Cohen L, Szuba MP, Burt VK, Gitlin M, Mintz J. Pharmacologic management of psychiatric illness during pregnancy: dilemmas and guidelines. *Am J Psychiatry* 1996; **153**:592–606.

6. Wisner KL, Gelenberg AJ, Leonard H, Zarin D, Frank E. Pharmacologic treatment of depression during pregnancy. *J Am Med Assoc* 1999; **282**:1264–9.

7. Robinson GE, Stewart DE. Postpartum psychiatric disorders. *CMAJ* 1986; **134**:31–7.

8. Georgiopoulos AM, Bryan TL, Wollan P, Yawn BP. Routine screening for postpartum depression. *J Fam Pract* 2001; **50**:117–22.

9. Ray KL, Hodnett ED. Caregiver support for postpartum depression (Cochrane Review). In: *The Cochrane Library*, Issue 4. Oxford: Update Software, 2001.

10. Appleby L, Warner R, Whitton A, Faragher B. A controlled study of fluoxetine and cognitive-behavioural counselling in the treatment of postnatal depression. *BMJ* 1997; **314**:932–6.

11. Lawrie TA, Herxheimer A, Dalton K. Oestrogens and progestogens for preventing and treating postnatal depression (Cochrane Review). In: *The Cochrane Library*, Issue 4. Oxford: Update Software, 2001.

12. D'Orban PT. Women who kill their children. *Br J Psychiatry* 1979; **134**:560–71.

Problems with Breastfeeding

Peter Thompson

INTRODUCTION

Although a physiological process, breastfeeding is an action that women perform for only a small part of their lives. For it to be successful, not only do the correct physiological processes have to occur, but both the mother and neonate need to adapt to this situation, and whereas some mothers and babies seem to be able to establish it without any problems, others do not. Increasing the proportion of women breastfeeding has been identified as a high priority for the government in their white paper 'Our Healthier Nation'.[1] Indeed, the World Health Organization recommends exclusive breastfeeding until the age of 4 months.[2] For these targets to be reached, interventions of proven benefit need to be employed throughout the health service. To achieve this and to provide consistency of information from all healthcare professionals, the government initiated the production of good practice guidance on breastfeeding to the National Health Service (NHS). This report promotes practices to improve the initiation and prolong the duration of breastfeeding.

DEFINITIONS

There are extensive data in the literature supporting the concept that the optimum food for babies is breast milk. The benefits bestowed upon the infant are pertinent in both the short and long term. Included in these benefits is reduced morbidity from respiratory, gastrointestinal, urinary tract and middle ear infections, as well as a decreased tendency towards atopy.[3] For the mother there are both health benefits, such as a decrease in the incidence of epithelial ovarian cancer and premenopausal breast cancer, and financial benefits. Therefore conditions that interfere with breastfeeding constitute important epidemiological health issues.

INCIDENCE

The last national audit in 1995 showed that following delivery approximately 62 per cent of women in England commence breastfeeding. Breastfeeding is much more common amongst women from social class I (90 per cent) than amongst those in social class V (50 per cent).[4] However, in the UK this falls to approximately 29 per cent by 4 months postpartum. (This last figure is corrected for both maternal age and the age at which full-time education was completed, and is therefore not directly comparable to the incidences quoted at delivery. Nevertheless it indicates a significant fall in the prevalence of breastfeeding with time.)

AETIOLOGY

The establishment of lactation is dependent upon a variety of influences, including the production of prolactin from the anterior pituitary gland and oxytocin from the posterior pituitary gland. These hormones stimulate milk production and ejection respectively. However, problems with lactation are rarely due to pituitary–hypothalamic axis dysfunction. Indeed, the main reasons why women neither initiate breastfeeding nor continue it as long as in other European countries appear to relate to social and cultural issues. This section does not attempt to discuss these, but concentrates on the management of mastitis, breast abscess formation, enforced separation of mother and baby, and poor infant feeding. Many of these problems are interrelated and it has been suggested that the majority can be avoided by using a technique of feeding on demand and attaching the baby to the nipple in the correct position from the first feed onwards.[5]

MANAGEMENT

Mastitis

Mastalgia is defined as painful breasts and, according to a recent survey in the UK, is the second most common cause cited by women for the discontinuation of breastfeeding.[4] The aetiology of this condition revolves around the imbalance between the production of milk and infant consumption that occurs in a small proportion of women. When milk production exceeds the infant's requirements, the alveolar spaces within the breasts become distended, with the breast feeling hot, swollen and tender. This swelling leads to compression of the capillaries, which in turn increases the arterial pressure to the breasts, causing compression of the connective tissues and a decrease in lymphatic drainage. This results in the formation of oedema and engorgement of the breast (obstructive mastitis), which may develop into infective mastitis.

Five factors have been associated with the development of breast engorgement: delayed initiation of feeds, infrequent feeds, time-limited feeds, a late shift from colostrum to milk production, and the habit of administering supplementary feeds.[6] Therefore avoidance of these will significantly decrease the incidence of this problem.

Many interventions have been proposed for the treatment of breast engorgement, some of which have been the subject of systematic reviews, which have examined both traditional and modern treatments. The most effective treatments tested involved the use of anti-inflammatory agents [II]. The agents tested are not available in the UK, and it is uncertain whether these results are applicable to similar agents. Interventions such as the topical application of cabbage leaves, the use of gel packs and ultrasound treatment all showed an improvement in symptoms, though not to a greater extent than placebo. It has been postulated that these improvements are secondary to warming and physically massaging the breast [Ia].[7]

As previously mentioned, breast engorgement may become complicated by infection, leading to infective mastitis. The most common causative organism is *Staphylococcus aureus*, with others occasionally being implicated, including *Staphylococcus epidermidis*, groups A, B and F betahaemolytic *Streptococcus*, *Haemophilus influenzae* and *Escherichia coli*. Management consists of the administration of an antibiotic that is effective against beta-lactamaseproducing bacteria and encouraging the mother to continue breastfeeding or manually expressing milk [II].

Breast abscess formation

Although uncommon, the exact prevalence of this condition is not well reported. The prevention of abscess formation is achieved by the avoidance of milk stasis.[8,9] However, unlike for infective mastitis, most authors would recommend that feeding from the affected breast ceases when pus is draining from the nipple [II]. Once formed, abscesses require surgical drainage, usually under general anaesthesia, with the administration of broad-spectrum antibiotics [II].[10] Choice of incision for the drainage is controversial; circumferential incisions give optimum cosmetic results, but radial incisions carry a smaller risk of damage to other lactiferous ducts. Therefore it would seem sensible to perform circumferential incisions to drain superficial abscesses, whereas deep abscesses should be drained via a radial incision [IV].

Enforced separation of mother and baby

Separation of mother and baby, usually secondary to the illhealth of one or both parties, may have a significant impact on the establishment of breastfeeding. The successful longterm establishment of breastfeeding is dependent upon frequent feeding,[6] and this is obviously complicated when the parties are physically separated or when one or other party is too ill to feed. However, systematic reviews have failed to show improved prevalence of long-term breastfeeding in groups of women who commence feeding early (within 30 minutes) when compared to those who commence feeding their infants between 4 and 8 hours post-delivery [Ia].[11]

If breastfeeding is to be established in these circumstances, the expression of breast milk, in place of frequent feeds, is essential [III]. This can be done by hand or mechanically, with collection of the milk in a container to feed the infant at a later date.

These problems are seen commonly in babies admitted to a neonatal unit and, because of the many advantages of breastfeeding such children, many units have established milk banks to store this milk. There are occasions when breastfeeding may be contraindicated, for example maternal human immunodeficiency virus (HIV) infection, or relatively contraindicated, for example severe maternal ill-health. In such conditions it may be appropriate to prescribe a dopamine antagonist such as cabergoline, which will cause the production of milk to stop.

Poor infant feeding

Poor infant feeding secondary to ill-health has already been considered above. Poor technique of breastfeeding is another cause of poor feeding. A systematic review of increased support for mothers by healthcare professionals has shown a significantly decreased risk of discontinuation of breastfeeding. In order to ensure one more woman exclusively breastfeeds because of this intervention, the number of women needed to treat is nine (95% confidence interval (CI) 6–21) [Ia].[3]

- Systematic reviews of randomized, controlled trials show that:
  - prolonged breastfeeding is not more prevalent in women who perform the first feed within 30 minutes of birth;
  - support from a professional person increases the likelihood of a woman exclusively breastfeeding;
  - the treatment of choice for breast engorgement is an anti-inflammatory agent.
- There are few randomized, controlled trials on the management of the other breast pathologies mentioned above, with most evidence coming from cohort or retrospective studies.

KEY POINTS

- Breastfeeding is beneficial to both mother and infant.
- A high proportion of women never commence breastfeeding and, of those that do, less than half will still be breastfeeding at 4 months.
- Women with obstructive and infective mastitis should continue to breastfeed.
- Women with breast abscesses should discontinue breastfeeding and will require surgical drainage.

KEY REFERENCES

1. Department of Health. *Our Healthier Nation*. London: HMSO, 1998.
2. Work Health Organization. The World Health Organization's infant feeding recommendations. *Epidemiol Rec* 1995; **70**:119–20.
3. Sikorski J, Renfrew MJ. Support for breastfeeding mothers (Cochrane Review). In: *The Cochrane Library*, Issue 3. Oxford: Update Software, 2001.
4. Foster K, Lader D, Cheesbrough S. *Infant Feeding 1995*. Office for National Statistics. London: HMSO, 1997.
5. Inch S, Renfrew MJ. Common breastfeeding problems. In: Iain Chalmers I, Enkin M, Keirse MJNC (eds). *Effective Care in Pregnancy and Childbirth*, Vol. 2. Oxford: Oxford University Press, 1989, 1375–89.
6. Moon JL, Humenick SS. Breast engorgement: contributing variables and variables amenable to nursing intervention. *J Obstet Gynecol Neonatal Nurs* 1989; **18**(4):309–15.
7. Snowden HM, Renfrew MJ, Woolridge MW. Treatments for breast engorgement during lactation (Cochrane Review). In: *The Cochrane Library*, Issue 4. Oxford: Update Software, 2001.
8. Thomsen AC, Hansen KB, Moller BR. Leukocyte counts and microbiologic cultivation in the diagnosis of puerperal mastitis. *Am J Obstet Gynecol* 1983; **146**: 938–41.
9. Thomsen AC, Espersen T, Maigaard S. Course and treatment of milk stasis, noninfectious inflammation of the breast, and infectious mastitis in nursing women. *Am J Obstet Gynecol* 1984; **149**:492–5.
10. Benson EA. Management of breast abscesses. *World J Surg* 1989; **13**:753–6.
11. Renfrew MJ, Lang S, Woolridge MW. Early versus delayed initiation of breastfeeding (Cochrane Review). In: *The Cochrane Library*, Issue 3. Oxford: Update Software, 2001.

PART THREE

Gynaecology

SECTION A

Reproductive medicine

Normal and Abnormal Development of the Genitalia

Catherine Minto

INTRODUCTION

Fetal development of the gonads, external genitalia, Müllerian ducts and Wolffian ducts can be disrupted at a variety of points, leading to a wide range of conditions with a large spectrum of clinical presentations. Intersex conditions occur when there is a disruption of either gonadal differentiation or fetal sex steroid production or action. Müllerian anomalies and Wolffian duct remnants occur when there is disruption of the embryological development of these systems. An understanding of embryology often helps to sort out the underlying problem. Some of these cases will present for the first time to the gynaecologist. Paediatric surgeons may have initially treated others. All may have co-existing medical problems and require thorough evaluation. As well as anatomical and fertility concerns for these patients, there are often many psychological issues. In some conditions the optimal management is still uncertain. For intersex conditions presenting in childhood, there is currently debate about genital surgery and sex assignment.

NORMAL EMBRYOLOGICAL DEVELOPMENT OF THE INTERNAL AND EXTERNAL GENITALIA

Genetic sex is determined at the moment of conception by the presence or absence of the Y chromosome, and after week 6 will guide the subsequent development of the fetus down one of two standard pathways – male or female. Until this time development is the same in all fetuses. Primordial germ cells can be seen at 3 weeks in the endoderm of the yolk sac wall. During weeks 5 and 6, they migrate by amoeboid movement to the genital ridge (future gonad), an area of mesenchyme medial to the developing mesonephros and Wolffian (or mesonephric) duct. During week 6, primitive sex cords form around the germ cells in the indifferent gonad. The two Müllerian (or paramesonephric) ducts also appear lateral to the Wolffian ducts. At the same time at the caudal end of the fetus, the cloacal membrane and folds are separated into the anterior urogenital and posterior anal parts. The urogenital section with the genital tubercle will become the future external genitalia, and by week 7 consists of a genital tubercle, urogenital membrane, urogenital folds and, more laterally, labioscrotal swellings. At the end of week 7, the urogenital membrane has degenerated and the urogenital sinus freely communicates with the amniotic fluid.

The first noticeable divergence in male and female fetuses is the differentiation of gonadal structure. The indifferent gonad has the potential for testicular or ovarian development. After gonadal differentiation has occurred, the presence or absence of gonadal hormone production and other fetal factors then guides the development of the

Müllerian ducts, Wolffian ducts and external genitalia. Testes secrete androgen, leading to male external genital development and differentiation of the bilateral Wolffian ducts into the vas deferens, seminal vesicle and epididymis. Testes also secrete anti-Müllerian hormone (AMH – also called Müllerian inhibiting substance, MIS), leading to active regression of the Müllerian ducts. The fetal ovaries do not secrete androgen or AMH, and therefore there is female external genital development, growth of the Müllerian ducts and spontaneous regression of the Wolffian ducts.

STANDARD MALE PATHWAY

In an XY fetus, activation of the *SRY* (sex-determining region of the Y chromosome) gene at the end of week 6 guides the indifferent gonad to commence development into a testis. Other autosomal genes (e.g. *WT1*, *SOX9*, *SF-1*) are also involved in this genetic cascade.[1] The medullary sex cord cells become Sertoli cells, surrounding the primitive germ cells. At puberty these will become the seminiferous tubules surrounding the spermatozoa. Sertoli cells produce AMH, which acts locally to cause apoptotic regression of the adjacent Müllerian ducts at weeks 8–10. The appendix testis and prostatic utricle are usually all that remain of the Müllerian ducts in the male.

At around weeks 8–10, Leydig cells appear in the testis and start to secrete testosterone. The control of testosterone production may be independent at first, and then under placental human chorionic gonadotrophin (hCG) control via the luteinizing hormone (LH) receptor. Later, fetal LH production controls testosterone production. Testosterone causes development of the Wolffian ducts into the vasa deferentia, and later the seminal vesicles and epididymides. Testosterone is also released into the circulation and undergoes peripheral conversion to dihydrotestosterone (DHT) in the cells of the external genitalia. There, DHT acting via the androgen receptor promotes development and growth of the genital tubercle, urogenital sinus, urogenital folds and labioscrotal swellings into the glans penis, penile shaft, urethral tube and scrotum respectively. The penis is similar in size to the clitoris at 14 weeks and, under the influence of DHT, continues growing until birth.

STANDARD FEMALE PATHWAY

In an XX fetus, absence of the *SRY* gene causes the indifferent gonad to commence ovarian differentiation at around week 7. Without *SRY* protein, the sex cord cells degenerate and secondary sex cords form and surround the primordial germ cells. Primordial follicles then arise after the germ cells have matured into oogonia and entered their first meiotic division, becoming primary oocytes. The presence of ovaries is not required for regression of the Wolffian ducts, and it is the absence of local testosterone that causes their regression at 10 weeks. The paroophoron, epoophoron and Gartner's cysts are all that may remain of the Wolffian ducts in the female. The absence of circulating testosterone also leads to an absence of peripheral DHT and directs the genital tubercle, urogenital sinus, urogenital folds and labioscrotal swellings to develop into the clitoris, lower vagina, labia minora and labia majora respectively.

As AMH is not produced by the fetal ovary, the Müllerian ducts continue to develop. These paired mesodermal ducts originate in week 5, lateral to the Wolffian ducts at the third to fifth thoracic segment. They are thought to be associated with the basement membrane of the Wolffian ducts and grow caudally down guided by them. The cranial ends of the Müllerian ducts are independent of the Wolffian ducts and remain separate as the fallopian tubes. At the pelvis, the Müllerian ducts cross the Wolffian ducts anteriorly to lie medially next to each other. At weeks 8–10, the pelvic Müllerian ducts have fused and subsequent breakdown of their medial walls leads to a single tube, which will become the upper vagina, cervix and the uterine epithelium and glands. Surrounding mesenchymal tissue will become the myometrium and stroma. At their caudal end, the fused Müllerian ducts form the Müllerian tubercle, which connects with a thickened area of the urogenital sinus that develops into the paired sinovaginal bulbs. This connection of the endodermal urogenital sinus and mesodermal Müllerian ducts forms the vaginal plate – a column of squamous tissue. It remains unknown how much of each tissue (and possibly some of the Wolffian duct) contributes to this developing vagina. Over weeks 10–16, the vaginal plate enlarges and develops a cavity, which is separated from the urogenital sinus by an endodermal membrane. Gradual change of the lower Müllerian duct epithelium from columnar to stratified squamous epithelium occurs, ending at the future external cervical os. By month 5, the urethra and vagina are separated by a septum, and the endodermal membrane between the vagina and urogenital sinus breaks down to form the hymen. The urogenital sinus forms the vaginal vestibule.

KEY POINTS

- The *SRY* gene directs the gonad to become a testis.
- The absence of the *SRY* gene allows the gonad to become an ovary.
- The presence or absence of androgen determines external genital development.
- The presence of gonadal testosterone production leads to Wolffian duct differentiation into vas deferens, epididymis and seminal vesicle.
- The presence of gonadal AMH production leads to Müllerian duct regression.

- The absence of gonadal AMH production allows Müllerian duct differentiation into the upper vagina, cervix, uterine glands and epithelium and fallopian tubes.
- The absence of gonadal testosterone production allows Wolffian duct regression.

ABNORMAL EMBRYOLOGICAL DEVELOPMENT – INTERSEX CONDITIONS

There is a wide range of intersex conditions, only the more common of which are considered here (Table 46.1). Traditional management models are now being re-evaluated due to recent debate on human gender development, new knowledge concerning fetal sexual differentiation and development, greater awareness and understanding of female sexual function and a more patient-centred emphasis on condition management. There are no randomized trials to inform intersex condition management, and currently expert opinion and a few small cohort studies and retrospective, uncontrolled trials form the basis of management.[2]

Definition

Intersex is defined as a mix or blend of the physically defining features associated with males or females, i.e. karyotype, gonadal structure, internal genitalia and external genitalia. Therefore 'intersex' covers a diverse range of conditions encompassing individuals with standard male or female genitalia, who may have a variety of internal genital organs and karyotypes, and also those with ambiguous external genitalia.

Various classifications of intersex conditions have been used in the past, for example true hermaphroditism, female pseudohermaphroditism (ovaries with male external genitalia) and male pseudohermaphroditism (testes with female external genitalia). With better understanding of the mechanisms of fetal sexual development and intersex aetiology, these older categories are now less useful and each intersex condition requires individual consideration.

Incidence

The incidence of intersex conditions in the UK is unknown. An estimate for intersex prevalence is 1 in 2000.[3] Conditions with autosomal recessive inheritance are more common in communities in which intermarriage is common.

Aetiology

Most intersex conditions occur due to a genetic or environmental disruption to the pathway of fetal sexual development. This disruption can be to gonadal differentiation or development, sex steroid production, sex steroid conversion or tissue utilization of sex steroids.

Presentation and investigation

Every intersex condition has a spectrum of severity and therefore may present in a variety of ways.

- Ambiguous genitalia at birth.
- Salt-losing crisis in neonatal life (congenital adrenal hyperplasia).

Table 46.1   Key points of intersex condition features

Intersex condition	Karyotype	External genitalia	Internal genitalia	Special features
Congenital adrenal hyperplasia (CAH)	XX	Masculinized	Uterus and ovaries	Co-existing glucocorticoid (and sometimes also mineralocorticoid) deficiency requiring steroid replacement therapy
Complete androgen insensitivity syndrome (CAIS)	XY	Female	Testes	Absent pubic and axillary hair; at risk of osteoporosis; gonadal malignancy risk small until after 50 years of age
Swyer's syndrome	XY	Female	Streak gonads and uterus	High risk of gonadal malignancy; poor breast development; normal axillary and pubic hair
5-α-reductase deficiency	XY	Female or ambiguous at birth, masculinizing at puberty	Testes	In those with testes in situ, 60–80% undergo change of gender from female to male at some point from late childhood onwards
17-β-hydroxysteroid dehydrogenase – type 3 deficiency	XY	Variable; often female or ambiguous at birth, masculinizing at puberty	Testes	In those with testes in situ, 60–80% undergo change of gender from female to male at some point from late childhood onwards
True hermaphroditism	71% XX 20% XX/XY 7% XY 2% other	Often ambiguous	Mix of ovary and/or testis and/or ovotestes; uterus or male ducts	Fertility described as both males fathering a child and females carrying a pregnancy

- Sibling history of intersex.
- Ambiguity of the genitalia developing in childhood or puberty.
- Inguinal hernia with unexpected gonad.
- Pelvic mass with gonadal tumour.
- Primary amenorrhoea or pubertal delay.
- Infertility.
- Sexual dysfunction.
- Part of a syndrome with other anomalies (e.g. renal anomalies in Drash syndrome).

Initial investigation will depend on presentation, but should include karyotype, testosterone, LH, follicle-stimulating hormone (FSH), 17-hydroxyprogesterone and pelvic ultrasound scan. Further investigation will depend on initial findings, external genital appearance and clinical presentation, and may include androstenedione, DHT, oestradiol, 24-hour urinary collection for steroid metabolites, hCG stimulation test, synacthen test, renal ultrasound scan, magnetic resonance imaging (MRI), and DNA for genetic testing.

Management

The areas to consider in intersex management are:

- accurate diagnosis,
- need for hormone replacement therapy,
- screening for associated medical conditions,
- provision of condition information,
- psychological treatments,
- genetic counselling for other family members,
- sex assignment for children,
- gonadal malignancy risk,
- fertility options,
- genital surgery options for ambiguous genitalia,
- vaginal enlargement options,
- access to peer support.

Accurate diagnosis at presentation is essential, and referral to an appropriate paediatric or adult multidisciplinary intersex service (endocrinology, gynaecology, surgery and psychology expertise), where available, is ideal. Individuals with different intersex conditions may require specific medical and surgical treatments; however, all should have access to experienced clinical psychologists and peer support via the relevant national support organizations. Over the past decade a major shift in management has been the recognition that all patients have a right to information concerning their condition details, and the provision of this information and the options available need sensitive communication in a supported environment. Ideally, this should be with the expertise of a trained clinical psychologist. It is no longer considered good practice to withhold condition details from the patient.[2] There is no evidence other than clinical experience and ethical evaluation on which to base this management, as there have been no studies evaluating long-term psychological outcomes with concealed or revealed diagnosis information. Gonadal malignancy and fertility options vary with the different intersex conditions.

Cases presenting at birth or in childhood may be seen by a paediatric gynaecologist as part of an intersex team, but more often will be under the care of a paediatric surgeon or paediatric urologist in an intersex team. The majority of these cases will have presented due to ambiguous genitalia. After thorough evaluation and diagnosis, sex of rearing is assigned and cosmetic genital surgery is considered where relevant. Currently, many neonates with ambiguous genitalia are assigned as females. Feminizing cosmetic surgery in early infancy is offered for the more severely virilized cases, with the theoretical aim of initially aiding parental acceptance of the child's assigned gender, and later improving the psychological outcomes for the child. This infant surgery was previously also thought to improve adult sexual function. All of these indications for genital surgery are now being re-evaluated, and there are only small, uncontrolled retrospective studies and cohort studies to provide data on outcomes. At present it remains unknown whether infant genital surgery has an effect on parental acceptance of assigned gender or on later psychological outcomes for the child. Small cohort studies suggest that the majority of infants undergoing genital surgery will require repeat genital treatment (surgery or vaginal dilatation therapy) at or after puberty, mainly for vaginal introital stenosis but also for cosmesis. Sexual function following feminizing genital surgery is unknown. Small retrospective, uncontrolled studies of children who have undergone clitoral reduction surgery have suggested that orgasm is not prevented;[4,5] however, cohort studies suggest that genital surgery may contribute to adult sexual dysfunction.[6,7]

Gynaecologists are more often involved in the care of the older child developing ambiguous genitalia at puberty, or in follow-up of adults who underwent feminizing genital surgery as children. In many subjects born with ambiguous genitalia, there will be vaginal hypoplasia or agenesis, and the gynaecologist will need to discuss the treatment options at the appropriate time. Where childhood surgery has been performed, there is a strong possibility that repeat surgery may be required for vaginal stenosis, hypoplasia or genital cosmesis. This treatment is indicated to improve psychological and sexual outcomes; however, there have been no studies to provide evidence that improvements in these outcomes are achieved.

Enlargement procedures for vaginal hypoplasia include self-dilatation therapy or surgical vaginoplasty. These interventions are offered to improve psychological and sexual outcomes. There is disagreement about both the optimal timing and the intervention to use. Vaginoplasty surgery is performed in childhood or after puberty. A working party statement from the British Association of Paediatric Surgeons has recommended that most vaginal interventions should be delayed until puberty or later.[8] There is some consensus now that vaginal dilatation therapy is the treatment of choice for vaginal hypoplasia due to the absence of surgical risk, including the later risk of malignancy in vaginal graft material. The success of dilators depends on the motivation of the patient, and the appropriate time to start treatment must be discussed on an individual basis. Concomitant psychological support may improve outcomes. Dilatation should not be used in children. The surgical vaginoplasty method depends on the genital configuration and surgeon's expertise. In some cases the aim of vaginoplasty is to open up the lower vagina, with the upper vagina being normally developed. A pull-through vaginoplasty with complete separation of the vagina from the urethra may be required where the vagina does not reach the perineum but instead has joined the urethra near to the bladder, forming a single urogenital perineal opening (the high confluence vagina). In conditions in which the entire vagina is hypoplastic or absent, there are many vaginoplasty techniques: laparoscopic tension via an external traction device, peritoneal grafting, amnion grafting, skin grafting, bowel grafting, muscle flaps, labial expansion flaps etc. Each method has different risks and benefits. The surgical risks include malignancy (in graft material), contracture leading to introital stenosis or loss of vaginal length, vaginal prolapse, dry vagina or excessive vaginal discharge.

Cosmetic genital surgery for ambiguous genitalia

- There is only minimal evidence to inform management.
- There have been no studies of psychological outcomes after childhood clitoral and genital surgery.
- Cohort studies suggest the cosmetic and anatomical outcomes of vaginal and clitoral childhood surgery may be poor.[9]
- Some uncontrolled, retrospective studies suggest that childhood cosmetic clitoral surgery does not prevent orgasm; however, no objective evaluation of adult female sexual function has been employed.[4,5]
- Cohort studies suggest that sexual function may be damaged by clitoral surgery.[6,7]

Vaginal enlargement procedures for vaginal agenesis or hypoplasia

- Retrospective studies show that childhood vaginal enlargement surgery may require revision in up to 90 per cent of cases.[9,10]
- There are no randomized, controlled trials of the outcomes of different vaginoplasty techniques.
- Retrospective uncontrolled studies have *not* shown one method of vaginoplasty surgery to have superior results to another method.

- Retrospective uncontrolled studies suggest that vaginal enlargement self-dilatation therapy is successful in up to 65 per cent of cases.[11]

Congenital adrenal hyperplasia

This intersex condition occurs in an XX fetus due to an enzyme deficiency (usually 21 hydroxylase) in the adrenal gland. The XX fetus proceeds down the female development pathway, with ovarian formation and development of the Müllerian ducts into uterus, cervix and upper vagina. Owing to the adrenal enzyme deficiency, cortisone production is deficient, and so the adrenal gland undergoes hyperplasia to try to produce sufficient cortisol. A by-product of this survival mechanism is the production of large quantities of androgens. These high circulating androgen levels lead to masculinizing effects at the external genitalia, and ambiguous genitalia or normal-looking male genitalia at birth.

This is one of the commonest intersex conditions, with a UK population prevalence estimated at 1 in 10 000. It is the only intersex condition that can be life threatening, as unrecognized cortisol deficiency can lead to a salt-wasting crisis in the neonate. Management aims to correct the cortisol deficiency and excess androgen production. Gender assignment at birth is usually female due to the presence of ovaries and uterus with fertility potential. Genital surgery to cosmetically feminize the appearance has been standard practice in the past, although there is now controversy concerning the benefits and risks of this procedure.[8] Adolescents and adults considering surgery to reduce the size of the clitoris, for cosmetic concerns or due to pain during sexual intercourse, are counselled that the risk of damage to clitoral orgasm is unknown, and the estimate of damage is 20–25 per cent. At puberty, a review of the vagina is necessary to identify obstruction, stenosis or hypoplasia.

Other causes of XX fetal virilization

In a manner similar to that of congenital adrenal hyperplasia, other exogenous causes of androgens (e.g. maternal androgen-secreting tumours or the use of virilizing drugs such as danazol in pregnancy) may rarely lead to masculinizing of the external genitalia in an XX fetus.

Complete androgen insensitivity syndrome

Complete androgen insensitivity syndrome (CAIS) occurs due to the complete inability of the body to respond to androgens. The cause is a disruption of the androgen receptor gene on the long arm of the X chromosome. Previously the condition was called testicular feminization, due to the erroneous assumption that the testes must be producing a feminizing factor. In this condition, an XY fetus proceeds initially down the pathway of male fetal sexual determination. The *SRY* gene leads to normal testicular development, and both AMH and testosterone are normally produced. The AMH ensures regression of the Müllerian duct; however, due to the lack of ability of all body cells to respond to androgen, female external genitalia develop and female central nervous system organization occurs. The result is an XY female with absent Müllerian structures, normal female genitalia, variable vaginal hypoplasia, absent pubic and axillary hair, normal breast development, normal female behaviour and gender identity and intra-abdominal testes that produce high levels of circulating testosterone.

Androgen insensitivity syndrome can also occur as a partial form (partial androgen insensitivity syndrome, PAIS) in which some response to androgens occurs. The aetiology of this condition is less well understood, although some cases have a disruption in the androgen receptor gene allowing some function. Presentation is a spectrum from ambiguous genitalia to a normal male phenotype with infertility. For those cases identified in early infancy, assignment of sex of rearing is difficult, with no data concerning outcome. Future sexual function as male or female is unknown, with physical growth of the genitalia being unpredictable and a lack of scientific knowledge about how sexual orientation and gender identity develop. It is likely that both male and female-type behaviours and gender identity are at least partly pre-programmed by the fetal sex steroid environment, and in PAIS the fetal sex steroid environment is unknown.

Swyer's syndrome (or complete XY gonadal dysgenesis)

In this condition, disruption at the very start of the male sex determination pathway causes an XY fetus to divert to the female development pathway. In 15–30 per cent of cases the fault lies with the *SRY* gene, and gonadal testicular differentiation does not occur. In the remaining cases, disruption of other testis-determining genes is assumed to be the cause. In the absence of *SRY* activation, ovarian determination probably occurs, but cannot be sustained due to the lack of a second X chromosome. The result is a dysgenetic (abnormally formed) streak gonad. As this gonad produces neither AMH nor testosterone, the external genital development is female and the Müllerian ducts develop into the vagina, uterus and cervix.

The streak gonad again fails to produce hormones at puberty, leading to the usual clinical presentation of primary amenorrhoea with poor breast development. In contrast to CAIS, these women have normal pubic and axillary hair and the presence of a normal uterus. Investigation will show raised gonadotrophins and low testosterone and

oestradiol levels. Menstruation usually commences with hormone replacement therapy (oestrogen and progesterone are necessary), and pregnancy is possible with donor oocytes. Gonadectomy is recommended due to the high malignancy risk of dysgenetic gonads.

Other forms of XY gonadal dysgenesis that can lead to intersex conditions are less well understood. Partial gonadal dysgenesis with some testicular function, and mixed gonadal dysgenesis (a unilateral testis and a contralateral streak gonad) are conditions that usually present with variable degrees of genital masculinization or ambiguity. Regression of each Müllerian duct depends on the local concentration of AMH produced by the fetal gonad on each side, and unilateral uterine development can occur if one gonad is more dysgenetic and hence produces less AMH than the contralateral gonad (see 'Intersex and karyotypic abnormalities').

5-Alpha-reductase type 2 deficiency and 17-beta-hydroxysteroid dehydrogenase type 3 deficiency

These two intersex conditions may present in a similar fashion with genital ambiguity at birth. In the past, most cases were assigned to a female sex of rearing; however, this management is currently under review and now each case is individually considered.[8] Both are autosomal recessive conditions in which an XY fetus initially starts down the male development pathway with normal testis development. However, there is a deficiency of enzymes involved in androgen synthesis, leading to mainly female external genital development. If left untreated in childhood, both conditions will result in increasing masculinization at puberty, and possibly a change in gender identity from female to male for some individuals. 5-Alpha-reductase-type 2 is the enzyme responsible for the peripheral conversion of testosterone to the more potent androgen DHT required for fetal genital masculinization. 17-Beta-hydroxysteroid dehydrogenase type 3 is the gonadal enzyme needed for the final step in testosterone production in the fetal testis, i.e. conversion of androstenedione to testosterone. Each of these enzymes has more than one isoenzyme, and it is likely that activation of other isoenzymes is responsible for the virilization seen at puberty.

Clinical presentation of both these conditions is usually mild ambiguity of the genitalia (clitoromegaly) at birth or early childhood in an XY female. However, the presentation can be variable. Müllerian structures are absent and Wolffian structures are present. The testes are intra-abdominal in childhood, and often descend to the inguinal canal or labioscrotal folds after puberty. Without childhood intervention, secondary sexual development is usually masculine, with poor breast development and normal pubic and axillary hair. The incidence of these conditions is unknown, but with the new scientific knowledge of these enzymes over the past decade, 17-beta-hydroxysteroid dehydrogenase type 3 deficiency is now being diagnosed in some cases previously labelled as CAIS. In cases diagnosed in childhood, the management and assignment of gender are difficult. There have been insufficient cohorts raised as either males or females from childhood to evaluate the outcomes of adult gender identity, sexual function, psychological outcomes and quality of life. Fertility may be possible as a male, although infertility is common.

True hermaphroditism

This condition is defined as the presence of both ovarian tissue with graafian follicles and testicular tissue containing distinct tubules in one person. It is said to be the rarest intersex condition, but has a higher prevalence in some areas, such as Africa. The gonads can be any mix of ovary, testes and ovotestes. The aetiology is unknown.

Most cases present with ambiguous genitalia, although clinical presentation is often very variable. The degree of genital masculinization is thought to be a reflection of the amount of functional testicular tissue. The spectrum of internal genital development is influenced by the composition of the adjacent gonad, with up to 80 per cent having internal female organs and therefore being potentially fertile. The karyotype is 46XX in the majority, with a smaller proportion having a mosaic XX/XY karyotype, and only a minority having a 46XY karyotype. At present there are insufficient data from cohort studies to advise on optimal management in terms of gender assignment in childhood.

ABNORMAL EMBRYOLOGICAL DEVELOPMENT OF THE MÜLLERIAN DUCTS AND PERSISTENCE OF WOLFFIAN STRUCTURES

Abnormal development of the Müllerian ducts can lead to a wide range of conditions. Many are subtle variations of normal Müllerian anatomy, and often remain asymptomatic or require no treatment. Others are transverse or longitudinal structural abnormalities or agenesis of parts of the Müllerian ducts, and may present to the gynaecologist in a variety of ways. An understanding of the timing and sequence of embryological development of the entire urogenital system helps in understanding the range of conditions that occur. Occasionally Müllerian anomalies may be associated with other conditions such as renal or spinal abnormalities or, more rarely, developmental defects of the cloaca such as bladder exstrophy, cloacal anomalies or anorectal anomalies. Ovarian development is independent of Müllerian duct development. Also considered in this section are lower transverse vaginal septae and the imperforate hymen (which derive from the urogenital sinus endoderm) and persistence of Wolffian duct remnants.

Müllerian anomalies

Definitions
There have been many attempts to classify Müllerian abnormalities, and the American Fertility Society classification is the most widely used (Figure 46.1). Congenital Müllerian

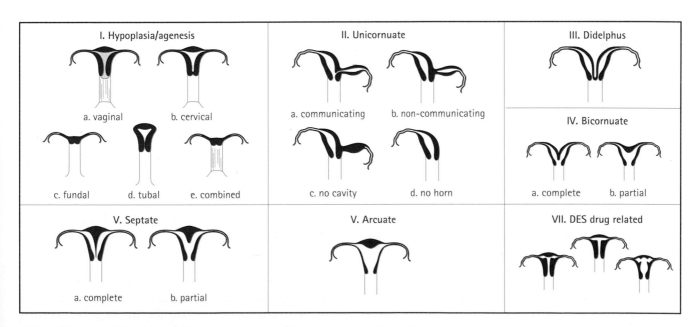

Figure 46.1 American Fertility Society classification of Müllerian anomalies. (From The American Fertility Society classifications of adnexal adhesions, distal tubal occlusion, tubal occlusion secondary to tubal ligation, tubal pregnancies, Müllerian anomalies and intrauterine adhesions. *Fertil Steril* 1988; **49**:944-55.) Reproduced with permission of the American Society for Reproductive Medicine. DES, diethylstilboestrol

Reproductive medicine

abnormalities generally fall into one of three groups: normally fused single Müllerian system with agenesis of one or more parts; unicornuate systems (unilateral hypoplasia or agenesis of one Müllerian duct); or lateral fusion failures (including didelphic and bicornuate anomalies). Rokitansky syndrome (agenesis of the uterus and vagina) is considered separately later in this section.

Incidence

The prevalence is thought to be 0.5 per cent in the female population.[12] The incidence in women with infertility is substantially higher. The commonest are septate and bicornuate anomalies.

Aetiology

The cause of Müllerian anomalies is unknown; they may be due to genetic errors or teratogenic events. Only a minority of cases appear to have a family history. It is assumed that there has been failure of fusion of the two Müllerian ducts, failure of one or both ducts to develop, or failure of resorption of the areas of Müllerian duct fusion. The causes of transverse vaginal septae are unknown.

Presentation and investigation

The spectrum of anomalies is wide and around 75 per cent of these women will remain asymptomatic. The remaining 25 per cent will present in a variety of ways. Secondary sexual development is normal as ovarian development and function are independent of Müllerian duct and urogenital sinus growth.

PRESENTATION OF MÜLLERIAN ANOMALIES
- Primary amenorrhoea.
- Cyclical abdominal pain (obstruction to menstruation).
- Severe dysmenorrhoea (obstruction to menstrual drainage from one Müllerian duct, e.g. the non-communicating rudimentary horn associated with a unicornuate uterus).
- Pelvic mass – haematocolpos (vagina distended with menstrual blood) or haematometra (uterus distended with menstrual blood).
- Menorrhagia.
- Dyspareunia (transverse or longitudinal vaginal septae).
- Infertility and recurrent miscarriage.
- Ectopic pregnancy.
- Obstetric complications, e.g. preterm birth, abnormal lie and uterine rupture.

INVESTIGATION OF MÜLLERIAN ANOMALIES
This includes an assessment of the internal and external uterine contours. Ultrasound, MRI and hysterosalpingogram are often used, sometimes in association with laparoscopy or hysteroscopy. Imaging of the renal tract is also indicated.

Management

Management of these anomalies depends on the type of anomaly and the presenting features. Symptomatic uterine and longitudinal vaginal septae can be resected hysteroscopically. The horns of a bicornuate uterus can be joined together into one cavity by an abdominal metroplasty. Any form of obstruction to menstrual flow requires surgery to relieve the obstruction and prevent pain and endometriosis. The didelphic uterus is often associated with vaginal septae that can lead to unilateral obstruction and requires careful vaginal surgery to remove the septum. Transverse vaginal septae can be of varying thicknesses, and complete removal is essential to try to prevent a stenotic ring at the site of surgery. For thick transverse vaginal septae, a combined abdomino-perineal procedure is often required.

The hymen usually opens after the fifth month of fetal life. An imperforate hymen presents either in neonatal life with a mucocolpos or at puberty with haematocolpos. A purple-blue bulge at the introitus associated with primary amenorrhoea is diagnostic. Surgery to create an adequate window for vaginal drainage cures the problem.

Rokitansky syndrome (also called Mayer–Rokitansky–Kuster–Hauser (MRKH) syndrome)

Definition and incidence

This condition is agenesis or hypoplasia of the vagina and uterus. The uterus is either absent or consists of a small central rudimentary uterine bud or bilateral uterine buds on the pelvic side walls. The incidence in the UK is estimated as between 1 in 4000 and 1 in 6000 females.

The aetiology remains unknown. The control mechanisms leading to Müllerian duct regression in males and Müllerian duct survival and growth in females are not well defined.

Presentation and management

The usual presentation is primary amenorrhoea with normal secondary sex characteristics. Occasionally the condition is identified in childhood. Investigation is as standard for primary amenorrhoea, and should exclude intersex conditions and include renal tract imaging due to the 30–40 per cent incidence of associated renal anomalies.

Management needs to encompass both psychological interventions, to help with aspects such as accepting the diagnosis, living with the condition, forming relationships and improving sexual function and quality of life outcomes, and interventions that can be used to enlarge or create the vagina. The aim of vaginal enlargement techniques (both surgical vaginoplasty and self-applied vaginal dilatation therapy) is to improve sexual function; however, there have been no studies to assess the effectiveness of these interventions on this outcome. Vaginoplasty surgery and dilators should not be used in childhood. Uterine transplant is not an option for the foreseeable future, although tissue engineering techniques may eventually provide new treatment options. As ovarian function is normal, fertility is possible via surrogacy.

Incomplete regression of the Wolffian system

Parts of the Wolffian duct may fail to regress completely in females, presenting as cysts lateral to the Müllerian duct. Usually these are incidental findings and most are asymptomatic, although they can grow to be large. The epoophoron and paraoophoron can be found beside the ovary in the mesosalpinx. Gartner's duct (the lower part of the Wolffian duct) cysts can occur anywhere from the broad ligament down to the vagina, and may present as vulval or vaginal masses. Wolffian remnants are also seen in the cervix. Very rarely, the Wolffian system may persist as the primitive mesonephric system draining functioning glomeruli, and an extra ureter can be found emptying into the vagina.

KEY POINTS

- Abnormalities of the Müllerian system are asymptomatic in 75 per cent of women.
- Imaging of the renal tract should be performed whenever abnormalities of the Müllerian system are found.

KEY REFERENCES

1. Warne GL, Zajac JD. Disorders of sexual differentiation. *Endocrinol Metab Clin North Am* 1998; **27**:945–67.

2. Creighton S, Minto C. Managing intersex. *BMJ* 2001; **323**:1264–5.

3. Blackless M, Charuvastra A, Derryck A, Fausto-Sterling A, Lauzanne K, Lee E. How sexually dimorphic are we? Review and synthesis. *Am J Hum Biol* 2000; **12**:151–66.

4. Randolph J, Hung W, Rathlev MC. Clitoroplasty for females born with ambiguous genitalia: a long-term study of 37 patients. *J Pediatr Surg* 1981; **16**:882–7.

5. Newman K, Randolph J, Parson S. Functional results in young women having clitoral reconstruction as infants. *J Pediatr Surg* 1992; **27**:180–3.

6. May B, Boyle M, Grant D. A comparative study of sexual experiences. *J Health Psychol* 1996; **1**:479–92.

7. Dittmann RW, Kappes ME, Kappes MH. Sexual behavior in adolescent and adult females with congenital adrenal hyperplasia. *Psychoneuroendocrinology* 1992; **17**:153–70.

8. Statement of the British Association of Paediatric Surgeons Working Party on the Surgical Management of Children Born with Ambiguous Genitalia, July 2001. Available at http://www.baps.org.uk/.

9. Creighton SM, Minto CL, Steele SJ. Objective cosmetic and anatomical outcomes at adolescence of feminising surgery for ambiguous genitalia done in childhood. *Lancet* 2001; **358**:124–5.

10. Alizai NK, Thomas DFM, Lilford RJ, Batchelor AGG, Johnson N. Feminizing genitoplasty for congenital adrenal hyperplasia: what happens at puberty? *J Urol* 1999; **161**:1588.

11. Robson S, Oliver GD. Management of vaginal agenesis: review of 10 years practice at a tertiary referral centre. *Aust N Z J Obstet Gynaecol* 2000; **40**:430–3.

12. Nahum GG. Uterine anomalies. How common are they and what is their distribution among subtypes? *J Reprod Med* 1998; **43**:877–87.

Karyotypic Abnormalities

Diana Fothergill

INTRODUCTION

There are a number of karyotypic abnormalities that may present to the gynaecologist with an initial complaint of primary amenorrhoea. Others will have been diagnosed in childhood but are referred on for further management by paediatricians and endocrinologists. Some karyotypic abnormalities have little impact on gynaecological problems, but those affecting the sex chromosomes are covered briefly. This is a rapidly changing field of medicine, and more sophisticated tests can lead to refinements in original diagnoses, so it may be appropriate to repeat genetic investigations or to test other cell lines.

TURNER'S SYNDROME (45X AND MOSAICS)

This is the commonest abnormality in females involving the sex chromosomes: 1 in 2000 live-born girls are affected, although most pregnancies with this abnormality are miscarried. It is estimated that 15 per cent of all miscarriages have a 45X karyotype. The incidence does not rise with increasing maternal age, but screening early pregnancies for increased nuchal thickness has led to more cases being diagnosed antenatally, as cystic hygroma and non-immune hydrops are frequently features of Turner's syndrome. Over half of these girls will have some form of mosaicism. The rate of detection is partly dependent on how hard it is looked for, as the cell lines may vary in different tissues.[1]

Physical abnormalities associated with Turner's syndrome

- Growth failure: low birth weight and short stature.
- Ovarian failure: no secondary sexual development in most cases, occasionally secondary amenorrhoea in mosaics.
- Inverted, widely spaced nipples, shield chest.
- Webbed neck.
- Puffy hands and feet in babies due to lymphoedema.
- Low hairline.
- Cubitus valgus.
- High, arched palate, micrognathia and defective dental development.
- Renal dysgenesis.
- Cardiac malformations, including coarctation of the aorta.
- Distortion of the Eustachian tube leading to otitis media.
- Nail dysplasia.
- Eye deformities.

Intelligence is usually normal. The phenotypic abnormalities result in most cases being diagnosed in infancy and childhood. The girls are then usually referred to a gynaecologist after optimal growth potential has been achieved for advice about long-term hormone replacement therapy (HRT). In most girls ovarian failure has occurred early in life; although they have a uterus and vagina, they will not develop any secondary sexual characteristics without hormonal supplements. A low dose of oestrogen is given initially to encourage steady growth of the breasts; this is usually started after the age of 12 years, as the administration of oestrogen promotes epiphyseal fusion, which stops further growth. The uterus will respond to oestrogen therapy, so it is necessary to add progestogens cyclically to produce regular endometrial shedding, or in a continuous combined regime to suppress endometrial development. Hormonal therapy may be by the oral or transdermal route. Many girls are maintained on oral contraceptive preparations that have the benefit of being socially acceptable as well as not incurring National Health Service (NHS) prescription charges.

When pregnancy is desired, women should be referred to an assisted conception unit for counselling about treatment with donor oocytes. Clinical pregnancy rates are reported to be comparable to those of other women with primary ovarian failure (up to 46 per cent per embryo transfer), but miscarriage rates are higher.[2] Spontaneous conceptions have been reported, usually in women with mosaicism or structural abnormalities of the X chromosome which have led to short stature but whose ovaries have been preserved. These pregnancies have a high rate of miscarriage and malformation, resulting in a healthy child being born in less than 40 per cent of pregnancies.[3]

There are a number of long-term health issues which affect women with Turner's syndrome:

- hypertension,
- structural defects in the aorta, which increase the incidence of dissecting aneurysm,
- diabetes – 25 per cent,
- hypothyroidism – 25–30 per cent,
- sensorineural hearing loss – 50 per cent,
- osteoporosis.

The gynaecologist may be the only point of regular medical contact and needs to be aware of these issues, particularly if pregnancy is desired. Hormone therapy should be continued at least until the age of 50 years.

Over two-thirds of Turner's syndrome cases result from loss of a paternal sex chromosome; in some there are fragments of a sex chromosome still present. If this is a Y chromosome, there is a 7–10 per cent risk of gonadoblastoma development, and gonadectomy is usually advised.[4] If this has not been performed, regular ultrasound examination of the gonad may be prudent.

- There is little published evidence on the effects of long-term HRT in Turner's women and on the optimal preparation to be used.
- Oestrogen therapy has been shown to increase bone mineral density.

Patients with Noonan's syndrome have a similar phenotypic appearance to Turner's, but this is an autosomal dominant trait with no abnormality of the sex chromosomes and there is no effect on ovarian function.

47XXX

These girls are not often referred to gynaecologists, although 47XXX occurs in about 1 in 1000 live-born females. They may have genitourinary abnormalities but are of normal height, and sexual development occurs normally. Academic performance is usually below average. The ovaries often fail prematurely and women may present with secondary amenorrhoea and require HRT. Somewhat surprisingly, most women give birth to chromosomally normal children, but prenatal diagnosis should be considered.

48XXXX, 49XXXXX

Almost all girls with these karyotypes are of subnormal intelligence. Ovarian dysfunction is quite common.

46XY

Characteristically, this diagnosis is made when a phenotypically normal girl presents with primary amenorrhoea or delayed puberty. There are a variety of conditions that are associated with this karyotype, which are described more fully earlier in this section.

In androgen insensitivity syndrome, the problem lies with the end-organ response to testosterone. The testes are functional and Müllerian inhibition factor is produced, so the uterus and vagina do not develop. Breast development usually takes place, as circulating testosterone is peripherally converted to oestrogen, but there is absent pubic hair due to the abnormal androgen receptors.

In Swyer's syndrome, or pure gonadal dysgenesis, there is a lack of functional gonadal tissue and, as a consequence, Müllerian structures persist and a normal uterus and vagina are found. Breast development does not normally occur and typically girls present above average height with delayed puberty. Pubic and axillary hair may be present due to the effect of peripherally produced androgens. Treatment is similar to that for Turner's syndrome, with oestrogen to develop the breasts and the addition of progestogens to cause withdrawal bleeds. Donor egg and embryo pregnancies have been reported.[5] Streak gonads may be present and there is concern that these have a high incidence of malignant change.[6]

STRUCTURAL ABNORMALITIES OF THE X CHROMOSOME

There are many abnormalities that can occur in the X chromosome. The commonest is an isochromosome for the long arm, most often found in mosaic form with 45X. Deletions of part of the long or short arm have variable effects depending on the level at which the deletion has occurred. If the short arm is missing, most girls will be of short stature; if the long arm is missing, there is usually gonadal dysgenesis. It is of interest to note that although one X chromosome is inactivated, it is necessary to have two normal X chromosomes to maintain fertility.

KEY POINTS

- Karyotypic abnormalities are a common cause of primary amenorrhoea.
- HRT is required in all patients with ovarian failure.
- Ovum donation may be an option for fertility.
- Turner's syndrome has long-term health implications.

KEY REFERENCES

1. Ranke MB, Saenger P. Turner's syndrome. *Lancet* 2001; 358:309–14.
2. Foudila T, Soderstrom-Anttila V, Hovatta O. Turner's syndrome and pregnancies after oocyte donation. *Hum Reprod* 1999; 14:532–5.
3. Tarani L, Lampariello S, Raguso G et al. Pregnancy in patients with Turner's syndrome: six new cases and a review of literature. *Gynecol Endocrinol* 1999; 12:83–7.
4. Gravholt CH, Fedder J, Naeraa RW, Muller J. Occurrence of gonadoblastoma in females with Turner syndrome and Y chromosome material: a population study. *J Clin Endocrinol Metab* 2000; 85:3199–202.
5. Sauer MV, Lobo RA, Paulson RJ. Successful twin pregnancy after embryo donation to a patient with XY gonadal dysgenesis. *Am J Obstet Gynecol* 1989; 161:380–1.
6. Lukusa T, Fryns JP, Kleczkowska A, Van Den Berghe H. Role of gonadal dysgenesis in gonadoblastoma induction in 46, XY individuals. The Leuven experience in 46,XY pure gonadal dysgenesis and testicular feminization syndromes. *Genet Couns* 1991; 2:9–16.

Menarche and Adolescent Gynaecology

Diana Fothergill

MRCOG standards

Theoretical skills
- Know the normal sequence of events in puberty to be able to recognize when investigation is appropriate.
- Know the causes of delayed puberty and how to establish the diagnosis.

Practical skills
- Be able to assess the stage of development of secondary sexual characteristics.
- Have observed consultations with the girl and mother, and be able to obtain the history and counsel about management.

INTRODUCTION

Puberty marks the change from childhood to adolescence, with the development of breasts and secondary sexual hair and the onset of menstruation. At the same time there is a period of accelerated growth. The gynaecologist is most often consulted when these events are delayed. The paediatrician will see more cases of precocious puberty.

Causes of precocious puberty

- Idiopathic.
- McCune Albright syndrome (café au lait spots and polyostotic fibrous dysplasia).
- Tumours of the adrenal or ovary producing steroids.
- Cerebral tumours.
- Ingestion of exogenous oestrogens.

The age at which the changes take place is variable, but it is abnormal for there to be no sign of secondary sexual development at the age of 14 years.

The trigger for the changes to start is an increasing frequency and amplitude of pulses of gonadotrophin release. The ovaries are then stimulated to begin to produce oestrogen, which acts on the breast tissue to promote growth. This usually begins at around the age of 9 and takes about 5 years to be completed. There is evidence to suggest that this is occurring at a younger age, particularly in African-American girls, prompting a reassessment of the age at which precocious puberty should be investigated.[1] Pubic hair growth is stimulated by androgens released by the ovary and theadrenal gland. Breast and pubic hair development is described in five stages following the classification by Marshall and Tanner (Table 48.1).[2] Growth charts indicate the range of normal ages at which these stages are attained. In most girls, breast development starts before the growth of pubic hair.

Even before these changes are obvious, there is acceleration of growth, which is frequently accompanied by a rapid increase in shoe size. The peak height velocity, of approximately 8 cm/year, occurs just before the onset of menses – on average around the age of 12 years. Oestrogen promotes closure of the epiphyses, so final height is usually attained about 2 years after menarche.

Table 48.1 Marshall and Tanner staging

Stage	Breast	Pubic hair
I	Pre-adolescent, elevation of papilla only	No pubic hair
II	Breast bud – elevation of breast and papilla as small mound; enlargement of areolar diameter	Sparse growth of long downy hair along the labia
III	Further enlargement but no separation of the contours	Hair coarser, darker and more curled; over mons
IV	Projection of the areola and papilla to form a secondary mound above the level of the breast	Adult-type hair but no spread to thighs
V	Mature; areola recessed to general contour of breast	Adult, with horizontal upper border and spread to thighs

Menarche occurs 2.3 ± 1 years after the onset of breast development. The average age of menarche has declined and is now 12.8 years in white girls and 12.16 years in African-Americans.[3] The factors involved include improved nutrition and genetic influences: daughters often undergo menarche at a similar age to their mothers. Initial menstrual cycles are usually anovulatory and often irregular for several years.

DELAYED PUBERTY

Most referrals to gynaecologists are because of concern about delay in the onset of menstruation. In order to determine the likely cause for this it is first important to establish whether puberty itself is delayed. A detailed history should be taken, asking about general health, the age at which breast and pubic hair development started, and if the girl has had a growth spurt or still appears to be growing. Any chronic illness may lead to constitutional delay in puberty. Teenage girls may be reluctant to answer questions and the mother frequently gives much of the history, but it is important to address the girl rather than talking directly to the mother. Examination should include accurate measurement of height, together with assessment of the stage of breast and pubic hair development, and these should be plotted on growth charts. The examination should be sensitively performed – ask the girl if she wishes her mother to be present, as some feel more embarrassed with the mother there – and only expose one part of the body at a time. An internal examination should not be performed; inspection of the external genitalia is all that is necessary, as further assessment of the internal organs will be achieved by ultrasound scanning of the pelvis.

Investigations usually include:

- measurement of gonadotrophins – follicle-stimulating hormone (FSH) and luteinizing hormone (LH) – and oestrogen,
- karyotyping,
- ultrasound scan of the pelvis to confirm the presence of the uterus and ovaries,
- possibly X-ray to determine bone age.

Additional biochemical tests to assess thyroid function, prolactin and 17-α-hydroxyprogesterone may also be appropriate.

ABSENT BREAST AND PUBIC HAIR

Hypogonadotrophic hypogonadism

The majority of girls with low gonadotrophins have constitutional delay in puberty. This may be secondary to chronic illness, for example cystic fibrosis. Improvement in the underlying condition usually results in catch-up growth.

Girls with anorexia nervosa have low levels of gonadotrophins and, if the problem starts at a young age, will have absent or poorly developed secondary sexual characteristics. A similar situation is found in many athletic girls, the classic example being gymnasts, who have a low body weight and very low body fat. This can lead to the 'female athletic triad', with disordered eating, amenorrhoea and osteopenia, and an increased risk of stress fractures.[4]

Congenital deficiency of gonadotrophins is more rarely encountered; this problem is more often seen in boys with delayed puberty. It may also be associated with anosmia due to hypoplasia of the olfactory lobes, when it is known as Kallman's syndrome. Brain imaging will be necessary to establish this diagnosis.

Acquired deficiency may follow damage to the hypothalamus or pituitary as a result of trauma, tumour such as a craniopharyngioma, irradiation, or infection – frequently secondary to hydrocephalus. Infiltration of these organs can also occur in haemochromatosis, which may be secondary to transfusions for sickle cell disease or thalassaemia and to Wilson's disease.

In all these conditions, ultrasound will confirm the presence of an immature uterus and small, inactive ovaries. The bone age will help to differentiate cases of constitutional delay, as it will be behind chronological and height age.

Treatment may be required if there are no signs of spontaneous onset of puberty, although most girls with constitutional delay will proceed to normal development if left untreated. A study conducted on untreated girls indicated that they experienced considerable distress, which affected their success at school, work or socially; 50 per cent would have preferred to receive treatment.[5] Pulsatile gonadotrophins have been used but are very difficult to sustain, as they require a subcutaneous injection attached to a portable pump for several months. The more widely used approach is to give low doses of ethinyl oestradiol 1-2 μg per day for 3–6 months. Frequently, spontaneous sexual maturation then occurs, but if not, the dose is gradually increased over several years.[6]

Hypergonadotrophic hypogonadism

This occurs when there is failure of gonadal development. The normal release of gonadotrophins occurs, but as there is no response from the gonad, there is no negative feedback to control gonadotrophin levels. The commonest cause is Turner's syndrome – 45X or other genetic problems (see Chapter 47). Other causes include damage to the ovaries by irradiation, surgery, chemotherapy or infection. Galactosaemia is also associated with ovarian failure and its management presents a challenge, as oral preparations of oestrogen and progesterone contain lactose. Autoimmune ovarian failure may be associated with other autoimmune disorders such as Addison's disease, vitiligo and hypothyroidism.

One of the less common causes of congenital adrenal hyperplasia is the deficiency of 17-α-hydroxylase. This enzyme is required to produce both oestrogen and testosterone, so virilization does not occur at birth, but there is also a failure of development of secondary sexual characteristics.

The treatment consists of gradually increasing levels of oestrogen replacement, combined with progesterone to induce withdrawal bleed once doses stimulate endometrial development.

NORMAL BREAST AND PUBIC HAIR DEVELOPMENT

Anatomical causes

If puberty has progressed normally but the girl has failed to menstruate, the commonest cause is an anatomical abnormality. It is uncommon for girls with an imperforate hymen or transverse vaginal septum to present to an outpatient clinic; they usually present as an emergency with cyclical abdominal pain, possibly with a palpable abdominal mass. The blockage prevents the flow of menstrual blood and there is usually a tense blue bulge seen at the introitus. Ultrasound scanning may show a distended vagina containing blood, and normal ovaries. Where there is a thin imperforate hymen, treatment is straightforward, as incision will allow the blood to drain and the mass will resolve. Treatment of a thicker and possibly higher septum is more complex and is best dealt with in a tertiary referral centre, as injudicious excision can result in stricture formation which is difficult to treat and will lead to considerable problems with intercourse.

The commonest cause is Müllerian agenesis, which is described in detail in the earlier part of this chapter.

Hyperprolactinaemia

This is more often a cause of secondary amenorrhoea, but can present as primary amenorrhoea and there may not be any galactorrhoea. A high prolactin level should prompt investigation for a pituitary adenoma. Treatment is the same as in the older female, with dopamine agonists such as cabergoline, which will result in the onset of menstruation.

Congenital adrenal hyperplasia

Menarche is often delayed in this condition, and when menstruation starts it may be erratic. Poor control of the condition, often due to poor compliance with treatment, may be the cause. The ovaries also often have a polycystic appearance on scan. Fertility rates in these women are poor for a number of reasons: infrequent ovulation, difficulties in achieving penetrative sex, and failure to form relationships.[7]

NORMAL BREAST BUT SCANTY OR ABSENT PUBIC HAIR DEVELOPMENT

This is the classical presentation of androgen insensitivity syndrome. The karyotype will be XY. Pubic hair fails to grow because of end-organ insensitivity to androgens, but breast development occurs due to peripheral conversion of androgens to oestrogen. No hormonal treatment is required.

MENORRHAGIA AND DYSMENORRHOEA

As initial menstrual cycles are usually anovular, they are normally painless, but bleeding may be prolonged.

Girls are often referred to gynaecologists because of concern about missing school, particularly when studying for state examinations, due to heavy and painful periods. Almost invariably they are accompanied by a mother who will tell you about the problems she had with her periods. It is very important to speak to the girl herself to try to establish if there is a genuine problem, and to make some effort to quantify the loss by the degree of soakage of the pads used. The number of pads used per day may be quite misleading, and as most women do not know what amount of loss is normal, it can be very difficult for a girl to know whether she is actually experiencing an abnormal amount of bleeding.

Excessive menstrual loss will usually result in a fall in the haemoglobin level, and occasionally the loss can be so great that emergency admission and transfusion are required. Many of these girls will have an underlying medical disorder. It is most important to exclude a coagulation disorder, such as von Willebrand's disease, or a platelet dysfunction, which may be present in a third of these cases.[8,9] There may be no previous personal or family history of bleeding symptoms. If such a disorder is found, it may be possible to treat the girl with desmopressin on a cyclical basis. The oral contraceptive pill is usually prescribed and, where blood loss is recurrently excessive, it can be helpful to prescribe this continuously for three or more cycles to reduce the frequency of withdrawal bleeds.

Occasionally girls present with life-threatening haemorrhage. The options for treatment include medroxyprogesterone acetate 5 mg orally every 1–2 hours for 24 hours and then 20 mg daily for 10 days, or oral oestrogen 1–2 mg every 4–6 hours. Intravenous oestrogen has also been used (40 mg 4-hourly for 24 hours) combined with a highly progestational oral contraceptive pill, but is not readily available in many pharmacies. It is rarely necessary to perform a diagnostic curettage.

- All girls with menorrhagia who are found to be anaemic should be investigated for a bleeding disorder, including testing for von Willebrand's disease and platelet function defects.

Reproductive medicine

Dysmenorrhoea usually responds to simple analgesia or oral contraceptives. However, where these measures fail, it is important to bear in mind the possibility of partial obstruction of menstrual flow. There are a number of reported cases of obstructed hemivagina and uterine horn associated with ipsilateral renal agenesis.[10] These usually present with severe cyclical pain and an abdominal mass due to a hemi-haematometra and haematocolpos. Removal of the occluded vaginal septum allows drainage and relief of symptoms. Endometriosis occurs in many of these patients, presumably secondary to the enforced retrograde menstrual flow.

There are many causes of chronic pelvic pain in young women, including psychosomatic factors. It is important to realize that endometriosis should be excluded in chronic pelvic pain that has not responded to simple measures. Laparoscopy may be indicated. The symptoms are often not those typically encountered in older women.[11]

KEY POINTS

- Secondary sexual characteristics have started to develop in most girls by the age of 14 years.
- Menarche normally occurs 2 years after breast development has commenced.
- Ovarian failure is the commonest cause of delayed puberty – karyotyping and gonadotrophins are essential investigations.
- Clotting studies should be performed for any girl with moderate to severe menorrhagia.
- Endometriosis can occur in teenagers.

KEY REFERENCES

1. Kaplowitz PB, Oberfield SE. Reexamination of the age limit for defining when puberty is precocious in girls in the United States: implications for evaluation and treatment. The Drug and Therapeutics and Executive Committees of the Lawson Wilkins Pediatric Endocrine Society. *Pediatrics* 1999; 104:936–41.

2. Marshall WA, Tanner JM. Variations in pattern of pubertal changes in girls. *Arch Dis Child* 1969; 44:291.

3. Herman-Giddens ME, Slora EJ, Wasserman RC et al. Secondary sexual characteristics and menses in young girls seen in office practice: a study from the Pediatric Research in Office Settings Network. *Pediatrics* 1997; 99:505–12.

4. Warren MP, Stiehl AL. Exercise and female adolescents: effects on the reproductive and skeletal systems. *J Am Med Womens Assoc* 1999; 54:115–20.

5. Crowne FC, Shalet SM, Wallace WH et al. Final height in girls with untreated constitutional delay in growth and puberty. *Eur J Pediatr* 1991; 150:708–12.

6. Albanese A, Stanhope R. Investigation of delayed puberty. *Clin Endocrinol* 1995; 43:105–10.

7. Mulaikal RM, Migeon CJ, Rock JA. Fertility rates in female patients with congenital adrenal hyperplasia due to 21-hydroxylase deficiency. *N Engl J Med* 1987; 316:178–82.

8. Smith YR, Quint EH, Hertzberg RB. Menorrhagia in adolescents requiring hospitalization. *J Pediatr Adolesc Gynecol* 1998; 11:13–15.

9. Bevan JA, Maloney KW, Hillery CA et al. Bleeding disorders: a common cause of menorrhagia in adolescents. *J Pediatr* 2001; 138:856–61.

10. Stassart JP, Nagel TC, Prem KA et al. Uterus didelphys, obstructed hemivagina, and ipsilateral renal agenesis: the University of Minnesota experience. *Fertil Steril,* 1992; 57:756–61.

11. Propst AM, Laufer MR. Endometriosis in adolescents. Incidence, diagnosis and treatment. *J Reprod Med* 1999; 44:751–8.

Ovarian and Menstrual Cycles

William L. Ledger

MRCOG standards

- Have a thorough understanding of the physiology of the menstrual cycle.
- Be able to explain disturbances in the cycle (e.g. anovulation, premature menopause) with reference to ovarian and uterine physiology.
- Understand the mechanism of action of drugs that affect the cycle.

INTRODUCTION

Efficient reproduction is essential to the continuance of any species and is the most basic drive to existence. Humans are relatively inefficient reproducers, but have still managed to over-populate the planet within only a few tens of thousands of years. Knowledge of the basic physiology of the processes by which the development of the ovarian follicle, ovulation, fertilization and implantation occur is an essential prerequisite to an understanding of the events which lead to malfunction of the system, for example in anovular infertility, premature ovarian failure and polycystic ovary syndrome.

THE OVARIAN CYCLE

The human premenopausal ovary consists of a central dense collagenous stroma surrounded by a thin outer cortex. The cortex contains thousands of primordial follicles, each containing a germ cell surrounded by a single layer of granulosa/theca cells. The germ cell is arrested at the diplotene stage of prophase of the first meiotic division. The primordial follicle may remain at this point for many years, until a change in the local environment within the ovary allows it to resume meiosis and grow. The primordial follicle will then develop into a **pre-antral** follicle in which the separate theca

and granulosa cell layers become discernable, and will then develop a cavity, or **antrum**, to become an **antral** follicle. The earliest stages of development of the follicle are independent of the gonadotrophins – luteinizing hormone (LH) and follicle-stimulating hormone (FSH) and may possibly be regulated by locally released **growth factors** within the ovary such as activin or GDF 9. The process by which individual primordial follicles re-enter the growth phase occurs throughout late fetal life, during childhood, through puberty and pregnancy and is not affected by drugs such as the oral contraceptive pill or gonadotrophin releasing hormone (GnRH) analogues. More than 99 per cent of all follicles will fail to ovulate, instead being destroyed and becoming **atretic** within the ovary, as a result of **apoptosis** (programmed cell death). The immutable nature of this process of **follicle depletion** helps in the understanding of the phenomenon of 'idiopathic' **premature ovarian failure** (premature menopause). A woman with early menopause probably received a lower than average number of primordial follicles during fetal life, leading to her 'running out' of her ovarian reserve more rapidly than others.

Each month, a cohort of antral follicles reaches the stage of sensitivity to FSH and LH at the time of the **intercycle rise** in FSH, the small but significant elevation in circulating FSH level that is seen during the menstrual phase of the cycle. One follicle (or occasionally two follicles) is at the correct stage of development to respond to FSH and LH by enlarging and continuing to grow. The outer **theca cell** layer of the follicle has receptors for LH and the necessary enzymes to synthesize androgens, whilst the inner **granulosa cell** layer, which is intimately connected to the oocyte, responds to FSH by developing **aromatase**, the enzyme which synthesizes oestrogens from androgens. Hence the theca/granulosa cell layers have to act in concert to synthesize oestrogens by responding individually to different gonadotrophins – the **two cell, two gonadotrophins theory**.

By secreting oestradiol into the circulation, the growing follicle reduces the circulating level of FSH by **negative feedback** on the hypothalamus and pituitary. Hence other follicles in the cohort are not exposed to a sufficiently high level of FSH to allow them to continue to develop, and they become atretic. Thus a single follicle each month becomes **dominant**, and is destined to ovulate some 10 to 12 days later. As the follicle grows, the granulosa cells secrete more oestradiol into the circulation and also secrete a complex mixture of peptide and glycoprotein growth factors into the oestrogen-rich **follicular fluid** that bathes the oocyte. As the follicular diameter reaches approximately 18 mm, the rising concentrations of oestradiol trigger a coordinated secretion of LH from the anterior pituitary – the **LH surge**. The LH surge triggers the final maturation of the oocyte, with completion of meiosis and extrusion of the first polar body, which contains one of the two haploid sets of chromosomes from the oocyte. At the same time, the LH surge also induces an inflammatory reaction within the wall of the follicle adjacent to the mouth of the fallopian tube. Rapid formation of new capillary blood vessels and release of interleukins, prostaglandins and other cytokines result in follicular rupture and ovulation some 38 hours after the initiation of the LH surge.

Following release of the oocyte, further neovascularization and enzyme induction within the luteinized theca/granulosa cells produce progesterone, which appears rapidly in the circulation after ovulation. Progesterone from the **corpus luteum** acts on the endometrium to induce secretory changes, and suppresses secretion of FSH from the pituitary, preventing development of a further dominant follicle. The processes of synthesis and secretion of progesterone are maintained by LH and later, if pregnancy occurs, by **human chorionic gonadotrophin (hCG)** from the trophoblast. In the absence of 'rescue' by hCG, the corpus luteum involutes after 12–14 days, resulting in a decline in concentrations of progesterone in the circulation, with concomitant menstruation as a result of progesterone withdrawal (Figure 49.1).

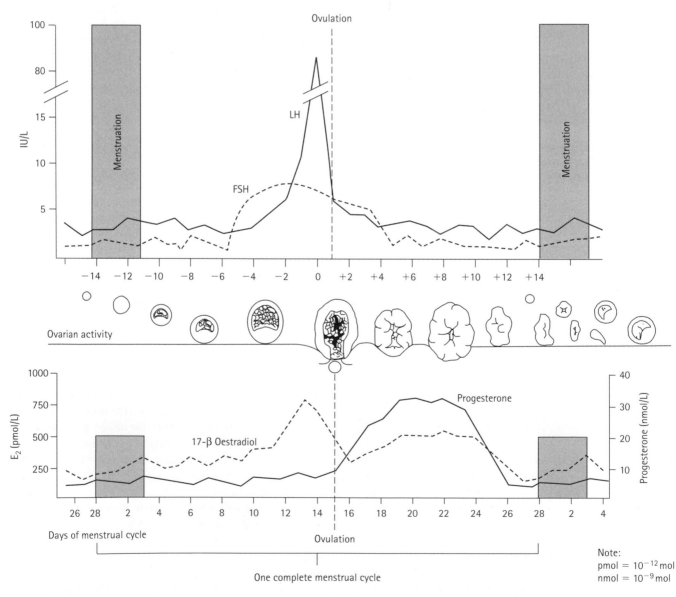

Figure 49.1   Ovarian and pituitary hormones and growth of endometrium during the cycle. LH, luteinizing hormone

THE MENSTRUAL CYCLE

Each month, the endometrium must become receptive to implantation of the early embryo at the correct time of the cycle, in coordination with the arrival of the newly fertilized embryo in the uterine cavity. The pattern of events during the menstrual cycle reflects the necessity for close coordination of ovulation, fertilization and endometrial receptivity. Initially, the endometrium must re-grow from the **basalis layer**, which remains after shedding of the more superficial layers of endometrium at menstruation. As the new endometrium grows, formation of **spiral arteries** provides the necessary vascular supply for later development of the maternal side of the placenta, should implantation occur. The **proliferative** endometrium grows in the first half of the menstrual cycle, being driven by oestradiol secreted into the circulation by the developing follicle. Hence follicular growth and endometrial growth are closely coordinated. After the LH surge, the follicle secretes large amounts of progesterone, which induces morphological changes in the endometrium. The glandular elements within the endometrium now proliferate and the superficial epithelial layer of the endometrium secretes a number of adhesion molecules, including **glycodelin** and **integrins**, which mediate the attachment, adhesion and initial stages of implantation of the embryo onto the endometrium. These proteins are only expressed for 1–2 days in the mid-luteal phase of the cycle, defining the **implantation window**.

The embryo attaches once it has hatched from the blastocyst, some 6 days after fertilization. Trophoblast cells invade into the endometrium to establish the early placenta, whilst the **inner cell mass** begins to differentiate into the new fetus. One of the earliest signs of the establishment of pregnancy is the identification of hCG from trophoblast in the maternal circulation. This hormone maintains the secretion of progesterone from the corpus luteum and thereby prevents breakdown of the endometrium, with menstruation. The presence of hCG is essential for the maintenance of early pregnancy, until the **luteo-placental shift** at 10–12 weeks' gestation, at which point the feto-placental unit becomes autonomous and luteal progesterone secretion is supplanted by production by placental cells.

INHIBINS IN THE OVARIAN CYCLE

Recently, a group of glycoprotein hormones termed inhibins has been observed to have co-regulatory effects on the hypothalamo–pituitary–ovarian axis. Inhibins are heterodimeric glycoproteins consisting of alpha and beta chains linked by disulphide bonds (Figure 49.2). They are secreted from the granulosa cell layer of the follicle and the theca/granulosa of the corpus luteum. Inhibin A, with alpha and beta A subunits, is secreted from the mature dominant follicle and in large amounts from the corpus luteum. Inhibin B, with alpha and beta B subunits, is released from the developing cohort of antral follicles in the early follicular phase of the cycle, and from the early dominant follicle. Inhibin B is not detectable in the luteal phase of the cycle or in pregnancy, whereas inhibin A secretion is maintained from the placenta during pregnancy and in labour. It seems likely that inhibin B from the dominant follicle acts with oestradiol to inhibit growth of other members of the cohort, preventing the risk of multiple pregnancy, while inhibin A may participate in the regulation of the LH surge and maintenance of the corpus luteum.

APPLICATIONS OF THE PHYSIOLOGY OF THE OVARIAN AND MENSTRUAL CYCLES

Investigation of anovular infertility

Accurate and rapid measurements of ovarian and pituitary hormones in peripheral blood samples have become the

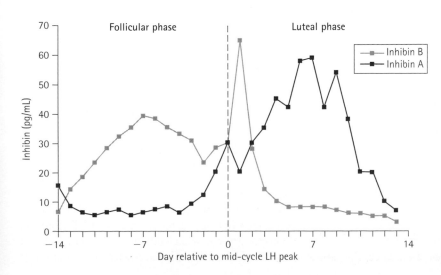

Figure 49.2   Inhibin A and B during the menstrual cycle. (Reproduced with permission from Groome NP, Illingworth PJ, O'Brien M et al. *JCEM* 1996; **81**(4):1401–5, copyright The Endocrine Society.)

mainstay of the investigation of anovulation. Women who are anovular generally report an irregular or absent menstrual cycle and may have stigmata of polycystic ovary syndrome, hyperprolactinaemia or anorexia. Pituitary function in such cases is usually assessed by measurement of LH, FSH, prolactin and thyroid function on day 2 or 3 of a menstrual period. If periods are absent or infrequent, menses can usually be induced by a short course of progestogen (e.g. 10 days of Provera, 10 mg twice daily). This regime will induce a **withdrawal bleed** if the endometrium is adequately oestrogenized. If no bleed occurs, the patient is pregnant, has damaged or absent basalis layer of the endometrium or lacks sufficient oestrogen to 'prime' the endometrium. Lack of oestrogen may result from hypogonadal hypogonadism or reduced circulating levels of FSH and LH commonly due to anorexia or over-exercise.

More commonly, levels of FSH and LH may be within the normal range, possibly with an elevation of LH. This will suggest a diagnosis of **polycystic ovary syndrome**, confirmed by measurement of serum androgens and sex-hormone-binding globulin and ovarian ultrasound. Patients with polycystic ovary syndrome may also exhibit mild elevation in levels of prolactin, but elevated levels of prolactin must always be assumed to be caused by a pituitary **prolactinoma** until proven otherwise. A clinical history of galactorrhoea and tunnel vision with amenorrhoea and headache should prompt imaging of the pituitary fossa, which is probably best done by magnetic resonance imaging (MRI).

If both FSH and LH are elevated, there is the possibility of **premature ovarian failure**. The patient may give a history of menopausal symptoms and may have a family history of early menopause. There may also have been exposure to pelvic irradiation or chemotherapy – more and more patients are surviving childhood cancers such as leukaemias and lymphomas, but at the cost of loss of ovarian function. A diagnosis of premature ovarian failure should always be confirmed by repeated measurement of gonadotrophins and oestradiol, a karyotype to rule out chromosomal abnormalities such as mosaic Turner's syndrome, and advice regarding hormone replacement therapy. Beware of results of measurements of LH and FSH being made in mid-cycle: samples may have been collected during the LH surge, possibly leading to a healthy ovular patient being erroneously diagnosed as having ovarian failure.

Principles of treatment of anovular infertility

A sound knowledge of the regulation of the ovarian cycle helps understanding of the principles of treatment of anovulation. Clomiphene citrate has been the first line of treatment for anovulation associated with polycystic ovary syndrome for many years. Clomiphene has a complex action on the ovary, being a mixture of two isomers, one strongly anti-oestrogenic and the other weakly pro-oestrogenic. In essence,

exposure to clomiphene citrate results in elevation of FSH levels in the circulation, by altering the set point of the feedback loop between oestradiol and FSH – a reduction in oestradiol caused by clomiphene resulting in an elevation in FSH. Higher levels of FSH may in turn induce a follicle to grow and ovulate, although at a cost of the risk of multiple pregnancy.

Similarly, daily injection of FSH can now be given to induce ovulation in clomiphene-resistant patients. This treatment over-rides the natural mechanism of follicle selection, which works by oestrogen and inhibin from the dominant follicle acting on the pituitary to reduce circulating levels of FSH, resulting in other members of the cohort of antral follicles becoming atretic. Maintenance of high levels of FSH by injection allows all members of the cohort to grow. In a young patient, more than 20 follicles may grow in synchrony, reflecting the large size of the antral follicle pool. Even larger numbers of follicles may be seen if FSH is given to a patient with polycystic ovary syndrome, leading to the risk of **ovarian hyperstimulation syndrome (OHSS)**. In older patients treated with similar doses of FSH, only two or three follicles may appear, demonstrating the decline in ovarian reserve that generally occurs after 35 years of age.

Measurement of inhibin B in the early follicular phase of the cycle may also be helpful in assessing ovarian reserve. A high level of inhibin B is suggestive of preservation of a large cohort of follicles, with 'good' ovarian reserve, whereas a low inhibin B suggests depletion of the follicle pool. A combination of high FSH and low inhibin B has been used in assisted conception to predict poor ovarian response to superovulation.

In the early days of superovulation with injected FSH, the hormone was derived from human pituitary, and later from the urine of postmenopausal women (who have high levels of FSH as a result of loss of ovarian oestradiol feedback on the pituitary). Such urinary preparations of FSH invariably also contain LH. More recently, the genes for the alpha and beta subunits of FSH have been transfected into a Chinese hamster ovarian cell line, which expresses human FSH protein in culture. Such 'recombinant' FSH is devoid of LH action. Most in-vitro fertilization (IVF) cycles are now conducted using FSH superovulation after pituitary down-regulation with a GnRH agonist, resulting in a profound suppression of endogenous LH production. Use of recombinant FSH following GnRH agonist down-regulation results in the growth of a cohort of follicles in an almost LH-free environment. The demonstration that such cycles generate healthy oocytes that can fertilize and produce pregnancies shows that only small amounts of LH are necessary for the maintenance of function of the theca cells in the follicle. However, studies with patients with Kallmann syndrome, who have essentially no LH, have shown that recombinant FSH will induce growth of follicles but not secretion of oestradiol, resulting in the absence of growth of the endometrium. Hence a basal secretion of LH is necessary for successful coordination of the ovarian and endometrial cycles, supporting the two cell, two gonadotrophin hypothesis.

Ovarian physiology in assisted reproduction

Progress in assisted reproduction has largely come about from an improved understanding of ovarian physiology and early embryology. Early IVF treatment required laparoscopic aspiration of the single dominant follicle present in the natural cycle, the development of which was followed by assay of metabolites of oestrogens in urine and LH in serum. As soon as the onset of the LH surge was detected, oocyte collection was undertaken, often at night-time or at weekends. The procedure was 'hit or miss', with many attempts failing to obtain an oocyte. Introduction of '**superovulation**' with FSH injection allowed the growth of a cohort of follicles, improving the chances of obtaining oocytes, but the high levels of oestradiol secreted from the multiple growing follicles produced the risk of a premature LH surge with loss of oocytes by ovulation before oocyte collection could be undertaken. The introduction in the mid-1980s of GnRH agonist pre-treatment before superovulation almost completely removed this risk. **Pituitary down-regulation** prevented the release of LH in response to rising levels of oestradiol, greatly improving the efficiency of superovulation and allowing day-time scheduling of oocyte collection.

Management of problems in early pregnancy

The principle of luteal 'rescue' by hCG secreted from the developing feto-placental unit resulting in maintenance of high circulating levels of progesterone has had considerable impact on the management of the luteal phase in down-regulated IVF cycles and on the treatment of recurrent early pregnancy failure. Measurement of hCG in serum or urine forms the basis of early detection of pregnancy, and sub-optimal rises or falls in hCG levels are associated with impending miscarriage or ectopic pregnancy. Pituitary down-regulation in IVF cycles has prevented the problem of premature LH surges but results in low levels of LH being present in the luteal phase of the cycle, with a negative effect on the function of the corpus luteum. '**Luteal phase** support' in the form of hCG injection or, more recently, progestogenic compounds given by injection or as vaginal pessaries is routinely given to IVF patients after embryo transfer, to overcome any adverse impact of low progesterone levels on the establishment of pregnancy. Similarly, patients with recurrent miscarriage have traditionally been given progesterone or hCG treatment in an attempt to prevent miscarriage, although the benefit of such an approach has not been demonstrated in randomized, controlled trials.

SUMMARY

This chapter outlines the events that regulate the ovarian and menstrual cycles. An understanding of the interplay between the pituitary gonadotrophins and ovarian steroids and glycoproteins has underpinned many of the recent developments in reproductive medicine. Knowledge of ovarian and uterine physiology helps the understanding of diagnostic and therapeutic approaches to patients with infertility and ovarian failure.

KEY POINTS

- The ovarian and uterine cycles are tightly coordinated in order to ensure receptive endometrium at the time at which the embryo is ready to implant.
- The pituitary hormones LH and FSH are regulated by feedback from the ovary by sex steroids (oestrogens and progesterone) and peptides (inhibins).
- Knowledge of pituitary–ovarian physiology has allowed rational development of drugs to influence the cycle, including GnRH agonists and antagonists to suppress the LH surge and prevent premature ovulation, and injectable gonadotrophins to stimulate multiple follicular development for IVF.
- The causes of anovulation can usually be elucidated quickly using timed measurements of FSH, LH, progesterone and oestradiol, sometimes with additional measurement of prolactin and thyroid function.

Contraception, Sterilization and Termination of Pregnancy

Louise Kenny

MRCOG standards

The established standards for this topic are:

- Have a thorough understanding of all methods of contraception; candidates are obliged to present evidence of practical experience.
- Understand the reasons for and the techniques and complications of performing therapeutic abortion.

We would suggest the following points for guidance.

Theoretical skills

- Revise the physiology and endocrinology of the menstrual cycle and the pharmacology of synthetic oestrogen and progesterone treatment.

Practical skills

- During the course of their training and prior to sitting Part II, candidates are required to receive instruction in at least eight sessions at family planning clinics. Candidates should be able to take an appropriate history and counsel patients requesting contraceptive advice, sterilization or termination of pregnancy.

INTRODUCTION

There is a wide and growing range of contraceptives available in the developed world. This chapter aims to give an overview of the knowledge of contraception and therapeutic abortion essential for candidates for the MRCOG examination.

GENERAL TERMINOLOGY

The **efficacy** of any method of contraception can be calculated and described in a variety of ways. The majority of modern studies and reviews present efficacy as the number of pregnancies experienced during 100 woman-years (HWY) of use of the method (a woman-year is defined as 13 cycles), and are standardized by 1-year, 2-year, 5-year (or much shorter or longer) cut-off points. This method of calculating efficacy is used in this chapter.

The **safety** of any method of contraception is of paramount importance to both the user and prescriber. The World Health Organization (WHO) has produced a classification system to aid selection of the most appropriate method. The suitability of different contraceptive methods is categorized in the presence of a specific illness or condition by weighing the health risks against the benefits of using a particular contraceptive method when any of these conditions are present. There are four categories.

1 A condition for which there is no restriction of the use of the contraceptive method.
2 A condition for which the advantages of using the method generally outweigh the disadvantages of using the method.
3 A condition for which the theoretical or proven risks usually outweigh the advantages of using the method.
4 A condition which represents an unacceptable health risk if the contraceptive method is used.

NATURAL METHODS

Natural family planning relies upon the fact that there are only certain days during the menstrual cycle when conception can occur. Following ovulation, the ovum is viable within the reproductive tract for a maximum of 24 hours. However, the life span of sperm is considerably longer, in the region of 3–7 days. Consequently, during a regular 28-day menstrual cycle, when ovulation occurs on day 14, it is possible to predict the most and least likely days for conception to occur following intercourse (calendar method). The success of this method is largely dependent upon the accurate prediction of ovulation, which can be extremely variable, and upon adherence to abstinence from intercourse during the potentially fertile period. In reality, this period of abstinence is on average 15–17 days each cycle, and the high failure rate of this method reflects the fact that many couples find it difficult to adhere to this.

Ovulation prediction can be enhanced by several complementary methods, including measuring basal body temperature (the rise in progesterone following ovulation produces a rise in the basal body temperature of approximately 0.2–0.4°C, which is maintained until the onset of menstruation) and detecting changes in the consistency of cervical mucus (Billings' method). Use of the latter method relies upon the fact that several days before ovulation occurs, cervical mucus assumes the appearances of raw egg white, i.e. clear, slippery and stretchy (spinnbarkheit). The final day of 'fertile mucus' is considered to be the day when ovulation is most likely to occur, and abstinence must be maintained from the day when fertile mucus is first identified until 3 days after the peak day. The end of the fertile period is characterized by the appearance of 'infertile mucus', which is scanty and viscous.

Personal fertility monitors (Persona, Unipath, UK) are small hand-held devices that are able to detect urine concentrations of oestrone-3-glucuronide (E3G) and luteinizing hormone (LH) and thus indicate the start and end of the fertile period. On potentially fertile days, a red light indicates the need for abstinence from intercourse. 'Safe' days are indicated by a green light, and a yellow light indicates that a urine sample is required. Following the urine test, a red or green light will be displayed, depending on the ratio of LH and E3G.

The efficacy of natural family planning methods varies widely. One large multicentre study suggested that, when strictly adhered to, the failure rate of the mucus method was 2.8 pregnancies per HWY [II]. This can be improved by combining the mucus method with the calendar and temperature methods to give a failure rate of 2.6 pregnancies per HWY [II]. Persona, when correctly used, is associated with a failure rate of 6.2 pregnancies per HWY. Aside from low and varying levels of efficacy, the main disadvantage of natural methods of family planning is that they provide no protection against the transmission of sexually transmitted infections (STIs).

BARRIER METHODS

Barrier methods of contraception prevent pregnancy by physically interrupting the progress of sperm in the female reproductive tract.

There are many types available, including condoms (worn by the male) and occlusive pessaries or caps, sponges and vaginal condoms in combination with spermicides (worn by the female).

Condoms

A large range of condoms is available in the UK. The majority are made of fine latex rubber. They are available in different sizes and textures and with and without additional spermicide. Condoms are a widely accessible and inexpensive form of reversible contraception which additionally provide a very high level of protection against STIs (including human immunodeficiency virus (HIV) infection) and carcinoma and pre-malignant disease of the cervix. The published efficacy of condoms ranges from 3 to 23 per HWY [III] and is highest when they are used correctly and consistently. The only absolute contraindication to condom use is latex allergy in either partner.

Occlusive pessaries

Four main occlusive pessaries are in current use: the diaphragm, cervical cap, vault cap and vimule. All devices are inserted into the vagina prior to intercourse to occlude the cervix and should be used in combination with spermicides to provide maximum protection.

Occlusive devices are available in a range of sizes and initially need to be fitted by trained personnel. They require a high degree of motivation for successful use and this is reflected in the varying rates of efficacy (4–20 per HWY) [III].

Female condom

The female or vaginal condom is a polyurethane sheath, which is inserted to and lines the vagina. It is widely available over the counter and has a reported failure rate of 5–21 per HWY [III].

Vaginal sponges

Vaginal sponges are made of polyurethane foam and are inserted with spermicide into the vagina to cover the cervix. They provide contraception by acting as a barrier, as a mechanism for absorbing semen and as a carrier for spermicide. They have a higher failure rate than the diaphragm and are consequently less popular.

The main advantage of barrier methods of contraception is the protection they afford against STIs. This is greatest for condoms, and their use should be encouraged in tandem with other contraceptive methods, particularly in groups perceived to be at high risk.

KEY POINTS

Barrier contraception:

- requires user motivation
- provides varying degree of protection against STIs
- has no systemic side effects.

COMBINED ORAL CONTRACEPTION

Combined oral contraception (COC) contains two steroid hormones, oestrogen and a progestogen (a synthetic progesterone). The oestrogen component of most modern COC is ethinyloestradiol (EE) in the dose range of 20–50 μg. The progestogen components vary in different preparations, but all are derivatives of 19-nortestosterone. They are divided into second generation (e.g. norethisterone and levonorgestrel) and third generation (e.g. desogestrel and gestodene). Third-generation progestogens have a higher affinity for the progesterone receptor and a lower affinity for the androgen receptor than second-generation compounds. This means that, in theory at least, they confer greater efficacy with fewer androgenic side effects. In addition, they also have fewer effects on carbohydrate and lipid metabolism than second-generation compounds, but, disappointingly, this has not translated into a reduction in the risk of arterial wall disease or acute myocardial infarction [Ia].

Dianette is an anti-androgen/synthetic oestrogen combination (cyproterone acetate 2 mg with ethinyloestradiol 35 μg). It is an effective treatment for acne and hirsutism (because of the anti-androgenic properties) and also provides good cycle control and effective contraception.

The efficacy of the COC is difficult to estimate accurately, as it is obviously user dependent. However, with 'perfect use', the efficacy approaches 100 per cent, and the UK Family Planning Association states that efficacy is 'over 99 per cent' with correct use.

Mechanism of action of combined oral contraception

- The oestrogen component inhibits pituitary follicle-stimulating hormone (FSH) secretion and thereby suppresses follicle growth, whilst the progestogen component inhibits the LH surge and thus prevents ovulation.
- Cervical mucus becomes scanty and viscous with low spinnbarkeit and thus inhibits sperm transport.
- The endometrium becomes atrophic and unreceptive to implantation.
- There are possibly direct effects on the fallopian tubes impairing sperm migration and ovum transport.

Combined oral contraception formulations are either fixed dose or phasic (the dose of oestrogen and progestogen changes once (biphasic) or twice (triphasic) in each 21-day course). Phasic preparations are designed to mimic the cyclical variations in hormone levels.

Non-contraceptive benefits of combined oral contraception

- Less dysmenorrhoea and menorrhagia.
- Reduced risk of carcinoma of the endometrium and ovary.
- Reduced incidence of benign breast disease.
- Reduced incidence of pelvic inflammatory disease (PID).
- Possible protective effect against rheumatoid arthritis, thyroid disease and duodenal ulceration.

Adverse effects of combined oral contraception

Metabolic effects

- Weight gain: this is associated with pills containing levonorgestrel but not desogestrel or gestodene.
- Carbohydrate metabolism: COC produces minor effects on insulin secretion.
- Lipid metabolism: the effect on the ratios of total and low-density lipoprotein (LDL) cholesterol to high-density lipoprotein (HDL) cholesterol depends on the relative doses of oestrogen/progestogen and the type of progestogen.

Cardiovascular effects

- Venous disease: EE causes an alteration in clotting factors, promoting coagulation and increasing the relative risk of venous thromboembolism (VTE) in current COC users by three–four-fold compared to women not taking COC. Combined oral contraceptives containing third-generation progestogens (desogestrel and gestodene) possibly carry a small additional risk of VTE beyond that of the second-generation compounds. The risk of VTE in COC users is increased by:
  - obesity
  - immobility
  - age
  - congenital and acquired thrombophilias.
- Arterial disease: the relative risk of myocardial infarction (MI) and haemorrhagic stroke in current users of COC with hypertension or who smoke is increased more than in non-smoking current users without hypertension, who are at no greater risk than non-users.

The relative risk of ischaemic stroke in normotensive current users of COC who do not smoke is increased about 1.5-fold compared to non-users. This risk increases with increasing oestrogen doses and is greatly elevated by hypertension and smoking.

Cancer and combined oral contraception use

Breast cancer

There is a small increase in the risk of developing breast cancer while women are taking COC and for a few years after discontinuing, diminishing to the background risk after 10 years [Ia].

Ovarian and endometrial cancer

There is a >50 per cent reduction in the risk of developing ovarian and endometrial cancer after 5 years of COC usage, which lasts for up to 15 years after the pill is stopped [Ia].

Cancer of the cervix

An observed increase in the incidence of both cervical intraepithelial neoplasia and cervical cancer in COC users may be related to greater sexual activity without the benefit of barrier contraception in these women [Ia].

Trophoblast disease

The regional centres in the UK, which monitor all cases of trophoblastic disease, recommend that all sex hormones should be avoided while hCG levels are raised. However, there are no data to suggest an increased risk of trophoblastic disease in pregnancies following COC use.

Absolute contraindications to combined oral contraception (WHO 4)

- Past or present circulatory disease
  1 Proven past arterial or venous thrombosis
  2 Ischaemic heart disease
  3 Severe or multiple risk factors for venous or arterial disease
  4 Focal migraine
  5 Transient ischaemic attacks
  6 Atherogenic lipid disorders
  7 Inherited and acquired thrombophilias
  8 Past cerebral haemorrhage
  9 Vascular malformations of the brain
  10 Significant structural heart disease
  11 Pulmonary hypertension
- Disease of the liver
  1 Active liver disease (i.e. with abnormal liver function tests)
  2 Liver adenoma or carcinoma
  3 Gallstones
  4 The acute hepatic porphyrias
- Other
  1 Pregnancy
  2 Undiagnosed genital tract bleeding
  3 Oestrogen-dependent neoplasm, e.g. breast cancer

  4 History of a serious condition known to be affected by sex steroids, e.g. pemphigoid gestationis

Relative contraindications to combined oral contraception (WHO 2 and 3)

- Undiagnosed oligomenorrhoea
- Cigarette smoking over age 35
- Diabetes
- Non-focal migraine
- Sickle cell disease (sickle cell trait is not a contraindication)
- Inflammatory bowel disease
- Obesity (if associated with other risk factors)

KEY POINTS

- Highly efficacious but user dependent
- Wide range of minor side effects
- Long-term use has both beneficial and possibly detrimental health effects
- Rapidly reversible

PROGESTOGEN-ONLY CONTRACEPTION

Mechanism of action

Progestogens have numerous actions throughout the reproductive tract. The most important in relation to contraception are thought to be:

- cervical mucus modification, which inhibits sperm penetration;
- endometrial modification to prevent implantation;
- variable local effects on the ovary, including suppression of follicular growth, inhibition of ovulation and suppression of luteal activity;
- variable hypothalamic and pituitary effects to inhibit cyclical release of FSH and LH, and hence suppression of follicular development and ovulation.

Advantages

Progestogen-only contraception has minimal adverse effects on the coagulation and fibrinolytic cascades and consequently does not induce or exacerbate VTE disease. Furthermore, progestogens have a minimal impact on lipid profiles and are not associated with the development of hypertension and may therefore be used in most cardiovascular diseases (with the exception of current severe arterial wall disease).

Reproductive medicine

Progestogen-only contraception has no impact upon milk production and can therefore be used by lactating mothers.

In addition, progestogen-only contraception has several non-contraceptive health benefits. There is evidence that depot medroxyprogesterone acetate (DMPA) provides protection against the development of endometrial cancer, acute PID and vaginal candidiasis. Progestogen methods also provide some symptomatic relief of dysmenorrhoea, premenstrual syndrome and Mittelschmerz, and may protect against the development of endometriosis, uterine myomas and ovarian cancer.

Disadvantages

The principal disadvantage of all progestogen-only methods is menstrual disturbance, which relates to the variable and unpredictable impact upon ovarian function. Amenorrhoea is particularly common with injectable methods, whereas low-dose progestogen-only methods may be associated with irregular and possibly prolonged spotting or bleeding. Although the majority of women experience a reduction in the total volume of blood lost each month, the erratic nature of the bleeding pattern may lead to dissatisfaction.

A small number of women using progestogen-only methods may develop functional ovarian cysts. These cysts, which are thought to be associated with luteinization of unruptured ovarian follicles, are usually asymptomatic but can occasionally result in pain and may mimic ectopic pregnancy.

Pregnancies in progestogen-only users are more likely to be ectopic than are pregnancies occurring in non-users. This is probably a relative increase, as progestogen-only methods protect against all pregnancies, but against intrauterine pregnancies to a greater extent. However, progestogens may modify tubal function and lead to a decrease in the rate of ovum transport. Therefore a history of a previous ectopic pregnancy is a relative contraindication for specific methods, such as the progestogen-only pill (POP), which may not universally inhibit ovulation.

Other minor side effects include acne (particularly with slightly androgenic progestogens such as levonorgestrel), headaches, breast tenderness and loss of libido.

Specific methods

Progestogen-only contraceptive pills

A variety of POPs is available in the UK consisting of various doses of levonorgestrel, norethisterone or ethynodiol diacetate. Pills should be taken at the same time every day and without a break, as this method relies primarily upon the effect on cervical mucus, which begins to wear off within the 24-hour period. However, there is also an extremely variable effect on ovulation, and this explains the principal side effect of menstrual disturbance. The efficacy of POPs is largely dependent on compliance. The overall failure rate is 0.3–4 per HWY (the lower rate applies to meticulous pill taking or POP contraception in combination with lactation).

Injectables

Two injectables are currently licensed in the UK: depot medroxyprogesterone acetate (DMPA, Depo-Provera) and norethisterone oenanthate (NET-EN, Norsterat, Norigest). DMPA is licensed for long-term general contraceptive use, whereas NET-EN is licensed only for short-term use (up to two injections) in conjunction with rubella immunization for the partners of men undergoing vasectomy or for postpartum women awaiting sterilization. Both are administered by deep intramuscular injection into the gluteal area; DMPA is usually given every 90 days, whereas NET-EN injections should be given 60 days apart. Both injectables work primarily by suppressing ovulation, supplemented by cervical mucous and endometrial effects, and consequently amenorrhoea is common. Both methods are highly effective; DMPA has a reported failure rate of <0.5 per HWY and NET-EN has a failure rate of <1 per HWY. Specific disadvantages of this method include a moderate delay in return to fertility following cessation of use, which in DMPA users may be 7–8 months, and weight gain, which is thought to occur through an increase in appetite.

Subdermal implants

Currently, the only subdermal implant licensed in the UK is Implanon™. It consists of a single rod of 68 mg of etonogestrel. It is licensed for 3 years and has an extremely high efficacy, with pregnancy rates approaching zero in clinical trials. It works primarily by suppressing ovulation, supplemented by cervical mucous and endometrial effects, and consequently amenorrhoea is common. Furthermore, past ectopic pregnancy is not a contraindication. The obvious disadvantage of any implant is the need for insertion and removal by trained personnel. However, following insertion, it requires no user motivation and hence compliance is not a problem.

Absolute contraindications to progestogen-only contraception (WHO 4)

- Known or suspected pregnancy.
- Undiagnosed vaginal bleeding.
- Current history of severe cardiovascular disease, e.g. ischaemic heart disease.
- Any serious side effect occurring on the COC and not clearly due to oestrogen or associated with past progesterone use, e.g. hepatic adenoma.
- Acute porphyria.
- Injectable methods should not be used in women with bleeding disorders or on anticoagulants.

Relative contraindications to progestogen-only contraception (WHO 2 and 3)

- The presence of *multiple* risk factors for arterial disease.
- Severe obesity, as it may reduce the efficacy of low-dose methods and may be exacerbated by injectables.

- Untreated breast cancer.
- Trophoblast disease.
- Concurrent use of enzyme-inducing drugs, which may interact, e.g. rifampicin.
- A history of recurrent functional ovarian cysts as low-dose methods, which do not inhibit ovulation, may exacerbate these.
- A past ectopic pregnancy, particularly in a young nulliparous women.

INTRAUTERINE CONTRACEPTIVE DEVICES

Intrauterine contraceptive devices (IUCDs) are the most commonly used reversible method of contraception worldwide, with about 127 million current users, most of them in China.

There are three types of IUCD: inert, copper bearing and hormone releasing. Inert devices are no longer available in the UK. Copper-bearing IUCDs consist of a plastic frame with copper wire round the stem and some have copper sleeves on the arms. The surface of the copper determines the effectiveness and active life of the device; most IUCDs are generally licensed for use over 5–10 years.

All IUCDs cause a foreign-body reaction in the endometrium, with increased prostaglandin production and leucocyte infiltration. This reaction is enhanced by copper, which affects endometrial enzymes, glycogen metabolism and oestrogen uptake and also inhibits sperm transport. The number of spermatozoa reaching the upper genital tract is reduced in copper-bearing IUCD users. Furthermore, alteration of uterine and tubal fluid impairs the viability of the gametes.

IUCDs are highly effective contraceptives. Newer devices have failure rates of <0.5 per cent.

The levonorgestrel-releasing intrauterine system (LNG-IUS, Mirena, Schering) consists of a plastic frame, similar in design to the Nova T series. This carries a reservoir of levonorgestrel, which is released following insertion at a rate of 20 μg per 24 hours over at least 5 years. In addition to the foreign-body effect common to all IUCDs, the intrauterine release of levonorgestrel from the LNG-IUS causes endometrial suppression and changes to the cervical mucus and utero-tubal fluid, which impair sperm migration. These effects combine to produce a highly efficacious contraceptive with a failure rate of 0–0.2 per HWY. Endometrial suppression also leads to a reduction in the amount and duration of blood loss experienced during menses and, consequently, Mirena is now licensed as a treatment for menorrhagia. Blood levels of levonorgestrel are generally low in Mirena users, and therefore side effects normally associated with progestogen administration, such as acne and depression, are rare. The main disadvantage of the LNG-IUS is the high incidence of irregular uterine bleeding in the months following insertion. This normally settles within 6 months, but it is important that women are adequately counselled prior to insertion.

Choice of device

Worldwide, the Copper T380 is the first choice, as it has the lowest failure rate and the longest life span. A woman who has a small uterine cavity or who has experienced pain or spontaneous expulsion with a framed IUCD should have a smaller IUCD such as GyneFix fitted. This IUCD is a frameless device that has six copper beads wound around a monofilament polypropylene thread. A knot at the upper end of the filament serves as an anchor, which is implanted into the fundal myometrium. A history of menorrhagia is an indication for LNG-IUS use.

Complications and their management

Dysmenorrhoea and menorrhagia

Intrauterine contraceptive devices may cause or exacerbate dysmenorrhoea and menorrhagia. Pain can be treated with non-steroidal anti-inflammatory drugs (NSAIDs). Intolerable menorrhagia that is resistant to treatment is an indication for removal of the IUCD and possibly changing to LNG-IUS.

Infection

Pelvic inflammatory disease associated with IUCDs is most likely to occur just after insertion. This risk can be minimized by screening patients prior to fitting. PID occurring in an IUCD user remote from fitting is usually associated with the acquisition of an STI. This should be managed routinely with full screening, contact tracing and appropriate antibiotic treatment. There is some controversy as to whether the IUCD should be removed. The acquisition of an STI may indicate that an IUCD is not the ideal contraceptive choice, but in any event the device should be removed if there is no response to treatment within 48 hours.

Actinomycosis is a serious and debilitating condition associated with granulomatous pelvic abscesses caused by *Actinomyces israelii*. This bacterium is occasionally detected by cytology in IUCD users. The presence of *Actinomyces* in the cervical smears of asymptomatic women is not thought to be clinically relevant, and opinion is divided as to whether the device needs to be replaced. However, if the patient is symptomatic, particularly if she has signs of pelvic infection, the device should be removed and sent for bacteriological examination immediately. High-dose penicillin for several weeks is the treatment of choice.

Pregnancy

Intrauterine pregnancy in the presence of an IUCD is rare. It is associated with a higher risk of spontaneous early or midtrimester pregnancy loss or premature labour if the device is left in situ. Therefore, if a pregnancy is confirmed in an IUCD user before 12 weeks' gestation and the threads are visible, the device should be removed.

After 12 weeks' gestation, the threads have usually been drawn up into the enlarged uterine cavity. Even if they are visible, there is a greater chance of the device being firmly wedged up alongside the conceptus and it should be left in place.

Although IUCDs are highly effective at preventing all pregnancies, they provide more protection against intrauterine than extrauterine pregnancy, and therefore the diagnosis of ectopic pregnancy should always be considered in a woman with an IUCD in situ and a positive pregnancy test.

Lost threads/devices

If the threads of an IUCD are not visible, it indicates that they have been drawn up into the cervical canal or the uterine cavity, or the device has been expelled or has migrated out of the uterus. If the threads cannot be located or retrieved, pelvic ultrasonography should locate the device. If the device is not visible on ultrasound, an X-ray of the abdomen should locate any device that has migrated from the uterus.

Spontaneous expulsion is most common in the first year after insertion and usually occurs during menstruation. For this reason, women should be advised to check for the presence of threads following each period.

Migration of the device from the uterus into the abdomen is rare and is usually a consequence of unrecognized partial perforation at insertion. Management depends on the clinical condition of the patient. If perforation is recognized at the time of insertion, laparoscopy should be performed and the device should be retrieved, as copper-bearing devices cause a sterile inflammatory reaction and rapidly become adherent to bowel and omentum.

Absolute contraindications to IUCD use (WHO 4)

- Known or suspected pregnancy.
- Undiagnosed vaginal bleeding.
- Suspected malignancy of the genital tract.
- Active or recent (within the past 3 months) STI or PID.
- Distorted uterine cavity that prevents proper insertion or placement (e.g. fibroids).
- Copper allergy or Wilson's disease (for copper-bearing devices only).

Relative contraindications to IUCD use (WHO 2 and 3)

- Menorrhagia and anaemia (an indication for LNG-IUS).
- Women perceived to be at high risk of STI.
- HIV infection, systemic corticosteroid treatment or immunosuppressive therapy.
- Benign trophoblastic disease.
- Valvular heart disease (risk of subacute bacterial endocarditis).
- Current anticoagulant therapy.

EMERGENCY CONTRACEPTION

Hormonal methods

The Yuzpe Regime (originally described by Albert Yuzpe) was marketed in the UK in 1984 as PC4 (Schering Health Care Ltd). It consists of ethinyloestradiol ($100\,\mu g$) and levonorgestrel ($500\,\mu g$) given twice, with the first dose taken within 72 hours of intercourse and the second taken 12 hours after the first. This method has recently been superseded by a progestogen-only form of emergency contraception. Levonorgestrel ($0.75\,mg$) (Levonelle-2, Schering) is given twice, again with the first dose taken within 72 hours of intercourse and the second dose taken 12 hours after the first. The mechanism of hormonal emergency contraception is probably multifocal. The Yuzpe Regime is thought to inhibit or delay ovulation, altering endometrial receptivity. Progestogen-only contraception also alters the characteristics of cervical mucus, impairing sperm transport and thereby preventing fertilization of an egg released within a few days after treatment. This may explain the greater efficacy of the progestogen-only method as compared with the Yuzpe Regime. If commenced within 24 hours of intercourse, PC4 will prevent 77 per cent of expected pregnancies, compared to 95 per cent prevented by Levonelle-2. However, the efficacy of both methods declines with time [Ia].

The commonest side effects of hormonal contraception are nausea and vomiting. These occur less frequently with the progestogen-only method, but it is common practice to offer an anti-emetic and to advise patients that if vomiting occurs within 2 hours of either dose, a further dose must be taken. Women using emergency contraception must also be advised that they may experience menstrual disturbance following treatment and that they must attend for a pregnancy test if their period does not occur within 1 week of expected menstruation.

Copper IUCDs

Copper IUCDs can be used as effective emergency contraception if inserted up to 5 days after the earliest calculated date of ovulation or up to 5 days after the first act of unprotected coitus. The mechanism of action is presumed to be through the spermicidal and blastocidal action of copper. There is no evidence of a rise in β-hCG following emergency use of IUCDs, so it is unlikely that implantation occurs. Levonorgestrel-releasing IUSs are not suitable for use as emergency contraception.

The copper IUCD has the lowest failure rate of any method of emergency contraception (<1 per cent). Age and nulliparity are not contraindications to fitting. Moreover, menorrhagia is not a contraindication, as the IUCD can be removed when the next menses occurs. However, the usual precautions for routine IUCD insertion also apply to emergency use. Women should be advised that there is an increased risk of

PID in the first month after fitting. It is therefore important to screen for infection and to prescribe antibiotics if indicated.

STERILIZATION

Sterilization is a common form of permanent, irreversible contraception in the UK, where approximately 30 per cent of couples include at least one sterilized partner, rising to over 50 per cent of those aged over 40.

Female sterilization

Female sterilization usually involves blocking both fallopian tubes during laparotomy, mini-laparotomy or, more commonly, laparoscopy. The RCOG has recommended laparoscopy and mechanical occlusion of the fallopian tubes with either clips or rings (as a day case wherever possible) as the procedure of choice in the UK.

Pre-sterilization counselling of a woman requesting sterilization should include exploring and ascertaining that she understands the irreversible and permanent nature of the procedure and the alternative methods of contraception available. The failure rate of the procedure should be discussed, and the RCOG recommends a rate of approximately 1 in 200 in the woman's lifetime as an appropriate level of risk. Furthermore, women should be informed of the increased risk of any post-procedure pregnancy being an ectopic pregnancy and of the risk that this can pose to her health.

Finally, women should be informed of the risks of laparoscopy and the chances of requiring laparotomy if there are problems with laparoscopy, particularly for those at increased risk from conditions such as previous abdominal surgery or obesity.

All women requesting sterilization should also be counselled with regard to male sterilization as a possible alternative option.

Vasectomy

The technique of vasectomy involves either division or removal of a piece of each vas, accompanied by fascial interposition or diathermy. This procedure can be performed on an outpatient basis, ideally under local anaesthetic whenever possible [IV]. Following the procedure, men should be advised to use effective contraception until there are two consecutive semen analyses showing azoospermia, 2–4 weeks apart, with the first test being at least 8 weeks after surgery [IV]. Provided these semen analyses are negative, the failure rate of vasectomy is approximately 1 in 2000. However, failure can occur up to 10 years after the procedure as a result of late recanalization [II].

Reports of an increase in the risk of developing testicular cancer following vasectomy have not been substantiated. However, several studies have highlighted the association of vasectomy with chronic testicular pain. This is probably due to distension and granuloma formation in the epididymis and vas deferens, and consequently men requesting vasectomy should be informed that, although there is no substantial long-term health risk associated with the procedure [II], there is a risk of developing chronic testicular pain [II].

INDUCED ABORTION

The conditions of the 1967 Abortion Act, as amended in 1990, state that abortion can be performed in the UK if two registered medical practitioners, acting in good faith, agree that the pregnancy should be terminated on one or more of the following grounds.

- The continuance of the pregnancy would involve risk to the life of the pregnant woman greater than if the pregnancy were terminated.
- The termination is necessary to prevent grave permanent injury to the physical or mental health of the pregnant woman.
- The pregnancy has not exceeded its 24th week and continuance of the pregnancy would involve risk, greater than if the pregnancy were terminated, of injury to the physical or mental health of the woman.
- The pregnancy has not exceeded its 24th week and continuance of the pregnancy would involve risk, greater than if the pregnancy were terminated, of injury to the physical or mental health of the existing children of the family of the pregnant woman.
- There is a substantial risk that if the child were born it would suffer from such physical or mental abnormalities as to be seriously handicapped.

The 1967 Abortion Act does not apply to Northern Ireland, where abortion is only legal under exceptional circumstances, for example to save the life of the mother.

Pre-abortion management

The decision to end an unplanned pregnancy is not an easy one for any woman to make. Pre-abortion management should include non-directive counselling to address the following issues.

- Alternatives to abortion, i.e. continuing with the pregnancy or having the baby adopted.
- Details of the method of abortion available and the possible complications.
- Future contraception.

The majority of women will come to a decision quickly. However, clinicians caring for women requesting abortion should try to identify those patients who require more support in decision-making than can be provided in a routine clinic setting; facilities for additional support, including access to social services, should be available [IV].

Pre-abortion assessment should include a pregnancy test. The gestation should be determined by menstrual history and a bimanual pelvic examination. Ultrasound scanning is not considered to be an essential prerequisite to abortion. However, all units should have access to ultrasound scanning, as it can be necessary in cases where there is doubt about the gestation or where ectopic pregnancy is suspected [IV]. If ultrasound scanning is performed, it should be done in a setting and manner that are sensitive to the woman's situation [IV].

A complete medical history should be taken and particular attention should be given to conditions such as cardiac or respiratory disease, which may influence the choice of method of abortion.

Blood should be taken for measurement of haemoglobin concentration, determination of ABO and rhesus blood groups, with screening for red cell antibodies and screening for other conditions such as haemoglobinopathies, HIV and hepatitis B if indicated on clinical grounds [II]. It is not cost effective routinely to cross-match women undergoing termination of pregnancy [Ib].

It is good practice to opportunistically obtain a cervical smear from those women who have not had one within their local screening programme, but mechanisms must be in place to ensure that the result is communicated to the women, acted upon appropriately and recorded within the local cervical cytology programme.

Methods of abortion

The most appropriate method of pregnancy termination is determined in part by the gestation of pregnancy (Table 50.1).

Vacuum aspiration

This technique involves dilating the cervix and passing a catheter or curette (up to 12 mm) into the cavity of the uterus. The uterine contents are usually aspirated using a mechanical pump. Cervical preparation is beneficial prior to suction termination and should be routine if the woman is aged under 18 years or at a gestation greater than 10 weeks [IV].

Table 50.1   Methods of termination of pregnancy

Gestation	Appropriate methods
Up to 9 weeks	Medical abortion
From 7 to 12 weeks	Vacuum aspiration
From 12 to 15 weeks	*Either* vacuum aspiration *or* medical abortion (see mid-trimester regime)
Greater than 15 weeks	*Either* dilatation and evacuation preceded by cervical preparation and undertaken by experienced practitioners *or* medical abortion (see mid-trimester regime)

In the UK, suction termination is mainly performed under general anaesthesia, although experience from other countries suggests that local anaesthesia may be sufficient and may be safer [IV].

The mortality from vacuum aspiration in the first trimester is <1/100 000, and is thus considerably less than the maternal mortality from continuing the pregnancy.

Conventional suction termination is an appropriate method at gestations between 7 and 15 weeks, although it is common practice to offer medical abortion at gestations over 12 weeks [IV].

Dilatation and evacuation

Mid-trimester abortion by dilatation and evacuation is not commonly performed in the UK. Nevertheless, when preceded by cervical preparation and performed by specialist practitioners with access to the necessary instruments and with sufficiently large caseloads to maintain their skills, it is a safe and effective method [Ia].

Medical abortion

A number of drugs, alone or in combination, can be used to induce abortion at various gestations.

Cervagem (gemeprost) is a synthetic derivative of the naturally occurring prostaglandin E_1. It causes strong uterine contractions and softening and dilatation of the cervix. It is widely used in early medical abortion, mid-trimester medical abortion and for the preparation of the cervix prior to surgical evacuation of the uterus. Misoprostol (also a prostaglandin E_1 analogue) given vaginally is a cost-effective, although as yet unlicensed, alternative to cervagem.

Mifepristone is a synthetic steroid that blocks the biological action of progesterone by binding to its receptor in the uterus and other target organs. Following withdrawal of the effect of progesterone, the uterus contracts and bleeding from the placental bed occurs, followed by abortion 2–5 days later. Mifepristone alone is only 60 per cent effective. However, the rate of complete abortion is increased to 95 per cent by the administration of a prostaglandin 36–48 hours after the administration of mifepristone.

In the UK, mifepristone is currently licensed for the induction of abortion up to 9 weeks' gestation, given as a single oral dose of 600 mg followed 48 hours later by 1 mg vaginal pessary of cervagem.

Recent evidence suggests that the dose of mifepristone can be reduced to 200 mg and misoprostol can be used as an alternative prostaglandin. Published regimens for early medical abortion therefore include:

- mifepristone 600 mg orally followed 36–48 hours later by cervagem 1 mg vaginally;
- mifepristone 200 mg orally followed 36–48 hours later by misoprostol 800 µg vaginally;*
- mifepristone 200 mg orally followed 36 hours later by cervagem 0.5 mg vaginally.*

*Regimens are unlicensed as described above.

Published regimens for mid-trimester medical abortion include:

- mifepristone 600 mg orally followed 36–48 hours later by cervagem 1 mg vaginally every 3 hours to a maximum of five pessaries;
- mifepristone 200 mg orally followed 36–48 hours later by misoprostol 800 µg vaginally, then review after 6 hours if not progressed. If necessary, repeat the dose of misoprostol 800 µg vaginally;*
- mifepristone 200 mg orally followed 36 hours later by cervagem 1 mg vaginally every 6 hours.*

*Regimens are unlicensed as described above.

Mifepristone binds to the glucocorticoid receptor and blocks the action of cortisol. Thus any patient on corticosteroids or who has suspected adrenal insufficiency should not be given mifepristone. Prostaglandins can cause bronchospasm: asthma is therefore an absolute contraindication to medical methods.

Complications

Complications that should be discussed prior to the procedure include the following.

Persistence of placental or fetal tissue

This is the commonest complication following abortion. Incomplete or missed abortion is commoner after medically induced abortion in the first trimester, and up to 5 per cent of women will require surgical evacuation within the first month. However, it can also occur after vacuum aspiration. Although an ultrasound scan and measurement of serum β-hCG may be helpful in diagnosing an ongoing pregnancy, the decision to intervene and perform surgical evacuation of the uterus is best made on clinical grounds, i.e. persistent or heavy bleeding from a bulky uterus in the presence of a dilated cervix.

Haemorrhage

Haemorrhage at the time of abortion is rare. It complicates around 1.5/1000 procedures overall and the incidence is lower at early gestations. Oxytocics are effective in reducing intraoperative blood loss.

Uterine perforation

This occurs in an estimated 1–4/1000 procedures. The rate is lower for abortions performed early in pregnancy and those performed by experienced clinicians. In cases of suspected perforation, laparoscopy is the investigation of choice.

Genital tract infection

Genital tract infection of varying degrees of severity occurs in up to 10 per cent of cases and in its severest form can lead to established pelvic infection. Abortion care should therefore encompass a strategy for minimizing the risk of post-abortion infective morbidity. Appropriate strategies include screening for lower genital tract organisms (e.g. chlamydia and gonorrhoea), with treatment of positive cases or the administration of prophylactic antibiotics to cover these organisms. The RCOG's suggested regimen is metronidazole 1 g rectally at the time of the abortion plus doxycycline 100 mg twice daily for 7 days, commencing post-abortion.

Cervical and vaginal trauma

These are rare complications, particularly when abortion is performed in the first trimester.

Aftercare

RhD-negative women

Anti-D immunoglobulin G (IgG) should be given to all non-sensitized RhD-negative women following abortion, whether by surgical or medical methods and regardless of gestational age [Ib].

Contraception

The very fact that a woman has had an abortion indicates that she also requires a review of her method of contraception. This discussion should ideally take place during pre-abortion counselling and certainly prior to discharge [IV]. All hormonal methods, including injectables and implants, can be safely initiated immediately following the abortion. It also safe and effective to insert an IUCD at this time [II]. Similarly, sterilization can be safely performed at the time of induced abortion. However, combined procedures are associated with higher rates of failure and of regret on the part of the woman [III], and consequently decisions about permanent methods of contraception are best left for some months. Regardless of the method chosen, it should be initiated immediately and the woman should leave hospital with adequate supplies.

Follow-up

A follow-up appointment (either within the abortion service or with the referring clinician) within 2 weeks of the procedure should be offered to each patient following abortion [IV]. At this visit, referral for further counselling should be made available for the small minority of women who experience long-term post-abortion distress. Risk factors for this include ambivalence before the abortion, lack of a supportive partner, a psychiatric history or membership of a cultural group that considers abortion wrong. However, it should be noted that there is no evidence of an increase in the incidence of serious psychiatric disorder following abortion. In contrast, the incidence of depression, suicide and child abuse is higher in women who have continued with the pregnancy because abortion was refused [III].

Endometrial Function

Christine P. West

INTRODUCTION

The main function of the endometrium is to receive a fertilized ovum (blastocyst) during implantation. As this occurs relatively infrequently, cyclical breakdown and regeneration of the endometrium during the menstrual cycle are its normal key events. These changes are under the control of the hypothalamo–pituitary–ovarian axis, with ovarian steroids acting directly within the endometrium via local intracellular receptors. Many other local mediators are involved in the complex and dynamic processes that take place within this metabolically highly active organ.

DEFINITION

Menstruation is the shedding of the superficial layer of the endometrium following the withdrawal of ovarian steroids secondary to failure of implantation. The development of the endometrium is secondary to the ovarian cycle; its proliferative phase corresponds to the ovarian follicular phase, with endometrial growth stimulated by rising oestrogen production by the dominant follicle. Following ovulation, the endometrium enters its secretory phase in preparation for implantation under progesterone domination, corresponding to the ovarian luteal phase. Equal in importance with the shedding of the endometrium is its regeneration, which commences 36 hours after the onset of bleeding and is normally completed by day 5–6 of the cycle.

MORPHOLOGICAL CHANGES

During the follicular phase of the cycle the endometrium proliferates from its basal layer in response to oestradiol. The developing glands are initially straight and tubular within a compact stroma but later become more convoluted. Following ovulation, exposure to rising levels of progesterone from the corpus luteum induces secretory changes in the endometrial glands. Sub-nuclear vacuoles appear initially, followed by evidence of glandular secretory activity. This is accompanied in the late luteal phase by oedema and predecidual changes in the stroma and increased coiling of the spiral arterioles, which supply the endometrium.

Failure of conception results in regression of the corpus luteum and an abrupt fall in circulating levels of oestrogen and progesterone. In the endometrium there is loss of tissue fluid, stromal infiltration of leucocytes and intense vasoconstriction of the spiral arterioles. Distal ischaemia and vasodilatation lead to tissue breakdown and bleeding from the damaged vessels. Thirty-six hours after the onset of bleeding, the process of endometrial regeneration commences in the basal layer.

MOLECULAR PROCESSES

These local events are controlled by changes in the circulating levels of oestrogen and progesterone that act via specific receptors in various cellular locations within the endometrium. These receptors are members of a large family of nuclear transcription factors that regulate the expression of numerous genes. Two subtypes of both the oestrogen (ER) and progesterone receptor (PR) have been described. Whereas ER is more specific, PR expression is controlled by both oestrogen and progesterone; the presence of oestrogen during the follicular phase up-regulates the synthesis of PR, which is subsequently down-regulated by progesterone during the luteal phase. While progesterone does not bind to ER, it inhibits oestrogen-mediated processes. This dual control is relevant to an understanding of both the endogenous and exogenous control of the endometrium by steroid hormones. Progesterone withdrawal seems to be the primary initiating event for the cascade of molecular and cellular reactions that lead to menstruation.

A host of other local factors are involved, although the exact mechanisms are poorly understood. The role of inflammatory cells is critical to the process of menstruation. Falling levels of progesterone trigger the influx of leucocytes and other inflammatory cells into the endometrial stroma during the late luteal phase. This process appears to be in part mediated by chemokines. Activation of lymphomyeloid cells releases a number of regulatory molecules, including cytokines and proteases. Matrix metalloproteinases (MMPs) are enzymes that play an important role in tissue breakdown at menstruation. Steroid hormones, growth factors and cytokines are all known to differentially regulate the genes for MMPs.

Other local mediators include vasoactive substances such as prostaglandins, endothelins and nitric oxide. Prostaglandins (Pgs) are locally released fatty acids, which act differentially on vascular and smooth muscle and platelet aggregation. Thromboxane A2 is a vasoconstrictor and stimulates platelet aggregation, while PgI2 (Prostacyclin) has opposite effects. PGF2a has vasoconstrictor and smooth muscle stimulating actions, in contrast to the vasodilator effects of PGE2. Endothelins are extremely potent vasoconstrictors that are produced in increased amounts during menstruation. The actions of these vasoactive substances are likely to stimulate the initial vasoconstriction of the spiral arterioles and to be involved later in the control of bleeding, by both vasoconstriction and increased platelet aggregation.

Rising levels of oestradiol stimulate endometrial repair, which involves regeneration of glandular, stromal and vascular elements mediated by a number of cytokines and growth factors. The process differs from other forms of adult wound healing in that it occurs without scarring.

CONTROL OF MENSTRUAL BLEEDING

Bleeding is controlled by a combination of factors that include platelet adhesion, spiral artery vasoconstriction and changes in the haemostatic and fibrinolytic systems. Increased fibrinolysis and decreased coagulation are demonstrable at the onset of menstrual bleeding; these processes are later reversed. Abnormalities in prostaglandin production have been demonstrated in women with menorrhagia and are also implicated in dysmenorrhoea. Endometrial repair is also critical to the control of menstrual bleeding. Knowledge of these mechanisms is the basis for current treatments for menorrhagia, and ongoing research into endometrial function is essential to the development of alternative therapeutic approaches.

KEY POINT

Knowledge of basic ovarian and uterine physiology is necessary to allow understanding of the principles of ovulation induction and superovulation for IVF, as well as to understand the physiological basis of disorders of the menstrual cycle.

Uterine Fibroids and Menorrhagia

Christine P. West

INTRODUCTION

Uterine fibroids are common in women of reproductive age. They are a frequent indication for gynaecological surgery, most commonly hysterectomy, although in the past many hysterectomies were carried out for asymptomatic fibroids because of concerns about the nature and consequences of a pelvic mass. Advances in imaging have facilitated the diagnosis of fibroids and enabled more women to be managed conservatively. Fibroids may be implicated in the causation of miscarriage and subfertility, but this chapter primarily addresses the evidence base for the management of menorrhagia associated with the presence of fibroids.

DEFINITIONS

Uterine fibroids, also known as myomas or leiomyomas, are benign tumours arising from the myometrium. They are composed of round whorls of smooth muscle and connective tissue and may be single, multiple or very numerous. Their site may be intramural, submucosal or subserous and their presentation and symptoms vary according to their size and site of origin. They are commonly asymptomatic and found incidentally during routine pelvic or ultrasound examination. Their commonest symptomatic presentation is with heavy menstrual bleeding or pressure symptoms.

INCIDENCE

Fibroids are present in up to 25 per cent of women of reproductive age.[1] In studies in which menorrhagia has been subjectively confirmed by blood loss measurements,[2] 40 per cent of women with losses >200 mL were found to have fibroids, compared with only 10 per cent whose losses were <100 mL. In a review of risk factors,[1] fibroids were reported to be commoner and to occur at a younger age in black women. They are also associated with nulliparity and are more common in women with a family history of fibroids. Smoking and the long-term use of the oral contraceptive pill and Depo-Provera are associated with a reduced risk. Fibroids regress in size and undergo degeneration after the menopause.

AETIOLOGY

Fibroids are hormone dependent and contain increased levels of receptors for both oestrogen and progesterone compared with normal myometrium.[3] The actions of steroid hormones on the uterus are mediated by a number of growth factors and it is likely that these are involved in fibroid growth. However, it is not clear how fibroids are initiated and there is no explanation for their heterogeneity in terms of numbers, size, site and behaviour within and between individuals. Although a causal relationship with menorrhagia has not been firmly established, it is likely that fibroids contribute to heavy bleeding if present submucosally or where intramural fibroids cause distortion of the endometrial cavity. There is little evidence that subserosal or pedunculated fibroids contribute to heavy blood loss.

MANAGEMENT

The management of uterine fibroids is covered in detail in a comprehensive evidence-based guideline.[4] Recommendations relevant to the management of menorrhagia associated with fibroids are also made in the Royal College of Obstetricians and Gynaecologists' (RCOG) evidence-based guidelines.[5,6] In common with all gynaecological disorders, the age and reproductive status of the individual woman and her preferences in relation to the various management options influence management.

Investigation

History and examination are supplemented by a full blood count.[5] Suspicion of fibroids is usually based on a palpably enlarged uterus on pelvic or abdominal examination. If the uterine enlargement is no greater than a 10-week size, medical management can be initiated within primary care without further investigation.[5] Failure to respond to medical therapy or uterine enlargement greater than a 10-week gestation size is an indication for further investigation [IV].

Investigation of abnormal bleeding is covered elsewhere and these recommendations apply to the investigation of suspected fibroids. Transvaginal ultrasound (TVS) should be the preliminary investigation [Ia],[4,6] combined with abdominal ultrasound where the uterine enlargement is in excess of a 12-week size [II]. It is important to visualize the ovaries and endometrium and, where possible, to document the size, number and position of individual fibroids as well as the overall uterine dimensions [IV]. Where submucosal fibroids are suspected, hysteroscopy or transvaginal sonohysterography (saline infusion sonography) should be undertaken [Ib],[4] depending on local facilities. Although its greater cost precludes its use as a routine tool, magnetic resonance imaging (MRI) scanning should be used if there is any doubt about the nature of a fibroid mass [II], in particular to distinguish benign fibroids from the rare condition of leiomyosarcoma[4,7] if conservative management is planned.

Endometrial biopsy should be carried out if there is irregular or intermenstrual bleeding or abnormal endometrial thickening on TVS [Ib].

Conservative management

First-line management of menorrhagia in the presence of fibroids should follow the standard protocol for menorrhagia outlined in the RCOG guideline.[5] Anaemia should be treated with oral iron [Ia]. Some women will wish to avoid further treatment, either medical or surgical, and this preference should be respected [IV]. The evidence for the symptomatic medical treatment of menorrhagia is based on trials in women with dysfunctional uterine bleeding, and the evidence supporting their use in women with fibroids is reviewed below.

Non-hormonal therapy

Non-steroidal anti-inflammatory drugs (NSAIDs) are not effective in the reduction of heavy bleeding secondary to the presence of fibroids [Ib].[4] There have been no randomized, controlled trials evaluating antifibrinolytics in the management of fibroid-associated menorrhagia, but in a non-random comparative study[8] there was a highly significant blood loss reduction of around 50 per cent in women with clinically diagnosed fibroids. This was similar to the response in women with normal-sized or slightly enlarged uteri. On the basis of this information, tranexamic acid should be used in preference to NSAIDs in the first-line management of fibroid-associated menorrhagia [II].

Combined oral contraceptives

There is no evidence that the oral contraceptive pill causes enlargement of fibroids; indeed, long-term use may be protective [II].[1] There have been no randomized trials of its use to control bleeding in women with fibroids, but one comparative study demonstrated a significant reduction in measured blood loss (around 50 per cent) with a high-dose combined oral contraceptive pill (COCP) in women with clinically diagnosed fibroids.[8] In women desiring contraception or for whom the use of the COCP is acceptable, this is a reasonable option in fibroid-associated menorrhagia [II].

Progestogens and antiprogesterones

Progestogens, even in high doses, do not shrink fibroids [II];[4] thus their use in fibroid-associated menorrhagia should be purely symptomatic and in a regimen that is effective for menorrhagia, i.e. for 21 days out of 28. The long-term use of depot medroxyprogesterone acetate (MPA) protects against the development of fibroids [II],[9] but its role in the symptomatic management of fibroid-associated menorrhagia is unknown. Similarly, the role of progestogen-releasing intrauterine systems has not been fully evaluated in women with fibroids. Users of the levonorgestrel-releasing intrauterine system (LNG-IUS) for contraception have a lower rate of development of fibroids compared with users of copper-containing devices [II].[4] Preliminary information from case reports and pilot studies of its use in women with symptomatic fibroids has been promising.[4] However, the incidence of spontaneous expulsion is stated to be higher in women with submucosal fibroids, which may limit its therapeutic use. Clearly more information is needed, but the use of the LNG-IUS can be considered in women with fibroid-associated menorrhagia where there is no significant cavity distortion [III].

Both the androgen danazol[4] and the androgenic antiprogesterone gestrinone[10] reduce fibroid size and blood loss during treatment. After cessation of gestrinone, fibroid regrowth is gradual, potentially increasing the usefulness of this therapy. Androgenic side effects are less with gestrinone compared with danazol and thus gestrinone is a potentially useful short-term management option [Ib].

The antiprogesterone mifepristone causes amenorrhoea and significant regression of fibroids[11] without having any detrimental effect on bone density. Currently it is not available for the treatment of fibroids, but antiprogesterones are likely to be an important future option.

GnRH analogues

Treatment with gonadotrophin releasing hormone (GnRH) agonists induces amenorrhoea and shrinkage of fibroids [Ia].[4] However, after cessation, regrowth is rapid. These changes are secondary to temporary ovarian suppression, and long-term treatment with GnRH agonists is contraindicated due to the risk of bone loss. Currently the role of these agents is largely limited to preoperative shrinkage of fibroids, although there is scope for their longer term use with the addition of hormonal add-back.

GnRH AGONISTS PRIOR TO HYSTERECTOMY AND MYOMECTOMY

Shrinkage of fibroids prior to hysteroscopic or conventional surgery has been advocated on the basis of reduced fibroid size and vascularity. Their use prior to hysterectomy or myomectomy has been the subject of a systematic review[12] that was based on 26 randomized, controlled trials. When used together with iron therapy, they are effective in the treatment of preoperative anaemia [Ia]. They significantly reduce intraoperative blood loss, particularly in women with very large uteri. With large uteri, they significantly increase the likelihood of a transverse abdominal incision or a vaginal rather than an abdominal hysterectomy [Ia]. However, their routine use for women who do not fall into these specific categories cannot be justified[4,12] unless particular surgical difficulty is anticipated [IV] and even then their cost-effectiveness has been challenged.[13]

There have been no randomized trials of their use prior to hysteroscopic myomectomy, although they are widely used in this situation. One non-randomized, controlled study[14] reported a significant reduction in operating time, blood loss, volume of distending medium and treatment failure following pre-treatment with a GnRH agonist [II].

GnRH AGONISTS PLUS HORMONAL ADD-BACK FOR LONGER TERM TREATMENT OF FIBROIDS

In women who have contraindications to or decline surgery and in whom other medical measures have failed, long-term relief of menorrhagia may be achieved with GnRH agonists in combination with low-dose hormone replacement therapy (HRT). The GnRH agonist should be administered alone for 3 months to obtain fibroid shrinkage [Ib][4] before addition of the HRT. Low-dose oral oestrogen–progestogen combinations, progestogens alone and tibolone have been tested in randomized, controlled trials.

The oestrogen estropipate 0.75 mg with cyclical norethisterone 0.7 mg was compared with continuous norethisterone

10 mg daily[15] in women treated with leuprolide acetate for a period of 2 years. Both add-back therapies prevented bone loss, but regrowth of the fibroids and a less favourable bleeding pattern occurred with the norethisterone. Continuous combined was compared with cyclical add-back HRT in a non-randomized study using very low-dose conjugated oestrogen 0.3 μg with continuous or cyclical MPA 5 mg.[16] Bone density showed a slight decline in both groups, while uterine shrinkage was maintained. Better control of both vasomotor and menstrual symptoms was achieved with the continuous add-back therapy. In a randomized, double-blind study,[17] tibolone was more effective than placebo in the relief of vasomotor symptoms and equally effective in reducing fibroid size and menstrual symptoms. Bone density was maintained in the group given tibolone, and irregular bleeding was a problem for only a minority of the patients in this group. On the basis of this limited evidence, tibolone is the treatment of choice for add-back therapy with GnRH agonists for the long-term treatment of fibroids [Ib].

HRT in menopausal women with fibroids

Conservative management is often offered to women with symptomatic fibroids who are perimenopausal on the basis that their symptoms will resolve spontaneously when they reach the menopause. It is therefore relevant to consider the effect of HRT on fibroids. Information from randomized trials is based on the use of continuous combined preparations and tibolone[4,18] in women with pre-existing fibroids and an established menopause. Use of transdermal oestradiol (50 μg) in combination with 5 mg MPA resulted in significant uterine enlargement, compared with 0.625 μg conjugated equine oestrogens (CEE) in combination with 2.5 mg MPA. However, symptomatic response and bleeding patterns were no different. The same dose of CEE combined with 5 mg MPA, when compared with tibolone,[18] caused less amenorrhoea and more irregular bleeding, but neither caused uterine enlargement. Information from these studies favours the use of oral HRT rather than the transdermal route and, in keeping with experience with add-back therapy, suggests that tibolone may be the treatment of choice in postmenopausal women with fibroids [Ib].

SURGICAL TREATMENT

Hysteroscopic surgery

Small submucous fibroids can be removed hysteroscopically.[4,6] However, assessment of the effectiveness of hysteroscopic resection has been based on retrospective reports from single centres.[4] The procedure is normally restricted to fibroids that are largely intracavitary and less than 5 cm in diameter, although removal of larger, partly intramural, fibroids has also been described.[4] The complications of hysteroscopic surgery include fluid overload, uterine perforation, haemorrhage and infection. One small study reported a reduction of menstrual blood loss after hysteroscopic resection of small fibroids of more than 70 per cent in all subjects. Life-table analysis of follow-up after hysteroscopic myomectomy[18] showed that the cumulative proportion requiring further surgery was 16 per cent after 9 years. Hysteroscopic myomectomy is thus an effective approach for the removal of small submucous fibroids [II].

Myomectomy

Myomectomy is a well-established alternative to hysterectomy for women wishing to preserve their fertility.[4,19] Improvement of menorrhagia in more than 80 per cent of women has been reported in retrospective case series. Recurrence of fibroids is common, with a 10-year recurrence of 27 per cent in one large follow-up study. Heavy blood loss is a potential problem at myomectomy, and techniques such as the use of occlusive clamps and tourniquets and vasopressin[19] have been described to reduce it, although there is no clear consensus as to which is most effective.[4,19] GnRH agonists can be used for the pretreatment of large uteri. Intramural fibroids smaller than 6 cm diameter may be removed successfully by laparoscopy in specialist centres, but this carries a greater risk of uterine rupture in subsequent pregnancies [III]. Laparotomy is the preferred route for most myomectomies and is associated with low morbidity and a favourable outcome for subsequent pregnancies [III].[4,19]

Hysterectomy

Hysterectomy offers a definitive cure for women with fibroid-associated menorrhagia who have completed childbearing. The abdominal route is most commonly used for large fibroids, although there are reports of use of the vaginal route by experienced operators.[19] The role of the preoperative use of GnRH agonists is discussed above. Hysterectomy is not recommended for the routine management of women with asymptomatic fibroids, even if they are very large [IV].[4]

Uterine artery embolization

This technique was initially performed for the control of postpartum haemorrhage but is now widely used for the treatment of fibroids. It is performed under radiological screening after selective catheterization of the uterine arteries via one or both femoral arteries. Polyvinyl alcohol particles are injected to embolize the uterine vascular bed.[4] It is carried out under local anaesthesia but requires hospitalization for opiate analgesia because of severe post-procedural ischaemic uterine pain. Complications are usually minor and include local haematomas at the puncture sites, urinary

retention, mild febrile reactions and delayed passage of infarcted submucous fibroids.[4,21,22] Severe complications have also been reported including overwhelming sepsis which has proved fatal. A complication-related hysterectomy rate of 1.5 per cent by 3 months after the procedure was reported in a prospective study of 555 women.[23]

Assessment of efficacy has largely been based on case series[4,22,24] although randomized clinical trials are now in progress. Follow-up has been limited in duration but early reports are encouraging with subjective symptomatic improvement in over 80 per cent of women followed up for between 6 months and 2 years. Fibroid shrinkage is gradual, reaching a mean of around 60 per cent at 6 months. There is a concern about future pregnancy outcome although reports to date have been encouraging.[25] The procedure is associated with a small risk of ovarian failure which largely but not exclusively affects women aged 45 years and over.[24,26]

Although early results support the use of uterine artery embolisation for symptomatic fibroids [III] there is a clear need for more information based on long-term outcome and on randomized trials comparing the procedure with hysterectomy and myomectomy.

These recommendations are based on three evidence-based clinical guidelines (only one of which was specific to the management of fibroids) and one systematic review of pre-surgical treatment. Many of the recommendations in these guidelines are based on information from uncontrolled, non-randomized and retrospective studies.

KEY POINTS

- Menorrhagia associated with uterine enlargement to less than 10-week size requires no investigation, except full blood count prior to the initiation of medical therapy [IV].
- Transvaginal ultrasound, combined with abdominal ultrasound for uteri larger than 12-week size, is the primary investigation for suspected fibroids [Ia].
- Both hysteroscopy and transvaginal sonohysterography (saline infusion sonography) are appropriate for the investigation of suspected submucosal fibroids [Ib].
- MRI scanning should be used if there is any doubt about the nature of a uterine mass [II].
- Tranexamic acid should be used in preference to NSAIDs in the first-line management of menorrhagia associated with fibroids [II].
- The COCP is not contraindicated in the presence of fibroids and may relieve menorrhagia [II].

- Progestogens do not shrink fibroids but may relieve menorrhagia at high doses if used continuously or for 21 days out of 28 [III].
- Progestogen-releasing intrauterine devices may be beneficial for menorrhagia associated with fibroids but have not been adequately evaluated [III].
- Gestrinone is a useful drug for the short-term symptomatic management of fibroids [Ib].
- GnRH agonists shrink fibroids and relieve menorrhagia [1a] and current evidence favours the use of tibolone [1b] as add-back therapy for long-term treatment.
- Oral administration of HRT is preferable to the transdermal route for postmenopausal women with fibroids [Ib].
- Small submucous fibroids (4 cm or less) should be removed by hysteroscopic surgery [II].
- Myomectomy is an alternative to hysterectomy for women with menorrhagia associated with fibroids who wish to retain their fertility [III].
- GnRH agonists are useful adjuncts to surgery in cases of anaemia, very large fibroids and where uterine shrinkage may result in a transverse abdominal incision or a vaginal rather than an abdominal hysterectomy [Ia].
- Hysterectomy is not recommended for the routine management of women with asymptomatic fibroids, regardless of their size [IV].
- Uterine artery embolization is a promising alternative to surgery for fibroids [III], but information based on randomized, controlled trials and longer term follow-up is required.

KEY REFERENCES

1. Vollenhoven B. The epidemiology of uterine leiomyomas. *Baillière's Clin Obstet Gynaecol* 1998; 12(2):169–76.
2. Rybo G, Leman J, Tibbin R. Epidemiology of menstrual blood loss. In: Baird DT, Michie EA (eds). *Mechanisms of Menstrual Bleeding*. New York: Raven Press, 1985, 181–93.
3. Nowak RA. Fibroids: pathophysiology and current medical treatment. *Baillière's Clin Obstet Gynaecol* 1999; 13(2):223–8.
4. Farquhar C, Arroll B, Ekeroma A et al. An evidence-based guideline for the management of uterine fibroids. *Aust N Z J Obstet Gynaecol* 2001; 41:125–40.
5. Royal College of Obstetricians and Gynaecologists. *The Initial Management of Menorrhagia*. Evidence-Based Clinical Guidelines No. 1. London: RCOG, October 1998.
6. Royal College of Obstetricians and Gynaecologists. *The Management of Menorrhagia in Secondary Care*. Evidence-Based Clinical Guidelines No. 5. London: RCOG, July 1999.
7. Schwartz LB, Zawin M, Carcangiu ML, Lange R, McCarthy S. Does pelvic magnetic resonance imaging differentiate among the histologic subtypes of uterine myomata? *Fertil Steril* 1998; 70:580–7.
8. Nilsson L, Rybo G. Treatment of menorrhagia. *Am J Obstet Gynecol* 1971; 10:713–20.
9. Lumbiganon P, Rugpao S, Phandhu-fung S, Laopaiboon M, Vudhikamraksa N, Werawatakul Y. Protective effect of depot-medroxyprogesterone acetate on surgically treated uterine leiomyomas: a multi-centre case-control study. *Br J Obstet Gynaecol* 1995; 103:909–14.
10. Coutinho EM, Goncalves MT. Long term treatment of leiomyomas with gestrinone. *Fertil Steril* 1989; 51:939–46.
11. Murphy AA, Morales AJ, Kettel LM, Yen SSC. Regression of uterine leiomyomata to the antiprog-esterone RU486: dose–response effect. *Fertil Steril* 1995; 64:187–90.
12. Lethaby A, Vollenhoven B, Sowter M. Pre-operative GnRH analogue therapy before hysterectomy or myomectomy for uterine fibroids (Cochrane Review). In: *The Cochrane Library*, Issue 4. Oxford: Update Software, 2001.
13. Farquhar C, Brown PM, Furness S. Cost effectiveness of pre-operative gonadotrophin releasing analogues for women with uterine fibroids undergoing hysterectomy or myomectomy. *Br J Obstet Gynaecol* 2002;109:1273–80.
14. Perino A, Chianchino N, Petronio M, Ciltadini E. The role of leuprolide acetate depot in hysteroscopic surgery: a controlled study. *Fertil Steril* 1993; 59:507–10.
15. Friedman AJ, Daly, M, Juneau-Norcross M, Gleason R, Rein MS, LeBoff M. Long-term medical therapy for leiomyomata uteri: a prospective randomized study of leuprolide acetate depot plus either oestrogen–progestin or progestin 'add-back' for 2 years. *Hum Reprod* 1994; 9:1618–25.
16. Maheux R, Lemay A. Treatment of perimenopausal women: potential long-term therapy with a depot GnRH agonist combined with hormone replacement therapy. *Br J Obstet Gynaecol* 1992; 99(Suppl. 7): 13–17.
17. Palomba S, Affinito P, Tommaselli GA, Nappi C. A clinical trial of the effects of tibolone administered with gonadotropin-releasing hormone analogues for the treatment of uterine leiomyomata. *Fertil Steril* 1998; 70:111–18.
18. de Aloysio D, Altieri P, Penacchioni P, Salgarello M, Ventura V. Bleeding patterns in recent postmenopausal outpatients with uterine myomas: comparison between two regimens of HRT. *Maturitas* 1998; 29:261–4.

19. Derman SG, Rehnstrom J, Neuwirth RS. The long-term effectiveness of hysteroscopic treatment of menorrhagia and leiomyomas. *Obstet Gynecol* 1991; **77**:591–4.

20. West CP. Hysterectomy and myomectomy by laparotomy. *Baillière's Clin Obstet Gynaecol* 1998; 12(2):317–35.

21. Spies JB, Ascher SA, Roth AR, Kim J, Levy EB, Gomez-Jorge J. Uterine artery embolization for leiomyomata. *Obstet Gynecol* 2001; **98**:29–34.

22. McLucas B, Adler L, Perrella R. Uterine fibroid embolization: non-surgical treatment for symptomatic fibroids. *J Am Coll Surg* 2001; **192**:95–105.

23. Pron G, Mocarski E, Cohen M, Colgan T, Bennett J, Common A, Vilos G, Kung R. Hysterectomy for complications after uterine artery embolization for leiomyoma: results of a Canadian multicenter clinical trial. *J Am Assoc Gynecol Laparosc* 2003;**10**:99–106.

24. Walker WJ, Pelage JP. Uterine artery embolisation for symptomatic fibroids: clinical results in 400 women with imaging follow up. *Br J Obstet Gynaecol* 2002;**109**:1262–72.

25. Ravina JH, Vigeron NC, Aymard A, Le Dref O, Merland JJ. Pregnancy after embolization of uterine myoma: report of 12 cases. *Fertil Steril* 2000;**73**:1241–3.

26. Spies JB, Roth AR, Gonsalves SM, Murphy-Skrzyniarz KM. Ovarian function after uterine artery embolization for leiomyomata: assessment with use of serum follicle stimulating hormone assay. *J Vasc Interv Radiol* 2001; **12**:437–42.

Heavy and Irregular Menstruation

Christine P. West

MRCOG standards

Theoretical skills
- Understand the causes of abnormal uterine bleeding.
- Know the principles of investigation and treatment of heavy periods.

Practical skills
- Be familiar with the practical skills of endometrial sampling, hysteroscopy, transvaginal ultrasound.
- Be familiar with the insertion of the levonorgestriel intrauterine system.
- Be familiar with techniques of endometrial ablation.
- Be familiar with surgical techniques of abdominal and vaginal hysterectomy.

INTRODUCTION

Regular menstruation is a feature of contemporary society. In the past, large family size, prolonged breastfeeding and reduced life expectancy limited the number of menstrual cycles experienced by women. Currently, women may experience more than 400 menstrual periods during reproductive life, and problems related to menstruation are a common cause of referral, both to general practitioners and to gynaecologists. Abnormal bleeding can be a consequence of pelvic pathology, including malignant disease, but the majority of women who present with bleeding problems have no underlying abnormality. Indeed, a significant proportion of women who complain of heavy bleeding are found to have normal menstrual loss if this is measured objectively. Concerns about the widespread use of hysterectomy in this situation have led to a well-developed evidence base for medical management. This, together with less invasive surgical methods, has increased the range of options available for the relief of menstrual bleeding problems.

DEFINITIONS

In their evidence-based guideline,[1] the Royal College of Obstetricians and Gynaecologists (RCOG) defined menorrhagia as heavy, regular blood loss occurring over several consecutive cycles. The accepted definition of heavy blood loss based on objective measurement is more than 80 mL per period, although a loss of 60 mL or more is associated with the development of anaemia.[2] Because of the practical difficulties of measuring menstrual blood loss, this is used only as a research tool, and a subjective diagnosis based on the history with or without pictorial charts is generally accepted as the basis for management. The term menorrhagia excludes intermenstrual or postcoital bleeding and should be distinguished from irregular bleeding or sudden changes in blood loss, all of which may be associated with underlying pathology. Regular heavy bleeding without an identified local cause is also known as dysfunctional uterine bleeding (DUB). It is useful to distinguish between ovulatory dysfunctional bleeding (regular cyclicity) and anovulatory dysfunctional bleeding. The latter usually occurs at the extremes of reproductive life and results in prolonged, irregular, sometimes heavy bleeding for which different management strategies are appropriate.

INCIDENCE

It has been estimated[3] that 5 per cent of women aged between 30 and 49 consult their general practitioner for excessive menstrual bleeding in a year. Excessive menstrual bleeding accounts for 12 per cent of gynaecology referrals and results in more than 80 000 surgical procedures (hysterectomy or endometrial resection) per annum in England and Wales. It was estimated in one study[4] that 1 in 5 women in the UK had undergone hysterectomy by the age of 55. Several studies have shown that rates of hysterectomy are inversely related to socio-economic class and educational achievement.[3] The reasons for this are not clear, but this is not a finding that can be justifiable on medical grounds.

AETIOLOGY

The aetiology depends on the pattern of abnormal bleeding and is also influenced by the age of the patient and other factors. Postmenopausal bleeding and abnormal bleeding secondary to contraceptives, hormone replacement therapy (HRT) or tamoxifen are not considered here.

Menorrhagia

Fibroids are the commonest structural cause of menorrhagia (see Chapter 51.2). Heavy bleeding associated with fibroids is often painless; painful heavy periods may be secondary to adenomyosis (see Chapter 51.6). Coagulation disorders are a rare cause of menorrhagia and usually present in young women in whom there is likely to be a history of other bleeding problems.

Ovulatory DUB is the commonest cause of subjectively reported menorrhagia. Studies involving objective measurement of blood loss have shown that in a high proportion of women reporting menorrhagia, blood loss is not abnormal.[2] However, a recent study of women referred to gynaecological clinics because of excessive menstrual loss showed that more than half did not perceive this as severe or as their main problem.[5] There was considerable overlap between problems related to bleeding and other menstrual problems such as pain and cyclical symptoms.

In cases of objectively confirmed menorrhagia (>60 mL blood loss per period), abnormalities in the local control of menstruation have been described.[6] These include abnormal levels of the vasoactive endometrial prostaglandins PGE2 and PGF2a and reduced activity of endothelins, which are potent vasoconstrictors. Abnormalities of the local coagulation mechanisms have also been described, including excess fibrinolytic activity and increased levels of endometrial plasminogen activator.

Heavy irregular bleeding

Anovulatory menstrual cycles are common following the menarche and in the lead up to the menopause, and abnormal bleeding is a consequence of prolonged stimulation of the endometrium by oestrogen, unopposed by progesterone. Bleeding is painless and in teenagers is usually limited to a few cycles. In the perimenopause, various histological abnormalities may occur, ranging from simple hyperplasia that is reversible by progestogens to severe atypia and malignancy. Anovulatory dysfunctional bleeding is also a well-recognized consequence of polycystic ovary syndrome. Irregular bleeding may be associated with other endocrine disorders, particularly thyroid disease, although the underlying mechanism is unclear.

Intermenstrual and postcoital bleeding

These two problems frequently co-exist and may have a common aetiology. While serious pathology, in particular cervical carcinoma, may be present, most cases are due to benign causes and often no cause can be found. Bleeding at mid-cycle is secondary to the mid-cycle oestradiol surge and is regarded as physiological. In young women, chlamydial infection[7] may present with intermenstrual or postcoital bleeding. On visualization of the cervix, benign cervical conditions such as polyps or ectopy may be present, but are more likely to be asymptomatic incidental findings. Similarly, the significance of abnormalities of the uterine cavity is uncertain. In a large retrospective review of outpatient hysteroscopies,[8] the incidence of endometrial polyps was increased in women presenting with intermenstrual bleeding or postcoital bleeding (16.8 per cent compared with the overall incidence of 11.3 per cent). The incidence of submucous fibroids was no higher in this group (20.4 per cent compared with a total incidence of 24.3 per cent). Although the incidence of both lesions rose with increasing age, they were present in all age groups.

MANAGEMENT

Decisions regarding both investigation and treatment are influenced by a number of factors, which include the age and reproductive status of the individual woman, the pattern and severity of her symptoms and the degree of disruption that she experiences. Many women may simply seek reassurance. A detailed and accurate history is essential in eliciting any relevant medical problems and in assessing the impact of the problem for each individual woman. As the assessment of the extent of the bleeding is subjective, this may be assisted by the use of calendars or pictorial charts [II].[9]

Investigation

Menorrhagia

Menorrhagia is covered in an RGOG evidence-based guideline[1] and falls within the scope of primary care. Abdominal and bimanual pelvic examinations should be performed, together with a cervical smear if due and a full blood count. If examination is normal, no additional investigations are required prior to the initiation of therapy [IV]. If the uterus is felt to be enlarged (>10–12-week size), an ultrasound scan will be helpful in delineating fibroids or excluding other causes of a pelvic mass [II]. If coagulation disorders are suspected, particularly in young women, a clotting screen should be carried out [II].[10] Where medical treatment has failed, or where there are specific risk factors for endometrial cancer (obesity, tamoxifen therapy, polycystic ovary syndrome),[1] more detailed evaluation of the endometrial cavity should be carried out[10] as described below.

Prolonged or irregular bleeding

Most cases will be associated with the perimenopause. Endocrine investigation is unnecessary unless there is clinical suspicion of thyroid disease or premature ovarian failure [II]. Endometrial assessment should be clinic based and includes endometrial sampling in combination with either transvaginal ultrasound (TVS) or outpatient hysteroscopy [Ia].[11,12] Biopsy alone will miss polyps or submucosal fibroids,[11] while TVS may not distinguish between the two [Ib].[11,12] Hysteroscopy is regarded as a gold standard for endometrial evaluation when used in combination with biopsy. However, it is costly and invasive and current guidelines[10,13] recommend that TVS should be used for the initial investigation of abnormal bleeding, with hysteroscopy as a back-up [Ib]. In centres where provision for outpatient hysteroscopy is limited, the ultrasound-based technique of saline infusion sonography (transvaginal sonohysterography)[13] is useful in delineating the uterine cavity [Ib]. Dilatation and curettage has no advantage over the clinic-based techniques described above for routine investigation [Ib].[10,11]

Intermenstrual and postcoital bleeding

Careful examination of the cervix is essential, and any suspicious findings are an indication for colposcopy. In young women, chlamydial infection should be excluded [II].[7] Where the bleeding is confined to mid-cycle, further investigation is not required. In many centres, intermenstrual or postcoital bleeding is an indication for outpatient hysteroscopy, but, as discussed above, TVS is a simpler and less invasive primary investigation in the detection of endometrial polyps or submusosal fibroids [Ib]. Although the incidence of polyps and endometrial abnormalities rises with increasing age,[8,12] submucosal fibroids are more common in younger women.[12] Thus such investigations should not be targeted to women in particular age groups [III].

MEDICAL MANAGEMENT

Non-hormonal therapy

For women with menorrhagia requiring non-hormonal treatment, antifibrinolytics (e.g. tranexamic acid)[14] or nonsteroidal anti-inflammatory drugs (NSAIDs; e.g. mefenamic acid)[15] are first-line drugs [Ia]. Both are used only during menstruation and are generally well tolerated. Reduction of blood loss is greater with the antifibrinolytic [Ia],[14] but associated menstrual pain is more effectively treated with NSAIDs (see Chapter 51.4). There is no evidence that the long-term use of antifibrinolytics increases the incidence of thrombosis.[14] As antifibrinolytics and NSAIDs have different mechanisms of action in menorrhagia, they may be effective when used in combination [IV], but there are no published data to support this. Ethamsylate (a drug that reduces capillary fragility) was used in the past for menorrhagia, but recent evidence[7] does not confirm its efficacy [Ib].

Combined oral contraceptive pill

For women requiring contraception or for whom hormonal agents are acceptable, combined oral contraceptive pill (COCP) preparations are effective in reducing menstrual bleeding, controlling cycle irregularities and relieving menstrual pain,[6] although reports of efficacy have largely been based on indirect evidence from contraceptive studies and one small randomized, controlled trial.[16] A 53 per cent reduction of menstrual blood loss was reported in one nonrandomized study.[6] There is some reluctance on the part of both professionals and consumers to use the COCP for the management of menorrhagia in older women. For nonsmokers who have no risk factors for vascular disease, there is no upper age limit for the use of the COCP, and current guidelines recommend its use as a first-line therapy for menorrhagia [Ib].[1]

Progestogens

Cyclical progestogens were commonly used in the past, but current evidence does not support their use for menorrhagia when given only during the luteal phase of the cycle [Ib].[17] They are effective when given at high doses between days 5 and 26 of the cycle (e.g. norethisterone 5 mg tid for 21 days out of 28) [Ib].[6] Long-acting high-dose progestogens (e.g. Depo-Provera) may be used to induce amenorrhoea [II].[1] However, the usefulness of these high-dose preparations may be limited by side effects.

Cyclical progestogens are traditionally the drug of first choice for the control of anovulatory dysfunctional bleeding.[18] They have been evaluated in two comparative studies.[18] In one small study, norethisterone 5 mg tid and medroxyprogesterone acetate 10 mg tid were both effective in reducing blood loss. In a larger study, cyclical norethisterone 5 mg tid and oral micronized progesterone 100 mg tid both induced regression of cystic hyperplasia and other histolo-gical abnormalities in the majority of subjects. This evidence, albeit limited, supports the use of cyclical progestogens for the control of anovulatory dysfunctional bleeding [Ib].

Progestogen-releasing intrauterine system

The levonorgestrel-releasing intrauterine system (LNG-IUS) is licensed in many countries for the relief of menorrhagia. The continuous exposure of the endometrium to progestogen induces progressive atrophy, with reduction of menstrual bleeding by more than 80 per cent after 3–6 months and more than 90 per cent at 12 months.[6,19,20] Spontaneous expulsion occurs in 3–6 per cent of women and there is an initial incidence of breakthrough bleeding as high as 25–55 per cent in the early months. Progestogenic side effects of bloating, breast tenderness, mood swings and acne may occur, and careful counselling is essential prior to insertion [IV].

The LNG-IUS has been compared in randomized trials and two systematic reviews[19,20] with other medical therapies, with endometrial resection and with hysterectomy. Reduction of menstrual blood loss was significantly greater than with tranexamic acid or an NSAID.[6] The side effects of breakthrough bleeding and breast tenderness were more common in women with the LNG-IUS compared with high-dose cyclical norethisterone,[6] but overall satisfaction was greater with the LNG-IUS.

In a study of women awaiting hysterectomy,[19] 64.3 per cent of those randomized to insertion of LNG-IUS cancelled their operation after 6 months, compared with 14.3 per cent in the control group. In a direct comparison with hysterectomy,[21] 20 per cent of the group assigned to the LNG-IUS opted for hysterectomy in the first year. However, quality of life assessment at 12 months was not significantly different in the two groups, with the exception of lower pain scores after hysterectomy. Costs were three times higher in the hysterectomy group. The LNG-IUS has also been compared with endometrial resection in three randomized trials[19,20,22] and with thermal balloon ablation.[23] Although reduction of blood loss was greater following resection and side effects were commoner with the LNG-IUS, overall satisfaction rates were similar.

These results indicate that the LNG-IUS is a highly effective treatment for menorrhagia [Ia] that has advantages over existing medical treatments and is a potential alternative to surgery.

Other medical therapies

Second-line drugs are available for the control of severe bleeding when simpler measures have failed and, as they reliably induce amenorrhoea, are useful in the management of severe anaemia or in the presence of medical disorders when surgery may be contraindicated. Androgens such as danazol and gestrinone induce amenorrhoea by a combination of negative feedback and direct effects on the endometrium, (see Chapter 51.5) while gonadotrophin releasing hormone (GnRH) agonists induce a hypogonadal state via their central action. While effective, these approaches are usually limited to short-term use because of their side effects [Ia]. They are also of value as endometrial-thinning agents prior to hysteroscopic surgery [Ia].[24] In cases of severe menorrhagia in which simple measures have failed, long-term therapy with a GnRH agonist plus hormonal add-back (see Chapter 51.5) can be considered if there are contraindications to surgery.

SURGICAL MANAGEMENT

While medical treatment should always be used as first-line therapy for menorrhagia [IV], limitations in efficacy and side effects will result in many women seeking a surgical solution for their problem. Traditionally, hysterectomy has been the principal surgical management for menstrual disorders. As the majority of hysterectomies are carried out for benign conditions or, in the case of dysfunctional bleeding, where no pathology is demonstrable, this policy has been called into question.[3] The use of the diagnostic techniques described above identifies some women with benign lesions (small submucosal fibroids or endometrial polyps) that are suitable for removal by hysteroscopic surgery [II].[10,13] Hysteroscopic methods of endometrial ablation are now well established as day case or outpatient procedures, and recent developments include 'second-generation' techniques that are simpler and safer than conventional methods. In common with all surgical procedures, adequate information and counselling are essential in the decision-making process [IV].[10]

Endometrial ablation

The object of endometrial ablation is the complete destruction of the endometrium down to the basal layer, resulting in fibrosis of the uterine cavity and amenorrhoea. In practice it is very difficult to achieve complete destruction, and rates of amenorrhoea are rarely in excess of 20–30 per cent.[25] However, patient satisfaction rates are over 70 per cent in the short term [Ia].[25] Life-table analysis of follow-up after endometrial resection[26] reported a cumulative hysterectomy rate of 27.4 per cent after 4 years. Favourable factors for the avoidance of hysterectomy included a more experienced surgeon and patient age over 45 years. There is some evidence that the presence of adenomyosis may be an unfavourable prognostic factor.

Established techniques carried out under direct hysteroscopic vision involve the use of fluid for distension and irrigation. These comprise:

- laser ablation,
- endometrial loop resection using electrodiathermy,
- rollerball electrodiathermy ablation.

Of these, laser ablation is limited by its costs to a very few centres. All three are operator dependent, time consuming and carry risks of systemic fluid absorption, haemorrhage and uterine perforation with heat damage to adjacent structures. The MISTLETOE Study,[27] a prospective national survey of more than 10 000 procedures in the UK, reported an overall immediate complication rate of 4.4 per cent. Complications were lower with laser and rollerball techniques, and highest with loop resection [II]. Complications were also related to the experience of the operator.

Newer techniques have been developed with the object of reducing operator dependency and minimizing risk. Of these, the best evaluated to date are microwave and thermal balloon ablation, both of which have been compared with conventional methods in randomized trials.[28] To date, they appear to have equivalent short-term efficacy with the advantage of shorter operating times and fewer complications [Ib]. Endometrial ablation should be offered as a treatment option to women with a history of failed medical treatment for menorrhagia [Ia], but until there is clear evidence favouring one method above others, the choice will depend on local factors such as the availability of equipment and individual experience.

Hysterectomy

Recent randomized trials comparing hysterectomy with endometrial ablation have highlighted the greater costs and morbidity of hysterectomy, together with its longer recovery time.[24] Satisfaction with the two methods appears to be similar in the short term. However, longer term follow-up shows satisfaction rates to be significantly greater following hysterectomy, with a gradual merging of the cost differential [Ia]. Satisfaction after hysterectomy is not universal; there may be long-term implications for bladder function, a recent systematic review[29] estimating a 60 per cent increase in the odds of developing urinary incontinence following hysterectomy.

Currently, there is interest in the optimal method of carrying out hysterectomy. This is partly motivated by short-term issues of hospital stay and recovery time, based on economic factors. This has accompanied the development of techniques such as laparoscopically assisted vaginal hysterectomy (LAVH) and an increased use of the vaginal route. However, while LAVH is associated with a shorter hospital stay, it is more expensive, takes longer than abdominal or vaginal hysterectomy and is associated with more complications, particularly bladder and ureteric injuries [Ib].[30–32] Despite great enthusiasm for LAVH, two recent randomized trials[31,32] have shown little difference in recovery time or patient satisfaction between the different techniques [Ib]. Vaginal hysterectomy has advantages in terms of cost and speed of recovery but, in common with LAVH, is dependent on the skill of the operator [II].[33] The role of subtotal hysterectomy has yet to be fully evaluated. Patient safety is the prime consideration, and the skill and experience of the individual surgeon should determine the method of hysterectomy in each individual case.

> These recommendations for the management of heavy and irregular menstruation are based on an Effective Health Care review, two evidence-based clinical guidelines, six systematic reviews of medical therapies and five systematic reviews relating to surgical management.

KEY POINTS

- The initial management of menorrhagia should take place within a primary care setting following pelvic examination and measurement of full blood count [IV].
- There is a poor correlation between subjective and measured blood loss. The use of pictorial charts may help to clarify the history [II].
- Clinical presentation with heavy menstrual bleeding may be influenced by the presence of other menstrual complaints [II].
- Young women presenting with intermenstrual or postcoital bleeding should be tested for chlamydia [II].
- Primary investigation of abnormal bleeding should be by TVS and endometrial biopsy followed by hysteroscopy if findings are abnormal or equivocal [Ib].
- NSAIDs and antifibrinolytics are effective in the management of menorrhagia [Ia], but ethamsylate is ineffective [Ib].
- The COCP is effective for menorrhagia provided there are no contraindications [Ib].
- Cyclical progestogens are effective for menorrhagia when given for 21 days out of 28 and for control of anovulatory dysfunctional bleeding [Ib].
- Continuous high-dose progestogens (e.g. depot preparations) may be useful if they induce amenorrhoea [II].
- The LNG-IUS device is highly effective in relieving menorrhagia, but adequate counselling is needed prior to insertion [Ia].
- Drugs that induce amenorrhoea are useful for the short-term management of severe menorrhagia or for endometrial thinning prior to endometrial ablation [Ia].
- Endometrial polyps and small submucous fibroids should be removed by hysteroscopic surgery [II].
- Endometrial ablation is cheap, safe and effective for the relief of menorrhagia in the short term [Ia] and outcome is best if it is carried out in women over the age of 45 [II].
- Newer techniques of ablation are as effective as older techniques and are simpler to perform [Ib].
- Long-term satisfaction is high with hysterectomy but it is associated with significant morbidity and mortality [Ia] and should be offered only if simpler alternatives have failed [IV].
- Laparoscopially assisted hysterectomy is more expensive than abdominal hysterectomy and carries a greater risk of serious complications, particularly in inexperienced hands [Ib].

- Vaginal hysterectomy may be more cost effective than the abdominal route but outcome is more dependent on the skill of the operator [II].
- The role of subtotal hysterectomy is unclear.
- The route selected for hysterectomy should be determined by the skill and experience of the individual surgeon [IV].

KEY REFERENCES

1. Royal College of Obstetricians and Gynaecologists. *The Initial Management of Menorrhagia*. Evidence-Based Clinical Guidelines No. 1. London: RCOG, October 1998.
2. Hallberg L, Hogdahl AM, Nilsson L, Rybo G. Menstrual blood loss – a population study. Variation at different ages and attempts to define normality. *Acta Obstet Gynaecol Scand* 1966; **45**:320–51.
3. *Effective Health Care. The Management of Menorrhagia*. NIH, University of Leeds & NHS Centre for Research & Dissemination, University of York Research Unit, Royal College of Physicians, 1995.
4. Vessey M, Villard-MacKintosh L, McPherson K, Coulter A, Yeates D. The epidemiology of hysterectomy: findings of a large cohort study. *Br J Obstet Gynaecol* 1992; **99**:402–7.
5. Warner P, Critchley HOD, Lumsden MA, Campbell-Brown M, Douglas A, Murray G. Referral for menstrual problems: cross sectional survey of symptoms, reasons for referral, and management. *BMJ* 2001; **323**:24–8.
6. Irvine GA, Cameron IT. Medical management of dysfunctional uterine bleeding. *Baillière's Clin Obstet Gynaecol* 1999; **13**(2):189–202.
7. Scottish Intercollegiate Guidelines Network. *Management of Genital Chlamydia trachomatis Infection. A National Clinical Guideline*. Edinburgh: SIGN Secretariat, Royal College of Physicians, 2000.
8. Nagele F, O'Connor H, Davies A, Badawy A, Mohamed H, Magos A. 2500 outpatient diagnostic hysteroscopies. *Obstet Gynecol* 1996; **88**:87–92.
9. Higham JM, O'Brien PM, Shaw RW. Assessment of menstrual blood loss using a pictorial chart. *Br J Obstet Gynaecol* 1990; **97**:734–9.
10. Royal College of Obstetricians and Gynaecologists. *The Management of Menorrhagia in Secondary Care*. Evidence-Based Clinical Guidelines No. 5. London: RCOG, July 1999.
11. Tahir MM, Bigrigg MA, Browning JJ, Brookes ST, Smith PA. A randomised controlled trial comparing transvaginal ultrasound, outpatient hysteroscopy and endometrial biopsy with inpatient hysteroscopy and curettage. *Br J Obstet Gynaecol* 1999; **106**:1259–64.
12. Farquhar C, Ekeroma A, Furness S, Arroll B. A systematic review of transvaginal ultrasonography, sonohysterography and hysteroscopy for the investigation of abnormal uterine bleeding in premenopausal women. *Acta Obstet Gynecol Scand* 2003; **82**:493–504.
13. Farquhar C, Arroll B, Ekeroma A et al. An evidence-based guideline for the management of uterine fibroids. *Aust N Z J Obstet Gynaecol* 2001; **41**:125–40.
14. Lethaby A, Farquhar C, Cooke I. Antifibrinolytics for heavy menstrual bleeding (Cochrane Review). In: *The Cochrane Library*, Issue 4. Oxford: Update Software, 2001.
15. Lethaby A, Augood C, Duckitt K. Nonsteroidal anti-inflammatory drugs for heavy menstrual bleeding (Cochrane Review). In: *The Cochrane Library*, Issue 4. Oxford: Update Software, 2001.
16. Ivor V, Farquhar C, Jepson R. Oral contraceptive pills for heavy menstrual bleeding (Cochrane Review). In: *The Cochrane Library*, Issue 4. Oxford: Update Software, 2001.
17. Lethaby A, Irvine G, Cameron I. Cyclical progestogens for heavy menstrual bleeding (Cochrane Review). In: *The Cochrane Library*, Issue 4. Oxford: Update Software, 2001.
18. Hickey M, Higham J, Fraser IS. Progestogens versus oestrogens and progestogens for irregular uterine bleeding associated with anovulation (Cochrane Review). In: *The Cochrane Library*, Issue 4. Oxford: Update Software, 2001.
19. Lethaby AE, Cooke I, Rees M. Progesterone/progestogen releasing intrauterine systems versus either placebo or any other medication for heavy menstrual bleeding (Cochrane Review). In: *The Cochrane Library*, Issue 4. Oxford: Update Software, 2001.
20. Stewart A, Cummins C, Gold L, Jordan R, Phillips W. The effectiveness of the levonorgestrel-releasing intrauterine system in menorrhagia: a systematic review. *Br J Obstet Gynaecol* 2001; **108**:74–86.
21. Hurskainen R, Teperi J, Rissanen P et al. Quality of life and cost effectiveness of levonorgestrel-releasing intrauterine system versus hysterectomy for treatment of menorrhagia: a randomised trial. *Lancet* 2001; **357**:273–7.
22. Istre O, Trolle B. Treatment of menorrhagia with the levonorgestrel intrauterine system versus endometrial resection. *Fertil Steril* 2001; **76**:304–9.
23. Barrington JW, Arunkalaivanan AS, Abdel Fattach M. Comparison between the levonorgestrel intrauterine system (LNG–IUS) and thermal balloon ablation in the treatment of menorrhagia. *Eur J Obstet Gynecol Reprod Biol* 2003; **108**:72–4.

Reproductive medicine

24. Sowter MC, Singka AA, Lethaby A. Pre-operative endometrial thinning agents before hysteroscopic surgery for heavy menstrual bleeding (Cochrane Review). In: *The Cochrane Library*, Issue 4. Oxford: Update Software, 2001.

25. Lethaby A, Shepperd S, Cooke I, Farquhar C. Endometrial resection and ablation versus hysterectomy for heavy menstrual bleeding (Cochrane Review). In: *The Cochrane Library*, Issue 4. Oxford: Update Software, 2001.

26. Pooley AS, Ewen P, Sutton CJ. Does transcervical resection of the endometrium for menorrhagia really avoid hysterectomy? Life table analysis of a large series. *J Am Assoc Gynecol Laparosc* 1998; **5**:229–35.

27. Overton C, Hargreaves J, Maresh M. A national survey of the complications of endometrial destruction for menstrual disorders: the MISTLETOE study. *Br J Obstet Gynaecol* 1997; **104**:1351–9.

28. Lethaby A, Hickey M. Endometrial destruction techniques for heavy menstrual bleeding: a Cochrane review. *Hum Reprod* 2002; **17**:2795–806.

29. Brown JS, Sawaya G, Thom DH, Grady D. Hysterectomy and urinary incontinence: a systematic review. *Lancet* 2000; **356**:535–9.

30. Meikle SF, Weston Nugent E, Orleans M. Complications and recovery from laparoscopy-assisted vaginal hysterectomy compared with abdominal and vaginal hysterectomy. *Obstet Gynecol* 1997; **89**:304–11.

31. Lumsden MA, Twaddle S, Hawthorn R et al. A randomised comparison and economic evaluation of laparoscopic-assisted hysterectomy and abdominal hysterectomy. *Br J Obstet Gynaecol* 2000; **107**:1389–91.

32. Ottosen C, Lingman G, Ottosen L. Three methods for hysterectomy: a randomised, prospective study of short term outcome. *Br J Obstet Gynaecol* 2000; **107**:1380–5.

33. Makinen J, Johansson J, Tomas E et al. Morbidity of 10 110 hysterectomies by type of approach. *Hum Reprod* 2001; **16**:1473–8.

Dysmenorrhoea

Christine P. West

INTRODUCTION

Pain during menstruation is an almost universal experience among women and, when severe, it has a significant economic impact through loss of time from work or education. Recognition of the consequences of this problem has led to several large-scale reviews of treatments for dysmenorrhoea, including alternative therapies. There is thus a well-founded evidence base for its management. Pain related to or exacerbated during menstruation or sexual intercourse may be a consequence of underlying pelvic pathology, although not all women with pelvic pain have a gynaecological disorder. This chapter is mainly concerned with gynaecological causes of cyclical pelvic pain but some reference is made to the multifactorial nature of the problem.

DEFINITIONS

Dysmenorrhoea is pain that occurs during menstruation. Primary dysmenorrhoea is also known as primary spasmodic dysmenorrhoea. This is a useful descriptive term for a condition of cramping lower pain that may radiate to the lower back and thighs, often associated with gastrointestinal and neurological symptoms. It typically lasts for between 8 and 72 hours, although young women almost universally experience milder manifestations.

Secondary dysmenorrhoea is menstrually related pain, which is secondary to identifiable pelvic pathology. It is characteristically associated with deep dyspareunia and the pain may precede the onset of menstrual bleeding. It is regarded as distinct from the condition of chronic pelvic pain in which pain of at least 6 months' duration is present continuously or intermittently, not associated exclusively with menstruation or sexual intercourse.[1] However, there is considerable overlap between the two conditions, and many women who present with chronic pain describe dyspareunia and/or premenstrual exacerbation.

INCIDENCE

In a large random sample of 19-year-old Swedish women[2] dysmenorrhoea was experienced by 72 per cent of the women. Fifteen percent reported limitation of daily activity and lack of relief from analgesics and 7.9 per cent reported repeated absence from work or school. Follow-up of the same cohort 5 years later[3] found that the prevalence and severity were reduced only in those who had completed a pregnancy or were pill users. It was unchanged in those who remained nulliparous or who had a history of early pregnancy loss or abortion. A systematic review[4] of published papers on pelvic pain in women in the UK estimated a prevalence rate of between 45 and 95 per cent for dysmenorrhoea. The studies did not distinguish between primary and secondary dysmenorrhoea, but 48 per cent of middle-aged women experienced pain during at least half their menses. The prevalence of chronic pelvic pain among women aged 18–50 years in a large community-based US study was 15 per cent.[5]

AETIOLOGY

Uterine myometrial hyperactivity has been demonstrated in women with primary dysmenorrhoea. This is likely to be secondary to increased uterine production of prostaglandins.[6] Other local mediators may also be involved, and increased circulating levels of vasopressin have been reported. These responses represent the extremes of the normal physiological response of the uterus to progesterone withdrawal, as primary dysmenorrhoea is not regarded as a pathological condition.

Severe dysmenorrhoea in young women is rarely due to any underlying abnormality. One exception is pain secondary to congenital abnormalities that are associated with obstruction to menstrual flow, for example cryptomenorrhoea in an accessory uterine horn.

Many of the conditions that cause secondary dysmenorrhoea may also present with chronic pelvic pain, in particular endometriosis, which occurs in around one-third of laparoscopies carried out for pelvic pain (Table 51.4.1). Adenomyosis is a cause of secondary dysmenorrhoea in older multiparous women. Uterine fibroids do not characteristically cause pain unless there is an acute complication such as torsion or expulsion. Chronic pelvic inflammatory disease and other causes of pelvic pain that are non-cyclical, such as adhesions or ovarian cysts, are not considered in this chapter.

Around one-third of laparoscopies carried out for the investigation of pelvic pain or secondary dysmenorrhoea are negative (see Table 51.4.1). This must not be interpreted as implying that the pain is psychogenic. Non-gynaecological conditions can be exacerbated or enhanced during menstruation. In particular, irritable bowel syndrome is commonly diagnosed following negative investigations for pelvic pain.[1] Pelvic pain may be musculoskeletal or nerve-related. Psychosocial factors are also important.[1] Factors such as personality traits, coping strategies, health beliefs and influences of family members may predispose an individual to the development of chronic pain. There is also a high prevalence in women with a history of physical or sexual abuse.[1]

Pelvic venous congestion is a condition described in multiparous women of reproductive age.[8] Chronic dull, aching pain is characteristically exacerbated perimenstrually, by activity and by sexual intercourse, and relieved by lying down. It is attributed to the presence of dilated veins in the broad ligament and ovarian plexus. Typical appearances have been described at venography and reported with

Table 51.4.1   Causes of pelvic pain

Normal findings	35%
Endometriosis	33%
Adhesions	24%
Chronic pelvic inflammatory disease	5%
Ovarian cyst	3%
Pelvic varicosities	1%
Fibroids	1%
Other	4%

Results of 1524 laparoscopies for pelvic pain (13 studies reviewed by Howard, 2000).[7]

both ultrasound and magnetic resonance imaging (MRI),[9] although studies reporting accuracy, sensitivity and specificity have not been undertaken. Indirect evidence for the existence of the condition was obtained from a small therapeutic study in which the vasoconstrictor dihydroergotamine[10] was more effective than placebo in relieving symptoms. However, the existence of the condition as an entity distinct from unexplained chronic pelvic pain is disputed.

MANAGEMENT

Investigation

Primary dysmenorrhoea does not require investigation [IV] and should be managed by the general practitioner or primary care physician. Referral for specialist advice is only required if there is a lack of response to standard therapies or if symptoms are atypical, giving rise to a suspicion of endometriosis or other pathology. Although a simple pelvic examination can provide reassurance, this is not indicated in a teenager who is not sexually active [IV]. A transabdominal ultrasound scan will exclude congenital uterine abnormalities or significant ovarian pathology [III][9] and should provide reassurance if negative. The role of ultrasound in the investigation of dysmenorrhoea and pelvic pain is not established, but it is sensitive in detecting uterine and ovarian pathology [II] and has the advantage of being non-invasive.[9]

For the purposes of this chapter, chronic pelvic pain that is exacerbated perimenstrually will be considered to be synonymous with secondary dysmenorrhoea. Abdominal and pelvic examination may be helpful in identifying tenderness and the presence of any masses. Areas of thickening or nodularity suggestive of endometriosis may be palpated in the pouch of Douglas. Indications for further investigation include symptoms suggestive of endometriosis and/or abnormal findings on pelvic examination or ultrasound scan. As endometriosis can only be diagnosed with certainty by laparoscopy [II], the nature and risks of the procedure require adequate discussion. In chronic pain, the value of laparoscopy as a routine investigation in the absence of abnormal clinical findings has been challenged.[11]

Management of primary dysmenorrhoea

Non-steroidal anti-inflammatory drugs

These drugs inhibit prostaglandin synthesis via inhibition of the enzyme cyclo-oxygenase. A systematic review of 56 clinical trials[12] concluded that naproxen, ibuprofen, mefenamic acid and aspirin are all effective in primary dysmenorrhoea [Ia]. Response rate ratios generally favour naproxen and ibuprofen, aspirin having the lowest response rate ratio. The overall incidence of side effects is low and generally related to the gastrointestinal tract. Naproxen causes more side effects than ibuprofen and mefenamic acid. The reviewers conclude that ibuprofen is superior in terms of its efficacy and favourable side effect profile [Ia].

Combined oral contraceptive pill

These preparations have been widely used for many years for the relief of primary dysmenorrhoea. The theoretical basis for their action is via inhibition of ovulation. Several population-based contraceptive studies[13] have reported their efficacy in relieving dysmenorrhoea [II]. However, there is a paucity of published information on the efficacy of the low-dose preparations in current use. In a recent systematic review,[13] combined oral contraceptive pills (COCPs) were found to be significantly more effective than placebo for pain relief [Ia]. Only four randomized, controlled trials met the criteria for inclusion in the review; all based on higher dose formulations than those in current use. Despite these reservations about the evidence base, the COCP should be regarded as a safe and effective therapy for the relief of primary dysmenorrhoea [Ia].

Surgical interruption of pelvic nerve pathways

Because of the chronic and recurrent nature of pelvic pain, surgical techniques have been described for division of the nerves which innervate the uterus. Sensory fibres from the lower uterus, cervix and upper vagina exit along autonomic nervous system pathways that run along the lower margins of the uterosacral ligaments. These pass superiorly via bilateral inferior hypogastric plexuses in the pararectal spaces to the superior hypogastric plexuses that lie over the bodies of L4 and L5 and the sacral promontory.[14] Presacral neurectomy (PSN) involves removal of the nerve bundles of the hypogastric plexus, a procedure traditionally done by laparotomy, but more recently laparoscopic methods have been described. Laparoscopic uterine nerve ablation (LUNA) is a simpler procedure that involves division of the uterosacral ligaments.

Two systematic reviews have assessed the role of these surgical interventions in primary and secondary dysmenorrhoea.[14,15] Both sets of reviewers criticized the quality of the data and the lack of randomized, controlled trials. The overall consensus from these reviews is that there is insufficient evidence to support the use of either procedure in the management of dysmenorrhoea, regardless of its cause [Ia]. Significant morbidity has been described following both procedures but is more common following PSN.

Alternative therapies

These are popular with the lay public and are widely used. There have been two Cochrane Reviews of alternative therapy in dysmenorrhoea. One reviewed five randomized, controlled trials of spinal manipulation[16] and found this to be ineffective [Ia]. The other[17] reviewed a number of herbal and dietary therapies that have been assessed by randomized, controlled trials. These comprised vitamin B1 (one large trial), vitamin B6 (one small trial comparing it with magnesium), vitamin E (in combination with ibuprofen), magnesium (three small trials), omega-3 fatty acids, and Japanese herbal combination. Although results were generally encouraging for all except vitamin E, the reviewers concluded that both magnesium and vitamin B1 are promising for the relief of dysmenorrhoea [Ib] but that insufficient evidence exists for the use of any of the other therapies.

New therapeutic approaches in primary dysmenorrhoea

Non-steroidal anti-inflammatory drugs (NSAIDs) in current use inhibit two different isoforms of the enzyme cyclo-oxygenase, known as COX-1 and COX-2. Selective inhibitors of the enzyme COX-2 may have similar analgesic efficacy but fewer of the side effects of the drugs in current use. However, these have not been assessed for their role in dysmenorrhoea. Transdermal administration of the smooth muscle relaxant glyceryl trinitrate is also under current evaluation.[6]

Secondary dysmenorrhoea and chronic pelvic pain

Management of secondary dysmenorrhoea will depend on its underlying cause. In cases of chronic pelvic pain where a diagnosis of endometriosis is suspected, laparoscopic confirmation of the diagnosis is unnecessary and a trial of medical therapy is justified provided that there are no other indications for surgery such as the presence of a suspicious adnexal mass [IV]. Interventions for the management of chronic pelvic pain have been the subject of a systematic review.[10] The main conclusion of the reviewers was that further studies of medical, surgical and psychological interventions are urgently needed.

Multidisciplinary approach

Even in the absence of positive factors suggestive of pelvic pathology such as endometriosis, there is a tendency to perform laparoscopy in order to exclude organic pathology. This approach has been challenged. One study[11] randomized women with chronic pelvic pain between routine laparoscopy followed by conventional management and an integrated approach. In the latter group, a gynaecologist, psychologist, physiotherapist and nutritionist assessed all the women and management was then directed as appropriate. Evaluation 1 year later showed a significantly greater improvement in daily activities and perception of pain in the latter group, although pain scores were not significantly different. Women with positive laparoscopic findings in the first group had other clinical features of pelvic pathology. Following negative laparoscopy, another study[10] compared expectant management with intervention comprising an ultrasound scan and an educational and counselling session. Interval reassessment showed a significant improvement in mood and pain scores in the intervention group. These studies highlight the importance of a multidisciplinary approach to chronic pelvic pain, such as that provided in a specialist pain clinic [Ib].

Antidepressants

In the absence of pelvic pathology, there is a tendency for chronic pain to be attributed to depression. Although symptoms of depression and sleep disturbances may be more prevalent among women with chronic pain,[1] the interaction is likely to be complex and not necessarily causative. A randomized comparison of the antidepressant sertraline (a serotonin reuptake inhibitor) with placebo in chronic pelvic pain sufferers[18] failed to show any difference in pain scores [Ib].

Progestogens for pain secondary to pelvic venous congestion

Although there is some dispute about the existence of the condition, treatment with continuous medroxyprogesterone acetate (MPA) has been advocated for women with chronic pelvic pain and dyspareunia attributed to the presence of pelvic varicosities. In a large randomized trial,[19] MPA 50 mg daily for 4 months was compared with placebo. In addition, both were used alone or in conjunction with psychotherapy. MPA was more effective than placebo for the duration of therapy, but the benefit was not sustained after completion [Ib]. Psychotherapy was no better than placebo. Despite these positive results, other methods of ovarian suppression have not been assessed in this group of women.

Hysterectomy for chronic pelvic pain

There are limited data based on prospective follow-up of women undergoing hysterectomy for pelvic pain. One review of five studies of women undergoing hysterectomy for chronic pain presumed to be of uterine origin[14] reported the relief of symptoms at 12-month follow-up in 83–97 per cent of women [II]. One of these studies was based on women with pelvic varicosities demonstrated by venography. However, the results of these studies showed that failure of pain relief was greatest among women with no demonstrable pelvic pathology [II], once again emphasizing the

importance of a multidisciplinary approach for women with unexplained pelvic pain.

> Recommendations for the management of primary dysmenorrhoea are based on six systematic reviews. The management of chronic pelvic pain has been the subject of one systematic review, which highlighted the need for further studies in this field.

KEY POINTS

- Primary dysmenorrhoea is experienced by more than two-thirds of women and a minority are severely incapacitated.
- Investigation is unnecessary unless there are atypical symptoms or abnormal findings on pelvic examination [IV].
- Ultrasound is a useful non-invasive method for the detection of pelvic abnormalities [II].
- NSAIDs are effective for the first-line management of primary dysmenorrhoea [Ia].
- COCPS are effective in primary dysmenorrhoea, although the evidence is based on higher dose formulations than those in current use [Ia].
- There is insufficient evidence to support the use of pelvic nerve interruption for the relief of primary or secondary dysmenorrhoea [Ia].
- Dietary supplements (magnesium, vitamin B1) may have a role in the management of dysmenorrhoea [Ib].
- There is considerable overlap between the causes of secondary dysmenorrhoea and chronic pelvic pain [II].
- Pain attributed to pelvic venous congestion is relieved by continuous high-dose MPA [Ib].
- Antidepressants are not effective in the management of chronic pelvic pain [Ib].
- Where possible, chronic pelvic pain should be managed in a multidisciplinary clinic [Ib].

KEY REFERENCES

1. Moore J, Kennedy S. Causes of chronic pelvic pain. *Baillière's Clin Obstet Gynaecol* 2000; **14**(3):389–402.
2. Andersch B, Milsom I. An epidemiological study of young women with dysmenorrhoea. *Am J Obstet Gynecol* 1982; **144**:655–60.
3. Sundell G, Milsom I, Andersch B. Factors influencing the prevalence and severity of dysmenorrhoea in young women. *Br J Obstet Gynaecol* 1990; **97**:588–94.

4. Zondervan KT, Yudkin PL, Vessey MP, Dawes MG, Barlow DH, Kennedy SH. The prevalence of chronic pelvic pain in women in the United Kingdom: a systematic review. *Br J Obstet Gynaecol* 1998; **105**:93–9.

5. Mathias SD, Kuppermann M, Liberman RF, Lipschutz RC, Steege JF. Chronic pelvic pain: prevalence, health-related quality of life and economic correlates. *Obstet Gynecol* 1996; **87**:321–7.

6. Facchinelti F, Sgarbi L, Piccinini F, Volpe A. A comparison of glyceryl trinitrate with diclofenac for the treatment of primary dysmenorrhoea: an open, randomized, cross-over trial. *Gynecol Endocrinol* 2002; **16**:39–43.

7. Howard FM. The role of laparoscopy as a diagnostic tool in chronic pelvic pain. *Baillière's Clin Obstet Gynaecol* 2000; **14**(3):467–94.

8. Beard RW, Reginald PW, Wadsworth J. Clinical features of women with lower abdominal pain and pelvic congestion. *Br J Obstet Gynaecol* 1988; **95**:153–61.

9. Cody RF Jr, Ascher SM. Diagnostic value of radiological tests in chronic pelvic pain. *Baillière's Clin Obstet Gynaecol* 2000; **14**(3):433–66.

10. Stones RW, Mountford J. Interventions for treating chronic pelvic pain in women. In: *The Cochrane Library*, Issue 4. Oxford: Update Software, 2001.

11. Peters AA, van Dorst E, Jellis B, van Zuuren E, Hermans J, Trimbos JB. A randomized clinical trial to compare two different approaches in women with chronic pelvic pain. *Obstet Gynecol* 1991; **77**:740–4.

12. Zhang WY, Po ALW. Efficacy of minor analgesics in primary dysmenorrhoea: a systematic review. *Br J Obstet Gynaecol* 1998; **105**:780–9.

13. Proctor ML, Roberts H, Farquhar CM. Combined oral contraceptive pill (OCP) as treatment for primary dysmenorrhoea (Cochrane Review). In: *The Cochrane Library*, Issue 4. Oxford: Update Software, 2001.

14. Vercellini P, De Giorgi O, Pisacreta A, Pesole AP, Vicentini S, Crosignani PG. Surgical management of endometriosis. *Baillière's Clin Obstet Gynaecol* 2000; **14**(3):501–23.

15. Proctor ML, Farquhar CM, Sinclair OJ, Johnson NP. Surgical interruption of pelvic nerve pathways for primary and secondary dysmenorrhoea (Cochrane Review). In: *The Cochrane Library*, Issue 4. Oxford: Update Software, 2001.

16. Proctor ML, Hing W, Johnson TC, Murphy PA. Spinal manipulation for primary and secondary dysmenorrhoea (Cochrane Review). In: *The Cochrane Library*, Issue 4. Oxford: Update Software, 2001.

17. Proctor ML, Murphy PA. Herbal and dietary therapies for primary and secondary dysmenorrhoea (Cochrane Review). In: *The Cochrane Library*, Issue 4. Oxford: Update Software, 2001.

18. Engel CC Jr, Walker EA, Engel AL, Bullis J, Armstrong A. A randomized double-blind crossover trial of sertraline in women with chronic pelvic pain. *J Psychosom Res* 1998; **44**:203–7.

19. Farquhar CM, Rogers V, Franks S, Pearce S, Wadsworth J, Beard RW. A randomized controlled trial of medroxyprogesterone acetate and psychotherapy for the treatment of pelvic congestion. *Br J Obstet Gynaecol* 1989; **96**:1153–62.

Endometriosis and Gonadotrophin Releasing Hormone Analogues

Christine P. West

MRCOG standards

Theoretical skills
- Understand the pathogenesis and clinical presentation of endometriosis.
- Know the principal medical therapies used in endometriosis–associated pain.
- Know the surgical principles underlying the conservative and medical approaches to endometriosis surgery.

Practical skills
- Be familiar with techniques of diagnostic laparoscopy and staging of endometriosis.
- Be familiar with conservative surgical techniques used in management of endometriosis and endometriomas.
- Be familiar with the advantages and possible complications of hysterectomy and oophorectomy for endometriosis.

INTRODUCTION

Endometriosis is a common condition with many diverse manifestations and a clinical course that is highly variable and unpredictable. It may be asymptomatic, but most commonly presents with pelvic pain that is usually cyclical and in severe cases there may be bowel or bladder involvement. The site of the lesions deep in the pelvis can cause dyspareunia and there is a well-recognized but poorly understood association with subfertility. Management is individualized and will depend on the patient's symptoms, her age and reproductive plans. This chapter deals mainly with the management of pain in endometriosis, which has attracted a large literature and for which evidence-based management is relatively well developed.

DEFINITION

Endometriosis is the presence of ectopic endometrial tissue in extrauterine sites, usually within the pelvis but very rarely at distant sites such as the lung. Endometriosis should be regarded as distinct from adenomyosis, in which endometrial tissue is present within the myometrium.

Endometriomas, also known as chocolate cysts, are retention cysts that develop as a consequence of ovarian endometriosis. They commonly form when adhesions develop between endometriotic deposits on the ovary and the pelvic side wall or may result from an inflammatory reaction to a superficial ovarian lesion, leading to adhesions developing around the lesion, producing progressive inversion of the surrounding cortex. Endometriomas may be multiple and very large, when they inevitably interfere with fertility by adhesion and distortion of the fallopian tubes.

In some women with endometriotic lesions predominantly affecting the uterosacral ligaments, marked fibrosis and scarring may develop, with infiltration of active endometriotic tissue into the rectovaginal septum. Dense adhesions involving the rectum may lead to partial or complete obliteration of the pouch of Douglas. Both processes may be associated with the development of tender nodules that are easily palpable on vaginal examination and are associated with bowel symptoms. Deep nodular lesions may also be visible as small, tender, bluish cysts in the posterior fornix. So-called deep infiltrating endometriosis may also be present on the uterovesical fold, leading to bladder involvement.

INCIDENCE

The widespread use of laparoscopy has led to increased detection of endometriosis. Reported prevalence has varied very widely within and between different societies and according to the indications for laparoscopy. In a prospective study of 1542 Caucasian women in a single Scottish centre,[1] endometriosis was visualized in 6 per cent of women undergoing sterilization, 21 per cent being investigated for infertility and 15 per cent being investigated for pelvic pain. However, in a review of 1524 laparoscopies for pelvic pain,[2] the prevalence of endometriosis was reported to be 33 per cent.

AETIOLOGY

It is generally accepted that endometriotic tissue reaches the pelvis by retrograde menstruation,[3] initiating a local inflammatory response. Failure of this response is believed to lead to implantation of the endometriotic tissue and its subsequent activity. Whether this failure is related to the volume of menstrual debris that reaches the pelvis or to a defect in the local peritoneal defence system remains unresolved. Retrograde menstruation occurs in the majority of women, but only a minority develop endometriosis. Factors that reduce menstruation, such as pregnancy and the use of oral contraceptives,[1,3] reduce its prevalence. Genetic factors also appear to be relevant and these may influence local response mechanisms and the subsequent course of the disease. Whatever the underlying mechanisms, it is evident that the progress of the disease differs considerably amongst individuals.[3] There is a suggestion that minimal or mild endometriosis is a natural condition that occurs intermittently in most women[3] but in a minority progresses to cystic ovarian endometriosis or deeply infiltrating disease.

The mechanism of pain in endometriosis is presumably by the release of inflammatory mediators such as prostaglandins from superficial lesions. Pain related to deep lesions may be caused by infiltration or constriction of nerves or may be secondary to adhesions.[4]

MANAGEMENT

Investigation

The commonest presentation of endometriosis is with pelvic pain (which is usually cyclical in nature) characteristically preceding the onset of menstruation and associated with deep dyspareunia. There may be tenderness on bimanual examination, with palpable nodules in the pouch of Douglas or ovarian lesions on ultrasound suggestive of endometriomas. More often, examination is unhelpful and the decision to carry out further investigation is based largely on the history and the wishes of the patient. There is no evidence that serum CA-125 is useful as a screening test [Ia],[5] although levels are likely to be raised in severe disease. Transvaginal ultrasound is of value in detecting ovarian endometriomas [Ia],[6] but these may be confused with haemorrhagic functional cysts. Negative ultrasound findings do not exclude the disease.

Magnetic resonance imaging (MRI) has greater sensitivity [II][5] and may assist in the evaluation of deep lesions.

The diagnosis of endometriosis is by laparoscopy [II]. This is an invasive procedure and in all cases its nature and risks must be fully discussed with the patient [IV].[7] Counselling must include discussion about the possible courses of action should endometriosis be diagnosed at the primary procedure. Initial management is likely to vary from centre to centre and will depend on whether there is associated infertility.

Laparoscopy must involve a two-port approach with careful inspection of the pouch of Douglas, the uterosacral ligaments, the pelvic side wall and the anterior surfaces of both ovaries [IV].[2] Where necessary, careful mobilization of the ovaries should be attempted in order to inspect their anterior surface, as the presence of adhesions is strongly suggestive of endometriosis. Where there is doubt about the nature of a lesion, this should be confirmed by biopsy [IV], but this procedure is not without risk and is not necessary as a routine. The operator must appreciate the varied appearances of endometriosis and be familiar with the American Fertility Society (AFS) classification.[8] Photographs are helpful in the documentation of disease extent, but otherwise use should be made of diagrams, in particular those based on the AFS classification, which should be available in all gynaecological theatres [IV].

Medical management of pelvic pain associated with endometriosis

Endometriosis-associated pain can be managed effectively by medical therapy [Ia]. The majority of therapies act by ovarian suppression and induction of amenorrhoea. Since this merely inactivates and does not remove local disease, symptoms recur after cessation in a proportion of patients and, for some, treatment may potentially be long term. As all the therapies discussed below have similar efficacy, their tolerability in terms of side effects and health risks is important when selecting the most appropriate treatment for an individual woman [Ia].[5]

In contrast to the important role that medical therapy has in the symptomatic management of endometriosis, it has no role in the management of endometriosis-associated infertility, and indeed delays rather than enhances fertility [Ia].[5] Medical suppression may be of temporary value in pain control, for example in women awaiting in-vitro fertilization (IVF) [IV].

Non-steroidal anti-inflammatory drugs

These offer a non-hormonal approach that is particularly useful in women trying to conceive. The evidence for efficacy is largely based on their use in the treatment of primary dysmenorrhoea, but evidence from small trials[5] also supports their use in endometriosis [Ib].

Combined oral contraceptives

Continuous use of low-dose combined oral contraceptive preparations (COCPs) is a common management strategy, although evidence to support it is lacking.[9] In a randomized trial comparing cyclical administration of a low-dose COCP with a GnRH agonist,[9] both were effective in the management of non-menstrual pain and dyspareunia. This evidence, albeit limited, supports the use of the COCPs as a first-line therapy [Ib]. In the absence of further information, the mode of administration, whether cyclical, tricyclical, 6-monthly or continuous, should be a matter for discussion between the clinician and the individual patient [IV]. Because of their relative safety for long-term use, COCPs may be suitable as adjuncts to maintain symptomatic relief following medical or surgical treatment [Ib].

Progestogens

Progestogens given continuously and at high dosage inhibit ovulation and have direct antiproliferative effects on endometriotic implants, causing decidualization and eventual atrophy. They have been widely used for the treatment of endometriosis and are the subject of two large reviews.[10,11] However, most published studies of their efficacy pre-dated the era of evidence-based medicine and their small scale and poor design limited critical evaluation. In randomized, controlled trials, both high-dose oral medroxyprogesterone acetate (MPA; 100 mg daily) and depot MPA (Depo-Provera 150 mg 3-monthly) were found to be effective in the relief of pain symptoms [Ib]. Considerably lower doses of MPA (30 mg, 50 mg) were effective in non-randomized trials [II].[11]

In a small study of women wishing to conceive, two doses of dydrogesterone, 40 mg and 60 mg, given cyclically during the luteal phase were compared with placebo.[10] Pain scores were significantly improved only in the women given the 60 mg dose, and there were no significant differences in AFS scores or pregnancy rates. Evidence from this study suggests that luteal phase use of high-dose progestogens may relieve endometriosis-related pain in women wishing to conceive [Ib].

The most commonly reported side effect of progestogens is breakthrough bleeding, with an overall incidence of around 33 per cent,[12] which is not dose related. Other side effects experienced by up to 10 per cent of women include weight gain, breast tenderness, bloating, headache and nausea. Progestogens, in particular long-acting depots, have an important role in the long-term management of endometriosis because of their low cost and good safety profile [Ib]. Limited information on the use of progestogen-containing intrauterine devices in the management of endometriosis[12] indicates that these may also be of value in relieving symptoms [III].

Gestrinone

Gestrinone is a 19-nortestosterone derivative that also has progestogenic and antiprogestogenic actions. Gestrinone has been compared in randomized trials[10] with placebo, with danazol and with a GnRH analogue. At a dose of 2.5 mg twice weekly for 6 months, gestrinone was as effective as danazol and a GnRH analogue in reducing pain scores [Ib], but both androgenic and hypo-oestrogenic side effects were less frequent with gestrinone. Clinical response was similar to that of a GnRH analogue, but hot flushes were more frequent with the GnRH analogue. Efficacy of gestrinone was maintained at a lower dose of 1.25 mg twice weekly but with reduced side effects [Ib].[10]

No direct comparison has been made between gestrinone and progestogens, but the reported incidence of breakthrough bleeding is much lower with gestrinone, making it a potentially useful alternative to progestogens, danazol or GnRH analogues [Ib]. However, there is a lack of information relating to its safety for long-term use.

Danazol

Previously, danazol was the most widely prescribed drug for endometriosis, but more recently it has been overtaken by GnRH agonists. It is an androgenic steroid, which acts both centrally and locally to suppress steroidogenesis and induce endometrial atrophy. It has also been the subject of a systematic review.[13] Compared with placebo, it significantly improves pain and AFS scores at doses of 400–600 mg daily. Androgenic side effects such as weight gain, limb tingling, acne, greasy skin, hirsutism and deepening of the voice are common, and atherogenic effects on lipid profiles have been reported. Although there is evidence that danazol suppresses endometriosis at low doses that are insufficient to suppress menstruation [II],[14] the dose selected is usually the lowest that will achieve amenorrhoea. Thus, while effective for the treatment of symptomatic endometriosis [Ia], danazol is not suitable for long-term use.

GnRH analogues

The GnRH analogues are derived from native hypothalamic GnRH by peptide substitutions that increase their potency and duration of action. Both agonist analogues and antagonists[15] have been developed, of which the agonists have been in established clinical practice for much longer. The antagonists act by competitive inhibition of pituitary GnRH receptors, with a rapid onset of action, whereas the agonists cause initial stimulation of gonadotrophin production followed by prolonged down-regulation. The antagonists have a clear advantage over the agonists for short-term pituitary suppression (e.g. during superovulation prior to IVF), but are unlikely to take over from agonists for longer term indications such as the management of endometriosis.

Down-regulation of pituitary GnRH receptors by GnRH agonists leads to the inhibition of follicle-stimulating hormone (FSH) and luteinizing hormone (LH) production and gonadal suppression. The GnRH agonists are thus useful in

Table 51.5.1 Gonadotrophin releasing hormone agonists for the treatment of endometriosis

Depot preparations		Intranasal preparations	
Goserelin	3.6 mg s.c.	Nafarelin	200 mcg bd
Leuprorelin	3.75 mg i.m. or s.c.	Buserelin	200 mcg tid
Triptorelin	3.75 mg i.m.		

the management of hormone-dependent conditions in both men and women. Administration of GnRH agonists is by nasal spray or depot injection (Table 51.5.1). The intranasal route tends to be less costly, while depot administration improves compliance.

Results of a systematic review of 26 randomized, controlled trials of GnRH agonist therapy have demonstrated its effectiveness in the treatment of pain associated with endometriosis [Ia].[16] In the only trial which was placebo controlled, 27 of 31 patients randomized to placebo discontinued because of poor efficacy. Comparison with gestrinone, a COCP and danazol (15 studies) demonstrated no significant differences in clinical response but expected differences in side effect profiles. The side effects of GnRH agonists include hot flushes, insomnia, vaginal dryness, reduced libido and headaches – all secondary to oestrogen suppression.

Various GnRH agonists were used in these studies (see Table 51.5.1), the majority for 6 months' duration. Comparison of different intranasal doses (600 vs 900 mcg buserelin; 400 vs 800 mcg nafarelin) showed no difference in symptomatic response and AFS scores, but side effects were reduced at the lower doses [Ib]. When 3 months of treatment was compared with 6 months, clinical response was similar, with the exception of deep dyspareunia, for which improvement was significantly greater after 6 months [Ib].

Like other medical treatments, GnRH agonists do not produce permanent disease regression. A life-table analysis of follow-up of women treated with various GnRH agonists for 6–9 months[17] reported a cumulative symptomatic recurrence rate of 53.4 per cent after 7 years [II]. For severe disease, the recurrence rate was 74.4 per cent, while for minimal disease it was 36.9 per cent.

Longer term use of GnRH analogues

The side effects of the GnRH analogues are largely related to oestrogen deficiency and are often well tolerated. However, loss of bone mineral density is a major concern and for this reason GnRH analogues should not be given as single agents for longer than 6 months [Ia]. In women needing longer term treatment, hormonal add-back therapy can be used with the object of reducing or preventing bone loss and minimizing other unwanted side effects. Several continuous combined regimens have been compared with placebo in patients treated with GnRH agonists for endometriosis.[16,18,19] These have included transdermal oestradiol 25 μg twice weekly plus oral MPA 5 mg daily; oral oestradiol 2 mg daily plus norethisterone (NET) 1 mg or 5 mg daily; conjugated equine oestrogens 0.625 mg daily plus NET 5 mg and tibolone. All were effective in sustaining pain relief while reducing side effects and

maintaining bone density [Ib]. However, a combination of conjugated equine oestrogens 1.25 mg with NET 5 mg was less effective in the relief of pelvic symptoms compared with a lower dose oestrogen combination or progestogen alone [Ib].

Progestogens have been studied as sole add-back agents.[16] NET at a dose of 5–10 mg daily was effective in reducing side effects and bone loss but was associated with atherogenic changes in lipid profiles [Ib].[16,19] For women who cannot tolerate hormonal add-back or for whom it is contraindicated, anti-resorptive agents, such as bisphosphonates, are effective in preventing bone loss [Ib].[20]

These results support the role of add-back therapy with GnRH agonists to suppress endometriosis-associated pain when given as continuous combined low-dose oestrogen–progestogen combinations or as tibolone [Ib]. Oestrogen should be given at low dosage in order to maintain symptomatic relief; incomplete suppression of vasomotor side effects may respond to an increase in the progestogenic component of the therapy [IV].

Although these preparations and combinations have been used for several years, very long-term follow-up data are lacking. Evidence from limited follow-up[19] indicates that bone density was preserved by a combination of a GnRH agonist and add-back hormone replacement therapy (HRT) over a 12-month period [Ib]. Further information based on longer term follow-up is clearly needed.

THE ROLE OF SURGERY IN ENDOMETRIOSIS-ASSOCIATED PAIN

Unlike medical therapies, there have been few comparative or controlled studies of surgical approaches,[21] although the latter have gained a large literature and surgical interventions are widely used. Because operative laparoscopy is associated with a significant risk of major complications and potential litigation [II],[7] such interventions are in urgent need of critical review.

Only one study has compared surgery, in this case laser laparoscopy, with expectant management in a randomized, double-blind trial.[22] Treatment comprised local ablation, adhesiolysis and laparoscopic utero-sacral nerve ablation (LUNA). Outcome was assessed in relation to the stage of the disease, but women with stage IV disease were excluded on ethical grounds. Women with mild and moderate disease (stages II–III) showed a significant improvement in pain scores at 6 months, with no improvement in those with minimal (stage I) disease. Overall, 62.5 per cent of those treated reported an improvement, compared with 22.6 per cent of controls. In a follow-up of the original study at 1 year,[23] which included second-look laparoscopy in women who remained symptomatic, 90 per cent of those who initially responded remained well, but only 29 per cent of the control women showed signs of disease progression.

This important but small-scale study, carried out in a nationally recognized laparoscopic surgery centre, supports

Reproductive medicine

the use of conservative laparoscopic surgery for the relief of pain in stage II and III endometriosis [Ib]. No serious surgical complications were reported, but these results may not be reproducible in a more general context, in terms of both efficacy and safety [IV]. The study does not support the use of surgical ablation for pain relief in minimal disease, although there is some evidence that the latter may be of benefit in women presenting with infertility [Ib].[5] Currently, there is insufficient evidence to support the use of LUNA as an adjunct to laparoscopic surgical treatment for pain in endometriosis [Ia].[24]

Surgical ablation of advanced disease, particularly where there are dense adhesions involving bowel, is a technically difficult procedure involving a high risk of bowel damage [III][25] and should only be carried out in specialist regional centres [IV] if it is to be attempted laparoscopically. Where issues of safety arise, laparotomy still has a role in the conservative management of advanced disease [II],[26] both for pain management and for enhancement of fertility.

Surgical management of endometriomas

Endometriomas do not resolve during medical suppression, although they may become asymptomatic. Simple drainage of an endometrioma is followed by rapid recurrence, even if it is fenestrated and irrigated [Ib].[27] Results of four comparative trials[28] have indicated a higher rate of recurrence following coagulation or laser vaporization of the inner lining of the cyst compared with stripping of the pseudocapsule [1a]. In practice, laparoscopic stripping may be difficult or incomplete and, as the available evidence does not support conversion to laparotomy for this indication alone [II], coagulation offers a reasonable alternative.

In cases of severe ovarian endometriosis where future fertility is an issue, ovarian tissue should be preserved where possible. With large and multiple endometriomata or where there is suspicion of malignancy, unilateral oophorectomy may be necessary. With severe bilateral disease, oophorectomy alone with preservation of the uterus will still leave the woman with a chance of pregnancy through oocyte donation [III].

Medical adjuncts to surgery

There is no evidence to support the use of medical adjuncts prior to conservative surgery for endometriosis [II], although they may be valuable in the control of symptoms prior to radical therapy. GnRH agonists administered for 6 months following conservative surgery for pain have been found significantly to prolong the duration of the symptom-free interval.[29,30] Similarly, 6 months of treatment with a low-dose cyclical COCP following surgical excision of endometriomas[31] was significantly more effective than placebo in reducing symptomatic and ultrasound evidence of recurrence at 12 months. However, this difference was not apparent at 24 and 36 months. Medical therapy is of value following conservative

surgery of endometriosis for pain [Ib], but the evidence suggests that it may need to be for longer than 6 months.

Long-term follow-up after surgery

Advocates of surgery claim that surgical excision of endometriotic lesions is more effective in the long term than medical therapy because of a reduced likelihood of recurrence. Symptomatic recurrence rates of between 15 and 57 per cent after 2 years have been reported in multicentre studies [Ib].[26,29,30] Such figures are likely to be dependent on both the severity of the disease and the experience of the operator. There are no randomized studies comparing medical and surgical therapies, in terms of either short-term efficacy or long-term recurrence.

Definitive surgery

In women with symptomatic endometriosis who have completed childbearing, hysterectomy offers a long-term cure, but only if combined with bilateral oophorectomy [III].[26] In advanced disease with dense bowel adhesions and deep lesions in the recto-vaginal pouch, complete removal of the disease will require a very radical approach [III], with careful consideration of the risks, especially if the symptoms are well controlled with medical therapy.

HORMONE REPLACEMENT THERAPY AND ENDOMETRIOSIS

Following hysterectomy with oophorectomy, HRT is mandatory in young women. Case reports have highlighted the potential risks of unopposed oestrogen [III][25] where there is residual endometriosis. Results of a small, randomized study[32] comparing oestrogen with tibolone in oophorectomized women with deep residual endometriosis favoured the use of tibolone [Ib]. Similarly, data on the use of HRT add-back in combination with GnRH agonists indicate that both tibolone and low-dose oestrogen continuous combined HRT preparations are suitable for the relief of menopausal symptoms and for bone preservation in women with severe endometriosis [Ib].

- Medical management of pain in endometriosis is supported by four systematic reviews based on a large number of randomized, controlled trials.
- Surgical management of pain in endometriosis is based on one small randomized, controlled trial and a systematic review of the use of pelvic denervation.
- There have been no randomized studies comparing medical with surgical management in the relief of endometriosis-associated pain.

KEY POINTS

- Adequate counselling is necessary prior to laparoscopy for suspected endometriosis [IV].
- Measurement of CA-125 is not helpful as an aid to diagnosis [Ia].
- Transvaginal ultrasound is useful in identifying endometriomas but lacks specificity [II].
- Medical therapy is effective in the management of pain associated with endometriosis [Ia] and selection should be determined by the relative side effect profiles [1a].
- COCPs, progestogens, danazol, gestrinone and GnRH agonists are all effective therapies [Ia].
- Because of a high recurrence rate of pain, treatment may need to be intermittent or long term [II].
- Levonorgestrel-releasing intrauterine systems may have a role in long-term pain control [III], but have not been adequately evaluated.
- If GnRH agonists are used for longer than 6 months, add-back therapy with low-dose continuous combined HRT or tibolone should be given [Ib].
- Laparoscopic surgery is effective in the treatment of pain secondary to endometriosis in experienced hands [Ib].
- There is insufficient evidence to recommend surgical pelvic nerve interruption for the relief of pain associated with endometriosis [Ia].
- Duration of response to surgery may be increased by postoperative medical suppression [Ib].
- Operative laparoscopy carries a significant risk, and cases of advanced disease should be referred to specialist centres for laparoscopic surgery [IV].
- Long-term outcome is similar with laparotomy and laparoscopy [II].
- If fertility is no longer an issue, hysterectomy with bilateral oophorectomy may provide a cure, but disease excision may be incomplete [III].
- Low-dose continuous combined HRT or tibolone is preferable to oestrogen-only HRT following hysterectomy with oophorectomy for severe endometriosis [Ib].

KEY REFERENCES

1. Mahmood TA, Templeton A. Prevalence and genesis of endometriosis. *Hum Reprod* 1991; 6:544–9.
2. Howard FM. The role of laparoscopy as a diagnostic tool in chronic pelvic pain. *Baillière's Clin Obstet Gynaecol* 2000; 14(3):467–94.
3. Wardle PG, Hull MRG. Is endometriosis a disease? *Baillière's Clin Obstet Gynecol* 1993; 7(4):673–85.
4. Moore J, Kennedy S. Causes of chronic pelvic pain. *Baillière's Clin Obstet Gynecol* 2000; 14(3):389–402.
5. Royal College of Obstetricians and Gynaecologists. *The Investigation and Management of Endometriosis.* Guideline No. 24. London: RCOG, 2000.
6. Moore J, Copley S, Morris J, Lindsell D, Golding S, Kennedy S. A systematic review of the accuracy of ultrasound in the diagnosis of endometriosis. *Ultrasound Obstet Gynecol* 2002;20:630–4.
7. Kalu G, Wright J. Laparoscopic surgery and the law. *Obstet Gynecol* 2001; 3(3):141–6.
8. American Fertility Society. Revised American Fertility Society classification of endometriosis. *Fertil Steril* 1985; 43:351–2.
9. Moore J, Kennedy S, Prentice A. Modern combined contraceptives for pain associated with endometriosis (Cochrane Review). In: *The Cochrane Library*, Issue 4. Oxford: Update Software, 2001.
10. Prentice A, Deary AJ, Bland E. Progestagens and anti-progestagens for pain associated with endometriosis (Cochrane Review). In: *The Cochrane Library*, Issue 4. Oxford: Update Software, 2001.
11. Vercellini P, Cortesi I, Crosignani PG. Progestins for symptomatic endometriosis – a critical analysis of the evidence. *Fertil Steril* 1997; 68:393–401.
12. Vercellini P, Aimi G, Panazza S, De Giorgio O, Pesole A, Crosignani PG. A levonorgestrel-releasing intrauterine system for the treatment of dysmenorrhoea associated with endometriosis: a pilot study. *Fertil Steril* 1999; 72:505–8.
13. Selak V, Farquhar C, Prentice A, Singla A. Danazol for pelvic pain associated with endometriosis (Cochrane Review). In: *The Cochrane Library*, Issue 4. Oxford: Update Software, 2001.
14. Vercellini P, Trespidi L, Panazza S, Bramante T, Mauro F, Crosignani PG. Very low dose danazol for relief of endometriosis-associated pelvic pain: a pilot study. *Fertil Steril* 1994; 62:1136–42.
15. Huirne JA, Lambalk CB. Gonadotropin-releasing-hormone-receptor antagonists. *Lancet* 2001; 358:1793–808.
16. Prentice A, Deary AJ, Goldbeck-Wood S, Farquhar C, Smith SK. Gonadotropin-releasing hormone analogues for pain associated with endometriosis (Cochrane Review). In: *The Cochrane Library*, Issue 4. Oxford: Update Software, 2001.
17. Waller KG, Shaw RW. Gonadotrophin-hormone releasing hormone analogues for the treatment of endometriosis; long term follow up. *Fertil Steril* 1993; 59:511–15.
18. Franke HR, van de Weijer PH, Pennings TM, van der Mooren MJ. Gonadotropin-releasing hormone agonist plus 'add-back' hormone replacement therapy for treatment of endometriosis: a prospective, randomized, placebo-controlled double-blind trial. *Fertil Steril* 2000; 74:534–9.

19. Hornstein MD, Surrey ES, Weisberg GW, Casino LA. Leuprolide acetate depot and hormonal add-back in endometriosis: a 12-month study. Leupron Add-Back Study Group. *Obstet Gynecol* 1998; **91**:16–24.

20. Mukherjee T, Baraad D, Turk R, Freeman R. A randomized placebo-controlled study on the effect of cyclic intermittent etidronate therapy on the bone mineral density changes associated with six months of gonadotropin-releasing hormone agonist treatment. *Am J Obstet Gynecol* 1996; **175**:105–9.

21. Jacobson TZ, Barlow DH, Garry R, Koninckx P. Laparoscopic surgery for pelvic pain associated with endometriosis (Cochrane Review). In: *The Cochrane Library*, Issue 4. Oxford: Update Software, 2001.

22. Sutton CJ, Ewen SP, Whitelaw N, Haines P. Prospective randomized, double-blind, controlled trial of laser laparoscopy in the treatment of pelvic pain associated with minimal, mild and moderate endometriosis. *Fertil Steril* 1994; **62**:696–700.

23. Sutton CJ, Pooley AS, Ewen SP, Haines P. Follow-up report on a randomized, controlled trial of laser laparoscopy in the treatment of pelvic pain associated with minimal to moderate endometriosis. *Fertil Steril* 1997; **68**:1070–4.

24. Vercellini P, De Giorgi O, Pisacreta A, Pesole AP, Vicentini S, Crosignani PG. Surgical management of endometriosis. *Baillière's Clin Obstet Gynaecol* 2000; **14**(3):501–23.

25. Magos A. Endometriosis: radical surgery. *Baillière's Clin Obstet Gynaecol* 1993; **7**(4):849–64.

26. Crosignani PG, Vercellini P, Biffignandi F, Constantini W, Cortesi I, Imparato E. Laparoscopy versus laparotomy in conservative surgical management for severe endometriosis. *Fertil Steril* 1996; **66**:706–11.

27. Donnez J, Nisolle M, Gillerot S, Anaf V, Clerckx-Braum F, Cananas-Roux F. Ovarian endometrial cysts: the role of gonadotropin-releasing hormone agonist and/or drainage. *Fertil Steril* 1994; **62**:63–6.

28. Vercellini P, Chapion C, De Giorgi O, Consonni D, Frontino G, Crosignani PG. Coagulation or excision of ovarian endometriosis? *Am J Obstet Gynecol* 2003;**188**:606–10.

29. Hormstein MD, Hemmings R, Yuzpe AA, Heinrichs WL. Use of nafarelin versus placebo after reductive laparoscopic surgery for endometriosis. *Fertil Steril* 1997;**68**:860–4.

30. Vercellini P, Crosignani PG, Fadini R, Radici E, Belloni C, Sismondi P. A gonadotropin-releasing hormone agonist compared with expectant management after conservative surgery for symptomatic endometriosis. *Br J Obstet Gynaecol* 1999; **106**:672–7.

31. Muzii M, Marana R, Caruana P, Catalano GF, Margutti F, Panici PB. Postoperative administration of monophasic combined oral contraceptives after laparoscopic treatment of ovarian endometriomas: a prospective, randomized trial. *Am J Obstet Gynecol* 2000; **183**:588–92.

32. Fedele L, Bianchi S, Rafaelli R, Zanconato G. Comparison of transdermal estradiol and tibolone for the treatment of oophorectomised women with deep residual endometriosis. *Maturitas* 1999; **32**:189–93.

Adenomyosis

Christine P. West

INTRODUCTION

Adenomyosis is implicated as a cause of both menorrhagia and dysmenorrhoea, but information about its prevalence among women presenting with these problems is lacking. Similarly, its incidence in a normal population is unknown. Most published information on adenomyosis is based on studies of hysterectomy specimens. This is because, until recently, the diagnosis has only been possible in retrospect. Recent advances in imaging have facilitated its diagnosis and led to greater opportunities for clinical trials of medical and conservative management. However, to date, such studies have been very limited and consequently the literature on adenomyosis is comparatively small, as is the evidence base for its management.

DEFINITION

Histologically, adenomyosis is characterized by the presence of endometrial glands and stroma in the myometrium, with adjacent smooth muscle hyperplasia,[1] the latter often resulting in significant uterine enlargement. The lesions are seen haphazardly and at varied depths within the myometrium, and the exact diagnostic criteria may be disputed.[2] Adenomyosis should be regarded as distinct from endometriosis in terms of its epidemiology, being most common in parous, middle-aged women. Although histologically both seem to have a common origin, the two conditions do not normally co-exist.

INCIDENCE

The incidence of adenomyosis is unknown. It is present in 15–30 per cent of hysterectomy specimens,[2–6] but its overall contribution to menstrual disorders is unclear. Studies based on findings at hysterectomy have yielded varied conclusions about the correlation between symptomatology and the presence of adenomyosis. Some have related the severity of dysmenorrhoea to the extent of adenomyosis and its depth of invasion into the myometrium,[7,8] but others have failed to find any relationship between its presence and individual symptoms[2] or the main indication for the hysterectomy.[4]

AETIOLOGY

Its cause remains speculative, but the adenomyotic tissue is presumed to be derived from the endometrium. It may be triggered by a weakness in the smooth muscle of the myometrium, by increased intrauterine pressure[1] or by surgical trauma. Among women undergoing hysterectomy, the incidence of adenomyosis is increased with increasing parity,[3,4] a history of miscarriage,[3] induced abortion[5,8] and caesarean section.[5] It is decreased in smokers compared with non-smokers.[3] A relationship between the presence of adenomyosis and both endometrial hyperplasia[1,2] and uterine fibroids[1,8] has been reported, but this may be related to the age and symptomatology of the women undergoing hysterectomy.

MANAGEMENT

Investigation

Available evidence suggests that women with symptomatic adenomyosis are likely to present with menorrhagia and dysmenorrhoea. Clinically, the uterus may be bulky and tender, but both the history and the clinical findings are very non-specific.

A large review of diagnostic techniques[9] concluded that transvaginal ultrasound (TVS) should be used as a primary screening modality for the diagnosis of adenomyosis [II]. Various sonographic appearances have been described,[10] including:

- diffuse echogenicity,
- myometrial cysts,
- subendometrial nodules,
- subendometrial linear striations,
- poor definition of the endometrial/myometrial border,
- asymmetric myometrial thickening.

However, TVS lacks specificity, in particular in distinguishing adenomyosis from fibroids.[9,11] In such cases, magnetic resonance imaging (MRI) should be used [II]. Both techniques, even when used in combination, may lack accuracy for the evaluation of very large uteri with a volume greater than 400 mL.[6]

Both hysteroscopic and laparoscopic myometrial biopsy techniques have been described,[12,13] but clearly have limitations when compared with non-invasive imaging.

Medical management

The current medical management of menstrual disorders includes non-steroidal anti-inflammatory drugs (NSAIDs), combined oral contraceptives, high-dose progestogens and the levonorgestrel-releasing intrauterine system (LNG-IUS). As most of these therapies are effective in the management of menorrhagia, dysmenorrhoea and endometriosis, they should theoretically be beneficial for adenomyosis [IV]. A small, uncontrolled study[14] showed the LNG-IUS to be effective in 23 out of 25 women with adenomyosis diagnosed at TVS and followed up for 12 months [III].

Surgical management

Where medical therapies fail, the presence or absence of adenomyosis may influence the choice of surgical treatment. There is some evidence that the presence of deep lesions of adenomyosis is associated with failure of endometrial ablation,[12,15] resulting in both regeneration of the endometrium and glandular activity within the myometrium [III]. However, at this stage it may not be possible to distinguish between pre-existing and iatrogenic lesions. On the basis of current evidence, use of the LNG-IUS may be preferred to endometrial ablation where a diagnosis of adenomyosis is suspected following TVS [III]. Hysterectomy is well established and, for the definitive treatment of adenomyosis, need not be accompanied by oophorectomy unless there are specific indications for the latter.

There is little supporting evidence for the advocated management plan, and the above text relies largely on small retrospective studies and descriptive studies.

KEY POINTS

- Adenomyosis is present in 15–30 per cent of hysterectomy specimens and is a cause of uterine enlargement.
- Its prevalence in the population is unknown and its role as a contributing factor to menstrual disorders is not well understood.
- TVS, backed up by MRI, is promising as a diagnostic tool [II].
- Medical therapy, including LNG-IUS, should be first-line management [IV].
- Endometrial ablation may carry a greater failure rate in the presence of adenomyosis [III].

KEY REFERENCES

1. Ferenczy A. Pathophysiology of adenomyosis. *Hum Reprod Update* 1998; 4:312–22.
2. Bergholt T, Eriksen L, Berendt N, Jacobsen M, Hertz JB. Prevalence and risk factors of adenomyosis at hysterectomy. *Hum Reprod* 2001; 16:2418–21.
3. Parazzini F, Vercellini P, Panazza S, Chatenoud L, Oldani S, Crosignani PG. Risk factors for adenomyosis. *Hum Reprod* 1997; 12:1275–9.
4. Vercellini P, Parazzini F, Oldani S, Panazza S, Bramante T, Crosignani PG. Adenomyosis at hysterectomy: a study on frequency distribution and patient characteristics. *Hum Reprod* 1995; 10:1160–2.

5. Valvis D, Agorastos T, Tzafetas J et al. Adenomyosis at hysterectomy: prevalence and relationship to operative findings and reproductive and menstrual factors. *Clin Exp Obstet Gynecol* 1997; **24**:36–8.

6. Dueholm M, Lundorf E, Hansen ES, Sorensen JS, Ledertoug S, Olesen F. Magnetic resonance imaging and transvaginal ultrasonography for the diagnosis of adenomyosis. *Fertil Steril* 2001; **76**:588–94.

7. Nishida M. Relationship between the degree of dysmenorrhoea and histologic findings in adenomyosis. *Am J Obstet Gynecol* 1991; **165**:229–31.

8. Levgur M, Abadi MA, Tucker A. Adenomyosis: symptoms, histology and pregnancy terminations. *Obstet Gynecol* 2000; **95**:688–91.

9. Arnold LL, Ascher SM, Schruefer JJ, Simon JA. The non-surgical diagnosis of adenomyosis. *Obstet Gynecol* 1995; **86**:461–5.

10. Atri M, Reinhold C, Mehio AR, Chapman WB, Bret PM. Adenomyosis: US features with histologic correlation in an in-vitro study. *Radiology* 2000; **215**:783–90.

11. Bazot M, Cortez A, Darai E et al. Ultrasonography compared with magnetic resonance imaging for the diagnosis of adenomyosis: correlation with histopathology. *Hum Reprod* 2001; **16**:2427–33.

12. McCausland AM, McCausland VM. Depth of endometrial penetration in adenomyosis helps determine outcome of rollerball ablation. *Am J Obstet Gynecol* 1996; **174**:1786–93.

13. Popp LW, Schwiedessen JP, Gaetje R. Myometrial biopsy in the diagnosis of adenomyosis uteri. *Am J Obstet Gynecol* 1993; **169**:546–9.

14. Fedele L, Bianchi S, Rafaelli R, Portuese A, Dorta M. Treatment of adenomyosis-associated menorrhagia with a levonorgestrel-releasing intrauterine device. *Fertil Steril* 1997; **68**:426–9.

15. Tresserra F, Grases P, Ubeda A, Pascual MA, Grases PJ, Labastida R. Morphological changes in hysterectomies after endometrial ablation. *Hum Reprod* 1999; **14**:1473–7.

Premenstrual Syndrome

Christine P. West

INTRODUCTION

Adverse emotional and physical symptoms are experienced by the majority of women in the lead-up to menstruation, although they are usually mild and regarded as a normal physiological response to cyclical hormone changes. However, a substantial number of women are sufficiently distressed by their symptoms to seek medical help and a minority are severely incapacitated by them. Hormonal treatments were commonly used in the past, but premenstrual syndrome (PMS) is no longer regarded as an endocrine disorder and first-line management includes non-hormonal approaches. However, the symptoms are triggered by the endocrine changes of the menstrual cycle and women with PMS continue to be referred to gynaecologists for consideration of hormonal suppression when other therapies have failed. Assessment of the efficacy of treatment for PMS is complicated by the subjective nature of the diagnosis and the strong placebo effect. Prospective methods of symptom assessment are now well established and there is an expanding literature of randomized, controlled trials covering various approaches to management, including several systematic reviews.

DEFINITIONS

Premenstrual syndrome is a cluster of menstrually related symptoms, which include:

- mood swings,
- tension, anger, irritability,
- headache,
- breast discomfort,
- bloating,
- increased appetite and food cravings.

These symptoms occur during the luteal phase of the cycle and are relieved with the onset of menstruation or soon afterwards. A minority of women with PMS suffer from premenstrual dysphoric disorder (PMDD), defined in the *Diagnostic and Statistical Manual of Mental Disorders, Fourth Edition* (DSM-IV). This is a more severe and disabling form of PMS in which mood symptoms predominate. Because no objective tests can confirm PMS or PMDD, the diagnosis is made on the basis of prospective daily symptom recording using various rating scales.[1]

Premenstrual syndrome and PMDD must be distinguished from premenstrual magnification/aggravation, in which symptoms are present throughout the cycle but are exacerbated premenstrually. There may also be premenstrual exacerbation of underlying psychiatric or medical disorders.

INCIDENCE

In a population-based questionnaire survey of 1083 women aged 18–46 in Goteborg,[2] 92 per cent experienced at least one adverse symptom in the lead-up to menstruation. Seventy per cent reported mental symptoms in combination with bodily swelling, and 30–40 per cent rated their symptoms as mild to moderate in intensity. Eleven per cent felt that their symptoms were severe enough to seek medical help. A study of 500 women from a UK-based general practice population[3] reported very similar findings. Such population-based studies rely on retrospective assessment and do not distinguish between PMS and premenstrual magnification, so that the true prevalence of PMS and PMDD is unclear. However, it is evident that cyclical symptoms contribute significantly to menstrual cycle morbidity.

AETIOLOGY

The frequency with which these symptoms are reported by women suggests that in their milder form they are a normal manifestation of the menstrual cycle, although it is likely that those at the more extreme end of the normal range have a pathological cause. Despite their relationship with the endocrine changes of the menstrual cycle, there is no evidence for any underlying disorder of the hypothalamo–pituitary–ovarian axis in women with PMS or PMDD. There have been many theories of aetiology, but current evidence suggests that PMS is a neuroendocrine disorder caused by serotonergic dysfunction,[4] which is supported by evidence that drugs that enhance serotonergic function are beneficial in its management.[5]

It is likely that there is a hormonally related trigger factor. Recent research indicates that this may be abnormal metabolism of progesterone to its metabolites allopregnenalone and pregnenalone, neuroactive steroids with differential effects on anxiety-related symptoms. Allopregnenalone has anxiolytic actions, whereas pregnenalone may promote anxiety.[4] However, the basis for any metabolic disorder remains unclear.

A study of prospective daily symptom self-assessment by women referred for specialist help because of cyclical symptoms found that PMS was confirmed in only one-third,[6] the remainder showing premenstrual magnification of ongoing psychological symptoms or symptoms exacerbated by menstruation itself. There was a significant relationship between menstrual and premenstrual magnification and previous psychiatric disorders, marital breakdown and increased parity.[6] Other studies have shown a relationship between self-reported PMS and personality disorders[3] and psychosocial stress.[7]

MANAGEMENT

Women with mild degrees of PMS are unlikely to seek medical help, but if they do, they should respond to reassurance and simple lifestyle and dietary advice (see below). Basic management lies within the scope of primary care. Referral for specialist help will depend on the severity of the problem, the experience of individual general practitioners and the expectations of the women involved. Most women

referred for specialist help will be experiencing disruption of family or professional life and have a history of previous treatment failures. Ideally, women with severe PMS should be seen in a specialist clinic or at least by a gynaecologist or a psychiatrist with a particular interest in the problem, preferably in a community-based clinic.

A diagnosis of PMS or PMDD based on retrospective history taking is unreliable, and prospective charting of symptoms for at least two menstrual cycles is essential in order to clarify the symptom pattern [Ia]. This must be preceded by a detailed medical, social and psychiatric history. Many methods of symptom assessment are available,[8] but as they are time consuming to analyse, most are only suitable for use in a specialist clinic or research setting. Simple pictorial charts are available for use in primary care.

All randomized, controlled trials of treatment for PMS have shown a very marked placebo response. This emphasizes the importance of critical appraisal of the evidence base before recommending specific therapies. The strength of the placebo effect in all trials of therapy for PMS may reflect the positive role of detailed history taking and a sympathetic approach.

Complementary and alternative therapies

These approaches are popular with patients and, given the high level of placebo response, are likely to be perceived as effective without the potential disadvantage of side effects associated with conventional medications. Many randomized trials have been reported using a variety of alternative therapies for PMS. There have been three systematic reviews of trials of such therapies: one covering a wide range of approaches,[9] one addressing dietary supplements,[10] and one on the use of vitamin B6.[11]

Dietary supplements

Vitamin B6, evening primrose oil, calcium, magnesium and vitamin E have all been compared with placebo in small-scale, randomized, controlled trials. Results showed a beneficial effect from calcium ($n = 2$), magnesium ($n = 3$) and vitamin E ($n = 2$) over placebo.[9,10] Only one of these, comparing calcium 1200 mg daily with placebo, was a large-scale multicentre study. Despite these positive results, the reviewers felt that weaknesses in methodology limited their recommendations of the value of such interventions [Ib]. Similarly, studies of nutritional supplements containing high doses of vitamins and other micronutrients have yielded inconclusive results.[9]

Dietary supplements are popular because they are perceived to have fewer side effects than conventional medicines. However, high-dose vitamin B6, used for many years for the treatment of PMS, was reported to have neurotoxic effects at doses above 200 mg daily.[11] A meta-analysis of ten randomized, controlled trials comparing various doses of vitamin B6 with placebo in 940 women[11] showed results significantly in favour of vitamin B6 for overall symptomatic response and for depression. There was no dose–response effect. Despite their comments on the methodological weaknesses of the studies, the authors concluded that 'doses of vitamin B6 up to 100 mg daily are likely to be of benefit in treating premenstrual symptoms and premenstrual depression' [Ia].

A meta-analysis of placebo-controlled trials of evening primrose oil[12] failed to find sufficient evidence to support its use for PMS [Ia], although at high dosage it is licensed for the relief of premenstrual mastalgia.

Despite the negative conclusions of the reviewers cited above, a recent Expert Consensus Group has endorsed the use of nutritional approaches for women with PMDD [IV].[13]

Herbal medicine

The fruit of the chaste tree (*Vitex agnus castus*) contains a mixture of iridoids and flavonoids and some compounds similar in structure to sex steroids. Initial controlled studies of its use were felt to be inconclusive.[9] A more recent, well-conducted, multicentre, randomized, controlled study[14] has shown the active treatment to be significantly more effective than placebo for the majority of the symptoms assessed (with the exception of bloating), with an overall response rate of 53 per cent for active treatment and 24 per cent for placebo. On the basis of this evidence, *Vitex agnus castus* fruit extract seems to be a potentially useful therapy for PMS [Ib].

Other alternative approaches

Massage, relaxation and aromatherapy are popular therapies for which benefit is likely to outweigh any possible harm [IV], although controlled studies of their use for PMS have yielded inconclusive results.[9] Chiropractic therapy has not been found to be effective. Similarly, although advice about graded exercise is useful for general health, there is no evidence for or against a specific benefit in PMS.

Support and self-help groups are commonly used for PMS. This approach has been evaluated in a controlled study. A package of strategies including self-monitoring, personal choice, self-regulation and environmental modification was administered within a peer support group with professional guidance. Comparison was with a control group waiting for the intervention. The active intervention was reported to be effective [Ib],[15] with a 75 per cent reduction in severity of PMS.

Cognitive therapy has also been evaluated by comparing immediate treatment with delayed treatment, showing a substantial improvement in the immediate treatment group [Ib].[16] However, such therapy is intensive, involving 12 weekly sessions of individual cognitive therapy, and thus not applicable for the majority of sufferers unless symptoms are very severe.

The Expert Consensus Group cited above[13] has endorsed the use of psychobehavioural approaches for women with PMDD [Ib].

HORMONAL MANIPULATION FOR THE MANAGEMENT OF PMS

Hormonal interventions for PMS fall into two main categories: supplementary cyclical progesterone or progestogens and therapies that suppress ovulation. There is current support for the latter approach on the basis that, although there is no identifiable underlying endocrine disorder, ovulation appears to act as a trigger factor and thus strategies that suppress ovulation or abolish the cycle altogether are likely to be beneficial.

Progesterone and progestogens

Luteal phase supplements of progesterone were widely used in the past, based on the unfounded assumption that PMS was secondary to a progesterone deficiency. In the UK, progesterone is available only for vaginal or rectal administration, hence the use of synthetic progestogens for this indication. However, evidence from hormone replacement therapy (HRT) studies indicate that these therapies might actually exacerbate PMS-type symptoms in susceptible individuals.[17]

A recent systematic review assessed 14 randomized, controlled trials of progesterone and four of progestogens in PMS.[18] Overall results of meta-analysis for progesterone showed no difference compared with placebo. There was a very small but significant benefit in the four studies that used oral micronized progesterone, while results favoured placebo in the eight studies that used progesterone suppositories. Results with progestogens were difficult to interpret due to the small number of studies and differences in the treatment protocols. Overall odds ratios were marginally but significantly in favour of progestogens for both physical and behavioural symptoms. The number of drop-outs due to side effects was high. The response to progestogens may have been influenced by the fact that two of the four studies used progestogens in an ovulation-suppressing regimen. However, this evidence does not support the use of either progesterone or progestogens in the management of PMS when given during the luteal phase of the cycle [Ia]. While the use of progestogens in ovulation suppressive doses (e.g. Depo-Provera) may be beneficial, there is insufficient evidence to support this approach.

Combined oral contraceptives

The occurrence of PMS symptoms in the post-ovulatory phase of the menstrual cycle and the observation that spontaneous anovulation causes the disappearance of cyclical symptoms in women with PMS[19] strongly suggest that any therapy that suppresses ovulation should relieve PMS. The combined oral contraceptive pill (COCP) has the advantage of being cheap and suitable for long-term use. Population and contraceptive studies have yielded varied results. Some have shown a reduction in the prevalence and severity of PMS with both older high-dose preparations[20] and new low-dose combinations.[21,22] Other studies have failed to show any difference in cyclical symptoms between COCP users and non-users amongst randomly selected women[23] or those self-selected because of reported PMS.[24] One study reporting a beneficial effect also showed that benefit was more marked in those with prospectively confirmed PMS compared with premenstrual aggravation,[21] illustrating the importance of distinguishing between the two groups.

Taken overall, this evidence suggests that a trial of therapy with a low-dose COCP is appropriate for women with no contraindications to its use [II].

Transdermal oestradiol

Transdermal oestradiol has been used in ovulation-suppressive doses in combination with cyclical luteal phase progestogen for the management of severe PMS. A dose of 200 μg twice weekly was found to be more effective than placebo in an initial cross-over study. Subsequently, a lower dose of 100 μg twice weekly was found to be as effective in the suppression of ovulation and symptom relief as the 200 μg dosage[25] but with fewer oestrogenic side effects. The authors did not comment on side effects related to the progestogen. Overall satisfaction at 8 months was around 50 per cent. These limited data support the role of ovulation-suppressive doses of transdermal oestradiol for the relief of PMS [Ib]. Its use in combination with the levonorgestrel-releasing intrauterine system for endometrial protection is an approach that merits future investigation.

Danazol

Several studies have supported the use of danazol for PMS. At a dose of 200 mg bd in a cross-over study,[26] 44 per cent of subjects on active therapy experienced a clinically significant improvement, compared with only 8 per cent of those treated with placebo. Although effective [Ib], the side effects and metabolic sequelae of danazol limit its usefulness for the long-term management of PMS.

GnRH agonists

Ovarian suppression with gonadotrophin releasing hormone (GnRH) agonists should eliminate PMS or PMDD when the diagnosis is confirmed by prospective assessment. However, results of placebo-controlled studies have emphasized the limitations of this approach. Whereas physical symptoms and some emotional symptoms such as irritability and fatigue respond well [Ib], severe premenstrual depression

may not be improved.[27] Women with premenstrual exacerbation of ongoing dysphoric symptoms do not experience symptom relief.[28] GnRH agonists therefore offer a useful means of further assessment in situations in which the diagnosis is unclear or, in particular, when oophorectomy is being considered.

In women with severe PMDD relieved by GnRH agonists, the use of hormonal add-back is necessary if treatment is to be long-term. In a double-blind, placebo-controlled study of the use of tibolone in women who had responded to leuprolide acetate,[29] symptomatic response was maintained in both groups [Ib]. However, in women who responded to a GnRH agonist, cyclical addition of oestradiol and progesterone caused symptom recurrence, which did not occur with placebo.[30]

The cost and potentially long-term nature of treatment of PMS with GnRH agonists when used with hormonal add-back should limit its use to women with severe symptoms that are socially disruptive and resistant to other forms of therapy [IV]. GnRH agonists alone may be used in the short term to clarify the pattern and nature of cyclical symptoms [IV].[30]

Oophorectomy

Although there have been reports of its efficacy in the literature,[31,32] oophorectomy is not recommended for the management of PMS unless the problem is very severe and has been confirmed by prospective assessment and there has been genuine failure of conservative therapies [IV].[31,32] It should not be considered unless supported by a trial of ovarian suppression with danazol[31] or, preferably, a GnRH agonist.[33] The latter also gives an opportunity to assess the response of the patient to add-back HRT. In the latter situation, the pros and cons of continuing medical suppression together with add-back HRT need to be carefully considered. Unless there are additional indications for hysterectomy, laparoscopic oophorectomy offers a less invasive surgical approach. In women undergoing hysterectomy for other indications, a history of PMS is not a sufficient indication for concurrent oophorectomy without careful assessment [IV],[33] as cyclical symptoms often improve following hysterectomy [II].[34] Indeed, improvement of PMS has been reported following endometrial ablation.[34]

Spironolactone

Spironolactone, a steroid receptor antagonist that has diuretic and anti-androgenic actions, has been used for the management of PMS with variable results. Originally it was used because of its diuretic actions, although there is no evidence that PMS symptoms are secondary to fluid retention. The most recent randomized, controlled trial[35] compared spironolactone 100 mg given during the luteal phase of the cycle with placebo using a six-cycle cross-over design. The results showed a significantly greater improvement in both somatic and mood symptoms with spironolactone, although its effect on the somatic symptoms of swelling and breast discomfort was more marked than on the psychological symptoms. Although the supporting evidence is limited, cyclical spironolactone may have a role in the management of PMS where physical symptoms predominate [Ib].

Selective serotonin reuptake inhibitors

Selective serotonin reuptake inhibitors (SSRIs) are now regarded as a first-line therapy for moderate to severe PMS, particularly in women who fulfil the criteria for PMDD. The use of SSRIs for PMS has been the subject of a systematic review.[5] Fifteen trials were included in the review. Various doses of fluoxetine ($n = 7$), sertraline ($n = 5$), citalopram ($n = 1$), paroxetine ($n = 1$) and fluvoxamine ($n = 1$) were used and whereas the majority used continuous therapy, some studied luteal-phase-only administration. The results strongly favoured active treatment over placebo for both behavioural and physical symptoms. The onset of effectiveness was rapid, and luteal-phase-only therapy seemed to be as effective as continuous treatment. The most commonly tested therapy was fluoxetine 20 mg daily, followed by sertraline 50–150 mg daily. Withdrawals due to side effects were 2.5 times more likely in the active treatment groups. Insomnia, gastrointestinal disturbances and fatigue were the most commonly reported side effects, reported by up to 20 per cent of subjects.

On the basis of this review, SSRIs, used continuously or cyclically, can be regarded as a first-line treatment for severe PMS [Ia]. They have the advantage of being suitable for long-term use. Despite this convincing evidence for their efficacy, side effects are a common reason for poor compliance, and 30–40 per cent of women with PMS fail to respond to SSRIs. High baseline symptomatology is one predictor of poor response.[36]

Other centrally active drugs

Selective serotinin reuptake inhibitors are significantly more effective than tricyclic antidepressants for PMS.[5] Alprazolam (a benzodiazepine) has been evaluated for its effectiveness in PMS and PMDD. Although initially results were positive, recent studies have failed to confirm its effectiveness [Ib].[37]

Venlafaxine is a selective inhibitor of both serotonin and noradrenaline reuptake. In a randomized, controlled trial of 164 women with PMDD,[38] venlafaxine at doses of 50–150 mg daily was significantly better than placebo in relieving both mood and physical symptoms. However, it remains unclear whether this drug has any advantage over existing therapies in specific groups of PMS sufferers or in the overall management of the condition.

MANAGEMENT OF WOMEN WITH PREMENSTRUAL MAGNIFICATION

There is now a wide evidence base for the management of PMS. However, eligibility for treatment trials included prospective confirmation of the diagnosis by daily self-rating, so that the majority excluded the group of women whose management tends to be most problematic – those with premenstrual magnification. The presence of high baseline postmenstrual symptom scores has been identified as one factor that leads to treatment failure with SSRIs[36] and GnRH agonists[28] and to poor response to the COCP.[21] Women with premenstrual magnification are therefore likely to be over-represented among those who present because of treatment failure. It is important that this group is identified and the nature of the problem and the limitations of management appreciated by both the clinician and the patient so that these women are not subjected to inappropriate and over-aggressive interventions such as hormonal manipulation or even surgery.

CONCLUSION

There is a wide range of therapies that have proven efficacy for PMS and PMDD. However, response rates to any individual therapy are rarely in excess of 60 per cent, and thus it is important that those involved in management are aware of these limitations and of different approaches to the problem. Ideally, women with severe symptoms and treatment failure should be managed in specialist multidisciplinary clinics. The importance of making a correct diagnosis based on adequate prospective daily symptom assessment cannot be over-emphasized.

- There are many published randomized, controlled trials covering various approaches to the management of PMS, but some of those relating to alternative therapies are open to methodological criticism.
- There have been five systematic reviews of PMS therapy, three of which relate to alternative or dietary approaches.

KEY POINTS

- Diagnosis of PMS should be confirmed by at least two cycles of prospective daily symptom rating [Ia].
- All treatment trials to date have demonstrated a strong placebo effect [Ia].

- Expert opinion is divided about the benefit of nutritional approaches [IV].
- Doses of vitamin B6 up to 100 mg daily are likely to be of benefit in treating premenstrual symptoms and premenstrual depression [Ia].
- *Vitex agnus castus*, a herbal therapy, is effective for the relief of the symptoms of PMS [Ib].
- Limited evidence supports the role of group support, lifestyle modification, cognitive therapy [Ib] and physical interventions such as relaxation [II].
- Progesterone or progestogens given during the luteal phase of the menstrual cycle are not effective for PMS [Ia].
- Suppression of ovulation with a COCP may be beneficial [II].
- Suppression of ovulation with transdermal oestradiol combined with progestogen for endometrial protection is effective in around 50 per cent of women [Ib].
- Danazol is effective for PMS but is not suitable for long-term use [Ib].
- GnRH analogues are effective for severe PMS and current evidence favours the use of continuous preparations such as tibolone for hormonal add-back [Ib].
- Oophorectomy should only be considered in severe PMS when medical measures have failed, and only if preceded by a trial of GnRH agonist therapy [IV].
- Used cyclically, spironolactone may have a role in the management of PMS where physical symptoms of breast discomfort and bloating predominate [Ib].
- SSRIs are effective for relieving both the physical and psychological symptoms of PMS [Ia].
- SSRIs are equally effective when given during the luteal phase of the cycle, and this is associated with fewer side effects [Ia].
- Tricyclic antidepressants and benzodiazepines (alprazolam) are not effective for PMS or PMDD [Ib].
- The presence of high baseline symptom scores (premenstrual magnification) is an important contributor to treatment failure [Ib].
- Women with severe PMS or PMDD, particularly those with a history of treatment failures, should be managed in a specialist clinic [IV].

KEY REFERENCES

1. Born L, Steiner M. Current management of the premenstrual syndrome and premenstrual dysphoric disorder. *Curr Psychiatry Rep* 2001; 3:463–9.

2. Andersch C, Wendestram L, Hahn L, Ohman R. Premenstrual complaints. 1. Prevalence of premenstrual symptoms in a Swedish urban population. *J Psychosom Obstet Gynecol* 1986; 5:39–49.

3. Coppen A, Kessel N. Menstruation and personality. *Br J Psychiatry* 1963; 109:711–21.

4. Berga SL. Understanding premenstrual syndrome. *Lancet* 1998; 351:465–6.

5. Dimmock PW, Wyatt KM, Jones PW, O'Brien PM. Efficacy of selective serotonin reuptake inhibitors in premenstrual syndrome: a systematic review. *Lancet* 2000; 356:1131–6.

6. West CP. The characteristics of 100 women presenting to a gynaecological clinic with premenstrual complaints. *Acta Obstet Gynaecol Scand* 1990; 68:743–7.

7. Warner P, Bancroft J. Factors related to self reporting of the premenstrual syndrome. *Br J Psychiatry* 1990; 157:249–60.

8. Steiner M, Streiner DL, Steinberg S et al. The measurement of premenstrual mood symptoms. *J Affect Disord* 1999; 53:269–73.

9. Stevinson C, Ernst E. Complementary/alternative therapies for premenstrual syndrome: a systematic review of randomized controlled trials. *Am J Obstet Gynecol* 2001; 185:227–35.

10. Carter J, Verhoef MJ. Efficacy of self-help and alternative treatments of premenstrual syndrome. *Women's Health Issues* 1994; 4:130–7.

11. Wyatt KM, Dimmock PW, Jones PW, Shaughan O'Brien PM. Efficacy of vitamin B6 in the treatment of premenstrual syndrome: systematic review. *BMJ* 1999; 318:1375–81.

12. Budeiri D, Li Wan Po A, Dornan JC. Is evening primrose oil of value in the treatment of premenstrual syndrome? *Control Clin Trials* 1996; 17:60–8.

13. Altshuler LL, Cohen LS, Moline ML, Kahn DA, Carpenter D, Docherty JP. The Expert Consensus Panel for Depression in Women. The Expert Consensus Guideline Series. Treatment of depression in women. *Postgrad Med* 2001; March: 1–107.

14. Schellenberg R. Treatment for the premenstrual syndrome with agnus castus fruit extract: prospective, randomised, placebo controlled study. *BMJ* 2001; 322:134–7.

15. Taylor D. Effectiveness of professional-peer group treatment: symptom management for women with PMS. *Res Nurs Health* 1999; 22:496–511.

16. Blake F, Salkovskis P, Gath D, Day A, Garrod A. Cognitive therapy for premenstrual syndrome: a controlled trial. *J Psychosom Res* 1998; 45:307–18.

17. Bjorn I, Bixo M, Nojd KS, Nyberg S, Backstrom T. Negative mood changes during hormone replacement therapy: a comparison between two progestogens. *Am J Obstet Gynecol* 2000; 183:1419–26.

18. Wyatt K, Dimmock P, Jones P, Obhrai M, O'Brien S. Efficacy of progesterone and progestogens in

management of premenstrual syndrome: systematic review. *BMJ* 2001; 323:776–80.

19. Hammarback S, Ekholm UB, Backstrom T. Spontaneous anovulation causing disappearance of cyclical symptoms in women with the premenstrual syndrome. *Acta Endocrinol (Copenh)* 1991; 125:132–7.

20. Andersch B, Hahn L. Premenstrual complaints II. Influence of oral contraceptives. *Acta Obstet Gynaecol Scand* 1981; 60:579–83.

21. Backstrom T, Hansson-Malmstrom Y, Lindhe BA, Cavalli-Bjorkman B, Nordenstrom S. Oral contraceptives in premenstrual syndrome: a randomized comparison of triphasic and monophasic preparations. *Contraception* 1992; 46:253–68.

22. Serfaty D, Vree ML. A comparison of the cycle control and tolerability of two ultra low-dose oral contraceptives containing 20 micrograms ethinyloestradiol and either 150 micrograms desogestrel or 75 micrograms gestodene. *Eur J Contracep Reprod Health Care* 1998; 3:179–89.

23. Sveindottir H, Backstrom T. Prevalence of menstrual cycle cyclicity and premenstrual dysphoric disorder in a random sample of women using and not using oral contraceptives. *Acta Obstet Gynaecol Scand* 2000; 79:405–13.

24. Bancroft J, Rennie D. The impact of oral contraceptives on the experience of perimenstrual mood, clumsiness, food craving and other symptoms. *J Psychosom Res* 1993; 37:195–202.

25. Smith RN, Studd JW, Zamblera D, Holland EF. A randomised comparison over 8 months of 100 micrograms and 200 micrograms twice weekly doses of transdermal oestradiol in the treatment of severe premenstrual syndrome. *Br J Obstet Gynaecol* 1995; 102:475–84.

26. Hahn PM, Van Vugt DA, Reid RL. A randomized, placebo-controlled, crossover trial of danazol for the treatment of premenstrual syndrome. *Psychoneuroendocrinology* 1995; 20:193–209.

27. Brown CS, Ling FW, Andersen RN, Farmer RG, Arheart KL. Efficacy of depot leuprolide in premenstrual syndrome: effect of symptom severity and type in a controlled trial. *Obstet Gynecol* 1994; 84:779–86.

28. Freeman EW, Sondheimer SJ, Rickels K. Gonadotropin-releasing hormone agonist in the treatment of premenstrual symptoms with and without ongoing dysphoria; a controlled study. *Psychopharmacol Bull* 1997; 33:303–9.

29. Di Carlo C, Palomba S, Tommaselli GA, Guida M, Di Spienzio Sardo A, Nappi C. Use of leuprolide acetate plus tibolone in the treatment of severe premenstrual syndrome. *Fertil Sreril* 2001; 75:380–4.

30. Schmidt PJ, Nieman LK, Danaceau MA, Adams LF, Rubinow DR. Differential behavioral effects of gonadal steroids in women with or without premenstrual syndrome. *N Engl J Med* 1998; 338:209–16.

31. Casson P, Hahn PM, Van Vugt DA, Reid RL. Lasting response to ovariectomy in severe intractable premenstrual syndrome. *Am J Obstet Gynecol* 1990; 162:99–105.

32. Casper RF, Hearn MT. The effect of hysterectomy and bilateral oophorectomy in women with severe premenstrual syndrome. *Am J Obstet Gynecol* 1990; 162:105–9.

33. Argent V, Woodward Z. Consent and the ovary. *Obstet Gynecol* 2001; 3(4):206–10.

34. Pinion SB, Parkin DE, Abramovich DR et al. Randomised trial of hysterectomy, endometrial laser ablation, and transcervical endometrial resection for dysfunctional uterine bleeding. *Lancet* 1994; 309:979–83.

35. Wang M, Hammarback S, Lindhe BA, Backstrom T. Treatment of premenstrual syndrome by spironolactone: a double-blind, placebo-controlled study. *Acta Obstet Gynaecol Scand* 1995; 74:803–8.

36. Freeman EW, Sondheimer SJ, Polansky M, Garcia-Espagna B. Predictors of response to sertraline treatment of severe premenstrual syndromes. *J Clin Psychiatry* 2000; 61:579–84.

37. Schmidt PJ, Grover GN, Rubinow DR. Alprazolam in the treatment of premenstrual syndrome. A double-blind placebo-controlled trial. *Arch Gen Psychiatry* 1993; 50:467–73.

38. Freeman EW, Rickels K, Yonkers KA, Kunz NR, McPherson M, Upton GV. Venlafaxine in the treatment of premenstrual dysphoric syndrome. *Obstet Gynecol* 2001; 98:737–44.

Normal Conception

Hany A.M.A. Lashen

INTRODUCTION

The fusion of the male and female gametes is the core event in reproduction. The genetic material in the two haploid gametes combines to produce a diploid zygote. In mammals the fusion of the gametes occurs within the female reproductive tract, and is followed by implantation and the development of the fetus in the uterus. Gametes are produced in the gonads, which also have endocrine functions that are essential for successful reproduction. It is important to explore the embryology, anatomy and some physiological aspects of the ovary and testis in order to understand conception and infertility.

THE OVARY AND FEMALE GAMETE

The functions of the ovary are to engineer the periodic release of gametes (oocytes) and to produce steroid and glycoprotein hormones. Both functions are integrated in the continuous process of growth and maturation of the Graafian follicle, containing the oocyte, followed by ovulation and formation of the corpus luteum, which then regresses if pregnancy does not occur. The ovary is a heterogeneous, ever-changing tissue whose cyclicity is measured in weeks. The human ovary consists of three major components:

1 the outer cortex, the outer part of which is the tunica albugenia, and the internal part consists of primordial follicles embedded in stromal tissue;
2 the inner medulla;
3 the rete ovarii (hilum), which is attached to the mesovarium and contains nerves, blood vessels and hilar cells, which have the potential to become active in steroidogenesis. The hilar cells are similar to the testosterone-producing Leydig cells of the testes.

The embryonic development of the ovary passes through four stages.

1 *The indifferent gonadal stage.* This stage lasts about 7–10 days and starts at approximately 5 weeks' gestation. It starts with the development of the gonadal ridges, which consist of consolidated coelomic projections overlying the mesonephros. At this stage the ridges are indistinguishable as testes or ovaries. The gonadal ridge is the only site where the germ cells (the direct precursors of the sperm and oocytes) can survive. By the sixth week, the indifferent stage is completed, leaving the indifferent gonads consisting of germ and supporting cells derived from the coelomic epithelium and the mesenchyme of the gonadal ridge.

2 *The stage of differentiation.* This occurs at 6–9 weeks if the gonad is destined to be a testis.

3 *The stage of oogonial multiplication and maturation.* This starts at 6–8 weeks and represents the first sign of ovarian differentiation. A rapid mitotic division of the germ cells takes place, giving rise to the oogonia, and by 10–12 weeks the number of oogonia reaches 6–7 million. This is the maximal oogonial content of the gonads. From this point onwards, the germ cell content will irretrievably decrease and will be exhausted approximately 50 years later. The germ cells undergo mitosis to produce the oogonia that enter the first meiotic division and arrest in the prophase to become oocytes. This process begins at 11–12 weeks, perhaps in response to a factor or factors produced by the rete ovarii.[1] Progression of meiotic prophase to the diplotene stage takes place throughout the rest of the intrauterine life. The completion of the first meiotic division occurs just before ovulation, and the second meiotic division takes place at sperm penetration. As a result of the two meiotic divisions, a single haploid ovum is produced and the excess genetic material is extruded as one polar body at the completion of each meiotic division.

There is a continuous loss of germ cells during all these events, as a result of several mechanisms: (a) follicular growth, atresia and regression during meiosis; (b) the follicles, which fail to become enveloped by granulosa cells, undergo atresia; (c) some germ cells migrate to the surface of the gonads and become incorporated into the surface epithelium or become eliminated into the peritoneal cavity. Once all the oocytes are incorporated into follicles (shortly after birth), the loss of oocytes will only take place as a result of follicular growth and atresia.

4 *The stage of follicular formation.* This starts at 14–20 weeks, when the entire follicle undergoes various stages of maturation leading to the production of the primary follicle before atresia takes place. However, ovulation does not occur in the fetal ovary.

At the onset of puberty, the germ cell mass, incorporated into primordial follicles, is usually reduced to approximately 300 000 follicles. These regularly undergo various stages of maturation, development and atresia. In all, less than 0.1 per cent of follicles will grow beyond the pre-antral stage and develop into a dominant follicle, which ovulates. This enormous attrition of primordial follicles forms part of the process of natural selection, by which only a tiny number of randomly selected germ cells pass through the reproductive cycle and form a new individual.

As the dominant follicle grows, it produces oestrogens, predominantly oestradiol, and inhibins, predominantly inhibin B. These hormones synchronize the development of the endometrial lining of the uterus with that of the follicle, and prepare the pituitary for eventual triggering of the luteinizing hormone (LH) surge. Once oestradiol production from the dominant follicle passes a threshold, a positive feedback is triggered at the pituitary and the LH surge occurs, leading to ovulation. Ovulation results in the physical release of the oocyte, allowing it to enter the fallopian tube, with potential for fertilization. The follicle then becomes blood filled and develops into the corpus luteum, the source of progesterone and inhibin A in the second half (luteal phase) of the cycle. Production of the sex steroids by the corpus luteum results in preparation of the uterus and the entire woman's body for the occurrence of conception. For this regular periodic process to occur, accurate communication between the ovary and the pituitary gland is essential.

THE TESTIS AND MALE GAMETE

The physiological responsibilities of the testis are, in principle, similar to those of the ovary, i.e. the production of gametes (spermatozoa) and sex steroids (testosterone). However, sex steroid production in the male is a continuous, non-episodic process, which is independent of the development of gametes. The early embryonic stages of testicular development also follow those of the ovary, starting from the indifferent gonad stage. However, at 6–7 weeks of embryonic life of the male fetus, the production of testes-determining factor (TDF) results in differentiation of the gonads to testes. TDF is the product of a gene located on the Y chromosome. However, the male phenotype is dependent on the production of anti-Müllerian hormone and testosterone. The absence of these two factors leads to the development of the female phenotype. Differentiation of the testis leads to the production of the spermatic cords, which include the Sertoli cells and primordial germ cells that later become the spermatogonia. The mature Sertoli cells produce androgen-binding protein and inhibin B. The former is responsible for maintaining the high local androgen environment necessary for spermatogenesis. The Leydig cells develop from the mesenchymal cells surrounding the spermatic cords. They produce testosterone, the secretion of which increases with the increase in the number of Leydig cells. The Leydig cell number reaches a peak at 15–18 weeks, after which they regress, leaving a few cells present at birth. These cells become responsive to gonadotrophins at puberty, leading to the production of testosterone and the initiation of spermatogenesis. The spermatogonia divide mitotically to produce primary spermatocytes, which then divide meiotically to produce the haploid secondary spermatocytes. Secondary spermatocytes undergo a maturation process to produce the spermatid, then the mature spermatozoon.

The Sertoli cells influence the process of spermatogenesis and are directed by genes on the Y chromosome. Approximately 74 days are required to produce a mature spermatozoon, of which about 50 days are spent in the seminiferous tubules. After leaving the testicle, the sperm takes 12–21 days to travel to the epididymis and appear in the ejaculate.

FOLLICULAR DEVELOPMENT, MATURATION AND OVULATION

Follicular development

This involves several stages, starting with the mobilization of the dormant primordial follicles to form a cohort of growing follicles, which progress through the pre-antral, antral, and pre-ovulatory stages to produce (usually) one dominant follicle that reaches ovulation. The mechanism determining which primordial follicles and how many will be released into the pool of growing follicles in each menstrual cycle is not known. However, this may be regulated by an intra-ovarian mechanism. The number of primordial follicles released from quiescence to enter the pool of growing follicles each cycle seems to be proportional to the size of the residual pool. Therefore, the reduction of the primordial follicle pool by total or partial unilateral oophorectomy, or towards the end of reproductive life, may result in a smaller cohort of growing follicles. The onset and the time span of folliculogenesis have been controversial. Mais et al.[2] suggested that the follicle destined to ovulate is recruited in the first few days of the cycle, whereas Gougeon[3] suggested that such a process occurs over a time span of several cycles, estimated to be 85 days to achieve a pre-ovulatory status. The initiation of follicular growth in the early stages is independent of pituitary control; however, without a rise in follicle-stimulating hormone (FSH), these follicles are destined for atresia.

Soon after the initial resumption of maturation, the follicle develops FSH receptors and becomes capable of responding to circulating FSH. This is known as the pre-antral stage, which starts to occur towards the end of the luteal phase of the preceding cycle. FSH, aided by other autocrine/paracrine factors, initiates steroidogenesis and granulosa cell proliferation, and is also responsible for up-regulation and down-regulation of its own receptors. Therefore the fate of each pre-antral follicle in the developing pool depends on its ability to convert an androgen microenvironment to an oestrogen microenvironment. This requires the development of aromatase within the granulosa cells that line the follicle. Once one follicle acquires sufficient aromatase to produce and secrete significant quantities of oestradiol, the remainder of the cohort stop growing and gradually become atretic.

The granulosa cell layer is separated from the stromal cells by a basement membrane called the basal lamina (lamina basalis). The surrounding stromal cells differentiate into concentric layers designated as the theca interna (closest to the basal lamina) and the theca externa (the outer portion).

As the follicle develops, the theca cells develop LH receptors, leading to LH stimulation of the production of androgens, which form the substrate for the production of oestrogen in the granulosa cell layer.

Under the influence of FSH and as the follicles grow, intrafollicular fluid secretion increases, to form a cavitated antral follicle. The intrafollicular fluid contains oestrogens and a variety of peptide growth factors, which provide the oocytes and the surrounding granulosa cells with an endocrine-rich environment essential for maturation and eventually ovulation.

The selection of a dominant follicle

In primates and humans, usually one follicle proceeds to ovulation and the rest of the cohort is destined for atresia. Oestradiol and inhibin B are produced in increasing amounts by the rapidly growing lead follicle in the cohort. These hormones exert a negative feedback on the pituitary, leading to a decrease in the circulating level of FSH. This in turn withdraws gonadotrophic support from the less developed follicles, but is sufficient for the continued growth of the most advanced follicle, which contains the highest number of FSH receptors. In the antral stage, the dominant follicle maintains the production of oestradiol and inhibin B, which further reduces the FSH level and seals the fate of the other less developed follicles in the cohort. The accumulation of a greater mass of granulosa cells is accompanied by advanced development of the thecal vasculature, which facilitates preferential delivery of gonadotrophins to the follicles, allowing the dominant follicle to maintain FSH responsiveness and continue to develop and function despite the decreasing levels of FSH.

In the pre-ovulatory stage, the granulosa cells enlarge, the theca become vacuolated and richly vascular, the oocyte resumes meiosis, and the oestradiol level continues to rise, reaching a peak approximately 24–36 hours prior to ovulation.[4]

Ovulation

The continuous production of oestradiol by the growing follicle leads to the surge in LH through a positive-feedback mechanism. The LH surge usually lasts 48–50 hours. Ovulation (follicular rupture and oocyte release) occurs 24–36 hours after the LH surge. The LH surge leads to several events essential for oocyte maturation and preparation of the endometrium for implantation. The oocyte resumes its first meiotic division, leading to the production and extrusion of the first polar body, and enters the second meiotic division, which will be completed on fusion of the sperm with the oocyte later on. This stage is essential for the oocyte to be fertilized by the sperm. Stimulation of the granulosa cells by LH leads to the production of progesterone necessary for converting the endometrium from the proliferative to the secretory phase. Furthermore, progesterone enhances the activity of proteolytic enzymes and prostaglandins to digest the follicular wall, leading to the rupture of the follicle and the release of the oocyte.

Fertilization

The oocyte released at the time of ovulation is surrounded by granulosa cells known as the cumulus oophorus, which is separated from the actual oocyte by a layer of glycoprotein known as the zona pellucida. Within 2–3 minutes of ovulation, the oocyte (surrounded by the cumulus) is within the ampullary part of the fallopian tube. The fertilizable life span of the human ovum is estimated to be 24–36 hours. Although several million sperm are deposited in the vagina, only about 200 will come in contact with the oocyte. For the sperm to bind with the zona pellucida, a receptor is required, which is species specific. The sperm has to undergo a process known as 'capacitation' in order to be able to bind with the receptor and penetrate the egg. The zona pellucida not only contains the receptors for the sperm, but also has a mechanism by which it prevents more than one sperm from entering the oocyte (polyspermy). This mechanism is known as the zona reaction.

IMPLANTATION

This is defined as the process by which the embryo attaches itself to the endometrial side of the uterine wall and gradually penetrates the epithelium to reach the circulatory system of the mother. This process requires preparation of both the endometrium and the embryo for a successful implantation to take place.

Embryo preparation

For the first post-fertilization week, the embryo prepares for implantation while dividing. Sufficient cell division needs to take place to produce the inner cell mass essential for the formation of the blastocyst. The embryo usually reaches the blastocyst stage by day 5 post-fertilization with a prominent inner cell mass and trophoblast. The two structures expand and hatch through the zona pellucida from day 7 onwards. The hatched blastocyst is capable of producing human chorionic gonadotrophin (hCG), which acts on the corpus luteum to maintain the production of progesterone and oestradiol. This prevents the onset of menstruation and allows the early pregnancy to continue. At the time of hatching, the trophoblast cells begin to differentiate into cytotrophoblasts and syncytiotrophoblasts. The expression of adhesion molecules in the trophoblast may be responsible for the initial attachment of embryo to the uterus. The embryo gradually develops its self-regulatory paracrine system and establishes a communication system with the endometrium. This leads to interaction with the uterine epithelium and decidua during apposition and invasion by the trophoblast.

Endometrial preparation

After ovulation, oestradiol and progesterone from the corpus luteum alter the molecular structure of the endometrium from proliferative to secretory. The individual components of the endometrium continue to grow, leading to tortuosity of the glands and coiling of the spiral arterioles. Intracytoplasmic glycogen vacuoles appear and transudation of plasma occurs, contributing to endometrial secretion. The peak secretory phase is reached by 7 days post-ovulation. At this point the endometrial cells are rich in glycogen and lipids. The receptivity of the endometrium is limited to days 16–19 (of a 28-day cycle), and it is essential that the hatched blastocyst impacts and adheres to the surface of the endometrium during this 'implantation window' if pregnancy is to occur.

KEY POINTS

- At the onset of puberty, the size of the primordial follicles pool is approximately 300 000 follicles.
- Once oestradiol production from the dominant follicle passes a threshold, a positive feedback is triggered at the pituitary and the LH surge occurs, leading to ovulation.
- The oestradiol level continues to rise, reaching a peak leading to the LH surge, which is followed 24–36 hours later by ovulation.
- The fertilization life span of the released ovum is 24–36 hours.
- The zona pellucida precludes more than one sperm entering the oocyte through a mechanism known as the zona reaction.
- The embryo usually reaches the blastocyst stage by day 5 post-fertilization with a prominent inner cell mass and trophoblast.
- The receptivity of the endometrium is limited to days 16–19 (of a 28-day cycle) and it is important that the hatched blastocyst adheres to the endometrium during this time if pregnancy is to occur.

KEY REFERENCES

1. Gondos B, Westergaard L, Byskov A. Inhibition of oogenesis in the human fetal ovary: ultrasound structural and squash preparation study. *Am J Obstet Gynecol* 1986; 155:189–95.

2. Mais V, Kazer RR, Cetel NS et al. The dependence of folliculogenesis and corpus luteum function on pulsatile gonadotrophin secretion in cycling women using a gonadotrophin-releasing hormone antagonist as a probe. *J Clin Endocrinol Metab* 1986; **62**:1250–5.

3. Gougeon A. Dynamics of follicular growth in the human: a model from preliminary results. *Hum Reprod* 1986; **1**:81–7.

4. Pauerstein CJ, Eddy CA, Croxatto HD et al. Temporal relationships of oestrogen, progesterone, and luteinizing hormone levels to ovulation in women and infrahuman primates. *Am J Obstet Gynecol* 1978; **130**:876–86.

Female Infertility

Hany A.M.A. Lashen

INTRODUCTION

Infertility is defined as the inability to conceive despite regular unprotected sexual intercourse over a specific period of time, usually either 1 or 2 years. The cumulative spontaneous pregnancy rate for a couple during a 2-year period is approximately 57 per cent after 3 months, 72 per cent after 6 months, 85 per cent after 1 year and 93 per cent after 2 years [III].[1] Accordingly, only 7 per cent of couples will conceive in the second year, which justifies starting investigations for infertility after 1 year. However, if the physician or the patient has a reason to suspect impaired fertility, the process should be started sooner. Furthermore, if the female partner is approaching 35 years of age, the investigations should not be delayed, given the rapid decline of female fecundity after this age. Over the past three decades the introduction of in-vitro fertilization (IVF) and the wide public interest in this aspect of infertility treatment, together with the increasing ease of obtaining information, have increased patients' expectations of infertility treatment.

EPIDEMIOLOGY

It has been estimated that infertility affects between 9 per cent and 14 per cent of couples, of whom 70 per cent suffer from primary infertility, i.e. no previous conception, and 30 per cent secondary infertility, i.e. have achieved a previous pregnancy (regardless of the outcome of that pregnancy). Figures from different studies are difficult to compare due to various definitions of the specified period of unprotected intercourse required to lapse before diagnosing infertility. Another question that has been difficult to answer is: 'Is the rate of infertility on the increase?'. The absence of reliable historical epidemiological data and the modern preference for deferring childbearing are among the confounding variables that deny a reliable answer to this question. The recent advances in infertility treatment and the access of patients to such information have led to early presentation of these patients and their request for treatment. This may give a false impression of an increasing infertility problem. However, there is concern that male fertility is declining due to environmental factors. This is discussed in detail in Chapter 52.3.

CAUSES OF INFERTILITY

For pregnancy to occur, there must be fertile sperm and egg, a means of bringing them together and a receptive endometrium to allow the resulting embryo to implant. A defect at any of these stages can lead to subfertility. It has been estimated that in 35 per cent of cases a male factor is the reason for infertility [II]. In the remaining 65 per cent of cases, a female factor is identified in 50 per cent of couples and no cause will be identified in the remainder [II]. The commonest causes of infertility in the female are tubal and ovulatory factors. Endometriosis in its moderate to severe forms has also been linked to infertility, despite a lack of clear understanding of the connection between the two phenomena [II]. Although failure of implantation will cause infertility, it is difficult to determine whether the embryo or the endometrium is at fault in such cases. The effect of age on female fertility is not a new concept, with a gradual decline in female fertility and an increase in the miscarriage rate being observed many years before the menopause [III]. As discussed earlier, women enter the reproductive age at puberty with a pool of primordial follicles of a predetermined size. The size of this pool and the rate of follicular depletion are the deciding factors in the timing of the menopause. Female fertility declines after the age of 35 and declines more rapidly after the age of 40 [II]. The rate of follicular loss is inversely proportional to the size of the primordial pool, i.e. the smaller the pool, the faster the rate. Delaying starting a family to the latter years of reproductive life also increases the risk of developing endometriosis and the risk of miscarriage.

Anovulatory infertility

Anovulation is a frequent cause of presentation to a infertility clinic. Negative-feedback and positive-feedback mechanisms allow the ovaries to interact with the hypothalamo–pituitary axis. The causes of anovulation can be classified according to the clinical findings when the level of disruption between the hypothalamic–pituitary axis and the ovary is assessed. This divides the causes of anovular infertility into three main categories – hypergonadotrophic hypogonadism, hypogonadotrophic hypogonadism and ovulatory dysfunction – with other less common causes considered separately.

Hypergonadotrophic hypogonadism
This occurs as a result of failure of the ovary to respond to gonadotrophic stimulation by the pituitary gland. The absence of negative feedback (by oestradiol and inhibin B) from a developing follicle results in excessive secretion of the gonadotrophic hormones, follicle-stimulating hormone (FSH) and luteinizing hormone (LH). Concentrations of these hormones reach postmenopausal levels. Hypergonadotrophic hypogonadism classically results from premature ovarian failure with exhaustion of the ovarian follicle pool. A variant of the condition, resistant ovary syndrome, describes the occurrence of elevated levels of serum gonadotrophins in the presence of a good reserve of follicles. Abnormalities in the FSH receptor may produce this picture. Neither premature ovarian failure nor resistant ovary syndrome is treatable by injection of FSH.

Hypogonadotrophic hypogonadism
Failure of the pituitary gland to produce gonadotrophins will lead to lack of ovarian stimulation. There are a number of disorders of the anterior pituitary gland that lead to failure of production of FSH. These include destruction of the anterior pituitary by a tumour (e.g. a benign non-functioning adenoma or craniopharyngioma), by a pituitary inflammatory reaction as in tuberculosis or following ischaemia as in Sheehan's syndrome. Rare congenital causes include Laurence–Moon–Biedl, Kallmann's and Prader–Willi syndromes. The pituitary can also be damaged by cranial irradiation or surgically at the time of hypophysectomy for a pituitary tumour.

Hypogonadotrophic hypogonadism will also occur if pulsatile secretion of gonadotrophin releasing hormone (GnRH) is slowed or stops. This is seen in hypothalamic dysfunction, commonly secondary to excessive exercise, psychological stress or anorexia nervosa.

Ovarian dysfunction
Once hypogonadotrophic and hypergonadotrophic states have been excluded, the likely cause of anovulation lies at the level of the ovary. Such normogonadotrophic anovulation is usually seen in polycystic ovary syndrome (PCOS). Levels of oestradiol and inhibin B approximate to normal follicular phase levels in PCOS, maintaining ovarian–pituitary feedback.

Other discrete causes
Endocrine disorders, most commonly hyperprolactinaemia and hypothyroidism, are possible causes of anovulation and should be excluded by appropriate biochemical testing.

Tubal infertility

Tubal damage underlies infertility in approximately 14 per cent of couples and 40 per cent of infertile women [II]. Any damage to the fallopian tube can prevent the sperm from reaching the oocyte or the embryo from reaching the uterine cavity, leading to infertility and tubal ectopic pregnancy respectively. The fallopian tube is more than just a 'tube': a number of key events occur within the tube, including capacitation of the sperm, fertilization and the early development of the zygote and embryo. Therefore, the fallopian tube may maintain its patency but lose the ability to promote these other functions. Currently accepted investigations can only test tubal patency.

The main causes of tubal damage are either pelvic inflammatory disease (PID) or iatrogenic causes. PID remains the major cause of tubal damage in the Western world, with *Chlamydia trachomatis* infection the prime pathogen in most cases. Pelvic infection or abscess caused by appendicitis, other bowel disorders or septic abortion is responsible for a lesser proportion of cases. Fallopian tubes can be damaged

Reproductive medicine

iatrogenically either directly, as in tubal ligation for sterilization, or indirectly as a consequence of pelvic surgery. Other rare causes of tubal damage include tuberculosis, schistosomiasis, viral infection and abdominal inflammatory disorders such as Crohn's disease.

Endometriosis

It is apparent that severe endometriosis can lead to mechanical tubal damage due to adhesion formation caused by the pelvic endometrial deposits. However, it is less certain whether the lesser degrees of endometriosis can lead to infertility. Both mild endometriosis and infertility are common, and may occur together as epiphenomena [II]. Endometriosis is discussed further in Chapter 51.5.

Uterine factors

Submucous leiomyomata, congenital uterine abnormalities, endometrial polyps and intrauterine adhesions are all potential causes of infertility. The presence of a fibroid that occludes or distorts the fallopian tubes will lead to tubal infertility [III]. Distortion of the uterine cavity, by a fibroid, a septum or in the T-shaped uterus following exposure of the female fetus to diethystilbestrol in utero, can lead to implantation failure and recurrent early miscarriage [III]. Such cases should be assessed individually and the likelihood of their contribution to infertility should be examined. Excessive uterine curettage after a miscarriage or abortion, especially in the presence of uterine infection, can lead to the destruction of the strata basalis endometrium. Intrauterine scarification and synechiae develop as a result, which is known as Asherman's syndrome. This condition can also result after caesarean section, uteroplasty or myomectomy.

It has been difficult to demonstrate a relationship between endometriosis and subfertility, except when the cause of endometrosis is tuberculosis. Tuberculous endometriosis is a rare (in UK) but increasing cause of infertility. The effect of chlamydial endometritis on implantation remains controversial, although there is evidence that patients with tubal disease undergoing IVF have significantly lower pregnancy and implantation rates.

Unexplained infertility

Completion of routine investigation of infertility fails to reveal a cause in 15–30 per cent of cases [II]. This does not indicate absence of a cause, but rather inability to identify it. The results of IVF have shown that there may be undiagnosed problems of oocyte or embryo quality or of implantation failure, neither of which can easily be tested unless IVF is undertaken. Unexplained infertility causes great distress to couples, who often find it harder to bear when a cause cannot be found.

INVESTIGATION OF THE FEMALE PARTNER

Investigation of infertility will usually be initiated in general practice, frequently followed by referral to a secondary or tertiary centre, where most treatments will take place. The RCOG has recently published guidelines for the management of infertility. These define the role of the medical practitioner at each level, and outline the evidence base for investigation and treatment.

History taking and examination

It is important to recognize that infertility is a problem that faces couples, and that both partners should be seen and investigated together whenever possible [IV]. Consultations involving infertility require tact and sensitivity on behalf of the clinician, a quiet, private environment and sufficient clinical time to allow exploration of the couple's anxieties and explanation of available treatments as well as classical history taking. A rapport must be established before more personal and sexual details can be sought.

Personal and social history

The couple's age, in particular that of the female partner, is important, as discussed earlier. The occupation of the couple, especially the male, can have an impact on their fertility. Exposure to high temperature, chemicals and ionizing radiation can seriously affect sperm production [III]. If either of the partners works away from home, this may affect the frequency of sexual intercourse around the time of ovulation. Smoking, alcohol and recreational drug use can also influence fertility. Appropriate advice should be given.

Menstrual history

The age of menarche and regularity of periods are important factors. Information about the frequency and length of the menstrual cycle and any associated problems such as dysmenorrhoea or heavy menstrual loss should be sought. Irregular menstrual cycles, oligomenorrhoea and amenorrhoea are all suggestive of anovulation. If amenorrhoea is reported, enquiries should be made about any menopausal symptoms, weight loss or gain, and symptoms of hyperprolactinaemia and hypothyroidism. These patients should be investigated in specialized centres [IV].

Obstetric history

The clinician should enquire about any previous pregnancies, both in the current and any previous relationship, as well as the outcome of these pregnancies. It may be wise to ask about breastfeeding and any sustained galactorrhoea at this stage. It is also important to establish if there were any difficulties encountered or treatment required prior to achieving a previous pregnancy.

Contraception

The use of the oral contraceptive pill and the long-acting progestogens can be followed by a period of amenorrhoea. In particular, use of long-acting progestogen-based contraceptives may be followed by delay in the resumption of ovulation [III]. The use of intrauterine contraceptive devices may increase the risk of pelvic infection, especially in young nulliparous women, leading to tubal disease [III].

Past medical history

It is important to establish any previous medical disorders that may affect either fertility or pregnancy. Preconceptional counselling may be necessary if a serious medical condition is identified. The possible impact of prescription medications on ovulation should be investigated: for example, some antidepressants can increase prolactin secretion and non-steroidal anti-inflammatory drugs can interfere with ovulation.

Sexual history

The clinician should enquire about the couple's frequency of sexual intercourse and associated problems such as dyspareunia or ejaculatory dysfunction. Regular intercourse (two to three times a week) is sufficient for most couples to achieve a pregnancy. It is frequently the case that infertile couples restrict their sexual activity to the period around mid-cycle and some use commercially available ovulation detection kits to time intercourse. There is no evidence that such practices can increase fecundability, and the increase in psychological stress that results from such practices is unhelpful [II]. Sensitive enquiry concerning sexually transmitted diseases should be made.

Other important points

The discussion should include advice concerning the use of folic acid and enquiry about rubella vaccination [Ia]. A cervical smear history should be taken and a smear offered if indicated [IV]. A family history, including enquiry concerning diabetes, endometriosis and PCOS, should be taken, as this information can be useful in the diagnosis and treatment of infertility [III]. A history of familial disorder should lead to an offer of genetic counselling before starting investigation and treatment [IV].

Examination of the female partner

Although the traditional teaching encourages thorough examination of patients presenting with infertility, the evidence base for this practice is lacking. Unless there is an indication from the patient's history that examination would be of any value in establishing the cause of infertility, there would seem to be little to be gained from routine examination.

Indications from the history, for example of cyclical pelvic pain or dyspareunia, should prompt pelvic examination. Other features of the physical examination, for example detection of an asymptomatic pelvic mass, have been supplanted by transvaginal ultrasound examination.

Assessment of body mass index is important, as both obesity and underweight can cause anovulation [II]. If the patient is found to be obese, regional obesity can be investigated by measuring the waist:hip ratio [II].

Laboratory investigations, endoscopy and imaging

The aim of these investigations is to assess ovulation, tubal patency and uterine factors.

Ovulation

A history of regular periods usually indicates ovulation. However, a reliable marker is useful to confirm that ovulation has occurred. After the release of the oocyte and the formation of the corpus luteum, progesterone levels rise sharply, reaching a peak level approximately 8 days after the LH surge. The detection of high levels of progesterone in serum or evidence of progesterone effect can be used as a secondary marker of ovulation. Historically, the effects of progesterone on basal body temperature, endometrial histology or cervical mucus were commonly used. Measuring serum progesterone at its peak in the mid-luteal phase is a reliable, safe and inexpensive test. Levels in excess of 30 nmol/L are diagnostic of ovulation [II]; however, lower (sub-optimal) levels may be due to incorrect timing of blood sampling or may be caused by a luteinized unruptured follicle. It is important to remember that the mid-luteal phase is approximately 7 days before the next expected period, i.e. day 21 and day 28 in 28-day and 35-day cycles respectively.

Commercially available urinary LH detection kits can detect the LH surge and can be used to time intercourse with ovulation induction or donor insemination treatments.

Tubal patency tests

Although the fallopian tube has functions other than as a conduit for the sperm, oocyte and embryo, it is not yet feasible to assess these functions in routine practice. Tubal patency can be assessed by three different methods: hysterosalpingography, laparoscopy and dye hydrotubation, and ultrasound scanning with hydrotubation. A fourth method, falloposcopy, has been introduced in order to assess both tubal patency and mucosa. However, the images of the tubal mucosa obtained at falloposcopy are not yet of sufficiently good quality to provide clinically useful information [III].

Hysterosalpingography

The principle of this test is to inject a radio-opaque contrast medium through the cervix into the uterus and take abdominal X-rays at intervals during and after the injection. The images should reveal the uterine outline and passage of contrast along the tubes, with free spill into the peritoneal cavity. Hysterosalpingography is usually carried out in the first 10 days of the menstrual cycle, to avoid disruption of an early pregnancy in the secretory phase of the cycle. It will cause period-like pain in most patients and may occasionally lead to a vasovagal attack. The main complication of hysterosalpingography is flare-up of PID. The overall risk of infection from this test in the normal population is approximately 1 per cent, rising to 3 per cent in high-risk patients. Therefore it is wise to carry out laparoscopy and dye test in high-risk patients and to use prophylactic antibiotics in suspected cases. The RCOG recommends the routine taking of cervical swabs for chlamydia in any patient before carrying out any intrauterine instrumentation [IV]. Hysterosalpingography is recommended by the RCOG as the primary screening procedure in low-risk patients [IV].

Laparoscopy and dye test

The principle of this procedure is to visualize the passage of methylene blue dye through the fallopian tubes. The procedure enables inspection of the fimbrial ends of the tubes and the pelvic structures for the presence of endometriosis or adhesions. Combining this procedure with electrocoagulation of any endometriotic spots or adhesiolysis adds therapeutic value. Hence it is advisable that such procedures are carried out in centres where the necessary expertise is available [IV].

Laparoscopy and dye test requires general anaesthetic and carries the risk of bowel or visceral injury. It is therefore not recommended as a first-line screening test [IV]. However, it should be considered in patients with a history suggestive of endometriosis, previous PID or previous pelvic surgery. Furthermore, if the hysterosalpingography reports abnormal results, verification should be carried out with diagnostic laparoscopy [IV]. Some clinicians hold the view that to diagnose unexplained infertility, both peritoneal factor and endometriosis should be excluded, even in patients with normal hysterosalpingography, by carrying out laparoscopic examination.

Visualization and assessment of the uterine cavity are not possible unless hysteroscopy is performed concurrently. However, the value of routine hysteroscopy is questionable [IV], as the frequency of asymptomatic intrauterine lesions that are not seen on transvaginal ultrasound is low. Hysteroscopy should probably therefore be reserved for cases where there is an indication from the history or previous investigations.

Ultrasound scan and hydrotubation

HyCoSy (hysterosalpingo contrast sonography) has recently been introduced as a method for studying tubal patency using ultrasonography. Ultrasonographic contrast medium is slowly injected into the uterine cavity under direct visualization, with imaging of the cavity and of flow along the fallopian tubes. This method does not require X-ray and allows the ultrasound assessment of the pelvic organs, i.e.

the uterus including the uterine cavity, tubes and ovaries. Nevertheless, the method has not been widely adopted, in part due to the cost of the contrast medium used and partly due to the occasional method failure that can occur even after appropriate training.

Assessment of the uterus

Uterine anatomy can be visualized by hysterosalpingography or hysteroscopy. Transvaginal ultrasound does not always provide a good quality image of the cavity, but this can be improved by injection of a small volume of saline. This may outline intrauterine polyps or synechiae. Endometrial biopsy, once the mainstay of the diagnosis of an adequate secretory phase, has fallen from favour due to its invasive nature and lack of reproducibility. Routine hysteroscopy for infertile patients has been discouraged by the RCOG [IV].

Postcoital test

The postcoital test provides information concerning the ability of the sperm to penetrate and survive in cervical mucus. However, reproducibility of the test is low and the false-positive rate is high. A diagnosis of an adverse cervical factor does not alter therapeutic decisions, as both 'cervical factor' and unexplained infertility are treated with intrauterine insemination or IVF. The RCOG guidelines on the management of infertility have not included the postcoital test as a routine test [II].

Management of female infertility

Any discussion about the management of infertility should begin with a description of the physiology of the cycle, with information about the 'fertile period'. Lifestyle issues, including advice on smoking, alcohol consumption and 'fitness for pregnancy', should be raised. Further planning of treatment protocols will depend on the presumed cause of the problem.

Management of tubal infertility

Tubal infertility can be treated with tubal surgery, IVF and embryo transfer (IVF-ET) or selective salpingography. Although tubal surgery is no longer recommended for severe tubal disease since the introduction of IVF-ET, it still has a place in less severe forms of the disorder.

Tubal surgery

Successful tubal surgery requires surgical skill and experience. The decline in the number of suitable cases has reduced training opportunities, and some advocate restriction of this practice to tertiary centres to allow concentration of expertise [IV]. This permits audit of outcome and estimation of realistic, single-centre pregnancy rates. Comparison between tubal surgery and IVF is difficult. The cost, success rate, complications and benefits must be assessed in every case individually. Decision-making may be altered in favour of IVF by the presence of other causes of infertility, particularly male factor and anovulation. The success rate after tubal surgery depends on the underlying disease, site of damage (proximal or distal) and patient's age. The cost of a single cycle of IVF has been calculated to be comparable to that of tubal surgery, and apart from patients with mild tubal disease, the cost-effectiveness argument is in favour of IVF-ET. However, tubal surgery, if successful, offers less risk of multiple pregnancy and ovarian hyperstimulation syndrome (OHSS), and avoids the ethical issues that fertilization in vitro can engender. Patients should be informed that the risk of ectopic pregnancy after tubal surgery is significantly higher than after IVF-ET [II].

Once tubal surgery is being contemplated, careful assessment of the tubes and pelvis with hysterosalpingography and laparoscopy should be carried out [IV]. The route of access should then be decided, i.e. laparotomy or laparoscopy. Laparoscopic surgery is less costly and offers less morbidity, more technical advantages and a marginally better pregnancy rate. If pregnancy does not occur within 6–12 months of tubal surgery, reassessment of the tubes with hysterosalpingography should be carried out. If the tubes remain blocked, IVF-ET is indicated. If the tubes remain patent, ovulation should be assessed and perhaps a short period of ovulation induction could be tried. This decision will depend on the patient's age and whether IVF-ET is affordable to the couple. The key issues here are to present the couple with all the available facts and to involve them in the decision-making process.

IVF-ET

Absent or irreparably damaged fallopian tubes were the main reason for the development of IVF-ET. A lower pregnancy rate after IVF-ET in tubal infertility couples compared to other causes of infertility has been reported. The reason is not entirely clear, but it is possible that fluid from a hydrosalpinx could be hostile to embryo development and implantation. Salpingectomy of an ultrasonographically visible hydrosalpinx should therefore be considered for some patients to improve the success rate of IVF treatment [II], although careful counselling is needed before performing salpingectomy for an infertile patient, even if the tubal damage is severe [IV].

Selective salpingography and tubal cannulation

These procedures can be carried out under image intensification or at hysteroscopy. These methods were originally developed for diagnostic purposes, but were subsequently proven to be useful in treating proximal tubal damage, for which surgery yielded disappointing success rates. The outcome of these procedures in terms of regaining tubal patency is immediately known. However, tubal function may not be restored, and failure of conception after tubal recannalization should lead on to IVF-ET.

Management of anovulatory infertility

A number of therapeutic interventions for the induction of ovulation are available. Selecting the most appropriate method depends on the cause of anovulation. Patients with ovarian failure and resistant ovary syndrome will not respond to ovulation induction and should be offered oocyte donation [II]. Normalization of body weight in underweight and obese patients can help to regain ovulation without the need for medical intervention [Ib]. Medical treatment of prolactinoma can also help regain normal ovulation [Ia]. Ovulation induction in patients with hypogonadotrophic hypogonadism can be achieved with the pulsatile administration of GnRH or by daily injection of gonadotrophin [II]. Ovulation induction in PCOS patients (80 per cent of anovular women) can be achieved by weight normalization in obese patients [II] (40–60 per cent of PCOS patients), medical or surgical methods. The medical methods include the use of GnRH, clomiphene citrate or gonadotrophins – discussed further under the 'Assisted conception' section. The surgical methods are either ovarian drilling or wedge resection. Stein and Leventhal suggested ovarian wedge resection in 1935. Their theory was that the thick tunica albugenia prevented the release of the ovum, hence the anovulation in PCOS patients. Although pregnancies resulted, the operation (performed by laparotomy) led to complications, including tubal damage and adhesion formation, and fell into disrepute. Ovarian drilling involves focal local destruction of the ovarian stroma with laser or diathermy, applied laparoscopically. The route of access reduces morbidity and postoperative complications. The value of ovarian drilling compared to medical ovulation induction in PCOS remains undecided. Ovarian drilling has less risk of multiple pregnancies, no risk of OHSS, and is less costly. On the other hand, the long-term advantages and risks of ovarian drilling require further assessment. Destroying ovarian tissue inevitably leads to destruction of primordial follicles and reduction of the ovarian reserve. These anxieties have partially been resolved by studies that demonstrate that a good therapeutic response can be achieved by minimal application of energy and after reduction of the number of diathermy burns from >20 to 4 per ovary. However, even if equal efficacy is assumed between surgical and medical methods of ovulation induction, the risks of surgery work in favour of the medical treatment.

Management of endometriosis-related infertility

This depends on the severity of the condition and the presence of any other infertility factors. The two main lines of treating endometriosis are medical and surgical. The medical methods are inappropriate in an infertile patient [Ia], as the medication either induces anovulation or carries a risk of teratogenicity. Meta-analysis of studies designed to test the efficacy of the medical management of endometriosis in resolving infertility has demonstrated that this approach is of no benefit.

Recent evidence suggests that conservative surgical treatment of minimal or mild endometriosis may improve natural conception rates postoperatively [Ib]. As many infertile patients will undergo diagnostic laparoscopy, diathermy to endometriosis can be delivered at the same session, alleviating the need for a further anaesthetic. Assisted reproduction has lent itself to treating endometriosis-related infertility. Except for cases with severe endometriosis, high pregnancy rates are seen after IVF-ET. Whether medical or conservative surgical treatment of endometriosis before carrying out IVF-ET can improve the ovarian response and pregnancy rates remains unclear.

Management of unexplained infertility

The lack of an identifiable reason for infertility in this category makes the treatment empirical. Conservative management, ovulation induction with or without intrauterine insemination, and IVF-ET are the main approaches to managing unexplained infertility. Approximately 60 per cent of couples with unexplained secondary infertility (diagnosed after 1 year) achieve a pregnancy within 3 years of conservative management [II]. Results are less good in primary infertility. However, the woman's age should be taken into consideration when advising this line of management. Ovulation induction (or, more properly, 'augmentation') with clomiphene citrate along with timed sexual intercourse has been used successfully in patients with unexplained infertility. The rationale is that by producing more eggs, the probability of fertilization and implantation can be improved. Furthermore, the presence of multiple corpora lutea may correct an underlying luteal phase defect in these patients. However, recent meta-analysis of studies in this area has not demonstrated benefit over the conservative approach [Ia], and treatment with clomiphene citrate carries a risk of multiple pregnancy.

A cumulative pregnancy rate of 40 per cent has been reported after controlled ovarian stimulation (COS) with gonadotrophins and intrauterine insemination (IUI) [II]. The pregnancy rates after IUI alone in couples with unexplained infertility have been disappointing. However, the advantage of IUI over timed sexual intercourse after COS has been controversial, and firm evidence is lacking. For logistic reasons, IUI may provide a better timing compared to sexual intercourse. Many centres advise two or three cycles of COS–IUI before moving to IVF-ET in this group. COS-IUI may be less stressful, less physically demanding and less costly per attempt than IVF.

In-vitro fertilization–embryo transfer in unexplained infertility has diagnostic as well as therapeutic value, as it provides information about fertilization and egg and embryo quality. Owing to its high cost, IVF-ET is usually seen as a last resort in unexplained infertility. The cost of three cycles of COS-IUI is comparable to that of one IVF-ET cycle, with the former offering a better pregnancy rate [III].

Gamete intrafallopian transfer (GIFT) used to be the treatment of choice for patients with unexplained infertility. However, IVF-ET, with its diagnostic potential, has superseded this modality. Although GIFT offered a high pregnancy rate, the ectopic pregnancy risk was also high [II], and the treatment requires general anaesthesia and laparoscopy in order for gametes to be placed within the ampulla of the fallopian tube. This method has largely been supplanted by IVF-ET.

Management of uterine factor infertility

Congenital defects, leiomyomas and intrauterine adhesions and polyps are the only treatable uterine factors. However, before offering surgical treatment, the impact of such findings on the couple's fertility should be carefully assessed [IV]. Myomectomy can be carried out either laparoscopically or by laparotomy with similar postoperative pregnancy rates [Ia]. Entry into the uterine cavity should be avoided if possible, and adhesion barriers and microsurgical technique should be used to reduce the risk of postoperative adhesions. The risk of a scar rupture during pregnancy is less if the endometrial cavity remains intact at myomectomy [III], although some fibroids cannot be removed without breach of the cavity. Postoperative adhesions can have a detrimental effect on tubal patency.

Submucous fibroids can successfully be resected hysteroscopically, depending on the size of the fibroid and its degree of protrusion into the uterine cavity. The risk of tubal damage with this procedure is minimal, but there is a risk of haemorrhage, uterine perforation and endometrial scarring leading to intrauterine adhesions. Hysteroscopic division of intrauterine adhesions and excision of polyps are usually straightforward, with low morbidity. Assisted reproductive technology is not applicable to uterine factor infertility. However, treatment of a uterine factor should be considered if failure of implantation seems to be the only cause of an unsuccessful IVF-ET treatment [IV].

- There is no evidence that ovulation detection kits and temperature charts increase the chance of conception.
- There is no evidence that thorough physical examination of every patient is necessary.
- The postcoital test is of limited value with regard to discriminating between couples achieving and not achieving a pregnancy.
- Drug treatment is ineffective in the treatment of endometriosis-related infertility.
- Ovarian stimulation and IUI is effective in the management of mild male factor and unexplained infertility.

KEY POINTS

- Infertility affects 9–14 per cent of couples, 70 per cent of whom suffer from primary infertility.
- Thirty-five per cent of the cases are due to male factor, while 65 per cent are due to female factor.
- Delaying starting a family until later life does not only reduce fertility, but also increases the risk of endometriosis and miscarriage.
- PCOS is the commonest cause of anovulatory infertility.
- Tubal disease is the commonest cause of female infertility.
- PID and iatrogenic causes are the main reasons for tubal infertility.
- *Chlamydia trachomatis* is the commonest pathogen leading to PID in the Western world.
- Unexplained infertility represents approximately 15–30 per cent of cases.

- Careful history taking is a very important starting point to the investigation of infertility.
- The mid-luteal phase is approximately 7 days from the next menstrual cycle, which is important when measuring serum progesterone levels for ovulation detection.
- Combining laparoscopy and dye test with electrocoagulation of minimal and mild endometriosis adds a therapeutic dimension to a diagnostic procedure.

KEY REFERENCE

1. Gutmacher AF. Factors affecting normal expectancy of conception. *J Am Med Assoc* 1956; **161**.855.

Male Infertility

Hany A.M.A. Lashen

INTRODUCTION

Other than in cases of absolute azoospermia or severe oligospermia/asthenospermia, the impact of the male factor on a couple's fertility is difficult to quantify. In other words, any man with motile normal spermatozoa in his ejaculate should be credited with some degree of fertility. Women undergoing donor insemination treatment have a higher probability of pregnancy if they are partners of azoospermic men than if they are partners of oligozoospermic men. This reflects that a degree of compensation can exist between the female and male partners. Accordingly, in most circumstances it is easier to define male fertility than infertility. The ability to make a woman pregnant or father a child can be considered evidence of the male's fertility. There are many causes of male infertility, although primary testicular disorders are most commonly responsible.

AETIOLOGY

Primary testicular disease

The majority of cases of male factor infertility lie in this category. The pathogenesis of testicular dysfunction is poorly understood, with no obvious predisposing factors being identifiable in more than 50 per cent of cases. Recent studies have linked azoospermia and severe oligospermia to microdeletions of genes on the Y chromosome, which appear to be involved in at least some cases of 'idiopathic' male infertility [III]. Other causes of failure of spermatogenesis include testicular maldescent, particularly if left uncorrected until puberty, testicular torsion, trauma or infection, neoplasm and effects of subsequent chemotherapy, haemosiderosis and Klinefelter's syndrome [III]. Mumps orchitis and severe epididymo-orchitis are the main inflammatory causes of testicular damage [III]. Other chromosomal anomalies can also lead to male infertility; however, Klinefelter's syndrome remains the only relatively commonly seen anomaly. Azoospermic and severely oligozoospermic men should have chromosomal karyotyping before their sperm are used for intracytoplasmic sperm injection (ICSI) in order to lessen the risk of transmission of a chromosomal disorder (commonly deletion or translocation) to the offspring [IV].

Obstructive male infertility

Obstruction can occur at any level of the male reproductive tract from the rete testis and the epididymis to the vas deferens. Obstruction can be due to congenital, inflammatory or iatrogenic causes. Desire for fertility following vasectomy is common. Congenital absence of the vas is also fairly common, being the cause of azoospermia in approximately 10 per cent of cases [III]. Bilateral congenital absence of the vas is seen in carriers of genes for cystic fibrosis [II], and pre-treatment screening of both partners is essential to avoid the possibility of cystic fibrosis in the offspring.

Endocrinological causes of male infertility

Endocrinopathies are rarely identified in cases of male infertility. The commoner conditions seen in this category include hypogonadotrophic hypogonadism, thyroid and adrenal disease [III]. Although rare, these conditions should be diagnosed, as their treatment is straightforward and can restore fertility. Hyperprolactinaemia in men can lead to impotence but has little effect on sperm production [II].

Autoimmune causes

Approximately 12 per cent of men have anti-sperm antibodies [II]. This can lead to decreased sperm motility and may impede the binding of the spermatozoon to the zona pellucida of the oocyte, hindering fertilization. Low levels of anti-sperm antibodies are not thought to have a significant impact on fertility [III]. The reason why some men develop anti-sperm antibodies is not known, although damage to the testis following trauma and surgery can be found in many cases.

Drugs

Drugs taken for medicinal and recreational purposes can affect sperm production and/or function. Alcohol, cigarettes, opiates and marijuana can suppress spermatogenesis and affect sperm function [III]. Anabolic steroids, antifungal drugs, sulfasalazine, corticosteroids and other classes of drugs also affect spermatogenesis. The effect of most of these drugs is reversible. In contrast, chemotherapy can cause permanent damage to spermatogenesis. Other drugs, including antidepressants, sedatives and anti-hypertensives, can lead to male infertility by causing erectile dysfunction.

Environmental factors

Exposure to heat, chemicals and ionizing irradiation can damage sperm production, and it is important to enquire about the male partner's occupation. Evidence for the extent of the effects of environmental toxins on male fertility is lacking. Although epidemiological studies have demonstrated a decline in sperm quality in the developed world, it is difficult to extrapolate from this population-based data to individual cases. However, it seems sensible to advise the avoidance of excessive heat and exposure to chemicals such as paints, organic solvents, lead-based products and pesticides in oligospermic/asthenospermic subfertile men.

Varicocele

A varicocele describes the presence of abnormally tortuous veins of the pampiniform plexus within the spermatic cord. Varicocele is more common on the left side of the pelvis, due to the direct insertion of the spermatic vein into the renal vein on this side. It occurs in both fertile and infertile men, although the incidence seems to be higher among infertile men [II]. The impact of varicocele on male fertility remains controversial. Increased testicular temperature (which is unfavourable for spermatogenesis) has been suggested as a mechanism of action in these cases, but surgical or radiological correction of the disorder is not thought to improve the chances of conception [Ia] and has fallen out of favour.

Ejaculatory disorders

Retrograde ejaculation, in which sperm enter the bladder rather than the penile urethra at ejaculation, can follow from neurological disorders, diabetes or bladder neck or prostate surgery. Failure of ejaculation due to neurological disorders, medication or psychological difficulties is a rare cause of male infertility.

INVESTIGATION OF THE MALE

All referrals to an infertility clinic should be seen as a couple, with concurrent investigation of the male and female partners. A routine semen analysis can be performed before seeing the couple in the clinic. A normal result can provide a degree of reassurance to the male partner, and erectile and ejaculatory problems can usually be excluded by a sensitively taken medical history. If the seminal parameters are abnormal, further investigations should be instigated. It is important to elicit from the history any of the causes of male infertility mentioned above. This should be followed by examination of genital development, the testicles, the epididymis and the vas deferens. Any of the aforementioned reversible causes can usually be corrected, and advice regarding smoking, alcohol and substance abuse should be given. Testicular cooling by wearing boxer shorts or taking cold baths is probably of little value, although occupational exposure to extreme heat should be avoided.

Semen analysis

The value of a diagnostic test depends on its sensitivity (ability to identify disease), specificity (ability to identify normality) and reproducibility (obtaining similar results each time the test is carried out). The wide overlap of the results of the various components of a semen analysis between fertile and infertile men reduces the sensitivity and specificity of

Table 52.3.1   Semen analysis reference values

Parameter	Reference value
Volume	2 mL or more
pH	7.2 or more
Sperm concentration	20 million/mL or more
Total sperm number	40 million or more per ejaculate
Motility	50% or more (grade a + b) or 25% with progressive motility
Morphology	See note below
Vitality	75% or more live
White cell count	Fewer than 1 million
Immunobead test	Less than 5% motile sperm with beads bound
MAR test	Less than 50% sperm with adherent particles

Note: Multicentre population-based studies utilizing the methods of morphology assessment in the manual are now in progress. Data from assisted reproduction suggest that fertilization rates drop if sperm morphology falls below 15% of the normal forms. MAR, mixed agglutination reaction.

Table 52.3.2   Sperm function tests

- Objective assessment of motility
- Hypo-osmotic swelling test
- Tests for sperm nuclear maturity
- Measure of acrosome status
- Acrosome reaction and acrosin activity
- Hamster zona-free oocyte penetration
- Human sperm zona binding and penetration

routine semen analysis as a test of infertility. Moreover, the large biological variation seen in the quality of sperm in repeated tests on the same individual limits the reproducibility of semen analysis as a diagnostic test. Routine semen analysis should be performed according to criteria established by the World Health Organization (WHO) in order to achieve standardization (Table 52.3.1). The test assesses several measures of sperm quality, some of which are more sensitive in identifying infertile men than others. The WHO-recommended method of semen analysis includes determination of the volume of ejaculate, concentration, motility and percentage of morphologically normal forms. Semen analysis can be carried out manually or using computer-assisted sperm analysis (CASA). Several population-based studies have produced statistical correlation between the different semen parameters and fertility potential in men. It is also important to remember that these values are not the minimum requirement to achieve a pregnancy; therefore they are referred to as 'reference' and not 'normal' values.

Many other tests of semen quality have been devised. These include biochemical analysis of the seminal fluid and detection of anti-sperm antibodies. Biochemical analysis of the seminal fluid can provide information about the prostate, seminal vesicles and epididymis. Zinc, fructose, carnitine and acid phosphatase have all been studied, but are not thought to impart useful diagnostic or prognostic information. The detection of anti-sperm antibodies using the immunobead or mixed antibody reaction (MAR) test may alter treatment and continues to be performed in most centres.

Sperm function tests

The functions of the sperm in vivo are to negotiate the cervical mucus, reach the ampullary part of the fallopian tube in sufficient numbers, undergo capacitation and finally fertilize the egg. However, routine semen analysis does not test these functions. Therefore several tests known as 'sperm

function tests' have been developed in tertiary centres. These tests are still of academic rather than practical value and have become less significant following the introduction of in-vitro fertilization (IVF) treatments, which circumvent most of the steps necessary for fertilization in vivo. Their role in routine infertility investigations has yet to be established. Some of these tests are listed in Table 52.3.2 and the interested reader can refer to the WHO manual for more details.

Other tests

Unexplained severe sperm abnormality including azoospermia merits further investigation. The objectives of such tests are to identify whether azoospermia is due to a primary testicular disorder or an outflow obstruction. Obstructive azoospermia is usually associated with normal concentration of follicle-stimulating hormone (FSH) in serum, as the testes continue to function normally. In contrast, disorders of spermatogenesis result in interruption of the gonadal–pituitary feedback loop with elevation of serum FSH. Measurement of FSH can thus be useful in the investigation of azoospermia. Invasive investigation using testicular biopsy can assess the extent of damage to the spermatogenesis and identify whether it is possible to obtain testicular sperm for use in ICSI, even if the patient is azoospermic. Karyotyping and cystic fibrosis gene screening are necessary if a chromosomal abnormality is suspected or to assess the carrier status for cystic fibrosis genes in patients with congenital absence of the vas. However, the modern management of male infertility has reduced the need for extensive investigations, especially in less severe cases of oligozoospermia or athenozoospermia. Where an endocrinologcial reason is suspected, the diagnosis should be made, as the treatment strategy in these cases differs from the usual treatment modalities for male infertility (Figure 52.3.1).

Examination of the male partner

Traditional teaching stipulates that examination of the male partner should be carried out as a matter of routine in all infertility cases. However, if there is a normal semen analysis, there is little to gain from examination of the male. In severe male factor infertility and especially in azoospermic men, examination is warranted to help establish the cause of

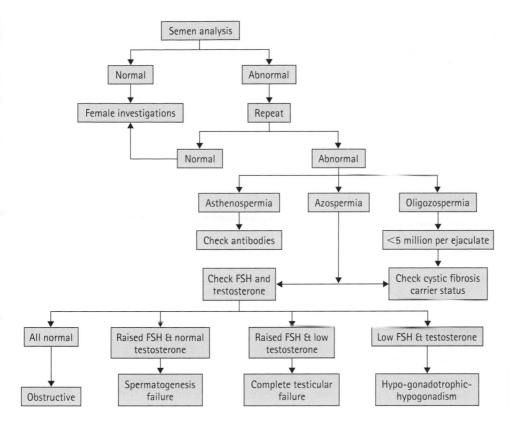

Figure 52.3.1 Investigations of male infertility. FSH, follicule-stimulating hormone

the problem. Both general and genital examinations should be undertaken. The objectives of the general examination are to assess the level of masculinization and to detect any stigmata of chromosomal abnormality, inguinal hernia or relevant surgical scars, gynaecomastia or evidence of systemic illnesses. This examination is frequently unrewarding, many such cases being discovered earlier in adolescence due to delayed onset of puberty. The genital examination should include assessment of the testes, epididymis and vas deferens and detection of any scrotal swellings or varicocele. If the history suggests penile or prostatic problems, it is advisable to refer for a urological opinion. The examination should be carried out in standing and supine positions in a warm private room. The testicular axis, volume and consistency should be assessed with a Prader orchiometer to measure the testicular volume. It should be noted that testicular volume is related to ethnic origin, weight and height and there is normally a small difference between the left and right testicles. For Caucasian men the normal volume is above 12 mL per testis. The consistency of the testicles can also be assessed. A soft consistency is associated with impaired spermatogenesis. Examination of the epididymis should assess its position in relation to the testicle, volume, any tenderness and any nodularity or swellings. Normally the epididymis is small and may not be palpable. The vas should have no thickenings or nodules. Careful examination for the presence of the vasa is essential in azoospermic men, especially if the testicular volume is normal. Scrotal examination for varicocele should be carried out in the standing position. If any other scrotal swelling is palpable, the patient should be referred for a urological opinion. Testicular maldescent in infancy is associated with an increased risk of testicular cancer in later life. Such patients may present to an infertility clinic for investigation of oligospermia. They should be appraised of this risk and taught to self-examine. Similarly, tissue collected at testicular biopsy that is used to obtain sperm for ICSI in azoospermic men should also be sent for histological examination.

MANAGEMENT OF MALE INFERTILITY

Until recently, men with primary testicular dysfunction or obstructive azoospermia were unable to reproduce. In vitro fertilization and micromanipulation of sperm now offers these men the opportunity to have children with their partners and has become the mainstay in the treatment of male factor infertility. The treatment of male factor infertility, including the use of donor insemination, is discussed in the chapter on assisted reproduction (Chapter 52.4). However, some more traditional methods of treatment merit consideration.

Varicocelectomy

This procedure refers to the ligation of varicocele, which was carried out both prophylactically and therapeutically for

Reproductive medicine

many decades. Some studies showed improvement in sperm motility or concentration after varicocelectomy, although this did not correlate with improvement in pregnancy rate. However, there is evidence that semen quality and pregnancy rates may improve in oligozoospermic men after treatment of a clinically apparent varcicocele [Ia]. The modern management of infertility has made the procedure redundant, removing the opportunity for further randomized trials to investigate its value.

Management of endocrine disorders

Hypogonadotrophic hypogonadism, often in association with Kallmann's syndrome, has been successfully treated with pulsatile GnRH or human menopausal gonadotrophins to restore spermatogenic drive and hence fertility. Initiation of spermatogenesis can take several months and treatment can become costly.

Management of anti-sperm antibodies

Many empirical therapies have been suggested for men with anti-sperm antibodies. The use of condoms and corticosteroids and intrauterine insemination of washed spermatozoa are some examples [Ia]. The value of all these modalities has been controversial, and IVF-ET and ICSI are currently the methods of choice in these cases. Donor insemination can be an alternative for financial reasons.

Reversal of vasectomy

Vasectomy reversal can be carried out successfully, with up to an 80 per cent chance of a subsequent pregnancy. The chance of success is inversely proportional to the length of time since the vasectomy was carried out. Although the integrity of the vas deferens can be restored in most cases, anti-sperm antibodies are common after vasectomy and reversal, and are probably the major bar to conception. In these cases and in those whose operation has failed, IVF with or without ICSI is the recommended treatment. A growing number of centres are offering collection and storage of sperm from the epididymis at the time of vasectomy reversal, for subsequent use in ICSI treatment if the reversal operation fails.

- The use of gonadotrophin drugs in hypogonadotrophic hypogonadal men is an effective treatment [Ib].
- The use of bromocriptine in men with sexual dysfunction as a result of hyperprolactinaemia is effective [Ib].
- Testicular biopsy should only be undertaken in tertiary centres [IV].
- Vasectomy reversal is an effective treatment [Ia].
- Anti-oestrogens, androgens and bromocriptine are not effective in improving sperm quality [II].
- The use of steroids in the treatment of anti-sperm antibodies is ineffective and further validation is required [Ib].
- Surgery on the male genital tract should be undertaken only in centres where expertise is available [IV].

KEY POINTS

- Semen analysis is an appropriate starting point in the investigations of the male partner.
- If a severe sperm abnormality is found, clinical examination and bacteriological and endocrinological tests should be undertaken.
- Tact and sensitivity are important when obtaining a history, examining patients and discussing abnormal results with them.
- If reversal of vasectomy is to be undertaken, efforts should be made to obtain epididymal sperm for freezing and future use in case of operation failure.
- There is a considerable variability in sperm quality when assessed in the same individual over time.
- Semen analysis, unlike many modern investigative tests, is operator dependent. Adequate training of the operator is therefore essential to minimize both intraobserver and interobserver variations.
- The andrology laboratory should be subject to external and internal quality control.

Assisted Reproduction

Hany A.M.A. Lashen

INTRODUCTION

The term assisted reproductive technology (ART) includes all methods of infertility treatment that require laboratory handling of gamete(s). Assisted reproduction originated from the practices of donor insemination and intrauterine insemination (IUI) by husband, which were practised long before in-vitro fertilization (IVF). The introduction of IVF and the later introduction of sperm micromanipulation were major developments in the management of infertility. Assisted reproduction technologies have opened many avenues for infertile couples, although not without financial cost and ethical concern. The first 'IVF child', Louise Brown, was the result of IVF of an oocyte obtained in a natural cycle, which was carried out by Patrick Steptoe and Robert Edwards in 1977. Advances in pharmaceuticals, vaginal ultrasound and laboratory practice have significantly improved the success rates of assisted reproduction since that time.

A typical cycle of ART passes through several steps: initial assessment and counselling, ovarian stimulation and monitoring, oocyte retrieval, IVF, embryo transfer (ET), pregnancy test and confirmation of viability with ultrasound. Variations on this theme may take place, depending on the modality of assisted reproduction. However, counselling is a common denominator in all ART modalities and is discussed first. The indications for the different forms of assisted reproduction have already been discussed under the individual causes of infertility.

COUNSELLING

Counselling in the context of IVF treatment refers either to information counselling, i.e. providing sufficient information to patients to allow them to take informed and considered decisions regarding treatment, or to therapeutic and preventative counselling. The former falls within the duties of the medical professional, whilst the latter should be carried out by trained counsellors and has different objectives. To avoid confusion, the roles of both the clinician and the counsellor are considered separately.

Counselling and the clinician

It is imperative for the clinician who deals with infertile couples to understand their feelings and the psychological and social stresses imposed on them. Infertile couples frequently report feelings of inadequacy, with low self-esteem, blame and social exclusion [II]. This significantly affects their social abilities, their marital relations and frequently their work performance [III]. The clinician should be able to assess these impacts, give the couple the opportunity to discuss their anxieties and direct them towards therapeutic counselling if appropriate. Establishing a rapport with the infertile couple is usually not difficult, as they are willing to put their hope in the clinician, who may help them to escape their childlessness. Seeing the couple together is essential [IV]. They should be made to feel at ease and that the doctor is sympathetic to their problem, and should be given ample opportunity to address all their points of concern. A clear plan of action should be agreed from the outset, along with a discussion of the reasons for undertaking all the proposed investigations. Providing the couple with written information and useful addresses is very important. The doctor should be prepared to discuss at length all aspects of the modalities of treatment available to them. It is not unusual to find that the couple have studied the literature and surfed the Internet looking for evidence, and that they are aware of the latest advances and the relevant statistics. Consequently, they may lose confidence if they sense any lack of knowledge on behalf of their doctor.

The counsellor

The counsellor plays a pivotal role in the success of assisted conception treatment. The adequate provision of counselling is a key aspect of HFEA inspection and licensing for any unit that proposes to provide assisted conception treatment. The diversity and versatility of the counsellor role require specific training and experience, as well as a great deal of understanding and compassion. The counsellor should be able to provide therapeutic and preventative counselling. The objective of the former is to alleviate the stresses imposed on the couple by infertility and to help them through the grieving process after a failed cycle or pregnancy loss. The latter modality should provide the couple with a means of dealing with potential stresses or ethical dilemmas that they may encounter during a particular form of treatment. Couples intending to undergo treatments involving gamete donation are particularly vulnerable and should spend time in discussion with the counsellor before starting the treatment cycle.

MODALITIES OF ASSISTED REPRODUCTION

The major forms of ART are IVF-ET, possibly including intra-cytoplasmic sperm injection (ICSI), gamete intrafallopian transfer (GIFT), zygote intrafallopian transfer (ZIFT), IUI, donor insemination (DI) and egg donation. Legal issues dominate practice in this area, and in the UK some of these treatments are regulated by the HFEA. The provision of GIFT and

IUI treatment does not require a licence from the HFEA. Micromanipulation of gametes for ICSI or assisted hatching is additional to basic IVF treatment. Micromanipulation refers to any technique that involves working with gametes or embryos microscopically. Currently, the most commonly used technique of micromanipulation is ICSI, which has revolutionized the management of male infertility and helped overcome fertilization difficulties. ICSI supplanted other, now obsolete, methods of improving sperm penetration into the oocyte, such as zona drilling (ZD) and subzonal sperm injection (SUZI). Assisted hatching as a micromanipulation technique refers to partial drilling or dissection of the zona pellucida to aid implantation of the embryo. The embryo has to 'hatch' by breaking through the zona pellucida before it can implant. Embryos resulting from IVF were thought to have a hardened zona, resulting in a low implantation rate. Weakening the zona mechanically or chemically was therefore thought to enhance embryo hatching and potentially aid implantation. Since the risk of damage to the embryo is increased, routine assisted hatching is not recommended, and this procedure is reserved for older patients and those with multiple cycle failures [IV]. Unlike ICSI, the efficacy of assisted hatching is unproven and many doubt that it is helpful [IV].

Pre-implantation genetic diagnosis (PGD) involves embryo micromanipulation for diagnostic rather than therapeutic purposes. The technique was developed initially to allow identification of the sex of the embryo and sex selection to prevent transmission of X chromosome-linked genetic disorders. However, in theory, any heritable disease for which the gene or chromosome defect is known can be identified in the embryo by PGD, with avoidance of transmission. Several single gene disorders are currently diagnosed using PGD, and the list is growing rapidly. The applicability of this technique for infertility treatment is limited and its real value is for patients who are carriers of genetic disorders [IV]. However, it is being applied as a means of aneuploidy screening, in an attempt to avoid the replacement of chromosomally abnormal embryos that may result in miscarriage. This application may be particularly relevant in improving live birth rates when 'older' women – i.e. those over 40 – are treated with IVF.

OVARIAN STIMULATION AND MONITORING

Although the first cycle of IVF was carried out in a natural ovulatory cycle, ovarian stimulation soon became the cornerstone of assisted conception treatment.

Controlled ovarian stimulation (COS) is now universally used in IVF in order to produce multiple mature oocytes capable of fertilization, implantation and pregnancy. A dazzling number of protocols have been developed using a combination of several agents to achieve this goal. The lack of uniformity amongst different centres in the regimens used reflects the lack of properly randomized studies and the shortage of knowledge regarding the regulation of ovarian function and folliculogenesis. This section reviews the available techniques of COS as well as the stimulating agents and ovarian monitoring.

Ovarian stimulatory agents

Several agents have been used individually and in combination to stimulate folliculogenesis and ovulation, with various degrees of success, as judged by the individual woman's response and the pregnancy rates achieved.

Human gonadotrophins

The use of gonadotrophins to stimulate ovulation was first described by Cole and Hart in 1930,[1] using pregnant mare serum gonadotrophins (PMSG) that could stimulate ovulation in hypophysectomized animals. In 1938 and 1939, two groups induced ovulation in humans using intravenous injection of purified gonadotrophic substance from pregnant mare serum.[2,3] In the 1950s, a variety of gonadotrophins of both human and animal origin was developed for the use of ovulation induction. However, these preparations lacked consistency, and monitoring of ovarian response was extremely basic, using basal body temperature, endometrial biopsy and daily vaginal smears, which were inaccurate and tedious. Others used human pituitary gonadotrophin to avoid the problem of antibody formation to animal proteins, but the availability of this preparation was limited by the difficulty in obtaining human pituitaries. A commercially available preparation of human gonadotrophin extracted from the urine of postmenopausal women was first described by Gemzell et al. in 1958.[4]

Human menopausal gonadotrophin (hMG) was used initially for ovulation induction in anovulatory women until the introduction of IVF led to its use to induce multiple ovulation so that a large number of follicles and oocytes could be obtained. Jones et al.[5] and Garcia et al.[6] used a low hMG dose (150 IU follicle-stimulating hormone (FSH)/day), and the ovarian response was monitored using ultrasound and serum oestradiol (E2) assay. Purified human urinary FSH preparations were later made available and successfully used to induce ovulation. The first IVF pregnancy using purified urinary human FSH was reported by Shaw et al. in 1985.[7] Several studies on the use of FSH alone, or in combination with hMG, have been reported and suggest that pure urinary FSH and hMG are equally effective in ovulation induction for assisted reproduction procedures [Ia].

Recombinant FSH

The production of urinary gonadotrophins requires the collection of vast amounts of urine from postmenopausal women. The difficulties associated with this collection and anxieties about the contamination of urinary FSH with other urinary excreted proteins led to the development of recombinant FSH (rec. FSH), which is >99 per cent pure FSH. Recombinant human FSH is produced from a Chinese hamster ovary cell line transfected with genes for the alpha and beta subunits of FSH. The polypeptide chain of rec. FSH is identical to the native molecule, although there are subtle differences in glycosylation and sialation. In a prospective, randomized study,[8] Out et al. reported that ovarian stimulation with rec. FSH and urinary FSH resulted in significantly more oocytes and embryos in favour of rec. FSH. However, the clinical pregnancy and live birth rates were similar in the two groups of patients.

Clomiphene citrate

Clomiphene citrate was first synthesized in 1956 and introduced for clinical trial use in 1960. It was first used successfully to induce ovulation in 1961 and continues to be the most commonly used drug for this purpose as well as in the empirical treatment of unexplained infertility. After early failure with the use of hMGs in COS for the purpose of IVF, attention turned to clomiphene citrate. Clomiphene citrate is a non-steroidal oestrogen designed as triphenylchloroethylene derivative and administered as a racemic mixture of cis and trans isomers. These isomers were re-labelled as enclomiphene (E) and zuclophene (Z) isomers. The racemic mixture used to induce ovulation comprises 38 per cent Z and 62 per cent E.

The exact mechanism of action of clomiphene citrate is not known. However, it has been suggested that it reacts with oestrogen receptors at the level of the hypothalamus and pituitary and its anti-oestrogenic action results in an increase in gonadotrophin secretion. The rise in FSH and luteinizing hormone (LH) results in the stimulation of follicular growth, and the subsequent ovulation results from the positive feedback of oestrogen produced by the growing follicles on the hypothalamus and pituitary. However, the cycle cancellation rate with clomiphene citrate or with combined clomiphene citrate and hMG was significant, mainly due to abnormal or poor ovarian response, poor follicular growth, or premature LH surge [II]. Consequently, most ART centres have moved away from this approach to COS.

Gonadotrophin-releasing hormone analogues

Native GnRH was first isolated from hypothalamic extracts and sequenced as a decapeptide by Schally et al.[9] Pharmaceutical modification of the amino acid sequence of the GnRH molecule resulted in the development of a large number of GnRH agonists, which are now widely used clinically. The administration of a GnRH agonist results in an initial agonistic effect, leading to the production of both FSH and LH, followed by a sustained decline in both pituitary response and gonadotrophin production, a process known as pituitary down-regulation. GnRH agonists are used with COS to improve the outcome of ovarian stimulation by allowing synchronous folliculogenesis and later to prevent premature luteinization by suppressing the endogenous LH surge. Suppression of the LH surge allows prolonged stimulation with FSH, producing a cohort of large ovarian follicles with mature oocytes.

Down-regulation protocols

Different protocols have been used to induce pituitary down-regulation, based on the timing of administration of the agonist.

- Most commonly, GnRH agonist treatment is begun in the mid-luteal phase of the preceding cycle. The woman will then experience a withdrawal bleed, after which FSH injection is started. This is known as the *long protocol*.
- The *short* or *flare-up protocol* involves agonist treatment being started 2–3 days before or concurrently with ovarian gonadotrophin stimulation. This protocol takes advantage of the initial endogenous release of stored pituitary gonadotrophin as a result of the agonistic effect of the GnRH agonist, followed by the direct stimulatory effect of the exogenous gonadotrophin.
- In the *ultra-short follicular phase protocol* GnRH agonist is administered for the first 3 days of the cycle only. This protocol has proved less popular and is rarely used in practice.

Although numerous reports have been published on different agonist regimes, there are few randomized studies that prospectively compare the efficacy of the various GnRH agonist protocols. Hughes et al.[10] carried out a meta-analysis of ten prospective, randomized trials on the use of GnRH agonists in IVF and concluded that the routine use of GnRH agonists in IVF was associated with a better ovarian response (higher number of oocytes and lower cycle cancellation rate) and greater clinical pregnancy rates [Ia]. They also commented that the available studies comparing the long and the short protocols did not demonstrate any significant difference in terms of cycle cancellation rate or clinical pregnancy rates. However, some concern about the possibility of adverse effects of increased follicular phase LH and progesterone levels seen in the flare-up protocol was later expressed.

Gonadotrophin-releasing hormone antagonists

The GnRH antagonists are synthesized from the native GnRH molecule by multiple amino acid substitutions. They are capable of immediate inhibition of pituitary gonadotrophin secretion and are likely to offer advantages over the currently available agonists due to the absence of the flare-up effect. The early development of these compounds was hampered by the side effects of histamine release and problems in developing a depot formation, with variable levels of absorption. However, these problems have been overcome and the results of large randomized clinical trials have been published. These suggest that pregnancy and live birth rates from GnRH antagonist-controlled IVF are equivalent to those seen in the 'traditional' long protocol [Ib]. The use of an antagonist avoids the prolonged pre-stimulation period of pituitary down-regulation, speeding up the cycle and removing the experience of menopausal side effects. There is also a suggestion that the incidence of OHSS is lower with this approach, although that has yet to be demonstrated in an adequately powered trial.

Monitoring of response to ovarian stimulation

Monitoring of the ovarian response to FSH stimulation is a critical part of good ART practice. Under-response may prompt cycle cancellation or an increase in FSH dosage, while over-response can lead to OHSS, with serious consequences. Both hormonal and ultrasonographic criteria have been used to monitor ovarian response to controlled stimulation and to manage the cycle. Serum concentrations of E2 reflect the growth and maturity of the follicle. The antral follicle produces increasing amounts of oestrogen while maturing, and the E2 concentration per follicle >15 mm in diameter should have reached 1000–1500 pmol/L. If these criteria are met, the presence of one or more pre-ovulatory oocytes is assumed. However, improvement in image quality of transvaginal ultrasound has resulted in a growing reliance on direct measurement of follicle growth, follicles of >16 mm mean diameter being regarded as 'mature'.

The aims of cycle monitoring are:

- to determine the optimum time to administer human chorionic gonadotrophin (hCG) to induce final oocyte maturation before egg collection;
- to predict and therefore prevent the severe forms of OHSS;
- to identify poor responders with a view to improving their response or cancelling the cycle.

In-vitro fertilization–embryo transfer

In-vitro fertilization refers to extracorporeal fertilization of an oocyte. However, the term has been more loosely applied to the whole treatment cycle in which fertilization in vitro is utilized. A typical IVF cycle begins with ovarian stimulation and final maturation of oocytes with a single hCG injection, followed by transvaginal ultrasound-guided oocyte collection, fertilization in vitro, incubation of embryos and ET.

Oocyte maturation in vivo

The oocyte will only become fertile if exposed to an LH surge, causing it to re-enter meiosis and extrude the first polar body. In an IVF cycle in which the endogenous LH surge is prevented by GnRH antagonist or agonist treatment, hCG is used to mimic the natural surge. Human chorionic gonadotrphin is usually given when three or more follicles are larger than 16 mm in mean diameter. Oocyte retrieval is then carried out 34–36 hours later – delay can lead to loss of oocytes due to ovulation.

Oocyte collection

Historically, oocyte collection was carried out laparoscopically, but this has been supplanted by transvaginal ultrasound-guided oocyte retrieval, an approach that offers simplicity and safety and yields more oocytes. Under ultrasound guidance, a 16–17 gauge needle is passed through the lateral vaginal fornix into the ovary to pierce the follicle and aspirate the intrafollicular fluid using a suction apparatus. The oocyte is then microscopically retrieved from the follicular fluid. The potential risks of transvaginal oocyte collection include ovarian infection (estimated at less than 1 per cent) and excessive vaginal bleeding, which can usually be controlled with pressure. Oocyte retrieval can be carried out under general anaesthesia or with local anaesthetic and sedation.

Laboratory procedures

The embryologist retrieves the oocyte from the follicular fluid, grades it for maturity and pre-incubates each oocyte before mechanically stripping the outer cumulus cells from the oocyte itself by repeated aspiration into a glass pipette. The sperm sample is prepared by washing and isolation of motile sperm by a swim-up technique, and a number of spermatozoa are added to each egg. Following incubation, the oocytes are examined microscopically for the presence of two pronuclei, confirming fertilization. The presence of more than two pronuclei indicates polyspermy, and the eggs are discarded as they contain excessive genetic material.

The fertilized eggs (zygotes) are then incubated for a further 1–2 days to allow for the development of the embryos. Embryos are then graded according to the size and number of their cells (blastomeres) and the presence of any fragmentation. The embryologist will select embryos for transfer, and 'spare' embryos can be cryopreserved at this stage if deemed suitable to withstand the freezing process.

Embryo transfer

The number of embryos routinely transferred varies in different countries. In the UK, a maximum of three embryos can be legally transferred. However, the HFEA and the British Fertility Society recommend transfer of a maximum of two embryos in all but exceptional cases, to reduce the risk of multiple pregnancy. Several reports have shown that the transfer of two embryos does not affect the pregnancy rate but significantly reduces the multiple pregnancy rate, which in turn considerably reduces neonatal morbidity and mortality [Ib].

The embryos are transferred transcervically into the uterine cavity using a soft polyethylene catheter. The procedure is usually painless and straightforward. Manipulation of the cervix by distending the urinary bladder or using a volsellum is occasionally required to facilitate a difficult ET.

Luteal phase support

The luteal phase is 'supported' until the pituitary gland recovers from pituitary suppression and produces the required LH to maintain the corpus luteum. This can be achieved by administering hCG to maintain the corpus luteum directly, or indirectly by administering progesterone to the patient. In earlier reports, the administration of hCG was held to have a marginal advantage over progesterone administration in terms of pregnancy rates, but with increas-esd risk of OHSS [Ia]. Recent evidence has not shown any difference in pregnancy rates between the two treatments

[Ia]. Progesterone can be administered in several forms; however, the intramuscular and transvaginal routes are most commonly used.

Pregnancy test and confirmation of a clinical pregnancy

If a pregnancy occurs, a positive urinary pregnancy test will be obtained approximately 14 days post-ET. Elevated serum levels of hCG can be detected earlier. The risk of ectopic pregnancy should be considered in all cases until an intrauterine pregnancy is later confirmed by ultrasound scan. If necessary, β-hCG levels should be serially measured to exclude ectopic pregnancy.

The definition of clinical pregnancy varies in different countries. The presence of fetal cardiac activity on ultrasound scan is important to make the diagnosis in most European countries, whereas in the USA the presence of a gestational sac is sufficient to diagnose a clinical pregnancy. A positive pregnancy test that is followed by a decline in the hCG levels without evidence of a clinical pregnancy is referred to as biochemical pregnancy.

- Infertility investigations and treatment cause significant stress to couples. Counselling services are an essential requirement if units are to be licensed by the HFEA.
- IVF is a suitable treatment for any cause of infertility.
- Transferring two instead of three embryos does not reduce the pregnancy rate, but significantly reduces the multiple pregnancy rate.
- The female partner's age, ovarian reserve, cause and duration of infertility and previous pregnancies affect the success rate of IVF treatments.
- Pituitary down-regulation prior to ovarian stimulation for the purpose of IVF treatment improves the pregnancy rate.
- The difference between urinary and high purity menopausal gonadotrophins with regard to pregnancy rates is in favour of the high purity, which yields clinical pregnancy rates similar to those of recombinant FSH.

ALTERNATIVES TO IVF

Intrauterine insemination

Washed partner or donor sperm can be inseminated into the uterine cavity using a polyethylene catheter. Intrauterine insemination of the partner's sperm without ovarian stimulation has been used to treat unexplained and cervical factor infertility, but with poor results. With the introduction of COS, this approach revived and has yielded good success rates in treating mild male factor and unexplained infertility. The presence of patent normal fallopian tubes is essential for this treatment. The majority of clinicians do not consider patients with a history of ectopic pregnancy to be suitable for this treatment, as tubal disease is the precipitating factor in most of these patients. Intrauterine insemination can be used in conjunction with ovarian stimulation with either clomiphene citrate or gonadotrophin. However, the results with gonadotrophins are generally better than with clomiphene citrate [II]. The success rates with this line of treatment have been discussed previously.

Use of donor gametes

Sperm from anonymous or known donors has been used to treat infertile couples for centuries. More recently, legislation has regulated this practice and recognized the need for careful counselling before treatment, particularly considering the welfare of the potential child. As IVF has grown, oocyte donation has also become feasible and is now widely practised. There are similarities between sperm and egg donation with regard to the screening of donors. Any potential donor should be interviewed and a thorough medical, social and family history taken. Donors have a legal obligation to divulge any previous history of medical illnesses and particularly any family history of congenital or hereditary diseases. Screening for human immunodeficiency virus (HIV), hepatitis (B and C), syphilis, cytomegalovirus, gonorrhoea and chlamydia should be conducted on every prospective donor. A negative HIV test should be repeated 6 months later. Donor insemination is now only carried out using quarantined frozen sperm, to reduce risk of HIV transmission.

Counselling

The counsellor's role is also to make sure that the couple have carefully considered the implications of their decision to undergo treatment, and to support them through a stressful time of their lives. Matching the physical characteristics of the donor with the recipient should also be discussed. This is usually straightforward if donor sperm is to be used, but more difficult given the smaller number of oocyte donors. The couple should also be informed that, despite careful screening of donors, the normal population risk of congenital anomalies still exists. Their plans to discuss the method of conception with the child should also be explored, as this can lead to conflict later.

Donor recruitment

It has been much easier to recruit male than female donors. An oocyte donor has to undergo ovarian stimulation and oocyte retrieval as described for IVF. Such risks and inconveniences do not apply to the male. Previous fertility, although desirable, is not always a prerequisite for accepting a donor. Some couples may choose to receive gametes from a known donor. However, the majority of couples prefer an anonymous donor, which is usually encouraged to avoid emotional and ethical complications. Given the rarity of volunteer female donors, the HFEA has recently allowed 'egg sharing', in which patients undergoing IVF for their own benefit donate a proportion of their oocytes in exchange for reduced treatment costs.

Indications for use of donated sperm

The uptake of donor insemination has fallen since the introduction of ICSI, which can be used for severely oligospermic males or for azoospermic males if sperm can be retrieved from a testicular biopsy. However, this is not always possible, and ICSI will fail to result in pregnancy in some couples. Testicular failure with complete absence of spermatogenesis, typically after chemotherapy, and the high cost of ICSI treatment are now the main indications for DI. Donor insemination is also used to remove the risk of transmission of inherited disorders and in the treatment of single women. It can be carried out intracervically or by IUI. Cumulative pregnancy rates of up to 80 per cent after 6–12 treatment cycles have been reported, much depending on the fertility and age of the female. IVF using donor sperm can be resorted to if the female partner has tubal disease or if insemination treatments fail.

Use of donor oocytes

Oocyte donation can be offered to women with ovarian failure or oocyte abnormalities, and also for the prevention of some hereditary disorders. Although initially used in cases of premature ovarian failure, the technique has now been controversially applied to women beyond natural menopause, and pregnancies with donated oocytes have been reported for women in their 60s and 70s.

Egg donation treatment is effectively carried out in an IVF cycle. The donor undergoes ovarian stimulation and oocyte collection, while the recipient undergoes the ET. The success rates from this treatment are similar to, if not slightly higher than, the average success rate expected from IVF treatment.

KEY POINTS

- Donor insemination is useful in cases of severe male factor infertility and genetic diseases in the male partner or rhesus iso-immunization.
- Unless the male partner is azoospermic and testicular sperm retrieval fails, the role of DI is becoming less evident in severe male factor infertility. However, financial constraints may force some couples to accept this form of treatment over ICSI.
- Intrauterine insemination using donor sperm with or without superovulation offers better pregnancy rates compared to intracervical insemination.
- Unless the female partner is anovulatory, DI treatment should be carried out in a natural cycle in the first place to avoid multiple pregnancies. The timing of introduction of ovarian stimulation in DI programmes is debatable. However, three to six natural treatment cycles need to be considered prior to starting ovarian stimulation.

COMPLICATIONS OF ASSISTED REPRODUCTION

Multiple pregnancy

In-vitro fertilization pregnancy rates are improved by the transfer of more than one embryo. However, the incidence of multiple pregnancy increases with the number of embryos transferred. Approaches to this problem vary around the world, but UK legislation and guidance restrict the number of embryos transferred to two, unless there are exceptional circumstances. Unfortunately, 'exceptional circumstance' has not been defined, leaving an obvious loophole for less scrupulous clinicians. Two-embryo transfer has been shown to offer good pregnancy rates without significant risk of multiple pregnancy, although late division of a transferred embryo can occasionally still produce a triplet pregnancy after a two-embryo transfer. Multiple pregnancy is clearly associated with higher maternal morbidity and both fetal mortality and morbidity [II]. Therefore, efforts should be made to reduce such risks and to counsel patients accordingly.

Ovarian hyperstimulation syndrome

This is a serious and potentially life-threatening complication of ovarian hyperstimulation. The incidence of significant OHSS complicating assisted conception is variably quoted as between 0.6 per cent and 14 per cent [III]. The underlying cause of OHSS is not known, but release of a vasoactive ovarian factor is likely to be involved. Several studies have reported that women with ultrasonographic or biochemical features of polycystic ovary syndrome are at higher risk of developing OHSS compared to those with normal ovaries. A link between lean habitus and OHSS has also been suggested.

The best approach to the management of OHSS is avoidance [II], as the syndrome only develops after the administration of hCG, and identifying those at high risk of developing OHSS can lead to prevention by cycle cancellation. This is costly and disappointing to patients and clinicians alike. The features used to identify 'high-risk' patients include a rapid rise in E2 in response to ovarian stimulation, high peak E2 level on the day of hCG administration, and the presence of large numbers of follicles on ultrasound. However, the predictive value of these commonly used criteria is low, and cases continue to occur in 'low-risk' women. If the risk is deemed excessive after hCG has been given, abandoning the embryo transfer, with elective cryopreservation of all embryos and later frozen embryo transfer, is effective in reducing the severity, but not the incidence, of symptomatic OHSS.

The clinical picture and the management of the syndrome depend on its degree of severity. It may present 3–7 days post-hCG injection (early presentation), or 12–17 days post-hCG (late presentation). The early presentation is an acute effect of the pre-ovulatory dose of hCG, whereas the late presentation is induced by the rising serum concentration of hCG produced by the pregnancy. A classification of OHSS based on the clinical signs is widely used to guide diagnosis and treatment. Golan et al.[11] described several degrees of severity of the syndrome. In the mild form, the clinical picture of OHSS includes abdominal distension, nausea and vomiting, diarrhoea and moderate ovarian enlargement (<12 cm in average diameter). The moderate form is similar to the mild but includes the presence of ascites on ultrasound scan. The severe form includes clinical evidence of ascites and/or hydrothorax, haemoconcentration and significant ovarian enlargement (>12 cm in average diameter).

In women with a mild/moderate form of OHSS (haematocrit value ≤44 per cent), bed rest and fluid replacement together with monitoring of the biochemical profile are all that is needed for their management. However, admission to the intensive therapy unit may be necessary in the severe form of the syndrome (haematocrit >44 per cent) and hospitalization is always mandatory. Paracentesis under direct ultrasound guidance is indicated in severely compromised patients and when respiration becomes difficult due to severe abdominal distension. It has also been reported that re-infusion of the ascitic fluid with or without ultrafiltration can be useful in some severe cases. Some reports suggest that albumin infusion can prevent severe OHSS. Owing to the potential risk of human albumin infusion, many units restrict its use to cases of biochemically proven hypoalbuminaemia.

Risk of ovarian cancer

Case reports of ovarian tumours in women undergoing infertility treatment led to concern about the potential neoplastic effect of ovarian stimulatory agents such as clomiphene citrate and gonadotrophins. Such an effect was hypothesized to occur because ovulation induction results in the development of a higher number of ovulatory follicles per cycle than occur naturally. Ovarian epithelial cells proliferate after ovulation to cover the exposed surface of the ovary. In some instances, epithelium may be incorporated into the ovarian stroma to form epithelial inclusion cysts. These inclusion cysts have been suspected to be the areas most likely to undergo malignant transformation. Anxiety concerning a possible effect of ovulation induction on the development of ovarian cancer was raised following publication of an analysis of pooled data from case-control studies in this area by Whittemore et al. in 1992.[12] It was reported that infertile women exposed to ovulation-inducing agents had a significantly higher risk of ovarian cancer compared to infertile women with no exposure. However, the study provided little information about the type of drug used, the duration of treatment and the dosage. The relative risk of the individual ovulation-inducing agents in causing ovarian cancer has also been studied. Rossing et al.[13] reported a significant association of clomiphene citrate use for 12 cycles or more and the diagnosis of ovarian tumour (relative risk 11.1, confidence interval 1.5–82.3). In the UK, the Committee on Safety of Medicines recommends that the use of clomiphene citrate should be restricted to 6 months per patient, although evidence that exceeding this limit for women who have conceived once using clomiphene citrate and wish to do so again is lacking. The 35th RCOG Study Group recommended that, as a part of shared decision making before treatment with any fertility drugs, women should be counselled regarding the possible risk of ovarian cancer after multiple treatments.

- The surest way of avoiding OHSS is to withhold the hCG injection.
- The use of clomiphene citrate should be restricted to 6 months to avoid the risk of ovarian epithelial neoplasia.
- More evidence is needed to establish any potential risk of ovarian neoplasia caused by externally administered gonadotrophins.

ETHICAL ISSUES

From the outset, human use of assisted conception technology brought with it numerous ethical concerns. A detailed review of this aspect of ART practice is beyond the scope of this chapter, but certain controversial areas stand out as frequently encountered ethical problems in clinical practice. These include problems of funding and access to treatment, payment for donors and the use of donated gametes, fetal reduction and human embryo research. These aspects are discussed here as examples of the ethical dilemmas that can occur.

Funding issues

In the UK, the limited resources of the National Health Service (NHS) have dictated the government position on funding infertility treatment. In some parts of the country, patients have limited access to NHS funding for IVF. Such funds are rationed by restrictive eligibility criteria, usually a mixture of factors relating to the chance of success (female age, normal body mass) and social criteria (neither partner should have a child already, no funding if either partner has been sterilized). The absence of a national policy on funding infertility treatment, coupled with overt rationing of access where some funds are available, has led to a protracted public debate. The National Institute for Clinical Excellence has now produced guidance in this area, which may help to resolve some of the discrepancies amongst regions.

Payment for donors

The HFEA Act (1990) stipulates that no money or other benefits should be given or received for supplying gametes or embryos, other than expenses and nominal fees. This has little effect on the number of volunteers offering to donate sperm, a procedure that is free of risk to the health of the donor. In contrast, oocyte donation carries significant risks of side effects of ovarian stimulation and oocyte recovery. Some have argued that oocyte donors should be allowed to receive payment to compensate them for the risk they encounter. To overcome the shortage of egg donors, egg sharing has also been allowed by the HFEA.

Fetal reduction

Assisted conception has increased the risk of multiple pregnancies, with the attendant increase in perinatal mortality and morbidity and cost to the health service. Even with a blanket two-embryo transfer policy, the risk of triplet pregnancy cannot be completely eliminated. If a higher order multiple pregnancy does occur, this can be reduced by selective fetal reduction. This is a difficult decision, made harder by the many years of unsuccessful treatment that may have led up to the pregnancy. The objective of fetal reduction is to reduce the perinatal mortality and morbidity associated with high-order multiple pregnancies. In most cases, triplets and quadruplet pregnancies are reduced to twins, but occasionally some couples request the reduction of twins to a singleton pregnancy. Selective fetal reduction is usually carried out at the beginning of the second trimester to allow for spontaneous miscarriage to take place. However, this is too early to screen for congenital anomaly. The procedure is not without risk, and complete miscarriage can be a very distressing consequence in about 15 per cent of cases. Careful, sympathetic counselling is obviously vital before selective reduction is undertaken.

Embryo cryopreservation

Cryopreservation of extra embryos allows more cycles of embryo transfer from one IVF cycle. Although the success rate for frozen embryo transfer is inferior to that for fresh cycles, such practice increases the potential success rate obtained from a single IVF cycle. So far, no risk has been linked to embryo freezing. The couple's consent should be obtained prior to freezing any embryos. Furthermore, the potential ethical issues that may arise should be carefully discussed with the couple, especially the fate of the embryos if either partner were to die.

Embryo research

Research on human embryos has been licensed by the HFEA since its inception in 1990. Study protocols are only approved if they ask questions that cannot be answered using other methods. Until recently, most human embryo research was directly linked to improving the outcomes of infertility treatment, for example in the development of PGD or the study of embryo and blastocyst culture conditions. The recent surge of interest in the therapeutic use of human embryonic stem cells has stimulated a heated debate on the ethics of using 'spare' IVF embryos for the creation of stem cell lines, resulting in a House of Lords' ruling that such research can be carried out within the UK within strict guidelines and governance.

HUMAN FERTILISATION AND EMBRYOLOGY AUTHORITY

The UK HFEA replaced the Voluntary Licensing Authority established by the Warnock Committee following passage of the Human Fertilisation and Embryology Act in 1990. The role of the HFEA is to monitor and licence centres that offer IVF treatment or deal with human gametes or embryos. The licence given to centres by the HFEA is subject to yearly renewal after the inspection of the relevant centre. The HFEA also regulates research on human embryos and gametes. The organization is largely funded by fees paid by couples undergoing treatment. The HFEA has a code of practice that guides licensed centres, and produces a yearly publication of the results of all centres that offer IVF and gamete donation along with a patient guide.

KEY POINTS

- Counselling is at the heart of ART treatment.
- IVF is effective in treating all types of infertility, with similar success rates.
- Two-embryo transfer is as effective as three-embryo transfer, without the risk of high-order multiple pregnancy associated with the latter.
- OHSS can be prevented by withholding hCG injection. However, its severity could be reduced by freezing all the embryos and not proceeding with fresh ET.
- OHSS is a potentially life-threatening condition; therefore, anticipation of its occurrence, early diagnosis and appropriate management are essential to avoid any fatalities.
- Clomiphene citrate should be given for a total period of no longer than 6 months.
- Every clinician should be aware of all the ethical issues surrounding ART, as it represents a key issue when counselling patients for such treatment modalities.

KEY REFERENCES

1. Cole HH, Hart GH. The potency of blood serum of mares in progressive stages of pregnancy in effecting the sexual maturity of the immature rat. *Am J Physiol* 1930; **93**:57–68.
2. Davis ME, Koff AK. The experimental production of ovulation in the human subject. *Am J Obstet Gynecol* 1938; **36**:183–99.
3. Siegler SL, Fein MJ. Studies in artificial ovulation with the hormone of pregnant mares' serum. *Am J Obstet Gynecol* 1939; **38**:1021–36.
4. Gemzel CA, Diczfalusi E, Tillinger G. Clinical effect of human pituitary follicle stimulating hormone (FSH). *J Clin Endocrinol Metab* 1958; **18**:1333–48.
5. Jones HW Jr, Jones SG, Andrews MC et al. The programme for in vitro fertilisation at Norfolk. *Fertil Steril* 1982; **38**:14–21.
6. Garcia J, Jones G, Acosta A et al. Human menopausal gonadotrophin–human chorionic gonadotrophin follicular maturation for oocyte aspiration: phase II 1981. *Fertil Steril* 1983; **39**:174–9.
7. Shaw RW, Ndukwe G, Imoedemhe DA et al. Twin pregnancy after pituitary desensitisation with LHRH agonist and pure FSH. *Lancet* 1985; 2:506.
8. Out HJ, Mannaerts B, Driessen S et al. Recombinant follicle stimulating hormone (rFSH: Puregon) in assisted reproduction: more oocytes, more pregnancies. Results from five comparative studies. *Hum Reprod Update* 1996; 2:162–71.
9. Schally AV, Kastin AJ, Arimura A. Hypothalamic FSH and LH-regulating hormone: structure, physiology and clinical studies. *Fertil Steril* 1971; **22**:703–21.
10. Hughes EG, Sagle MA, Fedorkow DM et al. The routine use of gonadotropin-releasing hormone agonists prior to in vitro fertilization and gamete intrafallopian transfer: a meta analysis of randomized controlled trials. *Fertil Steril* 1992; **58**:888–95.
11. Golan A, Ron-El R, Herman A et al. Ovarian hyperstimulation syndrome: an update review. *Obstet Gynaecol Survey* 1989; 6:430–40.
12. Whittemore AS, Harris R, Itnyre J, and the Collaborative Ovarian Cancer Group. Characteristics relating to ovarian cancer risk: collaborative analysis of 12 US case control studies. IV. The pathogenesis of epithelial ovarian cancer. *Am J Epidemiol* 1992; **136**:1212–20.
13. Rossing MA, Daling JR, Weiss NS et al. Ovarian tumours in a cohort of infertile women. *N Engl J Med* 1994; **331**:771–6.

Reproductive medicine

Polycystic Ovarian Syndrome

Enda McVeigh

INTRODUCTION

In 1935 Stein and Leventhal first described the polycystic ovary as a frequent cause of irregular ovulation or anovulation in women seeking treatment for subfertility. The initial management of the condition was surgical, with wedge resection of the ovary resulting in restoration of ovulation in the majority of cases.

However, a large group of women presented with symptoms of androgen excess, especially hirsutism, greasy skin and acne either in association with subfertility or as their main complaint, and were also found to have polycystic ovaries (PCO). With the availability of radioimmunoassay, it was recognized that many of these women had an increased ratio of luteinizing hormone (LH) to follicle-stimulating hormone (FSH) and this became a biochemical diagnostic criterion for the condition.

With the increased clinical use of ultrasound in the 1980s, it became clear that many women had the ultrasound characteristics of PCO, with or without the biochemical or clinical features of PCOS, and therefore that PCO were not associated with a single syndrome.

DEFINITIONS

The definition of PCOS has led to considerable debate. At a recent consensus meeting between the American Society of Reproductive Medicine (ASRM) and the European Society of Human Reproduction and Embryology (ESHRE) in Rotterdam in May 2003 it was agreed that the diagnostic criteria for PCOS should include the following.

- Evidence of hyperandrogenism, biochemical or clinical in the absence of non-classical adrenal hyperplasia. Most commonly hirsutism, acne and crown pattern baldness.
- Ovulatory dysfunction; amenorrhoea, oligoamenorrhoea.
- Morphological polycystic ovaries.

Women who have at least two of these three criteria are said to have PCOS. Polycystic ovaries should not be confused with the PCOS. Polycystic ovaries may be diagnosed in the absence of any clinical syndrome. The overlap in ultrasound, biochemical and clinical features of the syndrome and the realization that the condition is a continuum or spectrum leads to the difficulty in arriving at a precise definition (Figure 53.1).

Ultrasound is the gold standard for the diagnosis of PCO. The diagnostic criterion described by Adams et al.[1] of ten discrete follicles of $<10\,mm$, usually peripherally arranged around an enlarged, hyperechogenic central stroma, still holds today (Figure 53.2).

Previously it was thought not only to be essential to have an elevated level of LH, but the ratio of LH to FSH was also required to be elevated in order to define PCOS. Initially the

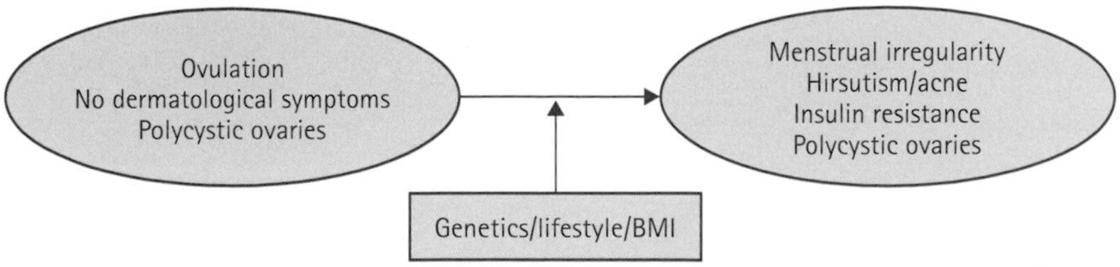

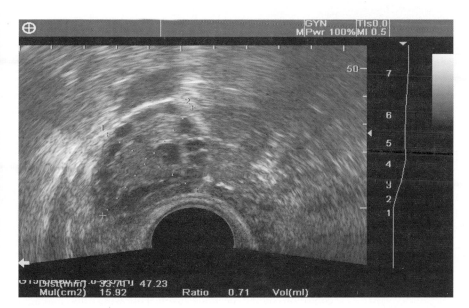

Figure 53.1 Concept of PCOS as a spectrum. BMI, body mass index

Figure 53.2 Ultrasound appearance of a polycystic ovary

ratio was 2:1, then 3:1. However, the idea of both elevated levels of LH and ratios being essential for the diagnosis of PCOS has now been abandoned. Similarly, elevated levels of androgens are unhelpful in defining the syndrome, as these levels are inconsistently elevated. Other limitations of the biochemical diagnosis of PCOS included the variable and imprecise nature of the assays and the dynamic nature of hormonal steroidal release from the ovaries.

INCIDENCE

Polycystic ovary syndrome is the most common female endocrine abnormality affecting women in their reproductive years. The prevalence of PCO in asymptomatic women is thought to be between 16 and 33 per cent (Table 53.1).[2] However, the percentage of women who have clinical manifestations (menstrual disorder, hirsutism and acne) in the presence of morphological PCO is as high as 90 per cent.

AETIOLOGY

Uncertainty still surrounds the exact aetiology of PCOS, although there is increasing evidence for genetic factors.[6]

Table 53.1 Incidence of PCO and PCOS in different populations

Reference	Setting	n	PCO (%)	PCOS (%)
Polson et al. (1988)[3]	Volunteers	258	23	76
Clayton et al. (1992)[4]	GP practice	190	22	30
Farquhar et al. (1994)[2]	Electoral roll	183	21	59
Michelmore et al. (1999)[5]	GP practice	224	34	65

PCO, polycystic ovaries; PCOS, polycystic ovary syndrome.

The syndrome clusters in families and prevalence rates in first-degree relatives are five to six times higher than in the general population. There is also a heritable component to pancreatic beta-cell dysfunction in PCOS families. An autosomal mode of inheritance has been postulated, but the most plausible theory is that PCOS is inherited as an oligogenic trait. In men, this genetic predisposition may be expressed as male pattern baldness.

There are a number of accepted pathophysiological events that contribute to the clinical syndrome of PCOS. One of the most significant is the elevated level of androgen production by the ovaries. This is the result of a series of complex biochemical processes that begins with disordered activity of the cytochrome P450c enzyme complex, which catalyses 17-hydroxylase and 17/20-lyase activities, the rate-limiting step in androgen production (Figure 53.3). Persistently elevated levels of LH will produce excessive

Reproductive medicine

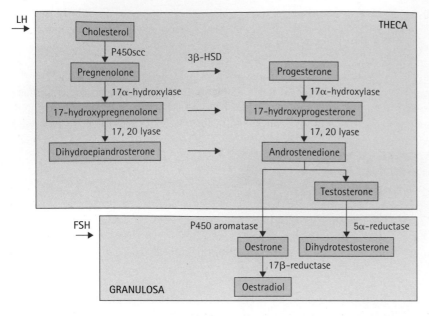

Figure 53.3   Steroid production in the ovary. LH, luteinizing hormone; HSD, hydroxysteroid dehydrogenase; FSH, follicle-stimulating hormone

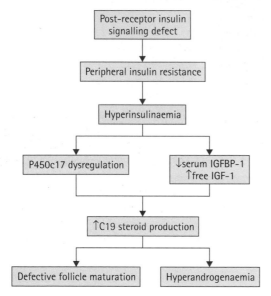

Figure 53.4   The insulin story. IGF-1, insulin growth factor 1; IGFBP-1, insulin growth factor binding protein 1

amounts of androstenedione by causing an increase in cytochrome P450 activity. However, this pathway cannot explain increased androgen levels in women who do not have elevated LH levels.

Insulin resistance occurs in 30–60 per cent of women with PCOS.[7] It is most prominent in women with a high body mass index (BMI). The resultant hyperinsulinaemia (and increased insulin-like growth factor, IGF-1) stimulates LH-induced androgen production from the ovaries. In the liver, the elevated insulin level causes a decreased production of sex hormone-binding globulin and IGF-1-binding protein, leading to elevated levels of biologically active androgens and IGF-1 in the circulation. It is through these processes that insulin may contribute to the overall free androgen excess seen in PCOS (Figure 53.4).

MANAGEMENT

The initial management of diagnosed PCOS will depend on the clinical presentation. Initially, an explanation of the condition should be undertaken. Following this, management will take the following form.

Lifestyle

Obesity is a common factor in the majority of women with PCOS. It is postulated that a woman may be genetically predisposed to developing PCOS but it is only the interaction of environmental factors (obesity) with the genetic factors that results in the characteristic metabolic and menstrual disturbances (see Figure 53.1). Weight loss, altered diet and exercise have been shown to be effective in the management of PCOS.

Anovulation and infertility

It is important that patients optimize their health before embarking on fertility therapy. The principle of the management of anovulatory infertility in women with PCOS is to induce regular unifollicular ovulation, whilst minimizing the risk of multiple pregnancy and ovarian hyperstimulation syndrome (OHSS). Ovulation induction strategies should begin with simple measures.

- *Weight loss*. Even moderate obesity (BMI >27 kg/m^2) is associated with a reduced chance of ovulation, with a body fat distribution leading to an increased waist:hip ratio (central obesity) appearing to be more important than body weight alone. The loss of as little as 10 per cent body weight may result in a return to regular ovuation.

- *Clomiphene citrate.* The anti-oestrogens clomiphene citrate and tamoxifen are effective treatments for anovulation in appropriately selected women. They block oestrogen receptors, with a resultant increase in endogenous FSH production. Ovulation induction with clomiphene citrate should only be performed in circumstances that allow access to ovarian ultrasound monitoring. If general practitioners are involved, there should be an agreed shared care protocol. There is no evidence to suggest an increased risk of ovarian cancer when clomiphene is used for fewer than 12 cycles, with the current recommendation being not to exceeding 6 months of continuous therapy. This 6-month therapy recommendation is based on cumulative conception data.

- *Gonadotrophin therapy.* Recombinant FSH and human menopausal gonadotrophin are both effective for ovulation induction in women with clomiphene-resistant PCOS – which accounts for about 20–30 per cent of women with PCOS. There is no advantage in routinely using gonadotrophin-releasing hormone (GnRH) analogues in conjunction with gonadotrophins for ovulation induction in women with clomiphene-resistant PCOS, as there is no increase in the pregnancy rate. Furthermore, their use may be associated with an increased risk of ovarian hyperstimulation.

- *Laparoscopic ovarian drilling* with either diathermy or laser is an effective treatment for anovulation in women with clomiphene-resistant PCOS. It has been shown to lead to ovulation in 80 per cent of patients, with a normalization of LH concentrations and good pregnancy rates with a low miscarriage rate. However, more research is needed into the long-term consequences of causing ovarian damage in this way. Laparoscopic ovarian diathermy should be considered for women who fail to respond to clomiphene citrate and who need a laparoscopic assessment of their pelvis or who live too far away from hospital to be able to attend for the intensive monitoring required on gonadotrophin therapy.

- The role of insulin resistance as a principal factor in the pathogenesis of PCOS has led to the use of *insulin-lowering agents* for its treatment. The most extensively studied insulin-lowering agent in the treatment of PCOS is metformin – an oral anti-hyperglycaemic agent used initially in the treatment of type 2 diabetes mellitus. A review of 23 prospective studies[8] addressing the effects of metformin on PCOS confirms a beneficial role of metformin in reducing insulin resistance in some women with PCOS. Other favourable biochemical effects include reduced free testosterone levels and increased sex hormone-binding globulin. Metformin may also improve menstrual regularity, leading to spontaneous ovulation, and may improve ovarian response to conventional ovulation induction therapies. There is, however, little evidence supporting the use of metformin to facilitate weight reduction or to improve serum lipids or hirsutism. Further evaluation is required to define the long-term effectiveness of metformin, who will benefit from metformin treatment, and the optimal duration of metformin therapy.

- Weight loss in women with an elevated BMI is an effective management strategy in PCOS [Ib].
- Clomiphene citrate is an effective treatment for anovulation in PCOS [Ia].
- Gonadotrophin therapy is an effective treatment for anovulation in clomiphene-resistant PCOS [Ia].
- Laparoscopic ovarian drilling is an effective treatment for anovulation in clomiphene-resistant PCOS [Ia].
- The use of metformin and other drugs that effect insulin resistance in the management of PCOS requires further evaluation.

SKIN MANIFESTATIONS AND HYPERANDROGENISM

Hirsutism, androgenic alopecia, seborrhoea and acne are all skin manifestations of androgen excess and may occur in the context of PCOS. Acanthosis nigricans is also a cutaneous marker of insulin resistance that is associated with PCOS.

Hirsutism

See Chapter 54.

Acne

Acne is a chronic inflammatory disorder of the pilosebaceous units. It is present in approximately 30 per cent of women with PCOS, although it affects up to 80 per cent of school-age children. It is caused by an increase in sebum production, abnormal keratinization of the pilosebaceous duct, abnormal microbial flora, in particular relating to *Propionibacterium acnes*, and inflammation. The sequence of events is that the increased androgen levels lead to an increase in size of the sebaceous glands, which in turn causes an increase in the active metabolites of androgens, which again leads to an increase in the gland size. These enlarged glands then produce more sebum, which promotes more *P. acnes*. The *P. acnes* then digest the sebum to a more viscous product, which leads to follicular plugging and subsequent formation of comedones, the initial lesions in acne.

Acne primarily affects the face and, less often, the back and chest. Comedones are non-inflamed lesions and are either open comedones (blackheads – black due to melanin) or closed comedone (whiteheads). Inflammatory lesions are either superficial (papules or pustules) or deeper pustules (nodules and cysts).

Treatment

Mild acne can be managed with topical agents, keratolytics, such as azalaic acid, retinoids or antibacterials, such as benzoyl peroxide, clindamycin 1 per cent lotion and erythromycin 2 per cent gel. More severe forms may require oral antibiotics such as tetracyclines or erythromycin.

The systemic androgen level may be lowered with the use of anti-androgens such as cyproterone acetate and spironolactone. The oral contraceptive pill (OCP) will also reduce the level of free androgen; however, it is important to choose an OCP with a low progestogenic effect.

For severe acne, isotretinoin is prescribed and produces remission in 70 per cent of cases. However, this drug is severely teratogenic and adequate contraception is necessary.

Acanthosis nigricans

Acanthosis nigricans is a mucocutaneous eruption characterized by hyperkeratosis, papillomatosis and increased pigmentation. It is primarily seen in patients with type 2 diabetes (insulin resistant). It occurs in up to 5 per cent of women with PCOS. Plaques are most often found in the axillae, the nape of the neck, under the breasts and in the flexures.

LONG-TERM HEALTH IMPLICATIONS OF PCOS

The long-term health implications of PCOS stem mostly from the insulin resistance and the long-term effect of unopposed oestrogen on the endometrium. Despite the clear relationship between the PCOS phenotype and risk factors for coronary heart disease (obesity, hyperinsulinism, elevated triglycerides and cholesterol, and increased prevalence of hypertension), a long-term follow-up in the UK[9] showed no significant increase in mortality rates form circulatory disease. This differs from women and men with type 2 diabetes, who have an increased incidence of coronary heart disease,[10] and may be due to an as yet unknown protective factor in the women with PCOS.

The epidemiological studies to date in this area are, however, fraught with the difficulty in accurately diagnosing PCOS retrospectively. Further epidemiological studies investigating the long-term health implications of PCOS are required.

KEY POINTS

- PCOS involves a spectrum of symptoms, which may change with changes in the patient's lifestyle and BMI.
- Management should be directed at the symptoms.
- If the patient's BMI is elevated, weight loss is central to successful management.
- The long-term health implications include:
  - increased incidence of multiple pregnancy, with subsequent increase in perinatal mortality and morbidity;
  - increased incidence of gestational diabetes (13 per cent in women with PCOS vs 5–10 per cent in the normal population);
  - increased incidence of pregnancy-induced hypertension independent of obesity and gestational diabetes;
  - bone metabolism is not affected, but there is a possibility of supernormal mineralization with androgens;
  - a five-fold increase in the incidence of endometrial cancer in PCOS;[11]
  - a 2.5-fold increase in ovarian cancer;[12]
  - no significant increase in mortality rates from circulatory disease.

KEY REFERENCES

1. Adams J, Franks S, Polson DW et al. Multifollicular ovaries: clinical and endocrine features and response to pulsatile gonadotrophin releasing hormone. *Lancet* 1985; 2:1375–9.

2. Farquhar CM, Birdsall M, Manning P, Mitchell JM, France TJ. The prevalence of polycystic ovaries on ultrasound scanning in a population of randomly selected women. *Aust N Z J Obstet Gynaecol* 1994; 34:67–72.

3. Polson DW, Adams J, Wadworth J, Franks S. Polycystic ovaries – a common finding in normal women. *Lancet* 1998; 1:870–2.

4. Clayton RN, Ogden V, Hodgkinson J. How common are polycystic ovaries in normal women and what is their significance for the fertility of the population? *Clin Endocrinol* 1992; 37:127–34.

5. Michelmore K, Balen AH, Dunger DB, Vezely MP. Polycystic ovaries and associated clinical and biochemical features n young women. *Clin Endocrinol* (Oxford) 1999; 51:779–86.

6. Kahsar-Miller MD, Nixon C, Boots LR, Go RC, Azziz R. Prevalence of polycystic ovary syndrome (PCOS) in

first-degree relatives of patients with PCOS. *Fertil Steril* 2001; **75**(1):53–8.

7. Marsden PJ, Murdoch AP, Taylor R. Tissue insulin sensitivity and body weight in polycystic ovary syndrome. *Clin Endocrinol (Oxf)* 2001; **55**(2): 191–9.

8. Awartani KA, Cheung AP. Metformin and polycystic ovary syndrome: a literature review. *J Obstet Gynaecol Can* 2002; **24**(5):393–401.

9. Peirpoint T, McKeigue PM, Isaac AJ, Wild SH, Jacobs HS. Mortality of women with polycystic ovary syndrome at long term follow up. *J Clin Epidemiol* 1998; **51**:581–6.

10. Abbasi F, Brown B, Lamendola C, McLaughlin T, Reaven G. Relationship between obesity, insulin resistance, and coronary heart disease risk. *J Am Coll Cardiol* 2002; **40**(5):937.

11. Dahlgren E, Friberg LG, Johansson S. Endometrial carcinoma; ovarian dysfunction – a risk in young women. *Eur J Obstet Gynaecol Reprod Biol* 1991; **41**:143–50.

12. Schildkrant JM, Schwingl PJ, Bastros E, Evanoff A, Huges C. Epithelial ovarian cancer risk among women with polycystic ovary syndrome. *Obstet Gynecol* 1996; **88**:554–9.

Chapter 54

Hirsutism and Virilism

Enda McVeigh

HIRSUTISM

Definition

Hirsuties may be defined as the growth of terminal hair on the body of a woman in the same pattern and sequence as that which develops in the post-pubertal male.[1]

Normal hair growth

The average person has about 2 million hair follicles, with 100 000 of these being on the scalp. There are two major hair types, vellus and terminal hair. Vellus hairs are fine and lightly pigmented and are present over most of the body and produced by smaller hair follicles. Terminal hairs are larger and pigmented and are found mostly on the scalp, eyebrows and eyelashes prior to puberty. Following puberty, terminal hairs are found in the axillae, pubic area and male beard. In addition, terminal hair becomes more abundant on the forearms and legs of women and men. In men, hairs also appear on the chest, shoulders and back.

Human hair grows in three phases:

1 anagen – the growing phase, which lasts for several months to 2–5 years on the scalp;

2 catagen – follows anagen and lasts for about 2 weeks; during this period the hair stops growing and the lower portion of the hair follicle involutes.

3 telogen – a resting phase that last about 3 months; at the end of this phase the hair is extruded from the follicle and the lower portion of the hair re-enters anagen.

Transformation of the vellus hair to terminal hair at puberty in the axillae, pubic and male beard areas is driven by systemic androgens. Hirsutism is the result of a change in the quality, size, degree of pigmentation and length of the hairs produced by individual follicles.

Incidence

The degree to which a female will report or complain of hirsutism will depend upon her cultural and racial norms. An estimation of the incidence of hirsutism in young females, taking account of racial and social norms, is approximately 9 per cent. Hirsutism should not be confused with hypertrichosis, which refers to non-androgen-dependent hair growth.

Pathogenesis

The dermal papilla's androgen receptors interact with dihydrotestosterone, the active metabolite of testosterone. This interaction results in an increase in the size of the hair follicle and the type of hair produced by the follicle. Hirsutism is associated with polycystic ovarian syndrome (PCOS), with approximately 60–70 per cent of women with PCOS being hirsute.

Clinical features

The patient's perception of the degree of hirsutism she suffers may differ from that clinically assessed. In order to maintain consistency of diagnosis and to monitor therapeutic intervention, it is important to have a standard grading system. The most common is the Ferriman and Gallwey grading system, which scores 11 areas of the body on a scale of 1 to 4 according to the degree of terminal hair growth. The scores are then added together.

Treatment

An explanation of the condition with a discussion about the expectation of successful treatment and the length of time (based on hair growth phases) that this may require is extremely important at the first consultation.

Physical methods of hair removal

- *Bleaching.* Hydrogen peroxide may be used to disguise pigmented facial hair. Occasionally, however, this may lead to discoloration of the skin.
- *Shaving.* This does not affect the rate of hair growth. Side effects include irritation and pseudofolliculitis.
- *Electrolysis.* This may be an effective means of permanent hair removal. However, the procedure is very operator dependent. Similarly, a laser may be used that produces monochromic light, which is specifically absorbed in the skin, and generates thermal energy to destroy hair follicles.
- *Weight loss.* Hirsutism is more common in obese women with PCOS than in thin women. Consequently, weight loss in obese women may result in a reduction in body hair.

Pharmacological methods (Table 54.1)

- *The oral contraceptive pill.* The oral contraceptive will suppress ovarian androgen activity and increase sex hormone-binding globulin (SHBG), thus decreasing free testosterone. Oral contraceptives containing norethisterone or levonorgestrel should be avoided, as they can potentially make the hirsutism worse. Combining the oral contraceptive pill with the anti-androgen cyproterone acetate (Dianette®) is more effective.

Table 54.1   Summary of drugs used for hirsutism

Drug	Mode of action	Note
Oral contraceptive pill	↓ Ovarian androgen	Avoid progestogens Add cyproterone acetate
	↑ SHBG	
Cyproterone acetate	Androgen receptor antagonist	Teratogenic
	Inhibits gonadotrophins	
Spironolactone	↑ Metabolic clearance of testosterone	↑ K⁺
	↓ 5-α reductase activity	
	Complexes with intracellular androgen receptor	
Flutamide	Anti-androgen	Hepatotoxicity Teratogenic
Finasteride	5-α reductase inhibitor	Teratogenic

SHBG, sex hormone-binding globulin.

- *Cyproterone acetate.* Cyproterone acetate will decrease hirsutism in two ways. It is an antagonist of the androgen receptor in the skin and it also has weak progestogen activity, which will inhibit gonadotrophin secretion, thereby decreasing ovarian androgen production. It should be administered along with an effective contraception (usually the oral contraceptive pill), as exposure in the first trimester of pregnancy can lead to feminization of a male fetus. The potential side effects include loss of libido, weight gain, fatigue, breast tenderness, gastrointestinal upset and headaches.
- *Spironolactone.* Spironolactone is an oral aldosterone antagonist with anti-androgenic properties. By increasing the metabolic clearance and reducing the cutaneous 5-alpha-reductase activity, it reduces the bioavailability of testosterone. It also works by complexing with the intracellular androgen receptor, forming a biologically inactive receptor. Owing to its potassium-sparing diuretic effect, the serum potassium level should be monitored at the start of treatment.
- *Flutamide.* Flutamide is a pure non-steroidal anti-androgen. Hepatotoxicity is an infrequent but serious side effect, and therefore liver function tests should be performed for the first few weeks. It must be used only in severe cases, under tertiary centre supervision.
- *Finasteride.* This is a 5-alpha-reductase inhibitor, which, as a result of its mode of action, is significantly teratogenic (potential feminization of male fetus), and therefore effective contraception must always be used. The use of finasteride should be limited to severe cases only, under tertiary centre supervision.

KEY POINTS

- Make a subjective evaluation.
- Explain the treatment regime and time scale to the patient.
- Weight reduction is central to the management of body mass index-related hirsutism.
- Be aware of the side effects of the drugs used.

VIRILISM

Whereas hirsutism may be the result of excessive androgen stimulation or excessive end-organ response, virilism is invariably due to excessive androgenic stimulation. The source of this excessive androgen will be either the adrenal cortex or the ovary. However, the stimulation for this excess production may lie elsewhere – in the hypothalamus, pituitary or even a bronchogenic carcinoma.

The clinical features of virilism are defeminizing secondary amenorrhoea, loss of subcutaneous fat, and breast atrophy and positive masculine features: (deepening of the voice, temporal recession of hair growth, clitoral enlargement and abnormal hair growth).

Causes of virilism

- Congenital adrenal hyperplasia.
- Iatrogenic virilization.
- Adrenal tumour.
- Masculinizing ovarian tumour.
- Cushing's syndrome.
- Acromegaly.
- Rarely, polycystic ovarian syndrome.

In order to differentiate between the various conditions that may lead to virilism, the following investigations should be performed.

- 17-Hydroxyprogesterone.
- Cortisol (morning and evening).
- Short Synacthen test.
- Dexamethasone suppression test.
- Magnetic resonance imaging (MRI) of adrenal glands.
- Testosterone.
- Adrenocorticotrophic hormone (ACTH).
- Androstenedione.
- Dehydroepiandrosterone (DHEA) and dehydroepiandrosterone sulphate (DHEAS).
- Chromosomal analysis.

In the adolescent, adrenal hyperplasia and the XY female are the most likely disorders to be encountered. Puberty is the time when most become evident, as the testis in the XY female becomes active and adrenal androgen activity in girls with adrenal hyperplasia increases.

The normal female produces 0.2–0.3 mg/day of testosterone. Approximately 50 per cent of testosterone is derived from the peripheral conversion of androstenedione, whereas the adrenal and the ovaries contribute approximately 25 per cent each to the circulating levels, except at midcycle, when the ovarian contribution increases by 10–15 per cent. DHEAS arises almost exclusively from the adrenal gland, whereas 90 per cent of DHEA arises from the adrenal. About 80 per cent of circulating testosterone is bound to a beta-globulin (SHBG), with androgenicity dependent mainly on the unbound fraction.

Androgen-producing tumours

A history of rapidly progressive masculinization should alert the clinician to the possibility of an androgen-producing tumour. This should lead to an MRI of the adrenal glands and the ovaries.

Adrenal hyperplasia

In the most common form, there is a 21-hydroxylase deficiency resulting in an increase in serum 17-hydroxyprogesterone and DHEAS. If urinary assays are used,

17-oxosteroids are always increased. In patients presenting after puberty, a distinction will need to be made between adrenal tumour and adrenal hyperplasia, and this can be done by a Synacthen test. This involves giving 250 µg of Synacthen between 8 a.m. and 9 a.m. and measuring the 17-hydroxprogesterone at 60 minutes. A positive result is a level >45.4 nM. In 3-beta-dehydrogenase deficiency, DHEA is also elevated.

If Cushing's syndrome is suspected, the initial test is a dexamethasone suppression test: 1 mg of dexamethasone at 11 p.m. followed by a plasma cortisol level at 8 a.m. the following morning. A cortisol level <138 nmol/L excludes the diagnosis. A level of <50 nmol/L is usual.

Drug induced

One of the most common drugs that can result in irreversible virilization is danazol. Women who are commenced on danazol should be advised about the potentially irreversible androgenic side effects of this drug.

Treatment

The treatment will depend upon the diagnosis and natural history of the condition. Treatment may involve hypophysectomy for Cushing's syndrome or acromegaly, removal of adrenal or ovarian tumours, or corticosteroids for virilizing adrenal hyperplasia.

KEY POINTS

- Virilism is usually pathological.
- Rapid onset may indicate an androgen-producing tumour.[2]
- If serum concentration of testosterone is >4.8 nmol/L further investigation should be undertaken.

KEY REFERENCES

1. Simpson N, Barht J. Hair patterns: hirsutism and baldness. In: Rook R, Dawber R (eds). *Diseases of Hair and Scalp*. Oxford: Blackwell Science, 1997, 71–126.
2. Ehrmann DA, Barnes RB, Rosenfield RL. Hyperandrogenism, hirsutism and the polycystic ovary syndrome. In: Groot LJ, Berse M, Burger HG et al. (eds). *Endocrinology*, 3rd edn, Vol. 3. Philadelphia: WB Saunders, 1994, 2093–112.
3. Balen AH, Conway GS, Kaltas G et al. Polycystic ovary syndrome: the spectrum of the disorder in 1741 patients. *Hum Reprod* 1995; **10**:2107–11.

Chapter 55

Amenorrhoea and Oligomenorrhoea

Enda McVeigh

DEFINITIONS

Amenorrhoea

Amenorrhoea is defined as the onset of menses by the age of 14 years in the absence of development of secondary sexual characteristics, or as the absence of the onset of menses by the age of 16 years regardless of the presence of normal growth and development with the appearance of secondary sexual characteristics (primary amenorrhoea). In a woman who has been menstruating, it is the absence of periods for a length of time equivalent to a total of at least three of the previous cycle intervals or six months of amenorrhoea (secondary amenorrhoea).

Oligomenorrhoea

Oligomenorrhoea is defined as an interval of more than 35 days between periods.

INVESTIGATION OF AMENORRHOEA AND OLIGOMENORRHOEA

In investigating these conditions, it is useful to consider the physiology of the events leading to menstruation and to employ diagnostic tests of each of the physiological areas of the body involved (Figure 55.1).

- *Step 1*. Exclude pregnancy and measure thyroid function (hypothyroidism is rarely a cause, but it is simple and rewarding when this diagnosis is made).
- *Step 2*. Progesterone challenge test – oral medroxyprogesterone acetate 10 mg bd daily for 5 days. The purpose of this test is to determine the level of endogenous oestrogen and the competence of the outflow tract. If the patient bleeds, a diagnosis of anovulation can be made with relative security. There are two rare exceptions: (i) the endometrium is already decidualized due to high androgen levels in polycystic ovarian syndrome (PCOS); and (ii) the endometrium is decidualized due to high progesterone levels associated with a specific adrenal enzyme deficiency.

  If the progesterone challenge test is negative (i.e. no withdrawal bleed), the outflow system and uterus can be further assessed by the administration of oestrogen followed by progesterone. If this does not result in a withdrawal bleed, an anomaly of the uterus or vagina (e.g. congenital absence of the uterus; imperforate hymen) is highly likely in primary amenorrhoea.
- *Step 3*. Gonadotrophin function – measurement of follicle-stimulating hormone (FSH) and luteinizing hormone (LH). This will determine whether the lack of oestrogen is due to a fault in the follicle or in the hypothalamic–pituitary axis. Table 55.1 shows possible diagnoses.

Causes of high levels of gonadotrophins

The measurement should be repeated at least 1–2 months apart to confirm the results.

- *Perimenopausal state*. It is normal for the gonadotrophin levels to rise before the date of the last menses. The increase in FSH is associated with a decrease in inhibin B.
- *Resistant or insensitive ovary syndrome*. This may be due to absent or defective gonadotrophin receptors on

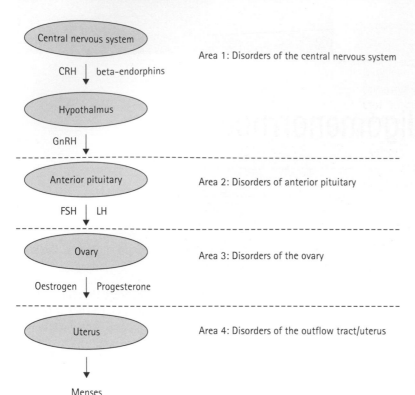

Area 1: Disorders of the central nervous system

Area 2: Disorders of anterior pituitary

Area 3: Disorders of the ovary

Area 4: Disorders of the outflow tract/uterus

Figure 55.1 Levels of disorders leading to amenorrhoea/oligomenorrhoea. CRH, corticotrophin-releasing hormone; GnRH, gonadotrophin-releasing hormone; FSH, follicule-stimulating hormone; LH, luteinizing hormone

Table 55.1 Differential diagnosis of amenorrhoea or oligomenorrhoea

Disorders of outflow
Asherman's syndrome
Müllerian anomalies
Müllerian agenesis
Androgen insensitivity (46XY)

Disorders of the ovary
Streak ovaries
   Turner's syndrome (XO)
   XX or mosaicism
   XY gonadal dysgenesis
Resistant ovary syndrome
Premature ovarian failure
Polycystic ovarian syndrome
Hormone-secreting ovarian tumour
Galactosaemia

Disorders of the anterior pituitary
Non-functional adenomas
Prolactin-secreting adenomas
Empty sella syndrome or compression of pituitary stalk
Sheehan's syndrome (acute infarction and necrosis of pituitary gland)

Disorders of the central nervous system
Hypothalamic amenorrhoea
Weight loss, anorexia, bulimia
Excessive exercise-induced amenorrhoea (decreased body fat and elevated endorphins and CRH)
Inherited genetic defects – Kallmann's syndrome (anosmia and amenorrhoea)

the follicles or to a post-receptor signalling defect. This condition is rare.

- *Premature ovarian failure due to autoimmune disease.* The ovaries contain normal-appearing primordial follicles, but the developing follicles are surrounded by nests of lymphocytes and plasma cells, with lymphocytic infiltration of the theca layer of cells.
- *Galactosaemia.* Fewer oogonia result as a direct result of the toxic effect of galactose metabolites on germ cell migration to the genital ridge.
- *Gonadotrophin-producing tumours* (rare).

All patients under the age of 40 who have been assigned the diagnosis of ovarian failure on the basis of elevated gonadotrophins should have a chromosomal analysis done. The presence of mosaicism with a Y chromosome will require the excision of the gonads due to the risk of developing a malignant tumour of the testicular tissue.

Deletion of the X chromosome (Turner's syndrome) can also result in a premature menopause. The majority of non-mosaic Turner's syndrome girls have primary amenorrhoea; however, those with a mosaic genotype may present with secondary amenorrhoea.

Normal or low gonadotrophins

This is a result of suppression of the hypothalamic–pituitary axis. The cause of this suppression may be a prolactin-secreting tumour of the pituitary or a tumour compressing the pituitary stalk and preventing dopamine transmission from the hypothalamus. Serum measurement of prolactin levels should be performed. If the level is greater than 1000 mU/L, a magnetic resonance image (MRI) scan of the pituitary is indicated.

Patients who have amenorrhoea without any of the above diagnoses may have hypothalamic amenorrhoea due to suppression of pulsatile gonadotrophin-releasing hormone (GnRH) secretion. This can be as a result of severe stress (elevated corticotrophin-releasing hormone (CRH) and beta-endorphin) or severe weight change, anorexia nervosa (weight loss of >15 per cent body weight) or bulimia (rapid fluctuations in weight).

Patients with oligomenorrhoea may be in a transient phase before entering into amenorrhoea for any of the reasons mentioned here. However, if they have a normal FSH level, they may have PCOS, as discussed above.

KEY POINTS

- Oligomenorrhoea and amenorrhoea are distressing symptoms that may arise from serious underlying medical conditions.
- Are there any life-threatening consequences of the diagnosis (e.g. Cushing's syndrome or androgen-insensitivity syndrome)?
- Are there any long-term health risks (e.g. eating disorders or premature ovarian failure with loss of bone mineral)?
- What are the fertility aspirations of the patient? Can these be achieved through simple ovulation induction or will oocyte donation or surrogacy be required?
- Investigate cause, both passively (serum hormonal levels) and activity (progesterone challenge test).
- Be systematic (in anatomical differentiation) in attempting to obtain a diagnosis.
- Treat the cause; be aware of potential systematic affect of premature ovarian failure.

Chapter 56

Menopause and Hormone Replacement Therapy

Michael E.L. Paterson

MRCOG standards

There are none available, but we would suggest the following guidelines.

Theoretical skills
- Understand the pathophysiology of the menopause.
- Understand the medication available.
- Be aware of the complications and contraindications.
- Be able to advise regarding the advantages and disadvantages of the different treatment modalities.

INTRODUCTION

The term menopause is derived from the Greek *menos* (month) and *pauses* (cessation), but the term has come to be used to describe the climacteric, which is again derived from the Greek *klimakter* (rung of a ladder). The dictionary definition of the climacteric is the period of life when fertility and sexual activity decline. The definition may be accurate but does not describe the profound changes that occur when the ovaries cease to function.

The average age of the menopause has not changed for centuries, but life expectancy has improved enormously, particularly in the last century. The life expectancy of women in Roman times was 29 years and, even by the late nineteenth century only 30 per cent of women survived to experience the menopause. Life expectancy among women is now almost 80 years and it has been estimated that there are 10 million postmenopausal women in the UK. The vast majority of women will reach the menopause and will spend one-third of their lives in this state. The long-term metabolic problems of the menopause are therefore becoming increasingly important.

PATHOPHYSIOLOGY

The number of primordial follicles declines even before birth and although the decline is dramatic just before the menopause, there are still a significant number present at the onset of the menopause. Hypothalamic–pituitary activity increases from about 10 years before the menopause. This is shown by the rising plasma levels of luteinizing hormone (LH) and, particularly, follicle-stimulating hormone (FSH). Closer to the menopause, anovulation occurs and luteal inadequacy becomes more frequent. There is a reduction in the production of progesterone and, as oestrogen levels do not decline as quickly, this may result in dysfunctional uterine bleeding and endometrial hyperplasia. Oestrogen levels decline dramatically at the menopause and menstruation ceases. The ovarian stroma still produces small quantities of androstenedione and testosterone, but the main postmenopausal oestrogen is estrone, which is produced in the peripheral fat from adrenal androgens. It is the lack of oestrogen that causes the majority of symptoms and pathology of the menopause.

SYMPTOMS

The characteristic symptoms of the menopause include hot flushes, night sweats, headaches, depression and lack of concentration and energy. The most obvious symptom is the hot flush. This is very different from a blush, which characteristically occurs over the face and chest. The hot flush, although it may start in the head or neck area, involves the whole body and is often followed by intense sweating and then by shivering. There is a rise in skin temperature of 1°C [Ib],[1] and although women feel very embarrassed, there is no obvious signs that they are having a hot flush. Hot flushes and sweats occur in 75 per cent of women and tend to be more severe following a surgical menopause. They will usually continue for more than a year, and 25 per cent will continue with hot sweats for more than 5 years [III].

Table 56.1   Menopausal symptoms

- Hot flushes
- Night sweats
- Palpitations
- Globus hystericus
- Formication
- Depression
- Anxiety
- Insomnia
- Headaches
- Loss of libido
- Loss of concentration
- Skin atrophy
- Joint pains
- Urge incontinence
- Myalgia

The diagnosis is straightforward when the patient is a year postmenopausal and has significant hot flushes and sweats, but if the patient is perimenopausal, the diagnosis may be much more difficult, particularly if her only symptom is that of depression. Depression is more common in the decade before the menopause than after it, and if the patient has a long history of depression, it is unlikely that her symptoms are due to oestrogen lack. Many women request oestrogens in the hope that other causes of depression may be helped. There are many other causes of depression at the time of the menopause, including loss of reproductive potential, lack of femininity, marital problems and the 'empty nest' syndrome. There have been studies to show the beneficial effects of oestrogen in the treatment of depression, but the main benefit seems to be amongst premenopausal women.

Many of the symptoms that can be related to ovarian failure are shown in Table 56.1, but it can be difficult to determine whether a particular symptom is caused by the menopause. If the diagnosis is uncertain, the only way of determining whether the symptom is oestrogen related is to prescribe a short course of hormone replacement therapy (HRT).

Cardiovascular disease

Coronary heart disease (CHD) is uncommon among premenopausal women, particularly if they do not smoke. There is a rapid increase in risk following the menopause and cardiovascular disease is now a leading cause of death among postmenopausal women. Even though the postmenopausal incidence increases, it does not reach the incidence in men at any age.

Why are premenopausal women given this protection? The mechanism is not clear, but the lipoprotein profile, with a higher high-density lipoprotein (HDL) and lower low-density lipoprotein (LDL) cholesterol concentration when compared with men, may in part be the answer. In post-menopausal women, the HDL:LDL ratio becomes much closer to the male ratio, but this may not explain all the differences, and oestrogen may well have a more direct effect on the vessel wall.

Oral oestrogens when given to postmenopausal women cause an increase in HDL and a lowering of LDL cholesterol concentrations, which should be beneficial. They also increase triglyceride levels, which are associated with an increased risk of cardiovascular disease. There have been a huge number of studies to try to find a drug with the ideal lipid profile but none has been conclusive. Until a definitive study is produced, it would be reasonable to assume that oestrogen-containing regimens may reduce the incidence of CHD in healthy women, but it is difficult to determine the magnitude of this reduction.

Early observational studies suggested that women taking or who have taken HRT have a lower CHD incidence and mortality by around 30 per cent, but there has been only one small randomized study [II], the Heart and Estrogen/Progestin Replacement Study (HERS). This showed no CHD benefit of taking HRT among women with stable CHD but a significant increased risk of thromboembolic events [Ib].[2] The study was surprising in view of all the previous epidemiological evidence, but the epidemiological studies could be criticized for possible selection bias and, on the other hand, there was a large number of drop-outs in the HERS. However, the picture has recently changed, owing to the publication of the US Women's Health Initiative (WHI) Trial, which has led to a reappraisal of the long-term use of HRT. This was the largest trial ever done in the field, with more than 16 000 women enrolled. The main aim of the study was to test whether postmenopausal use of HRT protected women against heart disease. The trial randomized women to receive continuous combined HRT in the form of 0.625 mg conjugated equine oestrogen (Premarin in UK) and 2.5 mg medroxyprogesterone acetate daily, or placebo. After 5 years of follow-up, the women taking HRT were found to have a higher incidence of breast cancer, myocardial infarction, stroke and pulmonary embolus, although there were reductions in the numbers of hip fractures and colorectal cancers. Part of the trial was then stopped early because of these events.

A second 'landmark' publication, the 'Million Women Study' has provided further high-quality evidence concerning the risks and benefits of HRT in women aged 50–64. This UK-based study collected data from women attending for breast screening as part of the National Health Service Breast Screening Programme. Women were classified according to their reported use of HRT, menopausal status, etc. Combined oestrogen/gestagen HRT use was associated with an increased number of breast cancers when compared with non-users. Users of oestrogen-only HRT (usually reserved for hysterectomized women) were at lower risk, and the risks to users of combined oestrogen/gestagen HRT only applied to current, not past, users.[3]

Following publication of these findings, the UK Committee on Safety of Medicines issued advice to prescribers of HRT, which can be summarized as follows.

- For short-term (e.g. 2–3 years) use of HRT for the relief of menopausal symptoms, the benefits outweigh the risks for most women.
- Longer term use of HRT is licensed for the prevention of osteoporosis. However, patients should be aware of the increased incidence of some conditions with long-term HRT use and of alternative options for the prevention of osteoporosis.
- The decision to use HRT should be discussed with each women on an individual basis, taking into consideration her history, risk factors and personal preferences.
- Individual risks and benefits should be regularly reappraised (e.g. at least annually) whilst using HRT.
- HRT should not be used for the prevention of CHD.

The results of this trial had a major impact on patterns of HRT used throughout the Western world. Other than the lack of a protective effect against heart disease, there was little new in the findings, but the study did re-emphasize the cautionary notes raised by earlier, smaller studies. Clearly, alternative strategies exist for protection against post-menopausal osteoporosis, including the use of selective oestrogen receptor modulators (SERMS) or bisphosphonates. The control of perimenopausal symptoms without resort to HRT is more problematic and it may be that many women will continue to use HRT for a few years during their early fifties. However, it seems likely that long-term use will decline over time.

- Recent epidemiological studies do not show a beneficial effect of HRT on CHD.
- One randomized trial showed no advantage of taking HRT for women with CHD.

Osteoporosis

Osteoporosis is a major cause of morbidity and mortality in women in the UK. Bone mass reaches a peak in women towards the end of their third decade. It then remains relatively constant until the menopause, after which the loss is lifelong. Seventy per cent of women over the age of 80 will have measurable osteoporosis. It is estimated that there are 60 000 hip fractures, 50 000 Colles fractures and 40 000 clinically apparent vertebral fractures a year in the UK. The clinical consequences are enormous, and women who have a fracture of the neck of femur have a 25 per cent of dying within a year and a 50 per cent chance of not being able to resume their social independence. The other fractures also cause significant morbidity, particularly as they often occur in elderly women who live alone and are just able to maintain their independence.

A minimum of 2 mg of oestradiol or equivalent is needed to increase rather than maintain bone mass. The combined oestrogen/progestogen preparations are effective, as is tibolone, a synthetic hormone preparation. There are plenty of randomized studies to show that HRT maintains bone mass, but no long-term study has shown a significant reduction in fractures. The major problem in running such a study is that there is a 30-year gap between the menopause and most of the fractures, and to sustain any such trial for that length of time is almost impossible. However, it does appear that bone density is maintained following treatment with combined preparations and that it will fall following cessation of treatment at the same rate as it does after the menopause [Ib].[4]

There are other treatments that may be useful in the treatment of osteoporosis. Calcium supplementation is of little value in younger, active patients but has been shown to be beneficial in elderly postmenopausal patients living in care. Bisphosphonates are also effective in the treatment of relatively elderly patients with established osteoporosis. Fluoride is not thought to be effective, but physical exercise is thought to be important in the prevention of osteoporotic fractures, mainly through improvement in posture, mobility and muscle function.

Urogenital system

Embryologically, the female genital tract and lower urinary system develop in close proximity, both developing from the primitive urogenital sinus. Vaginal discomfort, dyspareunia, dysuria, recurrent lower tract infections and urinary incontinence are all more common after the menopause. The urethra and vagina have a high concentration of oestrogen receptors and there is now significant evidence to support the use of oestrogens in the treatment of urogenital symptoms. Evidence exists that oestrogens relieve urogenital atrophic symptoms, induce an increase in lactobacilli in the vagina, prevent recurrent urinary tract infections, and alleviate urge incontinence, frequency and nocturia. In combination with alpha-adrenergic agonists, oestrogens improve stress incontinence [II].

Alzheimer's disease

The prevalence of dementia may be as high as 50 per cent by the age of 85. Alzheimer's disease accounts for 50–65 per cent of cases. Women are affected more commonly than men, with progressive symptoms over a decade until death intervenes from intercurrent illness.

Observational studies indicate that the risk of Alzheimer's disease may be reduced by one-third among women taking HRT. Oestrogens are known to have a beneficial effect on brain function, but as yet there are no randomized studies to confirm the observational data. It is likely that there is a benefit from HRT, but it may be some time before this can be accurately quantified [II].

DIAGNOSIS AND INVESTIGATION

The triad of hot flushes, amenorrhoea for a year and a raised serum FSH level of >15 IU/L makes the diagnosis easy and in the majority of cases it can be made on the history alone. The differential diagnosis includes depression, premenstrual syndrome, migraine and, very rarely, carcinoid syndrome. It can sometimes be more difficult when the patient has had a hysterectomy because this is associated with an earlier menopause, and a serum FSH level will often help to establish the diagnosis.

There are no essential investigations that must be carried out before commencing HRT, but it is a screening opportunity that should not be missed. This would include, if appropriate, breast self-examination, mammography, pelvic examination and cervical cytology. The patient should be weighed and her blood pressure checked before commencing treatment. Perceived weight gain is a common reason for discontinuing HRT, but randomized studies have not shown any significant gain in weight on HRT [Ib].

There is no indication to perform routine bone density measurements or endometrial biopsies. However, any erratic bleeding should be investigated before commencing HRT.

TREATMENT

Oestrogens

Oestrogens are effective at relieving menopausal symptoms and this has been confirmed by several randomized, double-blind studies [Ib].[5] For all women who have not had a hysterectomy, a progestogen should be added for at least 10 days each month to prevent endometrial hyperplasia and carcinoma [II]. This will result in a regular withdrawal bleed and, as many women find this unacceptable, continuous regimens of oestrogen and a progestogen have been introduced to reduce its incidence. The routes of administration are shown in Table 56.2. All these regimens are effective but have different side effects. This is important when prescribing HRT, because if the initial drug is ineffective, it is unlikely that changing to another route of administration will improve the symptoms. However, if the drug is effective but has

Table 56.2 Routes of administration of hormone replacement therapy

- Oral
- Patches
- Implants
- Vaginal ring
- Gel
- Nasal spray

unacceptable side effects, a different route of administration may well be more acceptable.

Oral preparations are by far the most common and they have the advantage of flexibility, a short half-life, ease of administration and lower cost. However, they do deliver a relatively high level of oestrogen to the liver, with an increased risk of gallstone formation and a tendency to increase triglyceride levels. The so-called sequential regimens that have oestrogen in the first half of the 28-day pack and oestrogen and a progestogen in the second half are particularly useful in treating patients close to the menopause, as they give better cycle control. Combined continuous therapy, which has progestogen every day, is useful for those women who are a few years past the menopause and who do not wish to have vaginal bleeding. There is now evidence that there is an increased risk of endometrial carcinoma if sequential regimens are taken for more than 5 years [II].[6] This is not seen with combined continuous regimens, and there may be a reduced risk of endometrial carcinoma [II]. Women should therefore consider changing after a few years from a sequential regimen to continuous combined therapy for long-term treatment.

Patches offer an alternative to oral preparations for those women who do not wish to take tablets or who have side effects. The matrix patch has removed most of the skin irritation problems, but there is a huge range of alternative routes of administration that are beneficial, including gels, vaginal rings, sprays and implants. Implants are useful in that as well as lasting for 6 months, they can also be used in combination with testosterone in those women who have loss of libido [II].[7] Implant may continue to release oestrogen for up to 2 years and if they are given too frequently, supra-physiological levels may occur [II].[8]

Side effects and complications

The main side effect is vaginal bleeding in patients with a uterus. This may be acceptable in women aged 50, but not 10 years later. The combined continuous preparations are associated with few bleeding problems in women over the age of 55, but erratic vaginal bleeding may be a problem close to the menopause. The addition of a progestogen may well cause many of the side effects, including bloating, fluid retention and mastalgia. Progestogens can be administered vaginally as a gel or pessary to try to reduce the severity of any side effects.

Breast disease

Hormone replacement therapy increases the rate of benign breast disease and increases the incidence of benign mastalgia and mammographic density. With the use of mammography to detect early breast cancer, HRT leads to an increase in the psychological and surgical morbidity because of the increased numbers of mammographically guided or open breast biopsies that have to be performed.

Table 56.3   The evidence against prescribing hormone replacement therapy (HRT) to women with breast cancer

- Oestradiol stimulates some breast cancer cells in culture
- Oophorectomy reduces rate of recurrence
- Breast cancer risk relates to age at menarche and menopause
- Stopping HRT may cause some breast cancers to regress
- Long-term HRT increases the risk of breast cancer

Table 56.4   Oestrogenic side effects

- Leg cramps
- Headaches
- Bloating
- Nipple sensitivity
- Nausea

Table 56.5   Progestogenic side effects

- Premenstrual syndrome
- Depression
- Poor concentration
- Acne
- Headaches
- Breast tenderness
- Fluid retention
- Dysmenorrhoea

There has been a large number of studies showing that HRT is associated with an increased risk of breast cancer. An analysis of 51 epidemiological studies [Ia][9] showed that the cumulative excess risk for women starting HRT at the age of 50 was 2 cases/1000 women after 5 years, 6/1000 after 10 years, and 12/1000 after 15 years. The background risk was 45/1000. This risk fell on discontinuing HRT, with no excess risk after 5 years. HRT does not increase mortality, and some studies have shown an improvement in prognosis [II].

Breast cancer has been regarded as an absolute contraindication to HRT and for that reason very few patients with breast cancer have been prescribed it. A study from Australia [III][10] involving more than 100 women with breast cancer was unable to find a significant increased risk of recurrence, but this was only 10 per cent of the total number with breast cancer treated in that institution. The case against prescribing HRT in women with breast cancer is still strong (Table 56.3). Great care needs to be taken before prescribing HRT to women with breast cancer, but the risks to women who have good-prognosis disease are probably small and the risks may be justified in women who have severe symptoms.

Venous thrombosis

There are marked haematological changes that occur secondary to the menopause, and users of HRT have further favourable and unfavourable changes. In the past it has been difficult to determine whether or not these changes indicate that women on HRT are at an increased risk. In 1996 and 1997, there was a total of five epidemiological studies of various study design showing that there was a very small increased risk for HRT users. The absolute risk years was 2/10 000 treatment-years for venous thrombosis, 0.6/10 000 treatment-years for pulmonary embolus and 2/million treatment-years for death. The first 12 months of treatment were associated with the highest risk [II].[11]

The risk of the occurrence of a venous thrombosis for any one individual is very small, but care needs to be taken before prescribing HRT for a patient with a history of deep vein thrombosis. HRT should be avoided in those patients who have had a serious proven event and in those who have ongoing risk factors.

Acceptability

Hormone replacement therapy is effective in relieving menopausal symptoms and is likely to reduce deaths from osteoporosis. One might expect a high uptake of the drug, but most studies have shown poor continuation rates on HRT. One study[12] showed that 31 per cent of women had discontinued HRT. Within 6 months, 51 per cent within 6 months and 75 per cent within 3 years, which is typical of the published data.

The reasons for stopping HRT are numerous and the reasons given in the study cited above are again fairly typical of many reported studies [III]: 36 per cent discontinued because of side effects, 24 per cent because of lack of efficacy, 18 per cent because the side effects were worse than the menopausal symptoms, 9 per cent because their symptoms had ceased, 9 per cent because of bleeding problems, and 18 per cent because of long-term risks.

Oestrogenic side effects are shown in Table 56.4 and progestogenic side effects in Table 56.5. The oestrogenic effects can be reduced by prescribing the lowest effective dose or by changing the route of administration. The progestogenic effects are often more troublesome, and may be improved by changing the progestogen, changing to a 3-monthly regimen or changing the route of administration.

The levonorgestrel intrauterine system has been used in combination with an oestrogen, and may be particularly useful in the perimenopausal woman with dysfunctional bleeding.

If the drug is not effective, the diagnosis should be reconsidered and perhaps one further type of HRT prescribed. If bleeding is the main problem, the progestogen can be changed and, for the older patient, combined continuous therapy or tibolone is available.

Alternative treatment

Norethisterone 5 mg daily has been shown to be effective in reducing hot flushes and sweats, but it has little effect on other menopausal symptoms [Ib].[13] Medroxyprogesterone acetate and megestrol acetate 40 mg daily are also effective and these drugs may be useful in women who have relative contraindications to HRT. Propranolol and clonidine have been used in the treatment of hot flushes but the effect is probably no better than placebo.

Vaginal oestrogen preparations can be used to treat atrophic vaginitis but repeated prescriptions can lead to systemic absorption.

Selective oestrogen receptor modulators are effective in the prevention of bone loss and are likely to have a cardiovascular benefit and reduce the incidence of breast cancer. They may increase hot flushes slightly and therefore are useful in those women whose hot flushes have settled but who are concerned about long-term osteoporosis.

Tibolone has been shown to be effective at relieving hot flushes and sweats and will prevent osteoporosis.

Naturally occurring oestrogens such as phytoestrogens occur in cereals, legumes and vegetables. Women living in countries that have a diet rich in phytoestrogens have fewer menopausal symptoms, but although a lifetime's use may be beneficial, these drugs have not yet been shown to be effective in randomized studies. Therefore, although these drugs are widely used, particularly in the USA, their efficacy needs to be established.

KEY POINTS

- Oestrogens are effective at relieving climacteric symptoms.
- Progestogens must be given if the patient has a uterus.
- There are few absolute contraindications.
- The long-term benefits, particularly in the prevention of osteoporosis, may be reduced because of the problems of compliance.

PUBLISHED GUIDELINES

Hormone Replacement Therapy and Venous Thromboembolism. RCOG Guideline No. 19. London: RCOG Press, April 1999.

KEY REFERENCES

1. Sturdee DW, Wilson KA, Pipili E, Crocker AD. Physiological aspects of menopausal hot flush. *BMJ* 1978; 2:79–80.

2. Hulley S, Grady D, Bush T et al. Randomized trial of estrogen plus progestogen for secondary prevention of coronary heart disease in postmenopausal women. *J Am Med Assoc* 1998; 280:605–13.

3. Million Women Study Collaborators. Breast cancer and hormone-replacement therapy in the Million Women Study. *Lancet* 2003; 362:419–28.

4. Christiansen C, Christensen MS, Transbol I. Bone mass in postmenopausal women after withdrawal of oestrogen/gestagen replacement therapy. *Lancet* 1981; I:459–61.

5. Campbell S, Whitehead M. Oestrogen therapy in the menopausal syndrome. *Clin Obstet Gynaecol* 1977; 4:31–7.

6. Beresford SAA, Weiss NS, Voigt LF, McKnight B. Risk of endometrial cancer in relation to use of oestrogen combined with cyclic progestogen therapy in postmenopausal women. *Lancet* 1997; 349:458–61.

7. Studd JWW, Chakravarti S, Collins WP et al. Oestradiol and testosterone implants in the treatment of psychosexual problems in postmenopausal women. *Br J Obstet Gynaecol* 1977; 84:314–15.

8. Ganger KF, Cust MP, Whitehead MI. Symptoms of oestrogen deficiency associated with supraphysiological plasma oestradiol concentrations in women with oestradiol implants. *BMJ* 1989; 299:601–2.

9. Collaborative Group on Hormonal Factors in Breast Cancer. Breast cancer and hormone replacement therapy: collaborative reanalysis of data from 51 epidemiological studies of 52,705 women with breast cancer and 108,411 women with breast cancer. *Lancet* 1997; 350:1047–59.

10. Dew J, Eden J, Beller E et al. A cohort study of hormone replacement therapy given to women previously treated for breast cancer. *Climacteric* 1998; 1:137–42.

11. Daly E, Vessey MP, Hawkins MM, Carson JL, Gough P, Marsh S. Case-control study of venous thromboembolism risk in users of hormone replacement therapy. *Lancet* 1996; 348:977–80.

12. Hope S, Wager E, Rees M. Survey of British women's views on the menopause and HRT. *J Br Menopause Soc* 1998; 4:33–6.

13. Paterson MEL. A randomised double blind crossover trial into the effect of norethisterone on climacteric symptoms and biochemical profiles. *Br J Obstet Gynaecol* 1982; 89:464–72.

Chapter 57

Problems in Early Pregnancy

Lawrence J. Mascarenhas

INTRODUCTION

The major groups of problems in early pregnancy are twofold, namely miscarriage and ectopic pregnancy. Few areas of gynaecological practice have seen such rapid recent changes as in the diagnosis and management of early pregnancy problems. The advent of transabdominal and latterly transvaginal ultrasound as well as the rapid assay of human chorionic gonadotrophin (hCG) have revolutionized diagnosis in this area, and the use of medical management for selected groups of women with either intrauterine or extrauterine non-viable pregnancies has equally revolutionized treatment. A clear understanding of the management of these common problems is essential for good gynaecological practice. While it is important to remember that there are many other causes of minor bleeding and abdominal pain in early pregnancy, the axiom that every

woman with such symptoms has an ectopic pregnancy until proven otherwise is as pertinent today as ever.

Most hospitals in the UK now have an early pregnancy assessment unit with access to transvaginal ultrasound and rapid hCG assay and trained nursing staff able to manage the majority of cases. Since not all patients seen in such units are pregnant, the management of non-pregnant patients with lower abdominal pain is summarized at the end of this chapter.

ECTOPIC PREGNANCY

Definition and incidence

The word ectopic comes from the Greek word *ektopos*, meaning out of place, and describes any implantation outside the uterine cavity. The most common site for an ectopic pregnancy is within the fallopian tube (98.3 per cent), followed by abdominal (1.4 per cent), ovarian (0.15 per cent) and cervical (0.15 per cent) sites. The incidence is around 1 in 100 of all pregnancies but increases to 1 in 30 pregnancies in high-risk populations. There is suspicion that rates of ectopic pregnancy are rising within the West, in parallel with the increasing number of cases of chlamydia infection.

Background

The management of ectopic pregnancy has changed dramatically over the years, from a surgical approach by laparotomy to either conservative, minimal access surgery or medical management.[1] Recent developments in the diagnosis and treatment of ectopic pregnancy have obliged us to re-evaluate our approach. Despite the existence of many treatments for ectopic pregnancy, only some are supported by randomized clinical trials.

The clinical history and examination should include a careful search for the risk factors for ectopic pregnancy that are present in 25–50 per cent of patients. Furthermore, any woman of childbearing age presenting with lower abdominal pain and/or vaginal bleeding and/or amenorrhoea should have a pregnancy test followed by appropriate investigations to locate the site of the pregnancy.

The level of evidence on which the studies are based uses the modified Canadian Task Force classification,[2] which consists of the following.

- *Classification I*: evidence obtained from a properly designed, randomized, controlled trial [Ib].
- *Classification II-1*: evidence obtained from a well-designed controlled trial without randomization [II].
- *Classification II-2*: evidence obtained from well-designed cohort or case studies, preferably from more than one centre or research group [II].
- *Classification II-3*: evidence obtained from comparisons between times or places with or without intervention, including dramatic results in uncontrolled experiments [III].
- *Classification III*: opinions of respected authorities, based on clinical experience, descriptive studies or reports of expert committees [IV].

Diagnosis (see Figure 57.1)

The two most important diagnostic tools are the determination of serum [beta]-hCG and transvaginal ultrasound (TVU) examination. They determine the clinical management of the patient.[3] TVU usually reveals an intrauterine pregnancy (IUP) when the serum hCG level exceeds 1500 mIU/mL. Combined IUP and extrauterine pregnancy (heterotopic pregnancy) is rare following spontaneous conception but is relatively common in pregnancy resulting from in-vitro fertilization (IVF). Accordingly, the finding of an intrauterine gestation on ultrasound almost always excludes the presence of an ectopic pregnancy unless IVF has been performed.

In those whose gestation is not visible on ultrasound, the measurement of endometrial thickness has not been helpful in establishing the diagnosis. The evaluation of gestational age by last menstrual period (LMP) is also not helpful (classification I).[4] The measurement of serum hCG remains the best diagnostic tool. Serum progesterone levels in women with viable IUP are also higher than in those with non-viable pregnancies, including ectopic pregnancy and IUP destined to abort (arrested pregnancy). However, the levels are not different in women with arrested pregnancy and in those with ectopic pregnancy.[3] Curettage as a diagnostic tool for ectopic pregnancy is rarely necessary, given the utility of non-invasive methods. However, histology of 'products of conception' should always be checked, with urgent recall of the patient if decidua only or Arias–Stella reaction is reported, as a misdiagnosis of miscarried IUP may have been made.

Identifying the risk factors of tubal rupture is important. In a population-based study in France (classification II-1) [II],[5] four factors were identified: a history of never having used contraception, a history of tubal damage and infertility, the induction of ovulation, and a high hCG level >10 000 mIU/mL. In that study, tubal rupture did not affect the subsequent IUP rate. Apart from the identification of these factors, a high index of suspicion and the use of TVU and hCG assays have enabled the early diagnosis of unruptured ectopic pregnancy, allowing conservative treatment.

Surgical management

Recently, three prospective, randomized trials [Ia] involving a total of 108 patients in the laparoscopy group and 123 patients in the laparotomy group have demonstrated that laparoscopic surgery is superior to laparotomy.[6] Whereas the laparoscopic approach has become the gold standard in haemodynamically stable patients, it has also been performed in the presence of haemoperitoneum by surgeons working in centres with excellence in this area of practice. Laparotomy remains the mainstay of management of the ruptured ectopic pregnancy if the patient is hypotensive, tachycardic or otherwise in a haemodynamically unstable condition.

The subsequent IUP and recurrent ectopic pregnancy rates after salpingotomy in studies involving 1514 patients were 61 and 15 per cent, respectively. Data from studies on salpingectomy showed an IUP rate of 38 per cent, which appeared to be lower than that after salpingotomy; however, this difference might be a reflection of the tubal status rather than of the choice of surgical procedure [III]. Dubuisson et al.[7] have reported that among 145 patients who underwent salpingectomy for ectopic pregnancy and a non-obstructed contralateral tube, the overall IUP and recurrent ectopic pregnancy rates were 50.3 and 15.2 per cent, respectively. In the subgroup of patients who had a normal contralateral tube and no history of infertility, the IUP and ectopic pregnancy rates were 75 and 9.6 per cent, respectively. In contrast, the subgroup of patients with an abnormal contralateral tube or a history of prior infertility had IUP and ectopic pregnancy rates of 36.6 and 18.3 per cent, respectively. The authors believe that salpingectomy would not compromise the IUP rate and would avoid the complication of persistent ectopic pregnancy. This study is probably the basis of the Royal College of Obstetricians and Gynaecologists (RCOG) guideline for removal of the tube containing the ectopic pregnancy when the contralateral tube is healthy.

Medical management

Single-dose methotrexate injection is the most widely studied medical treatment and its high success rates are not skill dependent. The method is straightforward and the success rate in properly selected patients is in the range of 86–94 per cent.[6] The dose of methotrexate is 50 mg/m^2 body

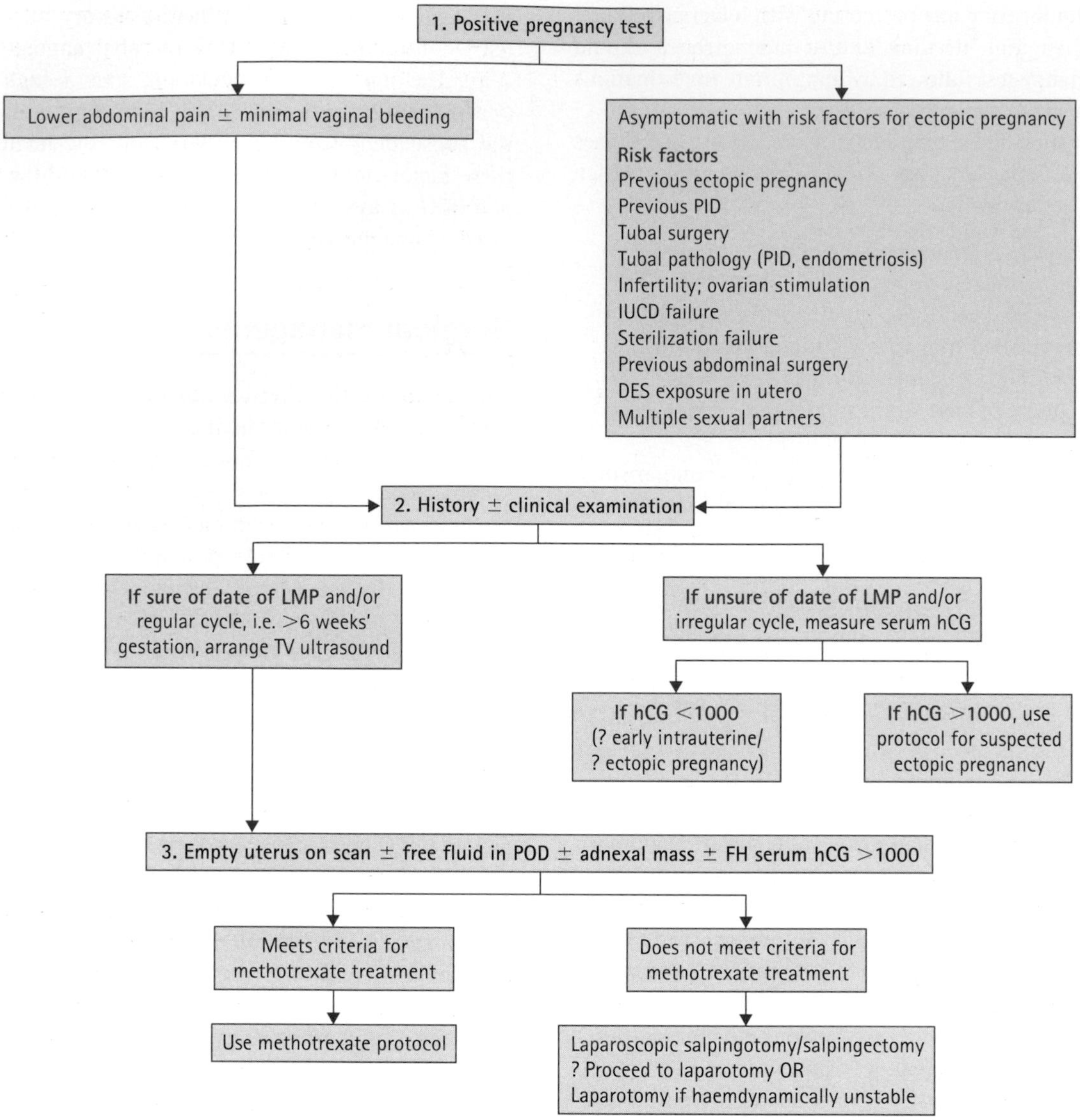

Figure 57.1   Ectopic pregnancy management algorithm. PID, pelvic inflammatory disease; IUCD, intrauterine contraceptive device; DES, diethylstilboestrol; LMP, last menstrual period; TV, transvaginal ultrasound scan; hCG, human chorionic gonadotrophin; POD, Pouch of Douglas; FH, fetal heart

surface or approximately 1 mg/kg body weight. The best candidates for methotrexate treatment are women with asymptomatic ectopic pregnancy, who have high compliance, serum hCG of <5000 mIU/mL, tubal size of <3 cm and no fetal cardiac activity on ultrasound.[3] The American College of Obstetricians and Gynecologists has issued guidelines for methotrexate administration.[8] Lipscomb et al. (classification II-1) [II][9] found that a high serum hCG level is the most important factor associated with the failure of methotrexate treatment. The treatment of ectopic pregnancy using a combination of mifepristone and methotrexate was investigated in a randomized, controlled trial (classification I).[10] Compared with methotrexate alone, the resolution time was shorter and a second injection or laparotomy was less likely to be needed in the combination group. Although the number of cases is small, the study

suggests that this combination has a more pronounced effect on the resolution of tubal pregnancy.

After medical treatment, it is not unusual to see an increase in serum hCG levels in the following 3 days and mild abdominal pain of short duration (1–2 days). However, the pain can also be severe. This could be as a result of tubal abortion or the formation of haematoma with tubal distension. Lipscomb et al. (classification II-2) [III][11] studied 53 patients with increased abdominal pain severe enough to be evaluated in the clinic or emergency room or requiring hospitalization. Only ten patients subsequently required surgery. Their report indicates that most patients who experience abdominal pain after methotrexate treatment do not require surgery. However, close observation is still needed.

There are currently several randomized studies confirming that medical treatment in selected cases of ectopic pregnancy is as effective as laparoscopic treatment (classification I) [Ib].[12,13] Both treatments are also equal in preserving tubal patency. As expected, the duration of time for hCG concentrations to decrease to undetectable levels is faster after laparoscopic surgery. A recent meta-analysis[14] revealed that the success rate of methotrexate treatment (87 per cent, range 75–90 per cent) is similar to that of laparoscopic salpingostomy (91 per cent, range 72–100 per cent).

However, medical treatment has a more negative impact on patients' health-related quality of life than surgical treatment (classification I) [Ib].[15] The possible risk of tubal rupture after medical treatment combined with a prolonged follow-up and a frequent initial rise in the serum hCG concentration are likely to cause distress. Abdominal pain several days after medical treatment also contributes to the patient's concern. A detailed informed consent before the administration of the treatment is important, and the ramifications of both treatments should be fully discussed. Mol et al. (classification I) [Ib][16] also found that systemic methotrexate was less costly than laparoscopy in women with initial serum hCG levels of <1500 mIU/mL. However, in women whose initial hCG levels were >3000 mIU/mL, methotrexate treatment was more expensive.

Many substances, such as hyperosmolar glucose, potassium chloride, and prostaglandin F2-alpha, have been used to treat ectopic pregnancy locally. Fernandez et al. (classification I) [Ib][17] compared the efficacy of local methotrexate administration with laparoscopic salpingostomy, and found that in selected cases the success rates were similar. However, after methotrexate treatment, the subsequent IUP rate was higher and the repeat ectopic pregnancy rate was lower than after surgical treatment. Tzafettas et al. (classification II-1) [II][18] treated unselected tubal pregnancy by local injection of 100 mg methotrexate transvaginally in 79 patients and laparoscopically in another 79. Methotrexate alone was effective in 79 per cent of cases. However, local treatment of ectopic pregnancy has some disadvantages. Compared with systemic treatment, it is operator dependent and it is probably preferable to remove the ectopic pregnancy once laparoscopy has been performed.

Expectant management

Most ectopic pregnancies probably resolve spontaneously, and the trend towards earlier diagnosis may be resulting in over-treatment. The overall efficacy of expectant management was 69.2 per cent in ten prospective studies.[6] Banerjee et al. (classification II-2) [III][19] followed 135 women with an unknown location of their pregnancy. Complete data sets were obtained in 127 cases. These included 34 (27 per cent) normal IUPs, 11 (9 per cent) miscarriages and 18 (14 per cent) ectopic pregnancies. A total of 64 (50 per cent) pregnancies resolved spontaneously. These data show that most pregnancies of unknown location are abnormal and many resolve spontaneously. On the other hand, the role of expectant

Table 57.1   Laboratory indices in diagnosis of ectopic pregnancy

Progesterone nmol/L	hCG IU/L	Diagnosis	Management
<20	<25	Reassuring	Blood/urine in 7 days
20–60	>25	High risk of ectopic	Blood in 2 days
>60	<1000	Low risk of ectopic	Repeat scan when hCG >1000 IU/L
>60	>1000	Ectopic	Repeat scan as soon as possible ± laparoscopy

hCG, human chorionic gonadotrophin.

management in those with known ectopic pregnancy is limited because of its risks compared with the high efficacy and accessibility of methotrexate or surgical treatment. The management of these cases can be greatly facilitated by using serum hCG in conjunction with serum progesterone as shown in Table 57.1.

Criteria for methotrexate treatment of ectopic pregnancy

Indications
- Haemodynamically stable, no active bleeding, no haemoperitoneum, minimal or no pain.
- No contraindications to methotrexate.
- Able to return for follow-up care for several weeks.
- Non-laparoscopic diagnosis of ectopic pregnancy.
- General anaesthesia poses a significant risk.
- Unruptured adnexal mass <4 cm in size on scan.
- No fetal cardiac activity on scan.
- hCG does not exceed 5000 IU/L (can be given up to 15 000 IU/L with consultant agreement).

Contraindications
- Breastfeeding.
- Immunodeficiency/active infection.
- Chronic liver disease.
- Active pulmonary disease.
- Active peptic ulcer or colitis.
- Blood disorder.
- Hepatic, renal or haematological dysfunction.

Side effects
- Nausea and vomiting.
- Stomatitis (sore mouth).
- Diarrhoea, abdominal discomfort.
- Photosensitivity skin reaction.
- Impaired liver function, reversible.

Reproductive medicine

- Pneumonitis (rare).
- Severe neutropenia (rare).
- Reversible alopecia (rare).
- Haematosalpinx and haematoceles.

Treatment effects

- Increase in abdominal pain (occurs in up to two-thirds of patients).
- Increase in hCG during first 3 days of treatment.
- Vaginal bleeding.

Signs of treatment failure and tubal rupture

- Significantly worsening abdominal pain, regardless of change in serum hCG (check full blood count if doubt).
- Haemodynamic instability.
- Levels of hCG that do not decline by at least 15 per cent between day 4 and day 7 post-treatment.
- Increasing or plateauing hCG levels after the first week of treatment.

Counselling

- Side effects and treatment effects discussed.
- Report:
  - severe abdominal pain,
  - heavy vaginal bleeding,
  - dizziness, syncope, tachycardia.
- Avoid sunlight, alcohol, vitamins, aspirin, non-steroidal anti-inflammatory drugs (NSAIDs) and sex.

Follow-up

Repeat hCG on day 5 post-injection:

- if <15 per cent decrease, consider repeat dose and recheck in 5 days,
- if >15 per cent decrease, recheck weekly until <25 IU/L.

Protocol for methotrexate

- Diagnosis as per guideline.
- Check criteria for medical management and discuss with the consultant responsible for the patient.
- Check full blood count, urea and electrolytes (U&Es), liver function tests (LFTs) U&Es, blood group (anti-D if Rhesus negative).
- Counsel patient, give written information and obtain written consent.

- Obtain patient's height and weight and calculate body surface area.
- Calculate methotrexate dose (50 mg/m^2 intramuscularly).
- Get methotrexate from pharmacy and administer intramuscularly.
- Arrange follow-up appointment between days 5 and 7 post-injection (repeat serum hCG).
- Review weekly clinically + serum hCG until hCG <25 IU/mL.

Follow-up

At follow-up, enquire specifically about pain and bleeding. Lower abdominal pain (separation pain) often worsens 2–6 days after methotrexate is given, but should resolve fairly quickly thereafter. Vaginal bleeding may occur for several days, but again should improve quickly thereafter. The woman's next period may occur before the hCG becomes undetectable, as the serum progesterone falls more quickly than hCG. Make sure that she is complying with contraceptive advice.

Levels of hCG typically rise up to day 4 but then start to fall. By day 7, the hCG should be at least 15 per cent less than the pre-treatment level and should fall substantially each week after that. Monitoring should continue until the hCG level is <25 IU/L, which usually takes 4 weeks or more.

Failed treatment is rare and is most common when the initial hCG is high (>5000 IU/L). Some centres use additional oral mifepristone 200 mg in these cases. If the hCG fails to fall or becomes static after an initial fall, a second dose of methotrexate can be given, with the same follow-up arrangements. The alternative is surgery.

Surgery should also be considered in all women presenting with pain in the first few days after methotrexate. Careful clinical assessment is required before assuming that a response to methotrexate is the cause of the pain, including signs of peritonitis and a full blood count. If there is significant doubt, surgery is the safest option.

SPONTANEOUS MISCARRIAGE

Definition and incidence

Pregnancy loss prior to viability occurs in 10–20 per cent of clinical pregnancies. The early use of ultrasound has resulted in earlier detection of non-viable pregnancy, leading to an apparent increase in incidence. However, the evidence that this is a real phenomenon is lacking.

Background

Spontaneous miscarriage can be classified as shown in Table 57.2.

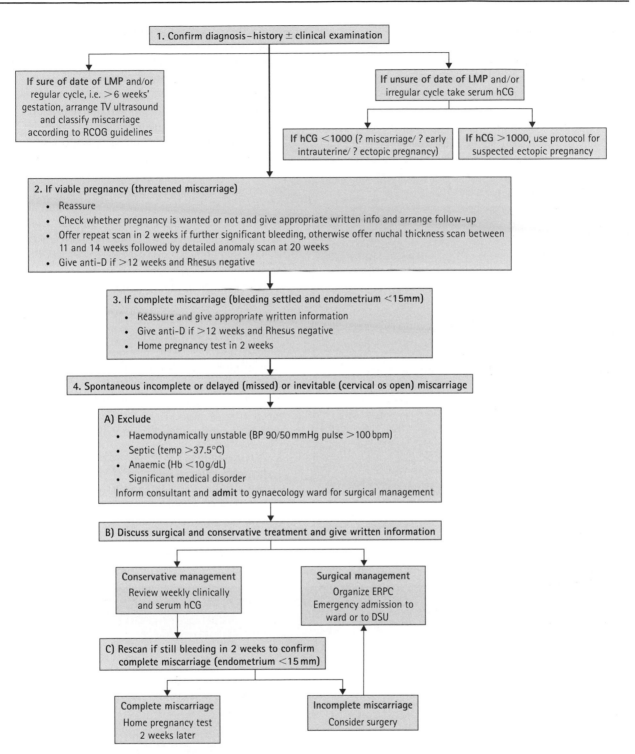

Figure 57.2   Miscarriage management algorithm. LMP, last menstrual period; TV, transvaginal; RCOG, Royal College of Obstetricians and Gynaecologists; hCG, human chorionic gonadotrophin; BP, blood pressure; ERCP, evacuation of retained products of conception; DSU, day surgery unit

Useful ultrasound landmarks include:

- mean sac diameter 1 cm at 5 weeks, 2 cm at 6 weeks and 2.5 cm at 7 weeks,
- yolk sac first seen between 5 and 6 weeks; normal yolk sac size 4–5 mm,
- fetal pole after 6 weeks,
- double decidual sign at 6–7 weeks,

- gestational age in days = 6 + crown–rump length (CRL) in mm.

Management (see Figure 57.2)

The available evidence[20] concerning the management of miscarriage can be summarized as follows.

Studies from primary care [IV]

In 1989 the Dutch College of General Practitioners issued a practice guideline based on the expectant management of spontaneous miscarriage. A revised guideline, issued in 1997, confirmed expectant management as the strategy of first choice.

Several observational studies [II] from the UK, Canada and the USA have also advocated expectant management

Table 57.2 Classification of spontaneous miscarriage at diagnosis as per RCOG guidelines

Classification	Vaginal bleeding	Scan endometrial thickness (mm)	Other scan findings
Complete miscarriage	No	<15	Midline echo or blood clot
Incomplete miscarriage	No/yes	Any	Heterogeneous tissues (with or without a gestational sac) distorting the endometrial midline echo
Delayed (missed) miscarriage	No/yes	Any	Fetal pole (crown–rump length >6 mm, no heart beat) or if crown–rump length ≤6 mm with no change on rescan 7 days later
Anembryonic pregnancy	No/yes	Any	Gestational sac (diameter >20 mm, no embryonic pole or yolk sac) or if diameter ≤20 mm with no change 7 days later

by doctors as a feasible option. These studies showed that a major proportion of women with spontaneous miscarriages – a quarter in the UK and almost half in the North American studies – were managed successfully by doctors, either in the general practice or at home. Additionally, these studies showed that virtually all women under specialist care were bound to undergo surgical evacuation. Through an education programme focusing on both doctors and patients in Vancouver, British Columbia, surgical evacuations were reduced from 46 per cent to 32 per cent, and the incidence of complications decreased during the study.

These studies do not allow any conclusions about the differences between expectant and surgical management or between the management in primary and secondary care, as it is likely that more serious cases were referred to hospital. They do, however, illustrate that expectant management is being practised widely in primary care, even in communities with a high rate of surgical intervention in the hospital environment.

Hospital-based studies

Several hospital-based, randomized, controlled trials [Ib] comparing the various management options for spontaneous miscarriage are now available and provide more solid ground for management decisions. Table 57.3 summarizes the results of these trials. Furthermore, two observational hospital-based studies [II] are of special interest.

1 A non-randomized study, performed by Cheung et al.[28] provides detailed information about short-term complications in a large series of patients. Women with complete abortions (n = 297) were managed expectantly, whereas those showing retained products

Table 57.3 Management of spontaneous miscarriage: randomized, controlled trials

Study	Type of patients	Retained products of conception	Comparison (A vs B)	Success of treatment (%) A	Success of treatment (%) B	P value	Complications (%) A vs B	P value
Nielsen and Hahlin (1995)[21]	Inevitable and incomplete abortion	15–50 mm	Expectant management vs surgery	81/103 (79)	52/52 (100)	>0.5	3 vs 11	>0.5
Chipchase and James (1997)[22]	Incomplete abortion	5–25 mm	Expectant management vs surgery	19/19 (100)	16/16 (100)	>0.5	0.5 vs 0.6	>0.5
De Jonge et al. (1995)[23]	Inevitable abortion	Uterine size <14 weeks	Medical treatment vs surgery	3/23 (13)	26/27 (96)	<0.05	?	–
Johnson et al. (1997)[24]	Missed and complete or incomplete abortion	?	Medical treatment vs surgery	17/17 (100)	12/12 (100)	>0.5	6 vs 8	>0.5
Hinshaw (1993)[25]	Missed and incomplete abortion	<24 mm and 24–77 mm	Medical treatment vs surgery	33/35 (94) and 54/64 (84)	70/72 (97) and 96/97 (99)	>0.5 and <0.05	3 vs 2	>0.5
Chung et al. (1999)[26]	Missed and incomplete abortion	>5 cm² (transverse) or >6 cm² (sagittal)	Medical treatment vs surgery	162/321 (50)	308/314 (98)	<0.05	4 vs 5 (short term) and 3 vs 7 (medium and long term)	<0.05 and <0.05
Nielsen et al. (1999)[27]	Missed and incomplete abortion	15–50 mm	Expectant treatment vs medical	47/62 (76)	49/60 (82)	>0.05	5 vs 2	>0.5

of conception on ultrasonography ($n = 470$) were treated surgically. Treatment complications after surgery occurred in 6 per cent of women – two cervical lacerations and four uterine perforations, for which two laparoscopies were performed – whereas another patient needed an emergency hysterectomy for uncontrollable pelvic bleeding. Short-term complications in those managed expectantly occurred in only 3 per cent of women and were less severe, but the difference did not reach statistical significance compared with those treated primarily by surgery.

2 In another observational study by Jurkovic et al.,[29] 221 asymptomatic women with a missed (delayed) miscarriage diagnosed by ultrasonography were offered a choice between surgical evacuation and expectant management. Among 85 women opting for expectant management, 25 per cent experienced a complete miscarriage, whereas 17 per cent needed surgical evacuation because of an incomplete miscarriage. The remaining 58 per cent requested surgical evacuation at some later stage, mostly for psychological reasons.

Finally, a recent observational study of expectant management of first trimester miscarriage by Luise et al.[30] showed that out of 1096 consecutive patients, 37 per cent had a complete miscarriage. Among the remaining women, 30 per cent chose surgical management and 70 per cent chose expectant management. For the women who chose expectant management, the rate of spontaneous completion was 91 per cent for incomplete miscarriage, 76 per cent for missed miscarriage and 66 per cent for anembryonic pregnancy.

In women facing the prospect of a first trimester spontaneous miscarriage, there is strong evidence to suggest that expectant management is a realistic alternative to surgical evacuation, whereas medical treatment does not seem to offer any advantage.[1] As mifepristone and misoprostol are associated with gastrointestinal side effects in up to 50 per cent of patients and increase costs, these drugs probably deserve no place in the management. Therefore, women with spontaneous incomplete or inevitable miscarriages in the first trimester should be counselled accordingly and offered a choice between expectant and surgical management. Obviously, patients' preferences should play a key part in these management decisions.

LOWER ABDOMINAL PAIN IN THE NON-PREGNANT WOMAN

Most cases seen in an early pregnancy assessment unit will result in a diagnosis of threatened, inevitable or complete or incomplete miscarriage, with a smaller percentage of ectopic pregnancies. However, a second (and increasing) group of patients seen within these units turn out not to be pregnant, but to have lower abdominal pain of another origin. The other possible diagnoses are therefore summarized below (with brief details of management) to allow easy reference for such cases.

Prior to referral to the emergency gynaecology unit, women arriving in the accident and emergency department should have had a urinary pregnancy test. All pregnant women follow the early pregnancy pathway (see previously). Those women who are not pregnant and present with lower abdominal pain should be referred to the emergency gynaecology unit.

Assessment of the patient should include a full history and examination (including vaginal and rectal examination (VE $\pm$ PR)) plus a specific assessment of the pain:

- severity,
- time of onset and chronology,
- relation to menstrual cycle,
- frequency (constant, intermittent),
- location,
- radiation,
- type (severe, crampy, achy, dull),
- relieving or exacerbating factors,
- treatments tried,
- associated symptoms.

The diagnoses to consider[31] are listed in Tables 57.4–57.7 according to:

- anatomical grouping,
- time of onset of symptoms,
- location of pain,
- age group.

Investigations

These should include:

- pelvic ultrasound scan,
- full blood count and C-reactive protein (CRP),
- urinalysis,
- high vaginal swab (charcoal swab), endocervical swab (Ames' transport medium).

Table 57.4 Causes of lower abdominal pain

Gynaecological	Pelvic inflammatory disease, mittelschmerz, ovarian torsion, endometriosis, dysmenorrhoea, fibroid uterus, endometritis, ovarian cysts, ovarian hyperstimulation syndrome, chronic undifferentiated pelvic pain, ovarian cancer
Urinary	Urinary tract infection, pyelonephritis, ureterolithiasis (calculi)
Abdominal	Appendicitis, gastroenteritis, diverticulitis, irritable bowel syndrome, constipation, inflammatory bowel disease
Miscellaneous	Inguinal or ventral wall hernia, aortic abdominal aneurysm, aortic dissection, herpes zoster, abdominal wall myositis

Table 57.5   Abdominal aetiologies and their time of onset

Onset minutes	Ovarian cyst rupture Ovarian torsion Tubo-ovarian abscess rupture Appendicitis Ureterolithiasis Abdominal aortic aneurysm Aortic dissection
Onset minutes to hours to a few days	Primary dysmenorrhoea Mittelschmerz Ovarian hyperstimulation Diverticulitis Gastroenteritis Herpes zoster
Onset days to weeks	Pelvic inflammatory disease Cystitis Pyelonephritis Diverticulitis Less commonly, appendicitis Neoplasms Abdominal wall myositis Aortic abdominal aneurysm
Onset weeks to months	Endometriosis Fibroids Chronic pelvic pain Neoplasms Sexual abuse Diverticular disease Irritable bowel syndrome Inflammatory bowel disease Abdominal wall myositis

Table 57.6   Locations of abdominal pain and anatomic origins

Mid-lower abdominal pain	Pain presenting just above the symphysis pubis, often from any organ in the pelvis, the bladder, the uterus, the rectum and lower colon; common disorders are urinary tract infection, primary dysmenorrhoea, fibroids, endometritis
RLQ pain only	Suggests late appendicitis
LLQ pain only	Suggests gastroenteritis, irritable bowel syndrome or irritable bowel disease, diverticulitis
Both right-sided and left-sided pain	Suggests more diffuse pain in early appendicitis, pelvic inflammatory disease, endometriosis, chronic pelvic pain, ovarian cancer
Pain on either one side or the other	Suggestive of ovarian cysts, ovarian torsion, aortic dissection, herpes zoster, myositis, abdominal wall muscle strain, inguinal hernias, bowel obstruction, regional enteritis, diverticulitis (more on LLQ), leaking abdominal aortic aneurysm, mittelschmerz, endometriosis, ureteral calculi, renal pain

RLQ, right lower quadrant; LLQ, left lower quadrant.

Table 57.7   Differential diagnoses grouped by age

Menarche to age 21	Primary dysmenorrhoea Pelvic inflammatory disease Ovarian torsion Ovarian cysts Appendicitis Irritable bowel disease
Age 21–35	Ovarian cysts Endometriosis Chronic pelvic pain Irritable bowel syndrome
Age 35–menopause	Fibroids Endometriosis Chronic pelvic pain Ovarian cancer Ureterolithiasis Irritable bowel syndrome Diverticulitis Hernias

Further investigations to consider include:

- group and save serum,
- amylase, LFTs, U&Es,
- abdominal films (kidney, ureter, bladder (KUB) view),
- abdominal/renal ultrasound.

KEY POINTS

- Ruptured ectopic pregnancy is a surgical emergency that requires prompt resuscitation and skilled surgery by laparotomy.
- Unruptured ectopic pregnancies are more frequently diagnosed due to technological improvements.
- Unruptured ectopic pregnancy may be treated medically, surgically or conservatively.
- Miscarriage is a common and distressing condition that demands sensitive counselling in addition to medical or surgical assistance.

KEY REFERENCES

1. Tulandi T, Sammour, A. Evidence-based management of ectopic pregnancy. *Curr Opin Obstet Gynecol* 2000; 12(4):289–92.
2. Woolf SH. Practical guidelines, a new reality in medicine. II. Methods of developing guidelines. *Arch Intern Med* 1992; 152:946–52.
3. Tulandi T. Current protocol for ectopic pregnancy. *Contemp Obstet Gynecol* 1999; 44:42–55.
4. Mol BW, Hajenius PJ, Engelsbel S et al. Are gestational age and endometrial thickness alternatives

for serum human chorionic gonadotropin as criteria for the diagnosis of ectopic pregnancy? *Fertil Steril* 1999; **72**:643-5.

5. Job-Spira N, Fernandez H, Bouyer J et al. Ruptured tubal ectopic pregnancy: risk factors and reproductive outcome: results of a population-based study in France. *Am J Obstet Gynecol* 1999; **180**:938-44.

6. Yao M, Tulandi T. Current status of surgical and non-surgical treatment of ectopic pregnancy. *Fertil Steril* 1997; **67**:421-33.

7. Dubuisson JB, Morice P, Chapron C et al. Salpingectomy – the laparoscopic surgical choice for ectopic pregnancy. *Hum Reprod* 1996; **11**:1199-203.

8. Anonymous. Medical management of tubal pregnancy. American College of Obstetricians and Gynaecologists. ACOG Practice Bulletin, No. 3. *Int J Gynaecol Obstet* 1999; **65**:97-103.

9. Lipscomb GH, McCord ML, Stovall TG et al. Predictors of success of methotrexate treatment in women with tubal ectopic pregnancies. *N Engl J Med* 1999; **341**:1974-8.

10. Gazvani MR, Baruah DN, Alfirevic Z, Emery SJ. Mifepristone in combination with methotrexate for the medical treatment of tubal pregnancy: a randomized, controlled trial. *Hum Reprod* 1998; **13**:1987-90.

11. Lipscomb GH, Puckett KJ, Bran D, Ling FW. Management of separation pain after single-dose methotrexate therapy for ectopic pregnancy. *Obstet Gynecol* 1999; **93**:590-3.

12. Saraj AJ, Wilcox JG, Najmabadi S et al. Resolution of hormonal markers of ectopic gestation: a randomized trial comparing single-dose intramuscular methotrexate with salpingostomy. *Obstet Gynecol* 1998; **92**:989-94.

13. Hajenius PJ, Engelsbel S, Mol BWJ et al. Randomised trial of systemic methotrexate versus laparoscopic salpingostomy in tubal pregnancy. *Lancet* 1997; **350**:774-9.

14. Morlock RJ, Lafata JE, Eisenstein D. Cost-effectiveness of single-dose methotrexate compared with laparoscopic treatment of ectopic pregnancy. *Obstet Gynecol* 2000; **95**:407-12.

15. Nieuwkerk PT, Hajenius PJ, Ankum WM et al. Systemic methotrexate therapy versus laparoscopic salpingostomy in patients with tubal pregnancy. Part I. Impact on patients' health-related quality of life. *Fertil Steril* 1998; **70**:511-17.

16. Mol BW, Hajenius PJ, Engelsbel S et al. Treatment of tubal pregnancy in the Netherlands: an economic comparison of systemic methotrexate administration and laparoscopic salpingostomy. *Am J Obstet Gynecol* 1999; **181**:945-51.

17. Fernandez H, Vincent SCY, Pauthier S et al. Randomized trial of conservative laparoscopic treatment and methotrexate administration in ectopic pregnancy and subsequent fertility. *Hum Reprod* 1998; **13**:3239-43.

18. Tzafettas JM, Stephanatos A, Loufopoulos A et al. Single high dose of local methotrexate for the management of relatively advanced ectopic pregnancies. *Fertil Steril* 1999; **71**:1010-13.

19. Banerjee S, Aslam N, Zosmer N et al. The expectant management of women with early pregnancy of unknown location. *Ultrasound Obstet Gynecol* 1999; **14**:231-6.

20. Ankum WM, Wieringa-deWaard M, Bindels PJE. Management of spontaneous miscarriage in the first trimester: an example of putting informed shared decision making into practice. *BMJ* 2001; **322**:1343-6.

21. Nielsen S, Hahlin M. Expectant management of first-trimester spontaneous abortion. *Lancet* 1995; **345**(8942):84-6.

22. Chipchase J, James D. Randomised trial of expectant versus surgical management of spontaneous miscarriage. *Br J Obstet Gynaecol* 1997; **104**(7):840-1.

23. de Jonge ET, Makin JD, Manefeldt E, De Wet GH, Pattinson RC. Randomised clinical trial of medical evacuation and surgical curettage for incomplete miscarriage. *BMJ* 1995; **311**(7006):662.

24. Johnson N, Priestnall M, Marsay T, Ballard P, Watters J. A randomised trial evaluating pain and bleeding after a first trimester miscarriage treated surgically or medically. *Eur J Obstet Gynecol Reprod Biol* 1997; **72**(2):213-15.

25. Hinshaw K, Cooper K, Henshaw R, el-Refaey H, Rispin R, Smith N, Templeton A. Management of uncomplicated miscarriage. Randomized trials are possible. *BMJ* 1993; **307**(6898):259.

26. Chung TK, Lee DT, Cheung LP, Haines CJ, Chang AM, Spontaneous abortion: a randomized, controlled trial comparing surgical evacuation with conservative management using misoprostol. *Fertil Steril* 1999; **71**(6):1054-9.

27. Nielson S, Hahlin M, Platz-Christensen J. Randomised trial comparing expectant with medical management for first trimester miscarriages. *Br J Obstet Gynaecol* 1999; **106**(8):804-7.

28. Cheung LP, Sahota DS, Haines CJ, Chang AMZ. Spontaneous abortion: short term complications following either conservative or surgical management. *Aust NZ J Obstet Gynaecol* 1998; **38**:61-4.

29. Jurkovic D, Ross JA, Nicolaides KH. Expectant management of missed miscarriage. *Br J Obstet Gynaecol* 1998; **105**:670-1.

30. Luise C, Jermy K, May C, Costello G, Collins WP, Bourne T. Outcome of expectant management of spontaneous first trimester miscarriage: observational study. *BMJ* 2002; **324**:873-5.

31. Robertson C. Differential diagnosis of lower abdominal pain in women of childbearing age. *Lippincott's Primary Care Practice. Gynaecologic and Other Women's Health Conditions.* 2 (3):210-29, May/June 1998.

SECTION B

Pelvic floor and lower urinary tract

SECTION B

Assessment of Lower Urinary Tract Function

James Balmforth

INTRODUCTION

Lower urinary tract symptoms are common and can be due to a wide variety of underlying mechanisms. It is therefore important to approach the investigation of such symptoms in a logical and objective manner. An accurate and detailed history and examination provide a framework for diagnosis. However, it is important to recognize that different underlying conditions can cause the same urinary symptoms and that the medical history alone is a poor predictor of pathophysiology. Diagnosis based on history and examination has been shown to be correct in only 65 per cent of women complaining of lower urinary tract symptoms.[1]

HISTORY

Although urinary symptoms alone do not lead directly to a diagnosis, this should in no way detract from the central importance of the medical history in assessing a woman who presents with urinary problems. Listening to any patient is important, and an appropriate history should be obtained in a targeted and methodical manner. Not only will this enable the woman's own words to be turned into a graduated list of symptoms, but it will also provide information about how the woman's quality of life is affected by the condition. There are a number of ways in which a woman can ameliorate her urinary symptoms through behavioural changes. When taking a history, it is important to elucidate these restrictions and adaptations in order to gain a proper impression of the morbidity of the disorder. For example, by severely restricting fluid intake and never venturing far from a toilet, it is possible that a woman could greatly reduce the number of episodes of leaking. However, these adaptations do not lessen the severity of the disorder, or the need for appropriate treatment that will reduce this social restriction.

Urinary symptoms are valuable in directing further management by guiding the investigator in his or her choice of additional tests. Investigations may produce a diagnosis that is inconsistent with the problems complained of by the woman. It is very important to establish which problems bother her most, so that management can be targeted at these problems. This can only be done by taking the time to listen to the patient's description of her urinary symptoms in her own words. To ensure that a complete picture of lower urinary tract symptoms is gained, it is often useful to question the patient about individual symptoms. This can take the form of a questionnaire or of a series of structured questions, and ensures that important features of the history are not omitted because the woman is unable to describe a symptom or is too embarrassed to mention it.

Lower urinary tract symptoms can be grouped into three main areas. These reflect disorders of different aspects of bladder and urethral function. That is, to store urine in a low-pressure reservoir until such time as it is socially convenient to void, when the bladder should be efficiently emptied to completion. The first group of symptoms reflects abnormal storage, the second group includes symptoms associated with abnormal voiding, and those in the final group comprise disorders of bladder sensation (Table 58.1).

Table 58.1   Classification of urinary symptoms into groups

Abnormal storage	Abnormal voiding	Abnormal sensation
Stress incontinence	Hesitancy	Urgency
Urge incontinence	Incomplete emptying	Dysuria
Frequency	Poor stream	Painful bladder
Nocturia	Post-micturition dribble	Loin pain
Nocturnal enuresis	Straining to void	Absent sensation

URINARY SYMPTOMS

Stress incontinence

Stress incontinence is the involuntary loss of urine on effort, associated with physical activities such as sneezing, coughing or lifting. The leakage of urine is usually in small, discrete amounts, coinciding with the physical activity. It is important to distinguish the subjective symptom of stress incontinence from the objectively demonstrated diagnosis of urodynamic stress incontinence, which can only be made following urodynamic assessment.

Urge incontinence

Urge incontinence is the involuntary loss of urine in association with a strong and sudden desire to void. It is frequently described as an inability to reach the toilet in time, and women suffering from this symptom often restrict their social activities to ensure that they are constantly near a toilet. Typical triggers for urge incontinence include hearing running water, opening the front door (latch-key incontinence) and sudden changes in temperature.

Frequency

Frequency is the number of times a woman voids during her waking hours. This should normally be between four and seven voids per day. Excessive frequency is therefore defined as more than seven daytime voids or voiding more often than every 2 hours.

Nocturia

Nocturia is rising from sleep to void at night. Up to the age of 70 years, more than a single void is considered abnormal. Thereafter one additional nocturnal void per decade is considered normal.

Nocturnal enuresis

Nocturnal enuresis is urinary incontinence during sleep. It can be primary or secondary. Primary nocturnal enuresis starts in infancy and can persist in adulthood. Secondary nocturnal enuresis occurs when the nocturnal incontinence restarts following a period of night-time continence. It is important to distinguish enuresis from night-time urge incontinence, in which the woman is awoken by urgency and leaks before making it to the toilet.

Hesitancy

Hesitancy is a delay in starting the urinary stream once the woman tries to initiate micturition. It is not uncommon for most women to experience this occasionally. Even in those women who complain of persistent hesitancy, only a small minority are found to be obstructed. The other causes of persistent hesitancy include poor detrusor contractility and a lack of co-ordination in the normal neurological control of micturition (detrusor sphincter dyssynergia).

Incomplete emptying

The sensation of incomplete bladder emptying is a similarly non-specific symptom. It does not always correlate with the presence of a significant urinary residual. Similarly, women with large residuals are often unaware of it. This sensation can also arise as a result of an open bladder neck, abnormal bladder sensation, and a cystocele acting as a urinary sump.

Poor stream

Urinary flow rate is dependent on the total volume voided, the pressure generated by the detrusor muscle, and outflow resistance. In order to differentiate between these causes, urodynamic investigations need to be undertaken. Bladder outflow obstruction is rare in women who have not undergone previous surgery. Other causes of poor urinary stream include an underlying neurological condition and a pelvic mass.

Post-micturition dribble

Post-micturition dribble is intermittent urinary loss after voiding has finished. This is not the same as intermittent voiding with terminal dribbling. This symptom is associated with a collection of fluid left in the bladder after voiding, such as is found with a cystocele. It is also seen where there is a separate reservoir of urine such as a urethral diverticulum, which fills up during voiding and subsequently drains.

Straining to void

Straining to empty the bladder is suggestive of voiding difficulty. Like the other symptoms in this category, it can be the result of a number of different disorders affecting bladder contractility as well as outflow resistance. Raising intra-abdominal pressure by a Valsalva manoeuvre exerts increased intravesical pressure to aid bladder emptying. The urinary flow produced is characteristically intermittent and prolonged.

Urgency

Urgency is a strong and sudden desire to void that is inapprospriate and, if not relieved, can result in urge incontinence.

Dysuria

Dysuria is pain experienced in the bladder or urethra on passing urine. It is most frequently associated with a urinary tract infection or urethritis, but can also be caused by inflammatory bladder conditions such as interstitial cystitis.

Painful bladder filling

Suprapubic bladder pain is a significant symptom and, if it persists, is an indication for cystocopy and bladder biopsy. Inflammation of the bladder, such as interstitial cystitis, as well as stones, bladder tumours, endometriosis and pelvic infections are associated with this symptom.

Loin pain

Loin pain is referred from the nerves innervating the kidney and urethra. If the ureter is involved, it often radiates around to the ipsilateral groin. There are many causes for this symptom and it is an indication for further assessment of the upper urinary tracts.

Absent sensation

Bladder hyposensitivity is usually due to denervation caused by spinal cord injury or pelvic trauma. It leads to infrequent micturition and a large-capacity bladder. It is often associated with overflow incontinence.

Haematuria

The presence of blood in the urine is always significant and should not be ignored. It warrants investigation of the upper urinary tracts with ultrasound or an intravenous urogram (IVU) and of the lower tract with cystoscopy and urine cytology.

PHYSICAL EXAMINATION

Abdominal and pelvic examinations form an essential part of the assessment of any woman who presents with urinary tract symptoms. Depending upon the medical history, there may be certain additional aspects of the physical examination that require particular attention. If there are any symptoms that point to a possible neurological cause, it is important to perform a screening neurological examination. The patient's mobility and mental state affect her ability to react to her symptoms and it may be appropriate to test these formally as part of the examination, as they will influence management. Similarly, an assessment of motivation and manual dexterity is important in determining the treatment most likely to prove effective.

As part of the gynaecological examination, the condition of the vulval skin should be noted. There may be signs of erythema and oedema from chronic exposure to urine. Vulval and vaginal atrophy may also be noted. Because of the close proximity of the lower urinary and genital tracts in the female, the presence of pelvic organ prolapse can have an important bearing on urinary symptoms and their management. This is best assessed in the left lateral position, using a Sims' speculum and asking the patient to cough and bear down. It is important to note that in order to demonstrate stress incontinence during examination, the bladder needs to be reasonably full, which is often not the case. Speculum examination should be complemented by performing a digital examination with the woman standing, legs abducted and performing a Valsalva manoeuvre. This gives a more accurate impression of the size and origin of any prolapse that is present. The grade of prolapse can be classified subjectively as mild, moderate or severe or graded according to the International Continence Society (ICS) Pelvic Organ Prolapse Quantification score (POP-Q). Whilst performing a vaginal examination in a woman who complains of leaking urine, it is important to assess the degree of anterior vaginal wall mobility and note any scarring that may be present, as this will influence the most appropriate choice of continence surgery. In addition, the anterior vaginal wall should be examined for any mass that may be a urethral diverticulum or cyst. Pelvic masses such as ovarian cysts or uterine enlargement can cause urinary symptoms and need to be excluded by bimanual examination. If this cannot be done with confidence, for example in the obese patient, a transvaginal ultrasound scan should be considered.

INVESTIGATIONS

The bladder has been described as an 'unreliable witness'. Although urinary symptoms provide a framework for diagnosis, they do not on their own allow an accurate impression

Table 58.2　Investigations of lower urinary tract disorders

Basic investigations	Midstream urine specimen
	Frequency–volume chart
	Pad test
Specialist investigations	Uroflowmetry
	Subtracted cystometry
	Videourodynamics
	Ambulatory urodynamics
	Urethral pressure profilometry
	Leak-point pressures
	Neurophysiological studies
	Radiological imaging
	Ultrasonography
	Endoscopy

to be formed of the underlying pathology. This may lead to inappropriate treatment being given and is especially important if surgical management is being considered, as the effects of surgery are irreversible. Investigations can be divided into basic tests, which all gynaecologists should be capable of interpreting, and more complex investigations that require specialist expertise to perform (Table 58.2).

Midstream urine specimen

A midstream urine specimen must be taken for microscopy, culture and sensitivity from all women presenting with urinary symptoms. Bacteriuria is considered to be significant if $>10^5$ organisms per millilitre of urine are reported. It is important to rule out a urinary tract infection before going on to perform more invasive investigations. The presenting lower urinary tract symptoms can be exacerbated or entirely caused by a bacterial infection, and effective treatment with appropriate antibiotics may be all that is required. If it proves necessary to proceed to urodynamic studies, it is important to ensure that there is not an infection already present, which would lead to unrepresentative findings and the risk of an ascending urinary infection of the upper tracts. In some situations, such as investigating a patient with recurrent urinary tract infections, it is necessary to request cultures for 'fastidious organisms' such as *Mycoplasma*, *Ureaplasma* and *Chlamydia*.

Frequency–volume chart

This is also known as a voiding diary or a volume-voided chart (Figure 58.1). The patient is asked to record on a standard time sheet the volume of all fluid consumed and of all urine passed, as well as indicating any episodes of urgency and incontinence. The value of this simple, non-invasive tool is often overlooked, which is unfortunate as it provides a good indication of fluid input and a natural volumetric record of bladder function.

An accurately filled out chart provides invaluable information about the patient's voiding function in her natural

King's College Hospital London
Frequency Volume Chart

Time	Day 1			Day 2			Day 3		
	In	Out	Wet	In	Out	Wet	In	Out	Wet
7 am		340						260	
8 am	300			400	330		350		
9 am		200						170	
10 am	200	150		150	200		200		
11 am			W		175			150	
12 am		200		150				50	
1 pm	150			150	200	W			
2 pm		175					320	200	
3 pm				200				200	
4 pm	450	150			220				W
5 pm		100					150		
6 pm		100	W	300			150	175	
7 pm	250	175		500	200 150				
8 pm	200	50		400	150 150	W	450	100	
9 pm	100				50	W		100	W
10 pm	350	180	BED	150			400	200	
11 pm					210	BED		210	BED
12 am									
1 am		270					200		
2 am	100					W			
3 am		300							
4 am					210				
5 am									
6 am									

Figure 58.1　Example of a 3-day frequency volume chart. If filled in conscientiously, this can prove an invaluable tool, providing useful information on fluid input and output, drinking habits, voided volumes and episodes of urgency and incontinence

environment and adds objectivity to the medical history (Table 58.3).

Frequency–volume charts can be completed prior to the initial hospital consultation to triage care and determine the urgency and complexity of the condition. In addition, they provide a useful form of feedback to the practitioner and the patient so that they can objectively evaluate the effectiveness of any therapy, for example in women undergoing

Table 58.3 Information that can be derived from a frequency–volume chart

- An idea of the normal functional bladder capacity, which should be fairly consistently around 300–500 mL. Frequent voids of variable amounts throughout the day imply bladder over-activity or behavioural adaptation to symptoms.
- A volumetric summary of diurnal urinary frequency and nocturia.
- Quantification of total fluid intake and its distribution throughout the day.
- A semi-objective evaluation of the severity of urinary incontinence and associated or provocative events.

bladder training for detrusor over-activity. A frequency-volume chart should always be completed prior to urodynamic testing so that the patient's functional bladder capacity is known. This prevents over-distension during filling cystometry. There is no standardized format for frequency-volume charts; the duration varies between 48 hours and 7 days in different centres. In addition to the standard volumetric information, the patient may be asked to quantitate incontinent episodes, note associated or provocative activities, and state the number of pads used per day.

Pad test

The objective demonstration of leaking is essential in reaching a diagnosis of urinary incontinence. It has been shown that a patient's subjective perception of the severity of incontinence correlates poorly with objective measures.[2] Pad testing provides a simple, non-invasive, objective method for detecting and quantifying urinary leakage. Various protocols exist for performing a pad test. To obtain a representative result, especially for those who have variable or intermittent urinary incontinence, the test should be as long as possible in circumstances that approximate those of everyday life. It should be conducted in a standardized fashion so that results are comparable and reproducible. This allows the effect of treatment to be objectively assessed in a non-invasive manner.

The ICS has produced guidelines for a standardized 1-hour pad test.[3] The patient wears a pre-weighed pad or sanitary towel, drinks 500 mL of water and rests for 15 minutes. She then performs 30 minutes of moderate exercise such as stair climbing and walking. The remaining 15 minutes are spent performing more provocative exercises, including coughing vigorously, bending over, hand washing and running. At the end of 1 hour, the pad is removed and re-weighed. An increase of >2 g is considered a significant loss. A weight gain of >10 g is categorized as severe incontinence.

The standard 1-hour ICS pad test has been shown to have good reproducibility, and reliably differentiates normal from abnormal continence mechanisms. However, the short period of study and lack of a standardized bladder volume before starting the test mean that there is a significant false-negative rate.

Long-term protocols also exist in which the patient is given several pre-weighed pads to be worn at home for periods of 12, 24 or 48 hours. The used pads are collected in sealed plastic bags and re-weighed at the end of the specified period to determine total urine loss. These longer tests have not as yet been subject to standardization, but have been found to be a valid method of detecting and quantifying incontinence. They are highly reproducible, show high sensitivity and a low false-negative rate. The extended pad test is particularly useful to confirm or refute leakage in those patients complaining of incontinence that has not been demonstrated on urodynamic studies.

Uroflowmetry

Uroflowmetry is the simplest and one of the most useful investigations in the assessment of voiding dysfunction. It consists simply of measuring urinary flow over time and allows a rapid and non-invasive analysis of the normality or otherwise of flow rate. When combined with the measurement of residual urine volume by ultrasound or catheterization, it provides information on the efficiency of micturition in emptying the bladder. One or more symptoms of voiding disorder are commonly described in women complaining of urinary tract disorders, and it is important to diagnose or eliminate voiding difficulty. This is particularly so when treatment is being considered for incontinence. Both surgical treatment of urodynamic stress incontinence and drug treatment for detrusor over-activity have the potential to cause voiding difficulty. Therefore pre-treatment uroflowmetry and the measurement of residual urine are essential.

Indications

Uroflowmetry should be regarded as a screening test for voiding difficulty in all women with symptoms of lower urinary tract dysfunction. It is important to appreciate that urinary flow is dependent upon a number of factors, including detrusor contractility, neurological co-ordination of sphincter relaxation and outflow patency. Uroflowmetry on its own cannot successfully distinguish between the causes of voiding dysfunction.

Methods

There are several different physical principles that can be utilized to provide an accurate assessment of flow. The following three methods are in common use.

- *Gravimetric method.* The rate of change of the weight of the voided urine in the collecting jug is converted into a flow rate (Figure 58.2).

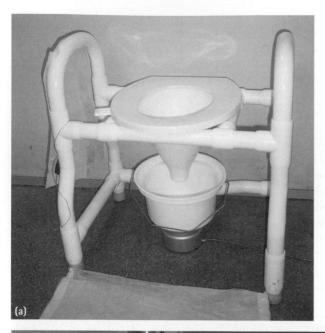

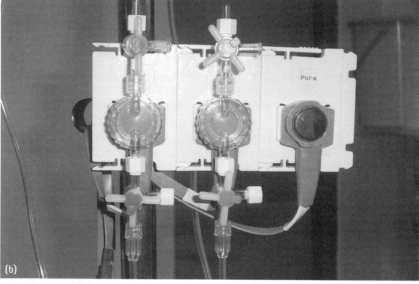

Figure 58.2 (a) Gravimetric flow meter. (b) External pressure transducers connected to the patient via fluid-filled lines inserted into the bladder and rectum. This allows accurate measurement of intra-vesical and intra-abdominal pressure

- *Rotating disc method.* A known amount of power is required to keep a rotating disc spinning at a constant rate. Voided fluid is directed onto the disc, increasing its inertia. The flow rate is proportional to the amount of extra power that is required to keep the disc spinning at a constant rate.
- *Capacitance dipstick.* A metal capacitor strip is attached to the side of the flowmeter. As urine accumulates in the container, the electrical capacitance of the dipstick changes and from this the rate of flow can be calculated.

It should be noted that the environment in which the woman performs the flow rate recording will have a considerable influence on the results. It is important that every

effort is made to make the patient feel as comfortable and relaxed as possible.

Interpretation

The definitions for urine flow rate measurements have been standardized by the ICS and should be expressed in millilitres per second (Figure 58.3).

The two most useful parameters are the maximum flow rate and the voided volume. The maximum flow rate is partially dependent on the voided volume, as this determines how distended the bladder muscle fibres are. For this reason, small voided volumes of <150 mL are insufficient to obtain an accurate impression of flow, and the test needs to be repeated.

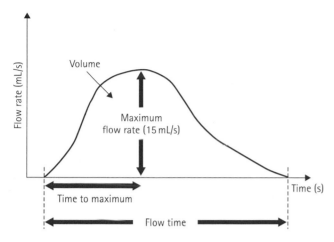

Figure 58.3 Diagrammatic representation of urinary flow rate with standardized International Continence Society (ICS) terminology. **Voided volume**: total volume expelled via the urethra; the area beneath the flow–time curve. **Maximum flow rate**: maximum measured value of the flow rate. **Flow time**: the time over which measurable flow actually occurs. If flow is intermittent, the time intervals between flow episodes are not included. **Average flow rate**: volume voided divided by the flow time. **Time to maximum flow**: elapsed time from onset of flow to maximum flow

Table 58.4   Cystometry

Phases of cycle	Urethra	Detrusor
Filling	Should remain closed and competent but can: • be incompetent due to physical stress, but without an associated rise in detrusor pressure (stress incontinence) • be incompetent as a direct result of an involuntary rise in detrusor pressure (detrusor over-activity)	Should remain relaxed/stable throughout filling but can: • show abnormal involuntary contractions (detrusor over-activity) • show a gradual rise in pressure with filling (low compliance)
Voiding	Should be appropriately relaxed but can: • be constricted, leading to outflow obstruction (obstructed cause)	Should contract efficiently under voluntary instruction but can: • be under-active or acontractile (possible neuropathic cause) • show high-pressure contractions (if over-active or needing to overcome an outflow obstruction)

The third major factor to consider when interpreting flow rate is the pattern of flow, in particular whether flow is continuous or intermittent. A normal flow curve is bell-shaped and characterized by a rapid rise to maximal flow. A prolonged, intermittent flow curve is suggestive of voiding dysfunction, with the patient using abdominal straining to achieve bladder emptying. The results must always be interpreted within the context of the clinical situation, and the limitations of the study should be recognized. More information concerning the cause of voiding difficulty is provided by the addition of simultaneous pressure measurements as part of cystometry.

Factors influencing urine flow rate

The maximum urine flow rate (MUFR) is highly dependent on voided volume, as has already been discussed. Most commonly, a minimum accepted MUFR of 15 mL/s is used, but nomograms have been constructed from healthy volunteers displaying flow rates in centile form for any given volume voided.[4] Urine flow rates are higher in women than in men for a comparable voided volume. Age and parity have not been shown to have a significant effect on urine flow rates in asymptomatic women. As might be expected, there is a progressive decline in flow rate with increasing grades of pelvic floor prolapse, especially uterine prolapse and cystourethrocele.

Altered detrusor function influences flow rate by determining the contractile force with which urine is expelled. In addition, bladder neck and urethral anatomy influence urine flow by affecting outflow resistance. To distinguish between these two major causes of voiding dysfunction, more complex urodynamic tests are required in which simultaneous pressure/flow measurements are taken.

Subtracted cystometry

Cystometry is the method by which the pressure/volume relationship of the bladder is assessed during filling and voiding. It involves the simultaneous measurement of intravesical and intra-abdominal pressures. Electronic subtraction of the intra-abdominal pressure from the intravesical pressure enables the detrusor pressure to be calculated and compared with changes in bladder volume and flow rate. Cystometry aims to characterize detrusor and urethral function during the filling and voiding phases (Table 58.4). It can be useful, when learning to interpret cystometrograms, to break down the functions of the detrusor and urethra by phases of the micturition cycle.

Indications

Ideally, cystometry should be performed on every woman who complains of lower urinary tract symptoms. As has been previously discussed, the assessment of urinary symptoms and basic investigations alone do not always allow the correct diagnosis to be made and appropriate treatment to be initiated.[5] However, when access to investigations is limited, it is reasonable to manage patients with clear-cut symptoms empirically with conservative treatment, provided that cystometry is subsequently performed in those in whom empirical treatment fails. Certainly surgical treatments should never be considered without urodynamic assessment, as the inappropriate selection of surgery can have disastrous and largely irreversible consequences for the patient.

If a policy of urodynamic screening on all women with lower urinary tract symptoms is not practised, selective testing should certainly be considered in the investigation of:

- symptoms that have failed to respond to empirical conservative measures,
- a patient being considered for any form of incontinence surgery,
- voiding difficulties,
- mixed symptoms (e.g. frequency, urgency and stress incontinence),
- previous unsuccessful incontinence surgery,
- suspected neuropathic bladder disorders.

The last two complex groups are better investigated by videourodynamics, as this yields valuable information about the anatomical structure of the urinary tract as well as the dynamic function.

Methods

It is important that cystometric diagnoses are related to the patient's symptoms and physical findings at the time of the investigation. The aim is to reproduce the presenting symptoms that cause the woman concern, so that a diagnosis can be made and appropriate treatment planned. Terminology and standards are defined by the ICS.[6] This allows cystometric data to be compared amongst different centres and used in research trials.

Modern multi-channel cystometry requires two pressure transducers (to measure the intra-abdominal and intra-vesical pressures), an electronic subtraction unit (to derive the detrusor pressure), an amplifying unit and a display or printout (Figure 58.4). Two types of pressure transducers are available: a fluid-filled pressure line inserted into the bladder or rectum and connected to an external transducer, and a solid micro-tip pressure transducer placed directly inside the body. The difference between the two is largely one of cost and convenience of use. All pressure measurements are made in centimetres of water (cmH_2O).

Prior to inserting the pressure catheters, the patient is asked to void on the flowmeter to allow the measurement of a free flow rate. The presence of any residual urine on subsequent urethral catheterization is noted. The pressure catheters are then inserted and calibrated. Quality control

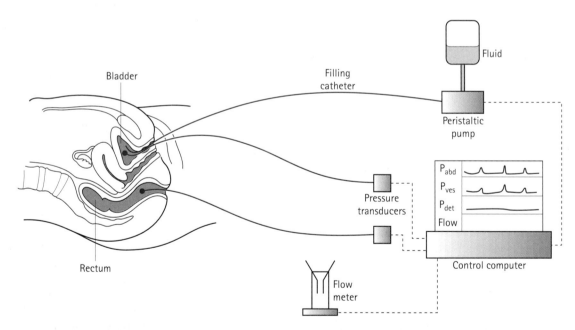

Figure 58.4   Schematic diagram showing the position of the pressure catheters and the measurements recorded during subtracted cystometry. The following measurements are made:

- Free-flow rate and residual urine are measured at the start of the test by means of a flow meter and subsequent urethral catheterization.
- Intra-abdominal pressure (P_{abd}) is measured with the rectal pressure catheter. Alternatively, this could be measured with a pressure catheter in the vagina or colostomy stoma.
- Intravesical pressure (P_{ves}) is measured with a pressure catheter in the bladder via the urethra or suprapubic route.
- Detrusor pressure (P_{det}) is derived from continuous electronic subtraction of abdominal from intravesical pressure ($P_{det} = P_{ves} - P_{abd}$) and displayed concomitantly.
- Filling volume is recorded by a peristaltic pump connected to the system or calculated manually.
- Flow rate is measured by a flow meter allowing simultaneous pressure-flow analysis.
- During filling, the patient is asked to indicate her first desire to void (FDV) and when she experiences a strong desire to void (SDV). This is taken as bladder capacity.
- In addition, it is important to explain to the patient the relevance of expressing her sensations (such as urgency) during the test so that the cystometry trace can be annotated. This helps to interpret the findings

is an essential part of performing cystometry if valid conclusions are to be drawn from the investigation. The system is checked for adequate subtraction by asking the patient to cough at regular intervals. An equal pressure rise should be observed in both the intra-abdominal and intravesical pressure traces, which should cancel out to leave the detrusor pressure unchanged. Once the integrity of the pressure readings has been checked and the system zeroed to atmospheric pressure, filling can commence.

Normal saline at room temperature is instilled into the bladder at a predetermined rate under the control of a peristaltic pump. This is usually in the range of 25–100 mL/min, depending on the indication for cystometry. This rate should be reduced to a slower filling rate closer to the normal physiological range when assessing patients with neuropathic bladders. During filling, the patient is asked to indicate her first desire to void (FDV) and when she experiences an uncontrollably strong desire to void (SDV). Any rise in detrusor pressure is noted and whether this is associated with the sensation of urgency or leaking. Filling is discontinued once there is a sustained SDV. This volume is taken as cystometric bladder capacity and is usually in the range 400–600 mL.

At the end of filling, the patient is asked to stand, to assess whether there is a postural rise in detrusor pressure, and to cough several times. More strenuous stimuli such as star jumps can be performed if leakage is not demonstrated by coughing in women who complain of this symptom in their history. The presence of any leakage is noted and whether a stable trace or an associated rise in detrusor pressure accompanies this. Provocative tests for detrusor overactivity are performed at this stage and the patient may be asked to listen to running water, wash her hands or heel bounce to try to induce leakage. Finally, the patient transfers back onto the flowmeter, with the pressure catheters still in situ. She is instructed to void and the detrusor pressure and urine flow rate are measured simultaneously to provide a simultaneous pressure/flow analysis.

Interpretation

As has been previously discussed, it is vital that the cystometric findings are evaluated in the light of the woman's symptomatology. The following are normal cystometric parameters.

- *Filling cystometry*:
  - residual urine <50 mL,
  - capacity (taken as SDV) >400 mL,
  - absence of systolic detrusor contractions during filling,
  - negligible rise in detrusor pressure on filling: this should be <15 cmH$_2$O for a filling volume of 500 mL.
- *Voiding cystometry*:
  - no leakage on coughing or performing exercise,
  - no provoked detrusor contractions as a result of precipitating factors such as postural changes, hand washing or coughing,

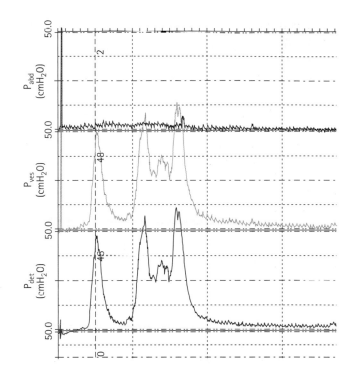

Figure 58.5   Part of a cystometrogram trace showing detrusor-overactivity. Note that intra-abdominal pressure is stable whilst the intra-vesical pressure line shows an involuntary detrusor contraction. Other abbreviations as Figure 58.4

  - a maximum voiding detrusor pressure of <50 cmH$_2$O, with a maximum flow rate >15 mL/s for a volume voided of >150 mL.

By considering urethral and detrusor function during the filling and voiding phases of cystometry, abnormalities can be systematically classified (Figure 58.5). The presence of involuntary systolic detrusor contractions during filling or on provocation that the patient cannot suppress is diagnostic of detrusor over-activity. If there is a gradual rise in detrusor pressure during filling to >15 cmH$_2$O, but without phasic contractions, this is termed low compliance. This can be artefactual owing to superphysiological, fast bladder filling. If there is a neurological condition present, such as multiple sclerosis, this is often accompanied by marked low compliance. If leakage occurs on coughing, with an associated rise in intra-abdominal pressure but in the absence of abnormal detrusor activity, urodynamic stress incontinence is diagnosed.

Videourodynamics

Videourodynamics offers the facility simultaneously to study the anatomical structure and the pressure/flow characteristics of the lower urinary tract. This is achieved by using contrast medium rather than saline to fill the bladder during cystometry, and screening the bladder and urethra intermittently throughout the procedure. The combination

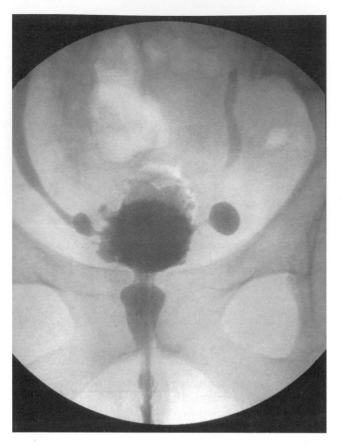

Figure 58.6 Additional anatomical and physiological information can be obtained with videourodynamics. Here bilateral vesico-uretic reflux and bladder diverticula are seen.

of these approaches results in the videocystourethrogram (VCU), which is regarded as the 'gold standard' for assessing lower urinary tract disorders. Most patients can be adequately investigated using simpler techniques, but VCU does offer several advantages over cystometry alone for the investigation of complex cases in tertiary centres. The addition of radiological screening provides valuable additional information relating to bladder morphology, the degree of bladder base support and function of the bladder neck during coughing, the presence of vesicoureteric reflux (which may be present in up to 7 per cent of incontinent patients) and the site of outflow obstruction (Figure 58.6). Clinical situations in which VCU offers significant advantages over plain cystometry include the following:

- Women in whom previous incontinence surgery has failed, as the position and mobility of the bladder neck can be assessed at rest and on straining. When combined with urethral pressure profilometry (UPP), an experienced investigator can infer information about the relative contributions of bladder neck hypermobility and sphincter deficiency as the causes of continued stress incontinence.
- Neurological lower urinary tract dysfunction. VCU is required to adequately assess the complex dysfunction

seen in neuropathic bladders and to provide a framework for treatment. It is important to look for the presence of vesicoureteric reflux in this group of women.
- Assessment of voiding difficulties or symptoms suggestive of an anatomical lesion such as a urethral diverticulum.

Technique

The technique is identical to that used for routine subtracted cystometry except that the investigation is performed in a room set up for radiological X-ray screening. Uroflowmetry, measurement of urinary residual and the insertion of pressure catheters are the same as for subtracted cystometry. Radio-opaque contrast is used to fill the bladder. X-ray screening takes place if the woman complains of leaking during filling and then during provocative coughing. This allows assessment of the degree of bladder neck opening, the severity of leakage and the extent of bladder-base descent. The presence of vesicoureteric reflux, bladder trabeculation and diverticulae is noted. The woman then commences voiding and, once flow is established, she is asked to interrupt it. This should result in cessation of flow and urine being 'milked back' from the proximal urethra into the bladder. Finally, the presence of a post-void residual can be determined.

Ambulatory urodynamic monitoring

Ambulatory urodynamic monitoring (AUM) is a relatively new diagnostic tool in the evaluation of lower urinary tract dysfunction. It is of particular use in the investigation of detrusor over-activity, where standard laboratory urodynamics have failed to replicate the symptoms that are experienced by the patient in her normal environment. Although laboratory urodynamics forms the standard method of objectively investigating bladder and urethral function, it is by design not physiological. This is because relatively fast retrograde filling of the bladder is employed rather than slower filling from the kidneys via the ureters. In addition, the environment in which the test is performed and the focus of attention directed towards the subject are far removed from her everyday activities. In an attempt to study bladder function in circumstances that more closely approximate those in which the subject normally finds herself, ambulatory urodynamics has been developed.

Ambulatory urodynamic monitoring uses natural anterograde bladder filling and allows the patient to reproduce her normal daily activities, including those that commonly provoke symptoms.

Technique

Ambulatory systems have three main components.

1 Micro-tip transducers are placed in the bladder and rectum in a way similar to that of laboratory urodynamics.

2 A portable recording system allows several channels of data to be recorded simultaneously. This should include an event marker, to enable the patient to mark particular activities on the trace, and a method quantifying urine leakage, such as an electronic pad.

3 An analysing system is needed to retrieve and process the data. All traces are interpreted with the patient present so that more information can be obtained about particular events.

The ICS has recently standardized the terminology and methodology of AUM[7] and this will allow comparison of results from different centres.

The investigation is usually carried out over a 4-hour time period. Once the transducers are inserted into the bladder and rectum and the system has been calibrated, the patient is encouraged to drink normally and perform normal activities. During the investigation, the patient is asked to keep a careful record of symptoms and events, and the position of the catheters is checked periodically. At the conclusion of the test, provocative manoeuvres are carried out with a full bladder prior to removing the transducers and analysing the results. Significantly more detrusor overactivity is diagnosed using AUM than with conventional laboratory urodynamics. However, it is uncertain at the present time whether this is due to a higher sensitivity or whether AUM simply has a high false-positive rate for diagnosing detrusor over-activity. Ambulatory urodynamics is subject to significant artefact, but this can be greatly reduced by rigorous methodology.

Urethral pressure profilometry

The relationship between the intravesical pressure and the urethral pressure is the key to maintaining continence. Normally, the urethral pressure exceeds the intravesical pressure at all times, except during voluntary relaxation of the bladder neck leading to micturition. Urethral pressure profilometry can assess this ability of the urethra to exert a positive closure pressure in order to prevent leakage. This is done by simultaneously measuring the intravesical and urethral pressures using a catheter with two pressure transducers set 6 cm apart.

Technique

The pressure catheter is inserted into the bladder with the distal pressure transducer inside the bladder and the proximal transducer near the bladder neck. It is then withdrawn at a standard speed by a mechanical retractor, allowing pressure measurements to be made along the functional length of the urethra to give a graph of pressure over distance travelled along the urethra. Two types of UPP may be measured:

1 resting UPP, with the patient at rest in a supine position,

2 stress UPP, with the patient coughing throughout the test to see if the intravesical pressure exceeds the urethral pressure during increases in intra-abdominal pressure – this would result in a negative closure pressure and leakage of urine per urethram.

Although the closure pressures in women with urodynamic stress incontinence are generally less than in their dry counterparts, this test is not sufficiently discriminatory to be used in the diagnosis of urodynamic stress incontinence. However, it is often useful in understanding the pathophysiology of urodynamic stress incontinence and in planning the most appropriate intervention, especially in women who have had previous failed surgery for incontinence. A low maximum urethral closure pressure correlates with a poor outcome for incontinence surgery. The other group of patients in whom UPP can be useful is women with voiding difficulties. An increased maximum urethral closure pressure indicates outflow obstruction, sometimes as the result of previous surgery or a stricture. In these women, urethral dilatation or urethrotomy may be appropriate.

NEUROPHYSIOLOGICAL INVESTIGATION

The normal co-ordinated functions of the bladder and urethra are controlled by a complex set of central and peripheral neurological reflexes. In an effort to understand these mechanisms better and to evaluate patients with lower urinary tract dysfunction, a whole range of neurophysiological tests has evolved. These techniques stimulate and record activity at different levels of the neurological pathways that control bladder and urethral function. The most commonly employed techniques in clinical neurophysiological testing are electromyography (EMG), in which recordings of bioelectrical potentials in muscles are studied, and nerve conduction studies. The latter examine the capacity of a nerve to transmit a test electrical stimulus along its length.

Electromyography

Electromyography is the study of bioelectrical potentials generated by the depolarization of muscle fibres. It is predominantly used to study striated muscle, in particular the urethral sphincter and the pelvic floor muscles. The functional unit studied is called a motor unit and consists of the muscle fibres innervated by branches from the motor neuron of a single anterior horn cell. The potential it generates during contraction is called the motor nerve unit potential (MUP). This can be measured by means of surface electrodes or various types of needle electrode. By measuring the amplitude, duration and number of phases of the action potential, the extent of neurological denervation and subsequent re-innervation in the target muscle can be inferred. Partial denervation of the pelvic floor following childbirth has been proposed as a factor in the subsequent development of incontinence and prolapse.[8] This is a highly specialist investigation and a skilled investigator is required to interpret the results. Whilst EMG studies have greatly improved our understanding of pelvic floor, lower urinary tract and bowel function in health and disease, the results to date have had little effect on clinical management. The main clinical indication for EMG studies is as an adjunct to videourodynamics to distinguish between striated and smooth muscle in neuropathic urethral obstruction.

Nerve conduction studies

A number of different techniques have been employed to study the conduction of central and peripheral nerve pathways to the bladder and urethra. These examine the capacity of a nerve to transmit a test electrical signal along its length. If the pathway being tested is damaged, there will be a delay in conduction time and thus a prolonged latency between the stimulus and the muscular response. In addition, the amplitude of the muscle response will be reduced. A wide range of neurological pathways has been investigated using variations of this technique, including the sacral reflex arc, pudendal terminal motor latencies, transcutaneous spinal stimulation and cortical evoked responses. As with EMG studies, these investigations have improved our understanding of the neurophysiological control of the normal and dysfunctional bladder, but are of limited use in the clinical investigation of most patients.

RADIOLOGICAL IMAGING

Radiological imaging of the urinary tract is not justified as a routine investigation in all women presenting with urinary symptoms, but instead should be targeted at specific indications. The diagnostic procedures available include plain abdominal films, intravenous urography and various contrast studies of the lower urinary tracts.

Plain X-ray

A plain abdominal film may be a useful screening investigation for a variety of conditions that affect lower urinary tract function. Foreign bodies and bladder calculi causing outflow obstruction can be diagnosed. Bladder wall calcification is rare in the UK, but is seen more frequently worldwide as a result of tuberculosis and schistosomiasis. Probably the most useful indication for plain radiographic films is to investigate spinal abnormalities, such as spina bifida or sacral agenesis, as a cause of neuropathic bladder disorder.

Intravenous urography

This is not a routine investigation of lower urinary tract dysfunction. It provides anatomical and some functional information on the kidneys, ureters and bladder. Intravenous urography (IVU) is indicated in women with neuropathic bladders, suspected congenital or acquired abnormalities (such as uterovaginal fistulae), haematuria and suspected ureteric compromise secondary to the effects of a pelvic mass or trauma.

Micturating cystourethrography

This investigation requires instillation of radio-opaque contrast medium into the bladder and then screening with fluoroscopy as the patient voids. It is similar to the X-ray screening performed as part of a videocystometrogram but without any pressure flow information. Its main value is to demonstrate bladder and urethral fistulae, vesicoureteric reflux and anatomical abnormalities of the lower tracts such as urethral diverticulae.

ULTRASONOGRAPHY

Ultrasound provides a relatively non-invasive method of imaging the urinary tract in real time, without exposing the patient to ionizing radiation. There is an ever-increasing range of applications for ultrasound imaging in the investigation of urinary tract dysfunction. As well as the lack of radiation exposure, ultrasound has the advantage of having significantly lower operating costs than comparable radiological investigation. The main disadvantage is that ultrasound waves do not penetrate as far and so the probe has to be held close to the target. The field of view is more limited than X-rays, so that only one part of the urinary tract can be viewed at a time. Ultrasound imaging depends on the different echogenicity of tissues to form a picture. It is especially well suited for visualizing fluid-filled and air-filled cystic structures.

Post-micturition residual volume

Ultrasonography is widely used to estimate residual urine volumes. This obviates the need for urethral catheterization, with its concomitant risk of infection. This is particularly useful in the assessment of women with voiding difficulties. It can also be used following postoperative catheter removal or in women in labour as an alternative to repeated catheterization to ensure that the bladder is not allowed to over-distend. Many methods of estimating bladder volume have been proposed,[9] most of which involve imaging the maximum cross-sectional area in two planes and measuring the antero-posterior, transverse and longitudinal diameters. These are then multiplied by a correction factor to approximate the volume of a sphere. This method has an accuracy of ±20 per cent.

Assessing lower urinary tract structure

Ultrasound offers an inexpensive, non-invasive method of assessing the structure of the lower urinary tract and is advocated as an alternative to cystourethroscopy for many indications. The arguments in favour of each technique are similar to those proposed for the use of transvaginal ultrasonography and hysteroscopy for the assessment of the reproductive organs. The sensitivity of ultrasonography and endoscopy in different disorders varies, largely according to the experience of the operator and the quality of the equipment used. The majority of bladder tumours are exophytic and papillary in shape and are well visualized by ultrasound. Similarly, bladder diverticulae and calculi are easily detected.

Transabdominal ultrasound does not provide satisfactory imaging of the bladder neck and urethra, owing to their position behind the symphysis pubis. These are visualized better with the use of a transvaginal, transrectal or perineal probe. Ultrasonography is a very sensitive method of detecting urethral diverticulae and their relation to the urethral sphincter. Differentiation from para-urethral cysts may be difficult if a connection cannot be visualized. Three-dimensional ultrasound has recently been used as a research tool to determine urethral sphincter volumes as part of the assessment of women presenting with incontinence.

Another technique that is currently not in widespread clinical use, but that shows promise, is the measurement of bladder wall thickness.[10] This is performed using the transvaginal approach when the bladder is empty and offers a reproducible, sensitive method of screening for detrusor over-activity.

CYSTOURETHROSCOPY

Cystourethroscopy enables the inside of the bladder and urethra to be visualized (Figure 58.7). It is an invasive but relatively low-risk procedure that can be undertaken for women of any age as a day case. The choice between a rigid or flexible cystoscope and the anaesthetic used will depend on the individual case and the preferences of the operator. Modern cystoscopes consist of at least three elements.

1 An optical system for transmitting the image to a video monitor with maximum clarity and resolution. In a

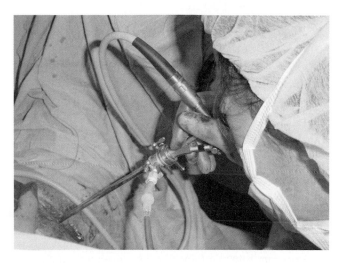

Figure 58.7   Rigid cystometry with multiple bladder biopsies being performed under general anaesthesia in a patient with a history of recurrent urinary tract infections.

rigid endoscope this is done by a rod-lens system, and in a flexible endoscope by a multifibre bundle of optical fibres.

2 Another system of optical fibres is needed to transmit light into the bladder.

3 An irrigating channel is needed to flush away blood and dilate the bladder under direct vision.

Most operating cystoscopes also have an outflow channel to carry debris away.

Cystourethroscopy is an invaluable tool in investigating the lower urinary tract, as it provides detailed anatomical information. It is not usually performed as part of the routine investigation of women with incontinence, but there are many indications for which direct visual inspection and targeted biopsies of the bladder and urethra are important in establishing a diagnosis.

Indications

- To investigate haematuria not related to urinary tract infection.
- When a reduced bladder capacity or painful filling is found at cystometry.
- To exclude bladder tumours and stones as a cause of recurrent or persistent urinary tract infection.
- If a lower urinary tract fistula is suspected.
- If interstitial cystitis is suspected.
- Following failed incontinence surgery when the patient complains of voiding difficulty, irritative symptoms or persistent incontinence.

Technique

The majority of cystourethroscopies undertaken by gynaecologists are performed under a general anaesthetic with a rigid scope. The advantages of a rigid cystoscope are that visualization is much clearer and more magnified, and that biopsies and other manipulative procedures are relatively easily carried out through the large instrument channel. Flexible cystoscopes offer the advantage of being able to be used in an outpatient setting, with topical anaesthetic only. However, the view is more limited, as is the instrumentation that can be used, making it difficult to take histologically valid biopsy specimens. Flexible cystoscopy is more often performed by urologists.

Rigid cystoscopes are available with several viewing angles, including 0 degrees (straight), 12 degrees, 30 degrees and 70 degrees. Angled telescopes have a field marker, which appears as a notch at the edge of the field of view and helps to maintain orientation. The choice of telescope depends on the procedure being performed and the operator's preference. The cystoscope is placed into the urethral meatus and advanced towards the bladder under direct vision with the irrigation fluid running. Sterile saline is usually used as the irrigating fluid unless diathermy is planned, in which case a non-ionic solution such as glycine is required. Once the bladder is sufficiently distended to allow inspection of the folds of mucosa (200–400 mL), the irrigation can be switched off. It is important to examine the bladder and urethra systematically so that no area is missed.[11] The careful inspection of the urethra is a vital part of the investigation and should not be neglected. This is most commonly done whilst withdrawing the instrument at the end of the procedure. The trigone and the position of the ureteric orifices should be noted. Next the mucosa is examined for colour, vascularity, trabeculation and abnormal lesions. Orientation is easily established by identifying the air bubble at the dome of the bladder. This serves as a landmark during inspection of the bladder mucosa, which is conventionally performed by going around clockwise in a series of 12 sweeps, coming back to the bubble after each one. Visualization of the bladder base can be difficult if a large cystocele is present. This is made easier by inserting a finger in the vagina to correct the prolapse.

QUALITY OF LIFE ASSESSMENT

In recent years there has been a growth of interest in quality of life (QoL) assessment of lower urinary tract disorders.[12] This employs carefully designed and validated patient-assessed health questionnaires to determine the impact of clinical problems. Traditionally doctors have categorized the severity of a condition using objective clinical measures. However, the impact of a disease and the success of any treatment should no longer be measured purely in terms of 'doctor-centred' clinical parameters alone. It is increasingly recognized that a patient's quality of life and psychosocial adjustment to an illness are equally as important as the status of their physical disease. Two major types of QoL questionnaire are available: generic questionnaires, which can be used across a range of medical conditions, and disease-specific questionnaires, which focus on the likely impacts of a particular disorder. It is very important that any questionnaires used for this form of assessment have been subjected to rigorous reliability testing and validation in order to derive meaningful data from them. Quality of life assessment is particularly useful in determining the response of patients to treatment. It gives useful information about therapeutic effects as seen from the patient's perspective across a range of different domains. This form of patient assessment has many applications. It is now widely used as an outcome measure in the evaluation of clinical practice and in research trials.

KEY POINTS

- Investigations of lower urinary tract dysfunction vary from simple tests that can easily be performed in an office setting, to complex investigations available in tertiary centres.
- As the correlation between lower urinary tract symptoms and underlying diagnosis is poor, early investigation is desirable so that a firm diagnosis can be established and rational treatment instigated.
- Thorough assessment, including urodynamics is mandatory prior to considering surgical treatment.
- The choice of investigations performed should be individualized according to the patient's presenting symptoms, and past medical history.

KEY REFERENCES

1. Sand PK, Ostergard DR. Incontinence history as a predictor for detrusor instability. *Obstet Gynecol* 1988; **71**:257–9.
2. Frazer MI, Hayden BT, Sutherst JR. The severity of urinary incontinence in women: comparison of subjective and objective data. *Br J Urol* 1989; **63**:14–15.
3. Bates P, Bradley W, Glen E et al. *Fifth Report on the Standardization of Terminology of Lower Urinary Tract Function*. Bristol: International Continence Society Committee on Standardisation of Terminology, 1983.
4. Haylen BT, Ashby D, Sutherst JR et al. Maximum and average urine flow rates in normal male and female populations – the Liverpool nomograms. *Br J Urol* 1989; **64**:30–8.
5. Shepherd AM, Powell PH, Ball AJ. The place of urodynamics in the investigation and treatment of female urinary tract symptoms. *J Obstet Gynecol* 1982; **3**:123–5.

6. Abrams P, Blaivas JG, Stanton SL et al. The International Continence Society Committee on Standardisation of Terminology; the standardisation of terminology of lower urinary tract function. *Scand J Urol Nephrol Suppl* 1988; **114**:5–19.

7. van Waalwijk van Doorn E, Anders K, Khullar V et al. Standardisation of Ambulatory Urodynamic Monitoring: Report of the Standardisation Sub-committee of the International Continence Society for ambulatory urodynamic studies. *Neurourol Urodyn* 2000; **19**:113–25.

8. Allen R, Hosker G, Smith A, Warrell D. Pelvic floor damage and childbirth: a neurophysiological study. *Br J Obstet Gynaecol* 1990; **97**:770–9.

9. Hartnell CG, Kiely EA, Williams G, Gibson RN. Real-time ultrasound measurement of bladder volume: a comparative study of three methods. *Br J Radiol* 1987; **60**:1063–5.

10. Khullar V, Salvatore S, Cardozo LD, Hill S, Kelleher CJ. Ultrasound bladder wall measurement – a non-invasive sensitive screening test for detrusor instability. *Neurourol Urodyn* 1994; **13**:461–2.

11. Robertson JR. Endoscopic examination of the urethra and bladder. *Clin Obstet Gynecol* 1983; **26**:347–58.

12. Kelleher CJ, Cardozo LD, Khullar V, Salvatore S. A new questionnaire to assess the quality of life of urinary incontinent women. *Br J Obstet Gynaecol* 1997; **104**:1374–9.

Chapter 59

Urinary Incontinence

Jane Rufford

INTRODUCTION

Urinary incontinence is a common problem throughout the world. Whilst many of the disorders of the lower urinary tract are not necessarily life threatening, they are very disruptive to the lives of the individuals and can have devastating effects, both socially and psychologically. In the UK alone, it has been estimated that there are more than 3.5 million sufferers.

Urinary incontinence is the complaint of any involuntary leakage of urine.[1] This chapter covers the different types of incontinence and their management.

THE CAUSES OF URINARY INCONTINENCE

- Urodynamic stress incontinence (USI).
- Detrusor over-activity.
- Overflow incontinence.
- Fistulae (vesicovaginal, ureterovaginal, urethrovaginal).
- Congenital (e.g. ectopic ureter).
- Urethral diverticulum.
- Other (e.g. urinary tract infection, faecal impaction, medication).
- Functional (e.g. immobility).

Urinary symptoms can be broadly divided. Detrusor over-activity is classically associated with frequency, urgency, urge incontinence, nocturia and nocturnal enuresis. Urodynamic stress incontinence is classically associated with involuntary leakage on effort or on exertion or on coughing or sneezing (see Table 59.1).

Table 59.1 Symptoms and definitions

Symptom	Definition
↑Daytime frequency	Complaint by the patient who considers that she voids too often by day
Urgency	Sudden and compelling desire to pass urine, which is difficult to defer
Urge urinary incontinence	Complaint of involuntary leakage accompanied by or immediately preceded by urgency
Mixed urinary incontinence	Complaint of involuntary leakage associated with urgency and also with exertion, effort, sneezing or coughing
Nocturnal enuresis	Complaint of loss of urine occurring during sleep
Continuous urinary incontinence	Complaint of continuous leakage
Stress urinary incontinence	Complaint of involuntary leakage on effort or exertion, or on sneezing or coughing

Continuous incontinence and/or post-micturition dribbling are more likely to be associated with neurological disorders, overflow, urethral diverticulae or a fistula. However, there are problems with making a presumptive diagnosis on the basis of symptoms alone. Many women complain of a mixture of symptoms. For instance those women who are found to have USI often complain of frequency, as they are going to the lavatory more often in order to avoid leaking. One study found that even an experienced clinician made the correct diagnosis only 65 per cent of the time when relying on symptoms only.[2]

URODYNAMIC STRESS INCONTINENCE

Definition

Urodynamic stress incontinence is noted during filling cystometry and is defined as the involuntary leakage of urine during increased abdominal pressure, in the absence of a detrusor contraction.

Incidence

Urodynamic stress incontinence is the commonest cause of incontinence in women. It is difficult to assess the true incidence, as many women suffer in silence and consider it an inevitable consequence of childbirth and ageing. However, conservative estimates are that 1 in 10 women will suffer from USI at some point in their lives.

Aetiology

There are various factors that are thought to predispose to the development of USI.

- Increased intra-abdominal pressure:
  - pregnancy
  - chronic cough
  - abdominal, pelvic mass
  - constipation
  - ascites.
- Damage to the pelvic floor:
  - childbirth
  - radical pelvic surgery.
- Fixed, scarred urethra:
  - previous surgery
  - radiotherapy.

Pathophysiology

The exact pathophysiology is unclear, but several hypotheses have been put forward.

- Failure of the supporting structures such as the pubourethral and pubovesical ligaments.
- Failure of the intrinsic sphincter mechanism as a result of damage to the rhabdosphincter, poor collagen or reduced urethral vascularity.
- Failure of the extrinsic sphincter mechanism as a result of weakness or damage to the pelvic floor musculature. This allows displacement of the bladder neck from within the intra-abdominal pressure zone.

KEY POINTS

- It is the most common cause of incontinence in women.
- The diagnosis is based on urodynamic assessment.
- Increased abdominal pressure, pelvic floor damage and urethral scarring all predispose to USI.

MANAGEMENT OF URODYNAMIC STRESS INCONTINENCE

Conservative management

Urodynamic stress incontinence interferes with a woman's quality of life but it is not a life-threatening condition and therefore conservative measures ought to be tried in every woman prior to resorting to surgical treatment. Conservative treatment is effective, has few complications and does not compromise further surgical procedures.[3] It is particularly useful in those women who are medically unfit for surgery, those who have not completed their family or are breastfeeding or less than 6 months postpartum.

Conservative measures include:

- pelvic floor exercises
- biofeedback
- electrical stimulation
- vaginal cones
- urethral devices.

In order to maximize the benefits that can be obtained using these techniques, it is vital to ensure that the treatment is tailored to the individual and that it is properly taught. Many women have no idea what or where their pelvic floor muscles are. The best people to teach these exercises are undoubtedly physiotherapists. Biofeedback is used to augment the effect of pelvic floor exercises. It can range in complexity from the very simple, such as a vaginal examination measuring the strength of the squeeze, which the woman can perform herself at home, to the much more sophisticated electromyography, which is usually used in a clinic. Biofeedback has not been shown to be superior to pelvic floor exercises alone.

Pelvic floor and lower urinary tract

Electrical stimulation uses an electrical pulse to augment the ability to produce a voluntary contraction. A probe is put into the vagina near the muscles of the pelvic floor and a pulse of electricity is passed. The pulse frequency is debated, but it is usually in the 35–40 Hz range. This method cannot be used in pregnancy or in those with an intrauterine contraceptive device (IUCD) in situ. It is not suitable for most women as it is excessively time consuming.

Vaginal cones or weights are now used infrequently, as the results are no better than those of pelvic floor exercises alone.

Many women find a tampon or an intravaginal device such as a Contigard very helpful. These devices elevate the bladder neck and in some cases partially obstruct the flow of urine. They are particularly suitable for women who find they are incontinent only at specific times, for instance during aerobics or playing tennis. Several urethral devices are available, but these are now very rarely used.

Pharmacological Management

Recently, there has been a lot of interest in a new drug called Duloxetine. It is a selective serotonin and noradrenaline reuptake inhibitor and increases contractility of the rhabdosphincter. Phase 3 studies have been completed and show encouraging results with a significant reduction in incontinence episode frequency when duloxetine was compared to placebo.[17] Whilst it is not currently available it will probably be launched in the near future.

Surgical procedures

More than 200 operative procedures for the treatment of USI have been described. Many of these are modifications of the same procedure, but there is not one definitive operation. The first operative procedure offers the best chance of cure and therefore it is very important to select the appropriate procedure for each patient.

Currently, the most commonly performed procedures are colposuspension, tension-free vaginal tape (TVT – which many consider to be a type of sling), other sling procedures and the use of peri-urethral bulking agents. Meta-analysis has shown poor long-term success rates for the anterior colporrhaphy, and therefore this should not be performed as a first-line treatment for USI and should probably be reserved as a primary procedure only for prolapse [Ia].

Colposuspension

The patient is placed in the modified lithotomy position using Lloyd–Davies stirrups. A Foley catheter is inserted into the bladder and allowed to drain freely. A low transverse incision is made just above the symphysis pubis (i.e. lower than a pfannenstiel). The retropubic space is dissected until the white paravaginal tissue lateral to the bladder neck is exposed. Two to four polydioxanone suture (PDS), Ethibond or polyglycolic acid sutures are inserted into the paravaginal fascia. Each suture is tied and the needle is then re-inserted into the ipsilateral iliopectineal ligament. The first suture is placed at the level of the bladder neck and the subsequent sutures are placed 1 cm laterally and 1 cm cranially (Figure 59.1). When all the sutures have been inserted, an assistant elevates the lateral fornix on each side to allow the sutures to be tied without tension. A suction drain is left in the retropubic space, a suprapubic catheter is inserted and the urethral catheter is removed (Figure 59.2).

The suprapubic catheter is left on free drainage for at least 2 days and then a clamping regimen is initiated. This usually entails clamping the catheter at a set time and allowing the patient to void normally. Initially, the residual

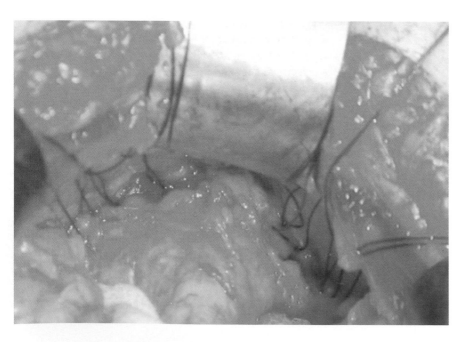

Figure 59.1   Colposuspension sutures

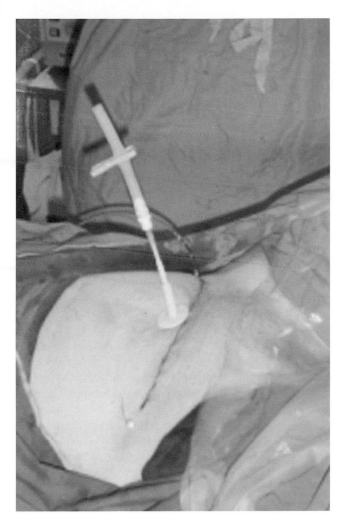

Figure 59.2   Suprapubic catheter and drain *in situ* at the end of a colposuspension

Table 59.2   Meta-analysis of the different procedures used to treat urodynamic stress incontinence

Procedure	Primary procedure mean (%)	Procedure for recurrent incontinence mean (%)
Bladder buttress	67.8	Not available
Marshall–Marchetti–Krantz	89.5	Not available
Burch colposuspension	89.8	82.5
Bladder neck suspension	86.7	86.4
Slings	93.9	86.1
Injectables	45.5	57.8

The values shown are the percentage of those who are continent following the procedure. Adapted from Jarvis (1994).[22]

colposuspension.[4] It seems to occur more commonly after previous continence surgery. It may be that a number of cases reflect pre-existing detrusor over-activity that went undetected at preoperative cystometry. Alternatively, the autonomic nerve supply may be damaged when the bladder is medially displaced at the time of surgery.[5]

A longer term complication is the development of prolapse. Enterocele and rectocele formation is thought to occur as a result of elevation of the anterior vaginal wall creating a posterior defect and causing intra-abdominal pressure to be transmitted directly to the posterior vaginal wall. The incidence is estimated to be between 7 per cent and 17 per cent.[6] It is unclear whether these represent new defects or merely a pre-existing defect becoming symptomatic once the support of the anterior vaginal wall has been rectified.

OUTCOME

Burch originally reported success rates of 100 per cent; however, objective cure rates determined on the basis of postoperative urodynamic testing are usually lower (Table 59.2). The colposuspension can be recommended, on current evidence, as the procedure that produces the best chance of long-lasting cure of urodynamic incontinence [Ib].

Whilst primary procedures have been shown to have the highest success rates, the colposuspension is still useful as a secondary procedure (see Table 59.2).

Laparoscopic colposuspension

In theory, a laparoscopic colposuspension should provide the long-term success rates of an open colposuspension, with low morbidity and shorter inpatient stay. Several techniques have been described, including an extraperitoneal approach and a transperitoneal approach. Only three randomized trials comparing laparoscopic and open approaches have been published to date. In each one, the objective results were lower in the laparoscopic group, possibly for the following reasons.

- The smaller size of the needle used to place sutures may result in less secure fixation of the tissues.
- At the open procedure, two to four sutures are usually inserted on each side, whereas laparoscopically only one or two are inserted.

is checked after each void or, if the patient experiences discomfort, the clamp is released and the residual measured. If the patient is passing good volumes of urine with small residuals, the time between unclamping can be extended to 12 hours and then 24 hours. When the residuals are persistently under 100 mL, the suprapubic catheter can be removed.

POSTOPERATIVE COMPLICATIONS

Voiding difficulties are the main complication following a colposuspension. In most studies the rate of voiding difficulties varies between 12 and 25 per cent. These women are initially managed by allowing them to go home with their suprapubic catheter in situ, leaving it on free drainage. Two weeks later they are re-admitted and a further trial of clamping is attempted. The majority of women will be able to void spontaneously at this stage. About 2 per cent will continue to complain of voiding difficulties, and these women are usually taught clean intermittent self-catheterization. Detrusor over-activity arises de novo in between 12 per cent and 18.5 per cent of women who have undergone a

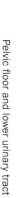

COMPLICATIONS OF LAPAROSCOPIC COLPOSUSPENSION

The incidence of urinary tract injury is higher during laparoscopic colposuspension than during the open operation. There appears to be a 1–10 per cent rate of bladder injury, and although the rate of ureteric injury or kinking is less than 0.1 per cent, this is significantly higher than at the open procedure, where it is very rare. Operative morbidity has been extensively studied: intraoperative blood loss, febrile morbidity and length of hospital stay are all higher in the open colposuspension group.[7] The cost aspect of laparoscopic surgery has also generated much discussion. Kholi et al. found that, despite a shorter inpatient stay, the costs of laparoscopic procedures were higher than those of a traditional approach, which was mainly due to the expense of the disposable instruments.[8]

A major disadvantage of laparoscopic surgery is the long learning curve required to gain proficiency. While laparoscopic colposuspension offers some promise for reducing operative morbidity, it has yet to be shown to be superior to open procedures.

At the time of writing, a large multicentre randomized trial of laparoscopic versus open colposuspension funded by the Medical Research Council (MRC) is underway. This will eventually provide evidence of the role of laparoscopic surgery in this area.

Tension-free vaginal tape

The tape itself is composed of a knitted prolene mesh and the aim of the procedure is to place the tape at the midurethra. The concept behind this is that USI results from the failure of the pubourethral ligaments at the level of the midurethra. The tape is inserted via a small vertical vaginal incision using two 5 mm trochars. The procedure was originally designed to be performed under local anaesthetic; however, it can be performed under local, regional or general anaesthesia. Data from the Austrian TVT Registry show that there is wide variation in practice: 43 per cent are put in under local, 43 per cent under regional and 13 per cent under general anaesthetic.[9] The patient is placed in the lithotomy position and the lower abdomen and vagina are prepared as a sterile operating field. Two small (1 cm) incisions are made in the abdominal wall, 5 cm apart, just above the superior rim of the pubic bone. A sagittal incision is made in the suburethral vaginal wall, starting 1 cm from the external urethral meatus. After minimal bilateral paraurethral dissection and hydrodissection of the retropubic space using saline or local anaesthetic (Figure 59.3), the tape (covered by a plastic sheath), is introduced with the help of the trochars. Each trochar perforates the urogenital diaphragm and is then passed through the retropubic space to emerge through the abdominal incision on the ipsilateral side (Figure 59.4). Following insertion of the trochars, a cystoscopy is carried out to ensure that there has been no damage to the bladder. It is obviously important that the surgeon performing the procedure has sufficient training in cystoscopy to recognize any complications, such as perforation of the bladder or urethra with a trochar.

The tape is then carefully pulled through and is left lying in a U-shape under the urethra (Figure 59.5). If the procedure is being carried out under local or regional anaesthetic, the tension of the tape can be adjusted by asking the woman to perform a series of coughs. The aim is to have the tape lying free at rest (hence 'tension free') whilst exerting sufficient pressure on the urethra during a cough to prevent leakage of urine. When the surgeon feels happy with the placement and tension of the tape, a repeat cystoscopy is performed, the plastic sheaths are removed and the tape is cut flush with the skin (Figure 59.6). Owing to the weave of the tape, it is self-retaining and requires no fixation. The incisions are sutured with appropriate suture material. A catheter is not usually left in at the end of the procedure. However, it is very important that if the woman does not void within 6 hours of the procedure, the residual volume is checked, by either catheterization or ultrasound.

COMPLICATIONS

The most common intraoperative complications include injury to the bladder at the time of trochar insertion and bleeding in the retropubic space. Postoperative complications include voiding difficulties, urinary tract infection and wound infection. Worrying long-term complications include the risk of tape rejection, tape erosion and long-term voiding difficulties.

OUTCOME

The preliminary results reported an 84 per cent cure rate, with no long-term voiding difficulties or de-novo detrusor over-activity.[10] A further study involving 131 women from multiple centres in Sweden showed a cure rate of 91 per cent.[11] These women had not had any previous surgery and were followed up for at least 12 months.

Long-term follow-up studies are only available from Scandinavia, where the procedure was developed. The 5-year data come from three centres: 85 patients had an objective cure rate of 84.7 per cent, whilst a further 10.6 per cent had improved and 4.7 per cent had failed. It was concluded from this that there is no increase in the failure rate over 5 years.[12] A recent randomized, multicentre study has been carried out in the UK comparing the TVT to colposuspension. The cure rate at 2 years was similar in each group, subjectively 61 per cent and 62 per cent and objectively 68 per cent and 66 per cent respectively.[13]

There have been several small studies looking at the TVT as a secondary procedure after previous failed incontinence surgery. From these small numbers it would appear that the TVT also performs very well as a secondary procedure.

Worldwide, there have been more than 210 000 TVTs inserted, in more than 30 different countries. There is an overall cure rate of 84–89 per cent and an improvement rate of 5 per cent.[14]

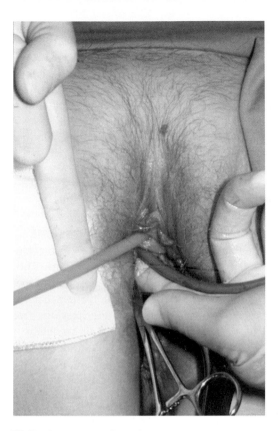

Figure 59.3   Para-urethral dissection

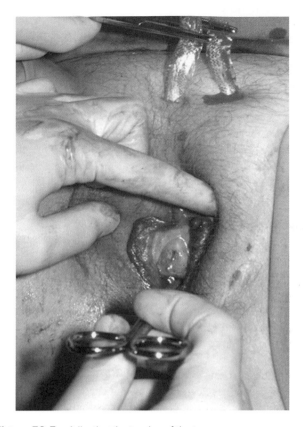

Figure 59.5   Adjusting the tension of the tape

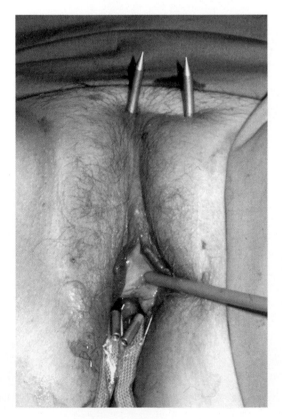

Figure 59.4   TVT trochars inserted

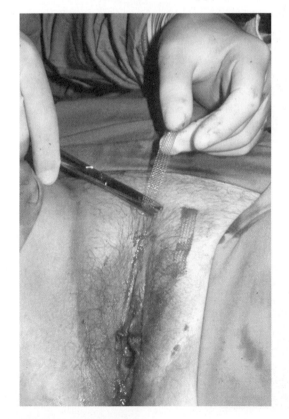

Figure 59.6   Cutting the tape

In conclusion, the short-term results for this procedure are very promising, but long-term data are still awaited.

Suburethral sling procedures

These are rarely used as a primary procedure (unless one considers the TVT a sling), mainly because of their high complication rate. The main complications are voiding difficulties, the development of detrusor over-activity and erosion of the sling through surrounding tissues. However, in expert hands the sling procedure can produce excellent results (see Table 59.2).

Sling procedures can be recommended as an effective treatment for USI [II].

Peri-urethral injections

The procedure can be performed under local, regional or general anaesthetic. The patient is placed in the lithotomy position and the vagina is prepared as a sterile operating field. The bladder neck is visualized cystoscopically with a 0 or 12 degree cystoscope. There are two ways of injecting the peri-urethral agents, using either a paraurethral or a peri-urethral approach. Whichever technique is used, the collagen or macroplastique bump should be visualized cystoscopically. Injection continues until 50 per cent of the urethral lumen has been occluded and then the procedure is repeated on the other side. The volume of collagen injected varies between 5 mL and 10 mL (Figure 59.7).

Which peri-urethral agent is used depends on the surgeon's preference, but it is usually either gluteraldehyde cross-linked bovine collagen (GAX) or a macroparticulate silicone.

This procedure often needs to be repeated, and it is usually reserved for those patients who are elderly and frail or who have had multiple continence procedures and are unsuitable for other conventional types of bladder neck surgery. Whilst the short-term success rates have been very encouraging, the published long-term data are less so (see Table 59.2).

The role of bulking agents is unclear, but they may have a role as a non-invasive form of treatment with a lower chance of cure and a lower risk of complications [II].

Endoscopic bladder neck suspensions

The Stamey and the Raz procedures were the most commonly performed bladder neck suspensions. The aim of these procedures is to pass a suture either side of the bladder neck, anchored by a buffer beneath the pubocervical fascia and tied above the rectus sheath. In the past, they were indicated for the treatment of primary or secondary incontinence, particularly in the elderly or frail, when an open procedure may have led to a higher morbidity. However, recent advances in other techniques such as the TVT have dramatically reduced their popularity.

There appear to be few, if any, indications to perform a needle suspension [Ia].

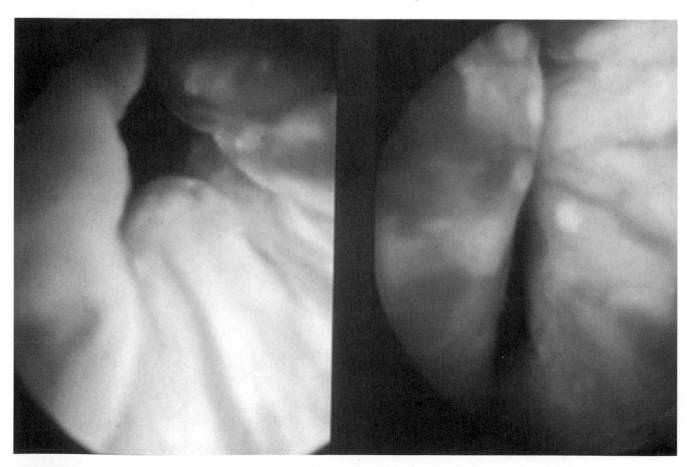

Figure 59.7   Peri-urethral bulking agent at bladder neck, before and after

Transobturator tape

This is a very new procedure that was first decribed in 2001.[15] A non-woven polypropylene tape is passed via a transmuscular approach, through the transobturator and puborectalis muscles. This aims to reproduce the natural suspension fascia of the urethra. The advantage of this approach is that the retropubic space is avoided and hence it is thought that the relatively high incidence of bladder perforations seen with the TVT should be avoided. The tape is covered with a fine silicone coating on the urethral surface which limits the shrinking of the polypropylene mesh and thereby forms a barrier to fibrosis extension around the urethra. It can be performed under local, regional or general anaesthetic. Because it has only recently been described there are very few published studies and no randomized controlled trials. However, early data suggest that this approach has similar success rates to the TVT.[16]

KEY POINTS

- Conservative measures should be offered prior to surgical intervention.
- Meta-analysis has shown poor long-term results following anterior colporrhaphy.
- Open colposuspension offers the best chance for long-term cure and is currently the first-choice procedure.
- Laparoscopic colposuspension appears to have a poorer objective outcome than the open procedure.
- TVT produces short-term results similar to those of colposuspension.
- Endoscopic sling procedures (Stamey, Ratz) are rarely indicated.

THE OVERACTIVE BLADDER SYNDROME

This is the term used to describe symptoms of urinary urgency, with or without urge incontinence, usually with frequency and nocturia. It is used to imply a possible underlying diagnosis of detrusor over-activity without the need to resort to urodynamic studies. It is treated in much the same way as detrusor over-activity.

DETRUSOR OVER-ACTIVITY

Detrusor over-activity is a urodynamic observation characterized by involuntary detrusor contractions during the filling phase which may be spontaneous or provoked. The detrusor is shown objectively to contract (either spontaneously or with provocation) during bladder filling whilst the subject is attempting to inhibit micturition.[18] Detrusor over-activity is a urodynamic diagnosis.

It usually presents with symptoms of frequency, urgency, urge incontinence, nocturia, nocturnal enuresis and sometimes incontinence at orgasm. However, in order to make the diagnosis, urodynamics must be performed (Figure 59.8).

Incidence

Detrusor over-activity is a common condition. In the adult female population, it is the second commonest cause of

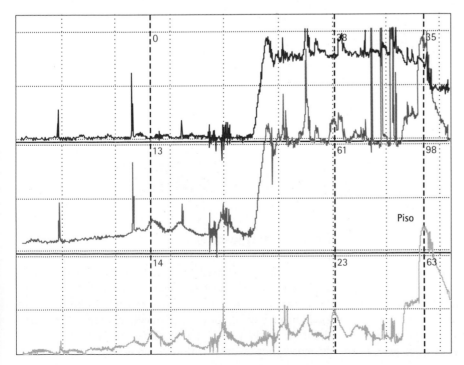

Figure 59.8 Urodynamic trace showing detrusor over-activity

urinary incontinence, accounting for 30–50 per cent of those investigated. However, amongst the elderly population it is the commonest cause and has been shown to exist in up to 80 per cent of those who present for urodynamic assessment.

Aetiology

The causes of detrusor over-activity include:

- idiopathic
- psychosomatic
- neuropathic
- incontinence surgery
- outflow obstruction.

Pathophysiology

The pathophysiology is uncertain and would appear to vary depending on the aetiology. It has been suggested that the common theme is a change in the property of the detrusor smooth muscle that predisposes the bladder to unstable contractions. It is postulated that this is caused by a reduction in the functional innervation of the bladder wall.

KEY POINTS

- Detrusor over-activity is the second most common cause of incontinence in women.
- It is the most common cause of incontinence in the elderly.
- The diagnosis is based on urodynamic assessment.
- Some type of underlying neuromuscular dysfunction is the likely cause.

MANAGEMENT OF DETRUSOR OVER-ACTIVITY

The treatment options are broadly divided into conservative, pharmacological and surgical. Surgery only plays a minor role in the treatment of detrusor over-activity and is used when all other measures have failed and some form of urinary diversion or bladder augmentation is being attempted.

Conservative measures include advice regarding fluid intake. It may be that simply cutting down on the volume of fluid consumed throughout the day or altering the times at which drinks are taken will be enough to reduce the symptoms and improve quality of life. Women should be advised to consume between 1 L and 1.5 L in any 24-hour period.

It is not advisable to restrict fluid intake severely, as a low urine output together with frequent voiding can lead to a reduction in the bladder's functional capacity. The best guide to ideal fluid intake is the colour of the urine. Caffeine and alcohol are well known to irritate the bladder, and women should be advised to try to avoid caffeine-based drinks or substitute them with decaffeinated drinks.

Bladder retraining

The principles of bladder retraining are based on the ability to suppress urinary urge and to extend the intervals between voiding. The regimen is generally initiated at set voiding intervals and the patient is not allowed to void between these predetermined times, even if she is incontinent. When she remains dry, the time interval is lengthened. This continues until a suitable time span is achieved, usually around 3–4 hours. Cure rates using bladder retraining alone and no pharmacological agents have been reported between 44 and 90 per cent. Many professionals advise the combined use of pelvic floor exercises with bladder retraining, as this can help suppress the symptom of urinary urgency.

Pharmacological intervention (Table 59.3)

There is a wide variety of therapeutic preparations available. It is difficult to compare the numerous preparations, as there is a high placebo effect (30–40 per cent), and since the response to any drug is likely to be in the region of 60 per cent, any differences detected will probably be small.

The aim of medical therapy is to:

- *inhibit bladder contractility*
  - anticholinergic agents
  - musculotrophic agents
  - tricyclic antidepressants
- *increase outlet resistance*
  - alpha-adrenergic agonists
- *decrease urine production*
  - desmopressin acetate (DDAVP)
- *improve local tissues*
  - oestrogens.

Anticholinergic drugs
BACKGROUND

Acetylcholine is released from postganglionic parasympathetic nerve terminals. It acts on muscarinic receptors in the detrusor muscle to initiate a bladder contraction. It is this mechanism that is thought to mediate both normal and abnormal bladder contractions. There are four subtypes of the muscarinic receptor within the body (M_{1-4}). M_2 receptors predominate in the bladder; however, the M_3 receptors appear to mediate the main part of bladder contraction. In addition, M_3 receptors are found in the salivary glands and the bowel, explaining some of the side effects associated with anticholinergic medication. Common side effects include dry eyes, dry mouth, constipation and tachycardia. Anticholinergics are contraindicated in women with narrow-angle glaucoma.

TOLTERODINE

Tolterodine is a competitive muscarinic receptor antagonist. It has no specificity for receptor subtypes; however, it does appear to target the bladder over the salivary glands. In randomized, double-blind, placebo-controlled trials it has been shown to have a similar clinical efficacy to oxybutynin but fewer adverse events, particularly dry mouth [Ia].[19] The usual dose is 2 mg twice a day, although it may be started at 1 mg twice a day if there is concern regarding adverse events, particularly in the elderly. Fortunately, it is usually very well tolerated and has now become one of the first-line treatments in the management of detrusor over-activity.

TROSPIUM

Trospium chloride is non-selective for muscarinic receptor subtypes. It has also been compared to oxybutynin in a randomized, double-blind, multicentre trial. Those taking trospium had a lower incidence of dry mouth (4 per cent vs 23 per cent) and were less likely to withdraw (6 per cent vs 16 per cent) when compared to the group receiving oxybutynin [Ia].[20] On balance, the evidence would suggest that trospium chloride is effective in suppressing uninhibited detrusor contractions and may be associated with fewer side effects than oxybutynin. The usual dose is 20 mg bd.

DARAFENACIN

Darafenacin is a selective muscarinic M3 receptor antagonist. It is currently undergoing phase 3 clinical trials and will probably be available in the near future.

SOLIFENACIN

Solifenacin is a long-acting muscarinic receptor antagonist which has been specifically developed to treat the overactive bladder. It is in the final phase of clinical trials and like darafenacin will probably be available in the near future.

Drugs with mixed actions
OXYBUTYNIN [IA]

Oxybutynin has long been recognized as an effective form of treatment for detrusor over-activity. It has antimuscarinic, direct muscle relaxant and local anaesthetic actions. The antimuscarinic adverse effects of oxybutynin are well documented and are often the dose-limiting factor. The major side effect is dry mouth, but other minor anticholinergic side effects may occur. To minimize the side effects and to maximize compliance, oxybutynin is often started at a low dose, for instance 2.5 mg three times a day, and if necessary increased to a maximum of 5 mg four times a day. It is possible to achieve higher local levels of oxybutynin whilst limiting the systemic adverse effects by changing the route of administration. Intravesical oxybutynin has been shown to increase bladder capacity and lead to a significant clinical improvement, and rectal administration has also been shown to be associated with fewer adverse effects when compared to oral administration. Recently, a controlled release oxybutynin preparation has been developed using an osmotic system (OROS®), which has been shown to have efficacy comparable to that of immediate-release oxybutynin but fewer adverse effects.[21]

In summary, the efficacy and safety of oxybutynin are well documented, although adverse effects frequently limit its clinical usefulness. Alternative routes of administration and the development of slow-release preparations may lead to an improved side-effect profile, producing better patient acceptability and compliance.

PROPIVERINE [IA]

Propiverine has been shown to combine anticholinergic and calcium channel-blocking actions. Significant common adverse effects are mainly antimuscarinic, including dry mouth and blurred vision. The usual dose is 15–30 mg bd.

Antidepressants
IMIPRAMINE [II]

Imipramine blocks the uptake of serotonin and noradrenaline and has been shown to have marked systemic anticholinergic effects. There are numerous side effects associated with the tricyclic antidepressants, some of which are potentially very serious, such as orthostatic hypotension and ventricular arrhythmias. Hence, imipramine is not a first-line treatment. However, it can be particularly useful in treating symptoms of nocturia and adult nocturnal enuresis. It is usually given at a dose of 75 mg at night.

Vasopressin analogues
DESMOPRESSIN (DDAVP)

Desmopressin, a synthetic vasopressin analogue, is widely used as a treatment for nocturnal enuresis in children. Its precise role in the treatment of detrusor instability needs further evaluation. Considerable caution needs to be taken when prescribing this drug. It should not be used in those with hypertension, renal or cardiac disease. The potentially serious side effects include fluid retention and hyponatraemia.

Oestrogens

Oestrogens have been used for many years to treat symptoms of urgency and urge incontinence, despite the fact that there are few clinical trials to support their use.

Pelvic floor and lower urinary tract

Table 59.3   Which symptom, which drug?

	Oxybutynin	Tolterodine	Propiverine	Trospium	Oestrogen	Imipramine	DDAVP
Frequency	✔	✔	✔	✔	✔		
Nocturia					✔	✔	✔
Urgency	✔	✔	✔	✔	✔		
Urge incontinence	✔	✔	✔	✔			
Stress incontinence						✔	
Enuresis						✔	✔
Coital incontinence						✔	✔

DDAVP, desmopressin acetate.

KEY POINTS

- Bladder retraining is safe but has a variable and unpredictable outcome.
- Surgical interventions such as diversion are reserved for cases for which no other treatment has succeeded and quality of life is poor.
- There is a marked placebo effect associated with all pharmacological interventions.
- Oxybutinin is effective, although it may have significant adverse side effects.
- More specific muscarinic blocking agents may achieve similar results to oxybutinin, with fewer or less severe side effects.
- Imipramine is rarely used as first-line treatment for detrusor overactivity, but may be of value in treating nocturia.
- Oestrogens are frequently prescribed, although there is little objective evidence to support their use.

URINARY FISTULAE

The development of a genitourinary fistula has profound effects on both the physical and psychological health of the woman. The most common simple genitourinary fistulae are (Figure 59.9):

- vesicovaginal (42 per cent)
- ureterovaginal (34 per cent)
- urethrovaginal (11 per cent)
- vesicocervical (3 per cent).

The development of a fistula following surgery has considerable legal implications. Whilst most gynaecologists accept that the development of a fistula is deeply regrettable, it was generally thought that this was, on occasion, unavoidable. However, more recent legal cases involving ureteric injury would seem to refute that. There is a body of opinion that holds the view that ureteric damage can always be avoided and that not to do so constitutes negligence.

Vesicovaginal fistulae

Aetiology

The most common cause of vesicovaginal fistulae in the developed world is gynaecological surgery. The procedure with the highest incidence of postoperative fistula formation is a hysterectomy, either abdominal or vaginal. This accounts for about 75 per cent of cases. Particular risk factors include distorted anatomy, for example previous surgery, fibroids or endometriosis. Other procedures associated with fistula formation include anterior colporrhaphy, laparoscopic pelvic surgery and urological surgery. Fistula formation has also been associated with pelvic malignancy, pelvic trauma and radiotherapy.

In the developing world, the most common cause remains obstetric trauma. It is estimated that the incidence is 1–3/1000 deliveries in West Africa.

Presentation

The majority of women with a vesicovaginal fistula present with continuous leakage of urine, both day and night. This leads to discomfort and excoriation in the genital region as the urine irritates the skin of the vulva and thighs. However, if the fistula is relatively small, a woman may just complain of increased vaginal discharge. The timing of presentation is variable, although the most common time to present is 5–10 days following surgery.

Diagnosis

A large fistula is usually obvious, and may easily be seen by examining the woman in the left lateral position using a Simms' speculum. Urine may be seen pooling in the vagina. If no fistula can be seen, useful diagnostic tests include the introduction of methylene blue into the bladder, via a urethral catheter. The blue dye may then be seen draining into the vagina. Alternatively, Bonney's 'three swab test', in which three swabs are placed in the vagina prior to instilling the dye, may help to locate the site of the fistula, which is indicated by the swab that emerges with the most dye. However, this may mask the presence of multiple fistulae. Intravenous urogram (IVU) is not usually helpful in the diagnosis of a vesicovaginal fistula, but it is mandatory to rule out a ureterovaginal fistula or ureteric obstruction,

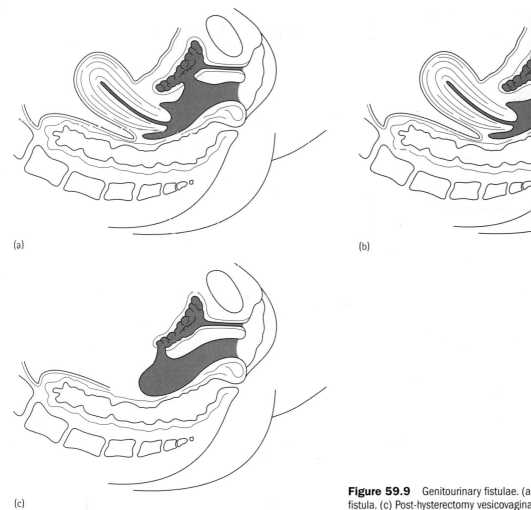

(a)

(b)

(c)

Figure 59.9 Genitourinary fistulae. (a) Mid-vaginal fistula. (b) Urethral fistula. (c) Post-hysterectomy vesicovaginal fistula

which is seen concurrently in as many as 12 per cent of cases and is obviously very important when planning future treatment. If an IVU has failed to elucidate the ureteric anatomy, retrograde ureteropyelography should be undertaken at the same time as a cystoscopy and examination under general anaesthesia.

When the woman is anaesthetized, it is often possible to palpate the vaginal opening of the fistula tract. The vesical opening may be seen at cystoscopy, usually on the posterior wall or at the bladder base. If the fistula is not related to recent gynaecological surgery for a benign condition, both the vaginal and the vesical openings should be biopsied to exclude the possibility of malignancy.

Treatment

Treatment options range from simple conservative measures to more complex surgical procedures and are outside the scope of this book. However, it is very important to give general advice regarding the management of symptoms experienced as a result of the fistula. Barrier creams may help prevent the skin becoming sore and excoriated. Advice about incontinence pads, the increased risk of urinary tract

infection and the need in some cases for prophylactic antibiotics may be required.

Urethrovaginal fistulae

In the developed world, these occur most commonly following an anterior repair with or without a vaginal hysterectomy. However, they may develop as result of a urethral diverticulum or its repair or following bladder neck suspension procedures. In the developing world, the overwhelming majority are again caused by childbirth.

Symptoms vary depending on the site of the fistula. With a fistula higher up in the urethra there may be continuous incontinence; a fistula nearer the bladder neck may present with stress incontinence and recurrent urinary tract infections; and one lower down may cause symptoms of spraying of urine at micturition or post-micturition dribble.

Again, the surgical treatment options are beyond the scope of this book and these unfortunate women ought to be referred to specialist centres.

Pelvic floor and lower urinary tract

KEY POINTS

- In the developed world, gynaecological surgery is the most common cause, with 75 per cent being attributable to hysterectomy.
- Obstetric trauma is the most common cause in the developing world.
- Most present between 5 and 10 days post-surgery.
- Presentation varies from a mild discharge with small fistulae to continuous urine loss with larger fistulae.
- IVU is mandatory as part of the assessment because of high ureteric co-morbidity.

OVERFLOW INCONTINENCE AND VOIDING DIFFICULTIES

Symptoms

These may be a result of the voiding difficulty, such as:

- poor stream
- prolonged voiding time
- double void
- incomplete emptying
- hesitancy
- frequency
- nocturia
- urgency
- pain
- abdominal distension

or may reflect the underlying disease:

- abdominal distension, due to a mass such as fibroids or an ovarian cyst
- pregnancy
- peri-anal pain
- peripheral paraesthesia
- herpetic rash

or a consequence of the voiding difficulties:

- recurrent urinary tract infections.

Aetiology

Neurological

The aetiology depends on the underlying neurological condition and the level at which the anatomy is affected. Central nervous system conditions that commonly cause voiding difficulties include multiple sclerosis, spinal injuries, cerebrovascular accidents and brain tumours. Peripheral lesions include lesions at the sacral outflow, for instance a prolapsed intervertebral disc or herpes zoster.

Myogenic

This usually results from ischaemia due to acute retention, for example after an epidural block or spinal shock.

Iatrogenic

Postoperative retention is relatively common and may be associated with long operation times, epidural anaesthesia, patient-controlled analgesia, high doses of opiates and large volumes of intravenous fluids. It may also be associated with obstructive outflow procedures such as those that are performed for USI.

Obstructive

This may be extrinsic, for example pregnancy or a large fibroid uterus, or intrinsic, such as a urethral stricture or foreign body. Alternatively, it may be as a result of kinking of the urethra, as can occur with a large prolapse.

Inflammatory

Any lesion may be sufficiently painful to inhibit the voiding reflex. This is seen, for instance, with vulval abscess or acute herpetic infections.

Diagnosis

Voiding difficulties should be suspected if a pelvic mass that is dull to percussion is palpable on clinical examination. The diagnosis can be confirmed using ultrasound. The patient is asked to empty her bladder and then an abdominal ultrasound scan can easily be performed to assess the residual urine. Alternatively, a urethral catheter can be inserted to assess the residual urine. In either case, it is very important that the residual volume is measured and accurately recorded.

MANAGEMENT OF OVERFLOW INCONTINENCE AND VOIDING DIFFICULTIES

It is vital that all clinicians are aware of the complications associated with an episode of acute retention and that all possible steps are taken to avoid it happening. If it does occur, catheterization should be undertaken as soon as possible and the catheter should be left in for at least 2 days, after which it is reasonable to undertake a trial without catheter, but only under strict supervision. If there is a further episode of retention, this should be managed with a suprapubic catheter and the bladder allowed to rest for a period of 2–6 weeks.

Medical therapy

Bethanechol, 25 mg tds, has been shown to enhance bladder emptying providing there is no evidence of outflow obstruction.

Surgery

If the voiding difficulties are a result of extrinsic compression, this is usually best treated by removing the underlying cause, for example a hysterectomy or myomectomy in the case of fibroids. However, in the case of pregnancy causing obstruction, supportive measures are usually used in the form of a urethral catheter until the uterus has grown a little more and the obstruction relieves itself.

If the obstruction is intrinsic, this may be treated by the removal of a foreign body or offending material. Alternatively, if a urethral stricture is suspected, a cystoscopy and an Otis urethrotomy may be required, in which case the patient would need to be counselled about having a urethral catheter on free drainage for 2 weeks on discharge from hospital and the possibility of postoperative urinary incontinence.

In the long term, intractable voiding difficulties may need to be treated with clean intermittent self-catheterization. The patient needs to be able to perform the technique, and this usually requires a degree of manual dexterity in addition to willingness to undertake it.

THE ELDERLY

All elderly women with urinary incontinence need assessment. Urinary incontinence in the elderly can be transient or established. It is important to think about the former, as it is often easily treatable.

Common causes of transient incontinence include:

- urinary tract infection
- confusional states
- faecal impaction
- oestrogen deficiency
- restricted mobility
- depression
- drug therapy.

Investigation of the elderly patient requires a gentle approach; many elderly women find it very difficult and embarrassing to discuss their problems. It is important to discuss what bothers them and always to remember to treat the individual not just the disease. What may be appropriate in a younger patient may be wholly inappropriate in someone older. All women who are incontinent should be asked about what pads or pants they are wearing. This is particularly important in the elderly, as they may not have access to shops and, once they have been properly assessed, suitable pads can be provided. This can help with some of the associated problems such as reducing skin excoriation.

All symptomatic women should have a urine specimen taken for microscopy, culture and sensitivity. Further investigation will usually take longer and it is very helpful if there are dedicated clinics specifically for this purpose, preferably with some input from the community continence advisors so that the women who are seen can be followed up at home.

In general, long-term catheterization should be avoided. The use of pads and pants with protective creams is usually preferable, as catheters generally increase the irritability of the bladder and the likelihood of infections and encourage stone formation. Prior to resorting to this type of management, all the reversible and treatable causes of incontinence should have been excluded.

KEY REFERENCES

1. Abrams P, Cardozo L, Fall M et al. The standardisation of terminology in lower urinary tract function. *Neurourol Urodyn* 2002; 21:167–8.
2. Jarvis GJ, Hall S, Stamp S, Miller DR, Johnson A. An assessment of urodynamic examination in incontinent women. *Br J Obstet Gynaecol* 1980; 87:893–6.
3. Berghmans LCM, Hendriks HJM, Bo K et al. Conservative treatment of stress urinary incontinence in women: a systematic review of randomised clinical trials. *Br J Urol* 1998; 82:181–91.
4. Alcalay M, Monga A, Stanton SL. Burch colposuspension: a 10–20 year follow up. *Br J Obstet Gynaecol* 1995; 102:740–5.
5. Cardozo LD, Stanton SL, Williams JE. Detrusor instability following surgery for GSI. *Br J Urol* 1979; 58:138–42.
6. Burch JC. Cooper's ligament urethrovesical suspension for urinary stress incontinence. *Am J Obstet Gynecol* 1968; 100:764–72.
7. Lyons TL, Winner WK Clinical outcomes with laparoscopic and open Burch procedures for urinary stress incontinence. *J Am Assoc Gynecol Laparosc* 1995; 2:193–8.
8. Kholi N et al. Open compared with laparoscopic colposuspension. A cost analysis. *Obstet Gynecol* 1997; 90:411–15.
9. Tamussino K, Hanzal E, Riss P. The Austrian TVT registry. *Int Urogynecol J* 2000; 11(Suppl.):S1–017.
10. Ulmsten U, Henriksson L, Johnson P, Varhos G. An ambulatory surgical procedure under local anaesthesia for treatment of female urinary incontinence. *Int Urogynecol J* 1996; 7:81–6.
11. Ulmsten U, Falconer C, Johnson P et al. A multicentre study of tension-free vaginal tape (TVT) for surgical treatment of stress urinary incontinence. *Int Urogynecol J* 1998; 9:210–13.
12. Nilsson CG, Kuava N, Falconer C, Rezapour M, Ulmsten U. Long-term results of the tension-free vaginal tape (TVT) procedure for surgical treatment of female stress urinary incontinence. *Int Urogynecol J* 2001; 12(Suppl. 2):S5–S8.
13. Ward K, Hilton P. Prospective multicentre randomized trial of tension-free vaginal tape and colposuspension

as primary treatment for stress incontinence. *BMJ* 2002; **325**:67–70.

14. Ethicon's own data.

15. Delorme E. Transobturator urethral suspension: mini invasive procedure in the treatment of stress urinary incontinence in women. *Prog Urol* 2001; **11**:1306–13.

16. Dargent D, Bretones S, George P, Mellier G. Insertion of a suburethral sling through the obturating membrane for teatment of female urinary incontinence. *Gynecol Obstet Fertil* 2002; **30**:576–82.

17. Dmochowski RR, Miklos JR, Norton PA, Zinner NR, Yalcin I, Bump RC. Duloxetine versus placebo for the treatment of North American women with stress urinary incontinence. *J Urol* 2003; **170**:1259–63.

18. Abrams P, Blavis JG, Stanton SL, Anderson JT. The standardisation of terminology of lower urinary tract function. *Br J Obstet Gynaecol* 1990; **97**(Suppl. 6): 1–16.

19. Abrams P, Freeman R, Anderstrom C, Mattiasson A. Tolterodine, a new antimuscarinic agent: as effective but better tolerated than oxybutynin in patients with an overactive bladder. *Br J Urol* 1998; **81**(6):801–10.

20. Madersbacher H, Stoher M, Richter R, Burgdorfer H, Hachen HJ, Murtz G. Trospium chloride versus oxybutynin: a randomized, double-blind, multicentre trial in the treatment of detrusor hyperreflexia. *Br J Urol* 1995; **75**(4):452–6.

21. Anderson RU, Mobley D, Blank B, Saltzstein D, Susset J, Brown JS. Once daily controlled versus immediate release oxybutynin chloride for urge urinary incontinence. OROS Oxybutynin Study Group. *J Urol* 1999; **161**(6):1809–12.

22. Jarvis G. Surgery for genuine stress incontinence. *Br J Obstet Gynaecol* 1994; **101**:371–4.

Chapter 60

Other Lower Urinary Tract Disorders

James Balmforth

MRCOG standards

Theoretical skills

- Understand the relevance of specific urinary symptoms and how appropriately to investigate these further.
- Understand the scientific basis of urogynaecological investigations and when to undertake them.

Practical skills

- Be competent in eliciting the relevant facts in a medical history and performing an appropriate physical examination.
- Be able to perform urethrocystoscopy and bladder biopsy when indicated and be able to interpret the findings.
- Have observed tertiary assessment of complex lower urinary tract disorders and have an appreciation of the role of the urologist in managing female urological complications.

INTRODUCTION

In the preceding chapters, the common urogynaecological disorders have been discussed together with the evidence-base that exists to guide clinicians in the management of these conditions. This chapter includes some less frequently seen disorders of the lower urinary tract. There is far less supporting evidence for the efficacy of different clinical interventions for these disorders, and the established management is based largely on non-randomized, observational data and expert opinion.

FREQUENCY, URGENCY AND PAINFUL BLADDER SYNDROMES

These are common urinary symptoms in women, which can be very distressing and have been shown to have a major adverse effect on social function and quality of life. Indeed, quality of life (QoL) scores for women suffering from these sensory symptoms have been shown to be poorer than for those complaining of other urinary symptoms, including incontinence.[1] The combination of irritative bladder symptoms (frequency, urgency, nocturia and dysuria) with pain and negative urine cultures gives rise to an ill-defined group of conditions known as painful bladder syndromes. In the majority of cases, the exact pathogenesis is uncertain and available treatments are largely empirical.

Incidence

Epidemiological data[2] suggest that up to 20 per cent of women complain of frequency and around 15 per cent of urgency. These figures increase only slightly with age. Associated pain on bladder filling or on micturition is a less common, but highly disabling, symptom.

Aetiology

There is a large number of disorders that can cause these symptoms, both in the lower urinary tract itself and also further afield. Some of the commoner causes are listed in Table 60.1.

A number of these conditions are dealt with elsewhere in this section on urogynaecological disorders. The group of conditions that cause bladder pain in association with frequency and urgency is considered below. This is a poorly defined collection of diseases, considered by some to be part

Table 60.1   Conditions causing urinary frequency and urgency (with or without pain)

Arising from the lower urinary tract	Outside the lower urinary tract
Detrusor over-activity	Excessive fluid intake
Urinary tract infection	Maladaptive learned behaviour
Functionally small bladder	Diuretic drugs
Radiation cystitis	Congestive cardiac failure
Chronic urinary residual	Pelvic mass
Cystocele	Diabetes mellitus
Oestrogen deficiency	Diabetes insipidus
Bladder calculus	Upper motor neuron lesion
Bladder tumour	Renal disease
Interstitial cystitis	Pregnancy
Sensory urgency	
Urethritis	

Table 60.2   Criteria for diagnosis of interstitial cystitis

Automatic inclusions	Automatic exclusions
Hunner's ulcer	<18 years of age
	Bladder tumour
	Radiation cystitis
	Tuberculous cystitis
Positive factors	
Glomerulations at cystoscopy	Bacterial cystitis
Low-compliance bladder	Cyclophosphamide cystitis
Pain on bladder filling/relieved	Vaginitis
on voiding	Urethral diverticulum
	Lower genital tract malignancy
	Active genital herpes
	Diurnal frequency <5 times
	Nocturia <2 times
	Bladder calculus
	Detrusor over-activity
	Capacity >400 mL

of a spectrum of 'painful bladder syndromes' that share common aetiologies. Exact classification is hampered by the lack of universally agreed definitions, poor understanding of the pathogenesis of these conditions and the absence of robust research evidence on which to base treatment.

Interstitial cystitis

This chronic inflammatory disorder of the bladder is notoriously difficult to manage and can result in considerable morbidity. A survey presented as part of a National Institute of Health Consensus Conference on Interstitial Cystitis found that 40 per cent of affected women were unable to work because of their disease, 58 per cent were unable to have intercourse, and 55 per cent had considered suicide. Quality of life scores in women with interstitial cystitis are consistently low.

Women between the ages of 40 and 60 years are most commonly affected. The condition occurs far more frequently in Caucasians and there is a 9:1 female predominance.[3] The aetiology remains obscure, but infection, autoimmune disease, epithelial cell dysfunction, allergy, psychosomatic disorders and an inability to repair the normal protective layer of glycosaminoglycans (GAGs) have all been postulated as mechanisms.

The diagnosis of interstitial cystitis is based on suggestive symptoms and characteristic cystoscopy findings. Typical symptoms include lower abdominal pain, frequency, urgency, dysuria and perineal pain, in the absence of bacterial cystitis. Often, voiding relieves the suprapubic discomfort, and drinking alcohol and caffeine-containing drinks frequently exacerbates the pain. Reported prevalence rates for this condition vary widely, as there is no universally accepted definition. In an attempt to standardize diagnosis, the National Institute of Arthritis, Diabetes, Digestive and Kidney Diseases published consensus criteria in 1988. These consist of a list of exclusion criteria together with some positive cystoscopic features (Table 60.2).

There is no universally agreed histological standard for diagnosing interstitial cystitis over-activity on bladder biopsy. However, biopsies are useful to exclude other pathology, including malignancy. Typical features of interstitial cystitis seen on cystoscopic examination include subepithelial petechial haemorrhages (glomerulations), splotchy haemorrhages, linear cracking of the mucosa, white urothelial scars and ulceration.

Sensory urgency

Sensory urgency is a diagnosis of exclusion made after urodynamic assessment. It consists of the symptom complex of frequency, urgency and occasionally urge incontinence, but with no evidence of detrusor over-activity on subtracted cystometry or other underlying intravesical pathology. The exact diagnostic criteria are rather vague. Some authors have suggested cystometric parameters that require the volume of first sensation to occur at <100 mL and the bladder capacity to be <400 mL. These criteria are not universally accepted and are heavily influenced by filling rate at cystoscopy. This makes it difficult to estimate the prevalence of this condition accurately, but it is reported at 5–10 per cent of women undergoing urodynamic assessment.

The aetiology of sensory urgency is poorly understood and it probably involves a group of women with more than one underlying pathology. Psychological factors may often play a role. Women with sensory urgency have been shown to have a heightened perception of bladder volume and to be more anxious than women with urodynamic stress incontinence or detrusor instability.[4] It is accepted that laboratory urodynamics can fail to detect detrusor over-activity during the comparatively brief period in which the patient in studied. Some patients who are labelled as having sensory urgency may therefore have unrecognized underlying detrusor over-activity, and ambulatory urodynamics may be an appropriate further investigation in these women.

Diagnosis of this disorder requires a detailed history and examination, a frequency–volume chart and subtracted cystometry. Having made the diagnosis, it is then important to undertake a cystoscopy and bladder biopsy to exclude other intravesical pathology.

Management

History

Patients presenting with frequency and urgency need to be carefully questioned about associated urinary symptoms. Associated urge incontinence and its severity are important, as is any associated dysuria or suprapubic pain. If haematuria is reported, this must be investigated further. The presence of a urinary tract infection, a bladder carcinoma, a calculus or a lesion of the upper urinary tracts needs to be excluded.

As there is such a wide-ranging differential diagnosis for possible causes of urinary frequency and urgency, conditions both within the urinary tract and further afield need to be considered. Information should be sought regarding any neurological symptoms, drinking habits and concomitant medication.

Examination

An abdominal examination will rule out a mass or large distended bladder. A neurological assessment is important to exclude an upper motor neuron lesion. The S2, S3, S4 nerve roots innervate the bladder and particular regard should be paid to these dermatomes.

On pelvic examination, a possible large fibroid uterus, ovarian mass or pregnancy should be considered. It is important to assess the degree and site of any pelvic organ prolapse that may be present. Tenderness on bladder palpation may be found in interstitial cystitis and other painful bladder syndromes. The urethra should be carefully inspected for local causes of irritative symptoms such as a urethral caruncle or signs of urethritis.

Investigations

These are described in more detail in the chapter on assessment of the lower urinary tract (Chapter 58). Initial investigation should always include a midstream urine sample for culture and sensitivity, and urine for cytology. Appropriate cultures for 'fastidious organisms' (*Mycoplasma*, *Ureaplasma* and *Chlamydia*), tuberculosis and schistosomiasis may be indicated. A completed frequency–volume chart is an invaluable tool, providing useful information on fluid input and output, drinking habits, voided volumes and the episodes of urgency and incontinence.

Where the cause for the symptoms is not revealed by the above assessment, the more specialist investigations should be considered. Ultrasound scan can be used to assess urinary residual volumes accurately, to measure bladder wall thickness and to give more information on any masses detected on pelvic examination. Once a urinary tract infection has been ruled out, subtracted cystometry may detect detrusor over-activity or sensory urgency. Cystourethroscopy should be performed for recurrent urinary tract infections:

- if haematuria is present,
- if pain is a significant symptom,
- if interstitial cystitis or a urethral diverticulum is suspected.

This can be undertaken with a flexible cystoscope under local anaesthetic and, more commonly, with a rigid cystoscope under a general anaesthetic. The latter allows far better biopsy samples to be taken for histological assessment, which is important in the diagnosis of many of these conditions. Although the histological appearance of biopsies taken from patients with interstitial cystitis is generally non-specific, the findings at cystoscopy are more characteristic. The bladder should be filled by passive gravity. The capacity under analgesia is usually <400 mL. The bladder is left distended for 1–2 minutes once filled to capacity. The irrigation fluid is then drained and the terminal fluid is typically seen to be blood tinged. On refilling the bladder for a second look, the characteristic features of glomerulations, splotchy haemorrhages, scarring and cracking of the mucosa are more readily seen.

Treatment

Treatment should be directed at the underlying cause of the urinary symptoms. This intervention may be well supported by evidence, such as a simple course of antibiotics for a urinary tract infection or bladder retraining and anticholinergic drug therapy for detrusor over-activity. In some of the less well-understood or rarer diseases, treatment may be largely empirical, with less chance of success, such as is often the case in women with interstitial cystitis.

Many different treatments have been tried for interstitial cystitis, with little sustained success. Proposed systemic treatments include antihistamines, heparin, amitriptyline and pentosan polysulphate, which is a synthetic analogue of glycosaminoglycan and augments the mucous protective layer of the bladder. Many patients with interstitial cystitis have been shown to have an improvement in symptoms following cystodistension. Unfortunately, any beneficial effects are short lived. The treatment that has most evidence to support its use is instillation therapy with dimethyl sulphoxide (DMSO), which is an industrial solvent. The treatment regimen is easy to perform on an outpatient basis, providing the patient can manage to self-catheterize, and is inexpensive. A significant improvement can be expected in more than 50 per cent of patients with early interstitial cystitis.[5] Finally, when other treatments fail and symptom severity is such that patient's quality of life is destroyed, a urological opinion should be sought and reconstructive surgery considered. Available options include partial cystectomy, augmentation cystoplasty and urinary diversion with or without cystectomy.

Bladder retraining is widely used to treat many of the disorders giving rise to symptoms of urinary frequency and urgency, including detrusor over-activity and sensory urgency. The patient is taught slowly to increase the interval between voiding episodes, so that frequency can be reduced and the functional cystometric capacity increases. This technique was used by Jarvis[6] to treat women with sensory urgency. He demonstrated that more than 50 per cent of these women were symptom free and objectively dry 6 months after treatment with bladder retraining.

KEY POINTS

- These are common urinary symptoms in women.
- There are numerous causes, both within and outside the urinary tract.
- Careful investigation is required to identify the underlying aetiology, as the treatments are very different.
- Some conditions, such as a urinary tract infection or poor habit, are easily rectified.
- Some of the other causes result in conditions that tend to run a chronic course, a number of which are very disabling.

URETHRAL PROBLEMS

The female urethra is a complex muscular tube, approximately 40 mm in length. It is composed of several layers of muscle, the richly vascular submucosa and the mucosa.

There is considerable debate as to the relative roles of different components of the muscles, both within the wall of the urethra and surrounding it, in maintaining continence. A number of changes occur to the urethra with age. The strength and the amount of urethral connective tissue fall as a result of oestrogen deficiency. This causes the support of the urethrovesical junction to weaken. In addition, urethral vascular pulsations in the submucosal plexus gradually decrease with age.

Urethritis

Urethritis is inflammation of the urethra leading to symptoms of frequency, urgency, dysuria and localized urethral pain. It is caused either by an infectious pathogen or by chemical irritation. Evidence of the use of causative chemical agents, such as bubble baths, vaginal deodorants and perfumed cosmetics, should be sought as part of the medical history in women with such symptoms. Responsible infectious agents include many of the micro-organisms associated with sexually transmitted infections such as herpes simplex virus, *Neisseria gonorrhoeae* and *Chlamydia*. The group of organisms that typically cause acute bacterial cystitis, such as *Escherichia coli*, may also cause urethritis.

Where urethritis is suspected, appropriate cultures should be taken from the urethra and vagina as well as a midstream urine culture. Urine microscopy typically shows evidence of pyuria and bacteria.

Acute urinary retention can occur secondary to urethritis and needs to be considered. Prompt treatment with an indwelling catheter until symptoms have resolved is important in order to prevent over-distension of the bladder. The initiation of treatment with the appropriate antibiotic usually results in a rapid recovery, but scarring of the urethra can result in strictures and subsequent voiding difficulties. Referral to a genitourinary medicine clinic for contact tracing and treatment of partners is important if sexually transmitted organisms are responsible. Cessation of the use of the offending chemical agent results in fairly rapid resolution of symptoms without the need for further treatment.

Urethral diverticulae

Urethral diverticulae are usually found in the distal third of the posterior urethral wall bulging towards the vagina. They are occasionally found congenitally, but thought to arise more often from repeated inflammation of the paraurethral glands and are found mainly in parous women. The incidence of this condition is unclear, but is probably of the order of 3 per cent. It is an increasingly encountered problem, which may be explained by the recent rise in the incidence of sexually transmitted infections.

The presenting symptoms vary, but usually include frequency, dysuria, dyspareunia, voiding difficulties and recurrent urinary tract infection. The classical symptom associated with this condition is post-micturition dribble, caused by the delay in the diverticulum draining after the voiding bladder has filled it up. On vaginal examination, it is sometimes possible to palpate a suburethral mass or even a calculus that has formed in the diverticulum. Tenderness can usually be elicited in this area and occasionally pus can be expressed from the urethral meatus. Alternatively, there may be no physical signs.

Often, urethral diverticulae are found incidentally as part of X-ray screening during videourodynamics (Figure 60.1). Similarly, they may be seen on transvaginal ultrasound examination. Urethral pressure profilometry shows a characteristic 'dip' in urethral closure pressure and gives useful information about the position of the opening of the diverticulum relative to the urethral sphincter and bladder neck. If a patient has symptoms suggestive of a diverticulum and a diagnosis is required, a voiding cystourethrogram or a positive-pressure double-balloon urethrography using a Trattner catheter will give useful information about the size and position of the defect prior to surgery. These lesions are not always easy to see on cystourethroscopy unless the opening into the diverticulum is large.

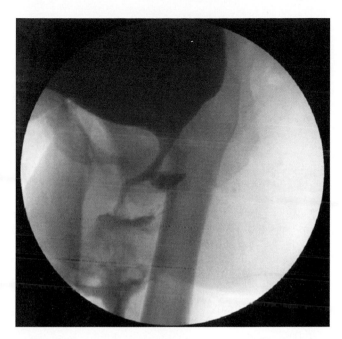

Figure 60.1   A urethral diverticulum is clearly seen during the voiding phase of videourodynamic assessment

Surgical repair is usually undertaken if the patient displays related symptoms, such as suffering from recurrent urinary infections. The techniques described include marsupialization and vaginal diverticulectomy. There are no good long-term studies to guide clinicians as to the best surgical techniques for treating urethral diverticulae. Recurrence is fairly common, especially if there has been failure to remove the whole sac. If the diverticulum is small and not causing any problems, it is better left alone.

Urethral caruncles

These are commonly seen lesions in elder women. They appear as a small red mass at the urethral meatus, usually on the posterior aspect. It is thought that oestrogen deficiency plays a role in their aetiology. The caruncle consists of well-vascularized transitional epithelium and is sometimes uncomfortable during voiding, but more often does not give rise to any urinary symptoms. The patient may alternatively present with postmenopausal 'spotting'.

Initial treatment is with topical oestrogen therapy. If the lesion does not respond to this, it is important to biopsy it to exclude more serious pathology. Once malignancy is ruled out, it can be treated by either excision or cautery. There is a high rate of recurrence.

IATROGENIC URINARY TRACT INJURY

Damage to the urinary tract at the time of pelvic surgery is an important consideration for all gynaecological surgeons.

It is estimated to occur in 0.5–2.5 per cent of routine pelvic operations and in as many as 30 per cent of radical pelvic procedures for malignancy.[8] Although relatively uncommon, when it does occur, it presents a difficult challenge both to identify the injury and then to repair the damage. A good understanding of female pelvic anatomy and how this may be altered as the result of previous surgery or pelvic pathology is essential in order to minimize the risk of inadvertently damaging the urinary tract. Prompt recognition of the injury and the early involvement of an experienced urologist are important in ensuring a good outcome.

Aetiology

There are three common sites of ureteric injury during gynaecological surgery:

1 at the point where the ureters cross over the pelvic brim and enter the pelvis in close proximity to the ovarian vessels;
2 as the ureters course medially in the base of the broad ligament with the uterine artery crossing directly over the top of them; this is the site at which the ureters may be crushed by a clamp or divided whilst taking the uterine pedicle at hysterectomy;
3 at the ureterovesical junction as the ureters sweep medially to enter the bladder.

Any disease process that alters the normal anatomical course of the ureters or that makes their intraoperative identification more difficult increases the risk of injury. Malignant disease, advanced stage endometriosis and previous abdominal surgery or radiotherapy all make it more difficult to predict the path of the ureters. Similarly, the normal anatomical relations of the bladder are often distorted in these circumstances. It is often wise to consider the use of a preoperative intravenous urogram or the placement of ureteric stents at cystoscopy before proceeding to pelvic surgery. The path of the ureters should always be identified prior to any extensive pelvic dissection.

Management

A keen awareness of the proximity of the lower urinary tract during gynaecological surgery is the key to preventing these injuries. Such damage is largely preventable and forms an ever-increasing source of medical litigation. The success of managing these problems once they occur is largely dependent on whether the injury was detected at the time of operation and on close liaison with urological colleagues.

Most bladder injuries are relatively straightforward to repair, provided they are identified intraoperatively. Methylene blue dye instilled into the bladder via a urethral catheter can aid in the identification of bladder injuries. If damage is found, associated ureteric injury should also be borne in mind.

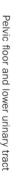

The bladder can be satisfactorily repaired with two layers of absorbable suture and left to drain freely with an indwelling catheter for at least 7 days. The bladder heals well and the prognosis for such repairs is extremely good.

If ureteric injury is suspected intraoperatively, the advice of a urologist should be sought. The course of the ureter above and below the area of concern needs to be demonstrated. Indigo carmine dye can be given intravenously to aid in checking the integrity of the ureters. The most appropriate method of repairing damage to the ureters depends largely on the site of the injury and should only ever be undertaken by an experienced surgeon with appropriate urological training. It is not appropriate for a gynaecologist who has not received such training to embark on these procedures. The most commonly employed techniques are summarized in Table 60.3.

In those cases in which injury to the lower urinary tract goes unnoticed at the time of operation, the patient is likely to develop symptoms and signs within a few days postoperatively. These may include fever, abdominal or loin pain, abdominal distension, sepsis, decreased urine output and rising serum creatinine. These result from the extravasation of urine into the peritoneal cavity or from ureteric obstruction. However, the presentation may be delayed and the patient later on complains of persistent discharge from a fistula or abdominal wound. Sometimes ureteric obstruction is only discovered many years later as an incidental finding.

If damage to the bladder or ureters is suspected postoperatively, an intravenous urogram is the diagnostic study of choice.[9] Repair of the damaged bladder is dependent upon the extent of urinary leakage. Extraperitoneal injuries and small leaks in women who are still voiding spontaneously can be managed with a trial of catheter drainage for 7–10 days in order to rest the bladder. In patients with more extensive bladder damage, intraperitoneal injuries with physical signs and in those in whom conservative management has failed, surgical exploration and repair of the defect are required. In cases where ureteric injury is recognized postoperatively, it is important to identify the site of damage in order to plan the most appropriate course of action. A retrograde pyelogram can give more information regarding the precise location of the injury. If the patient is septic or not well enough to undergo immediate surgical re-exploration,

a nephrostomy tube can be inserted to improve renal function to the point at which surgery is a more realistic alternative. In a small minority of cases where ureteric obstruction is caused by suture entrapment, nephrostomy drainage alone may resolve the damage. More often, surgical intervention is required. The techniques available are the same as those discussed previously for performing an intraoperative repair at the time of the initial injury.

KEY POINTS

- The ureters and bladder should always be accorded great respect by gynaecologists operating in the pelvis.
- A thorough knowledge of their anatomical relationships and of how these may be modified by pathological processes is important in order to minimize the risk of inadvertently damaging the lower urinary tract.
- The possibility of such an injury should always be borne in mind, both at the time of surgery and in the postoperative period.

KEY REFERENCES

1. Kelleher CJ, Cardozo LD, Khullar V et al. Symptom scores and subjective severity of urinary incontinence. *Neurourol Urodyn* 1994; 13:373–4.
2. Bungay G, Vessey MP, McPherson CK. Study of symptoms in middle life with special reference to the menopause. *BMJ* 1980; 281:181–3.
3. Parsons CL. Interstitial cystitis. In: Kursh ED, Mcguire EJ (eds). *Female Urology.* Philadelphia: Lippincott, 1994; 421–38.
4. Macauley A, Stanton S, Holmes D. Micturition and the mind: psychological factors in the aetiology of urinary disorders in women. *BMJ* 1987; 294:540–3.
5. Perez-Marrero R, Emerson LE, Feltis JT. A controlled study of dimethyl sulphoxide in interstitial cystitis. *J Urol* 1988; 140:36–9.
6. Jarvis GJ. The management of urinary incontinence due to primary vesical sensory urgency by bladder drill. *Br J Urol* 1982; 54:374–6.
7. Neuman M, Eidelman A, Langer R et al. Iatrogenic injuries to the ureter during gynecologic and obstetric operations. *Surg Gynecol Obstet* 1991; 173:268–72.
8. Spence H, Duckett J. Diverticulum of the female urethra: clinical aspects and presentation of a simple operative technique for cure. *J Urol* 1970; 104:432–7.
9. Mann WJ. Intentional and unintentional ureteral surgical treatment in gynecologic procedures. *Surg Gynecol Obstet* 1991; 17:453–6.

Table 60.3 Repair of ureteric injuries

Position of ureteric injury	Possible methods of repair
Mid-ureter	Boari flap
	Primary ureteric anastomosis (uretero-ureterostomy)
	Ureteric anastomosis to the contralateral ureter (transuretero-ureterostomy)
Lower ureter (distal 4 cm of the ureter)	Primary ureteric anastomosis (uretero-ureterostomy)
	Psoas hitch
	Ureteric re-implantation into the bladder

Lower Urinary Tract Infections

Dudley Robinson

MRCOG standards

Theoretical skills
- Have comprehensive knowledge of the infectious diseases affecting pregnant and non-pregnant women.
- Know the epidemiology of lower urinary tract infections.
- Be aware of the various diagnostic techniques used.
- Understand and have knowledge of the prophylaxis and treatment of lower urinary tract infections.

Practical skills
- Be able to manage bladder symptoms.
- Be able to diagnose, investigate and manage urinary tract infection.

PREVALENCE

Lower urinary tract infections remain an important cause of morbidity worldwide, accounting for 6 million consultations a year in the USA and for between 1 per cent and 6 per cent of visits to general practitioners in the UK.

Women are more prone than men to developing urinary infections, with 20 per cent of women aged 20–65 years suffering one episode a year. Approximately 50 per cent of women will develop a urinary infection during their lifetime,[1] the prevalence being 5 per cent per year.

DEFINITIONS

Bacteriuria

This is used to describe the presence of small numbers of bacteria in the urine. In a clean-catch freshly voided sample, this represents <10 000 colony-forming units (cfu) per mL.

Significant bacteriuria

This describes bacteria multiplying in the urine and represents a count of >100 000 cfu per mL,[2] although a single culture has a 20 per cent chance of representing contamination only.[3] However, 20–40 per cent of women with symptomatic urinary tract infections may present with bacterial counts of <100 000 cfu per mL. In addition, bacterial counts of only 100–10 000 cfu per mL have been associated with symptoms of cystitis, although this may simply represent the early phase of infection. In order to clarify the situation, more recent work has suggested that a threshold of 100 cfu per mL in symptomatic women is significant and should be treated, this giving both high specificity and sensitivity.[4]

Asymptomatic bacteriuria

This is the term used to describe the condition in which there is significant bacteriuria although the patient remains asymptomatic. It is found in approximately 5 per cent of young women and increases with age, reaching a prevalence of 22–43 per cent in elderly women. In general it is not thought to be of clinical significance, except in certain clinical circumstances such as pregnancy, instrumentation of the lower urinary tract and renal transplant patients. It is more likely to be present in those patients with a chronic indwelling catheter.

Recurrent urinary tract infection

This is the term used to describe a symptomatic infection that follows the resolution of a previous urinary tract infection, generally after treatment. It occurs in 12–27 per cent of women after their first urinary tract infection and in 48 per cent of women who have had a previous urinary tract infection. The ratio of recurrent urinary tract infection to pyelonephritis has been estimated to range between 18:1 and 28:1.

Recurrent infection may be due to relapse of the original organism or to re-infection with the same or a different organism. As it is often difficult to differentiate between relapse and re-infection, a relapse is defined as a recurrent urinary tract infection caused by the same organism, and a re-infection as a recurrent urinary tract infection caused by a different organism. Around 80–90 per cent of recurrent infections are due to re-infections, with one-third being with the same organism.

Complicated lower urinary tract infections

This is used to describe infections that may be related to other pathology (Table 61.1). One of the most common forms of complicated urinary tract infection is related to the use of catheterization. The incidence of bacteriuria associated with an indwelling urinary catheter is 3–10 per cent per day, and the duration of catheterization is the most important risk factor for developing infection of the lower urinary tract. Whereas less than 5 per cent of catheter-induced episodes of bacteriuria result in bacteraemia, they represent a huge reservoir of resistant bacteria in the hospital environment.

Pregnancy also represents a special case of complicated lower urinary tract infections, although pregnant women are not at greater risk of asymptomatic bacteriuria. However, there is an increased risk of perinatal complications such as premature delivery and developing a symptomatic infection and pyelonephritis in later pregnancy.

Table 61.1 Conditions associated with complicated lower urinary tract infection

Structural	Urolithiasis
	Malignancy
	Ureteric stricture
	Urethral stricture
	Bladder diverticulae
	Renal cysts
	Fistulae
	Urinary diversions
Functional	Neurogenic bladder
	Vesicoureteric reflux
	Voiding difficulties (incomplete bladder emptying)
Foreign bodies	Indwelling catheter
	Ureteric stent
	Nephrostomy tube
Other	Diabetes mellitus
	Pregnancy
	Renal failure
	Renal transplant
	Immunosuppression
	Multi-drug resistance
	Hospital-acquired (nosocomial) infection

PATHOGENESIS

The urinary tract is usually sterile above the level of the distal urethra, although bacteria do gain access to the bladder, generally from neighbouring sites. The faecal–perineal–urethral route of infection is well documented, and *Escherichia coli* is the main causative organism, with the rectal flora serving as the main reservoir.[5] Other sites include the bowel, perineum, vaginal vestibule, urethra and paraurethral tissues.

Ascending infection along the urethra occurs most commonly and may be spontaneous or facilitated by sexual intercourse or catheterization. In addition, infection may also be via lymphatic spread or blood borne on rare occasions. The method of entry is not fully understood, although it has been proposed that bacteria may reflux into the bladder following a void or may ascend against the urinary stream because of turbulent flow or milk back into the bladder.

Host defences

The bladder has a number of mechanisms to resist infection. The most important is the hydrokinetic or 'washout' effect in which diuresis and voiding dilute the bacterial load and wash away infecting organisms. Consequently, the risk of infection will depend on the number and multiplication rate of the organisms in addition to the urinary residual, urine flow rate and frequency of voiding. Extremes of urine pH, osmolarity and high urea concentration tend to be protective.

The bladder mucosa is also thought to have a bactericidal action and produces a surface layer of mucus, providing an antibacterial barrier. The lamina propria of the bladder wall and urethra has also been shown to synthesize immunoglobulin A (IgA), and this also has a bactericidal effect by preventing bacterial adherence. Finally, Tamm–Horsfall protein, a mucoprotein shed from the renal tubular cells and excreted in the urine, has been shown to bind and trap *E. coli* and to be increased in patients with pyelonephritis and vesicoureteric reflux.

Virulence factors

Uropathogens have the ability to survive and multiply in the bladder, as well as being able to adhere to the bladder epithelium. This is supported by the findings of one study in which women with recurrent urinary tract infections had increased receptivity of urothelial cells for bacteria and increased frequency of vaginal colonization and subsequent infection when compared to a control population.[6] Adherence of the organism to the bladder wall triggers an acute inflammatory response by the activation of cytokines. These in turn stimulate the production of an intracellular adhesion molecule, which, by leucocyte adhesion, causes migration of cells to the point of infection. This prevents the organisms from being 'washed out' and, by increasing their nutrient supply, they divide more efficiently.

The structure of bacteria is also known to be important when considering virulence and pathogenicity. Pili and fimbriae are found on the outer membrane of some bacteria and promote binding, using an adhesion molecule on their tip. P-fimbriae mediate adherence to the glycolipids in the urothelium whilst Type I fimbriae confer the ability to adhere to the mucous layer within the bladder. Enterobacteriaceae have an antigenic structure that induces an antibody immune response. The outer cell membrane contains O antigens, which, together with endotoxins, initiate the immune response in the bladder wall by stimulating cytokine production. Capsular (K) antigens on the surface of the bacteria help to inhibit phagocytosis and IgA and IgG in the urothelium. Finally, some bacteria are able to break down bladder mucin and invade the urothelium beneath.

RISK FACTORS FOR URINARY TRACT INFECTION

These predisposing factors can be considered in terms of congenital anomalies and acquired causes (Table 61.2).

The congenital risk factors for urinary tract infection are as follows.

- *Urethra*
  - hypospadias
  - epispadias.
- *Bladder*
  - vesico-ureteric reflux
  - ectopic ureters
  - obstructive mega-ureter.

Table 61.2   Acquired causes of urinary tract infection

Traumatic	Surgery (urinary diversion, clam cystoplasty)
	Sexual intercourse
	Sexual abuse
	Foreign bodies (catheters, stents)
	Contraceptive diaphragm
Inflammatory	Vulvo-urethritis
	Chronic inflammation (tuberculosis, syphilis, schistosomiasis)
	Interstitial cystitis
	Radiotherapy
	Fistula
Metabolic	Calculi
	Diabetes mellitus
Drugs	Cyclophosphamide
	Tioprofenic acid
Anatomical	Cystocele
	Urethral diverticulum
Functional	Detrusor hypotonia
	Detrusor dyssynergia
	Constipation
Malignancy	Bladder tumours
	Other pelvic tumours (cervix, uterus, ovary)

- *Pelvis*
  - pelvic–ureteric junction obstruction.
- *Central nervous system*
  - meningomyelocele
  - tethered cord syndrome.

CAUSATIVE ORGANISMS

Community infections

The commonly occurring organisms in community practice[7] differ when compared to those found within the hospital enviroment (Table 61.3).[7]

Table 61.3   Common uropathogens in general practice and hospital

Organism	Community (%)	Hospital (%)
Escherichia coli	77.5	62.9
Proteus mirabilis	4.5	4.5
Klebsiella–Enterobacter spp	4.7	9.3
Enterococcus spp	4.9	9.2
Staphylococcus spp	1	2.7
Others (*Ureoplasma, Mycoplasma, Chlamydia*)	7.4	7.6
Pseudomonas aeruginosa		3.8

ANTIBIOTIC SENSITIVITIES

Community infections

The antibiotic sensitivities of uropathogens in the community (Table 61.4) also differ from the sensitivities of the same organisms within the hospital.[7]

Table 61.4   Comparison of the sensitivities to antibiotics in the community and in hospital

Antibiotic	Community (%)	Hospital (%)
Amoxycillin/ampicillin	56.9	48.8
Cephaloradine	86.9	73.1
Ciprofloxacin	90.3	83.3
Co-trimoxazole	86.8	74.1
Nalidixic acid	85.7	73.5
Nitrofurantoin	88.4	79.3
Sulphonamide	64.5	55.5
Tetracycline	65.0	57.9
Trimethoprim	74.0	64.9

CLINICAL SYMPTOMS

Women with lower urinary tract infections typically complain of symptoms of cystitis, i.e. dysuria, suprapubic discomfort, frequency and nocturia. There may also be associated microscopic or macroscopic haematuria. Of these women, approximately 30 per cent will also have an upper urinary tract infection, which may present as loin pain and tenderness. In the elderly, urinary tract infections may present with atypical symptoms such as confusion and falls, whilst young children may present with general malaise and pyrexia.

INVESTIGATIONS

In the majority of women with simple acute cystitis, there is no need for further investigation. However, some cases do warrant further investigation in order to exclude an underlying cause.

Indications for investigation include:

- children,
- proven recurrent urinary tract infection,
- adults with a childhood history of urinary tract infection,
- haematuria,
- atypical infection,
- atypical organism,
- persistent infection,
- failure to respond to antibiotic therapy.

Women presenting with symptoms suggestive of simple acute urinary infection should be investigated using dipstick urinalysis prior to a midstream, clean-catch sample being sent for microscopy, culture and sensitivity.

In those women who have recurrent or complicated urinary infections, renal function should be assessed with serum creatinine, urea and electrolytes. In addition, urine should be sent for culture of fastidious organisms (*Mycoplasma hominis, Ureaplasma urolyticum, Chlamydia tracomatis*) to rule out the more unusual causes of infection.

Ultrasound of the upper urinary tract will exclude renal causes such as hydronephrosis or calculi, whilst a postmicturition scan will rule out a significant urinary residual. An alternative is radiological imaging using an intravenous urogram, although this involves exposure to ionizing radiation and has not been shown to influence treatment in the majority of cases. In addition, a transvaginal ultrasound should be performed to exclude the possibility of a pelvic mass.

Cystourethroscopy and bladder biopsy will exclude an intravesical lesion such as a bladder tumour and also anomalies such as diverticulae and calculi. A bladder biopsy may show evidence of chronic follicular or interstitial cystitis.

TREATMENT

The management of lower urinary tract infection is aimed at treating the current infection and preventing further recurrences. The aims of treatment may be summarized as follows:

- symptomatic relief,
- clinical cure,
- microbiological cure,
- detection of predisposing factors,
- prevention of upper urinary tract involvement,
- management of recurrence,
- prevention of recurrence.

General measures: prophylaxis

Primary prevention consists of general advice regarding hygiene, fluid intake and frequency of voiding. In women complaining of recurrent infections related to sexual intercourse, postcoital voiding should be encouraged and they should also be advised to avoid using a diaphragm and condoms with nonoxynol 9, as both of these may increase the risk of recurrent infection. Appropriate advice regarding bladder emptying, such as timed voiding or double-voiding, may also help those with mild voiding difficulties. Should these not be successful, self-catheterization or a long-term suprapubic catheter may be the only option.

General measures: treatment

Patients with cystitis should be encouraged to increase their fluid intake in order to achieve a short voiding interval and a high flow rate, which will help to dilute and flush out the infecting organism. Using potassium citrate preparations may provide symptomatic relief. With such measures, spontaneous remission of symptoms may occur in up to 40 per cent of women.

Cranberry juice has also been shown to be an important factor in the prevention of lower urinary tract infections. Regular intake of at least 300 mL a day has been associated with a reduced risk of urinary tract infections. The incidence of bacteriuria in those taking cranberry juice was 42 per cent of those in the control group and they were also found to be four times more likely to clear bacteria spontaneously.[8] Cranberry juice is thought to act by reducing bacterial adherence to the bladder wall.

Antimicrobials

When treating urinary tract infections, an antimicrobial should be selected that has the appropriate sensitivity and is also able to achieve a high concentration within the urinary tract. Drugs should be safe and efficacious, have a broad spectrum of activity and few side effects (Table 61.5). Ideally, the drugs should be rapidly absorbed and not induce bacterial resistance.

Table 61.5   Common antibiotic sensitivities

Gram-negative bacilli	Norfloxacin
Staphylococci	Ciprofloxacin
Streptococci	Gentamycin
	Sulphonamides
	Co-trimoxazole
	Trimethoprim
	Nitrofurantoin
Pseudomonas	Norfloxacin
	Ciprofloxacin
	Gentamycin

Duration

Compliance with therapy may be improved by using shorter courses of antimicrobial therapy or, ideally, by using a single-dose regimen, which also has the advantage of reducing the effect on faecal and vaginal flora and may help in reducing the emergence of resistant organisms. A large number of studies have assessed the use of single-dose therapy and found it to be effective, although better results have been reported using a short-term (3-day) regimen. There is no evidence to show that protracted courses are more effective. At present, trimethoprim, co-trimoxazole and the fluoroquinolones (ciprofloxacin, norfloxacin) are the preferred single-dose agents; amoxycillin has been shown to be less effective.

Antimicrobial sensitivities

Antimicrobial therapy should ideally be based upon culture and sensitivity results from a midstream specimen of urine, although initially treatment often needs to be on a 'best guess' basis.

Community-acquired infections often have a different range of sensitivities from those found in the hospital setting (see Table 61.4). Some antimicrobials are particularly useful when treating urinary infections. Nitrofurantoin is specific to the urinary tract and therefore has little effect on bowel and vaginal flora. It is bactericidal to most common uropathogens and is particularly useful as a prophylactic measure. It is safe to use in pregnancy, although contraindicated in cases of renal failure. Trimethoprim, whilst primarily bacteriostatic, is also useful in the treatment of urinary tract infection, and a recent survey has shown it to be the most commonly used agent in general practice.[9]

When considering acute, uncomplicated cystitis, short-term (3-day course) therapy would appear to be preferable. Trimethoprim, norfloxacin, ciprofloxacin and ofloxacin are appropriate.

Oestrogens

Endogenous oestrogen withdrawal following the menopause is thought to increase the risk of lower urinary tract symptoms as well as of urinary infections. Oestrogen therapy has been shown to increase vaginal pH and to reverse the microbiological changes that occur in the vagina following the menopause. A meta-analysis of oestrogen therapy in the management of recurrent lower urinary tract infections[10] has concluded that vaginal oestrogen seems to be effective in the prevention of recurrent urinary tract infections in postmenopausal women, although other routes of administration were not shown to be useful.

PROPHYLAXIS

Antimicrobials may be used as prophylaxis for recurrent urinary tract infections. Short-term and long-term low-dose prophylaxis as well as intermittent and postcoital therapy may be used, depending on the clinical situation. The most effective drugs include norfloxacin, nitrofuantoin and trimethoprim. In addition, cephalexin may be used as effective prophylaxis against recurrent infections in sexually active women. Overall, prophylactic therapy has been shown to reduce recurrence rates by up to 95 per cent when compared to placebo, with re-infection rates being reduced from 2–3 per patient-year to 0.1–0.4 per patient-year.[11]

LOWER URINARY TRACT INFECTIONS IN PREGNANCY

Asymptomatic bacteriuria occurs in 4–7 per cent of pregnancies. It is associated with the development of acute cystitis, pyelonephritis, preterm labour and low birth weight. If untreated, up to 30 per cent of women will develop acute cystitis, although this can be reduced to 3 per cent with effective treatment.

There is also an increased risk of developing pyelonephritis in pregnancy and of these women, up to 20 per cent may develop serious complications such as septic shock. Several authorities have suggested that there may be an association between positive urine cultures for group B streptococci and preterm delivery, although this remains unproven. There is, however, a clear association between elevated levels of urinary antibodies to group B streptococci and *E. coli* antigens and preterm delivery. This suggests that a local inflammatory response to urogenital infection may be important in stimulating preterm labour.[12] The treatment of asymptomatic bacteriuria has been shown to reduce preterm delivery.

The increased susceptibility in pregnancy may be due to incomplete emptying and the presence of a chronic residual due to the pressure of the gravid uterus. Progesterone is also known to increase stasis in the urinary tract by causing ureteric relaxation, which will also increase the risk of ascending infections. In addition, bacterial growth would appear to be enhanced in pregnancy, with the bacterial count of *E. coli* being twice that of non-pregnant women.

A review of randomized, controlled studies has found good evidence that urine culture and dipstick testing for leucocytes and nitrites reduced the risk of pyelonephritis and was cost effective, thus offering a rationale for screening.[13]

Treatment

When treating lower urinary tract infections in pregnancy, penicillins and cephalosporins have been shown to be safe in the first and second trimesters. As it is a folate antagonist, trimethoprim should be avoided in the first trimester, although it may be used safely in late pregnancy. Conversely, nitrofuantoin and sulphonamides are safe in early pregnancy, although they should be avoided in the third trimester when the former may cause a haemolytic anaemia and the latter hyperbilirubinaemia and kernicterus. Tetracyclines should be avoided because of their chelating action, which will lead to hypoplasia and staining of the teeth. Whilst in general erythromycin is considered safe, the estolate salt may be associated with cholestatic jaundice. Finally, fluoroquinolones may affect fetal cartilage formation, and chloramphenicol may be associated with neonatal cardiovascular collapse.

KEY POINTS

- Lower urinary tract infections are a common cause of morbidity, accounting for up to 6 per cent of consultations in primary care.
- A significant number of women may develop recurrent lower urinary tract infections which may be due to relapse or re-infection.
- Community acquired infections may be caused by different organisms from those acquired in hospital.
- In the majority of women with uncomplicated cystitis there is no indication for further investigation.
- Antimicrobial therapy should be based upon culture and sensitivity results although often initial treatment is on a 'best guess' basis.
- Short and low dose antibiotics may be used as prophylaxis and reduce infection rates by 95 per cent compared with placebo.
- Urinary tract infection in pregnancy may be associated with pyelonephritis, preterm delivery and low birth weight.

KEY REFERENCES

1. Asscher AW. Urinary tract infections. *J R Coll Physicians Lond* 1981; **15**:232–8.
2. Kass EH. Asypmtomatic infections of the urinary tract. *Trans Assoc Am Phys* 1956; **69**:56–64.
3. Kass EH. The role of asymptomatic bacteriuria in the pathogenesis of pyelonephritis. In: Quinn EL, Kass EH (eds). *Biology of Pyelonephritis*. Boston: Little, Brown, 1960, 399–406.
4. Stamm WE, Counts GW, Running KR et al. Diagnosis of coliform infection in acutely dysuric women. *N Engl J Med* 1982; **307**:463–8.
5. Yamamoto S, Tsukamato T, Terai A et al. Genetic evidence supporting the faecal–perineal–urethral hypothesis in cystitis caused by *Escherichia coli*. *J Urol* 1997; **157**:1127–9.
6. Kozody NL, Harding GK, Nicolle LE et al. Adherence of *Escherichia coli* to epithelial cells in the pathogenesis of urinary tract infection. *Clin Invest Med* 1985; **8**:121–5.
7. Gruneberg R. Pathogenesis and microbiology. In: Stanton SL, Dwyer PL (eds). *Urinary Tract Infection in the Female*. London: Martin Dunitz, 2000, 19–33.
8. Foxman B, Geiger AM, Palin K, Gillespie B, Koopman JS. First time urinary tract infection and sexual behaviour. *Epidemiology* 1995; **6**:162–8.
9. Brumfitt W, Hamilton-Miller JM. Consensus viewpoint on management of urinary infections. *J Antimicrob Chemother* 1994; **33**:147–53.
10. Cardozo L, Lose G, McClish D, Versi E, de Koning Gans H. A systematic review of oestrogens for recurrent urinary tract infections. Third report of the HUT Committee. *Int Urogynecol J Pelvic Floor Dysfunct* 2001; **12**:15–20.
11. Nicolle LE, Ronald AR. Recurrent urinary tract infections in adult women: diagnosis and treatment. *Infect Dis Clin North Am* 1987; **1**:793–806.
12. McKenzie H, Donnet ML, Howice PW et al. Risk of preterm delivery in pregnant women with group B streptococcal urinary infections or urinary antibodies to group B and *E. coli* antigens. *Br J Obstet Gynaecol* 1994; **101**:107–13.
13. Villar J, Bergsjo P. Scientific basis for the content of routine antenatal care. *Acta Obstet Gynaecol Scand* 1997; **76**:1–14.

Chapter 62

Urogenital Prolapse

Dudley Robinson

INTRODUCTION

Urogenital prolapse occurs when there is a weakness in the supporting structures of the pelvic floor allowing the pelvic viscera to descend and ultimately fall through the anatomical defect.

Whilst usually not life threatening, prolapse is often symptomatic and is associated with a deterioration in quality of life and may be the cause of bladder and bowel dysfunction. Increased life expectancy and an expanding elderly population mean that prolapse remains an important condition, especially since the majority of women may now spend a third of their lives in the postmenopausal state. Surgery for urogenital prolapse accounts for approximately 20 per cent of elective major gynaecological surgery and this increases to 59 per cent in elderly women. The lifetime risk of having surgery for prolapse is 11 per cent; a third of these procedures are operations for recurrent prolapse.

The economic cost of urogenital prolapse is considerable, with figures from the USA revealing a total expenditure of $1012 million in 1997: vaginal hysterectomy accounted for 49 per cent, pelvic floor repairs for 28 per cent and abdominal hysterectomy for 13 per cent of costs.[1]

EPIDEMIOLOGY

Age

The incidence of urogenital prolapse increases with increasing age, with approximately 60 per cent of elderly women having some degree of prolapse and up to half of all women over the age of 50 years complaining of symptomatic prolapse. In a study of women with severe vaginal vault prolapse following hysterectomy, 60 per cent were over the age of 60.

Parity

Urogenital prolapse is more common following childbirth, although it may be asymptomatic. Studies have estimated that 50 per cent of parous women have some degree of urogenital prolapse and, of these, 10–20 per cent are symptomatic. Only 2 per cent of nulliparous women are reported to have prolapse.

Race

Prolapse is generally thought to be more common in Caucasian women and less common in women of Afro-Caribbean origin. However, a study examining racial differences in North America has shown that this may not be the case, as there was little racial variation noted, although this may simply reflect cultural differences in reporting.

CLASSIFICATION

Urogenital prolapse is classified anatomically depending on the site of the defect and the pelvic viscera that are involved.

- *Urethrocele*: prolapse of the lower anterior vaginal wall involving the urethra only.
- *Cystocele*: prolapse of the upper anterior vaginal wall involving the bladder. Generally there is also associated prolapse of the urethra and hence the term cystourethrocele is used.
- *Uterovaginal prolapse*: this term is used to describe prolapse of the uterus, cervix and upper vagina.
- *Enterocele*: prolapse of the upper posterior wall of the vagina, usually containing loops of small bowel. A traction enterocele is secondary to uterovaginal prolapse, a pulsion enterocele is secondary to chronically raised intra-abdominal pressure, and an iatrogenic enterocele is caused by previous pelvic surgery. An anterior enterocele may be used to describe prolapse of the upper anterior vaginal wall following hysterectomy.
- *Rectocele*: prolapse of the lower posterior wall of the vagina involving the anterior wall of the rectum.

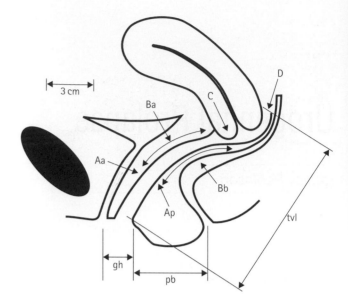

Figure 62.1   International Continence Society (ICS) Prolapse Scoring System (POPQ)

GRADING OF UROGENITAL PROLAPSE

- *First degree*: the lowest part of the prolapse descends halfway down the vaginal axis to the introitus.
- *Second degree*: the lowest part of the prolapse extends to the level of the introitus and through the introitus on straining.
- *Third degree*: the lowest part of the prolapse extends through the introitus and lies outside the vagina. Procidentia describes a third-degree uterine prolapse.

PROLAPSE SCORING SYSTEM

Recently, the International Continence Society (ICS) produced a standardization document in order to assess urogenital prolapse more objectively.[2] The ICS Prolapse Scoring System (POPQ) allows the measurement of fixed points on the anterior and posterior vaginal walls, cervix and perineal body against a fixed reference point, the genital hiatus (Figure 62.1). Measurements are performed in the left lateral position at rest and at maximal valsalva, thus providing an accurate and reproducible method of quantifying urogenital prolapse.

ANATOMY OF THE PELVIC FLOOR

The pelvic floor provides support to the pelvic viscera and consists of the levator ani muscles, urogenital diaphragm, endopelvic fascia and perineal body. The levator ani, when

considered with its associated fascia, is termed the pelvic diaphragm.

The muscle fibres of the pelvic diaphragm are arranged to form a broad U-shaped layer of muscle with a defect anteriorly. This physiological defect is the urogenital hiatus and allows the passage of the urethra, vagina and rectum through the pelvic floor.

Pelvic floor musculature

The muscles of the pelvic floor are composed of the levator ani and coccygeus, which form a cradle within the bony pelvis supporting the pelvic organs. The levator ani originate on each side from the pelvic sidewall, arising anteriorly just above the arcus tendineus fasciae pelvis (the white line) and inserting posteriorly into the arcus tendineus levator ani. The arcus tendineus fasciae pelvis and arcus tendineus levator ani fuse near the ischial spine; the levator ani unite in the midline to form the anococcygeal raphe (Figure 62.2).

The levator ani has three divisions: the pubococcygeus, iliococcygeus and puborectalis muscles (Figure 62.3). The iliococcygeus and pubococcygeus arise from the arcus tendineus levator ani fascia overlying the obturator internus and insert into the midline anococcygeal raphe and the coccyx, whilst the latter forms the inner fibres of the pelvic floor musculature inserting into the rectum and perineal body. Posteriorly, the coccygeus arises from the ischial spine and sacrospinous ligament and inserts into the coccyx and sacrum.

The striated muscle of the pelvic floor is composed of both slow and fast twitch muscle fibres. The slow twitch fibres provide muscle tone over a long period of time, thus supporting the pelvic viscera, whilst the fast twitch fibres react to sudden increases in intra-abdominal pressure.

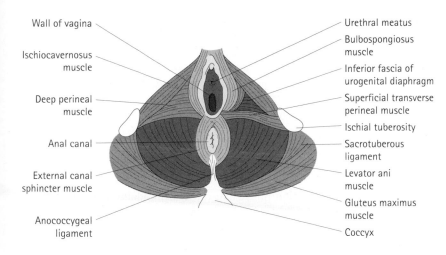

Wall of vagina
Ischiocavernosus muscle
Deep perineal muscle
Anal canal
External canal sphincter muscle
Anococcygeal ligament

Urethral meatus
Bulbospongiosus muscle
Inferior fascia of urogenital diaphragm
Superficial transverse perineal muscle
Ischial tuberosity
Sacrotuberous ligament
Levator ani muscle
Gluteus maximus muscle
Coccyx

Figure 62.2   Anatomy of the pelvic floor

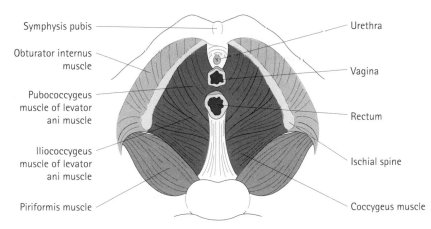

Symphysis pubis
Obturator internus muscle
Pubococcygeus muscle of levator ani muscle
Iliococcygeus muscle of levator ani muscle
Piriformis muscle

Urethra
Vagina
Rectum
Ischial spine
Coccygeus muscle

Figure 62.3   Anatomy of the pelvic floor showing the divisions of levator ani

Urogenital diaphragm

The urogenital diaphragm (perineal membrane) is a triangular sheet of dense fibrous tissue spanning the anterior half of the pelvic outlet, which is pierced by the vagina and urethra. It arises from the inferior ischiopubic rami and attaches medially to the urethra, vagina and perineal body, thus supporting the pelvic floor.

Perineal body

The perineal body lies between the vagina and the rectum and provides a point of insertion for the muscles of the pelvic floor. It is attached to the inferior pubic rami and ischial tuberosities through the urogenital diaphragm and superficial transverse perineal muscles. Laterally it is attached to the fibres of the pelvic diaphragm; posteriorly it inserts into the external anal sphincter and coccyx.

Pelvic fascia

The endopelvic fascia is a meshwork of collagen and elastin that represents the fused adventitial layers of the visceral

structures and pelvic wall musculature. Condensations of the pelvic fascia are termed ligaments and these have an important part in the supportive role of the pelvic floor.

Uterine support

The parametrium, composed of the uterosacral and cardinal ligaments, attaches the cervix and upper vagina to the pelvic sidewall. The uterosacral ligament forms the medial margin bordering the pouch of Douglas; the cardinal ligaments attach the lateral aspects of the cervix and vagina to the pelvic sidewall over the sacrum. The former is composed mostly of smooth muscle, whereas the cardinal ligaments contain mostly connective tissue and the pelvic blood vessels. The round ligaments are not thought to have a role in supporting the uterus, although they may help to maintain anteversion and anteflexion; the broad ligaments are simply folds of peritoneum and provide no support.

Vaginal support

Support to the upper third of the vagina is provided principally by the downward extension of the cardinal ligaments;

the middle third is supported by lateral attachments to the arcus tendineus fasciae pelvis, a condensation of the obturator and levator fasciae. These supports suspend the anterior vaginal wall across the pelvis, the layer of fascia anterior to the vagina being called the pubocervical fascia. Postero-laterally the vagina is attached to the endopelvic fascia over the pelvic diaphragm and sacrum by the rectovaginal septum (fascia of Denonvilliers), which extends caudally into the perineal body and cranially into the peritoneum of the pouch of Douglas. The lower third is attached anteriorly to the pubic arch by the perineal membrane, posteriorly to the perineal body and laterally to the medial aspect of levator ani.

Urethral support

The proximal urethra is supported by a sling of endopelvic fascia and the anterior vaginal wall, which is stabilized by lateral attachments to the arcus tendineus fasciae pelvis, and medial border of the levator ani. Contraction and relaxation of the levator muscles allows elevation or descent of the urethra respectively, which is important in the control of voiding. In addition, an increase in intra-abdominal pressure causes compression of the urethra against the fixed anterior vaginal wall, thus maintaining continence. Bladder neck mobility and the stress continence mechanism are thus dependent on fascial integrity and connective tissue elasticity.

AETIOLOGY

Pregnancy and childbirth

The increased incidence of prolapse in multiparous women would suggest that pregnancy and childbirth have an important impact on the supporting function of the pelvic floor. Damage to the muscular and fascial supports of the pelvic floor and changes in innervation contribute to the development of prolapse.

The pelvic floor may be damaged during childbirth, causing the axis of the levator muscles to become more oblique and creating a funnel that allows the uterus, vagina and rectum to fall through the urogenital hiatus. In addition, the proportion of fascia to muscle within the pelvic floor tends to increase with increasing age, and thus once damaged by childbirth, muscle may never regain its full strength. This is supported by studies showing decreased cellularity and increased collagen content in 70 per cent of women with urogenital prolapse, compared to 20 per cent of normal controls.

Mechanical changes within the pelvic fascia have also been implicated in the causation of urogenital prolapse.

During pregnancy, the fascia becomes more elastic and thus more likely to fail. This may explain the increased incidence of stress incontinence observed in pregnancy and the increased incidence of prolapse with multiparity.

Denervation of the pelvic musculature has been shown to occur following childbirth, although gradual denervation has also been demonstrated in nulliparous women with increasing age. However, the effects were greatest in those women who had documented stress incontinence or prolapse.[3] Furthermore, histological studies have revealed changes in muscle fibre type and distribution, suggesting denervation injury associated with ageing and also following childbirth. In conclusion, it would appear that partial denervation of the pelvic floor is part of the normal ageing process, although pregnancy and childbirth accelerate these changes.

The biochemical properties of connective tissue may also play an important role in the development of prolapse. Changes in collagen content have been identified, the hydroxyproline content in connective tissue from women with stress incontinence being 40 per cent lower than in continent controls. In addition, changes in collagen metabolism may be associated with the development of urogenital prolapse, increased levels of collagenases being associated with weakened pelvic support and stress incontinence.

Hormonal factors

The effects of ageing and those of oestrogen withdrawal at the time of the menopause are often difficult to separate. Rectus muscle fascia has been shown to become less elastic with increasing age, and less energy is required to produce irreversible damage. Furthermore, there is also a reduction in skin collagen content following the menopause. Both of these factors lead to a reduction in the strength of the pelvic connective tissue.

More recently, oestrogen receptors, alpha and beta, have been demonstrated in the vaginal walls and the uterosacral ligaments of premenopausal women, although the beta receptor was absent from the vaginal walls in postmenopausal women. However, a further study was unable to identify oestrogen receptors in biopsies from the levator ani muscles in urinary incontinent women participating in pelvic floor exercises. In conclusion, it would appear that oestrogens, and oestrogen withdrawal, have a role in the development of urogenital prolapse, although the precise mechanism has yet to be established.

Smoking

Chronic chest disease resulting in a chronic cough leads to an increase in the intra-abdominal pressure and thus exposes the pelvic floor to greater strain. Over a period of time this will exacerbate any defects in the pelvic floor musculature and fascia, leading to prolapse.

Constipation

Chronically increased intra-abdominal pressure caused by repetitive straining will exacerbate any potential weaknesses in the pelvic floor and is also associated with an increased risk of prolapse.

Obesity

Although obesity has been linked to urogenital prolapse due to a potential increase in intra-abdominal pressure, there has been no good evidence to support this theory.

Exercise

Increased stress placed on the musculature of the pelvic floor will exacerbate pelvic floor defects and weakness, thus increasing the incidence of prolapse. Consequently, heavy lifting and exercise as well as sports such as weight lifting, high-impact aerobics and long-distance running increase the risk of urogenital prolapse.

Surgery

Pelvic surgery may also have an effect on the occurrence of urogenital prolapse. Continence procedures, whilst elevating the bladder neck, may lead to defects in other pelvic compartments. At Burch colposuspension, the fixing of the lateral vaginal fornices to the ipsilateral ileopectineal ligaments leaves a potential defect in the posterior vaginal wall that predisposes to rectocele and enterocele formation. In a 5-year follow-up study of women, 36 per cent had cystoceles 66 per cent rectocele, 32 per cent enterocele and 38 per cent uterine prolapse. A further study of 109 women with vaginal vault prolapse reported that 43 per cent had previously undergone Burch colposuspension. Overall, 25 per cent of the women who had had Burch colposuspension required further surgery for prolapse.

Needle suspension procedures such as the Pereyra or Stamey endoscopically guided bladder neck suspension are also associated with an increased incidence of recurrent cystocele, although this is not the case following sling procedures. In addition, there is an increased incidence of posterior compartment defects, such as enterocele and rectocele, after Manchester repair, caused by the anterior plication of the uterosacral and cardinal ligaments, which leaves a large posterior hiatus.

The association between prolapse and prior hysterectomy is not as clear. One large study reported that 37 per cent of women had the onset of symptoms more than 37 years following hysterectomy, although 39 per cent of these women became symptomatic within 2 years. However, other factors such as the ageing process and oestrogen withdrawal following the menopause may also have an important role. Prolapse of the vaginal vault may present following either vaginal or abdominal hysterectomy, although the incidence is low, with only 0.5 per cent of women who have had a hysterectomy requiring further surgical intervention for vaginal vault prolapse.

CLINICAL SYMPTOMS

Most women complain of a feeling of discomfort or heaviness within the pelvis in addition to a 'lump coming down'. Symptoms tend to become worse with prolonged standing and towards the end of the day. Women may also complain of dyspareunia, difficulty in inserting tampons and chronic lower backache. In cases of third-degree prolapse, there may be mucosal ulceration and lichenification, which results in a symptomatic vaginal discharge or bleeding.

A cystocele may be associated with lower urinary tract symptoms of urgency and frequency of micturition in addition to a sensation of incomplete emptying, which may be relieved by digitally reducing the prolapse. Recurrent urinary tract infections may also be associated with a chronic urinary residual. Whilst less than 2 per cent of mild cystoceles are associated with ureteric obstruction, severe prolapse may lead to hydonephrosis and chronic renal damage. Between 33 per cent and 92 per cent of cases of complete procidentia are associated with some degree of ureteric obstruction.

A rectocele may be associated with difficulty in opening the bowels, some women complaining of tenesmus and having to digitate to defecate.

CLINICAL SIGNS

Women are generally examined in the left lateral position using a Simms' speculum, although digital examination when standing allows more accurate assessment of the degree of urogenital prolapse and, in particular, vaginal vault support. An abdominal examination should also be performed to exclude the presence of an abdominal or pelvic tumour that may be responsible for the vaginal findings.

Differential diagnosis includes:

- vaginal cysts,
- pendunculated fibroid polyp,
- urethral diverticulum,
- chronic uterine inversion.

INVESTIGATION

In women who also complain of concomitant lower urinary tract symptoms, urodynamic studies or a post-micturition bladder ultrasound should be performed in order to exclude a chronic residual due to associated voiding difficulties. In such cases, a midstream specimen of urine should be sent for culture and sensitivity.

Subtracted cystometry, with or without videocysto-urethrography, will allow the identification of underlying detrusor instability, which is important to exclude prior to surgical repair. In cases of significant cystocele, stress testing should be carried out by asking the patient to cough whilst standing. Since occult urodynamic stress incontinence may be unmasked by straightening the urethra following anterior colporrhaphy, this should be simulated by the insertion of a ring pessary or tampon to reduce the cystocele. If stress incontinence is demonstrated, a continence procedure such as colposuspension or insertion of tension-free vaginal tape (TVT) may be a more appropriate procedure.

In cases of severe prolapse in which there may be a degree of ureteric obstruction, it is important to evaluate the upper urinary tract with either a renal tract ultrasound or an intravenous urogram.

Although a cystocele itself may be responsible for irritative urinary symptoms, if these are unusually severe cystoscopy should be performed to exclude a chronic follicular or interstitial cystitis.

MANAGEMENT

Prevention

In general, any factor that leads to chronic increases in intra-abdominal pressure should be avoided. Consequently, care should be taken to avoid constipation, which has been implicated as a major contributing factor to urogenital prolapse in Western society. In addition, the risk of prolapse in patients with chronic chest pathology such as obstructive airways disease and asthma should be reduced by effective management of these conditions. Hormone replacement therapy may also decrease the incidence of prolapse, although to date there are no studies that have tested this effect.

Smaller family size and improvements in antenatal and intrapartum care have also been implicated in the primary prevention of urogenital prolapse. The role of caesarean section may also be important, although studies examining the outcome in terms of incontinence and symptomatic prolapse have had mixed results. Equally, antenatal and postnatal pelvic floor exercises have not yet been shown conclusively to reduce the incidence of prolapse, although they may be protective.

Physiotherapy

Pelvic floor exercises may have a role in the treatment of women with symptomatic prolapse, although there are no objective evidence-based studies to support this. Education about pelvic floor exercises may be supplemented with the use of a perineometer and biofeedback, allowing quantification of pelvic floor contractions. In addition, vaginal cones and electrical stimulation may also be used, although again, whilst they have been shown to be effective in the treatment of urodynamic stress incontinence, there are no data to support their use in the management of urogenital prolapse.

In summary, physiotherapy probably has a role in cases of mild prolapse in younger women who find an intravaginal device unacceptable and are not yet willing to consider definitive surgical treatment, especially if they have not yet completed their family.

Intravaginal devices

The use of intravaginal devices offers a further conservative line of therapy for those women who are not candidates for surgery. Consequently they may be used in younger women who have not yet completed their family, during pregnancy and the puerperium, and also for those women who may be unfit for surgery. Clearly this last group of women may include the elderly, although age alone should not be seen as a contraindication to surgery. In addition, a pessary may offer symptomatic relief whilst awaiting surgery.

Ring pessaries made of silicone or polythene are currently most frequently used. They are available in a number of different sizes (52–120 mm) and are designed to lie horizontally in the pelvis with one side in the posterior fornix and the other just behind the pubis, hence providing support to the uterus and upper vagina. Pessaries should be changed every 6 months; long-term use may be complicated by vaginal ulceration and therefore a low-dose topical oestrogen may be helpful in postmenopausal women.

Ring pessaries may be useful in the management of minor degrees of urogenital prolapse, although in severe cases, and for vaginal vault prolapse, a shelf pessary may be more appropriate. These may be difficult to insert and remove and their use is becoming less common, especially as they preclude coitus.

SURGERY

Surgery offers definitive treatment of urogenital prolapse. As in other forms of pelvic surgery, patients should receive prophylactic antibiotics to cover both Gram-negative and Gram-positive organisms, as well as thromboembolic prophylaxis in the form of low-dose heparin, and thromboembolic deterrent (TED) stockings.

All patients should also have a urethral catheter inserted at the time of the procedure unless there is a particular history of voiding dysfunction, in which case a suprapubic catheter may be more appropriate. This allows the residual urine volume to be checked following a void without the need for re-catheterization.

Patients having pelvic surgery are positioned in lithotomy with the hips abducted and flexed. To minimize blood loss, local infiltration of the vaginal epithelium is performed using 0.5 per cent xylocaine and 1/200 000 adrenaline, although care should be taken in patients with co-existent cardiac disease. A vaginal pack may be inserted at the end of the procedure, and removed on the first postoperative day.

Anterior compartment defects

Anterior colporrhaphy
INDICATION
Correction of cystourethrocele.

PROCEDURE
A midline incision is made in the vaginal epithelium from 1 cm below the urethral meatus to the cervix or vaginal vault. The cystocele is dissected off the overlying epithelium using sharp and blunt dissection and is secured using two polyglycolic (Vicryl, Ethicon) or polydioxanone (PDS, Ethicon) purse-string sutures. The redundant skin edges are then trimmed and the epithelium and fascia closed using interrupted polyglycolic (Vicryl, Ethicon) sutures.

In patients who have mild concurrent stress incontinence, a 'Kelly' mattress suture[4] may be placed under the urethrovesical junction, although colposuspension is preferable in cases of severe stress incontinence and will also cure a mild to moderate cystocele.

Lower urinary tract injury is uncommon. However, should a bladder or urethral injury occur, the defect can be repaired in layers using absorbable sutures and the bladder left on free drainage for 10 days.

Paravaginal repair
INDICATION
Correction of cystourethrocele.

PROCEDURE
First described in 1909, this offers an abdominal approach to correct an anterior compartment defect. The retropubic space (cave of Retzius) is opened through a Pfannenstiel incision and the bladder swept medially, exposing the pelvic sidewall. The lateral sulcus of the vagina is elevated with the overlying pubocervical fascia and re-attached to the pelvic sidewall using interrupted polydioxanone (PDS, Ethicon) sutures from the pubis to just anterior to the ischial spine. Long-term follow-up in a series of 800 patients reported a cure rate of more than 95 per cent.[5]

Posterior compartment defects

Posterior colporrhaphy
INDICATION
Correction of rectocele and deficient perineum.

PROCEDURE
Two Allis forceps are first placed on the perineum at the level of the hymenal remnants, allowing the calibre of the introitus to be estimated. Following infiltration, the perineal scarring is excised and the posterior vaginal wall opened using a longitudinal incision. The rectocele is mobilized from the vaginal epithelium by blunt and sharp dissection and secured using two or more polyglycolic (Vicryl, Ethicon) or polydioxanone (PDS, Ethicon) purse-string sutures. The redundant skin edges are then trimmed, taking care not to remove too much tissue and thus narrow the vagina. The pararectal and rectovaginal fasciae from each side are approximated using interrupted polyglycolic (Vicryl, Ethicon) sutures incorporating the vaginal epithelium, and the posterior wall is closed with a continuous polyglycolic (Vicryl, Ethicon) suture. Care should be taken not to create a constriction ring in the vagina, which will result in dyspareunia. Finally, a perineoplasty is performed by placing deeper absorbable sutures into the perineal muscles and fascia, thus building up the perineal body to provide additional support to the posterior vaginal wall and lengthening the vagina.

Injury to the rectum is unusual, but should be identified at the time of the procedure so that the defect can be closed in layers using an absorbable suture and the patient managed with prophylactic antibiotics, low-residue diet and faecal softening agents to avoid constipation.

Pelvic floor surgery may also have an adverse effect on sexual function. Following pelvic floor repairs with or without vaginal hysterectomy, 50 per cent of women reported sexual dysfunction, nearly half of the cases being due to shortening of the vagina, dyspareunia or fear of injury.[6] These findings have been confirmed more recently in a follow-up study of women undergoing posterior repair.[7] This series reported an increase in sexual dysfunction from 11 per cent preoperatively to 27 per cent following surgery. In addition, 22 per cent of women complained of vaginal pain, 11 per cent had incontinence of faeces and 33 per cent had constipation.

Enterocele repair
INDICATION
Correction of enterocele.

PROCEDURE
An enterocele repair is normally performed using a vaginal approach similar to that of posterior colporrhaphy. The vaginal epithelium is dissected off the enterocele sac, which is then secured using two or more polyglycolic (Vicryl, Ethicon) or polydioxanone (PDS, Ethicon) purse-string sutures. It is

not essential to open the enterocele sac, although care should be taken not to damage any loops of small bowel that it may contain. The posterior vaginal wall is then closed as described for posterior colporrhaphy.

An abdominal approach may also be used, although this is much less common. The Moschowitz procedure[8] is performed by inserting concentric purse-string sutures around the peritoneum in the pouch of Douglas, thus preventing enterocele formation.

Uterovaginal prolapse

Vaginal hysterectomy
INDICATION
Uterovaginal prolapse. This procedure may be combined with anterior and posterior colporrhaphy.

CONTRAINDICATIONS (RELATIVE)
- Uterine size >14 weeks' gestation although morcellation[9] or uterine bisection may be used.
- Two or more caesarean sections.
- Endometriosis.
- Pelvic inflammatory disease.
- Suspected malignancy (uterine or ovarian).

PROCEDURE
A cervical incision is performed and the uterovesical fold and pouch of Douglas opened. The uterosacral and cardinal ligaments are divided and ligated first, followed by the uterine pedicles and finally the tubo-ovarian and round ligament pedicles. In cases of procidentia, care should be taken to avoid kinking of the ureters, which are often dragged into a lower position than normal. After closure of the pelvic peritoneum, the upper pedicles are tied in the midline to provide support for the vaginal vault, whilst the uterosacral ligaments are tied posteriorly to obliterate the potential enterocele space. In addition, a McCall suture[10] may be performed, bringing the two uterosacral ligaments together in the midline as a further precaution against enterocele formation. Inclusion of the upper posterior vaginal wall also provides additional vault support. The vaginal epithelium is then closed with interrupted sutures.

Manchester repair (Fothergill repair)
INDICATION
Uterovaginal prolapse with preservation of fertility.

PROCEDURE
This procedure is only rarely performed nowadays. Cervical amputation is followed by approximating and shortening the cardinal ligaments anterior to the cervical stump and elevating the uterus. This is combined with an anterior and posterior colporrhaphy. The operation has fallen from favour, as the long-term complications include fertility problems in

addition to recurrent uterovaginal prolapse and enterocele formation.

Vaginal vault prolapse

Vaginal vault prolapse occurs equally commonly following vaginal or abdominal hysterectomy, with an incidence of approximately 5 per cent, although only 0.5 per cent of women require further surgery.

Sacrospinous ligament fixation
INDICATION
Vaginal vault prolapse.

PROCEDURE
A longitudinal posterior vaginal wall incision is performed to expose the rectovaginal space. The right ischial spine is then identified and exposed using sharp and blunt dissection. The sacrospinous ligament may then be palpated running from the ischial spine to the lower aspect of the sacrum. An absorbable braided polyglycolic suture (Dexon, Davies+Geck) is passed through the ligament using a Miya hook ligature carrier and then through the vaginal vault. Care must be taken to avoid the sacral plexus and sciatic nerve, which are superior, and the pudendal vessels and nerve, which are lateral to the ischial spine. Once the enterocele has been secured using two purse-string sutures, the upper third of the vagina is closed as previously described. The sacrospinous sutures are then tied to support the vaginal vault from the sacrospinous ligament, following which a perineorrhaphy is performed.

Success rates of 98 per cent have been reported,[11] although posterior fixation of the posterior vaginal wall increases the incidence of anterior compartment defects. For this reason it should not be performed routinely at vaginal hysterectomy. As the vaginal axis is changed by the procedure, there is a risk of postoperative dyspareunia and development of stress incontinence.

Abdominal sacrocolpopexy
INDICATION
Vaginal vault prolapse.

PROCEDURE
This procedure may be performed through a lower midline or Pfannenstiel incision after packing the vagina. The apex of the vagina and sacral promontory are identified and a retroperitoneal tunnel is created between the two just to the right of the midline and medial to the right ureter. A strip of Mersilene tape is then passed through the peritoneal tunnel and sutured to the vaginal vault and posterior vaginal wall using interrupted, non-absorbable ethylene sutures (Ethibond, Ethicon). Once the other end of the tape has been secured to the periosteum overlying the sacral promontory, the sutures are tied, allowing gentle elevation of the vaginal vault towards the sacrum but without tension. The peritoneum

is then closed over the vaginal vault and sacral promontory. Complications include bleeding from the presacral venous plexus and sacral artery and damage to the right ureter and sigmoid colon.

A 93 per cent success rate has been reported,[12] although associated cystocele or rectocele may still require a vaginal colporrhaphy. In addition, since the vaginal axis is changed, there is also the risk of developing dyspareunia and stress incontinence following the procedure. Mesh erosion into the vagina, and rarely into the bladder or bowel, is a possible late complication.

Posterior intravaginal slingplasty

INDICATION

Vaginal vault prolapse

PROCEDURE

The posterior intravaginal slingplasty (IVS), using an 8 mm polypropylene tape, has been described as a minimally invasive procedure for the treatment of vaginal vault prolapse. Under tension a 5 cm transverse full thickness incision is made in the posterior vaginal wall 1.5 cm below the scar line at the vaginal vault. Adjacent rectocele and enterocele are than dissected out so as to avoid accidental damage whilst passing the IVS tunneller (Tyco Healthcare, USA) needle. Bilateral 1 cm perineal skin incisions are then made 2 cm lateral and below the external anal sphincter at the 4 and 8 o'clock positions.

Next the IVS tunneller is advanced 4 cm into the ischirectal fossa before being turned inwards and guided using a finger through the rectovaginal fascia so as to exit through the transverse vaginal incision. The procedure is then repeated on the contralateral side and a rectal examination performed to exclude bowel injury. The tape is then secured to the vaginal vault using polydioxanone (PDS, Ethicon) and the vagina closed with interupted polyglycolic (Vicryl, Ethicon) sutures. A posterior colpoperineorrhaphy is then performed as previously described. Finally the polypropylene tape is pulled posteriorly through the bilateral buttock incisions pulling the vaginal vault in a postero-superior direction. The tape is then cut flush with the skin and incisions closed using interrupted sutures.

To date only one retrospective series of posterior intravaginal slingplast has been reported[13] with symptomatic cure rates of 91%. However there were five cases of tape rejection, one rectal tape erosion and one rectal perforation. Consequently, whilst early data would appear to be encouraging, more studies are required to determine its role in the management of vaginal vault prolapse.

Recurrent urogenital prolapse

Approximately one-third of operations for urogenital prolapse are for recurrent defects. Recurrent prolapse may occur following both abdominal and vaginal hysterectomy, previous vaginal repairs and continence surgery. In addition, women with intrinsically weak connective tissue, such as patients with Elhers Danlos syndrome, are at increased risk.

In such cases the vaginal epithelium may be scarred and atrophic, making surgical correction technically more difficult and increasing the risk of damage to the bladder and bowel. The risk of postoperative complications such as dyspareunia secondary to vaginal shortening and stenosis is also increased. In those women who have had a previous continence operation, such as colposuspension, there is an increased risk of recurrent incontinence that may require further surgical correction.

The use of synthetic mesh is becoming increasingly common in patients with recurrent defects, and may offer further support in cases in which the endopelvic fascia and vaginal epithelium are felt to be deficient. The ideal mesh should be strong and flexible, allowing ease of use. In addition, woven meshes should have an adequate pore size to allow the ingrowth of fibroblasts so as to minimize the risks of erosion and rejection. At present, Mersilene (Ethicon) mesh is commonly used, although currently Vypro (Ethicon) mesh is under evaluation. As this is a combination weave of an absorbable suture – Vicryl (Ethicon) – and a non-absorbable – Prolene (Ethicon) – it may offer an improvement in terms of outcome. A further alternative is the use of porcine collagen harvested from pig intestine or pig dermis although these too are currently undergoing clinical evaluation. Dyspareunia is a common complication associated with the use of synthetic mesh and may be associated with erosion into the vagina, lower urinary tract and rectum. Although the use of mesh is becoming more common, it should be reserved for those patients with recurrent defects in specialist pelvic floor reconstructive surgery units.

CONCLUSION

Although not life threatening, urogenital prolapse is responsible for a significant degree of morbidity and impairment of quality of life. With approximately half of elective gynaecological operations being performed for correction of urogenital prolapse, the economic considerations are also considerable. In common with continence procedures, the initial procedure offers the greatest probability of success, and therefore patients should be carefully assessed with regard to their symptoms and investigations prior to surgery.

Although conservative measures may be useful in the management of mild symptomatic prolapse, surgery offers the definitive treatment. The number of surgical procedures described is indicative of the fact that there is no perfect solution, and this is reflected in the number of patients who complain of recurrent prolapse. Such women should be managed in tertiary units by surgeons with a specialist interest in pelvic floor reconstructive surgery.

KEY POINTS

- Urogenital prolapse is a common condition associated with a high degree of morbidity.
- Incidence increases with increasing age and parity.
- Lifetime risk of surgery for urogenital prolapse is 11 per cent.
- Urogenital prolapse may be associated with concomitant urinary and faecal incontinence.
- Conservative management involves pelvic floor exercises and the use of vaginal pessaries.
- Surgery should be tailored to the needs of the individual patient.
- The use of synthetic mesh should be reserved for re-do procedures only.
- There is a high risk of recurrence following surgery, with a third of women requiring a further procedure.
- Complicated or recurrent cases are best managed using a multidisciplinary approach.

KEY REFERENCES

1. Subak LL, Waetjen E, van den Eeden S, Thom DH, Vittinghoff E, Brown JS. Cost of pelvic organ prolapse surgery in the United States. *Obstet Gynecol* 2001; 98:646–51.
2. Abrams P, Blaivas JG, Stanton SL, Andersen JT. The International Continence Society Committee on Standardization of Terminology. The standardization of terminology of lower urinary tract function. *Scand J Urol Nephrol* 1988; 114S:5–19.
3. Smith ARB, Hosker GL, Warrell DW. The role of partial denervation of the pelvic floor in the aetiology of genitourinary prolapse and stress incontinence. A neurophysiological study. *Br J Obstet Gynaecol* 1989; 96:24–8.
4. Kelly HA. Incontinence of urine in women. *Urol Cutan Rev* 1913; 17:291–7.
5. Richardson AC. Paravaginal repair. In: Benson JT (ed.). *Female Pelvic Floor Disorders*. New York: Norton, 1992, 280–7.
6. Francis WJA, Jeffcoate TNA. Dyspareunia following vaginal operations. *Br J Obstet Gynaecol* 1961; 68:1.
7. Kahn MA, Stanton SL. Posterior colporrhaphy: its effects on bowel and sexual function. *Br J Obstet Gynaecol* 1997; 104:82–6.
8. Muschovitz AV. The pathogenesis, anatomy and cure of prolapse of the rectum. *Surg Gynecol Obstet* 1912; 15:7.
9. Magos A, Bournas N, Sinha R, Richardson R, O'Connor H. Vaginal hysterectomy for the large uterus. *Br J Obstet Gynaecol* 1996; 103:246–51.
10. McCall ML. Posterior culdoplasty. *Obstet Gynecol* 1957; 10:595.
11. Shull BL, Capen CV, Riggs MW, Kuehl TJ. Pre-operative and post-operative analysis of site-specific pelvic support defects in 81 women treated with sacrospinous ligament suspension and pelvic reconstruction. *Am J Obstet Gynecol* 1992; 166:1764–71.
12. Addison WA, Livergood CH, Parker RT. Post hysterectomy vaginal vault prolapse with emphasis on management by transabdominal sacral colpopexy. *Post Grad Obstet Gynaecol* 1988; 81.
13. Farnsworth BN. Posterior intravaginal slingplasty (infracoccygeal sacrocolpopexy) for severe posthysterectomy vaginal vault prolapse – a preliminary report on efficacy and safety. *Int Urogynecol J* 2002; 13:4–8.

Infection and Sexual Health

Melanie C. Mann

PELVIC INFLAMMATORY DISEASE

This section covers the diagnosis, treatment and follow-up of PID. PID is important because it can have serious long-term sequelae such as pelvic pain, ectopic pregnancy and infertility. It is the result of post-infection scarring that is normally associated with healing. The virulence of the infection and the host immune factors both determine the extent of the damage caused. There may be complete tubal closure, extensive peritubal adhesions, intratubal adhesions, mucosal and cilial damage, all of which can cause ectopic pregnancy and infertility (including interference with ovum transport and sperm migration). In a large, multicentre World Health Organization (WHO) study of more than 8000 couples in 25 countries investigated for infertility, approximately 32 per cent of diagnoses were tubal factor infertility in the female.[1]

Incidence

The incidence of PID is unknown, as many cases go unnoticed until investigations for infertility are performed. There is no record of cases of PID held nationally apart from diagnosed records of all attendances at genitourinary (GUM) clinics (KC 60 returns).

Aetiology

Neisseria gonorrhoeae and *Chlamydia trachomatis* are the most important organisms, although *Gardnerella vaginalis*, anaerobes and other organisms such as mycoplasmas commonly found in the vagina may also be implicated.

Other factors associated with PID include:

- young age (<25 years)
- multiple sexual partners
- past history of STI (in the patient or her partners)
- termination of pregnancy
- insertion of an intrauterine contraceptive device in the past 6 weeks
- hysterosalpingography
- in-vitro fertilization procedure
- postpartum endometritis
- bacterial vaginosis
- a recent new sexual partner (within the previous 3 months).

Diagnosis

Pelvic inflammatory disease can be symptomatic or asymptomatic. Even in symptomatic patients, clinical symptoms and signs lack sensitivity and specificity. The positive predictive value of a clinical diagnosis is 65–90 per cent compared to laparoscopic diagnosis in experienced hands.[2,3] The symptoms suggestive of PID include:

- lower abdominal pain
- dyspareunia
- unscheduled vaginal bleeding
- abnormal vaginal discharge.

The signs associated with PID are usually also non-specific. Pyrexia may be present, but not exclusively. Lower abdominal and adnexal tenderness on bimanual examination as well as cervical excitation (cervical motion tenderness) on bimanual examination are indicative of acute inflammation affecting the pelvic peritoneum. However, they are not specific for PID. Other conditions that should be considered when assessing lower abdominal pain in a young woman include:

- ectopic pregnancy
- acute appendicitis
- endometriosis
- complications of an ovarian cyst (torsion or rupture)
- constipation
- functional pain (pain of unknown origin).

Investigation of suspected pelvic inflammatory disease

Testing for gonorrhoea and chlamydia in the lower genital tract is recommended, as positive results support a diagnosis. However, the absence of infection at this site does not exclude PID. Absence of cultured organisms may be due to poor sampling technique, inadequate storage and/or transportation of swabs or the presence of organisms that cannot easily be cultured in the laboratory, such as mycoplasmas. An elevated erythrocyte sedimentation rate (ESR) or C-reactive protein (CRP) can support the diagnosis.

Laparoscopy may strongly support the diagnosis of PID but is not justified routinely on the basis of cost and invasiveness. Furthermore, even laparoscopy lacks the sensitivity to identify mild intratubal inflammation or endometritis reliably.

Endometrial biopsy and ultrasound scanning may also be helpful when there is diagnostic difficulty, but there is insufficient evidence to support their routine use at present.

Management

It is likely that delay in treatment increases the risk of the development of long-term sequelae of PID such as ectopic pregnancy, pelvic pain and infertility. Owing to this, and to the lack of definitive diagnostic criteria, it is recommended that clinicians have a low threshold for treating empirically.

It is also important that women are not labelled with the wrong diagnosis just because they appear to be in a high-risk group for having PID. Effort must be made to confirm the correct diagnosis, particularly in difficult or recurrent episodes of lower abdominal pain. It is also important in the gynaecological setting *not* to forget to investigate and treat the sexual partner(s), in order to prevent re-infection.

General measures

- Rest is advised for severe disease (preferably as an inpatient for observation to check that there is resolution of symptoms and signs) [II].
- A pregnancy test should be performed [II].
- Appropriate analgesia is advised [II].
- Parenteral therapy as an inpatient is advised for those with severe disease [II].
- Patients should avoid sexual intercourse until they and their partners have been fully treated and contact traced [II].

A full explanation should be given to the patient regarding the short-term and long-term issues associated with PID. Leaflets to clarify and back-up verbal explanation should be given to the client and her partner, if present.

All patients should be offered full STI screening and human immunodeficiency virus (HIV) testing at some point in the management [II]. Good links with local GUM clinics are essential.

Antibiotic treatment

Broad-spectrum antibiotics are needed that will cover gonorrhoea and chlamydia. There is a lack of evidence regarding antibiotic use and the prevention of long-term complications and fewer data on oral than parenteral regimens. There are important factors to be considered when choosing a regimen:

- local antimicrobial sensitivities (especially gonorrhoea),
- local epidemiology of infections (knowing where there are high-prevalence areas for gonorrhoea),
- cost,
- patient preference and likelihood of compliance,
- severity of disease.

When considering selection for inpatient treatment, the uncertainty of the diagnosis and severity of the disease will usually be sufficient to identify those who require inpatient observation. Other cases for which inpatient supervision is advised include women who have failed to respond to orally administered outpatient therapy, those who are suspected of having a tubo-ovarian mass and those who are unable to tolerate oral therapy. Two special subgroups might also be considered for inpatient treatment: those known to have an immunodeficiency problem (where a much more severe disease situation can develop quickly) and those who are pregnant – PID can occur up to about 12 weeks of pregnancy.

Recommended regimens

The following are evidence based. Intravenous therapy should be continued until 24 hours after clinical improvement and then switched to oral treatment [Ib].

OUTPATIENT REGIMENS

- Oral ofloxacin 400 mg twice daily plus oral metronidazole 500 mg twice daily for 14 days.
- Intramuscular (i.m.) ceftriaxone 250 mg single dose or i.m. cefoxitin 2 g single dose with oral probenecid 1 g followed by oral doxycycline 100 mg daily plus metronidazole 400 mg twice daily for 14 days.

INPATIENT REGIMENS

- Intravenous (i.v.) cefoxitin 2 g four times daily (or i.v. cefotetan 2 g twice daily) plus i.v. doxycycline 100 mg twice daily (oral doxycycline may be used if tolerated) followed by oral doxycycline 100 mg twice daily plus oral metronidazole 400 mg twice daily for a total of 14 days, **or**
- i.v. clindamycin 900 mg three times daily plus i.v. gentamycin (2 mg/kg loading dose followed by 1.5 mg/kg three times daily – a single daily dose may be substituted) followed by either oral clindamycin 450 mg four times daily or oral doxycycline 100 mg twice daily to complete 14 days, plus oral metronidazole 400 mg twice daily to complete 14 days.

If the above regimens are not available, 14 days' therapy to cover *N. gonorrhoeae* (quinolones, cephalosporins, penicillin – bearing in mind sensitivities locally), *C. trachomatis* (tetracyclines, macrolides) and anaerobic bacteria (metronidazole) should be used.

Other important situations

Women with HIV may have more severe disease and so i.v. therapy may be preferable.

Pregnant women should ideally receive i.v. therapy, as PID is associated with higher maternal and fetal morbidity. None of the regimens above is of proven safety in this group. There is insufficient evidence in pregnant women to suggest one treatment over another as long as the appropriate organisms are covered for 14 days' treatment and this is parenteral if possible.

Fitz–Hugh–Curtis syndrome comprises right upper quadrant pain associated with perihepatitis, which occurs in up to 10–20 per cent of women with PID and may be the most obvious symptom. There is insufficient evidence to recommend laparoscopic adhesiolysis in this situation.

Management of partners should be by testing and treatment, ideally in a GUM clinic. Empirical treatment should be given anyway if testing cannot be done. Contact tracing of all partners in the previous 6 months is recommended.

Follow-up

All patients should be followed up at 3 days to check improvement and exclude the need for parenteral or surgical treatment. Further review at 4 weeks is recommended to check resolution of symptoms and to discuss long-term issues. It is also an ideal time to check up on partner notification and treatment.

SEXUALLY TRANSMITTED INFECTIONS

This section focuses generally on the management of women, but one should not forget to consider partners and to think about them when talking about this aspect of gynaecology. Talking about these very personal aspects of a woman's life is very important and all gynaecologists need to be able to talk about sex sensitively and non-judgementally in order to do the best for the patient. It is therefore important that clinicians practise taking a sexual history to achieve this (see below).

Sexually transmitted infections are an important part of the everyday work of a gynaecologist and these conditions can have long-term sequelae for the patient if not managed promptly and thoroughly. The majority of large towns and cities in the UK have a department of GUM with at least one specialist employed. It is good practice to develop strong links with this local department to improve the overall management of STIs within each gynaecology unit. This will ensure that patients receive optimum evidence-based treatment and that contact tracing and partner notification are performed according to approved guidelines.

Taking a sexual history to assess the risk of STI

Preface by warning the patient that you need to ask some personal questions to do with her relationships with partners.

I need to ask you some personal questions now.
Are you in a sexual relationship?

You need to find out if this is a heterosexual or homosexual relationship. This is one of the most difficult questions. You can ask the first name of the partner and then clarify whether male or female if the first name is equivocal, e.g. Nicky or Chris. Or you can say, *Can I just check, is your partner male or female?*

How long have you been with your partner?

Avoid the term 'steady' or 'long term' as these have different meanings for different people.

Do you or your partner have any other partners, as far as you are aware?

In some situations it is important to ask about different sexual practices such as oral or anal sex. Sometimes patients may volunteer the information that sex in a particular position causes discomfort, so it is important to be able to discuss this openly.

Basic tenets of GUM

- The patient's confidentiality is paramount and patient details are not given to other patients or other healthcare professionals without the patient's informed consent.
- If a patient has a STI, at least one other person is also carrying it and needs to be sought, treated and contact traced.
- If a patient has one STI, she must be at risk of all other STIs. She should therefore be offered screening for all other infections. This will often be carried out in a GUM clinic.
- When swabs for STI are taken, it is important to obtain informed consent about the nature of the tests and explain what the follow-up procedure will be if the test is positive for a STI.
- Patients diagnosed with a STI should be advised not to have sexual intercourse until they and their partners have completed treatment and follow-up. This is to minimize further spread or re-infection.
- Patients should be given a detailed account of their condition, with particular emphasis on the long-term implications for themselves and their partner(s). This should be reinforced with clear and accurate written information.

Terms used in GUM clinics

Partner notification

Contact slips, with a nationally agreed code for each STI, are given to patients to pass on to their sexual contacts. Contacts can then present the slip at any GUM clinic in the UK, where the infection will be managed appropriately. This is because there is communication between GUM clinics regarding partner notification.

Contact tracing

This involves finding the sexual contacts of the index patient carrying an infection and managing them appropriately, including ongoing partner notification if possible.

Health advisors

These are specially trained professionals whose job is to educate patients in the GUM clinics about STIs, including pre-test counselling for HIV. They are also responsible for most partner notification and contact tracing.

Gonorrhoea

Gonorrhoea is a sexually transmitted infection caused by the Gram-negative diplococcus *N. gonorrhoeae*. The primary sites of infection are the mucous membranes of the urethra, endocervix, rectum, pharynx and conjunctiva. Transmission occurs as a result of direct inoculation of secretions from one mucous membrane to another. Vertical transmission from mother to fetus may also occur during labour.

Clinical features

Up to 50 per cent of women are asymptomatic. In those who do have symptoms, the most common are an increased or altered vaginal discharge (up to 50 per cent) and lower abdominal pain (up to 25 per cent). Urethral infection may cause dysuria (12 per cent) but not usually frequency. Gonorrhoea is a rare cause of intermenstrual bleeding or menorrhagia and this is due to infection of the endometrium (endometritis). Infection in the pharynx is usually asymptomatic.

In men, the infection may also be asymptomatic (<10 per cent) but generally causes urethral discharge (80 per cent) or dysuria (50 per cent).

Clinical signs

Less than 50 per cent of women will present with mucopurulent endocervical discharge and easily induced endocervical bleeding, and less than 5 per cent will present with pelvic or lower abdominal tenderness. Commonly no abnormal findings are present on clinical examination. In men, there is usually a purulent urethral discharge present. Epididymal tenderness or balanitis, although reported, is rare.

Gonorrhoea is also transmitted vertically to the fetus. It can cause severe conjunctivitis (ophthalmia neonatorum) and this is a notifiable disease in the UK. Neonatal infections can be severe and should be managed systemically by a paediatrician/ophthalmologist.

Complications

Transluminal spread of *N. gonorrhoeae* may occur, causing PID (<10 per cent) and epididymo-orchitis (<1 per cent) in men. Haematogenous dissemination can also occur, causing skin lesions, arthralgia, arthritis and tenosynovitis. Disseminated gonococcal infection is rare (<1 per cent).

Diagnosis

The most reliable diagnosis is achieved by identification by culture of the organism from an infected site. Specimen collection in women should be from the endocervix and urethra, with the swab being rotated to obtain purulent secretions, if present. Infection of the cervix is present in 90 per cent of women with gonorrhoea, and the use of cervical culture as a single screening test for gonorrhoea has a sensitivity of 85 per cent.

Management

All patients should be treated if they have a positive test result or if a recent partner has confirmed gonococcal disease and testing of the patient is not possible. Referral to GUM is highly recommended [Ib].

Recommended treatment in uncomplicated infection in adults (i.e. not PID)

- Ciprofloxacin 500 mg orally as a single dose [Ia], **or**
- Ofloxacin 400 mg orally as a single dose [Ia], **or**
- Ampicillin 2 g or 3 g plus probenecid 1 g orally as a single dose where regional prevalence of penicillin-resistant *N. gonorrhoeae* is <5 per cent [Ib].

Chosen treatment regimens must take into account the local sensitivities and should eliminate infection in at least 95 per cent of those presenting in the local community. Continued surveillance of resistance is important, as this may change over time. This is another reason why all cases should be referred to GUM in the UK.

Treatment of gonorrhoea when pregnant or breastfeeding

Pregnant women should not be treated with quinolone or tetracycline antimicrobial.

Recommended regimes
- ceftriaxone 250 mg i.m. as a single dose [Ia], **or**
- cefotaxime 500 mg i.m. as a single dose [Ia], **or**
- spectinomycin 2 g i.m. as a single dose [Ia], **or**
- ampicillin 2 g or 3 g plus probenecid 1 g orally as a single dose where regional prevalence of penicillin- resistant *N. gonorrhoeae* is <5 per cent [Ib].

In the case of allergy, the above regimes can be used.

Co-infection with *C. trachomatis* is common (up to 40 per cent of women) and therefore screening and, if positive, treatment should always be performed. Partner notification and contact tracing should be performed as described previously [Ib].

Follow-up

At least one follow-up visit is recommended to confirm compliance with therapy, resolution of symptoms and partner notification. A test of cure is usually performed in UK practice, which entails obtaining cultures at least 72 hours after the completion of therapy [II]. If infection is identified after treatment, this usually indicates re-infection rather than treatment failure.

Chlamydia trachomatis

Chlamydia trachomatis genital infection is common; in UK general practice it affects 3–5 per cent of sexually active women. The chlamydia opportunistic screening pilot studies involving women under the age of 25 in Portsmouth and the Wirral are reporting a higher prevalence of approximately 10 per cent (interim information), which may reflect the age group screened.[4] Infection is sustained by unrecognized and untreated, symptomless chlamydial infection. It is now thought that overall the complication of this infection costs at least £50 million annually in the UK.

Clinical features

Eighty per cent of infected women are asymptomatic. When symptoms are present they include postcoital or intermenstrual bleeding, lower abdominal pain, purulent vaginal discharge, mucopurulent cervicitis and/or contact bleeding. Fifty per cent of men are asymptomatic, with urethral discharge and dysuria being the most common symptoms. The risk factors associated with chlamydial infection include young age (<25 years), new sexual partner or more than one sexual partner in recent years. There is also an association with contraceptive practice, with infection being less common in barrier contraception users and more common in those using combined oral contraception. Women undergoing termination of pregnancy also appear to have a higher association with chlamydial infection.

Complications

One of the immediate complications is developing PID. In chlamydial PID, perihepatitis can also occur; this is known as Fitz–Hugh–Curtis syndrome. As with other types of PID, the long-term sequelae include tubal damage resulting in an increased risk of infertility and ectopic pregnancy and chronic pelvic pain. Chlamydia can be transmitted to the neonate at the time of delivery, causing neonatal conjunctivitis and pneumonia. Less common outcomes include adult conjunctivitis and sexually acquired reactive arthritis or Reiter's syndrome. This is more common in men who have chronic chlamydial infection.

Specimen collection

Chlamydia is an obligate intracellular parasite; it is therefore imperative that samples contain cellular material. Cervical swabs are ideally the best; these should be inserted inside the cervical os and firmly rotated against the endocervix. Pus on the swab is not useful for chlamydial tests, and inadequate specimens reduce the sensitivity of all diagnostic tests. There is no consensus on how to take a urethral swab in women. It is now also possible to test first-pass

Pelvic floor and lower urinary tract

urine specimens and vulvo-vaginal swabs and there is some recent evidence that testing for *C. trachomatis* may be more accurate if it is performed in the latter part of the menstrual cycle.[5]

Laboratory tests for *C. trachomatis*

This is a rapidly developing and somewhat complex field. There is currently a Chlamydia Screening Study (ClaSS) underway which will investigate which specimen and which test are the most cost effective for diagnosing chlamydial infection. Originally, diagnosis depended on cell culture, but this is now done in only very few laboratories in the UK. It has high specificity, which is essential for medicolegal work, but sensitivities can be as low as 40 per cent. In addition, it is expensive, labour intensive and requires expertise.

Enzyme immunoassays (EIAs) have a high specificity (>99 per cent) when combined with a confirmation assay. However, their sensitivity is variable and assay dependent and can be as low as 50–60 per cent, yet in other assays as high as 99 per cent. EIA is cheap, automatable and therefore suitable for large numbers of tests. Positives are often confirmed by direct fluorescent antibody (DFA) tests.

Direct fluorescent antibody testing is highly sensitive in experienced hands but is labour intensive and so is not suitable for large numbers. It can be used for confirmation of other assays. The sensitivity is 50–90 per cent and the specificity is >95 per cent.

Nucleic acid amplification techniques (NAATs) are the newest and most expensive tests. They have very high sensitivity and specificity (56–100 per cent and >99 per cent respectively). However, the sensitivity of the test may be influenced by transportation, storage and pregnancy. It seems likely that this test will revolutionize large-scale screening, as it functions with urine and vulvo-vaginal swabs and with time will become more available and less expensive.

It is recommended that chlamydial tests should have an ideal sensitivity >90 per cent and specificity >99 per cent. NAATs come closest to this ideal. If EIA is used, it should be confirmed by DFA or NAAT.

Treatment

The recommended treatment of uncomplicated chlamydial infection is with doxycycline 100 mg twice a day for 7 days or azithromycin 1 g orally in a single dose [Ia]. Alternative regimens include erythromycin 500 mg four times a day for 7 days or erythromycin 500 mg twice a day for 14 days. The majority of studies are flawed in design, small and give no details regarding the treatment of sexual partners. Doxycycline and azithromycin have been the most rigorously tested. Quinolones and tetracyclines should not be used in pregnancy; the safety of azithromycin in pregnancy and breastfeeding has not yet been fully evaluated.

Follow-up of chlamydial infection is recommended to check partner notification, re-inforce health education, assess treatment efficacy and exclude re-infection [Ib].

Trichomonal infection

The causative organism is *Trichomonas vaginalis*. This is a flagellated protozoon, which is found in the vagina, urethra and paraurethral glands. Transmission is almost exclusively sexual in adults. It can be acquired perinatally and occurs in 5 per cent of babies born to infected mothers. If infection is found after the first year, sexual contact is implied, although other modes of transmission are postulated.

Clinical features

Between 10 and 50 per cent of women are asymptomatic [Ib]; amongst the remainder, the commonest symptoms are vaginal discharge, vulval itching, dysuria and offensive odour. Occasionally, lower abdominal pain may be present. Seventy per cent of infected women have a vaginal discharge, which can vary in consistency from thin and scanty to profuse and thick. The classical frothy yellow discharge occurs in 10–30 per cent. Vulvitis, vaginitis and cervicitis are associated with trichomonal infection. A 'strawberry cervix' appearance is visible to the naked eye in approximately 2 per cent of cases and in more women on colposcopy. No abnormalities are found in 10–15 per cent of women.

Complications

There is increasing evidence that trichomonal infection can have a detrimental effect on pregnancy and is associated with preterm delivery and low birth-weight infants [Ib].

Diagnosis

Direct observation of a wet smear from the posterior fornix will diagnose 40–80 per cent of cases, whereas culture of the organism will correctly diagnose 95 per cent of infected women. Trichomonads are sometimes reported on cervical cytology, the sensitivity being about 60–80 per cent, but the false-positive rate is about 30 per cent, so that if a cervical smear report suggests trichomonad infection, it is worth confirming the diagnosis by the above two methods. Diagnostic tests based on the polymerase chain reaction (PCR) have recently been developed and sensitivities and specificities approaching 100 per cent have been reported.

Treatment

Systemic chemotherapy is recommended, as urethral and paraurethral glands are frequently infected. Most strains of *T. vaginalis* are highly sensitive to metronidazole and related drugs (approximately 95 per cent cure rate). There is a spontaneous cure rate in 20–25 per cent.

The recommended regimens for treating trichomonal infection include metronidazole 2 g orally in a single dose or metronidazole 400–500 mg twice daily for 5–7 days [Ia]. The single dose is cheaper with better compliance, but there is evidence that there may be a higher failure rate, especially if partners are not treated concurrently. Patients should be advised not to drink alcohol for the duration of and for 48 hours after completion of treatment due to the disulfiram-like effect (severe sickness).

Treatment failures should be referred to GUM to assess the possible reasons, such as poor compliance, re-infection, co-infection and/or resistance.

Metronidazole is relatively contraindicated in the first trimester of pregnancy and its safety is not established. However, the published data suggest no association with increased teratogenic risk [Ia].[6] Local treatment such as clotrimazole pessaries (100 mg daily for 7 days) can be used in symptomatic patients in the first trimester, but systemic treatment will eventually be required. High-dose treatments are best avoided in pregnancy and breastfeeding.

Genital herpes

Genital herpes is acquired by sexually transmitted infection with either herpes simplex type 1 virus (HSV-1) – which is the usual cause of oro-labial herpes – or herpes simplex type 2 virus (HSV-2). The infection may be primary or non-primary and disease episodes may be initial or recurrent and symptomatic or asymptomatic.

After childhood, symptomatic primary infection with HSV-1 is equally likely to occur in the genital or oral areas.

After primary infection, the virus becomes latent in local sensory ganglia, periodically reactivating to cause symptomatic lesions or asymptomatic but infectious viral shedding. This may be important in the acquisition of infection in long-term relationships where there has been primary infection with no history of a new partner.

New diagnoses of genital herpes are equally likely to be caused by HSV-1 or HSV-2; however, HSV-2 is more likely to recur than HSV-1. Median recurrence rates per month after a first episode are 0.34 for HSV-2 and 0.08 for HSV-1.[7] Recurrence rates generally reduce over time.

Clinical features of genital herpes in women
(Table 63.1.1)
The most common symptoms are those of vulval pain, which is usually associated with ulcers that are preceded by blisters. In a primary attack this can be quite severe and the whole vulva can become swollen, ulcerated and infected. This in turn can cause discharge and dysuria and in severe cases urinary retention. The cervix may also become ulcerated. Inguinal lymphadenopathy is also a feature of the

Table 63.1.1   Clinical features of acute herpes infections in women

Symptoms	Signs
Painful ulceration, dysuria, vaginal discharge Fever, myalgia (flu-like symptoms) - more common in primary infections May be asymptomatic	Blistering and ulceration of vulva ± cervix, preceded by vesicles Inguinal lymphadenopathy

primary infection, although this may be the result of secondary infection.

More generalized features of a viral illness may also be present, particularly in primary infections. These include fever and myalgia. Herpetic infection can be asymptomatic; this is more likely in recurrent episodes.

Complications
Urinary retention can occur as a result of autonomic neuropathy, or because of the severe pain engendered by the local reaction around the urethra and vulva. It has also been postulated that chronic vulval pain may also be a result of post-herpetic neuralgia.

Diagnosis
Herpes simplex virus confirmation and typing are important for diagnosis, prognosis and counselling [II].

Swabs must be taken from the base of a lesion, kept cold and transported directly to the laboratory in the viral culture medium. Serology is not commonly used to make the diagnosis. Given the implications of the diagnosis and potential for recurrent infections, it is vital that an accurate diagnosis be made at the outset. It cannot be assumed that vulval ulceration is herpetic until so proven by viral culture.

Management
PRIMARY GENITAL HERPES
General advice includes saline bathing and analgesia with a combination of non-steroidal anti-inflammatory agents and topical anaesthetic gels. Antiviral drugs are indicated if commenced within 5 days of the start of the episode and if lesions are still developing. Aciclovir (200 mg five times daily), valaciclovir (500 mg twice daily) and famciclovir (250 mg three times daily) all reduce the severity and duration of episodes [Ia], but they do not alter the natural history of the infection. Topical agents are less effective than oral agents, and intravenous therapy is only indicated when the patient cannot tolerate oral medication.

MANAGEMENT OF COMPLICATIONS
Hospitalization may be required because of urinary retention, meningism and severe constitutional symptoms. If catheterization is required, it is recommended that the suprapubic approach be used [II] to prevent the theoretical risk of ascending infection, reduce the painfulness of the procedure and allow normal micturition to take place without multiple attempts at re-catheterization.

RECURRENT GENITAL HERPES
Recurrent attacks of genital herpes are generally less severe than primary attacks and are self-limiting. It is important to make management decisions together with the patient, and advice should be given with regard to sexual activity whilst potentially infective. However, not all patients will be aware of their potential infective state, particularly those who do not have symptoms or a prodrome (disordered local vulval

sensations prior to the onset of a recurrent attack). Supportive and episodic antiviral therapy may be given [Ia], but if individuals suffer more than six attacks each year, suppressive therapy using antiviral agents and under the supervision of a genitourinary physician should be considered. Counselling may be required for those with problems adapting to the diagnosis.

Management in pregnancy

FIRST-EPISODE GENITAL HERPES

First and second trimester acquisition

Management should be as above, with oral or intravenous aciclovir in standard doses. Aciclovir is not licensed in pregnancy but there is substantial clinical evidence supporting its safety. Unless there are other complications, vaginal delivery can be anticipated. Continuous aciclovir in the last 4 weeks of pregnancy reduces the risk of both clinical recurrences at term and the need for caesarean section [Ia].[8]

Third trimester acquisition

Caesarean section should be considered for those developing symptoms after 34 weeks, as the risk of viral shedding during labour is very high, and thus also the risk of vertical transmission to the neonate. Caesarean section for the prevention of neonatal herpes has not been evaluated in randomized, controlled trials (RCTs) and may not be completely protective against neonatal herpes. If vaginal delivery is unavoidable, aciclovir treatment of the mother and baby may be indicated.

RECURRENT GENITAL HERPES

Sequential cultures in late pregnancy do not predict viral shedding at term. If there are no lesions at delivery, caesarean section should not be performed, even if there has been a brief recurrence during the third trimester. Continuous aciclovir in the last 4 weeks of pregnancy may be cost effective compared with no therapy or caesarean section. It may not reduce the risk of caesarean section, as it does not eliminate viral shedding completely. There is no proven benefit of taking swabs for viral cultures at delivery to assess asymptomatic shedding.

GENITAL LESIONS AT DELIVERY

The current consensus is that a caesarean section should be performed, despite lack of evidence for its effectiveness. The risks for the fetus at vaginal delivery may be small and need to be compared to the risks to the mother of caesarean section.

Prevention of acquisition of infection [II]

All women should be asked about genital herpes in themselves or in their partners. The asymptomatic female partners of men known to have genital herpes should be advised to avoid sexual contact during recurrences. Conscientious use of condoms during pregnancy may reduce the risk of acquisition, but this is unproven. Pregnant women should be advised about the risk of oro-genital contact for acquiring HSV-1.

The identification of susceptible women by means of type-specific antibody testing has not been shown to be cost effective.

All women, not just those with a history of genital herpes, should undergo careful inspection of the vulva at the onset of labour to look for clinical signs of herpes infection.

Mothers, staff and other relatives and friends with active oral lesions should be advised about the risk of postnatal transmission.

Bacterial vaginosis

Bacterial vaginosis is characterized by an overgrowth of predominantly anaerobic organisms (*Gardnerella vaginalis*, *Prevotella* sp., *Mycoplasma hominis*, *Mobiluncus* sp.) in the vagina. This leads to replacement of lactobacilli and an increase in pH from a normal of 4.5 to 7. Bacterial vaginosis can arise and remit spontaneously in sexually active and non-sexually active women. It is more common in black than in white women, in those with an intrauterine device and in those who smoke cigarettes.

Bacterial vaginosis is not regarded as a sexually transmitted infection and its aetiology is unknown. It is the commonest cause of vaginal discharge in women of childbearing age. The reported prevalence varies from 5 per cent in a group of asymptomatic college students to 50 per cent of women in Uganda. It has been reported in 12 per cent of pregnant women[9] and in 30 per cent of women undergoing termination of pregnancy in the UK.[10]

Clinical features

In approximately 50 per cent of confirmed cases there are no volunteered symptoms. Those with symptoms usually complain of an offensive, fishy-smelling vaginal discharge, not usually associated with vulvo-vaginitis. There is also a thin, white, homogeneous discharge coating the walls of the vagina and vestibule.

Complications

Although the incidence of bacterial vaginosis is high in women with PID, there are no prospective studies investigating whether treating asymptomatic women for bacterial vaginosis reduces their risk of developing it subsequently. The condition is common in some populations of women undergoing elective termination of pregnancy and is associated with post-termination endometritis and PID [Ia]. In pregnancy, bacterial vaginosis is associated with late miscarriage, preterm birth, preterm premature rupture of the membranes and postpartum endometritis [Ia]. It has been associated with an increased incidence of vaginal cuff cellulitis and abscess formation following transvaginal hysterectomy [Ib]. It is unclear how important this is in the UK, where antibiotic prophylaxis is routine practice. There are no studies investigating the role of bacterial vaginosis in the development of PID following intrauterine device insertion.

Diagnosis

> **Amsel's criteria for diagnosing bacterial vaginosis**
>
> At least three out of the four should be present for the diagnosis to be confirmed.
>
> - Thin, white, homogeneous discharge.
> - Clue cells on microscopy.
> - pH of vaginal fluid >4.5.
> - Release of a fishy odour on adding alkali (10% potassium hydroxide).

Routine use of a high vaginal swab may not be useful, as culture of *G. vaginalis* can be possible in more than 50 per cent of normal women [Ib]. However, criteria can be used to judge whether a vaginal smear that has been Gram-stained shows features consistent with a diagnosis of bacterial vaginosis.

Management

Initially, simple advice should be offered; this includes advice against the practice of vaginal douching, use of shower gels and antiseptic bath agents [II].

Antibiotic treatment is recommended for symptomatic women [Ia], women undergoing surgical procedures [Ia] and some pregnant women [Ia]. Using the oral route of administration, recommended regimens for treating bacterial vaginosis include metronidazole 400–500 mg twice daily for 5–7 days [Ia] or metronidazole 2 g as a single dose [Ia]. An alternative approach is to use the vaginal route, with intravaginal metronidazole gel (0.75%) once daily for 5 days [Ia] or intravaginal clindamycin cream (2%) once daily for 7 days [Ia]. All these treatments have been shown to achieve cure rates of 70–80 per cent after 4 weeks in controlled trials using placebo or comparing with oral metronidazole.

No reduction in relapse rates has been reported in studies in which the male partners were treated, and therefore there is no indication to treat the male partners of women with bacterial vaginosis.

Follow-up is only required if symptoms recur, although a more cautious approach should be employed in pregnancy where recurrent infection may be associated with adverse outcomes.

The optimal management of those who have recurrent episodes of bacterial vaginosis remains unresolved.

Pregnancy and bacterial vaginosis

Meta-analyses have concluded that there is no evidence for teratogenicity from the use of metronidazole in pregnancy [Ia].

The results of clinical trials investigating the value of screening for and treating bacterial vaginosis in pregnancy are conflicting, and it is therefore difficult to make firm recommendations. In summary, three RCTs have shown a reduction in the incidence of preterm birth following screening and treating bacterial vaginosis in women with a history of prior preterm birth or second trimester loss. However, this conclusion was based on subgroup analysis in two studies, and all three studies used different treatments.[11–13] The largest multicentre RCT randomized 1953 asymptomatic women with bacterial vaginosis to receive 2 g metronidazole or placebo, taken under supervision in the clinic and repeated at home 2 days later. The course was repeated 4 weeks later. There was no difference in gestational age at delivery between the two groups or in the subgroup of women with a prior preterm birth. The possible limitations to this study were that treatment was commenced at a relatively late gestational age (20–24 weeks), the short course of metronidazole given and the high number of women screened positive for bacterial vaginosis who were not randomized.[14] One study did show a benefit from treatment with oral clindamycin 300 mg twice a day for 7 days. This was a cohort design rather than a randomization, which is limiting in terms of making recommendations.[15] The use of clindamycin cream to treat bacterial vaginosis in the second trimester of pregnancy did not reduce preterm birth in two studies [Ia].

> **Bacterial vaginosis in pregnancy**
>
> All symptomatic pregnant women with bacterial vaginosis should be treated in the normal way [Ib]. Asymptomatic pregnant women with a history of preterm birth or second trimester loss, of unknown cause, may be screened and treated with oral metronidazole 400 mg twice daily for 7 days, but current evidence does not support routine screening for bacterial vaginosis.

Anogenital warts

Aetiology

Warts are benign epithelial skin tumours that are caused by the human papillomavirus (HPV), of which there are more than 90 genotypes. The mode of transmission is most often sexual, but it may be transmitted perinatally and also from digital lesions (more commonly in children). Although the majority are benign and caused by HPV subtypes 6 and 11, others may contain oncogenic subtypes that are associated with genital tract dysplasia and cancer. Warts are just one manifestation of HPV infection of the genital tract, as there may also be subclinical and latent infection. Anogenital warts are the commonest sexually transmitted infection in the UK (65 000 new diagnoses in GUM clinics in England and Wales in 1999).[16]

Clinical features

Anogenital warts may cause irritation but generally present as 'lumps' which women find disfiguring and psychologically distressing. They can occur at any site in the genital area including peri-anally, which does not imply anal intercourse.

Occult lesions may also occur in the vagina and cervix. Extragenital lesions may occur on the oral mucosa, larynx, conjunctiva and nasal cavity. Warts may be exophytic, single or multiple, keratinized and non-keratinized, broad based or pedunculated, and some are pigmented.

Diagnosis is mainly by naked-eye examination, although any doubt about the diagnosis should prompt biopsy under local anaesthetic. Speculum examination should be performed to look for cervical and vaginal lesions.

Management

GENERAL ADVICE
Condom usage with regular partners has not been shown to affect the treatment outcome of anogenital warts.[17] However, using condoms may result in both partners feeling more comfortable and may prevent the transmission of HPV to uninfected partners and therefore should be encouraged.

TREATMENT
Treatment is generally uncomfortable and can be painful, and patients should be made aware that all treatments have significant failure and relapse rates. The choice of treatment depends on the morphology, number and distribution of the warts. First-line and second-line treatments are not based upon robust evidence.

Soft, poorly keratinized warts respond well to podophyllin, podophyllotoxin and trichloroacetic acid, whereas keratinized lesions are better treated with physical ablative therapies such as cryotherapy, excision and electrocautery. Imiquimod, an immune modulating agent, may be suitable for both types. Podophyllotoxin is usually administered over a 4-week cycle and imiquimod for up to 16 weeks, and both are suitable for self-application at home after appropriate instruction and screening for other sexually transmitted diseases. This is best supervised from a GUM clinic, as are most anogenital wart treatments. Adequate contraception must be ensured prior to the use of podophyllin-type chemicals because of the known teratogenic effect in animals.

Anogenital warts in pregnancy
Podophyllin and podophyllotoxin should be avoided because of their possible teratogenic effects, and currently imiquimod does not have approval for use in pregnancy. The objectives of treatment in pregnancy are to minimize the number of lesions present at delivery and to reduce neonatal exposure to the virus. Potential problems in the neonate are the development of laryngeal papillomatosis and anogenital warts. Very rarely, a caesarean section is indicated due to blockage of the vaginal outlet.

Cervical cytology
The National Health Service Cervical Screening Programme (NHSCSP) recommends no changes to the screening intervals for women with anogenital warts. Furthermore, developing anogenital warts prior to the age when screening would normally start is not an indication to commence cervical screening.

Immunosuppressed women
This category includes women with impaired cell-mediated immunity (renal transplant patients and those infected with HIV), who are likely to have poor treatment responses, increased relapse rates and dysplasia. Careful follow-up is required.

Syphilis

Aetiology
Treponema pallidum, the spirochaete responsible for sexually acquired syphilis, causes one type of treponemal disease'. The pathological strains also cause non-sexually transmitted tropical diseases such as yaws, endemic syphilis, bejel and pinta. These organisms are serologically and morphologically similar and cannot be grown on artificial media. Occasionally, saprophytic strains, found in the mouth in dental sepsis, can cause diagnostic confusion.

Syphilis is transmitted sexually, and vertically in pregnancy; therefore the condition can be acquired and congenital.

Epidemiology
Syphilis first became widespread and epidemic at the end of the fifteenth century in Europe. Syphilis and gonorrhoea were recognized as STIs in the eighteenth century, but were thought to be the same disease until they were finally shown to be separate infections in the mid-nineteenth century. Until recently, syphilis was in a steady decline in the West, but over the last 10 years the incidence has begun to increase together with HIV infection.

Classification
Acquired syphilis can be divided into early and late infections. Early syphilis is further subdivided into primary, secondary and early latent (<2 years' infection). The subdivisions of late infection include late latent (>2 years) and tertiary, which includes gummatous, cardiovascular and neurological involvement. Cardiovascular and neurological involvement is sometimes classified as quaternary syphilis.

Congenital syphilis is divided into early (first 2 years) and late, which includes the classical stigmata of congenital syphilis.

Clinical features
Primary syphilis is characterized by an ulcer (the chancre) and regional lymphadenopathy. The chancre is classically a single, painless and indurated ulcer with a clean base discharging clear serum and is usually found in the anogenital region. However, it may also be atypical, multiple, painful, purulent, destructive and occur at extragenital sites. The ulcer(s) of primary syphilis should not be confused with other genital ulcerative disorders.

Aetiology of anogenital ulceration

- Herpes simplex
- Syphilis
- Chancroid
- Lymphogranuloma venereum
- Donovanosis
- Candidiasis (severe)
- Behçet's disease
- Scabies-excoriated

Secondary syphilis is characterized by multisystem involvement occurring within the first 2 years of infection. The features include a generalized polymorphic rash, often affecting the palms and soles, condylomata lata, mucocutaneous lesions, generalized lymphadenopathy and other rare multisystem manifestations. Early latent syphilis is characterized by positive serological tests for syphilis with no clinical evidence of treponemal infection, again within the first 2 years of infection.

In cases testing positive serologically for treponemal infection in the absence of clinical signs, it is important to exclude other infections such as yaws, particularly in those of Caribbean origin.

All women with positive treponemal serology should be investigated and treated in a GUM department.

Diagnosis

The diagnosis can be made by direct demonstration of *Treponema pallidum* from lesions or infected lymph nodes in early syphilis by dark field microscopy, direct fluorescent antibody testing and tests based upon the PCR. Serological tests include:

- cardiolipin (reaginic) tests: Venereal Diseases Research Laboratory (VDRL),
- carbon antigen test/rapid plasma reagin (RPR) test,
- specific tests: treponemal EIA to detect IgG, IgG and IgM, *T. pallidum* haemagglutination assay (TPHA) and others.

Treatment

The mainstay of treatment is parenteral penicillin, as it is given under supervision, therefore ensuring compliance, and has bioavailability guaranteed. Suitable approaches include procaine penicillin or Jenacillin or long-acting Biclinicillin i.m. for 10 days [Ib]. Doxycycline may also be given. All patients should be offered screening for other STIs, including HIV.

Pregnancy

Seventy to 100 per cent of the infants of pregnant women with untreated early syphilis will be infected and one-third will be stillborn. Patients should be jointly managed with GUM physicians and treated as above but substituting erythromycin for doxycycline. All neonates should be treated at birth.

Congenital syphilis

Babies of mothers with positive serology for syphilis and treated antenatally should be managed jointly by a GUM physician and a paediatrician. Laboratory blood tests should be performed on the infant's (not cord) blood. In view of the highly treatable nature of the disease and the high perinatal morbidity and mortality of congenital syphilis, it is extremely important to continue with antenatal testing.

Human immunodeficiency virus

There are two strains of HIV, types 1 and 2, of which HIV-1 is responsible for most HIV infections. The human immunodeficiency virus carries its genetic code as RNA; this is translated by an enzyme present in the virus (reverse transcriptase) into DNA, which then integrates into the host's target cells, including CD4 T-cell lymphocytes, and other cells of the immune system. This results in a decline in CD4 cells and progression to acquired immunodeficiency syndrome (AIDS). HIV infection can cause a decline in CD4 counts from a normal level of about $1000/\mu L$ to $<200/\mu L$. The infected person then becomes susceptible to the opportunistic infections and malignancies characteristic of AIDS.

Human immunodeficiency virus disease is an extremely important, fatal disease worldwide. It is currently estimated that approximately 40 million people are infected. HIV infection increases the susceptibility to other infectious diseases, such as tuberculosis, with a huge impact on morbidity and mortality. HIV is most prevalent in economically deprived areas in the developing world where people are less likely to be able to afford the expensive antiretroviral drugs that can limit disease progression and spread. HIV is transmitted sexually, in blood products and to the fetus vertically and through breastfeeding. In developed countries such as the UK, infected people have access to the latest evidence-based treatments and are managed by GUM physicians.

With the currently available antiretroviral agents, eradication of HIV infection is not likely to be possible. The aims of treatment are to prolong life and improve quality of life by maintaining suppression of virus replication for as long as possible. Treatment is recommended for patients with primary HIV infection, asymptomatic HIV infection and symptomatic HIV infection or AIDS. However, treatment is not indicated in patients with asymptomatic HIV infection with a CD4 count that is high (>350 cells/μL) [Ia]. Data are lacking to support decisions on when to start therapy, but it should be started before the CD4 count drops to less then 200 cells/μL. There is overwhelming evidence from cohort studies to show that the dramatic fall in AIDS-related mortality seen in the developed world coincided with the introduction of highly active antiretroviral therapy (HAART). HAART regimens should be individualized to achieve the best potency, minimize toxicity and avoid drug interactions.

HAART consists of three drugs, which can be from a variety of types: protease inhibitors, non-nucleoside reverse transcriptase inhibitors or nucleoside reverse transcriptase inhibitors. There have been no definitive controlled trials to demonstrate the clinical superiority of any one HAART regimen used as initial therapy. Issues to be considered during therapy are adherence, toxicity, resistance, long-term safety, clinical trial data and stage of disease. Change of therapy is advocated for virological failure diagnosed by viral load testing. There may be sex differences in the use of antiretroviral drugs, although the data are limited. The menstrual cycle may have a small influence on HIV RNA levels. There is no change in treatment guidelines for women.

HIV and contraception

It is important that HIV-positive women are open about their infection so that they receive the best advice. Safer sex is to be encouraged, with the concomitant use of condoms as well as a reliable hormonal method to prevent pregnancy.

Women should be advised that there is decreased efficacy of the oral contraceptive pill with protease and non-nucleoside reverse transcriptase inhibitors. This is also important with progestogen-only methods such as the progestogen-only pill (POP), depot and implant delivery systems.

HIV AND INTRAUTERINE CONTRACEPTIVE DEVICES

There has been controversy about the use of the intrauterine contraceptive device (IUCD) in HIV-positive women due to their risk of PID. IUCDs also increase menstrual blood loss and therefore may increase the risk of HIV transmission. Insertion may cause transient inflammatory reaction in the endometrium, which may facilitate virus entry. However, for women on HAART with relatively intact immune systems and for whom the use of a hormonal method may not be reliable, an IUCD may be acceptable. STI screening should be carried out and the use of prophylactic antibiotics to cover insertion might be considered.

HIV and cervical screening, colposcopy and cervical cancer

Cervical cancer is an AIDS-defining illness. Women with HIV need to have regular cervical cytology and all women with cervical cancer should be offered an HIV test. The current NHSCSP guidelines on screening suggest that HIV-positive women should have an annual smear, although the evidence for this is weak. Any cytological abnormality, however minor, should be taken as an indication for colposcopy. As there is a higher incidence of inflammatory vagino-cervical disorders in HIV-positive women, the accuracy of both cytology and colposcopy is less than in non-HIV-infected women.

Women with proven cervical intraepithelial neoplasia (CIN) require treatment, although the results of treatment of CIN are significantly worse than in non-HIV women. Data also suggest that HIV-positive women with normal CD4 counts have better outcomes than those who have low CD4 counts. This observation supports the concept that the host cell-mediated immune system is implicated in the eradication of CIN following local treatments.

HIV infection and pregnancy

The prevalence of HIV in pregnancy varies hugely over the UK. For example, in 1999, the prevalence in London was 1 in 400 live births, whereas elsewhere in the country it was 1 in 4500. There was a total of 380 births to infected women in 1999. The risk of transmission is related to maternal health, obstetric factors and infant prematurity. There appears to be a linear correlation between maternal viral load and risk of transmission, but the evidence to show that transmission never occurs below a certain threshold does not exist.

Obstetric factors that consistently show an association with risk of transmission are mode of delivery and duration of membrane rupture. Delivery before 34 weeks has been shown to be associated with an increased risk of transmission. In 1992, the association of breastfeeding and increased transmission was shown, and formula feeding is advocated in the UK. Elsewhere in the world, where formula feeding poses extra risks to the infant because of unsafe water, breastfeeding is recommended. Caesarean section has been shown in both a meta-analysis and a RCT to be protective in terms of transmission.[18] There is an untreated vertical transmission risk of 25 per cent. The findings of the first RCT in 1994 showed that the use of zidovudine (AZT) could reduce transmission from 25 per cent to 8 per cent. This has since been confirmed by multiple smaller observational studies. Only AZT is specifically indicated for use in pregnancy; the use of most other antiretroviral drugs in pregnancy is cautioned against. Standard treatment in the UK is with at least three antiretroviral drugs (antiretroviral therapy (ART) or combination therapy), so the management of many pregnant women requires consideration of the woman's own health needs, the need to reduce transmission and the possible adverse effects of ART.

Pregnant women with HIV need a great deal of psychosocial support in order to make informed decisions about taking treatment, both for their own health and also to reduce vertical transmission in pregnancy. There is very little evidence and few studies relating current drug therapies to treat HIV to pregnancy outcomes, making it difficult for the physician to advise. There should be clear local referral pathways for HIV pregnant women, including specialist nurses and social workers where available. Information for the woman concerning follow-up for the baby needs to be given.

Women with HIV are probably at a small increased risk of adverse pregnancy outcome such as spontaneous abortion, stillbirth and intrauterine growth restriction.

Preconception and fertility management in men and women with HIV

There are three groups to consider:

1 HIV-positive men and negative female partners.
2 HIV-negative men and positive female partners.
3 HIV-infected couples.

All three groups may have fertility problems, but for the first two groups there is also the risk of HIV transmission.

POSITIVE MAN, NEGATIVE WOMAN

The risk of transmission to the woman is approximately 1:500 per sexual encounter and until recently this was the only way couples could conceive. Limiting exposure to the most fertile period only has been shown to reduce the risk of transmission. In one study, 4 of 103 women seroconverted using this method. In 1992, Semprini invented the technique of 'sperm washing' – a process whereby spermatozoa are removed from the surrounding seminal plasma.[19] (HIV is found in the seminal plasma but not bound to the spermatozoa themselves.) There have not so far been any seroconversions of women after they have been inseminated with washed sperm. The technique of sperm washing is only available in a few centres in the UK and not on the NHS.

NEGATIVE MAN, POSITIVE WOMAN

Couples are advised to use condoms and then to practise artificial insemination around ovulation to minimize the risk of transmission to the man.

POSITIVE COUPLES

These couples are recommended to practise safer sex (condoms) in order to reduce the risk of transmission of viral variants. They are advised to have unprotected sex around ovulation. There has been considerable debate concerning HIV-infected couples and in-vitro fertilization (IVF): it is now ethically acceptable as the vertical transmission rate is less than 1 per cent and there is an increased life expectancy for parents on treatment.[20]

KEY POINTS

- PID is most commonly caused by *Chlamydia trachomatis* and *Neisseria gonorrhoeae*; the long-term sequelae include infertility, ectopic pregnancy and chronic pelvic pain.
- The symptoms and signs of PID can be non-specific and treatment may have to be initiated empirically.
- PID should be considered as a sexually transmitted disease and therefore contact tracing, treating partners and liaison with GUM are important features of management.
- Gynaecologists should take sexual histories where indicated and apply the basic tenets of GUM practice.
- Many patients will have concurrent sexually transmitted diseases; therefore genitourinary screening is recommended.
- For better patient care, it is recommended that each clinician should have a thorough understanding of the chlamydia test used in his/her clinical setting.
- Testing for chlamydial infection should be considered when undertaking any procedure that

entails instrumentation of the upper genital tract, such as hysteroscopy and IUCD insertion, because of the serious possible complications.

- The only way to assess risk of infection is to take a sexual history, as outlined above.
- The vulva should be carefully examined in all women – not just those at high risk of genital herpes – at the onset of labour.
- The aetiology of bacterial baginosis is unknown; it is not sexually transmitted.
- Anogenital warts are the most common STI in the UK; they do not indicate the need for cervical screening outwith the NHSCSP.
- All women with positive tests for syphilis should be referred to GUM to confirm or exclude neurological, cardiovascular and ophthalmic involvement.
- There has been a significant improvement in survival and quality of life for HIV-infected women treated with HAART.

PUBLISHED GUIDELINES

National Guideline for the Management of Pelvic Infection and Perihepatitis. Ross J for Clinical Effectiveness Group: Association for Genitourinary Medicine and the Medical Society for the Study of Venereal Diseases, 2002.

National Guideline for the Management of Gonorrhoea in Adults. Bignell C for Clinical Effectiveness Group: Association for Genitourinary Medicine and the Medical Society for the Study of Venereal Diseases, 2002.

National Guideline for the Management of Chlamydia trachomatis *Genital Tract Infection.* Horner PJ and Caul EO for Clinical Effectiveness Group: Association for Genitourinary Medicine and the Medical Society for the Study of Venereal Diseases, 2002.

National Guideline for the Management of Trichomonas vaginalis. Sherrard J for Clinical Effectiveness Group: Association for Genitourinary Medicine and the Medical Society for the Study of Venereal Diseases, 2002.

National Guideline for the Management of Bacterial Vaginosis. Hay P for Clinical Effectiveness Group: Association for Genitourinary Medicine and the Medical Society for the Study of Venereal Diseases, 2002.

National Guideline for the Management of Anogenital Warts. Maw R for Clinical Effectiveness Group: Association for Genitourinary Medicine and the Medical Society for the Study of Venereal Diseases, 2002.

National Guideline for the Management of Early Syphilis. Goh B for Clinical Effectiveness Group: Association for

Pelvic floor and lower urinary tract

Genitourinary Medicine and the Medical Society for the Study of Venereal Diseases, 2002.

National Guideline for the Management of Late Syphilis. French P for Clinical Effectiveness Group: Association for Genitourinary Medicine and the Medical Society for the Study of Venereal Diseases, 2002.

National Guideline for the Management of Genital Herpes. Herpes simplex Advisory Panel for Clinical Effectiveness Group: Association for Genitourinary Medicine and the Medical Society for the Study of Venereal Diseases, 2002.

Ross JD. European guideline for the management of pelvic inflammatory disease and perihepatitis. *Int J STD AIDS* 2001; **12**(Suppl. 3):84–7.

Templeton A. (ed.) *Recommendations Arising from the 31st Study Group: The Prevention of Pelvic Infection in The Prevention of Pelvic Infection.* London: RCOG Press, 1996.

All the guideliness are available at <www.agum.org.uk>.

KEY REFERENCES

1. Rowe PJ. Workshop on the standardised investigation of the infertile couple. In: Harrison RF, Bonnar J, Thompson W. (eds), *Fertility and Sterility*. Lancaster: MTP Press, 1984, 427–42.

2. Bevan CD, Johal BJ, Mumtaz G, Ridgway GL, Siddle NC. Clinical, laparoscopic and microbiological findings in acute salpingitis: report on a United Kingdom cohort. *Br J Obstet Gynaecol* 1995; **102**:407–14.

3. Morcos R, Frost J, Hnat M, Petrunak A, Caldito G. Laparoscopic versus clinical diagnosis of acute pelvic inflammatory disease. *J Reprod Med* 1993; **38**:53–6.

4. Tobin JM, Harindra V, Tucker LJ. The future of chlamydia screening. *Sex Transm Infect* 2000; **76**:233–4.

5. Moller JK, Andersen B, Oleson F, Lignell T, Ostergard L. Impact of menstrual cycle on the diagnostic performance of LCR, TMA, and PCE for the detection of *Chlamydia trachomatis* in home obtained and mailed vaginal flush and urine samples. *Sex Transm Infect* 1999; **75**:228–30.

6. Burtin P, Taddio A, Adburnu O, Einarson TR, Koren G. Safety of metronidazole in pregnancy: a meta-analysis. *Am J Obstet Gynecol* 1995; **172**:525–9.

7. Benedetti JK, Zeh J, Corey L. Clinical reactivation of genital herpes simplex virus infection decreases in frequency over time. *Ann Intern Med* 1999; **131**:14–20.

8. Scott LL, Sanchez PJ, Jackson GL et al. Acyclovir suppression to prevent cesarean delivery after first-episode genital herpes. *Obstet Gynecol* 1996; **87**:69–73.

9. Hay PE, Lamont RF, Taylor-Robinson D, Morgan DJ, Ison C, Pearson J. Abnormal bacterial colonisation of the genital tract and subsequent preterm delivery and late miscarriage. *BMJ* 1994; **308**: 295–8.

10. Blackwell AL, Thomas PD, Wareham K, Emery SJ. Health gains from screening for infection of the lower genital tract in women attending for termination of pregnancy. *Lancet* 1993; **342**:206–10.

11. McDonald HM, O'Loughlin JA, Vigneswaren R et al. Impact of metronidazole therapy on preterm birth in women with bacterial vaginosis flora (*Gardnerella vaginalis*): a randomised, placebo controlled trial. *Br J Obstet Gynaecol* 1997; **104**:1391–7.

12. Hauth JC, Goldenberg RL, Andrews WW, DuBard MB, Copper RL. Reduced incidence of preterm delivery with metronidazole and erythromycin in women with bacterial vaginosis. *N Engl J Med* 1995; **333**:1732–6.

13. Morales WJ, Schorr S, Albritton J. Effect of metronidazole in patients with preterm birth in preceding pregnancy and bacterial vaginosis: a placebo-controlled, double-blind study. *Am J Obstet Gynecol* 1994; **171**:345–7.

14. Carey JC, Klebenhoff MA, Hauth JC et al. Metronidazole to prevent preterm delivery in pregnant women with asymptomatic bacterial vaginosis. *N Engl J Med* 2000; **342**:534–40.

15. McGregor JA, French JI, Parker R et al. Prevention of premature birth by screening and treatment for common genital tract infections: results of a prospective controlled evaluation. *Am J Obstet Gynecol* 1995; **173**:157–67.

16. Sexually transmitted disease quarterly report: anogenital warts and anogenital herpes simplex virus infection in England and Wales. *CDR Weekly Communicable Disease Report* 30 June 2000; **10**(26):230–2.

17. Krebs H-B, Helmkamp BF. Treatment failure of genital condylomata acuminata in women: the role of the male sexual partner. *Am J Obstet Gynecol* 1991; **165**:337–9.

18. The European Mode of Delivery Collaboration. Elective caesarian section versus vaginal delivery in the prevention of vertical HIV-1 transmission: a randomised clinical trial. *Lancet* 1999; **353**:1035–9.

19. Semprini AE, Levi-Setti P, Bozzo M, Ravizza M, Taglioretti A, Sulpizio P, Albani E, Oneta M, Pardi G. Insemination of HIV-negative women with processed semen of HIV-positive partners. *Lancet* 1992, Nov 8; **340**(8831):1317–9.

20. Gilling-Smith C, Smith RJ, Semprini AE. HIV and infertility: time to treat. *BMJ* 2001; **322**:566–7.

Dyspareunia and Other Psychosexual Problems

Melanie C. Mann

MRCOG standards

The established standards relevant for this topic are:

Theoretical skills

- Understand the classification and causes of dyspareunia.
- Be able to manage the individual causes of dyspareunia.
- Understand the different types of psychosexual conditions in women and how they affect gynaecological patients.

Practical skills

- Be able to take an appropriate sexual history with regard to dyspareunia.
- Be able to perform a clinical examination to diagnose the cause of dyspareunia.
- Be able to ask about sexual relationship problems related to the dyspareunia, either as a result of the dyspareunia or causing the dyspareunia, i.e. be able to take a related psychosexual history.

DYSPAREUNIA

This is recurrent genital pain associated with sexual activity, usually penetration, although it can refer to any genital stimulation. Dyspareunia can be primary, where pain has always occurred, or secondary, where it occurs after a period of pain-free sexual activity. It is important to classify it further in terms of the site of pain: superficial or deep.

Dyspareunia can itself lead to relationship difficulties due to the cycle of fear. Pain at intercourse can lead to problems of sexual arousal, causing further sexual pain and then avoidance of sexual activity.

Talking to patients about the exact site, nature and other features of the pain is important. It is also important to be comfortable talking about aspects of the sexual act, especially as some dyspareunia may be position related. Remember that patients are usually more embarrassed mentioning these aspects to us and may expect us to bring up the subject.

Main causes of superficial dyspareunia (superficial vulval and vaginal pain at intercourse)

- Vulvitis and vulvovaginitis (infection, hypo-oestrogenic)
- Vulvar vestibulitis syndrome
- Essential vulvodynia
- Topical irritants/dermatitis
- Urethral disorders and cystitis
- Vaginismus
- Lack of vaginal lubrication (arousal problems)
- Obstetric perineal trauma, mainly episiotomy
- Radiation vaginitis

Main causes of deep dyspareunia

- Pelvic inflammatory disease
- Endometriosis
- Genital or pelvic masses, e.g. ovarian cyst
- Pelvic congestion syndrome
- Urinary tract infection
- Retroverted uterus in some women
- Irritable bowel syndrome
- Psychosexual issues

Most of these causes are dealt with in more detail in other sections of this book.

It is important to confirm diagnoses as far as possible with diagnostic tests such as pelvic ultrasonography, microbiological swabs, laparoscopy or vulval biopsy where appropriate. Some diagnoses or problems are best dealt with by general practitioners or other specialists such as gastroenterologists.

If an organic cause for dyspareunia is found, it does not necessarily exclude emotional and/or psychological sequelae for the woman. The aetiology of dyspareunia should be viewed on a continuum from primarily physical to primarily psychological, with many women exhibiting components of both.

PSYCHOSEXUAL PROBLEMS

Psychosexual problems may present to the gynaecologist as part of general history taking for a variety of presenting complaints, and it is sometimes difficult to disentangle how much of the gynaecological complaint is due to the psychosexual problem or whether the gynaecological problem has caused the psychosexual issue. It is therefore extremely important that the clinician feels comfortable asking about sexual problems, especially in relation to gynaecological problems, for which there is a good chance of concomitant psychosexual issues such as vulval disorders and dyspareunia. However, there may also be circumstances in which it is important to establish sexual habits and issues, for example prior to gynaecological surgery when any interference with sexual function can cause problems within a sexual relationship.

Psychosexual history taking

Each clinician needs to find his/her own words that feel comfortable to use when talking about sex with the patient. There is no substitute for practice, and the more you use the words and ask the difficult questions, the more comfortable you will feel. Open-ended questions are useful in order to encourage the patient to talk, for example. 'Tell me a little bit about...'. The clinician's body language is also extremely influential to the way the patient will feel about opening up in this very intimate part of history taking. For example, sitting back in the chair, putting down your pen and not having a large expanse of desk between you and the patient will go a long way towards making her feel more comfortable.

Typical questions for use in psychosexual history taking

Not all the questions need to be asked or are appropriate to ask every time.

- 'Are you in a sexual relationship?'
- 'Is sex comfortable for you?'
- 'Are there any problems with sex?'
- 'Do you get any pain with sex?'
- 'Where exactly does it hurt during sex – on the outside or the inside?'
- 'Is there anything that makes the pain worse, any position, for example?'
- 'Are you able to have an orgasm during sex?'
- 'Have you ever masturbated? Do you get an orgasm during masturbation?'
- 'Tell me a little bit about your relationship with your partner.'

- 'Tell me a little bit about what happens when you try to have sex with your partner.'

Most gynaecologists would refer a patient on to an expert in psychosexual medicine for further treatment. There will be local variation in availability and waiting time.

SEXUAL PAIN DISORDERS

Dyspareunia

This is the only sexual disorder in which physical factors are thought to play a major aetiological role. However, the psychological and interpersonal factors are significant.[1] The organic causes for this condition are discussed above. In addition to gynaecological treatment approaches, most women require an adjunctive course of cognitive–behavioural sex therapy to ensure good outcomes.[2]

Vaginismus

Vaginismus is the involuntary spasm of the pubococcygeal and associated muscles causing painful and difficult penetration of the vagina, during sex, tampon insertion or clinical examination. Primary vaginismus occurs when a woman has never experienced vaginal penetration; secondary vaginismus is diagnosed when the problem occurs after previous successful vaginal penetration.

The patient may present with a painful vulva at intercourse. The differential diagnosis is then of organic vulval disorders such as vulval vestibulitis. However, there is likely to be some degree of vaginismus in all women with organic vulval disease. The skill is in trying to work out whether the vaginismus is the primary problem or is a result of organic disease. The 'Q-tip' test can be helpful to elucidate the exact site of pain and whether it is in the contracted muscles or in the tender epithelium of the vestibule. (The 'Q-tip' test involves the use of a moistened cotton bud to elicit the exact site and degree of discomfort of vulval pain.) The other main form of presentation is admission of non-consummation of a relationship in the fertility clinic setting.

Aetiology

Vaginismus is a conditioned (learned) response that often results from associating sexual activity with pain and fear. It can occur together with a phobia of all sexual contact or as the only problem within an otherwise normal sexual relationship. Typical phrases used by the patient include: 'There's a block', 'He just can't seem to get it (his penis) in', 'It's as if it is too small (her vaginal opening)'.

Sometimes the doctor may be able to feed back to the patient that she appears to be disassociated from that area of her body, and further questioning often confirms that she does not touch that area much herself due to concerns with cleanliness, smell or religious beliefs.

> **Causes of vaginismus**
>
> - Sexual abuse
> - Physical abuse
> - Painful medical procedure in the perineal area
> - Painful first intercourse
> - Relationship problems/anger between couples ('I won't let him in'– subconsciously)
> - Fear of pregnancy/labour
> - Religious orthodoxy
> - Poor sexual education
> - Sexual inhibition

Treatment

There needs to be discussion around the main issues in the relationship and how the woman feels about touching her own genitalia. Behavioural therapy comprising systematic desensitization, pubococcygeal muscle training and the use of vaginal trainers works well. The response to this therapy for this group is good, with complete resolution for most couples, especially if the origin is uncomplicated in nature.[3] The phobia of penetration needs to be explored so that the woman reaches a situation in which she feels in control of her vagina and can enjoy sex when and how she wishes.

- Discussion and education about sex and the condition.
- Teaching the location and control of the vaginal (pubococcygeal) muscles.
- Self-examination of the vulva and vagina when alone and relaxed, e.g. in the bath (beginning of systematic desensitization).
- Insertion of her own finger, then fingers or plastic vaginal trainers.
- Doing the above in a sexual situation with her partner present.
- The woman inserting her partner's finger, then penis with her in control.
- Insertion of the penis with her partner in control, but with the woman on top so that it is less threatening.
- Sexual intercourse as the couple would wish.

> There have been no randomized, controlled trials. Observational studies indicate that treatment is generally very successful for women with vaginismus.

SEXUAL DESIRE DISORDERS

This usually presents as loss of libido (loss of interest in sex). The prognosis is variable, but is better when it is the female with the initial problem. One study examined 60 couples presenting with the female partner's loss of interest as the major problem. There was only modest success, with 56 per cent experiencing a relatively good outcome at the end of treatment.[4] These problems are usually the symptom of a generally poor relationship overall, and the sexual disorder is only part of the whole problem.

SEXUAL AROUSAL DISORDER

It is difficult to separate sexual arousal disorder from sexual desire disorder and female orgasm disorder due to the close relationship of the three conditions in women. Additionally, the widespread use of vaginal lubricants may mask the disorder. There are no studies considering this as a separate entity.

FEMALE ORGASMIC DISORDER (ANORGASMIA)

Definition

This is the term used for failure to achieve orgasm due to inhibition of the orgasmic reflex or poor sexual technique/ignorance.

Aetiology

There may be fear of losing control, holding back. It may be situational, in that the woman can achieve orgasm by masturbation or with the aid of sex toys but not during sexual intercourse. Sometimes, realistic ideas and the discussion of what most women achieve are necessary. For example, many women do not experience orgasm by penetration alone and do need other clitoral stimulation at the same time. Education regarding sexual positions to enhance clitoral stimulation and education about the clitoris itself may be required. There may be unrealistic expectations on the part of the partner, who may equate the female orgasm with his own and will not be happy unless his female partner also has one during penetration. This pressure on the female can lead to faking of orgasm to keep the partner happy and a premature end to the sexual act and frustration on the part of the female, who has not actually achieved orgasm.

Treatment of anorgasmia

- Encourage self-exploration and what is pleasurable when she is alone.
- Sensate focus–concentration on the sensual pleasure of touching her partner but avoiding the genitals.

- Masturbation.
- Use of sex toys such as vibrators, if helpful; use of videos to help arousal and provide ideas (e.g. *The Lovers' Guide* series by Dr Andrew Stanway, Pickwick Video).
- Discussion and resolution of unconscious fears of orgasm, if present.
- Heightening sexual arousal so that the woman is close to orgasm before penetration.

Hysterectomy and orgasm

There is debate in the literature about the role of hysterectomy in sexual function. This has become more important now that women are more involved in their own treatment choices and feel more able to demand a good outcome from surgery. It has also become more pertinent since there have been more non-surgical (e.g. the levonorgestrel intrauterine system) and less-complicated procedures (e.g. endometrial destruction methods) to treat one of the commonest reasons for hysterectomy, namely menorrhagia. There has been a steady rise in the number of supracervical hysterectomies performed for benign conditions.[5] This may reflect the changing attitudes of surgeons and women towards a less invasive procedure, which has reduced operative morbidity and reduced the risk of urinary and sexual dysfunction. Various mechanisms have been proposed to explain why cervical conservation may have a less detrimental effect on sexual function than total abdominal hysterectomy. Early pioneering work[6] described elevation of both the cervix and uterus during excitement and the plateau phase, followed by fundal uterine contractions progressively involving the lower uterine segment as orgasm developed. Cervical os dilatation occurred immediately afterwards, implicating a role for the cervix in the female sexual response. Another theory postulates that the ability to achieve orgasm depends on the nerve endings of the uterovaginal (cervical) plexus of Frankenhauser.[7] This plexus is a matrix of nerve fibres intimately surrounding the cervix. Stimulation of the cervix may contribute to a pleasurable sensation ultimately experienced as orgasm.

Studies examining sexual function after hysterectomy are contradictory. Several studies show a decrease in sexual function after hysterectomy and others show an increase. The studies that show an increase in sexual functioning after hysterectomy[8] may reflect the relief from dyspareunia and bleeding problems with excision of the uterus. There has been a paucity of evidence to show which sorts of hysterectomy cause more sexual dysfunction than others. One study showed that there was a statistically significant reduction in orgasm frequency among total abdominal hysterectomy patients compared to supracervical hysterectomy patients.[9] Another small retrospective questionnaire study comparing supracervical to total abdominal hysterectomy showed that patients who had the latter reported worse postoperative sexual outcome (statistically significant) than supracervical

hysterectomy patients with respect to intercourse frequency, orgasm frequency and overall sexual satisfaction.[10] Irrespective of type of hysterectomy, a proportion of women undergoing bilateral salpingo-oopherectomy with hysterectomy experienced worse overall sexual satisfaction compared to those who underwent hysterectomy alone. Further prospective studies are required, as the data available showing a better outcome for supracervical hysterctomy are from small studies in which there may have been other confounding variables.

PLACES TO REFER WOMEN/COUPLES WITH PSYCHOSEXUAL PROBLEMS

- Relate – the national agency previously known as The Marriage Guidance Council – provides counselling for all relationship and psychosexual problems. (There may be a fee.)
- Local contraceptive/reproductive healthcare services may have a psychosexual service (contact your local consultant).
- Local hospital-based psychosexual services – may be within urology, gynaecology, genitourinary medicine or psychiatry departments.
- Private sex therapists (contacted via the British Association for Sexual and Marital Therapists or the British Association for Counselling).
- Doctors trained by the Institute of Psychosexual Medicine (contact the institute directly).

KEY POINTS

- It is important to classify further into site of pain: superficial or deep.
- Pain at intercourse can lead to problems of sexual arousal causing further sexual pain and then avoidance of sexual activity.
- If an organic cause for dyspareunia is found it does necessarily exclude emotional and/or psychological sequelae for the woman.
- In assessing gynaecological problems, where there is a good chance of concomitant psychosexual issues, such as vulval disorders and dyspareunia, it is extremely important that the clinician feels comfortable to ask about sexual problems.
- Dyspareunia is the only sexual disorder in which physical factors are thought to play a major aetiological role. However the psychological and interpersonal factors are significant.
- Observational studies indicate that treatment is generally very successful for women with vaginismus.

KEY REFERENCES

1. Rosen RC, Leiblum SR. The treatment of sexual disorders in the 1990s: an integrated approach. *J Consul Clin Psychol* 1995; **65**:877–90.
2. Schover LP, Youngs DD, Cannata R. Psychosexual aspects of the evaluation and management of vulvar vestibulitis. *Am J Obstet Gynecol* 1992; **167**:630–6.
3. Hawton K, Catalan J, Martin P, Fagg J. Long term outcome of sex therapy. *Behav Res Ther* 1986; 24:665–75.
4. Hawton K, Catalan J, Fagg J. Low sexual desire: sex therapy results and prognostic factors. *Behav Res Ther* 1991; **47**:832 8.
5. Sills E, Saini J, Steiner CA, McGee M, Gretz HF. Abdominal hysterectomy practice patterns in the United States. *Int J Gynecol Obstet* 1998; **63**:277–83.
6. Masters WH, Johnson VE. *Human Sexual Response.* Boston: Little, Brown, 1966.
7. Hanson HM. Cervical removal at hysterectomy for benign disease, risks and benefits. *J Reprod Med* 1993; 38:781–90.
8. Rhodes JC, Kjerrulff KH, Langenberg PW, Guzins GM. Hysterectomy and sexual functioning. *J Am Med Assoc* 2000; **283**(17):2238–9.
9. Kilkku P, Gronroos M, Hirvonen T, Rauramo L. Supravaginal uterine amputation versus hysterectomy: effects on libido and orgasm. *Acta Obstet Gynecol Scand* 1983; **62**:147–52.
10. Saini J, Kucccczynskii E, Herbert F, Gretz M, Scott Sills E. Supracervical hysterectomy versus total abdominal hysterectomy: perceived effects on sexual function. *BMC Women's Health* 2002; 2(1):1.

Child Sex Abuse

Melanie C. Mann

MRCOG standards

There are no established MRCOG standards for this topic, but we would suggest the following guidance points.

- Be able to define child sex abuse.
- Be aware of the different types and levels of abuse
- Be able to take a history relating to child sex abuse without causing mental or physical harm to the child.
- Be aware of referral pathways and support infrastructure for suspected cases of child sex abuse.

INTRODUCTION

The management of these problems requires special skill and sensitivity. It also requires knowledge of the legal issues surrounding allegations of child sexual abuse and the proper procedures that need to be followed. The skills required have a wide overlap with those necessary to deal with paediatric gynaecological problems and adult psychosexual problems.

The Children's Act 1989 defines a child as 'a person who has not yet reached 18 years of age'. In England and Wales the present age of consent for sexual intercourse is 16 years.

All health professionals play a part in ensuring that young people receive the care, support and services they require to promote their development. Sexual abuse is one form of child abuse. The others are emotional abuse, physical abuse and neglect.

Nature of sexual acts in child sex abuse

- **Exposure:** the viewing of sexual acts, pornography and exhibitionism.
- **Molestation:** fondling the genitals of the child or asking the child to fondle or masturbate the adult's genitals.
- **Sexual intercourse:** vaginal, oral or anal intercourse without excessive force, often chronic.
- **Rape:** vaginal sexual intercourse without consent, often with threats or the use of violence, which may occur on an acute basis.

DEFINITION

Child sex abuse is the involvement of dependent, developmentally immature children and adolescents in sexual activities that they do not fully comprehend, are unable to give informed consent to, and that violate the social taboos of family roles. It may occur over a wide range of ages and can involve single incidents perpetrated by strangers or frequent contacts by a family member or friend.

DETECTION OF CHILD SEX ABUSE

Occasionally a child may present to a gynaecologist for investigation of symptoms and there may be a query about sexual abuse. It is important that the gynaecologist is able to bear the risk of child sex abuse in mind during the history and examination without causing mental or physical harm to the child.

The recognition of penile or digital penetration is very difficult in certain age groups and should always be referred to a paediatrician. Ideally, all children should be examined in a child-friendly environment with a paediatric-trained nurse present. All Trusts in the UK have a child protection policy and it is the duty of all healthcare professionals working with children to be aware of the local referral pathways. Each Trust has a named doctor and nurse who take a professional lead for child protection matters within the Trust. This will ensure that each suspected case is treated promptly in the best interests of the child.

DETECTION OF A SEXUALLY TRANSMITTED INFECTION IN A CHILD

In children under 3 years old, the possibility of vertical transmission must always be considered and investigated.

In children aged 12 years or older, the possibility of consensual sexual intercourse should be considered. The proportion of young people who are sexually active before the age of 16 is increasing. The co-existence of drug or alcohol misuse and the increased vulnerability of those living away from home/accommodated by the local authority must be considered and addressed. The possibility of the young person being a commercial sex worker must also be considered.

Liaison with local social workers, paediatricians and genitourinary physicians is mandatory. There are specific medicolegal methods for the investigation of sexually transmitted infections (STIs) that need to be followed. See 'chain of evidence', as described in Chapter 63.5.

The confidentiality of young people attending for advice is very important. In practice, a clinician must take into account both the need of the young person for a confidential sexual health service and the need to protect that young person from sexual abuse and sexual exploitation. The clinician also has a duty to consider the possibility that other young people may be at risk of abuse. This means that the clinician must work with the young person to obtain her confidence and inform her if and when confidentiality may have to be broken.

KEY POINT

Liaison with local Child Protection Team is mandatory.

ADULT SEQUELAE OF CHILD SEX ABUSE[1]

Recent prevalence studies show that about 1 in 3 adult women have had sexual contact with an older person as a child. Sexual abuse is a serious mental health problem and often results in impairment as adults, but less than 20 per cent of affected women show serious psychopathology.

There can be many manifestations of child sex abuse that has taken place in the past, and these can be mild or can cause havoc in the adult's life and can be revealed during history taking or examination. Sensitivity and care must be exercised in all consultations to ensure that the woman is enabled to reveal the intimate secret and can be directed to appropriate help as required. Occasionally, just a sympathetic attitude and 'believing her' are all that is required. The adult sequelae of child sex abuse include the following.

- Depression: the commonest symptom, coinciding with low self-esteem, anxiety and sleep disorders.
- Pelvic pain: several studies have shown an association with pelvic pain and other gynaecological complaints.
- Sexual adjustment problems: these vary from retreat to apparent preoccupation with sexual matters and promiscuity.
- Interpersonal relationship problems: victims are more likely to have physically violent partners – 'continuing victims'.
- Social functioning: there is link between child sex abuse and later prostitution; there is also evidence for increased alcohol and drug abuse in this group.

There is no clear-cut evidence as to which factors lead to a negative outcome for child sex abuse survivors, but there are trends. It would appear that the worse-case scenario is regular abuse, with force, by a close, older member of the family, such as father to daughter.

Adult survivors should be referred to an appropriately trained counsellor. The referral pathways differ locally.

KEY POINTS

- Sensitivity during history taking and examination will aid the diagnosis of previous child sex abuse.
- The patient can then be referred to an appropriate counsellor.
- Child sex abuse is a serious mental health problem often resulting in impairment in adulthood.

PUBLISHED GUIDELINES

Thomas A, Forster G, Robinson A, Rogstad K.
National Guideline on the Management of Suspected Sexually Transmitted Infections in Children and Young People. Clinical Effectiveness Group (AGUM and MSSVD) 2003. <www.mssvd.org.uk>.

KEY REFERENCE

1. Sheldrick C. Adult sequelae of child sexual abuse. *Br J Psych* 1991; **158**(Suppl. 10):55–62.

Pelvic floor and lower urinary tract

Rape and Rape Counselling

Susan J. Houghton

MRCOG standards

The are no established standards relevant for this topic. The following are suggested.

Theoretical skills
- Understand the definitions of types of sexual assault.
- Be aware of the signs of sexual trauma on general and genital examination.
- Be aware of the holistic needs of the victims of sexual assault.

Practical skills
- Be aware of how to conduct a forensic examination and what forensic evidence needs to be collected.

INTRODUCTION

It is estimated that between 1 in 4 and 1 in 6 women will be raped during their lifetimes [II].[1,2] Drug-assisted assault is becoming increasingly common. Rape and sexual assault can be associated with physical harm, infection, unwanted pregnancy and severe psychological damage. The aim of this chapter is to highlight the role of the examining doctor in the assessment of victims of sexual assault (the complainants). It defines rape, details the forensic medical examination and what forensic evidence should be obtained, and what is required in the witness statement. Ideally, all victims of sexual assault should be examined by forensic medical examiners who have received specific training in forensic gynaecology (police surgeons).

DEFINITIONS

Rape is defined as 'unlawful sexual intercourse by a man with a woman, by force, fear or fraud' (Sexual Offences Act, 1956, England).

Either the man must know that the woman did not give consent or he was reckless (i.e. did not care) whether she gave consent or not (Sexual Offences (Amendments) Act, 1976, England).

Unlawful means without valid consent (due to no consent being given or invalid consent, if the victim is below the age of consent, or mentally deficient).

Sexual intercourse refers to any degree of vaginal or anal penetration (from entry of the tip of the penis to full penetration).

Force, fear or fraud includes actual bodily violence, threat of violence to self or third party, use of drugs or alcohol to subdue the woman, a medical claim that intercourse is a form of treatment, impersonation of the woman's husband in darkness.

The age of consent in Britain is 16 years; below this age, sexual intercourse is always unlawful. In 1994 a man could be charged with raping his wife (R v RIAC 599 House of Lords).

Indecent assault includes unproven rape, a male masturbating over the complainant, insertion of objects into an orifice, fondling of breasts, thighs and perineum, and putting a hand up a woman's skirt.

MANAGEMENT

The examination of an alleged rape victim should take place as soon as possible after the alleged assault and in an appropriate environment, preferably in a specifically designed 'rape suite' in a police station or hospital. A trained woman police officer should be present, if the complainant requests police involvement, and the complainant should choose the gender of the examining doctor.

Management of the immediate medical needs of the complainant

The management of injuries requiring immediate medical attention takes priority over forensic sampling. Up to 80 per cent of rape victims have some form of physical injury [III],[3] with up to 5 per cent having major non-genital injuries [II].[4] A minority of rape victims sustain genital injury, with <30 per cent of premenopausal and <50 per cent of post-menopausal victims having demonstrable genital injury [III].[5] Injury is much more likely if forced anal intercourse has occurred.

Accurate history taking of the alleged incident to determine which forensic samples should be taken

Prior to the medical examination, the police officer should obtain a detailed investigative history, or 'first account', from the complainant to establish if an offence has been committed. The forensic medical examiner (FME) should ask direct questions based upon the first account (Table 63.5.1) and the questions and answers should be recorded verbatim in the medical records. The complainant's name, age and date of birth; the date, time and place of the examination; persons present at the examination and their relationship to the victim; and details of the victim's general practitioner should be clearly documented.

Relevant medical and sexual history

This is necessary to assist with the interpretation of the medical findings and to identify any medical problems that may be attributable to the assault (Table 63.5.2).

Informed consent for the forensic medical examination

Consent must be obtained for a medical examination (non-genital and genital), the collection of forensic evidence, the retention of relevant items of clothing for forensic examination and the disclosure of details of medical records to the police and/or Crown Prosecution Service (CPS).

Thorough medical examination

The examination should be performed with the use of a Sexual Offences kit, which contains all the necessary equipment, such as swabs, gloves, disposable speculum, specimen and blood bottles, plastic and brown-paper bags,

Table 63.5.1 Assault history to be taken by forensic medical examiner

Details of the assault
Date and time of assault
Time lapse from assault
Name of assailant (if known)
Relationship of assailant to victim
History of assault
Source of history
Events preceding the assault
Place of assault
Drugs or alcohol consumed by the victim
Details of the assault – to direct forensic sampling
Damage or disruption to clothing
Site and mechanism of injuries – to include details of any
weapons or implements used
Defence used by victim
Relative position of parties
Any loss of consciousness
Exact nature of assault
Digital/vaginal – yes/no
Oral/vaginal – yes/no
Oral/penile – yes/no
Penile/vaginal – yes/no (If yes, did ejaculation occur?)
Penile/anal – yes/no (If yes, did ejaculation occur?)
Digital/anal – yes/no
Lubricant used?
Condom used?
Events following assault
Description of what occurred following the assault, to include details of:
changing of clothes
washing the genital area
taking a shower or bath
washing of hair
cleaning of teeth
micturition or defecation
vomiting
ingestion of food or drink
any medical treatment received since assault

Table 63.5.2 Relevant medical and sexual history

Gynaecological history	
Age at menarche	
Last menstrual period – forensic analysis cannot distinguish between	
menstrual blood and that related to injury	
Menstrual cycle	
Any gynaecological problems:	
current	
past history	
Obstetric history:	
pregnant - presently/previously/never	
outcome of previous pregnancies	
Sexual history	
Sexually active - presently/previously/never?	
Last coitus:	
date	
time	
use of lubricant	– yes/no
Genital problems	– past/present
Sexually transmitted diseases	– yes/no
General medical history	
History of serious illness	– past/present
Psychiatric problems	– yes/no
Previous operations	– yes/no
Bruising tendency	– yes/no
Skin problems	– yes/no
Social history	
Current occupation	

labels, scissors, combs, gown, a sheet of brown paper, information sheet and medical examination record.

External examination

The general appearance and emotional state of the complainant are assessed for evidence of alcohol/drug intoxication, damage or staining of clothes, hair, face, hands and fingernails, and evidence of the acute phase of rape trauma syndrome. Clothing should be removed by the complainant whilst standing on a sheet of brown paper (shiny side up) to catch any falling debris. Each item is inspected and described in detail before the police officer places it into a labelled brown-paper bag and submits it for forensic examination. The complainant is carefully examined for any injuries, and an estimate made of the timing of these injuries. All injuries should be described according to the Crane classification [IV][6] and documented on a body chart. Complex injuries should be photographed. Bite marks should be swabbed to obtain samples of the assailant's saliva and photographed by a forensic odontologist.

Genital and internal examination

The forensic samples taken are listed in Table 63.5.3. The samples must be clearly labelled and documented before transport to the forensic science laboratory. Anonymous samples may be sent, with consent, in cases where the complainant does not want to report the assault to the police.

Table 63.5.3   Forensic samples to be taken at forensic medical examination

Non-intimate samples
Control swabs – wet and dry
Buccal swab – for DNA analysis if venesection refused
Saliva specimen – if oral assault
Skin swab – at site of kissing/sucking/ejaculation/bite (moistened if necessary)
Head hair combings
Head hair cuttings
Right and left nail scrapings – if visible debris or if victim scratched assailant
Nail cuttings – if broken nails or if victim scratched assailant
Nail filings – to recover blood samples or skin fragments

Intimate samples
Pubic hair combings
Pubic hair cuttings
Vulval swabs
Introital swabs
Low vaginal swabs
Cervical swabs – should be taken if vaginal intercourse has taken place more than 48 hour ago
Anal and rectal swabs – a proctoscope may need to be used in cases of anal penetration
High vaginal swabs – preferably four swabs should be taken
Blood samples – for DNA analysis, blood typing, alcohol estimation, toxicology screen
Tampon or sanitary towel – if used, can be analysed for semen and body fluids
Urine sample – for alcohol and toxicology testing
Examination gown should be sent for analysis

A photographer of the same gender as the victim must take any genital or intimate photographs. Colposcopy is not routinely used in the UK for the assessment of rape victims.

Management of the sexual and mental health of the victim

Preventing and treating sexually transmitted infections

Sexually transmitted infections occur in between 4 and 56 per cent of women following sexual assault.[7] Screening for gonorrhoea, chlamydia, trichomoniasis and syphilis should be performed at initial presentation.[8] If screening is not possible, or is declined, empirical antibiotic prophylaxis should be offered:

- ciprofloxacin 500 mg plus doxycycline 100 mg twice daily for 7 days, **or**
- ciprofloxacin 500 mg plus azithromycin 1 g **or, if pregnant or breastfeeding,**
- amoxycillin 3 g plus probenecid 1 g or erythromycin 500 mg twice daily for 14 days.

Hepatitis B vaccination should be offered up to 3 weeks after sexual assault to all victims who are not known to be immune.[8] The risk of contracting human immunodeficiency virus (HIV) infection as a result of rape is unknown, but is thought to be very low in areas of low prevalence, such as the UK. The risk may be higher in cases of genital trauma.[9] Individual risk is assessed and post-exposure prophylaxis (PEP) with zidovudine and lamivudine plus nelfinavir or indinivar is offered to those with a negative baseline HIV ELISA test. PEP should be continued for 28 days and involves pre-HIV test counselling, informed consent and monitoring by an HIV specialist.

A repeat infection screen should be performed at 2 weeks' follow-up if antibiotic prophylaxis was not given initially. At 3 months, HIV, hepatitis B and syphilis tests should be repeated with hepatitis C testing, if thought to be at risk.

Pregnancy

Rape-related pregnancy occurs in up to 5 per cent of women [II].[10] Postcoital contraception with Levonelle-2 (within 72 hours) or an intrauterine contraceptive device (within 5 days) should be offered and a pre-existing pregnancy excluded. Counselling and support, with referral to specialist agencies, should be offered to those who become pregnant.

Psychological support

It is estimated that over half of all women who are raped suffer from post-traumatic stress disorder (PTSD). Following the rape, symptoms of anxiety, depression, tearfulness, flashbacks, humiliation, self-blame, disbelief, anger, fear, powerlessness and physical revulsion are common [III].[11] Long-term problems with social adjustment, sexual relationships, physical health and substance abuse can occur [II].[12] Verbal and written advice concerning support and counselling agencies should be given.

> - Victim Support, Crammer House, 39 Brixton Road, London SW9 6WQ, Tel: 020 7735 9166; <www.victimsupport.com>
> - Survivors UK Ltd, PO Box 2470, London SW9 6WQ, Tel: 020 7613 0808; <www.survivorsuk.co.uk>
> - Rape Crisis Federation Wales & England, 7 Mansfield Road, Nottingham NG1 3FB, Tel: 0115 934 8474; <www.rapecrisis.co.uk>

Completion of a witness statement

The 'professional' witness statement should include details of the history of the assault and relevant medical, surgical and psychiatric history, document all of the normal and abnormal findings of the examination, list the forensic specimens taken, and give details about any medical treatment given and post-examination arrangements. The FME should give an opinion as to the degree of certainty about the likely cause of the injuries.

The statement should have a professional appearance, must be carefully checked for errors, and must include a statutory declaration, with the date and signature at the bottom of each page and at the end of the declaration. A witness should also sign each page. The FME should state his or her qualifications, appointment and relevant experience and it is advisable for new examining doctors to discuss the case and statement preparation with an experienced FME. Many police forces have standard statement forms for the FME to complete.

SUMMARY

Any doctor involved in the care of a rape victim must be sensitive, sympathetic and highly professional. With advances in forensic science, it is essential that forensic samples are taken in an attempt to identify DNA for profiling. A meticulous examination, detailed medical records and an accurate and detailed statement are essential in the management of victims of sexual assault.

> The supporting evidence for the advocated management plan (and the above text) relies on observational data, cohort studies, retrospective descriptive studies and 'expert opinion'. Given the nature of the condition, it is unlikely that evidence based upon more robust methodologies will be forthcoming.

KEY POINTS

- Be sympathetic and professional.
- Attend to immediate medical needs.
- Examine in an appropriate and comfortable environment.
- Obtain consent for examination.
- Take an accurate history.
- Clearly document findings and carefully label samples.
- Give appropriate medical, prophylactic and psychological treatment.
- Advise on counselling and support agencies.

KEY REFERENCES

1. Walch AG, Broadhead WE. Prevalance of lifetime sexual victimisation among female patients. *J Fam Practice* 1992; **35**:511–16.
2. Roberts R. Rape crisis management. *Diplomate* 1994; **1**:6–11.
3. Bowyer L, Dalton ME. Female victims of rape and their genital findings. *Br J Obstet Gynaecol* 1997; **104**:617–20.
4. Marchbanks PA, Liu KJ, Mercy JA. Risk of injury from resisting rape. *Am J Epidemiol* 1990; **132**:540–9.
5. Cartwright PS and the Sexual Assault Study Group. Factors that correlate with injury sustained by survivors of sexual assault. *Obstet Gynecol* 1987; **70**:44–6.
6. Crane J. Injury. In: McClay WDS (ed.). *Clinical Forensic Medicine*. London: Greenwich Medical Media, 1996, 143–62.
7. Lamba H, Murphy SM. Sexual assault and sexually transmitted infections: an updated review. *Int J STD AIDS* 2000; **11**:487–91.
8. Clinical Effectiveness Group. *National Guidelines on the Management of Adult Victims of Sexual Assault.* Association of Genitourinary Medicine and the Medical Society for the Study of Venereal Diseases, 2001. Available on: <http://www.mssvd.org.uk> [September 2001].
9. Claydon E. Rape and HIV. *Int J STD AIDS* 1991; **2**:200–1.
10. Holmes MM, Resnick HS, Kilpatrick DG, Best CL. Rape-related pregnancy: estimates and descriptive characteristics from a national sample of women. *Am J Obstet Gynecol* 1996; **175**:320–5.
11. Hampton HL. Care of the woman who has been raped. *N Engl J Med* 1995; **332**:234–7.
12. Mezey GC, Taylor PJ. Psychological reactions of women who have been raped: a descriptive and comparative study. *Br J Psych* 1988; **152**:330–9.

SECTION C

Lower genital tract

Chapter 64

Benign Vulval Problems

Charles Redman

INTRODUCTION

Many women have vulval symptoms but only a fraction will seek medical advice. Of these, only a selected few will be referred for a specialist opinion. Some may be advised to attend a genitourinary medicine (GUM) clinic, whilst others will be referred for a gynaecological opinion. This chapter primarily relates to women attending gynaecological or vulval clinics.

ANATOMICAL CONSIDERATIONS

Vulval skin comprises stratified squamous epithelium as in other parts of the body. The mons pubis and labia majora contain fat, sebaceous, apocrine and eccrine sweat glands and blood vessels, which can develop varicosities. However, whereas the labia minora are rich in sebaceous glands, there are few sweat glands and no hair follicles. The epithelium of the vestibule is neither pigmented nor keratinized, but contains eccrine glands. These glands and epithelial appendages are a source of vulval lumps.

Deep to the posterior parts of the labia majora are the Bartholin's or greater vestibular glands, whose ducts open into the posterior part of the vagina, just behind the mid-point and superficial to the hymenal ring. The glands and ducts can be the site of infection or cyst formation.

ASSESSMENT

Extrinsic and intrinsic causes

Whereas benign vulval disease has relatively few symptoms (pruritus, burning, pain, lumps), there are a myriad of causes. It is helpful when assessing a case to consider whether the problem arises from the skin itself or from the variety of factors that it comes into contact with, such as moisture (sweat, urine, vaginal discharge, infection, allergens and irritants). The key to making a diagnosis is clinical assessment from a careful history and, in particular, examination.

History

It is important accurately to ascertain the nature of the presenting problem and the pattern of the symptoms in terms of periodicity and aggravating and relieving factors. It is vital to ask about what treatments have been used in the past as well as about current and previous medications and general health.

Examination

This should include a survey of the whole of the skin and other systems as indicated. An examination of the rest of the lower genital tract should always be considered, though it is by no means always necessary.

Table 64.1 International Society for the Study of Vulvar Diseases (ISSVD) classification of non-neoplastic epithelial disorders of the vulva

Lichen sclerosus
Squamous cell hyperplasia
Other dermatoses
Primary irritant dermatitis
Allergic dermatitis
Seborrhoeic dermatitis
Psoriasis
Lichen planus
Hidradenitis suppuritiva
Behçet's syndrome

Vulval biopsy

Biopsy is frequently necessary to confirm the diagnosis, if not clear, and to assess or confirm whether or not a lesion is pre-invasive or malignant. It is important to biopsy chronic dermatoses that do not respond to medical treatment. By and large, vulval biopsies can be performed in the clinic using disposable biopsy punches with local anaesthesia.

NON-NEOPLASTIC EPITHELIAL DISORDERS

The group of conditions once referred to as vulval dystrophies is now termed non-neoplastic epithelial disorders, classified by the ISSVD in 1987 (Table 64.1).

Lichen sclerosus

Definition

Lichen sclerosus is characterized by epithelial thinning, inflammation and distinctive histological changes in the dermis. It can affect both sexes and can occur at any age, but it is typically found in the anogenital region in postmenopausal women.

Lichen sclerosus can be asymptomatic, but the most common presentation is intractable itching (pruritus vulvae) and vaginal soreness with dyspareunia. Burning and pain are uncommon symptoms and should arouse suspicion of alternative or concomitant conditions.

The clinical findings are distinctive but variable. The lesions may be characterized by a crinkled or parchment-like appearance that usually extends around the anal area in a figure-of-eight configuration. There is often loss of the normal vulval architecture, with atrophy of the labia minora, constriction of the vaginal orifice, and the development of adhesions, ecchymoses, telangiectasia and fissures.

Incidence

The prevalence of lichen sclerosus is unknown, but this group of patients usually constitutes the largest single diagnostic group in a hospital-based vulval clinic.

Aetiology/risk factors

The cause is unknown.

Prognosis

Lichen sclerosus can occur in children and in about two-thirds of cases the lesions will clear at puberty.[1] In adults, lichen sclerosus is a chronic condition that can be considered to be pre-malignant, with a reported incidence of progression to squamous vulval cancer ranging from 0 to 9 per cent.[2,3]

Management

The aims of management are to control the symptoms and to detect changes suggestive of malignant change.

GENERAL MEASURES

It is important to reassure patients that lichen sclerosus is a well-recognized condition, which, although unlikely to disappear, can almost always be satisfactorily controlled with simple measures.

Bland emollients should be used liberally and can provide significant relief [II]. The high response rates noted when these are used as the placebo arm in randomized, controlled trials (RCTs) are thought to be more than a placebo effect.[4]

TOPICAL STEROIDS

Three RCTs have found that potent topical steroids (e.g. clobetasol propionate) provided significant symptom control, particularly in the short term [Ia], and that they are more effective than topical testosterone or petroleum jelly. Few, if any, adverse effects have been noted in association with the use of clobetasol propionate, even when used on an 'as-required basis' for maintenance therapy for 1–3 years [II].[4]

Testosterone is no more effective than petroleum jelly [Ib], but can be associated with virilization, hypertrichosis, pruritus and pain.

RETINOIDS

One small RCT has found acitretin to be more effective that placebo [Ib]. Acitretin is associated with severe peeling of palms and soles and with hair loss [Ib], as well as with congenital abnormalities in women exposed during the first trimester of pregnancy. It is therefore contraindicated in the reproductive age group.

Surgery

In general, surgery should be avoided unless there is malignant change [IV]. There is no systematic review, RCTs or good-quality observation studies demonstrating the benefits of surgery for symptomatic relief in lichen sclerosus. Three studies reported re-operation rates after vulvectomy of 23–50 per cent for recurrence of symptoms, malignant change or introital stenosis [III].[2]

Squamous cell hyperplasia

Definition

This is a diagnosis of exclusion. Histologically there is hyperkeratosis (greater than is seen in lichen sclerosus) and lengthening and distortion of the rete pegs (acanthosis). Cellular elements of the epithelium proliferate but maturation is normal. An inflammatory response in the dermis usually occurs, consisting of lymphocytic and plasma cell infiltration.

The skin is thickened with white hyperkeratotic patches, excoriation and fissures.

Incidence

The incidence is unknown, but squamous cell hyperplasia is less commonly seen than lichen sclerosus in vulval clinics.

Aetiology/risk factors

Squamous cell hyperplasia may be the result of repetitive surface irritation and trauma from irritants that cause scratching and rubbing.

Prognosis

The risk of developing vulval cancer has been estimated to be 1–5 per cent.

Management

In general terms, the management of squamous cell hyperplasia is the same as for lichen sclerosus, although the long-term use of potent topical steroids has more adverse sequelae [II].[5]

Lichen sclerosus/squamous cell hyperplasia symptom control

- Bland emollients are more effective than placebo.
- Three RCTs suggest that potent steroids are safe and effective in controlling symptoms and that testosterone is no more effective than placebo.
- No evidence supports the use of surgery.

Lichen planus

Definition

This can be an acute or chronic condition affecting the skin or mucous membranes or both.

On keratinized skin, lichen planus is characterized by flat-topped, violaceous, shiny papules. On the vulva, the appearance ranges from delicate, white reticulated papules to an erosive, desquamating process. Large denuded areas may lead to profuse discharge and scarring.

Incidence

Lichen planus is uncommon.

Aetiology

The aetiology is unknown, but the evidence suggests that it is immunologically mediated.

Prognosis

Vulval lesions tend to disappear after weeks or months. Erosive lesions heal poorly and may be pre-malignant.

Management

The diagnosis is confirmed by biopsy.

Initial treatment consists of topical high-potency corticosteroid ointments. Short courses of systemic corticosteroids may be needed for severe symptoms [III].

Inflammatory dermatoses

Definition

Inflammatory dermatoses can be classified as either contact or primary irritant dermatitis or allergic dermatitis. It can be difficult to differentiate between the two.

Typical findings are diffuse reddening of the involved skin with excoriation and ulceration. Secondary infection may occur. The main differential diagnosis is vulval candidiasis.

Aetiology

Irritants such as perfumed soaps, feminine hygiene deodorants, bubble baths, urine and tight clothing [III] cause irritant dermatitis, a common cause of vulval irritation.

In atopic individuals, non-irritant substances that include iatrogenic factors such as local anaesthetic creams cause allergic dermatitis.

Incidence

The population-based incidence is unknown, but inflammatory dermatoses account for about 25 per cent of new vulval clinic patients [III].[6]

Management

Once the causative factor has been identified and exposure to it avoided, symptomatic control can be instigated using either oral antihistamines or a topical corticosteroid. Fluorinated steroid creams may be used, but for short periods only as atrophy can be associated with their long-term use [II].

Seborrhoeic dermatitis

Definition

This occurs in areas of the skin where sebaceous glands are active, such as the face, scalp, body folds and, less commonly, the genitalia. When the vulva is involved, the labia majora and mons pubis are affected. The lesions are scaly, orange-pink in colour and can be secondarily infected.

Incidence

Seborrhoeic dermatitis is an uncommon vulval problem.

Aetiology

It is associated with *Malassezia ovalis* infection, a yeast that plays a central role in the pathogenesis of seborrhoeic dermatitis.

Management

The treatment of choice is an antifungal agent such as 2 per cent miconazole or 2 per cent ketoconazole cream or shampoo. Antifungal treatment is more effective than hydrocortisone creams or placebo [Ib].[7,8]

Psoriasis

Aetiology

Psoriasis is a hereditary skin disorder that affects 1–2 per cent of the general population.

Incidence

Genetic and environmental factors are both important. About a third of people with psoriasis have a family history, but physical trauma, acute infection and selected medications are commonly viewed as triggers [III].

Definition

A well-defined, smooth erythematous lesion with a sharp outline is characteristic.

Prognosis

There are no long-term prognostic studies and at present there is no cure for psoriasis.

Management

There are no systematic reviews or publications on the specific management of vulval psoriasis. In general terms, the aim of management is to achieve short-term suppression of symptoms with minimal adverse effects.

As several trigger and perpetuating factors for psoriasis have been recognized, management of lifestyle might have been thought to be helpful. However, there is no good evidence to support this view or the use of non-drug treatment.

Emollients and keratolytics have no proven benefit [Ia] and tar preparations should be avoided, as they are irritating [III].

In psoriasis in general, topical steroids are beneficial in the short term [Ia], but prolonged use should be avoided. Vitamin D derivatives may be as effective as steroids, but without the risk of skin atrophy, although irritation may be a problem [Ia].[9]

Hidradenitis suppurativa

Definition

This is a chronic, suppurative, inflammatory disorder of the apocrine glands. It is characterized by deep, painful subcutaneous nodules that may ulcerate and drain, leading to open sinuses and extensive scarring. On the vulva, the disease primarily affects the labia majora and intercrural folds, but may also involve the mons pubis, labia minora and clitoris.

Incidence

Hidradenitis suppurativa is a common condition, particularly in black women. It is rare before puberty and less common after the climateric.

Aetiology

The aetiology is unknown.

Management

Multiple therapies, including topical and systemic antibiotics and oral contraceptives, steroids and isotretinoin, have been used with limited success [II]. Surgery remains a mainstay in the treatment of this disorder, and wide excision of the involved areas may be necessary [II].

Ulcerative dermatoses

Definition

The ulcerating lesions of the vulva in this condition may be solitary or multiple, painful or non-tender.

Incidence

The lesions are uncommon in a standard vulval clinic, but are seen more often in a GUM clinic.

Aetiology

The ulcers that arise from vesicles are typical of herpes simplex virus (HSV). The ulcers arising from papules are characteristic syphilis, chancroid, granuloma inguinale and lymphogranuloma venereum. Solitary, non-tender ulcers are characteristic of syphilis, lymphogranuloma venereum and neoplasia. Multiple painful ulcers occur in HSV, Behçet's disease and Crohn's disease.

Management

Laboratory evaluation including serological testing and culture is often necessary, and there should be a low threshold for seeking the opinion of the GUM team. When a single ulcer is present, biopsy is important [IV].

Treatment is dependent on the diagnosis. The vulval manifestations of Behçet's disease can be treated by topical fluorinated corticosteroid creams [III].

Vulval dermatoses other than lichen sclerosus and squamous cell hyperplasia

The evidence relating to the management of this group of conditions is limited. A number of non-randomized studies indicate that topical steroids are useful in certain conditions, but the following points should be noted.

- *Seborrhoeic dermatitis.* A number of uncontrolled studies have confirmed the effectiveness of antifungal treatment and one small RCT indicates that it is more effective than hydrocortisone creams.
- *Psoriasis.* No vulva-specific evidence has been found. More than 30 RCTs have shown that topical steroids are beneficial in the short term, but prolonged use should be avoided. One systematic review has demonstrated that vitamin D derivatives may be as effective as steroids.

KEY POINTS

Benign vulval skin conditions

- Comprehensive clinical assessment is essential.
- Multidisciplinary assessment can be useful.
- Biopsy when symptoms are refractory or there is suspicion of atypia.
- Simple measures, such as the use of emollient creams, are often effective.
- In lichen sclerosus, potent corticosteroids are effective and safe.
- In general, the prolonged use of potent corticosteroids is to be avoided.
- With the exception of hidradenitis suppurativa, surgery is best avoided.

VAGINAL DISCHARGE

A vaginal discharge resulting from cervical and vaginal secretion is normal in women in the reproductive age group. Vulval soreness and irritation can be secondary to excessive vaginal discharge, the causes of which are listed in Table 64.2. Vaginal discharge arising as a result of a sexually transmitted infection is covered in Chapter 63.1.

Management is based on diagnosis, which is reached by systemic clinical enquiry and examination, supplemented by appropriate investigation.

Physiological discharge can be increased in pregnancy and in oral contraception users. Heavy vaginal loss can be associated with a large cervical ectropion. Although bacterial vaginosis is at least twice as common as vulvovaginal

Table 64.2   Causes of excessive vaginal discharge

Physiological

Infective
Bacterial vaginosis
Monilial vaginosis
Trichomonal vaginosis

Malignant
Endometrial cancer
Cervical cancer
Vaginal cancer

Miscellaneous
Foreign body, e.g. retained or 'lost' tampon, vaginal ring

candidiasis,[10] it does not usually cause vulvitis, although it may co-exist with thrush. In the context of a vulval clinic, recurrent vulvovaginal candidiasis is an important condition.

Candidal vulvovaginosis

Definition

Vulvovaginal candidiasis is a mycotic disease, which is usually caused by the dimorphic yeast *Candida albicans*, a commensal of the genital and digestive tracts. A minority of cases are caused by the non-albicans species, such as *Candida glabrata* and *Candida tropicalis*. The clinical features caused by albicans and non-albicans species are indistinguishable.

The condition is characterized by vulval itching, although burning and soreness may occur; however, none of these symptoms is specific. Typically, the vulva is red, dry and fissured. A white, curdish discharge that adheres to the vaginal walls and cervix is classically described.

Acute infection is confirmed by the presence of candidal pseudohyphae or budding yeast forms, but this is a relatively insensitive test. Culture of a vaginal swab is the most sensitive test; the presence of more than ten yeast colonies supports the diagnosis.

Recurrent vulvovaginal candidiasis is defined as four or more episodes of symptomatic candidiasis annually.

Incidence

The prevalence of *Candida albicans* in healthy young women is 20–25 per cent. Uncomplicated vulvovaginal candidiasis affects about 75 per cent of women at least once in their lifetime. Recurrence is said to occur in <5 per cent of cases.

Aetiology

Most episodes occur without an obvious cause. A relatively small proportion of women treated with broad-spectrum antibiotics subsequently develop vulvovaginal candidiasis, usually as a result of prior colonization. There is a strong association with sexual activity. There are a number of other well-recognized risk factors, including:

- diabetes mellitus
- immunosuppression

- pregnancy
- oral contraceptive pill
- cunnilingus.

Prognosis

Uncomplicated vulvovaginal candidiasis is usually self-limiting.

Management

Patients should avoid local irritants and tightly fitting synthetic garments [II].

Topically applied azoles (clotrimazole, econazole, miconazole) are effective in treating symptoms; they should always be used with vaginal pessaries. There is no evidence to suggest that asymptomatic women need treatment [Ia].[11] Four-day courses will cure just over half of infections, whereas a 7-day course cures more than 90 per cent. Pregnant women should be offered longer courses of treatment than non-pregnant women [Ia].[11] There is no evidence that any one imidazole is more effective than another. There are no reliable studies concerning the safety or efficacy of any complimentary therapies for prevention or cure (e.g. live yoghurt), and such treatments cannot therefore be recommended.

No differences exist in terms of the relative effectiveness (measured as clinical and mycological cure) of antifungals administered by the oral and intravaginal routes for the treatment of uncomplicated vaginal candidiasis, and no definitive conclusion can be made regarding their relative safety, although pregnant women should not be given oral treatment [Ib]. The oral route of administration is the preferred route for antifungals for the treatment of vulvovaginal candidiasis [Ia].[12] in women who are not pregnant.

In women with recurrent symptoms, it is important to exclude diabetes. There are a number of studies that have demonstrated the effectiveness of either an oral or topical antifungal maintenance therapy, which can be continued for about 6 months [Ib].

Vulvovaginal candidiasis

Summary of Cochrane database systematic review.

- Asymptomatic infection does not warrant treatment.
- Topical and oral antifungal azoles are both highly effective.
- The treatment of partners is ineffective.

KEY POINTS

Vaginal discharge

- Excessive vaginal discharge is a common gynaecological complaint and can cause vulval symptoms.

- Comprehensive clinical assessment is essential.
- Vulvovaginal candidiasis is highly responsive to antifungal treatment; the persistence of symptoms throws doubt on the diagnosis.
- Recurrent vulvovaginal candidiasis, which can occur in 5 per cent of cases, can be palliated by prolonged antifungal maintenance therapy.

Vulval lumps (Table 64.3)

Definition

Cysts are either congenital or arise from obstructed glands. Mucous cysts arise from mesonephric duct remnants and may be found at the introitus or labia minora. A cyst of the canal of Nuck (processus vaginalis peritonei) that fills with fluid can give rise to a hydrocele within the labia majora (associated with a concurrent inguinal hernia in 30 per cent of cases). The clinical manifestations are either due to the cyst itself or to infection, as in a Bartholin's abscess.

Vulval skin is subject to the same range of lesions that can occur on skin in other parts of the body. Most cause no symptoms other than compromising cosmesis.

Incidence

Vulval lumps of one sort or another are common and usually benign. Bartholin's cysts are the most common cystic lesions. Vulval varicosities are more common during pregnancy. Pigmented vulval skin lesions occur in 10 per cent of women, of which lentigo is the most common. Fibromata and fibromyomata are the most common of the benign solid tumours, usually developing along the insertion of the round ligament into the labia majora, and lipomata are the second most common solid tumours.[13]

Prognosis

By and large, benign vulval neoplasms behave like similar lesions elsewhere. It has been suggested that vulval naevi may be more likely to undergo malignant transformation than elsewhere, but the likelihood of this occurring is small.

Table 64.3 Types of benign vulval lumps

Cystic	Solid	Anatomic
Bartholin's cyst	Lentigo	Varicosities
Congenital mucous cysts	Seborrhoeic keratosis	Herniae
Skene's duct cyst	Fibroepithelial polyp	
Cyst of the canal of Nuck	Papillomatosis	
Epidermal inclusion cyst	Fibroma	
Furunculosis	Dermatofibroma	
Sebaceous cysts	Lipoma	
	Condylomata	
	Hidradenoma	

Management

Most vulval lumps are benign and can be treated conservatively. Cysts can be drained and/or marsupialized, particularly if symptomatic. Solid tumours are better excised for histological assessment [IV].

KEY POINTS

Benign vulval lumps

- Most vulval lumps are benign and can be treated conservatively.
- Excisional biopsy is indicated in solid lesions or when the diagnosis is uncertain.
- Cysts can be drained without risk to vulval cosmesis.

KEY REFERENCES

1. Wallace HJ. Lichen sclerosus et atrophicus. *Transactions of the St John's Hospital Dermatological Society* 1971; **57**:9–30.

2. Abramov Y, Elchalal U, Abramov D, Goldfarb A, Schenker JG. Surgical treatment of vulval lichen sclerosus: a review. *Obstet Gynecol Surv* 1996; **51**:193–9.

3. Tidy JA, Soutter WP, Luesley DM, MacLean AB, Buckley CH, Ridley CM. Management of lichen sclerosus and intraepithelial neoplasia of the vulva in the UK. *J R Soc Med* 1996; **89**:699–701.

4. Thomas E, Murphy D, Redman C. Premalignant vulval disorders. In: *Clinical Evidence*, Issue 6. London: BMJ Publishing Group, 2001, 1461–6.

5. Clark TJ, Etherington IJ, Luesley DM. Response of vulvar lichen sclerosus and squamous cell hyperplasia to graduated topical steroids. *J Reprod Med* 1999; **44**:958–62.

6. Ball SB, Wojnarowska F. Vulvar dermatoses: lichen sclerosus, lichen planus, and vulvar dermatitis/lichen simplex chronicus. *Semin Cutan Med Surg* 1998; **17**:182–8.

7. Faergemann J. Seborrhoeic dermatitis and *Pityrosporum orbiculare*: treatment of seborrhoeic dermatitis of the scalp with miconazole-hydrocortisone (Daktacort), miconazole and hydrocortisone. *Br J Dermatol* 1986; **114**:695–700.

8. Skinner RB, Noah PW, Taylor RM et al. Double-blind treatment of seborrheic dermatitis with 2% ketoconazole cream. *J Am Acad Dermatol* 1985; **2**:52–6.

9. Ashcroft DM, Li Wan Po A, Williams HC, Griffiths CEM. Systematic review of comparative efficacy and tolerability of calcipotriol in treating chronic plaque psoriaisis. In: *Clinical Evidence*, Issue 6. London: BMJ Publishing Group, 2001, 963–7.

10. Barbone F, Austin H, Lou WC, Alexander WJ. A follow-up study of methods of contraception, sexual activity and rate of trichomiasis, candidiasis and bacterial vaginosis. *Am J Obstet Gynecol* 1990; **163**:510–14.

11. Young GL, Jewell D. Topical treatment for vaginal candidiasis (thrush) in pregnancy (Cochrane Review). In: *The Cochrane Library*, Issue 4. Oxford: Update Software, 2001.

12. Watson MC, Grimshaw JM, Bond CM, Mollison J, Ludbrook A. Oral versus intra-vaginal imidazole and triazole anti-fungal treatment of uncomplicated vulvovaginal candidiasis (thrush) (Cochrane Review). In: *The Cochrane Library*, Issue 4, Oxford: Update Software, 2001.

13. Hopkins MP, Snyder MK. Benign disorders of vulval and vagina. In: Curtis MG, Hopkins MP (eds). *Glass's Office Gynecology*, 5th edn. Baltimore: Wilkins & Wilkins, 1999, 417–26.

Chapter 65

Vulval Pain Syndromes

David Nunns

INTRODUCTION

The vulval pain syndromes incorporate vulval vestibulitis and dysaesthetic vulvodynia. They are separate conditions, although there are many clinical overlaps.[1] Before a diagnosis of vulval pain syndrome can be made, infections and vulval dermatoses should be excluded (see Chapter 64).

PAIN PATHOPHYSIOLOGY

Clinical pain can either be inflammatory or neuropathic in origin. Inflammatory pain is associated with tissue damage or injury and clinically exhibits sensory hypersensitivity, which is characterized by hyperalgesia and allodynia. Hyperalgesia is the exaggerated response to noxious substances through a general increase in the responsiveness of tissues. Allodynia is the production of pain by stimuli that do not usually cause pain by a reduction in the sensory threshold of neurons. Hence, inflammatory pain seen with vulval vestibulitis is associated with pain on light touch and is usually localized. Neuropathic pain is usually caused by damage to either the central or peripheral nervous system and produces a diffuse burning, aching pain with intermittent flare-ups. Hyperalgesia and allodynia may not necessarily be present.

ASSESSMENT

History

An accurate pain history is essential to differentiate between the two conditions. In addition to the nature of the pain, one should record any aggravating and relieving factors, with particular reference to sexual intercourse. Any past treatments should also be recorded to avoid duplication. A psychosexual history is essential, as many women have significant dysfunction and may require a psychosexual referral [II].[2]

Examination

Identifying sites of vulval tenderness and discomfort can help in making a diagnosis. Clinical examination should also exclude other vulval conditions that can produce similar symptoms. Inflammatory vulval diseases such as lichen sclerosus and seborrhoeic dermatitis can cause vulval pain and soreness through excoriation, splitting and fissuring of the vulval skin, as well as itching. Some conditions may not be manifest at the time of examination, such as a tight posterior fourchette and the fragile fissured vulval syndrome.[3] Symptomatic dermographism is a rare cause of vulval pain, but this may be suggested by dermographism evident at other body sites.[4] Other less common causes of vulval pain are worth considering, including aphthous ulceration, erosive lichen planus and herpes simplex infections.

VULVAL VESTIBULITIS

Definition

Vulval vestibulitis is a cause of superficial dyspareunia and is characterized by vestibular tenderness on light touch.[5] This hyperaesthesia can be generalized throughout the vestibule or can be more focal, involving the opening of the ducts of the major vestibular glands or the posterior fourchette (focal vestibulitis).[6]

Clinical features

Affected women are usually Caucasian, aged between 20 and 40 years, and present with a history of provoked pain such as superficial dyspareunia, tampon intolerance and pain during gynaecological examinations.[5,7] There is often a delay between the onset of symptoms and receiving a diagnosis, which varies from months to years. A 6-month period of time has been arbitrarily suggested from the onset of symptoms to making a diagnosis of vulval vestibulitis so as to exclude women recovering from acute vulval inflammation from other causes.[6]

As the condition is frequently chronic, a high level of psychological morbidity is common. Some patients are prone to stress and anxiety, which may play a role in developing symptoms [III].[2] Sexual dysfunction is common and frequently reported.[8] Reduced sexual arousal, more negative sexual feelings and less spontaneous interest in sex (not elicited by a partner) have all been described in vulval vestibulitis. These are all risk factors for significant psychosexual dysfunction such as vaginismus and anorgasmia, the management of which usually requires psychosexual input [III] (see Chapter 63.3).

Clinically, simply using a Q-tip applicator can identify vestibular tenderness. A defining feature of vulval vestibulitis is that the labial skin is non-tender. Vestibular erythema is a subjective finding that is often present on normal examination and is usually not helpful in making the diagnosis of vulval vestibulitis or in planning management.[9] The application of diluted acetic acid to the vulva does not assist in making a diagnosis [II].

Incidence

The incidence within gynaecology clinics in the UK remains unknown. However, the prevalence of vulval vestibulitis was 1.3 per cent of women attending a Central London genitourinary medicine clinic.[10] Misdiagnosis is common.

Aetiology/risk factors

This remains unknown, but is likely to be multifactorial. It is often difficult to identify a cause, as symptoms usually develop insidiously. Recurrent attacks of vaginal candidiasis are frequently cited, but this may be due to initial misdiagnosis.

Prognosis

Up to 30 per cent of women with vulval vestibulitis may experience resolution of their symptoms without treatment and in 50 per cent of these, resolution can occur within 12 months [II].[6]

Management

The aims of management are to reduce vestibular tenderness and to identify the potential need for input from other disciplines, for example psychosexual counsellors.

General measures

Reassurance and an explanation of the condition are essential, and providing written information is helpful [II].[11] Strict vulval hygiene measures should be practised to reduce the chance of contact sensitivity [III].

Only one randomized, controlled trial (RCT) exists which addresses surgery, group therapy and biofeedback.[12] Good evidence for effective treatment is lacking. Many studies are methodologically flawed, for example low study numbers, short follow-up times.

Topical agents and vaginal dilators

No RCTs have compared topical agents. Local anaesthetic gel/ointment prior to sex and emollients are worthy of mention as first-line treatment [III]. Lignocaine gel together with the use of vaginal dilators can help desensitize the pelvic floor for patients who are fearful of sex and where secondary vaginismus may exist [II].[13]

Other topical agents include steroids and antifungal creams, which have been used with variable results, but no control arm existed in these studies.[14] Long-term empirical prescribing of topical medicaments should be discouraged, as it places the woman at unnecessary risk of irritancy and contact allergy.

Pain management and psychosexual counselling

A cognitive–behavioural assessment has been suggested to complement the physical treatments [Ib].[12] Over a series of sessions, a clinical psychologist can teach patients coping mechanisms and pain management strategies such as the pain-gate theory, and can address the patient's expectations of treatment, which might not necessarily be a cure for pain, but rather the ability to have penetrative sex. For many women with vulval vestibulitis, sexual rehabilitation may be required and this can be structured over several sessions with a psychosexual counsellor, preferably with the woman's partner. Improving physical non-coital sexual contact, helping to overcome pelvic floor muscle hypertonia using sensate focus therapy, and addressing secondary psychosexual dysfunction such as low libido and anorgasmia will be of help to many.[8]

Surgery

The modified vestibulectomy is the procedure of choice, involving excision of a horseshoe-shaped area of the vestibule and inner labial fold followed by dissection of the posterior vaginal wall [II]. The vaginal tissue is then advanced to cover the skin defect. The complete response rate is

59 per cent. Women who respond to lignocaine gel prior to sex have a more successful outcome.[15] The response rate can be further improved with postoperative psychosexual counselling, which is likely to help overcome the fear of sex after surgery [II].[13]

In a RCT, 78 women with vulval vestibulitis were randomized to one of three arms: (1) group cognitive–behavioural therapy (12 weeks' duration), (2) pelvic floor biofeedback therapy (12 weeks' duration), and (3) vestibulectomy.[12] At follow-up at 6 months, all patients reported significant improvements in pain scoring. Sexual functioning with surgery had the highest success rates; however, one concern was the high number of participants randomized to surgery who declined to be included in the study. The study did support both non-surgical treatments for vulval vestiulitis and suggested that patients prefer a behavioural approach to treatment than a surgical one.

Other treatments

Biofeedback therapy using surface electromyographic (sEMG) signals from the pelvic floor has been used successfully to help overcome pelvic floor muscle dysfunction in women with vulval vestibulitis [II].[16] Using portable home machines with a special vaginal skin sensor, 78 per cent of patients with apareunia had resumed penetrative sex and there was an objective improvement in the sEMG reading of the pelvic floor; however, many of these patients were also treated with amitryptyline. The system is not routinely available and experience in the UK is lacking.

No evidence exists that dietary manipulations can improve outcome in vulval vestibulitis.

Vulval vestibulitis

- Topical agents are commonly used, but the evidence supporting a specific application is lacking.
- Surgery is of benefit in well-selected patients.
- One RCT showed a benefit of vestibulectomy above biofeedback therapy and group cognitive–behavioural therapy.
- Biofeedback is effective, but UK experience is limited.

DYSAESTHETIC VULVODYNIA

Definition

Dysaesthetic vulvodynia is a cutaneous dysaesthesia causing non-localized vulval pain. Unlike vulval vestibulitis, in which pain is provoked, women with dysaesthetic vulvodynia have more constant neuropathic-type pain in the vulva and occasionally the peri-anal area.[17]

Clinical features

The affected women are typically perimenopausal or post-menopausal and, like women with vulval vestibulitis, can present with a long history of multiple, inappropriate use of topical agents prior to a diagnosis.[18] Superficial dyspareunia is not consistently reported, as many women are less sexually active.[5] In addition, many experience rectal, perineal and urethral discomfort and there may be an overlap with other perineal pain syndromes.[17] Psychological morbidity is likely to be high as a consequence of chronic pain.

Clinical examination of the vulva is normal.

Incidence

The incidence is unknown, but, as with vulval vestibulitis, misdiagnosis is likely.

Aetiology/risk factors

These remain unknown.

Prognosis

The prognosis also remains unknown.

Management

The aims of treatment are pain relief and identification of the potential need for input from other disciplines.

General measures

Reassurance and an explanation of the condition are essential, and providing written information is helpful.[11] Strict vulval hygiene measures should be practised to reduce the chance of contact sensitivity.

No RCTs have been carried out to assess the management of this group of patients, and only case-controlled studies exist, which frequently contain small numbers of women.

Tricyclic antidepressants and neuroleptics

Amitryptyline (a tricyclic antidepressant) is of benefit and addresses the central and peripheral components of neuropathic pain seem in dysaesthetic vulvodynia [II].[16] A dose of 10 mg/day, increasing every week until the pain is controlled, has been suggested. The average dosage is 60 mg/day, although up to 150 mg/day can be used. Side effects may affect compliance. The duration of treatment is debatable, but 3–6 months has been suggested. Patients intolerant of the side effects can try dothiepin or nortryptyline. The neuroleptic gabapentin can be used as a second-line agent. In the only series to date of 17 patients with dysaesthetic vulvodynia, the complete response rate was 41 per cent with a follow-up period of 26 months [II].[19]

Table 65.1 The multidisciplinary approach to vulval pain syndromes

Health professional	Treatments offered
Clinician	Topical agents Tricyclic antidepressants/ neuroleptics Modified vestibulectomy
Clinical psychologist	Cognitive-behavioural therapy Pain management Coping strategies
Psychosexual counsellors	Treatment of secondary sexual dysfunction Sensate focus therapy Increasing non-coital sexual activity
Physiotherapist	Biofeedback Pelvic floor muscle rehabilitation

Surgery

Surgery is contraindicated in this group.

Other treatments

Acupuncture has shown limited promise in cases refractory to standard medical treatments. In one study including only 12 patients with dysaesthetic vulvodynia, two were completely cured [II].[20]

Dysaesthetic vulvodynia

- Tricyclic antidepressants and gabapentin are of benefit.
- Surgery is contraindicated.

CONCLUSION

Women with vulval pain syndromes form a heterogeneous group, with the clinical presentation reflecting physical, psychological and psychosexual factors. As with other chronic pain syndromes, a specific cause remains elusive and is probably multifactorial. A multidisciplinary approach to the syndromes is likely to be of benefit to address the many complex issues surrounding vulval pain (Table 65.1). For some women who fail to respond to treatment, living and coping with pain become key issues in management.

KEY POINTS

- A good history and clinical examination are essential to distinguish between vulval vestibulitis and dysaesthetic vulvodynia.
- Surgery is only suitable for well-selected patients with vulval vestibulitis.

- Amitryptyline/gabapentin are treatments for dysaesthetic vulvodynia.
- A multidisciplinary approach can be helpful.
- Good evidence for effectiveness is lacking.

KEY REFERENCES

1. Ridley CM. Vulvodynia. Theory and management. *Sex Trans Dis* 1998; **16**(4):775–8.
2. Nunns D, Mandal D. Psychological and psychosexual aspects of vulval vestibulitis. *Genitourinary Med* 1997; **73**(6):541–4.
3. Harrington C. Presidential address. In: Proceedings of the British Society for the Study of Vulval Disease Biennial Meeting, Oxford, UK, 1999.
4. Lambiris A, Greaves MW. Urticaria: increasingly recognised but not adequately highlighted cause of dyspareunia and vulvodynia. *Acta Derm Venereol (Stockh)* 1996; **77**:160–1.
5. Friedrich EG. Vulvar vestibulitis syndrome. *J Reprod Med* 1987; **32**:110–14.
6. Peckham BM, Mak DG, Patterson JJ. Focal vulvitis: a characteristic syndrome and a cause of dyspareunia. *Am J Obstet Gynecol* 1986; **154**(4):855–64.
7. Marinnoff SC, Turner MLC. Vulvar vestibulitis syndrome: an overview. *Am J Obstet Gynecol* 1991; **165**:1228–33.
8. Schover LR, Youngs DD, Cannata RN. Psychosexual aspects of the evaluation and management of vulval vestibulitis. *Am J Obstet Gynecol* 1991; **167**(3):630–6.
9. Van Beurden W, van der Vange N, de Craen AJM et al. Normal findings in vulvar examination and vulvoscopy. *Br J Obstet Gynaecol* 1997; **104**:320–4.
10. Denbow ML, Byrne MA. Prevalence, causes and outcome of vulval pain in a genitourinary medicine clinic population. *Int J STD AIDS* 1998; **9**:88–91.
11. The Vulval Pain Society, PO Box 7804, Nottingham, NG3 5ZQ (send a s.a.e.).
12. Bergeron S, Binik YM, Khalife S, Pagidas K et al. A randomised comparison of group cognitive-behavioural therapy, surface electromyographic biofeedback and vestibulectomy in the treatment of dyspareunia resulting from vulvar vestibulitis. *Pain* 2001; **91**:297–306.
13. Abramov L, Wolman I, David MP. Vaginismus: an important factor in the evaluation and management of vulvar vestibulitis syndrome. *Gynaecol Obstet Inv* 1994; **38**:194–7.
14. Friedrich EG. Therapeutic studies on vulval vestibulitis. *J Reprod Med* 1988: **33**(6):515–18.
15. Kehoe S, Leusley D. An evaluation of modified vestibulectomy in the treatment of vulvar

vestibulitis: preliminary results. *Acta Obstet Gynecol Scand* 1996; **75**:676–7.

16. Glazer HI. Treatment of vulval vestibulitis syndrome with electromyographic biofeedback of pelvic floor musculature. *J Reprod Med* 1995; **40**(4):283–90.

17. McKay M. Dysaesthetic vulvodynia. *J Reprod Med* 1993; **38**(1):9–13.

18. McKay M. Subsets of vulvodynia. *J Reprod Med* 1987; **32**:110–14.

19. Ben-David B, Friedman M. Gabapentin therapy for vulvodynia. *Anesth Analg* 1999; **89**:1459–60.

20. Powell J, Wojnarowska F. Acupuncture for vulvodynia. *J R Soc Med* 1999; **92**:579–81.

Chapter 66

Pre-invasive Disease

Ian J. Etherington

MRCOG standards

The established standards relevant for this topic are:

Theoretical skills
- Understand the central role of human papillomavirus in the aetiology of cervical intraepithelial neoplasia.
- Understand the principles of organizing population screening.
- Be confident about interpreting cervical cytology reports and counselling women accordingly.

Practical skills
- Be able to carry out a colposcopic examination of the lower genital tract under indirect supervision.
- Be able to perform a large loop excision of the transformation zone of the cervix under supervision.

INTRODUCTION

Worldwide, cervical cancer is the most common cancer affecting women after breast cancer. Of the estimated 371 000 new cases in 1990, around 77 per cent were in developing countries, where about 200 000 women die each year from the disease. In developed nations, the figures for invasive cervical cancer are much lower. The disease has a relatively long natural history, and intervention and treatment in the pre-malignant phase is highly effective. The accessibility of the cervix and the availability of a simple test for the presence of pre-malignancy make it suitable for mass screening. Other malignancies and pre-malignancies of the lower genital tract are much less common and therefore most of this chapter focuses on the cervix.

CERVICAL INTRAEPITHELIAL NEOPLASIA AND CERVICAL SCREENING

Definitions (Table 66.1)

Pre-cancer of the cervix was first described at the end of the nineteenth century. Areas were described where the whole thickness of the epithelium was replaced by neoplastic cells that had not breached the basement membrane. They were referred to as carcinoma-in-situ (CIS). Retrospective studies found CIS lesions in women who subsequently went on to develop cervical cancer, and so the precursor nature of CIS came to be established. Subsequent prospective studies have confirmed these findings.[1,2] After exfoliative cytology was introduced, lesser degrees of change, not amounting to CIS, were recognized and termed 'dysplasia'. In order to rationalize the classification to encompass all degrees of change, the term cervical intraepithelial neoplasia (CIN) was introduced.[3] Pre-invasive changes were divided into grades 1, 2 and 3. Grades 1 and 2 corresponded to mild and moderate dysplasia respectively, and grade 3 combined severe dysplasia and CIS into one category. The definition implied a continuum of change from CIN1 through to CIN3 and invasive cancer. As knowledge of the natural history of pre-malignancy has grown, the concept of a continuum of change has been challenged. For practical purposes, there is now a two-stage grading, with CIN1 becoming low-grade CIN (in which there is a significant chance of regression), and CIN2 and CIN3 being grouped together as high-grade CIN. In North American and some European countries, this grouping has been formalized as The Bethesda Classification, consisting of low-grade squamous intraepithelial lesions (LSIL) and high-grade squamous intraepithelial lesions (HSIL).

Incidence

The UK has the second highest recorded incidence of CIN in the European Community. In 1997 there were 2740

Table 66.1   Glossary of terms

Term	Explanation
CIN	Cervical intraepithelial neoplasia, graded 1–3 depending on severity
VaIN	Vaginal intraepithelial neoplasia, graded 1–3 depending on severity
VIN	Vulval intraepithelial neoplasia, graded 1–3 depending on severity
AIS	Adenocarcinoma-in-situ, pre-invasive disease of glandular tissue
CIGN	Cervical intraepithelial glandular neoplasia, pre-invasive disease of glandular tissue graded low and high grade; high-grade CIGN = AIS
Pap smear	Cervical smear – cytological test described by Papanicolaou
ASCUS	Atypical squamous cells of uncertain significance – Bethesda System grade equating to borderline nuclear abnormalities
LSIL	Low-grade squamous intraepithelial lesion – Bethesda System grade equating to mild dyskaryosis/CIN1
HSIL	High-grade squamous intraepithelial lesion – Bethesda System grade equating to moderate and severe dyskaryosis/CIN2 and CIN3
Dyskaryosis	A cytological term describing the nuclear abnormalities – not synonymous with dysplasia
Squamo-columnar junction (SCJ)	Where squamous and columnar tissue meet; this is not fixed but is affected by metaplasia
Metaplasia	A physiological process whereby columnar epithelium is replaced by squamous tissue in response to the acid environment of the vagina
Transformation zone	That area on the cervix that has undergone metaplasia; it is bounded by the original SCJ and the present SCJ
Dysplasia	A histological term describing architectural abnormalities within tissue
LLETZ	Large loop excision of the transformation zone
LEEP	Loop electrosurgical excision procedure
DLE	Diathermy loop excision: taking a cone biopsy with an electrosurgical loop

new cases of invasive cervical cancer in England and Wales, which is a 26 per cent fall in incidence over the previous 5 years, with 9.3 cases per 100 000 women. It is difficult to estimate the total numbers of cases of CIN, as cancer registries only record cases of CIN3, but there are around 19 000 cases of CIN3 in England and Wales each year, with the peak incidence being between 25 and 29 years of age. According to work performed by the Imperial Cancer Research Fund (now a part of Cancer Research UK), cervical screening prevents between 1100 and 3900 cases of cervical cancer each year.[4]

Aetiology

Human papillomavirus (HPV) infection is the essential pre-requisite for the development of cervical malignancy. The most recent data on Dutch archived cervical cancer specimens, using sensitive methods of detecting HPV DNA, call into question whether HPV-negative cervical cancers actually exist: the estimated prevalence of HPV in cervical cancers is 99.7 per cent.[5] On the other hand, population-based studies have shown that genital HPV infection is extremely common and, in the overwhelming majority of cases, will not lead to the development of cancer. Progression or regression depends on several factors that interfere with the host's ability to clear the virus. The cell-mediated arm of the adaptive immune response is responsible for clearing HPV. If cell-mediated immunity is impaired, such as in transplant patients or in HIV-positive women, the virus will not be cleared and abnormalities will develop as the cells undergo immortalization and transformation. Smoking is a recognized co-factor for the development of disease: local immunity within the cervix appears to be suppressed in women who smoke. The major histocompatibility complex is responsible for presenting viral antigen to the host's immune system and there is limited evidence to suggest that women with particular human leucocyte antigen (HLA) types may have increased susceptibility to disease.

Cervical pre-cancer has a long natural history, which is one of the reasons why it is suitable to screen for it. If a cancer is going to develop at all, it will take several years to do so, even from a CIN3 lesion. It is unclear why some CIN3 lesions become invasive while others stay as intraepithelial disease, and it is not known how many CIN3 lesions will become invasive, as prospective studies are unethical. However, the best prospective data suggest that at least 36 per cent of women with CIN3 would develop invasive cancer if left untreated.[2]

More than 40 per cent of women with minor cytological abnormalities will revert to normal without treatment.[6] However, it should be noted that women with mild dykaryosis have a 16–47 times increased incidence of invasive disease compared with the general female population.[7]

Screening for cervical intraepithelial neoplasia

The programme

By definition, a screening test is not diagnostic but identifies a subgroup of the reference population at increased risk of the disease for which further tests should be carried out. Screening is always a trade-off between sensitivity and specificity. In this case, the reference population being screened comprises healthy, asymptomatic women.

No randomized trials have been undertaken to establish whether screening actually reduces mortality from cervical cancer. Evidence in support of screening has been extrapolated from reducing trends in incidence and mortality in those areas where screening has been introduced. This is most strikingly illustrated by considering data from Scandinavia: Iceland, Finland, Sweden and Denmark noted reductions in incidence and mortality soon after their screening programmes achieved target coverage of the population in the

1960s. Norway, on the other hand, with no organized programme in the 1960s, continued to show increasing incidence rates into the 1970s.[8]

A nationwide, organized (as opposed to opportunistic) cervical screening programme was introduced in England and Wales in 1988 with a national computerized call-and-recall system. The regions still have a degree of autonomy in planning their screening programme, but there is now a National Co-ordinating Network to ensure the adoption of common standards and working practices. Regions are required to offer screening to women aged 20–64 on a maximum 5-yearly cycle. Some regions screen 3 yearly, but the emphasis is on coverage rather than frequency: it is far better to screen 100 per cent of eligible women every 5 or even 10 years than to screen 50 per cent every 2 or 3 years. In other words, the women who do not get screened are likely to be those at most risk of the disease. Nationwide coverage is now around 85 per cent. Over 4.5 million smears are assessed annually in England to detect pre-invasive changes and, hopefully, reduce the 3700 cases of invasive cervical cancer and the 1300 deaths each year.

If maximum coverage for a 5-yearly programme is achieved, it has been estimated that 84 per cent of cases of invasive cancer could be prevented; the figure for a 3-yearly programme is 91 per cent and the incremental gains become less and less thereafter with increasing screening frequency. Therefore, in terms of cost–benefit, there is little justification for reducing the screening interval to less than 3 years. Because of the extremely low incidence of invasive cervical cancer in women under 20 years and because of the high prevalence of HPV infection at this age, screening of women under the age 20 is not justified. Similarly, at the other end of the spectrum, provided a woman has been adequately screened, and provided she has not recently changed her partner, there is no justification for continuing with screening after the age of 65 years if the smear history is normal. Indeed, some authors have questioned the validity of screening such women beyond the age of 50 years.[9]

The test

The Papanicolaou (Pap) smear test is used worldwide to screen for pre-cancerous cellular changes from the cervix. More than 90 per cent of cervical cancers develop within the transformation zone, the upper limit of which is the squamo-columnar junction, so it is important that this area is adequately sampled. A variety of spatulae and brushes is used for sample collection. The traditional Ayre's spatula is less effective at collecting endocervical cells than extended-tip designs such as the Aylesbury spatula. Smears that contain endocervical cells are more likely to detect dyskaryosis. However, the most effective method of collection appears to be a combination of an extended-tip spatula with an endocervical brush.[10]

Test performance

Cervical cytology is not a perfect test: there are false-positive results (i.e. no disease is actually present) and false-negative results (i.e. genuine disease is missed). False-positive rates vary from 7 to 27 per cent and false-negative rates from 20 to 50 per cent.

About 92 per cent of the smears taken are adequate for diagnosis, and just under 10 per cent of adequate smears are 'not normal'. Most smear abnormalities are at the minor end of the spectrum.

Overall test outcomes of smears are as follows:

- 4.3 per cent are reported as borderline changes,
- 2.5 per cent are reported as mild dyskaryosis,
- 1 per cent are reported as moderate dyskaryosis,
- 0.7 per cent are reported as severe dyskaryosis,
- 0.15 per cent are reported as suspected invasion or glandular neoplasia.

In general, the proportion of normal smears increases in older women, but so does the proportion of abnormalities representing invasive cancer. Borderline changes and mild dyskaryosis are very common in young women; the proportion of moderate dyskaryosis is highest for women aged 20–29; and the proportion of severe dyskaryosis is highest in women aged 25–34.[11]

Traditionally, the cytology sample from the cervix is spread on a glass slide at the time of collection. Each slide will therefore have only a proportion of the cells collected from the cervix. Liquid-based cytology collects the whole sample from the sampling device in a liquid medium that is sent to a laboratory for processing. Cells are transferred from the transport liquid to a slide as a monolayer for examination. This technique reduces the proportion of inadequate smears and increases the detection of true dyskaryosis. It is more expensive than conventional cytology and its role within the screening programme has recently been evaluated.[12] The conclusions so far are that liquid-based systems should be implemented and become the standard test.

Management

Colposcopy

Further investigation of smear abnormalities is by colposcopy. A colposcope is a low-power binocular microscope that allows magnification from around 4× to 25×. In the UK, colposcopy is a secondary investigation; in other countries that do not have organized cytological screening it may be used as a primary tool.

The current indications for colposcopy referral are detailed in Table 66.2.

It is important to recognize that the screening programme has the ability to generate considerable psychological morbidity.[13] Appropriate counselling at the time of or before colposcopy is important, and the vast majority of women can be reassured prior to the examination that they are extremely unlikely to have cancer: this is very important to emphasize.

Table 66.2　Interpretation and management plans for different smear grades

Smear result	Interpretation	Management plan
Negative	No cellular abnormalities detected	Routine recall after 3–5 years
Borderline changes	Cellular appearances that cannot be described as normal	Repeat smear in 6–12 months and refer for colposcopy if any abnormality persists
Mild dyskaryosis	Cellular appearance consistent with underlying CIN1	Repeat smear within 6 months and refer for colposcopy if any abnormality persists
Moderate dyskaryosis	Cellular appearance consistent with underlying CIN2	Refer for colposcopy
Severe dyskaryosis	Cellular appearance consistent with underlying CIN3	Refer for colposcopy
Suspicious of invasive cancer	Possibility of invasive cancer	Refer for colposcopy
Glandular neoplasia	Cellular appearance suggests an abnormality in the endocervical canal or endometrium	Refer for colposcopy and gynaecological assessment
Inadequate	The smear is unable to be interpreted in the laboratory; it may be poorly prepared at the point of collection, obscured by blood or inflammatory cells or may not contain the right type of cells	Repeat the smear; if infection is suspected as the reason for the inadequate smear, treat this first

CIN, cervical intraepithelial neoplasia.

Table 66.3　Treatment modalities for cervical intraepithelial neoplasia

Excisional techniques	Ablative techniques
LLETZ – removal of the transformation zone using an electrodiathermy loop; requires local or general anaesthesia	**Radical electrodiathermy** – burning the transformation zone; usually requires general anaesthesia
Laser cone – removal of the transformation zone using the laser; requires local or general anaesthesia	**Cold coagulation** – destroying the transformation zone by applying a probe heated to 100–120°C; usually requires local anaesthesia
Knife cone biopsy – taking a cone with a knife; usually requires general anaesthesia	**Cryocautery** – freezing the tissue; does not require any anaesthesia
Hysterectomy – may be suitable if the woman has other gynaecological problems	**Laser** – vaporizing the tissue; requires local or general anaesthesia

LLETZ, large loop excision of the transformation zone.

The cervix is first examined at low magnification (4–6×). A saline-soaked cotton-wool ball is then applied, which moistens the epithelium, allowing the underlying blood vessels to be examined under higher magnification (preferably 16× or even 25×). A green filter may be used as it makes the capillaries stand out more clearly. The shapes of the capillaries are studied and the intercapillary distances estimated. Acetic acid (3 per cent or 5 per cent) is then applied to the cervix. Areas of CIN will appear as varying degrees of whiteness. This is termed acetowhiteness, in contrast to areas of hyperkeratosis or leukoplakia, which appear white before application of acetic acid. The exact reason why CIN tissue turns white with acetic acid is not fully understood. The cytoplasm becomes dehydrated, so in areas of abnormality, where there is a high nuclear:cytoplasmic ratio in the cells, the nuclei become crowded and the light from the colposcope is reflected back. Such areas will therefore appear white. However, not all areas of high nuclear density are abnormal and so not all acetowhiteness necessarily correlates with CIN: areas of regenerating epithelium, subclinical papillomavirus infection and immature metaplasia

may also appear acetowhite. One of the challenges facing the colposcopist is to decide which areas of acetowhiteness truly represent pre-malignancy and to avoid treating benign conditions. The classical vessel patterns of CIN are punctation and mosaicism. Bizarre-shaped vessels suggest cancer.

Another test used in the colposcopy clinic involves the application of Lugol's iodine solution to the cervix. Normal squamous epithelium contains glycogen and stains dark brown when Lugol's iodine is applied. Conversely, premalignant and malignant squamous tissue contains little or no glycogen and does not stain with iodine. This is Schiller's test: areas that are non-staining with iodine are referred to as Schiller positive and those that take up iodine as Schiller negative. The test may be used following acetic acid colposcopy.

Treatment

High-grade lesions (CIN2/3) should be treated, but there is some debate about whether and when CIN1 should be treated, as a proportion will resolve spontaneously. If it is decided that treatment is needed, there is a variety of options. Abnormal tissue can be removed (excisional techniques) or it can be destroyed (ablative techniques) (Table 66.3). Removing the entire transformation zone has the advantage of allowing a large specimen to be examined: the pathologist can comment on the most severe abnormality and can assess whether all the abnormal tissue has been removed. Destroying the transformation zone does not allow this, so it is mandatory to establish the diagnosis by taking a small biopsy before treatment. However, punch biopsy has been shown to be an inaccurate investigation when compared with subsequent loop excision from the same cervix.[14]

The success of treatment is usually defined as negative cytology 6 months following intervention. Randomized trial data on the different methods of treating CIN do not point to one overwhelmingly superior technique.

Cryotherapy is cheap and easy to use, with low morbidity. It should be used as a double freeze–thaw–freeze technique.

Success rates for treating CIN3 vary between 77 per cent and 93 per cent. Cryotherapy is a reasonable option for the treatment of low-grade disease but not of high-grade disease. It may be suitable in resource-poor situations. All of the other ablative and excisional methods achieve cure (or success) rates of 90–98 per cent.[15]

Current treatments rely on the destruction or excision of affected tissue. However, with expanding knowledge about the role of HPV and the body's immune response to it, new immunological methods of disease prevention and therapy have been proposed. These aim to address the cause of the disease (i.e. HPV infection) and to either prevent (prophylactic vaccination) or treat (therapeutic vaccination) it. Prophylactic vaccination targets the viral capsid and aims to prevent infection or the early spread of infection through the production of neutralizing antibody. Therapeutic vaccines aim to boost the host's cell-mediated immune arm to attack established infection. Both are experimental, but, if successful, prophylactic vaccination would appear to offer significant hope on a worldwide scale as a weapon to fight the spread of cervical cancer.

Screening for human papillomavirus infection

As HPV infection is so strongly implicated in the genesis of CIN and cervical cancer, it is logical to ask whether viral detection could improve the screening process. Two methods of detecting HPV that are suitable for population screening are the polymerase chain reaction (PCR) and the hybrid capture system. Data from studies using earlier methodology can be disregarded. Applications of HPV testing can be at a primary or secondary level. Most published data refer to HPV testing as an adjunct to cytology and test the hypothesis that HPV detection improves the accuracy of cytology alone.[16] Qualitative identification of HPV in women presenting with a high-grade smear is pointless, as the vast majority will be high-risk HPV-positive anyway. It is becoming apparent that the same is true for women who have true mild dyskaryosis (or LSIL). However, in women with a borderline smear (roughly equivalent to atypical squamous cells of undetermined significance (ASCUS)), it may be more discriminatory. This is particularly so in situations in which the background prevalence of infection is lower (such as in women over 30 or 35 years of age). Quantitative HPV estimation has been suggested as being more discriminatory than qualitative estimation.[17] Methods of quantification vary and have limited reproducibility. Furthermore, recent data suggest that viral load varies in the natural history of disease and may be of limited predictive value.[18] There is a large multicentre, randomized trial (TOMBOLA) currently recruiting in the UK to evaluate the role of HPV testing in women with minor smear abnormalities. Results from the trial can be expected in 2006. HPV testing remains an experimental procedure that should not be offered to women outwith the confines of a clinical trial.

Glandular pre-invasive disease

Adenocarcinoma-in-situ (AIS), or high-grade cervical intraepithelial glandular neoplasia (CIGN) of the cervix is a rare condition. It presents a particular challenge to the colposcopist, who may only see one case per year. Cytology screening is unsatisfactory, and the disease has no reliable colposcopic features. Diagnosis is often made by chance during the treatment of squamous pre-invasive disease, which commonly co-exists with AIS. Although the entire endocervical canal can be the site of disease, most lesions lie within 1 cm of the squamo-columnar junction. Skip lesions are rare, making fertility-sparing surgery a possibility, provided that endocervical margins are clear of disease. Recurrent disease occurs in 14 per cent of cases when cone margins are free of disease and rises to more than 50 per cent if the margins are involved. The method of conization is immaterial provided that a large enough specimen is taken and that the endocervical margins can be evaluated by the pathologist. There are no guidelines on the optimal follow-up of conservatively managed women; however, most would recommend that regular endocervical cytology be performed in addition to conventional cytology and colposcopy.[19]

Cervical intraepithelial neoplasia

- Virtually all cervical cancer is related to HPV infection [Ib].
- Cervical sampling devices that extend into the endocervical canal are superior to traditional Ayre's spatula [Ia].
- The treatment methods (other than cryotherapy) to eradicate CIN are all equally effective [Ia].

KEY POINTS

- HPV is an extremely common infection that rarely causes cancer [II].
- Organized cervical cytology programmes have been shown to reduce the incidence of invasive cancer [II].
- The screening of teenagers cannot be justified [IV].
- Screening for HPV infection is not yet routinely recommended.
- Neither Pap smear nor colposcopy is a reliable method for detecting glandular disease [III].

VAGINAL INTRAEPITHELIAL NEOPLASIA

Pre-invasive disease of the vagina is extremely uncommon (about 150 times less common than CIN). In 70 per cent of cases of vaginal intraepithelial neoplasia (VaIN) there will be associated CIN. The average age of the woman with VaIN tends to be higher than for CIN. The major predisposing factor is the same, namely oncogenic HPV, but the reason for the lower incidence is the relative stability of the epithelium compared with the metaplastic cervical epithelium. Women exposed to stilboestrol in utero have a higher incidence of VaIN as here the areas of metaplastic transformation extend on to the vagina. Around 25 per cent of women with VaIN will have had a hysterectomy previously, for either CIN or a benign condition. Like CIN, VaIN is graded 1–3, but in common with vulval intraepithelial neoplasia (VIN), the invasive potential is less than for CIN. Treatment of VaIN3 is by surgical excision, which may necessitate a combined abdominovaginal approach to excise the vaginal vault. Chemosurgery using 5-fluorouracil prior to diathermy ablation is an experimental treatment that has shown some promising results. Radiotherapy is an alternative treatment for women who may not be suitable for surgery. Lower grades of disease can be observed. For women who have had a hysterectomy in which VaIN is seen at the vaginal vault, there may still be disease buried above the vault in the cuff that was closed over at hysterectomy. In view of this, if high-grade VaIN is detected at the vault of the vagina, it should be treated by excision rather than destruction.

KEY POINTS

- VaIN is very uncommon and there is little evidence base on the subject.
- It usually co-exists with CIN [III].
- The risk factors are similar to those for CIN [III].
- In-utero diethylstilboestrol exposure increases the risk of VaIN [III].

VULVAL INTRAEPITHELIAL NEOPLASIA

Pre-malignant disease of the vulva is much less common than its cervical counterpart. Human papillomavirus infection is recognized as a major factor in the aetiology of most, though not all, vulval intraepithelial neoplasia (VIN). The HPV types most commonly associated with VIN are HPV 16 and 33. HPV-associated VIN is increasing in incidence, particularly in younger women.[20] This increase may be explained by a number of factors, such as increased awareness amongst medical practitioners leading to improved detection, increased smoking by younger women, or changing sexual attitudes and increased exposure to HPV. These women should be examined for other intraepithelial neoplasia of the anogenital tract.

The pre-malignant potential of VIN has been estimated to range from 4 per cent for treated cases[21] to 80 per cent

Table 66.4 Comparison of characteristics of vulval intraepithelial neoplasia grade 3 (VIN3) and cervical intraepithelial neoplasia grade 3 (CIN3)

	VIN3	CIN3
Proportion of cases of disease adjacent to malignancy	25%	>90%
Invasive potential	Low (<10%)	Significant (40%)
Time to progress to invasion	20–30 years	10–15 years
Spontaneous regression	Up to 40%	Low

for untreated cases.[22] Most published series estimate a risk of 10 per cent or less.

Vulval intraepithelial neoplasia affects mainly the labia minora and the perineum. It can take a variety of forms and can be difficult to diagnose. Up to 60 per cent of affected women may complain of itching, soreness and burning,[23] but many are asymptomatic and the abnormality can be a chance finding on examination. The lesions may extend to the perianal and anal mucosa. Diagnosis is made by examining the vulva with a good light source such as the colposcope at low magnification, and by taking representative biopsies. Like CIN, VIN is graded 1–3 in increasing severity of abnormal cell maturation and stratification. However, there are some striking differences between VIN and CIN (Table 66.4).

Current treatments for VIN are suboptimal in terms of their poor clinical response rates, high relapse rates and associated physical and psychological morbidities. The high recurrence rates following many therapies may reflect the fact that they fail to remove the reservoir of HPV present in the vulval skin. Low-grade VIN should be observed. VIN3 lesions can be treated by local excision or laser vaporization. Recurrences of 39 per cent and 70 per cent have been described after surgical excision and laser ablation respectively.[24,25]

A topical immunomodulator called imiquimod may be of use in the management of women with VIN, although it remains experimental at present.

KEY POINTS

- VIN is uncommon and there is little evidence base on the subject.
- VIN in younger women is strongly associated with HPV [II].
- The commonest presenting symptom is pruritus [III].
- Lesions may be multifocal and have a variety of appearances.
- Multicentric disease should be considered when VIN is diagnosed.
- Conservative surgery is currently the basis of treatment [IV].
- Long-term follow-up is essential as recurrence is common [III].

MULTICENTRIC INTRAEPITHELIAL NEOPLASIA

There is a small group of women in whom intraepithelial neoplastic changes can be detected at more than one site in the lower genital tract. The sites involved are the cervix, vagina, vulva, perineum, anal canal and natal cleft. Although the number of women affected by multicentric intraepithelial neoplasia (MIN) is small, the number appears to be increasing, which may be a true reflection of more disease or it may be a result of increased awareness and detection. The aetiology of MIN is a combination of HPV infection and host immunosuppression of varying degrees. Patients in whom cell-mediated immunity is compromised, such as women who have had organ transplantation or who carry the human immunodeficiency virus (HIV), often have recognizable HPV-associated changes in numerous sites in the lower genital tract. Conversely, women with humoral immunodeficiency do not have an increased risk of HPV-associated lesions.

Multicentric intraepithelial neoplasia may be detected in a woman who has repeated abnormal smears despite treatment for CIN, or in a woman being assessed for VIN. Genitourinary physicians who perform colposcopy may also encounter MIN in HIV-positive women under their care.

At the time of writing, there are no national guidelines for the management of women with MIN. Such cases are often complex and become chronic, the women sometimes having repeated surgery over several years. It is therefore important to be aware that these women may suffer adverse psychological sequelae as a result of their condition. As their numbers are small, women with MIN should be managed in large centres to concentrate experience and expertise. Investigations should be individualized, but may include multiple colposcopically directed biopsies, HPV typing, HIV testing and tests of T-cell function. Management aims to exclude invasive cancer and control symptoms whilst preserving anatomical and functional integrity where possible. The treatments of lesions of the vagina and vulva are described above. Lesions of the perineum and anal canal may require an initial colostomy prior to skin grafting. Such cases require a multidisciplinary team comprising a gynaecologist, colorectal surgeon, plastic surgeon, stoma nurse and possibly a psychologist.

New immunomodulating therapies currently under investigation, such as therapeutic vaccination and imiquimod, hold out some hope for women affected with MIN. At present, they remain the subjects of research.

KEY POINTS

- MIN is a rare condition and there is no evidence base.
- There is an association with conditions in which cell-mediated immunity is impaired [III].

- It is often a chronic, relapsing condition [III].
- The key aim of management is to do the least required to exclude invasion and control symptoms [IV].

SUMMARY

Lower genital tract pre-malignancy is an important area of gynaecology. Most of the pre-cancers in this area have an association with HPV, but HPV infection is extremely common and causes no problems in the majority of individuals affected. Organized national screening seems to have been effective in reducing the incidence and mortality from cervical cancer, but there has been a cost to pay in terms of over-investigation and treatment of women who have very minor changes that are unlikely ever to progress to cancer. Pre-cancers of the vagina, vulva and perineum are much less common but require specialized skills for accurate diagnosis and appropriate management. Current treatment modalities for the pre-cancers involve destruction or excision. As our knowledge of the aetiology of lower genital tract pre-malignancy expands, it may be possible to target the underlying cause more accurately through the use of therapeutic and prophylactic vaccinations.

PUBLISHED GUIDELINES

Guidelines for Clinical Practice and Programme Management, 2nd edn. NHSCSP Publication No. 8, 1997.
Achievable Standards, Benchmarks for Reporting and Criteria for Evaluating Cervical Cytopathology. NHSCSP Publication No. 1, 2000.
Standards and Quality in Colposcopy. NHSCSP Publication No. 2, 1996.
All guidelines from <www.cancerscreening.nhs.uk/cervicalpublications>.

KEY REFERENCES

1. Koss LG, Stewart FW, Foote FW et al. Some histological aspects of the behaviour of epidermoid carcinoma in situ and related lesions of the uterine cervix. *Cancer* 1963; 16:1160.
2. McIndoe WA, McLean MR, Jones RW, Mullins PR. The invasive potential of carcinoma in situ of the cervix. *Obstet Gynecol* 1984; 64:451–8.
3. Richart RM. Natural history of cervical intraepithelial neoplasia. *Clin Obstet Gynecol* 1968; 10:748.

Lower genital tract

4. Sasieni PD, Cuzick J, Lynch-Farmery E. Estimating the efficacy of screening by auditing smear histories of women with and without cervical cancer. The National Co-ordinating Network for Cervical Screening. *Br J Cancer* 1996; **73**:1001–5.

5. Walboomers JMM. Human papillomavirus is a necessary cause of invasive cervical cancer worldwide. *J Pathol* 1999; **189**(1):12–19.

6. Robertson JH, Woodend BE, Crozier EH, Hutchinson J. Risk of cervical cancer associated with mild dyskaryosis. *BMJ* 1988; **297**:18–21.

7. Soutter WP. The management of a mildly dyskaryotic smear: immediate referral to colposcopy is safer. *BMJ* 1994; **309**:591–2.

8. Laara E, Day NE, Hakama M. Trends in mortality from cervical cancer in the Nordic countries: association with organised screening programmes. *Lancet* 1987; I:1247–9.

9. Van Wijngaarden WJ, Duncan ID. Rationale for stopping cervical screening in women over 50. *BMJ* 1993; **306**:967–7.

10. Martin-Hirsch P, Jarvis G, Kitchener H, Lilford R. Collection devices for obtaining cervical cytology samples (Cochrane Review). In: *The Cochrane Library*, Issue 4. Oxford: Update Software, 2001.

11. *NHS Cervical Screening Programme Review* 2001, <www.cancerscreening.nhs.uk/cervical publications/ 2001review>.

12. National Institute for Clinical Excellence Technological Appraisals. *Cervical Smear Tests – Liquid Based Cytology*, No. 5. <www.nice.org.uk>

13. Marteau TM, Walker P, Giles J, Smail M. Anxieties in women undergoing colposcopy. *Br J Obstet Gynaecol* 1990; **97**:859–61.

14. Buxton EJ, Luesley DM, Shafi MI, Rollason T. Colposcopically directed punch biopsy: a potentially misleading investigation. *Br J Obstet Gynaecol* 1991; **98**:1273–6.

15. Martin-Hirsch PL, Paraskevaidis E, Kitchener H. Surgery for cervical intraepithelial neoplasia (Cochrane Review). In: *The Cochrane Library*, Issue 4. Oxford: Update Software, 2001.

16. Bavin PJ, Giles JA, Deery A et al. Use of semi-quantitative PCR for human papillomavirus DNA type 16 to identify women with high grade cervical disease in a population presenting with a mildly dyskaryotic smear report. *Br J Cancer* 1993; **67**:602–5.

17. Cuzick J, Terry G, Ho L, Hollingworth T, Anderson M. Type-specific human papillomavirus DNA in abnormal smears as a predictor of high-grade cervical intraepithelial neoplasia. *Br J Cancer* 1994; **69**:167–71.

18. Woodman CB, Collins S, Winter H et al. Natural history of cervical human papillomavirus infection in young women: a longitudinal cohort study. *Lancet* 2001; **357**:1831–6.

19. Etherington IJ, Luesley DM. Adenocarcinoma in situ of the cervix – controversies in diagnosis and treatment. *J Lower Genital Tract Dis* 2001; **5**(ii):94–8.

20. Jones RW, Baranyai J, Stables S. Trends in squamous cell carcinoma of the vulva: the influence of vulvar intraepithelial neoplasia. *Obstet Gynecol* 1997; **90**:448–52.

21. Iversen T, Tretli S. Intraepithelial and invasive squamous cell neoplasia of the vulva: trends in incidence, recurrence and survival in Norway. *Obstet Gynecol* 1994; **6**:969–72.

22. Jones RW, Rowan DM. Vulvar intraepithelial neoplasia 3: a clinical study of the outcome in 113 cases with relation to the later development of invasive vulvar cancer. *Obstet Gynecol* 1994; **5**:741–5.

23. Campion MJ, Singer A. Vulvar intraepithelial neoplasia: clinical review. *Genitourinary Med* 1987; **63**:147–52.

24. DiSaia PJ, Rich WM. Surgical approach to multifocal carcinoma in situ of the vulva. *Am J Obstet Gynecol* 1981; **140**:136–45.

25. Townsend DE, Levine RU, Richart RM, Crum CP, Petrilli ES. Management of vulvar intraepithelial neoplasia by carbon dioxide laser. *Obstet Gynecol* 1982; **60**:49–52.

SECTION D

Gynaecological oncology

Endometrial Cancer

Margaret E. Cruickshank

MRCOG standards

The established standards relevant for this topic are:

Theoretical skills

- Revise your knowledge of pelvic anatomy.
- Understand the epidemiology and aetiology of endometrial cancer.
- Understand the principles of carcinogenesis and pathology.
- Be able to describe the diagnostic and staging techniques of endometrial cancer.
- Be able to describe the management of early and advanced/recurrent disease.

Practical skills

- Be confident to perform outpatient endometrial biopsy.
- Be able to stage endometrial cancer and counsel patients with direct supervision.
- Be able to recognize, assess and manage surgically and non-surgically carcinoma of the endometrium.
- Be able to evaluate response to oncology treatment and counsel regarding prognosis.
- Be able to manage palliative care in liaison with an expert team.

INTRODUCTION

Endometrial cancer usually arises in postmenopausal women. The incidence continues to increase in many developed countries. It is the second most common gynaecological cancer in the UK. Seventy-five per cent of women present with stage I disease and for most of them the treatment is surgical and the prognosis is relatively good.

INCIDENCE

Endometrial cancer is the fifth most common cancer in women in the UK. In 1997, there were 4850 new cases, or 13.8 per 100 000 women per year. This compares with 3912 new cases in 1992 and 4446 in 1995 (Office of National Statistics), demonstrating an upward trend in the incidence. The 5-year age-standardized relative survival is 70 per cent (CRC CancerStats for England and Wales 1971–1995),[1] but for stage I disease, there is an overall 5-year survival of 85 per cent. The incidence increases between the ages of 40 and 55, thereafter reaching a plateau. It is rare in women before the age of 40, at less than 2 per 100 000 women.

AETIOLOGY

Women with relatively high levels of circulating oestrogens or prolonged oestrogen influence are a recognized high-risk group for endometrial cancer. This is seen in the following situations:

- obesity due to the peripheral conversion of androgens in adipose tissue,
- tamoxifen therapy,
- oestrogen therapy unopposed by progestogens,
- polycystic ovarian syndrome (PCOS),
- early menarche and late menopause.

Endometrial hyperplasia results from protracted oestrogen stimulation. Those cases without atypia are benign, but when cellular atypia is present this is considered to be pre-malignant.

OESTROGEN REPLACEMENT

The use of unopposed oestrogen replacement therapy (ERT) is clearly linked to endometrial cancer and more than doubles the risk (relative risk (RR) 2.3 for users compared with non-users, 95% confidence interval (CI) 2.1–2.5) [Ia].[2] This meta-analysis of 30 studies found significant heterogeneity between the studies analysed, which was mostly due to differences in the dose and duration of oestrogen. Higher doses of oestrogen and duration of use of 10 or more years have a relative risk of 9.5 (95% CI 7.4–12.3). The risk does reduce after discontinuation of ERT, but interrupted use does not lower the risk compared with daily use.

The highest risk of hormone replacement therapy (HRT) is for atypical endometrial hyperplasia, but there is also an effect on advanced cancer and mortality. The concurrent use of a progesterone reduces the relative risk to almost that of a non-ERT-user (RR 0.8, 95% CI 0.6–1.2), but the direction of this effect does vary between case-control and cohort studies. Unopposed ERT increases the rate of irregular bleeding and non-adherence to treatment [Ia].[3] The addition of progesterone, whether cyclical or sequential, prevents the development of endometrial hyperplasia and improves compliance. Irregular bleeding is more likely with a continuous than a sequential preparation (odds ratio (OR) 2.3, 95% CI 2.1–2.5), but with longer duration of therapy, continuous is more protective than sequential in preventing endometrial hyperplasia.

GENETIC PREDISPOSITION

Endometrial cancer in women under the age of 45 may be associated with Lynch Type II familial cancer syndrome, which is known as hereditary non-polyposis colorectal cancer (HNPCC). There does not appear to be a site-specific inherited form of endometrial cancer, but it is associated with a genetic predisposition as a component of the HNPCC syndrome. Families affected with this syndrome have a predisposition to bowel cancer and also to ovarian tumours.

HRT and endometrial cancer

- A meta-analysis of 30 observational studies to estimate the risk of endometrial cancer for ever use of postmenopausal oestrogen and for ever use of oestrogen combined with progesterone found the data for risk of women on combined HRT to be limited and conflicting. This analysis clearly showed that there is a substantial risk from unopposed ERT and this should only be used for hysterectomized women.
- A systematic review of 18 randomized, controlled trials (RCTs) shows that combined HRT, either cyclical or sequential, reduces the rates of endometrial hyperplasia and improves treatment compliance.

PATHOLOGY

The uterine corpus lies above the level of the internal cervical os and is composed of the fundus above the tubal ostiae and the body below. The blood supply is the uterine artery, a branch of the internal iliac artery. The lymphatic drainage passes with the artery to the internal, external and common iliac nodes and para-aortic nodes.

The International Federation of Gynecology and Obstetrics (FIGO) Committee on Gynaecologic Oncology recommends that endometrial cancer is surgically staged.[4] This includes histological verification of the tumour grading and the extent of tumour. The degree of tumour differentiation has an important impact on the natural history of the disease and on treatment selection. Ninety-five per cent of uterine cancers are adenocarcinomas arising from the endometrium. They are graded with regard to the degree of cell differentiation (Table 67.1).

Table 67.1 Grading of tumour differentiation

G1	5% or less of a non-squamous or non-morular solid growth pattern
G2	6–50% of a non-squamous or non-morular solid growth pattern
G3	>50% of a non-squamous or non-morular solid growth pattern

Notable nuclear atypia that is inappropriate for the architectural grade raises it to the next tumour grade.

Nuclear grading takes precedence in serous and clear-cell adenocarcinomas.

Histopathological reporting should include:

- depth of myometrial invasion,
- tumour grade,
- histological subtype,
- presence or absence of hyperplasia in adjacent non-neoplastic endometrium; vascular space invasion,
- lymph node involvement,
- the status of peritoneal washings taken at surgery.

There are clearly recognized risk factors for lymph node involvement, distant metastasis and poor survival. These are tumour grade, tumour subtype and the depth of myometrial invasion. Papillary serous adenocarcinomas and clear-cell carcinomas are high-risk subtypes and they are associated with about 50 per cent of all relapses. Their 5-year survival is 27 per cent and 42 per cent respectively. Mucinous, squamous and undifferentiated tumours are rare.

Histopathology by World Health Organization/International Society of Gynaecological Pathology Classification

- Endometrioid carcinoma.
- Adenocarcinoma.

- Adenocanthoma (adenocarcinoma with squamous metaplasia).
- Adenosquamous carcinoma (mixed adenocarcinoma and squamous cell carcinoma).
- Mucinous adenocarcinoma.
- Papillary serous adenocarcinoma.
- Clear-cell adenocarcinoma.
- Adenosquamous carcinoma.
- Undifferentiated carcinoma.
- Mixed carcinoma.

PRESENTATION AND DIAGNOSIS

Endometrial cancer usually presents with vaginal bleeding in postmenopausal women. Postmenopausal bleeding (PMB) is defined as bleeding from the genital tract 1 or more years after a woman's last period. Women who continue to menstruate after the age of 55 also need to be investigated. Up to 8 per cent of women with PMB will have an endometrial carcinoma. The incidence of endometrial cancer has now been seen to plateau with age; the likelihood of an underlying cancer increases with age at presentation.

INVESTIGATION OF POSTMENOPAUSAL BLEEDING

Most women with PMB can be investigated rapidly and accurately as outpatients.

Transvaginal ultrasound scanning (TVS) is an accurate method of excluding endometrial cancer [Ia]. Women can be assessed quickly and triaged for endometrial biopsy on the basis of the scan findings. This restricts the use of endometrial biopsy to women with an endometrial thickness of >4–5 mm, an irregular endometrial outline or fluid in the uterine cavity. The majority of women will have a thin, regular endometrium and can be reassured at a first visit without further investigation. The sensitivity for detecting endometrial cancer is 94–100 per cent and the specificity 43–81 per cent, depending on the cut-off point taken for endometrial thickness. The negative predictive value is almost 100 per cent in excluding endometrial cancer, which allows successful triage of women for biopsy. This reduces the need for further intervention, service costs and patient anxiety and provides rapid reassurance for those women with a normal result.

There are a number of devices for taking outpatient endometrial biopsies which have been compared in prospective studies. There is no RCT evidence of outpatient biopsy compared with dilatation and curettage (D&C). The Novak and Vabra aspirators and the Karman curette appear to be as accurate as D&C for diagnosis [II]. The Karman curette has 100 per cent sensitivity and can be used in an outpatient setting for 80 per cent of women referred with PMB

[II]. Samples taken by Pipelle are comparable with the Vabra and Novak aspirators in terms of specimen adequacy and diagnostic accuracy. In addition, this method produces less patient discomfort. D&C should only be used when outpatient biopsy is unsuccessful [IV].

Hysteroscopy is often used to investigate PMB, as it allows direct inspection of the endometrium. It can detect 95 per cent of intrauterine abnormalities and is a sensitive means of identifying polyps and submucous fibroids [II]. It can be used in the outpatient setting, and outpatient hysteroscopy is highly acceptable to women [II].

Dedicated postmenopausal bleeding clinic

Many centres now provide a dedicated service for the investigation of women with PMB. A common clinic protocol is to provide TV scanning by appropriately trained staff. Women who meet the criteria of PMB can be fast-tracked to this service, with written information provided in primary care prior to their visit. The diagnosis of cancer can be excluded for most women at their first visit. Endometrial biopsy and outpatient hysteroscopy should be provided for those women with an abnormal scan result at their first assessment. The majority of consultant gynaecologists in a Scottish audit supported such outpatient investigation [II].

Presentation of endometrial cancer

- A meta-analysis of 35 studies found TVS scanning to be an accurate means of excluding endometrial cancer.
- Initial assessment of PMB should be provided as an outpatient service and TVS used to assess the endometrium.
- Seven prospective studies have evaluated TVS in women with PMB, comparing it against D&C or outpatient endometrial biopsy.
- There are no RCTs comparing D&C with outpatient biopsy for women with PMB.
- The cost effectiveness and clinical effectiveness of outpatient investigation of PMB have not been evaluated.

WOMEN ON TAMOXIFEN

Tamoxifen is a non-steroidal oestrogen antagonist, which is used widely as adjuvant treatment for postmenopausal women who have breast carcinoma. The absolute improvement in recurrence is greatest during the first 5 years of treatment [Ia].[5] Tamoxifen has been shown to decrease the overall progression of the disease and to prevent disease in the contralateral breast. Long-term tamoxifen use is controversial due to its oestrogenic effects on the endometrium. Although it acts as an anti-oestrogen on breast cancer cells, it has a mild oestrogenic effect on the endometrium, bone and cardiovascular system.

Long-term use is associated with proliferative endometrium, and a spectrum of benign and malignant changes of the endometrium has been reported, including hyperplasia, polyps and carcinoma. The incidence of endometrial carcinoma in postmenopausal women taking tamoxifen is significantly higher than in women not on tamoxifen [Ia].[5] However, the absolute decrease in contralateral breast cancer is twice as large as the absolute increase in endometrial cancer, and overall the benefits of tamoxifen are greater than the risks.

Postmenopausal women who have a uterus and are taking tamoxifen should be advised of these effects. Abnormal bleeding needs to be investigated fully and promptly. A Pipelle biopsy is appropriate as the first line of investigation, but a negative result is not conclusive. Women with a negative result still require hysteroscopy. Transvaginal ultrasound scan can be useful in triaging the urgency of further investigation. The fact that the ultrasonic appearances can be misleading needs to be considered. Tamoxifen has a sono-translucent effect on both the endometrial stroma and myometrium. This can give rise to false-positive reports in cases of cystic atrophy, which appears as thickened cystic endometrium on scan. Histology confirms this to be multiple cystic spaces lined by atrophic epithelium within a dense fibrous stroma. Hysteroscopy may be the investigation of choice in this situation as it allows direct inspection of the endometrium, and full-thickness biopsies can be taken at the same procedure.

There is no evidence that asymptomatic women on tamoxifen should be screened for endometrial changes [II]. Asymptomatic women taking tamoxifen have a greater endometrial thickness on TVS scan. Comparatively, those who present with bleeding have a significantly thicker endometrium and are more likely to have endometrial pathology [II],[6] and women with endometrial pathology are also more likely to present with symptoms. Outpatient hysteroscopy, although a good screening tool, is not as useful when biopsies are necessary. A randomized, cross-over study comparing TVS with outpatient hysteroscopy found the former together with sonohysterogram more sensitive, specific and acceptable to women.[7] There is no clinical or cost-effectiveness evidence to support the endometrial screening of asymptomatic women on tamoxifen [II], and the benefit in terms of breast cancer mortality far outweighs the risk to the endometrium. However, the evidence is less clear for healthy women taking tamoxifen to reduce their risk of breast cancer. The International Breast Cancer Intervention Study (IBIS), which started in 1992, will provide data on the risk:benefit ratio of tamoxifen preventative treatment. This trial aims to look at 7000 women randomized to 5 years of tamoxifen or placebo. An earlier US trial, The Breast Cancer

Prevention Trial (BCPT-P-1), was stopped early when a 45 per cent decrease in new breast cancers was reported in the tamoxifen arm. There was also an increase in endometrial cancers. Newer selective oestrogen receptor modulators (SERMs) have a similar profile to tamoxifen without the uterotrophic effects. Long-term data on the endometrium are awaited.

Tamoxifen and the endometrium

- A systematic review of 55 RCTs of adjuvant tamoxifen versus no tamoxifen before recurrence and with at least 5 years of follow-up data shows that tamoxifen substantially improves the 10-year survival of women with oestrogen-receptor-positive breast cancer. It also found that the incidence of endometrial cancer increases by a factor of 2 at 1–2 years and by a factor of 4 after 5 years of tamoxifen treatment.
- There is no evidence to support the screening of asymptomatic women on tamoxifen for endometrial abnormalities.

STAGING

The staging of endometrial cancer is surgical/pathological. Tumour grade and the depth of myometrial involvement are the main determinants of extrauterine spread. These two pathological criteria are often used to determine the risk of recurrence and to select women for postoperative radiotherapy. Metastatic spread occurs characteristically to the pelvic and para-aortic lymph nodes. Distant metastasis is uncommon at presentation. The most common sites of distant spread are the vagina and lungs, but the inguinal and supraclavicular lymph nodes, liver and brain may also be involved. When surgery is not appropriate or feasible, the clinical staging adopted by FIGO in 1971 is applied (Table 67.2), but selection of this staging system should be noted.

Radiological imaging

Preoperative evaluation and planning for treatment require clinical staging. The risk of pelvic and para-aortic lymph node involvement depends on the stage, grade and myometrial invasion. Twelve per cent of women with stage I disease will have lymph node metastasis. With grade 3 disease, this rises to 18 per cent, and when there is deep myometrial involvement to 22 per cent. Without proper assessment and a treatment plan based on the risk of nodal disease, the prognosis is poorer [III].

Endometrial biopsy will already have confirmed the diagnosis and given information on the tumour grade.

Table 67.2   International Federation of Gynecology and Obstetrics
(FIGO) classification

Stage 1	Carcinoma confined to the corpus
1A	No invasion into the myometrium
1B	Invasion <50% of the myometrium
1C	Invasion >50% of the myometrium
Stage II	Carcinoma confined to the corpus and the cervix but has not extended outside the uterus
IIA	Endocervical glandular involvement only
IIB	Cervical stromal invasion
Stage III	Extends outside of the uterus but is confined to the true pelvis
IIIA	Invades serosa and/or adnexa and/or positive peritoneal cytology
IIIB	Vaginal metastasis
IIIC	Metastasis to pelvic and/or para-aortic lymph nodes
Stage IV	Involves bladder or bowel mucosa or has metastasized to distant sites
IVA	Invasion of bladder and/or bowel mucosa
IVB	Distant metastasis including intra-abdominal and/or inguinal lymph nodes

Myometrial invasion can be assessed by TVS or magnetic resonance imaging (MRI). Transvaginal ultrasound can assess the depth of myometrial invasion and can be used to triage women for appropriate management at a cancer centre or cancer unit. Although TVS is quicker and relatively cheap, it is less accurate than MRI. Magnetic resonance imaging appears to be the optimum method of evaluating the soft-tissue structures of the pelvis, including myometrial invasion and the status of the pelvic lymph nodes. Computerized tomography (CT) scanning is less useful in imaging these soft tissues. The results are similar in predicting nodal disease but less accurate at assessing the depth of myometrial invasion [II] and cervical involvement. The role of MRI assessment is being evaluated as part of the ASTEC trial.[8] A chest X-ray should also be performed for staging, as the lungs are a common metastatic site.

Endometrial cancer imaging

- MRI is the imaging method of choice for pre-treatment staging.
- There are no RCTs.
- There are eight prospective non-controlled studies on MRI, five prospective comparative studies of MRI and TVS and two prospective comparative studies of MRI and CT scanning.

MANAGEMENT

Women with disease localized to the corpus are usually curable by surgery. When there is deep myometrial invasion or grade 3 disease, the prognosis with standard surgery alone is poorer because of the risk of nodal disease and recurrence.

Early stage disease

Most women present with early stage disease, and primary surgery is fundamental to achieving a cure. The treatment of choice is total abdominal hysterectomy and bilateral salpingo-oopherectomy (TAH/BSO), with peritoneal washings taken on opening the abdominal cavity for staging cytology. It is not necessary to remove a vaginal cuff or parametrial tissue [III]. Recurrence at the vaginal vault is related to the recognized risk factors of tumour grade, myometrial invasion and particularly cervical involvement – factors that reflect lymphatic vessel involvement.

Stage IIa disease should be treated the same as stage I disease by TAH/BSO. Where there is cervical stromal involvement, the treatment options are radical hysterectomy with pelvic lymphadenectomy or TAH/BSO with or without lymphadenectomy followed by postoperative radiotherapy. The choice of treatment depends on the tumour site and size and the fitness of the patient when considering the feasibility of extirpative surgery. Laparoscopic studies have shown the feasibility of laparoscopic lymphadenectomy [III] but there has been no contemporaneous controlled assessment of these procedures and no measurement of long-term clinical outcome.

Women with endometrial cancer are often elderly with other medical problems, and preoperative assessment for fitness for an anaesthetic and surgery is essential. However, survival rates are reduced by 20 per cent when primary surgery is not feasible.

Role of lymphadenectomy

The role of pelvic lymphadenectomy remains controversial. In the USA, it is used to improve surgical staging, but there is no clear evidence as to whether it improves survival. Available data are limited to a case-control study and retrospective case series. In a retrospective review, node dissection did not appear significantly to increase overall morbidity from hysterectomy in a selected series of patients [III].[9] A case-control study found a lower relative risk of recurrence for both high-risk and low-risk cases with lymphadenectomy [II].[10] However, case-mix and non-surgical treatment could have influenced the results in both these studies. Lymphadenectomy can rationalize the use of radiotherapy by excluding extrauterine disease, but in fact there is now little evidence to support adjuvant radiotherapy for low-risk and intermediate-risk disease (see below).

There are recognized complications, especially when lymphadenectomy is combined with postoperative radiotherapy, such as leg and lower abdominal oedema. There have been no RCTs of lymphadenectomy to measure its clinical effectiveness without bias from patient and surgical factors. Currently, the selection of women for lymphadenectomy is guided by preoperative assessment of risk factors for nodal involvement and patient fitness for additional anaesthetic time and surgery. There has been no rigorous evaluation of the selection of patients. A RCT (ASTEC) has been initiated by the Medical Research Council.[7] This is a multicentre RCT of lymphadenectomy and of external-beam radiotherapy in endometrial cancer. It opened in 1998 and is currently recruiting women from UK centres.

Who should perform surgery?

Endometrial cancer categorized as low risk following full preoperative assessment can be safely treated by TAH/BSO by a general gynaecologist. High-risk disease with a risk of cervical or pelvic node involvement should be referred to a specialist gynaecological oncologist.

Role of radiotherapy

Endometrial cancer is radiosensitive [III] and cure can be achieved with early stage disease. There have been no RCTs comparing surgery and primary radiotherapy. Currently, women with stage I disease considered to be at increased risk of recurrence are often given postoperative radiotherapy. This is usually based on tumour grade and depth of myometrial invasion. However, there are currently no accepted criteria for the triage of women into risk groups.

Vault brachytherapy is used to prevent vault recurrence, and external-beam therapy to the pelvis is used to treat the parametrium and pelvic sidewalls. However, it should be remembered that there is no evidence to show that radiotherapy improves survival in an unselected patient population. The role of postoperative radiotherapy for early stage endometrial cancer has been undefined due to the low rate of relapse and the lack of data from adequately powered randomized trials. Pelvic irradiation will reduce the incidence of local and regional recurrence, but improved survival has not been shown [Ib]. An earlier randomized trial compared intracavity therapy alone with external-beam combined with intracavity therapy. Aalders et al. suggested that, despite lower pelvic recurrence rates in the combined group, there was no overall survival benefit.[11] A more recent multicentre, prospective, randomized trial of postoperative radiotherapy for women with TAH and BSO without lymphadenectomy for low-risk or intermediate-risk stage I endometrial carcinoma (PORTEC) confirmed this, again showing that locoregional recurrences are reduced but that there is no impact on overall survival.[11] The survival was better in women below the age of 60 years than in those over 60 years.

Currently, women are selected with care for postoperative radiotherapy because of the impact of the treatment regime and the associated complications related to quality of life. The incidence of bowel complications is 3 per cent and can be higher after pelvic lymphadenectomy. The postoperative radiation therapy in endometrial carcinoma (PORTEC) trial[12] reported treatment-related complications in 25 per cent of

radiotherapy patients, although a fifth of these were grade 1. Most of the complications were associated with the gastro-intestinal tract. The symptoms resolved after some years in 50 per cent of women. Grade 1–2 genitourinary symptoms occur in 8 per cent of women treated by surgery and radiotherapy, compared with 4 per cent of women treated by surgery alone. Two per cent of women discontinued radiotherapy due to acute related symptoms. In addition, patients with acute morbidity have an increased risk of late radiotherapy complications, including rectal bleeding, fistulae or radiation damage to the small or large bowel.

The prognosis for most women with endometrial cancer is good, and therefore any impact of radiotherapy on survival will come from salvaging the small number of patients who would otherwise develop a pelvic recurrence. This requires a sufficiently large RCT powered to detect the effect on survival. There is no RCT on the role of radiotherapy in women who have also undergone pelvic lymphadenectomy, but this is currently being evaluated in the ASTEC trial, which has been designed to measure the effect independently of lymphadenectomy and postoperative radiotherapy on survival.

Progesterone therapy

Progesterone therapy for women who have had surgery for early stage endometrial cancer is not recommended, as overall survival is not improved [Ia].[13] Although deaths from endometrial cancer (OR 0.88, 95% CI 0.71–1.01) and the rate of disease relapse are reduced (OR 0.81, 95% CI 0.65–1.01), non-endometrial cancer-related deaths are more common (OR 1.33, 95% CI 1.02–1.73) [Ia].

Hormone replacement therapy

Traditionally, ERT has not been advocated in the first 2 years following surgery for endometrial cancer because of the concern of activating any residual disease. However, there is no evidence to support this, and the benefits of ERT may outweigh any theoretical risks [II]. The use of HRT following the treatment of endometrial cancer is currently being investigated by prospective randomized trials in the USA and Europe.

Advanced stage disease

In general, women with stage III disease are treated with surgery and radiation or radiotherapy alone. Laparotomy will allow staging and tumour-reductive surgery including hysterectomy if possible. However, sidewall extension will prevent tumour resection. Radiotherapy is used when surgery is inappropriate or incomplete. This may be a combination of intracavity and external-beam radiation, and cure rates of

30 per cent and 20 per cent for stage III and IV disease respectively have been reported. If the woman is not fit for surgery or irradiation, progesterone therapy is appropriate [II]. If radiotherapy achieves significant tumour shrinkage, 'adjuvant' surgery should be considered if the woman is fit.

With stage IV disease, the tumour site and the resultant symptoms will dictate management. Bulky pelvic disease or heavy vaginal bleeding may be controlled by radiation, either intracavity or external beam, or in combination. Local radiation can palliate symptomatic metastasis (e.g. to the lung, brain or bone). The role of chemotherapy is discussed below.

Recurrent disease

Women with recurrence limited to the pelvis who have not previously received radiotherapy may be salvaged by radiotherapy, with a 5-year survival of about 25–50 per cent. Para-aortic lymph nodes may be palliated by radiotherapy and, with localized pelvic recurrence, this can be curative when there has been no previous irradiation. The prognosis for distant metastatic endometrial cancer is poor. Progesterones will produce a clinical response in about 20 per cent of women with recurrent disease [II] and appear to be more effective in women with a long disease-free interval prior to recurrence. Standard agents are megestrol and medroxyprogesterone.

Role of chemotherapy

There is no evidence that chemotherapy has an adjuvant role in primary treatment, but it may have a limited palliative role for women with advanced or recurrent disease not amenable to radiation. There is no standard chemotherapy regime due to the lack of reliable evidence on clinical effectiveness. Combinations containing doxorubicin and epirubicin have been shown to have some anti-tumour activity. Paclitaxel and platinum-based regimens have about a 20 per cent response rate, but there is no evidence to show improved survival or quality of life. Median survival is still less than 1 year for these women. Combination regimens can produce higher response rates, but at the cost of increased toxicity and only minimal effect on survival. Current research into chemotherapy regimens is limited to Phase 1 and Phase 2 trials in the UK and USA. There is no evidence to date for adjuvant chemotherapy in primary treatment.

Table 67.3 Five-year survival rates for endometrial adenocarcinoma by stage

Stage	5-year survival
Stage I	80%
Stage II	65%
Stage III	30%
Stage IV	10%

Treatment of endometrial cancer

- There are no published surgical RCTs relating to endometrial carcinoma. Two retrospective studies suggest that lymphadenectomy may improve survival.
- Cases-series reports have shown that laparoscopic surgery is feasible, but there is no evidence concerning its clinical effectiveness over abdominal hysterectomy.
- Two RCTs have shown adjuvant radiotherapy reduces the rate of pelvic recurrence but have not been able to show any improvement in overall survival. The available evidence is that adjuvant radiotherapy should not be offered to women under the age of 60 with low-risk or intermediate-risk disease.
- A meta-analysis of six RCTs and a large RCT have both shown no reduction in death rates for endometrial cancer with progesterone therapy.
- The use of chemotherapy is limited to Phase I and II clinical trials.

PROGNOSIS

Survival is related to stage at presentation and grade of tumour (Table 67.3). There is a wide variation in rates of recurrence with early stage disease, from <10 per cent in low-risk women (Stage Ia G1 disease) to almost 50 per cent in high-risk women (Stage Ic G3 disease). When the only evidence of extrauterine spread is positive peritoneal washings, the influence on outcome is unclear, and there is no evidence that adjuvant therapy is of value unless extrauterine disease is present [III].[14]

KEY POINTS

- Investigation of PMB should be provided as a rapid-access outpatient service.
- The benefits of tamoxifen in breast cancer treatment outweigh the increased risk of endometrial cancer. Any abnormal vaginal bleeding while on tamoxifen requires full investigation.
- Surgery offers good prognosis in early stage disease, but the role of pelvic lymphadenectomy is still not clearly defined.
- Endometrial carcinoma is radiosensitive, but the benefits of locoregional control need to be balanced against treatment-related morbidity.
- Adjuvant radiotherapy should be restricted to intermediate disease in women over 60 years of age and high-risk disease.

SUMMARY

Endometrial cancer usually presents with PMB at an early stage. Staging is surgical/pathological, and preoperative imaging should include a chest X-ray and imaging for depth of myometrial penetration. Early stage disease should be managed by TAH and BSO, with peritoneal washings for staging. The role of pelvic lymphadenectomy is currently being investigated. Postoperative radiotherapy will reduce the number of local recurrences but may not give any survival advantage. The role of adjuvant progestogen therapy is limited to advanced or recurrent disease.

PUBLISHED GUIDELINES

Reviewers for the NHS Centre for Reviews and Dissemination. Endometrial cancer. *Effective Health Care*, June 1999; 5(3).

NHS executive. *Good Practice, Improving Outcomes in Gynaecological Cancers, The Manual*. London: Department of Health, 1999.

NHS executive. *Good Practice, Improving Outcomes in Gynaecological Cancers, The Research Evidence*. London: Department of Health, 1999.

Recommendations Arising from the 37th Study Group: Hormones and Cancer. RCOG Study Group Recommendations. London: RCOG Press, November 1999; <www.rcog.org.uk/study/hormones>.

KEY REFERENCES

1. Coleman MP, Babb P, Damieki P et al. Cancer survival trends in England and Wales 1971–1995. Deprivation and NHS region. London: HMSO, 1999.
2. Grady D, Gebretsadik T, Kerlikowske K, Ernsster V, Petitti D. Hormone replacement therapy and endometrial cancer risk: a meta-analysis. *Obstet Gynecol* 1995; 85(2):304–13.
3. Lethaby A, Farquhaar C, Sarkis A, Roberts H, Jepson R, Barlow D. Hormone replacement therapy in postmenopausal women: endometrial hyperplasia and irregular bleeding. *Cochrane Database of Systematic Reviews*, Issue 2. Oxford: Update Software, 2001.
4. Creasman WT, Odicino F, Maisonneuve P et al. Carcinoma of the corpus uteri. *J Epidemiol Biostat* 2001; 6(1):45–86.
5. Early Breast Cancer Trialists' Collaborative Group. Tamoxifen for early breast cancer. In: *The Cochrane Library*, Issue 2. Oxford: Update Software, 2001; 24.
6. Marconi D, Exacoustos C, Cangi B et al. Transvaginal sonographic and hysteroscopic findings in postmenopausal women receiving tamoxifen. *J Am Assoc Gynecol Laparosc* 1997; 4(3):331–9.
7. Timmerman D, Deprest J, Bourne T, Van den Berghe I, Collins WP, Vergote I. A randomized trial on the use of ultrasonography or office hysteroscopy for endometrial assessment in postmenopausal patients with breast cancer who were treated with tamoxifen. *Am J Obstet Gynecol* 1998; 179(1):62–70.
8. MRC Protocol. ASTEC: A Study of the Treatment of Endometrial Cancer: A randomised trial of lymphadenectomy and of adjuvant external beam radiotherapy in the treatment of endometrial cancer. 1998; ncrn.org.uk/portfolio.
9. Homesley HD, Kadar N, Barrett RJ et al. Selective pelvic and periaortic lymphadenectomy does not increase morbidity in surgical staging of endometrial carcinoma. *Am J Obstet Gynecol* 1992; 167(5):1225–30.
10. Kilgore LC, Partridge EE, Alvarez RD et al. Adenocarcinoma of the endometrium: survival comparisons of patients with and without pelvic lymph node sampling. *Gynecol Oncol* 1995; 56:29–33.
11. Aalders J, Abeler V, Kolstad P et al. Postoperative external radiation and prognostic parameters in stage 1 endometrial carcinoma. *Obstet Gynecol* 1980; 58:419–27.
12. Creutzberg CL, van Putten WLJ, Koper PC et al. Surgery and postoperative radiotherapy versus surgery alone for patients with stage I endometrial carcinoma: multicentre randomized trial. *Lancet* 2000; 355:1404–11.
13. Martin-Hirsch PL, Lilford RJ, Jarvis GJ. Adjuvant progesterone therapy for the treatment of endometrial cancer: review and meta-analysis of published randomised controlled trials. *Eur J Obstet Gynecol Reprod Biol* 1996; 65:2201–7.
14. Kadar N, Homesley HD, Malfetano JH. Positive peritoneal cytology is an adverse factor in endometrial carcinoma only if there is other evidence of extrauterine disease. *Gynecol Oncol* 1992; 46(2):145–9.

Chapter 68

Cervical Cancer

Pierre L. Martin-Hirsch

MRCOG standards

The established standards relevant for this topic are:

Theoretical skills
- Revise the anatomy of the cervix, blood supply and lymphatics.
- Understand the epidemiology and pathology of disease.
- Know the optimum pre-treatment assessment.
- Know how to manage surgically and non-surgically.

Practical skills
- Be able to recognize suspicious cervical lesions.
- Be able to take appropriate diagnostic biopsies.
- Be able to counsel patients with regard to diagnosis, management options and prognosis.

EPIDEMIOLOGY

Cervical cancer is the most common form of cancer in women in developing countries and the second most common form of cancer in the world as a whole. Three-quarters of affected women live in developing countries and it is estimated that up to 450 000 new cases of invasive cancer of the cervix occur per year in these countries. Cervical cancer accounts for 6 per cent of all malignancies in women. There are an estimated 16 000 new cases of invasive cancer of the cervix and 5000 deaths in the USA each year. In England and Wales in 1992, there were 3400 registrations, and 1225 deaths in 1997. Although cervical screening has been carried out in the UK since the 1960s, the benefits of screening are only now becoming apparent, following the reorganization of the service in 1988. The incidence of

cervical cancer has fallen in the UK by 26 per cent since 1992, and mortality from 7.1 per 100 000 in 1988 to 3.7 per 100 000 in 1997, a decrease of almost 50 per cent. This decrease is almost certainly due to the widespread coverage of screening, which has risen from less than 35 per cent in 1988 to 85 per cent in 1998 through the introduction of an effective call–recall system for cervical screening. The reduction of deaths is due to a reduction in both incidence and the proportion of advanced disease.

Epidemiological studies convincingly demonstrate that the major risk factor for the development of pre-invasive and invasive carcinoma of the cervix is human papillomavirus (HPV) infection, which far outweighs other known risk factors such as high parity, increasing number of sexual partners, young age at first intercourse, low socioeconomic status, and positive smoking history. In an international study consisting of 1000 specimens collected from patients with invasive cervical cancer in 32 hospitals in 22 countries, HPV DNA was present in 99.7 per cent of cervical cancers.[1] HPV 16 was the predominant type in all countries except Indonesia, where HPV 18 was more common.[1] The role of HPV in cervical carcinogenesis is expanded on in Chapter 66.

PATHOLOGY

Squamous cell and adenosquamous carcinomas comprise approximately 85 per cent and adenocarcinoma approximately 15 per cent of cervical cancers. Squamous carcinomas are large-cell keratinizing, large-cell non-keratinizing and small-cell types. The small-cell neuroendocrine-type typically behaves like similar disease arising from the bronchus. Adenocarcinomas can be pure or mixed with squamous cell carcinomas, the adenosquamous carcinoma. About 80 per cent of cervical adenocarcinomas are made up of cells of the endocervical type with mucin production. The remaining tumours are populated by endometroid, clear, intestinal or a mixture of more than one type of cell.

KEY POINTS

- Cervical cancer is the most common form of cancer in women in developing countries.
- The incidence of and deaths from cervical cancer are decreasing in the UK due to cervical screening.
- HPV DNA is present in the vast majority of cervical cancers.
- Squamous cell and adenosquamous carcinomas comprise approximately 85 per cent and adenocarcinomas approximately 15 per cent of cervical cancers.

CLINICAL MANAGEMENT

The goals of the management of cervical cancer are to stage the disease and to treat both the primary lesion and other sites of spread. Cervical cancers spread by direct spread into the cervical stroma, parametrium and beyond and by lymphatic metastasis into parametrial, pelvic sidewall and para-aortic nodes. Blood-borne spread is unusual. Among the major factors that influence prognosis are:

- stage
- volume
- grade of tumour
- histological type
- lymphatic spread
- vascular invasion.

In a large surgico-pathological staging study of patients with clinical disease confined to the cervix, the factors that predicted lymph node metastases and a decrease in disease-free survival were capillary–lymphatic space involvement by tumour, increasing tumour size and increasing depth of stromal invasion.[2,3] A similar study of 626 patients with locally advanced disease demonstrated that para-aortic and pelvic lymph node status, tumour size, clinical stage, patient age and performance status were all significant prognostic factors for a reduction in progression-free interval and survival.[4] The incidence of para-aortic and pelvic lymph node disease according to stage is illustrated in Table 68.1.

Staging

Women should be fully staged using the International Federation of Gynaecology and Obstetrics (FIGO) system (Table 68.2). FIGO staging is based largely on clinical assessment, chest X-ray and cystoscopy. Radiological staging, particularly by magnetic resonance imaging (MRI), which permits more accurate determination of disease extent,[11] also permits assessment of lymph node status. Routine use of imaging enhances the selection of women in whom surgery alone is likely to be curative.

Table 68.1 Incidence of nodal disease in cervical cancer according to stage[5-10]

Stage	n	Positive pelvic lymph nodes (%)	Positive para-aortic lymph nodes (%)
Ia1 (<1 mm)	23	0	0
Ia1 (1–3 mm)	156	0.6	0
Ia2 (3–5 mm)	84	4.8	<1
Ib	1926	15.9	2.2
IIa	110	24.5	11
IIb	324	31.4	19
III	125	44.8	30
IVa	23	55	40

Table 68.2 International Federation of Gynecology and Obstetrics (FIGO) staging

Stage I	
Stage I	Carcinoma strictly confined to the cervix; extension to the uterine corpus does not affect the stage.
Stage Ia	Invasive cancer identified only microscopically. All gross lesions, even with superficial invasion, are stage Ib cancers. Invasion is limited to measured stromal invasion with a maximum depth of 5 mm and no wider than 7 mm.
Stage Ia1	Measured invasion of the stroma no greater than 3 mm in depth and no wider than 7 mm diameter.
Stage Ia2	Measured invasion of stroma greater than 3 mm but no greater than 5 mm in depth and no wider than 7 mm in diameter.
Stage Ib	Clinical lesions confined to the cervix or pre-clinical lesions greater than stage Ia.
Stage Ib1	Clinical lesions no greater than 4 cm in size.
Stage Ib2	Clinical lesions greater than 4 cm in size.
Stage II	
Stage II	Carcinoma that extends beyond the cervix but has not extended onto the pelvic wall. The carcinoma involves the vagina, but not as far as the lower third.
Stage IIa	No obvious parametrial involvement. Involvement of up to the upper two-thirds of the vagina.
Stage IIb	Obvious parametrial involvement, but not onto the pelvic sidewall.
Stage III	
Stage III	Carcinoma that has extended onto the pelvic sidewall. On rectal examination, there is no cancer-free space between the tumour and the pelvic sidewall. The tumour involves the lower third of the vagina. All cases with a hydronephrosis or non-functioning kidney should be included, unless they are known to be due to other causes.
Stage IIIa	No extension onto the pelvic sidewall but involvement of the lower third of the vagina.
Stage IIIb	Extension onto the pelvic sidewall or hydronephrosis or non-functioning kidney.
Stage IV	
Stage IV	Carcinoma that has extended beyond the true pelvis or has clinically involved the mucosa of the bladder and/or rectum.
Stage IVa	Spread of the tumour onto adjacent pelvic organs.
Stage IVb	Spread to distant organs.

Treatment

Specialized gynaecological oncology teams should determine the management of women with cervical cancer. Decisions about how best to treat early disease in young women in particular require considerable experience. Both surgery and radiotherapy are effective in early stage disease, whereas locally advanced disease relies on treatment by radiation or chemoradiation. Surgery does provide the advantage of conservation of ovarian function.

Factors that influence the mode of treatment include stage, age and health status. Radiation can be used for all stages, whereas surgery should only be considered an option for early disease; stage I and stage IIa. A large randomized trial reported identical 5-year overall and disease-free survival rates when comparing radiation therapy with radical hysterectomy, but women who had surgery and adjuvant radiotherapy suffered significantly higher morbidity than those who had either surgery or radiotherapy alone [Ib].[12]

There are clear advantages to surgery in women at low operative risk. Surgery permits conservation of ovarian function in premenopausal women and also reduces the risk of chronic bladder, bowel and sexual dysfunction associated with radiotherapy. Complications in the hands of skilled surgeons are uncommon. Surgery also permits the assessment of risk factors, such as lymph node status, that will ultimately influence prognosis. Complications of surgery include fistulae (<1 per cent), lymphocyst, primary haemorrhage and bladder injury. Chronic bowel and bladder problems that require medical or surgical intervention occur in up to 8–13 per cent of women[13] due to parasympathetic denervation secondary to surgical clamping at the lateral excision margins.

Stage Ia disease

Micro-invasive disease is one in which neoplastic cells invade from the epithelium to a maximum depth of 5 mm and a maximum horizontal spread of 7 mm. Any invasion beyond these dimensions upstages the disease to Stage Ib. The identification of early disease allows the selection of a group of women who are not at risk of lymph node disease and can be treated with less aggressive and, importantly, fertility-sparing therapy.

Micro-invasive disease comprises 20 per cent of invasive cancers. Stage Ia1 disease (invasion <3 mm) is rarely associated with lymph node metastases (see Table 68.1). This disease should be formally diagnosed by cone biopsy or diathermy excision. Knife cone biopsy does not cause any thermal damage, and the extent of disease may be more accurately assessed than on a loop excision specimen. If the disease and any associated intraepithelial neoplasia are removed with clear margins, no further treatment is necessary. If disease is present at the margins, further excision or hysterectomy is required. A simple abdominal total hysterectomy is sufficient, as there is no risk of parametrial involvement. Because invasive disease of <3 mm invasion is associated with a very low risk of lymph node disease (see Table 68.1), lymphadenectomy is not indicated. Lymphadenectomy should, however, be considered for Stage Ia2 (invasion 3–5 mm) disease as the rate of node involvement reaches 5 per cent, particularly if the tumour is poorly differentiated.

Stage Ib–IIa

Stage Ib is divided into Ib1 (<4 cm diameter) and Ib2 (≥4 cm diameter); stage IIa means upper vaginal but not parametrial involvement.

Surgical therapy for Stage Ib and IIa tumours <4 cm across usually involves radical hysterectomy and pelvic lymphadenectomy. Radical hysterectomy involves removing the tumour with adequate disease-free margins. This involves excising the parametrial tissue around the cervix and upper vagina, with removal of part or all of the cardinal and utero-sacral ligaments, depending on the extent of the dissection. More radical dissections are associated with a higher incidence of perioperative morbidity and chronic bladder and bowel dysfunction with no survival advantage [Ib].[14] The lymph node dissection should include obturator, internal, external and common iliac nodes. In the absence of suspicious pelvic nodes, para-aortic lymphadenectomy is not mandatory, but it should be performed in the presence of involved pelvic nodes or if there is clinical suspicion of para-aortic node involvement. If there is any suspicion about the nature of the para-aortic nodes, they should be removed and subjected to frozen section. Confirmed para-aortic disease at the start of surgery is a contraindication to radical pelvic surgery. Lymphadenectomy may result in lymphocyst formation. Lymphoedema following pelvic lymphadenectomy can occur, although its incidence increases if adjuvant radiotherapy is given.

In cases in which positive nodes are encountered, there are differing views. Some would advocate abandoning surgery in favour of radical chemoradiation. Others would argue that, if possible, radical surgery should be completed to achieve an adjuvant setting for radiotherapy. If suspicious nodes are identified and confirmed to be diseased at frozen section, it is probably best to remove resectable nodes and treat with chemoradiation, including brachytherapy, which requires the uterus to be in situ. Radical surgery followed by radical radiotherapy is associated with increased morbidity.

Adjuvant radiotherapy is normally recommended for women with resected positive pelvic nodes to reduce the risk of recurrence. Patients with 'close' vaginal margins (<0.5 cm) may also benefit from pelvic irradiation.[15] Indirect evidence from non-randomized studies suggests it can improve pelvic control, but there is no firm evidence of increased survival [II].[16,17] Careful preoperative radiological imaging reduces the risk of encountering unexpected lymphadenopathy or unexpectedly large tumours.

Because bulky Ib tumours have a higher risk of positive nodes and close surgical margins, these are now regarded by many as being better treated with chemoradiation as opposed to surgery or radiotherapy alone. Some women with small-volume stage Ib disease who wish to conserve their fertility might be suitable for trachelectomy (radical excision of the cervix) combined with either laparoscopic or open lymphadenectomy. This technique is still under evaluation. Some surgeons recommend the insertion of an abdominal isthmic cervical cerclage to reduce the risk of late miscarriage. Indeed, in selected cases of Ib1 disease that are just greater than 7 mm in horizontal spread, a large cone biopsy may be adequate for central control, even though it may need to be combined with lymphadenectomy.

Stage IIb and above

It is not feasible to perform surgery with curative intent in these advanced stages of disease. Radical radiotherapy and chemoradiation are the only modalities of treatment that offer the potential for cure. One randomized trial has suggested that preoperative chemotherapy to shrink disease followed by radical surgery may be superior to radical radiotherapy, but this has not been confirmed.[18] It is inevitable that preoperative chemotherapy followed by surgery will still require some women to undergo adjuvant or non-adjuvant radiotherapy that is likely to result in unacceptable toxicity.

Radical radiotherapy

Radical radiotherapy is indicated for women unfit for surgery, bulky stage Ib2 disease and more advanced disease. The goals of such treatment are to treat primary disease and to control metastatic pelvic lymph nodes. The radical dose is delivered by external-beam (teletherapy) and intracavitary treatment (brachytherapy). The standard technique now is of remote after-loading (e.g. using the Selectron). Intracavitary treatment is designed to give high doses locally to the primary site. Teletherapy is designed to treat any pelvic spread. The challenge in administering radiotherapy is in achieving an optimal dose throughout the primary tumour and pelvic sidewall without causing high morbidity. The peripheral field of treatment of intracavitary radiotherapy delivers an insufficient dose to treat the pelvic sidewalls. The dose-limiting normal tissues within the pelvis are the rectum posteriorly, the bladder anteriorly, and any loops of small bowel within the pelvic radiation fields.

Prescribing rules have been devised for determining the precise dose of radiotherapy within the pelvis, and improved planning by computerized tomography (CT) has enabled more accurate targeting of external-beam radiation in particular. An example is the Manchester system. This uses a number of predetermined source sizes and radioactive loadings such that a constant dose rate is delivered to a point A. Point A is defined as a point 2 cm lateral to the central axis of the uterus and 2 cm from the lateral fornix. A second point (B) lying in the same plane 3 cm lateral to point A is used to determine the dose to parametrial tissues. Following the insertion of the sources for each patient, a dose distribution is calculated. The total dose is a product of the dose rate and treatment time. The usual doses delivered are 70–80 Gray to point A and 60 Gray to point B, limiting the bladder and rectal dose to <60 Gray. To achieve this, it is necessary to have adequate packing to keep the bladder and bowel away from the intracavitary source. External-beam radiation

is usually given 2–3 weeks after intracavitary treatment to allow for involution of the primary disease. External-beam radiotherapy is fractionated over 20–30 days' treatment, as this technique allows a cancericidal effect while enabling normal tissue recovery between fractions.

Routine extended field radiotherapy designed to include para-aortic nodes has not been proven to improve survival compared with pelvic radiotherapy alone, and it is associated with significantly more gastrointestinal complications [Ib].[19] While there does not appear to be significant benefit from extended field irradiation for all cases, para-aortic node irradiation is appropriate in cases of proven para-aortic node involvement as indicated by diagnostic imaging or surgical staging.

Chemoradiation

Five recent randomized trials from the USA[20–24] have shown an overall survival advantage for cisplatin-based therapy given concurrently with radiation therapy [Ib]. The patient populations in these studies included women with FIGO stages Ib2–IVa cervical cancer treated with primary radiation therapy and women with FIGO stages I–IIa disease found to have poor prognostic factors (metastatic disease in pelvic lymph nodes, parametrial disease, or positive surgical margins) at the time of primary surgery. Although the trials vary somewhat in terms of stage of disease, dose of radiation, and schedule of cisplatin and radiation, they all demonstrate significant survival benefit for this combined approach, the risk of death from cervical cancer being decreased by 30 per cent. These trials reported higher rates of short-term and medium-term complications with chemoradiation, and although longer follow-up is required to examine the true morbidity of this treatment regimen, there is now international acceptance that chemoradiation is superior to radiation alone.

Recurrent cervical cancer

Treatment for recurrent cervical cancer depends on the mode of primary therapy and the site of recurrence. Women who have had initial treatment by surgery should be considered for radiotherapy, and those who have had radiotherapy should be considered for exenterative surgery, provided the recurrence is central and there is no evidence of distant recurrence. These women require very careful preoperative assessment and counselling in order to understand the consequences of defunctioning surgery. Exenterative surgery in carefully selected cases can result in 5-year survival of 50 per cent [III]. Positive nodes at the time of attempted salvage surgery and positive resection margins are associated with a poor prognosis. Anterior exenteration requires excision of the bladder and most of the vagina en bloc with the recurrence, and posterior exenteration requires excision of the sigmoid rectum with formation of a colostomy. Sometimes a combination of the two is required. This type of surgery should only be undertaken by teams of highly skilled pelvic surgeons. Relapse within 2 years of primary treatment, the presence of hydronephrosis and symptoms of pain are all associated with poorer outcomes in terms of exenterative surgery.

Palliation of progressive cervical disease

Chemotherapy is palliative and should be reserved for patients who are not considered curable by the other two treatment modalities. Urinary tract symptoms are particularly common in advanced cervical disease. Ureteric obstruction with subsequent pain, infection and ultimately impaired renal function are common features. Mechanical diversion by nephrostomy or ureteric stenting is only usually justified as part of treatment with curative intent. Fistulae can occur in late stage disease and can cause intolerable symptoms. If there is a prospect of surviving more than 8 weeks, palliative surgery should be offered in order to divert faeces or urine.

In progressive late stage disease, there is usually ureteric obstruction, which heralds a terminal phase. Pain can be particularly distressing due to infiltration of the lumbosacral nerve plexuses. Meticulous attention to pain control and psychological and emotional support are essential.

The preventative nature of cervical cancer, its involvement of young women, and the difficulties associated with recurrence require a meticulous and highly skilled approach to all aspects of its management.

KEY POINTS

- Early micro-invasive disease can be treated by cone biopsy or excisional treatment alone [II].
- Surgery and radiotherapy for Stage Ib/IIa disease have similar 5-year overall and disease-free survival rates, but women who have had surgery and adjuvant radiotherapy combined have significantly higher morbidity than those who have had either surgery or radiotherapy alone [Ib].
- Preoperative imaging with MRI scans may reduce the number of women undergoing both modalities of treatment [II].
- Chemoradiation increases survival over radiotherapy alone for advanced disease, but toxicity is increased [Ib].

KEY REFERENCES

1. Walboomers JM, Jacobs MV, Manos MM et al. Human papillomavirus is a necessary cause of invasive cervical cancer worldwide. *J Pathol* 1999; **189**:12–19.

2. Delgado G, Bundy BN, Fowler WC et al. A prospective surgical pathological study of stage I squamous carcinoma of the cervix: a Gynecologic Oncology Group study. *Gynecol Oncol* 1989; **35**:314–20.

3. Zaino RJ, Ward S, Delgado G et al. Histopathologic predictors of the behavior of surgically treated stage IB squamous cell carcinoma of the cervix. A Gynecologic Oncology Group study. *Cancer* 1992; **69**:1750–8.

4. Stehman FB, Bundy BN, DiSaia PJ, Keys HM, Larson JE, Fowler WC. Carcinoma of the cervix treated with radiation therapy. I. A multi-variate analysis of prognostic variables in the Gynecologic Oncology Group. *Cancer* 1991; **67**:2776–85.

5. Boyce, Fruchter R, Nicastri AD, Ambiavagar P-C, Renis MS, Nelson JH. Prognostic factors in stage I carcinoma of the cervix. *Gynecol Oncol* 1981; **12**:154–65.

6. Inoue T, Okumura M. Prognostic significance of parametrial extension in patients with cervical carcinoma Stages IB, IIA, and IIB. A study of 628 cases treated by radical hysterectomy and lymphadenectomy with or without postoperative irradiation. *Cancer* 1984; **54**:1714–19.

7. Lohe KJ. Early squamous cell carcinoma of the uterine cervix. *Gynecol Oncol* 1978; **6**:10–30.

8. van Nagell J, Donaldson ES, Wood EG, Parker JC. The significance of vascular invasion and lymphocytic infiltration in invasive cervical cancer. *Cancer* 1978; **41**:228–34.

9. Tinga DJ, Timmer PR, Bouma J, Aalders JG. Prognostic significance of single versus multiple lymph node metastases in cervical carcinoma stage IB. *Gynecol Oncol* 1990; **39**:175–80.

10. Nahhas WA, Sharkey FE, Whitney CW, Husseinzadeh N, Chung CK, Mortel R. The prognostic significance of vascular channel involvement and deep stromal penetration in early cervical carcinoma. *Am J Clin Oncol* 1983; **6**:259–64.

11. Scheidler J, Hricak H, Yu KK, Subak L, Segal MR. Radiological evaluation of lymph node metastases in patients with cervical cancer. A meta-analysis. *J Am Med Assoc* 1997; **278**:1096–101.

12. Landoni F, Maneo A, Colombo A et al. Randomised study of radical surgery versus radiotherapy for stage Ib–IIa cervical cancer. *Lancet* 1997; **350**:535–40.

13. Fujikawa K, Miyamoto T, Ihara Y, Matsui Y, Takeuchi H. High incidence of severe urologic complications following radiotherapy for cervical cancer in Japanese women. *Gynecol Oncol* 2001; **80**:21–3.

14. Landoni F, Maneo A, Cormio G et al. Class II versus class III radical hysterectomy in stage IB–IIA cervical cancer: a prospective randomized study. *Gynecol Oncol* 2001; **80**:3–12.

15. Estape RE, Angioli R, Madrigal M et al. Close vaginal margins as a prognostic factor after radical hysterectomy. *Gynecol Oncol* 1998; **68**:229–32.

16. Soisson AP, Soper JT, Clarke Pearson DL, Berchuck A, Montana G, Creasman WT. Adjuvant radiotherapy following radical hysterectomy for patients with stage IB and IIA cervical cancer. *Gynecol Oncol* 1990; 37:390–5.

17. Kinney WK, Alvarez RD, Reid GC et al. Value of adjuvant whole-pelvis irradiation after Wertheim hysterectomy for early-stage squamous carcinoma of the cervix with pelvic nodal metastasis: a matched-control study. *Gynecol Oncol* 1989; 34:258–62.

18. Sardi JE, Giaroli A, di Paola G et al. Long-term follow-up of the first randomized trial using neoadjuvant chemotherapy in stage Ib squamous carcinoma of the cervix: the final results. *Gynecol Oncol* 1997; 67:61–9.

19. Haie C, Pejovic MH, Gerbaulet A et al. Is prophylactic para-aortic irradiation worthwhile in the treatment of advanced cervical carcinoma? Results of a controlled clinical trial of the EORTC radiotherapy group. *Radiother Oncol* 1988; 11:101–12.

20. Whitney CW, Sause W, Bundy BN et al. Randomized comparison of fluorouracil plus cisplatin versus hydroxyurea as an adjunct to radiation therapy in stage IIB–IVA carcinoma of the cervix with negative para-aortic lymph nodes: a Gynecologic Oncology Group and Southwest Oncology Group study. *J Clin Oncol* 1999; 17:1339–48.

21. Morris M, Eifel PJ, Lu J et al. Pelvic radiation with concurrent chemotherapy compared with pelvic and para-aortic radiation for high-risk cervical cancer. *N Engl J Med* 1999; 340:1137–43.

22. Rose PG, Bundy BN, Watkins EB et al. Concurrent cisplatin-based radiotherapy and chemotherapy for locally advanced cervical cancer. *N Engl J Med* 1999; 340:1144–53.

23. Keys HM, Bundy BN, Stehman FB et al. Cisplatin, radiation, and adjuvant hysterectomy compared with radiation and adjuvant hysterectomy for bulky stage IB cervical carcinoma. *N Engl J Med* 1999; 340:1154–61.

24. Peters WA 3rd, Liu PY, Barrett RJ 2nd et al. Concurrent chemotherapy and pelvic radiation therapy compared with pelvic radiation therapy alone as adjuvant therapy after radical surgery in high-risk early-stage cancer of the cervix. *J Clin Oncol* 2000; 18:1606–13.

Benign and Malignant Ovarian Masses

Karina Reynolds

MRCOG standards

The established standards relevant for this topic are:

Theoretical skills

- Revise your knowledge of anatomy as applied to surgical procedures undertaken by the gynaecological oncologist.
- Understand the epidemiology and aetiology of ovarian tumours.
- Understand the indications for referral for genetic screening.
- Know how to assess and stage ovarian cancer.
- Understand the indications for referral to a gynaecological oncologist.
- Know the principles of treatment: surgery, chemotherapy and radiotherapy.
- Understand the principles of managing palliative care in concert with an expert team.

Practical skills

- Be able to competently manage the adnexal mass presenting as an emergency.
- Be able to competently manage the adnexal mass at low risk of malignancy.
- Be able to evaluate the response to oncological treatments.
- Have seen laparotomy, staging and cytoreductive surgery for the management of primary ovarian cancer.
- Have completed a 'Breaking Bad News' course.

INTRODUCTION

By the age of 65, 4 per cent of women will have been admitted to hospital with an ovarian cyst, making this the fourth most common gynaecological cause for hospital admission in England. Among premenopausal patients, more than

Table 69.1 Incidence (1996) and mortality (1998) of the common gynaecological malignancies in England and Wales

Cancer	Incidence	Crude rate/ 100 000	Mortality	Crude rate/ 100 000
Ovarian	6570	21.9	4520	15.1
Uterine	4520	15.1	1230	3.1
Cervical	3320	11.1	1330	4.4
Vulval	800	2.5	340	1.29

From *Cancer Trends in England and Wales 1950–1999*, cancer@ons.gov.uk.

90 per cent of surgically managed cases are benign, as opposed to just 60 per cent in the postmenopausal population. Although differentiating malignant from benign disease is critical in optimizing management for the individual, non-invasive diagnosis continues to be elusive. Prompt identification and appropriate treatment of cancer of the ovary are essential if the survival rates are to be optimal. In England and Wales, it is not just the commonest gynaecological malignancy, it also continues to kill more women than all other gynaecological cancers together (Table 69.1).

HISTOPATHOLOGY AND CLASSIFICATION OF OVARIAN MASSES

An ovarian mass may be neoplastic or physiological, and most adnexal masses are benign. The current edition of *International Classification of Tumours*, published by the World Health Organization (WHO),[1] provides a classification of ovarian tumours that has been universally accepted. Epithelial tumours are derived from the surface epithelium of the ovary and are further classified as benign, borderline or malignant, according to cell type and behaviour (Figures 69.1 and 69.2).[1]

Epithelial tumours account for 60–65 per cent of all ovarian tumours and approximately 90 per cent of those that are malignant. Sex-cord stromal tumours are, as their

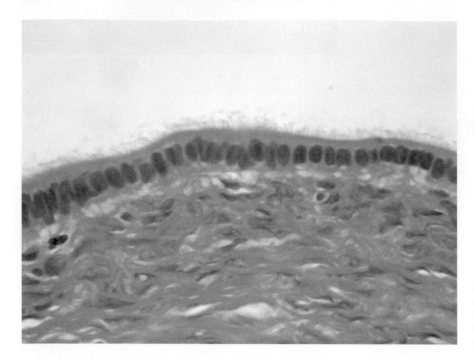

Figure 69.1   Haematoxylin and eosin staining of a section of tumour demonstrating the typical epithelium of a benign serous cystadenoma – note single layer and bland appearance

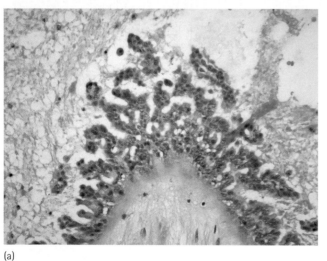

(a)

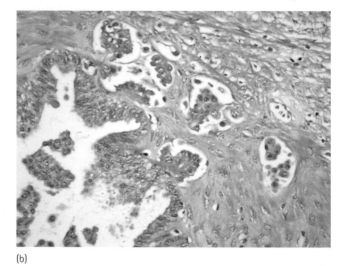

(b)

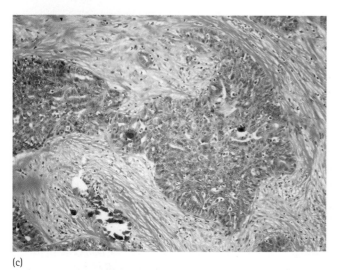

(c)

Figure 69.2   Haematoxylin and eosin sections from borderline, microinvasive and malignant ovarian tumours demonstrating increasing architectural complexity and nuclear pleomorphism. (a) Borderline serous ovarian tumour. (b) Borderline serous ovarian tumour with microinvasion. (c) Invasive serous cystadenocarcinoma

name suggests, derived from the sex cords and stroma of the ovary and account for approximately 8 per cent of all ovarian tumours. Germ-cell tumours, derived from the germ cells, account for 30 per cent of ovarian tumours, largely in the form of mature cystic teratomas (dermoid cysts). Although germ-cell tumours account for only 1–3 per cent of all ovarian malignancies, they represent more than 60 per cent of ovarian cancers in children and adolescents.

Note: the term **ovarian cancer** is used in this chapter to include not only epithelial ovarian malignancies, but also malignant sex-cord stromal and germ-cell neoplasms.

Epithelial ovarian tumours

The ovary first appears in fetal life as an aggregation of cells covered with primitive coelomic epithelium. Subsequently, germ cells migrate from the yolk sac into the gonadal area. The coelomic epithelium that covers the ovary also gives rise to a variety of epithelia of Müllerian origin, which line the genital tract structures, including the Fallopian tubes, the uterus and the cervix, and are similar to those found in epithelial tumours of the ovary. Well-differentiated serous carcinoma resembles epithelium of the Fallopian tube, whereas the cell type in endometrioid tumours has a similar appearance to the cells found in endometrial glands. The WHO classification of epithelial ovarian tumours is based on this similarity in cell type (Table 69.2).

The serous tumours are the most common in this group (40–50 per cent). Mucinous tumours (10 per cent) may reach an enormous size and may be associated with pseudomyxoma ovarii and peritoneii. More than 10 per cent of primary endometrioid ovarian carcinomas are associated with carcinoma of the endometrium (coincidental primaries in most cases). Endometrioid carcinomas account for approximately 20 per cent of malignant epithelial tumours, but Brenner tumours make up a very small proportion, as 99 per cent are benign. Clear-cell carcinomas account for between 5 and 10 per cent and have a worse prognosis than the other histological types. Bilaterality of epithelial ovarian malignancies is common.

Although endocrine function is most commonly a feature of sex-cord stromal tumours, it may also occur in association with epithelial ovarian tumours. Paraneoplastic syndromes are a rare feature of these tumours.

Table 69.2   Epithelial ovarian tumours – simplified classification

Serous tumours
Mucinous tumours
Endometrioid tumours
Clear-cell tumours
Transitional cell (Brenner) tumours
Mixed epithelial tumours
Undifferentiated and unclassified tumours

Sex-cord stromal tumours

These tumours are composed of granulosa cells, theca cells, Sertoli cells, Leydig cells, fibroblasts or the precursors of these cells in varying proportions. The classification of these tumours (based on the WHO classification) is shown in Table 69.3. They may be associated with an oestrogenic, androgenic or (more rarely) progestogenic effect, but functional activity does not correlate with the appearance of the cell. Many of these tumours are benign and most of the clinically malignant forms are granulosa cell tumours. Fibromas are well known for their association with ascites and right hydrothorax, reported by Meigs in 1937 (Meigs syndrome).

Table 69.3   Sex-cord-stromal tumours – simplified classification

Granulosa-stromal cell tumours
Sertoli–stromal cell tumours
Gynandroblastoma
Sex-cord tumour with annular tubules
Unclassified sex-cord tumours
Steroid cell tumours

Germ-cell tumours

Approximately 30 per cent of benign and malignant ovarian tumours are of germ-cell origin (Table 69.4). However, as only a small proportion is malignant, they account for less than 5 per cent of all ovarian cancers. Nonetheless, they are the commonest ovarian malignancy in the first two decades of life.

Dysgerminoma is the commonest germ-cell malignancy, and 75 per cent of cases present with stage I disease. In contrast with other malignant germ-cell tumours, 10–15 per cent are bilateral, with contralateral involvement usually being microscopic. Five to 10 per cent occur in phenotypic females with abnormal gonads (the androgen insensitivity syndrome or gonadal dysgenesis).

Teratomas are tumours that are composed of tissue derived from two or three embryonic layers. The mature cystic teratoma is the commonest ovarian germ-cell tumour and is usually benign. Most are unilateral, but 15–20 per cent are bilateral. They are the commonest ovarian tumours leading to torsion. Hair and teeth may be present in the cysts, the latter resulting in the classical appearance on plain abdominal X-ray. Malignant transformation is reported in up to 2 per cent,

Table 69.4   Ovarian germ-cell tumours – simplified classification

Dysgerminoma
Teratoma (immature, mature and monodermal)
Yolk sac tumour (endodermal sinus tumour)
Embryonal carcinoma
Polyembryoma
Choriocarcinoma
Mixed germ-cell tumours

squamous carcinoma being the commonest malignancy to develop. A diagnosis of struma ovarii is made when these tumours are predominantly composed of thyroid tissue. Primary ovarian carcinoid tumours are also variants of monodermal teratomas and usually have a favourable prognosis. However, secondary carcinoids (not associated with a monodermal teratoma) are usually metastatic from the gastrointestinal tract and have a poor prognosis.

Immature teratoma is the second commonest germ-cell malignancy and accounts for approximately 20 per cent of ovarian malignancies in females under 20 years of age. Virtually all immature teratomas are unilateral and they are currently classified according to a grading system that is based on the degree of differentiation and the quantity of immature tissue.

Embryonic markers

Most patients with ovarian yolk sac tumours have elevated levels of alpha-fetoprotein (AFP), but normal levels do not exclude this diagnosis. Embryonal carcinomas are extremely rare. They usually secrete beta-human chorionic gonadotrophin (β-hCG) and may secrete AFP. Ovarian choriocarcinoma secretes β-hCG and polyembryoma secretes β-hCG and AFP. These are also very rare tumours. The commoner immature teratoma and pure dysgerminoma do not secrete these tumour markers.

Gonadoblastoma

This rare tumour consists of admixed germ-cell and sex-cord stromal elements. This is usually a tumour of the second decade of life and rarely occurs in normal ovaries. Eighty per cent occur in phenotypic females who are virilized, and 20 per cent in phenotypic males with developmental abnormalities of the external genitalia. The most common karyotypes are 46XY and 45XO/46XY (mosaic).

Secondary ovarian malignancies

Up to 10 per cent of ovarian masses are metastases from some other organ and in many cases the ovarian metastases are detected before the primary tumour. The most common metastatic cancers are those arising from the colon, stomach, breast and, of course, the female genital tract. Bilaterally enlarged ovaries that contain signet-ring cells on microscopic assessment have been named after Krukenberg, who described these ovarian tumours in patients with metastatic gastric or (less commonly) colonic cancer.

Primary peritoneal carcinoma

Primary peritoneal carcinoma is a highly malignant tumour arising from the peritoneum and resulting in signs and symptoms very similar to those of primary epithelial ovarian cancer. Rare benign and borderline variants have been described. Thus a patient who has previously had both ovaries removed may develop a condition that clinically simulates ovarian cancer. Management is essentially as for advanced primary epithelial ovarian cancer.

Primary fallopian tube cancer

This rare cancer accounts for approximately 0.3 per cent of all female genital tract cancers. The classical presenting triad consists of:

- a prominent watery discharge (hydrops tubae profluens)
- pelvic pain
- a pelvic mass.

It is similar to primary epithelial ovarian cancer in histological appearance and clinical behaviour. Management is therefore essentially the same.

Rare ovarian tumours

Rare ovarian tumours include primary small-cell carcinoma and various types of sarcoma, all having a poor prognosis. Lymphoma or extramedullary leukaemia may also manifest initially as an ovarian tumour.

KEY POINTS

- The mature cystic teratoma is the commonest ovarian germ-cell tumour and the commonest ovarian tumour leading to torsion.
- 90 per cent of malignant ovarian tumours are epithelial, but germ-cell tumours account for 60 per cent of ovarian cancers in adolescents and children.
- Bilaterality of epithelial ovarian malignancies is common.
- Up to 10 per cent of ovarian masses are secondary to metastases from some other organ.

EPIDEMIOLOGY, INCIDENCE AND AETIOLOGY OF EPITHELIAL OVARIAN CANCER

In England and Wales, ovarian cancer is the commonest gynaecological malignancy and accounts for more deaths in these countries than the other gynaecological malignancies together (see Table 69.1). The incidence and mortality rates are influenced by country of origin and race. In general, epithelial ovarian cancer is most common and most lethal in industrialized countries (excepting Japan) and has the lowest rates in the non-industrialized world. In contrast, germ-cell tumours represent up to 15 per cent of ovarian cancers in black and oriental populations, in whom epithelial ovarian cancers are less common.

Approximately 40 per cent of ovarian tumours in post-menopausal women are malignant, but less than 10 per cent are malignant in the premenopausal population. Most epithelial ovarian cancers occur in postmenopausal women, with less than 1 per cent affecting females under the age of 21 years. In this age group, more than 60 per cent of ovarian malignancies are of germ-cell origin.

Aetiology

Environmental factors

The cause of ovarian cancer is unknown. Various associations between environmental factors and the development of ovarian cancer have been reported and reviewed.[2] High-fat diets have been associated with an increased risk of ovarian cancer, as has a diet low in fibre and vitamin A. Perineal dusting with talcum powder has also been shown to increase the risk of subsequent development of this cancer. The risks of a high caffeine intake and of exposure to asbestos or radiation are unclear. The role of certain viral infections (mumps, rubella and influenza) has been studied, with inconclusive results.

Reproductive and hormonal factors

The effects of reproductive and hormonal factors on ovarian cancer risk have also been extensively documented and summarized.[3,4] It is generally accepted that populations with small families have an increased risk of ovarian cancer. It has been postulated that this is at least in part due to an increased risk of ovarian cancer related to nulliparity per se. Nonetheless, the published data are consistent, showing that pregnancy is protective, increasing protection occurring with increasing parity. Greatest protection is afforded by the first pregnancy, and breastfeeding also reduces the risk. The data on associations between the timing of menarche and menopause and ovarian cancer risk are less consistent. Tubal ligation has been reported by American and Australian investigators to decrease the risk of ovarian cancer, and all but one European study supports their conclusion that hysterectomy (with ovarian conservation) is also protective (six studies) [II].[3,4]

Based on the results of case-control studies, it is now widely accepted that use of the combined oral contraceptive pill is protective; increasing duration of use increases the level of protection afforded [II]. By contrast, the association between the use of fertility drugs and ovarian cancer risk has resulted in an international controversy initiated by a report of an increased risk of borderline and malignant ovarian tumours in users [II]. Data suggesting that the use of clomiphene for 12 or more cycles significantly increased the risk of borderline ovarian tumours followed [II]. Two more recent studies found an association between the use of fertility drugs and development of borderline and malignant ovarian tumours [II], but the association was due to the effect of nulliparity alone. At the present time, evidence of a causal association between the use of ovulatory stimulants and the subsequent development of epithelial ovarian tumours is lacking.

One model that helps to explain much of the above is the concept of hormonal stimulation resulting in proliferation followed by epithelial injury on ovulation. This offers the opportunity for genetic damage. Factors that limit the number of ovulations are associated with reduced risk of ovarian cancer. Conversely, 'incessant ovulation' is associated with increased risk.

Genetic factors

The concept that there is a familial predisposition to ovarian cancer was initially suggested by epidemiological studies that have consistently documented an increased relative risk for ovarian cancer associated with a family history of the disease. Three hereditary ovarian cancer syndromes have been described in which members of these families are at increased risk of developing ovarian cancer:

1 site-specific ovarian cancer, in which ovarian cancer is expressed in multiple female members of the genetic lineage, consistent with the presence of an autosomal dominant gene of high penetrance;
2 hereditary breast – ovarian cancer syndrome, in which breast and/or ovarian cancers are present in family members;
3 Lynch syndrome II (hereditary non-polyposis colon cancer, HNPCC), in which a genetic tendency to develop ovarian, endometrial and colon cancers can be demonstrated in the pedigree.

Hereditary ovarian cancers are unlikely to represent more than 10 per cent of all ovarian cancers. The role of hereditary factors in ovarian cancer has been eloquently reviewed.[5]

In 1994, following intense linkage analysis, a large gene was cloned and sequenced and confirmed to be the *BRCA1* – BReast CAncer 1 – gene. Confirmatory studies have identified more than 100 mutations. It has been estimated that *BRCA1* is responsible for approximately 5 per cent of ovarian cancers in women less than 40 years of age. Although the estimated risk of developing either ovarian or breast cancer by the age of 70 is 82 per cent, most carriers do not develop both diseases, and thus the penetrance for development of ovarian cancer is lower and estimated at 42 per cent. Mutations in the *BRCA2* gene also increase the risk of ovarian cancer in carriers, the site of mutation possibly correlating with risk, as in the case of *BRCA1*.

Hereditary non-polyposis colon cancer has been classified into two syndromes termed Lynch I and II. The latter has an association with cancers at other sites, including the ovary and endometrium. The genes responsible for HNPCC have now been identified. The lifetime risk of ovarian cancer among gene carriers has not been precisely documented but may be as high as seven times that of non-carriers.[5]

Narod and colleagues have reported in a case-control study that women from families with hereditary ovarian cancer syndromes reduce their risk of developing ovarian cancer by ever use of the combined oral contraceptive pill [II]. More recently, they have demonstrated that tubal ligation is protective in *BRCA* mutation carriers [II].[6]

Aetiology of ovarian cancer

- Tubal ligation and hysterectomy (with ovarian conservation) decrease the risk of ovarian cancer [III].
- The use of the combined oral contraceptive pill is protective, increasing duration of use increasing the level of protection afforded [II].
- Women from families with hereditary ovarian cancer syndromes reduce their risk of developing ovarian cancer by ever use of the combined oral contraceptive pill [II].
- Tubal ligation is protective in *BRCA* mutation carriers [II].

KEY POINTS

- Pregnancy, breastfeeding, tubal ligation, hysterectomy and the combined oral contraceptive pill protect against the development of epithelial ovarian cancer.
- Evidence of a causal association between the use of ovulatory stimulants and the subsequent development of epithelial ovarian tumours is currently lacking.
- Three hereditary ovarian cancer syndromes have been described.
- Hereditary ovarian cancers are unlikely to represent more than 10 per cent of all ovarian cancers.
- *BRCA1* is responsible for approximately 5 per cent of ovarian cancers in women aged less than 40 years.
- HNPCC has an association with cancer of the ovary and endometrium.

SCREENING FOR OVARIAN CANCER

The possibility of pre-symptomatic genetic testing raises a number of medical, psychological, ethical, legal and social issues. Due to the limitations of genetic testing at the present time, it is imperative that it is offered only to high-risk individuals in cases for which the result of the test will affect medical management. In this context it must be remembered that a woman with a single affected relative has a lifetime risk of developing ovarian cancer of only 3–4 per cent (see 'Published guidelines').

Women who are at high risk for developing ovarian cancer (i.e. >10 per cent lifetime risk based on family history) may be offered ovarian screening. Participation in the NCRI (formerly UKCCCR) prospective, non-randomized trial of ovarian cancer screening should be encouraged. However, data regarding the efficacy or potential morbidity of ovarian screening in the asymptomatic population are lacking. A prospective multicentre, randomized, controlled trial of asymptomatic women without a significant family history is ongoing (the United Kingdom Collaborative Trial of Ovarian Cancer Screening – UKCTOCS). Screening this population is contraindicated until such time as studies show that it is justified (see 'Published guidelines').

MANAGEMENT OF THE ADNEXAL MASS

An adnexal mass may present either as a result of symptoms, which may be severe in the case of a cyst accident, or as an incidental finding when performing a pelvic examination or radiological investigation. Cyst accidents include torsion, haemorrhage and rupture. Pelvic pain radiating down the inner aspect of the leg is a common presenting symptom, and torsion classically presents as severe pain associated with vomiting. Although rupture of a small cyst may be asymptomatic with few associated signs, the abdomen of a patient experiencing a cyst accident is usually tender, with guarding and rigidity. Rupture of a large cyst may produce signs of peritonitis, particularly if the cyst contents are irritant (e.g. endometriotic cyst or dermoid cyst), and the patient may be shocked in cases of extensive rupture or continuing haemorrhage.

Investigation

A complete history and examination are essential, as the diagnosis is usually based on clinical findings. The history should include information about the duration and growth of the mass. Symptoms, past history or family history increasing the likelihood of malignancy should be sought. The duration of use of combined oral contraception should be noted. General, abdominal, vaginal and rectal examinations are mandatory.

Full blood count, group and save, serum amylase, urea, electrolytes and liver function tests should be performed. Tumour markers should be measured if the mass is complex – if this information is not available, serum may be stored until histopathology has been reported. Pregnancy must be excluded and urinalysis performed. A midstream specimen of urine should be sent for culture and sensitivity. Other investigations may be indicated by the patient's condition, for example cross-match and coagulation screen in cases of haemorrhage.

A pelvic ultrasound, preferably transvaginal, will reveal the dimensions and morphology of the mass and is the single most important investigation in predicting whether an ovarian mass is benign or malignant. Most ovarian masses are cystic, but the presence of solid areas makes a tumour most likely and a malignancy possible. However, some benign tumours are solid, for example thecoma, fibroma and Brenner tumours. Thickened walls and septae are other features of malignancy. The results of colour Doppler imaging have been disappointing, and this technique has not proven superior to morphological assessment.

Measurement of CA 125 may be misleading, as normal levels are found in 50 per cent of stage I ovarian cancers. However, Jacobs and colleagues included ultrasound findings and menopausal status with CA 125 in an algorithm termed the 'Risk of Malignancy Index' (RMI) and reported 87 per cent sensitivity, 89 per cent specificity and 75 per cent positive predictive value (given an RMI cut-off value of 200).[7] The RMI is the product of the serum CA 125 level (in units per millilitre), the ultrasound score (0, 1 or 3) and the menopausal status (1 if premenopausal, 3 if postmenopausal). The ultrasound score is calculated by giving one point for each of the following findings:

- multilocular cyst
- solid areas
- bilateral lesions
- metastases
- ascites.

The RMI provides a means of triaging women for referral to a gynaecological oncologist – those cases likely to have benign disease can have their surgery performed by general gynaecologists.

Conservative and surgical management

Management depends on the presentation (cyst accident or asymptomatic finding) and the risk of malignancy. Surgical intervention is usually required when an ovarian cyst presents with acute symptoms, although a conservative approach may be taken in mild cases where the findings indicate a low risk of malignancy. Most functional cysts can be managed conservatively and disappear spontaneously within two cycles if managed with combined oral contraceptives or observation alone.[8] Patients with peritonitis or hypovolaemic shock require prompt resuscitation.

The benefits of laparoscopic surgery are widely reported, and large studies have been published demonstrating the safety and efficacy of this approach (see 'Published guidelines'). However, specialized and skilled gynaecologists

performed the surgery in these series, and the unfortunate consequences of laparoscopic management of undiagnosed ovarian cancers have been reported. If an adequate preoperative assessment indicates that the risk of malignancy is low, a laparoscopic approach should be considered. However, laparoscopic aspiration of cysts should not be performed to make a diagnosis of cancer, as the negative predictive value of cyst fluid cytology is low in most departments and aspiration adversely affects the prognosis of a stage I malignancy. Furthermore, therapeutic aspiration of ovarian cysts is usually ineffective, as most recur.

Patients at intermediate risk of malignancy may also be considered for laparoscopic assessment when the operator is skilled, there is a safe method of retrieval of the mass and there are facilities for prompt frozen section analysis. In this situation, access to immediate surgical staging must be available. All patients with obvious malignancy should be referred to a gynaecological oncologist for further management. The role of laparoscopy in the management of ovarian cancer is currently under evaluation.

At laparoscopy, a careful assessment is performed and washings taken. If the findings are suspicious for malignancy, a biopsy is taken if metastases or surface excrescences are identified. An appropriate procedure is then rescheduled following the results of histopathology (see below). If there are no suspicious findings, the surgeon may proceed to cystectomy or oophorectomy as indicated.

KEY POINTS

- At the present time, there is no role for ovarian screening in the asymptomatic population.
- All women presenting with vague pelvi-abdominal symptoms warrant a complete history and examination, including vaginal and per-rectal examination.
- The RMI may be used to identify cases for referral to a gynaecological oncologist.

CLINICAL MANAGEMENT OF OVARIAN CANCER

Clinical presentation and diagnosis

Primary ovarian cancer is most common in women in the seventh decade of life. Hereditary cancers usually present in younger women, occurring approximately 10 years earlier. Most women with ovarian cancer are asymptomatic and when symptoms do occur they are often non-specific and vague. A complete history and examination are essential to make the diagnosis, to identify patients with secondary ovarian malignancy and to assess fitness for surgical and non-surgical management.

Symptoms

When the tumour is confined to the ovary, the patient may present with pressure symptoms (urinary frequency, constipation, pelvic pain/pressure, dyspareunia) and, rarely, symptoms of a cyst accident. In advanced stage disease, symptoms are usually due to metastases affecting the bowel and mesentery, and ascites. Resulting symptoms (bloating, constipation, early satiety, loss of appetite) may be misinterpreted as irritable bowel syndrome. Symptoms due to pressure effects in the pelvis may also occur. Abnormal vaginal bleeding (in premenopausal and postmenopausal women) is a less common presenting feature.

Clinical signs

Assessment should include examination of supraclavicular, axillary and inguinal nodes, breast examination, chest examination (pleural effusion) and abdominal examination, including assessment of liver size. In women presenting with the above symptoms, a pelvic examination (including per-rectal examination) is mandatory. The presence of a solid, irregular mass is highly suspicious, particularly when associated with an upper abdominal mass (omental cake).

Investigations

Investigations are performed to assess the likelihood of malignant disease, to assess fitness for anaesthesia and surgery, and to plan the extent of surgery. Ultrasonography (see above) should include assessment not just of the pelvis but also of the kidneys and liver. Liver metastases increase the likelihood of a non-ovarian primary, and significant hydronephrosis should be identified preoperatively. Chest X-ray is essential. CA 125 (see above) and carcinoembryonic antigen (CEA) levels should be measured, the latter to identify primary gastrointestinal malignancy. In young women, AFP and β-hCG levels should also be measured, as germ-cell tumours are the commonest gynaecological malignancy in the first two decades of life. Full blood count, urea, creatinine, electrolytes and liver function tests (including total protein and albumin) should also be done.

Magnetic resonance imaging and computerized tomography are not usually indicated. Nonetheless, the former may assist surgical planning in patients with a fixed pelvic mass and the latter is useful in assessing the upper abdomen. In patients with abnormal vaginal bleeding, full assessment of the cervix and uterus, including outpatient endometrial biopsy, should be considered – an ovarian mass may be the site of secondary spread from a primary cervical or endometrial carcinoma. Endoscopy of the upper or lower gastrointestinal tract is indicated in women whose symptoms suggest a primary gastrointestinal malignancy.

Table 69.5 International Federation of Gynecology and Obstetrics (FIGO) staging and 5-year overall survival* of ovarian cancer

Stage	Description	5-year survival (%)
I	**Confined to one/both ovaries**	
Ia	Limited to a single ovary; no ascites; capsule intact with no surface tumour	89.9
Ib	Limited to both ovaries; no ascites; capsule intact with no surface tumour	84.7
Ic	One or both ovaries have ruptured capsule or surface tumour; malignant ascites or positive peritoneal washings	80
II	**Extension to pelvic structures**	
IIa	Extension to uterus or fallopian tubes	69.9
IIb	Extension to other pelvic tissues	63.7
IIc	As for IIA or IIB but one or both ovaries have ruptured capsule or surface tumour; malignant ascites or positive peritoneal washings	66.5
III	**As for stage I/II but also with peritoneal implants outside pelvis or with positive retroperitoneal lymph nodes**	
IIIa	Histologically confirmed microscopic seeding of abdominal peritoneal surfaces and negative retroperitoneal lymph nodes	58.5
IIIb	Histologically confirmed implants of abdominal peritoneal surfaces <2 cm and negative retroperitoneal lymph nodes	39.9
IIIc	Histologically confirmed implants of abdominal peritoneal surfaces >2 cm or positive retroperitoneal lymph nodes	28.7
IV	**Distant metastases (including liver parenchyma/positive pleural fluid cytology)**	16.8

*FIGO Annual Report on the Results of Treatment in Gynaecological Cancer, 24th volume. International Federation of Gynecology and Obstetrics, Milan 2000.

Staging of primary ovarian cancer

Ovarian cancers are staged according to the International Federation of Gynecology and Obstetrics (FIGO) recommendations (Table 69.5). Staging is based on findings at laparotomy, but preoperative assessment is required to assess extraperitoneal spread. Accurate staging is of paramount importance, as it determines not only prognosis but also to a large extent the requirement for adjuvant treatment. FIGO report the 5-year survival of patients with stage I disease as 70 per cent. This is in contrast to survival rates of more than 90 per cent reported in studies on patients with properly staged disease, and suggests that a significant proportion of women are not undergoing careful surgical staging.

Technique for surgical staging

A midline incision is essential to allow adequate access for thorough surgical staging and should be performed

Table 69.6   Metastases in apparent early stage epithelial ovarian carcinoma presented as percentages

	Percentage of cases with occult metastases
Diaphragm	7.6
Omentum	7.1
Cytology	18.8
Peritoneum	9.8
Pelvic lymph nodes	8.9
Para-aortic lymph nodes	12.3

Adapted with permission from: Moore DH. Primary surgical management of early epithelial ovarian carcinoma. In: Rubin CR, Sutton GP (eds). *Ovarian Cancer*, 2nd edn. Philadelphia: Lippincott Williams and Wilkins, 2001, 201–18.

whenever an ovarian malignancy is anticipated. A systematic exploration of all peritoneal surfaces and viscera is performed. The staging laparotomy involves the following steps.

- Sending ascites or peritoneal washings for cytological assessment.
- Performing a total abdominal hysterectomy and bilateral salpingo-ophorectomy (TAH/BSO).
- Omentectomy.
- Peritoneal biopsies of all suspicious areas or multiple random sampling if all surfaces are apparently normal.
- Diaphragmatic biopsies or scrapings for cytological assessment.
- Sampling of pelvic and para-aortic lymph nodes.

The rationale for TAH/BSO is the high incidence of bilateral tumours (metastatic or primary) and metastases to the uterus. Furthermore, the endometrium may be the site of a coincidental primary carcinoma, particularly in the case of endometrioid carcinoma of the ovary. The omentum is removed, as it is the major site of abdominal metastases. An infra-colic omentectomy is most universally performed, but a supracolic procedure may be preferable and, indeed, is often essential to achieve adequate cytoreduction of gross omental disease. Washings may be positive in apparent stage Ia disease, substantially altering decision making with regard to adjuvant treatment. Table 69.6 illustrates the rate of occult metastases when adequate surgical staging is performed by combining results from 13 published series involving a total of over 1000 cases.

Appendicectomy has not yet been universally accepted as part of the standard procedure but is currently under consideration. However, the appendix is commonly the site of metastases in advanced stage disease and is reported to be a site of occult disease in a significant proportion of apparent stage I disease as well. Furthermore, the ovary may be a site of secondary disease in the rare case of an appendiceal primary and may be associated with pseudomyxoma peritoneii.

SURGICAL AND NON-SURGICAL MANAGEMENT OF OVARIAN CANCER

The management of ovarian cancer is discussed below in seven consecutive sections.

Primary surgery: early epithelial ovarian cancer

In cases of early stage disease, the surgical objective is to identify occult metastases through meticulous systematic exploration. The commonest pattern of metastatic spread of epithelial ovarian cancer is transcoelomic. The cells disseminate and implant along the peritoneal surfaces following the circulatory path of peritoneal fluid. Lymphatic dissemination to pelvic and para-aortic nodes is also common and may occur in apparent early stage disease. Haematogenous spread is uncommon at the time of diagnosis, but the liver and lung are the preferred sites. The importance of adequate surgical staging in apparent early disease cannot be overemphasized. In the mid-1970s, a 5-year survival rate of 60 per cent was reported for stage I disease and many of these cases did not receive chemotherapy.

The standard surgical procedure for early stage disease has already been described. However, when operating on a young patient for whom fertility is important, it is advisable to perform an adequate staging procedure while minimizing the risk to future fertility. Although frozen section may be useful if it produces a definitive diagnosis of malignancy, the heterogeneity and size of ovarian malignancies result in under-diagnosis in a considerable proportion of cases. Delaying a sterilizing procedure until the final histopathology is available allows a decision regarding further surgical management to be made in consultation with the patient. An initial procedure in such a case would involve complete surgical staging as described, but the uterus and contralateral ovary would be left in situ following careful inspection. A decision regarding completion of surgery and adjuvant treatment should then be made in consultation with the patient and based on the advice of the cancer centre's multidisciplinary team.

Laparotomy is currently the gold-standard surgical procedure for the diagnosis and staging of early ovarian cancer. The role of laparoscopy is undefined and it should only be used as part of well-designed prospective clinical trials.

Primary surgery: advanced epithelial ovarian cancer

In contrast with early ovarian cancer, the surgical emphasis in advanced disease is on tumour cytoreduction. Cytoreductive surgery typically involves performing a TAH/BSO, complete omentectomy and resection of any metastases.

The principal goal of cytoreductive surgery is to remove all primary cancer and, if possible, all metastatic disease. If this is not possible, the surgeon aims to reduce the tumour load to achieve 'optimal' status. Griffiths, who suggested in 1975 that residual nodules should be no greater than 1.5 cm in maximum diameter, first introduced this concept. His results have been substantiated by almost every subsequent large series reported. In 1983, Hacker et al. showed that patients with residual disease of 5 mm or less had a median survival of 40 months, compared with 18 months for those with lesions <1.5 cm, and only 6 months for patients with nodules >1.5 cm.[8] Primary cytoreductive surgery has become established as the standard management of patients with advanced ovarian cancer.

Resectability of disease depends not only on the skill of the surgeon, but also on the site of disease. Optimal cytoreduction is unlikely if there is extensive disease on the undersurfaces of the diaphragms or affecting the liver, porta hepatis or root of the small bowel mesentery. Retrospective data suggest that this type of surgery is feasible in 70–90 per cent of cases when performed by a gynaecological oncologist.[9] Major morbidity is approximately 5 per cent and operative mortality 1 per cent. Although prognosis depends on the extent of residual disease following surgery, it is also determined by the patient's age, the volume of ascites and performance status (independent prognostic variables). In planning management, these factors must be taken into consideration.

It is possible that the biology of the disease determines resectability and prognosis. In 1992, a systematic review of surgery in advanced ovarian cancer questioned whether surgical intervention of this type provided the patient with an advantage[10] and suggested that cytoreductive surgery has only a small effect on the survival of women with advanced ovarian cancer. Indeed, the evidence for aggressive primary surgery has never been demonstrated in a randomized trial, and is based on retrospective case-control studies at best [II]. The only prospective randomized trial of cytoreductive surgery [Ib][11] has demonstrated a survival advantage for patients randomized to a second resection of disease as an interval procedure. The performance of cytoreductive surgery remains the current gold standard of care, but trials of primary surgery versus neoadjuvant chemotherapy with interval surgery are planned.

KEY POINTS

- The importance of adequate surgical staging in apparent early stage ovarian cancer cannot be overemphasized.
- Primary cytoreductive surgery followed by chemotherapy is the current gold standard of care for patients with advanced ovarian carcinoma.

CHEMOTHERAPY

In general, it is agreed that patients with (adequately staged) low-grade stage Ia and Ib disease have a very good prognosis and do not require adjuvant treatment [Ia]. A number of publications and a systematic review of chemotherapy effects in ovarian cancer support this approach.[12]

However, patients with early stage disease and poor prognostic factors *may* benefit from adjuvant treatment, as they have a substantial risk of micrometastases. Two large randomized trials addressing this issue (ICON 1 and ACTION – over 900 patients studied) demonstrate a statistically significant improvement in recurrence-free survival and overall survival in women receiving adjuvant chemotherapy.[13,14] A multivariate analysis of studies of prognostic variables involving 1545 patients found that degree of differentiation and cyst rupture were independent poor prognosticators [II].[15] This topic has recently been reviewed by Winter-Roach et al.[16]

Adjuvant radiotherapy for ovarian cancer involves either whole abdominal radiotherapy or the administration of intraperitoneal radiocolloid (P^{32}). Whole abdominal radiotherapy is the standard treatment in some North American institutions for patients with optimal cytoreduction. Neither approach has been shown to have an advantage over chemotherapy, nor have these techniques become widely established. Pelvic radiation alone is not as effective as adjuvant treatment but may be used to palliate isolated pelvic recurrence, for example a bleeding mass at the vaginal vault.

Single chemotherapeutic agents active in epithelial ovarian cancer include:

- alkylating agents (e.g. cyclophosphamide),
- platinum compounds (cisplatin and carboplatin),
- anthracyclines (e.g. epirubicin),
- taxanes (paclitaxel and docetaxel) and others.[17]

Most of these agents are administered intravenously, some orally. At the present time, the role of intraperitoneal chemotherapy is unclear.

Alkylating agents were the mainstay of treatment before the 1970s and produced response rates of 40–50 per cent. With platinum-based chemotherapy, response rates rose to more than 70 per cent. Forty-nine trials involving 8763 women have been systematically reviewed. The available evidence suggests that platinum-based therapy is better than non-platinum therapy [Ia]. There is some evidence that combination therapy improves survival compared with platinum alone [Ia]. No difference in effectiveness between cisplatin and carboplatin has been shown [Ia]. In most regimens, carboplatin has now been substituted for cisplatin, as it has the advantage of producing less gastrointestinal, renal and peripheral neurological toxicity.

In two prospective randomized trials in advanced ovarian cancer,[18,19] paclitaxel in combination with cisplatin provided a survival benefit over cyclophosphamide/cisplatin (the previous standard of care). Both studies reported a significant improvement in clinical response rate, median progression-free interval and overall survival in the paclitaxel arm [Ia]. Based on these trials, paclitaxel and a platinum analogue became the new standard of care; however, the large ICON 3 study, which involved more than 2000 patients, failed to identify an advantage for the use of paclitaxel/carboplatin over single-agent carboplatin alone, challenging the new gold standard.[20] Three randomized trials have compared carboplatin/paclitaxel and cisplatin/ paclitaxel but are not yet fully reported and no differences in outcome have yet been identified.[12]

Currently, standard treatment for patients with high-risk early stage disease involves adjuvant chemotherapy: either carboplatin/paclitaxel or carboplatin alone, for six cycles. The latter is usually preferred in less-fit patients. For the treatment of advanced stage ovarian cancer, combination chemotherapy with carboplatin and paclitaxel, or carboplatin alone, for six cycles is recommended.

It has been suggested that patients with advanced disease not amenable to optimal cytoreduction should be offered primary chemotherapy rather than primary surgery (neo-adjuvant chemotherapy). The rationale for this approach is that a proportion of patients would be rendered optimally debulkable. Furthermore, it has been reported that patients treated in this way have outcomes comparable to those of patients treated with primary surgery.[21] However, these data conflict with reports that primary surgery confers benefit. A prospective randomized, controlled trial under the auspices of the European Organisation for Research and Treatment of Cancer (EORTC) is currently addressing this issue, and a UK NCRI trial (CHORUS) will begin in 2004.

KEY POINTS

- Additional therapy may be considered for patients who have early stage disease associated with high-risk factors.
- Standard adjuvant therapy for ovarian cancer involves intravenous chemotherapy.
- Paclitaxel and a platinum analogue have become the new standard of care for women with advanced ovarian cancer.
- Response rates to second-line chemotherapy are much lower than for primary treatment.

Second-line chemotherapy is indicated in cases of recurrent or progressive disease. Response rates are much lower than for primary treatment (15–35 per cent versus 80 per cent), although better response rates are found in women with longer disease-free intervals before recurrence. In patients with platinum-sensitive disease (i.e. women with a progression-free interval of at least 12 months since platinum-based therapy), re-treatment with platinum or paclitaxel is appropriate. In platinum-resistant cases, an

agent without cross-resistance is required. These include alkylating agents (liposomal doxorubicin), anthracyclines, topoisomerase inhibitors (etoposide, topotecan) and others (hexamethylmelamine, tamoxifen). There is some evidence from observational studies that tamoxifen may produce a response in a modest proportion of women with relapsed ovarian cancer. Single-agent regimens are often adopted due to ease of administration and low toxicity.

KEY POINTS

- Patients with low-grade stage Ia and Ib disease do not require adjuvant treatment [Ia].
- In stage I invasive epithelial ovarian carcinoma, degree of differentiation, capsular penetrance, surface excrescences, malignant ascites and cyst rupture are independent poor prognosticators [Ia].
- Platinum-based therapy is better than non-platinum therapy [Ia].
- There is some evidence that combination therapy improves survival compared with platinum alone [Ia].
- No difference in effectiveness between cisplatin and carboplatin has been shown [Ia].
- Paclitaxel in combination with cisplatin may provide a survival benefit over cyclophosphamide/cisplatin [Ib].

SECONDARY CYTOREDUCTIVE SURGERY

As optimal primary cytoreductive surgery is associated with improved outcomes in patients with advanced ovarian cancer, it has been suggested that there is a role for debulking in patients with persistent or recurrent disease. This group of patients is highly heterogeneous, but may be broadly categorized as follows:

- patients undergoing second-look laparotomy (see below) who are found to have macroscopic disease;
- patients with persistent disease following completion of primary treatment;
- patients with recurrent disease after completion of primary treatment;
- patients for whom primary surgery was not optimal who undergo a further attempt at cytoreduction after several cycles of chemotherapy (interval debulking surgery).

Patients undergoing second-look laparotomy

Second-look laparotomy was part of standard treatment in the 1970s and 1980s. Asymptomatic patients who had completed a course of chemotherapy following primary surgery were offered a systematic laparotomy to determine the results of treatment. The patients selected for this procedure had no clinical evidence of persistent disease. The rationale for this approach was that a negative second-look procedure would indicate that adjuvant treatment (usually in the form of prolonged courses of alkylating agents) should be discontinued.

However, there is a significant recurrence rate after negative second-look laparotomy and no effective salvage therapy for women found to have persistent disease. Secondary cytoreduction is likely to benefit a small proportion of these women only, and there is significant concern about the negative effect of laparotomy on the quality of life of these patients. Furthermore, modern chemotherapeutic regimens are quite different from those used when this operation was introduced. As a result, this procedure is no longer used by most gynaecological oncologists and does not play a role in the modern management of ovarian cancer.

Patients with persistent or recurrent disease following completion of primary treatment

Patients whose disease progresses during chemotherapy, those with persistent disease at the completion of chemotherapy and those who develop recurrence early have a limited median survival. Treatment should therefore be directed at optimizing quality of life. As a result, cytoreductive surgery is rarely indicted in these groups. However, patients who have had complete clinical responses to primary treatment and who develop localized recurrences after a disease-free interval of 24 months or more may benefit from cytoreductive surgery.

Patients selected for interval debulking surgery

Van der Burg et al. published the results of a randomized, controlled trial of cytoreductive surgery.[11] In this study, women who had completed three cycles of adjuvant chemotherapy (cisplatin/cyclophosphamide) were randomized to either surgery or no surgery. All patients had had suboptimal primary surgery (residual disease volumes >1.0 cm). This group reported that patients having interval debulking had longer progression-free and overall survival and a reduced risk of dying of disease.

Although the results of this report are encouraging, there is limited experience with this approach. Furthermore, these data are in conflict with the results of a more recent study from the USA. Nonetheless, it appears that women who have optimal interval cytoreduction have outcomes equivalent to those of patients who have optimal surgery performed as a primary procedure. Therefore, in cases in which initial surgery has involved biopsy only, with no attempt at cytoreduction of advanced disease, it is reasonable to consider definitive surgery after three cycles of chemotherapy, with three further cycles being given following surgery.

PALLIATIVE SURGERY

The most common indication for palliative surgery is bowel obstruction, which is a common feature of recurrent disease but may also be the presenting feature in undiagnosed patients. Most patients have small-bowel obstruction, approximately one-third have large-bowel obstruction and a minority have both. However, in many cases of small-bowel obstruction due to ovarian cancer, the site of obstruction is not single and on occasions the entire small bowel is rendered dysfunctional due to extensive peritoneal and mesenteric involvement (carcinomatous ileus). As these latter cases are not amenable to surgery, careful case selection is the essence of good management. Surgery may involve bowel resection, but most commonly intestinal bypass and/or stoma formation is required.

The median survival for patients undergoing palliative surgery for bowel obstruction is 3–12 months. Those who are young, with a good nutritional status (normal albumin levels) and who do not have rapidly accumulating ascites have the best prognosis. Reported morbidity and mortality rates are 30 per cent and 10 per cent respectively.

MANAGEMENT OF RARER TUMOUR TYPES

Borderline ovarian tumours

Approximately 15 per cent of epithelial ovarian tumours are borderline (tumours of low malignant potential). They affect younger women than primary epithelial ovarian cancers and may present in pregnancy. They are usually of low stage and have a very good prognosis. Surgical resection is the primary modality of treatment, as there are no prospective data suggesting that adjuvant treatment prolongs survival. Premenopausal women who wish to preserve fertility may be treated by conservative surgery (recurrence rate is <10 per cent in these patients). Nonetheless, it should be emphasized that a small subgroup of these patients has rapidly progressive disease and a poor prognosis. Long-term follow-up is advised, as late recurrences do occur.

Germ-cell tumours of the ovary

Adequate surgical staging, cytoreduction and adjuvant chemotherapy is current standard therapy for germ-cell tumours of the ovary. As these malignancies usually occur in young women, conservation of the contralateral ovary and uterus is appropriate. However, the importance of a complete and thorough staging procedure cannot be underestimated – patients with stage Ia dysgerminoma and stage I, grade 1 immature teratoma require no further therapy if comprehensively staged. All other patients should be treated with three or more cycles of combination chemotherapy (bleomycin, etoposide and cisplatin). Most patients with these tumours are cured of disease and most survivors can anticipate normal menstrual and reproductive function. Tumour markers are often useful in monitoring disease and planning management.

Sex-cord stromal tumours

Although they are reported to be most common among postmenopausal women, these tumours often affect children and young adults. They are the most hormonally active of all ovarian tumours and there is an association with hyperplasia and well-differentiated adenocarcinoma of the endometrium. Surgery is the cornerstone of management, but early stage disease may be managed by unilateral oophorectomy and endometrial biopsy when fertility sparing is important. Late recurrence is the hallmark of these tumours.

Pseudomyxoma peritoneii

This condition involves the accumulation of gelatinous material in the peritoneal cavity. It occurs in association with mucinous tumours of the appendix and/or ovary. It is extremely rare and has a very poor prognosis. Cases should be referred for specialist opinion as early as possible. A histopathological diagnosis of pseudomyxoma ovarii would warrant such a referral.

QUALITY OF LIFE

Most patients with ovarian cancer present late and die of disease. Cure is the ultimate goal of patient and oncologist, but is not achieved for the majority. Therefore a careful balance must be struck between the pursuit of that goal and optimization of the quality of the period of life remaining. Specific treatments and their potential impact on disease must be weighed against the morbidity of each therapy. The optimum balance between these opposing aims will be different for each patient. The informed patient's voice is critical to finding the best compromise for her and should be heard. Management decisions should be made with the balance of probabilities and the patient's desires clearly in focus.

CONCLUSION

The management of ovarian cancer represents a major challenge and requires close multidisciplinary team working amongst medical, clinical and surgical oncologists, radiologists, pathologists, clinical nurse specialists and specialists in palliative care. The Calman-Hine Report, *A Policy Framework for Commissioning Cancer Services* and the subsequent report 'Improved Outcomes' recommended changes in the provision of gynaecological cancer services in England and Wales.[22] These developments are designed to improve compliance with management guidelines, provide specialist training and treatment and consequently improve patient care and outcomes and are particularly pertinent to the care of women with ovarian cancer. The centralization of gynaecological cancer services should also facilitate the running of large clinical trials, the development of translational research strategies and audit. Cancer networks are currently emerging to facilitate these changes.

Data are accruing to support this approach. A prospective, controlled study in Scotland of more than 1800 women with ovarian cancer found a survival advantage for those women operated on by subspecialist gynaecological oncologists compared to those operated on by either general gynaecologists or general surgeons.[23] The gynaecological oncologists saw more women with advanced disease, advanced age and ascites. In spite of this selection bias, there was a 25 per cent improvement in the 3-year survival for patients with stage III disease treated by gynaecological oncologists as compared to those treated by general gynaecologists. This finding is further supported by retrospective data from the West Midlands.[24]

PUBLISHED GUIDELINES

BRCA1 Genetic Screening. Rockville: Kaiser Permanente, 1998: helen.stallings.org.

Drouin P, Dubuc-Lissoir J, Ehlen T et al. Guidelines for the laparoscopic management of the adnexal mass. *SOGC Clinical Practice Guidelines* 1998; **76**: www.g-o-c.org.

Ferrini R. Screening asymptomatic women for cancer. *Am J Prev Med* 1997; 13(6):444–6: www.acpm.org.

KEY REFERENCES

1. Scully RE, Sobin LN. Histological typing of ovarian tumors. In: *World Health Organization International Classification of Tumors*, 2nd edn. Berlin: Springer-Verlag, 1999, 28–36.

2. Daly M, Abrams GI. Epidemiology and risk assessment for ovarian cancer. *Semin Oncol* 1998; 25:255–64.

Gynaecological oncology

3. Fox H. Origins of ovarian cancer. In: Kavanagh JJ, Singletary SE, Einhorn N, DePetrillo AD (eds). *Cancer in Women.* London: Blackwell Science, 1998, 406–14.

4. Look KY. Epidemiology, etiology and screening of ovarian cancer. In: Rubin SC, Sutton GP (eds). *Ovarian Cancer.* Philadelphia: Lippincott Williams and Wilkins, 2001, 167–80.

5. Lynch HT, Casey MJ, Shaw TG, Lynch JF. Hereditary factors in gynecologic cancer. *Oncologist* 1998; 3(5):319–38.

6. Narod SA, Sun P, Risch H. Ovarian cancer, oral contraceptives, and *BRCA* mutations. *N Engl J Med* 2001; **345**:1706–7.

7. Davies AP, Jacobs I, Woolas R et al. The adnexal mass: benign or malignant? Evaluation of a risk of malignancy index. *Br J Obstet Gynecol* 1993; 100:927–31.

8. Hacker NF, Berek JS, Lagasse LD, Nieberg RK, Elashoff RM. Primary cytoreductive surgery for epithelial ovarian cancer. *Obstet Gynecol* 1983; 61:413–20.

9. Heintz AM, Hacker NF, Berek JS, Rose T, Munoz AK, Lagasse LD. Cytoreductive surgery in ovarian carcinoma: feasability and morbidity. *Obstet Gynecol* 1986; 67:783–8.

10. Hunter RW, Alexander NDE, Soutter WP. Meta-analysis of surgery in advanced ovarian carcinoma: is maximum cytoreductive surgery an independent determinant of prognosis? *Am J Obstet Gynecol* 1992; 166:504–11.

11. Van der Burg ME, van Lent M, Buyse M et al. The effect of debulking surgery after induction chemotherapy on the prognosis of advanced epithelial ovarian cancer. *N Engl J Med* 1995; **332**:629–34.

12. Hogberg T, Glimelius B, Nygren P. A systematic overview of chemotherapy effects in ovarian cancer. *Acta Oncol* 2001; **40**:340–60.

13. Colombo N, Guthrie D, Chiari S et al. International Collaborative Ovarian Neoplasm trial 1. A randomized trial of adjuvant chemotherapy in women with early-stage ovarian cancer. *J Natl Cancer Inst* 2003; 95:125–32.

14. Trimbos JB, Vergote I, Bolis G et al. Impact of adjuvant chemotherapy and surgical staging in early-stage ovarian carcinoma: European Organisation for Research and Treatment of Cancer-Adjuvant Chemotherapy in Ovarian Neoplasm trial. *J Natl Cancer Inst* 2003; **95**:113–25.

15. Vergote I, De Brabanter J, Fyles A et al. Prognostic importance of degree of differentiation and cyst rupture in stage I invasive epithelial ovarian carcinoma. *Lancet* 2001; **357**:176–82.

16. Winter-Roach B, Hooper L, Kitchener H. Systematic review of adjuvant therapy for early stage (epithelial) ovarian cancer. *Int J Gynecol Cancer* 2003;13:395–404.

17. McGuire WP, Harris WL. Chemotherapy of epithelial ovarian cancer. In: Deppe G, Baker VV (eds). *Gynecologic Oncology.* New York: Oxford University Press, 1999, 212–40.

18. McGuire WP, Hoskins WJ, Brady MF et al. Cyclophosphamide and cisplatin compared with paclitaxel and cisplatin in patients with stage III and stage IV ovarian cancer. *N Engl J Med* 1996; **334**:1–6.

19. Piccart MJ, Bertelsen K, James K et al. Randomized intergroup trial of cisplatin–paclitaxel versus cisplatin–cyclophosphamide in women with advanced epithelial ovarian cancer: three-year results. *J Natl Cancer Inst* 2000; **92**(9):699–708.

20. Harper P. A randomized comparison of paclitaxel and carboplatin versus a control arm of single agent carboplatin or CAP (cyclophosphamide, doxorubicin and cisplatin): 2075 patients randomized into the 3rd International Collaborative Ovarian Neoplasm Study (ICON-3). *Proc Am Soc Clin Oncol* 1999; 18:A1375.

21. Schwartz PE, Rutherford TJ, Chambers JT, Kohorn EI, Thiel RP. Neoadjuvant chemotherapy for advanced ovarian cancer: long-term survival. *Gynecol Oncol* 1999; **72**:93–9.

22. Calman-Hine. *A Policy Framework for Commissioning Cancer Services.* London: NHS Executive, Department of Health, 1995.

23. Junor E, Hole D. Specialist gynaecologists and survival outcome in ovarian cancer: a Scottish National Study of 1866 patients. *Br J Obstet Gynaecol* 1999; **106**(11):1130–6.

24. Kehoe S, Powell J, Wilson S et al. The influence of the operating surgeon's specialisation on patient survival in ovarian carcinoma. *Br J Cancer* 1994; **70**(5):1014–17.

Chapter 70

Vulval and Vaginal Cancer

John Tidy

MRCOG standards

Theoretical skills
- Understand the relevant anatomy of the vulva, vagina and perineum.
- Know the epidemiology and aetiology of vulval and vaginal cancer.
- Understand the importance of histological type.
- Understand the routes of spread and natural history of different types of vulval cancer.
- Understand the principles upon which treatment is based.

Practical skills
- Be able to perform a competent examination of the perineum and lower genital tract and regional groin nodes.
- Be able to recognize areas that are suspicious of malignancy or pre-malignancy.
- Be able to take appropriate diagnostic biopsies.
- Know how to arrange for appropriate investigations to accurately plan subsequent management.
- Be able to counsel patients and their carers with regard to disease, management and outcome.

INTRODUCTION

Vulval and vaginal cancers are rare, accounting for about 1000 new cases per year in the UK. It is important to recognize the symptoms and signs associated with these cancers to make an early diagnosis. As in all cancers, appropriate treatment at an early stage in the disease will lead to a better outcome for the patient, as reported by a population-based study of a series of 411 women in the West Midlands [Ib].[1] Most of the evidence for the management of these cancers is derived from case-controlled series, and the rarity of these tumours is a major obstacle in undertaking randomized trials.

VULVAL CANCER

Vulval cancer is a disease primarily of the older age group, with the majority of cases presenting between the ages of 60 and 75. Some young women do present with this disease and therefore this diagnosis must always be borne in mind. Approximately 800 new cases of vulval cancer are diagnosed in the UK each year. The incidence has remained steady over the past three to four decades despite the increasing recognition of patients with vulval intraepithelial neoplasia (VIN). The majority (90–95 per cent) of vulval carcinomas are of squamous origin, although adenocarcinomas can arise from the Bartholin's gland and also in conjunction with Paget's disease of the vulva. Melanoma of the vulva is the second most common malignancy arising in the vulva, accounting for 4–9 per cent of cases. Basal cell and verrucous carcinomas also occur in the vulva.

Aetiology

Pathology
Certain pre-existing vulval dermatoses are known to be associated with the development of vulval carcinoma. Vulval intraepithelial neoplasia is often found in association with vulval cancer and VIN3 is regarded as a pre-invasive condition. The risk of this condition progressing to invasive cancer is highly variable, according to the literature. In women who have previously been treated for VIN, the risk is estimated at between 7 and 8 per cent,[2] whereas in one study in which women remained untreated, the progression rate of VIN to invasive cancer was 80 per cent at 10 years [III].[3] Lichen sclerosus is a common vulval inflammatory dermatosis affecting older women and is generally thought to carry an increased chance of malignant progression, although the exact risk is unknown because the ascertainment of lichen

sclerosis is inexact. Extramammary Paget's disease of the vulva is a rare form of VIN and is occasionally associated with cancer of the apocrine gland.

Molecular biology

Approximately 30 per cent of all vulval cancers are associated with human papillomavirus (HPV) and about 80–90 per cent of vulval cancers develop in women under the age of 50. Variations in the cell-cycle regulatory protein p53 are reported in approximately 30 per cent of cancers and for the remainder there currently appears to be no aetiological or molecular biological event. Recent studies have shown similar molecular changes, including alterations in p53, to be present in both vulval cancer and the surrounding lichen sclerosus.

Smoking may be an important co-factor in the development of HPV-related VIN and is linked to a lower survival rate for women with vulval cancer.

KEY POINTS

Vulval cancer: epidemiology and pathology

- Vulval cancer is uncommon and most evidence arises from observational studies and case series.
- Population-based observational studies confirm better outcomes with early detection.
- There appear to be different aetiologies: one linked to infection with oncogenic HPV and another linked to pre-existing vulval maturation disorders.
- The reported malignant potential of VIN varies between 5 and 80 per cent. This probably reflects the variations in the observational studies rather than a widely varying biological effect.

Diagnosis

Women with vulval cancer usually present with symptoms, although an asymptomatic mass may be an unusual presentation. The associated symptoms are usually vulval soreness and itching and there may be a mass that is painful and bleeds. Investigation of postmenopausal bleeding should always include examination of the vulva. The most common site of involvement is the labium majus (about 50 per cent of cases). The labium minus accounts for 15–20 per cent of cases. The clitoris and Bartholin's glands are less frequently involved. In the majority of cases, a vulval cancer is obvious to the alert clinician, but very early cancers may be clinically indistinguishable from florid warty VIN.

Investigations

When women present with vulval symptoms, a full clinical examination should be performed, paying particular attention to palpation of the groins for lymphadenopathy. A full-thickness biopsy should be taken from the tumour and should include the interface between the apparent normal surrounding tissue and the cancer. This allows for the most accurate histological interpretation and for the depth of invasion to be assessed, which is important in determining the future management. The cervix should be visualized to exclude a cervical cancer, which may occasionally co-exist. Assessment of the inguinal glands is not absolutely reliable with any imaging technique at present, but should there be a clinical or radiological suspicion of inguinal lymph node enlargement, a computerized tomography (CT) or magnetic resonance (MR) assessment of the pelvis should be undertaken to exclude obvious pelvic lymphadenopathy.

Treatment

There is increasing emphasis placed on the individualization of treatment for women with vulval cancer. In deciding the optimum treatment, it is best to consider early and advanced vulval cancers separately and to manage the primary lesion and the regional lymph glands on individual merit. Because of the rarity of vulval cancer, and the need for careful assessment to optimize both vulval preservation and care, these women should be managed by specialized gynaecological oncologists in cancer centres. In addition to imaging, the pathological assessment of these tumours is extremely important in forming decisions about adjuvant treatment.

Early stage vulval cancer
PRIMARY LESION

Treatment of the primary lesion is in part determined by the risk of local vulval recurrence and the risk of groin node involvement at the time of diagnosis. A retrospective surgical-pathological study of 135 cases found that if a pathological disease-free margin of 8 mm can be achieved, the risk of local recurrence is zero [III].[4] Therefore the primary lesion should be excised with a 1 cm disease-free margin including the deep margin. The 1 cm margin will allow for tissue shrinkage due to fixation of the specimen. In most early cancers this can be achieved by a wide radical local excision and will allow for the preservation of non-involved structures. If the primary lesion is associated with a vulval maturation disorder or VIN, this may be removed as well. However, if the VIN is very widespread, this could necessitate a very large excision requiring myocutaneous flaps. Under these circumstances it may not be considered essential to remove all VIN as part of the primary surgical procedure to remove a carcinoma.

REGIONAL LYMPH NODES

Depth of invasion is the best predictor of risk of nodal metastasis in vulval cancer.

The most recent staging criteria for vulval cancer (Table 70.1) has recognized the concept of micro-invasive or

Table 70.1   Staging of vulval cancer

FIGO	Description	TNM
Ia	Lesion confined to vulva with <1 mm invasion, superficially invasive vulval carcinoma	$T_1aN_0M_0$
Ib	All lesions confined to the vulva with a diameter <2 cm and no clinically suspicious inguinal lymph nodes	$T_1bN_0M_0$
II	All lesions confined to the vulva with a maximum diameter >2 cm and no suspicious inguinal nodes	$T_2N_0M_0$
III	Adjacent spread to the lower urethra and/or vagina and/or anus	$T_3N_0M_0$
		$T_3N_1M_0$
	Lesions of any size confined to the vulva and having unilateral node metastases	$T_1N_1M_0$
		$T_2N_1M_0$
IVa	Lesions with bilateral inguinal node metastases	$T_1N_2M_0$
	Lesions involving mucosa of rectum, bladder, upper urethra or involving bone	$T_2N_2M_0$
		$T_3N_2M_0$
		T_4, any N, M_0
IVb	All cases with pelvic or distant metastases	Any T, any N, M_1

FIGO, International Federation of Gynecology and Obstetrics classification; TMN, tumour, nodes, metastases, Union Internationale Contre le Cancer (UICC).

superficially invasive vulval cancer (Stage Ia), as the risk of nodal involvement in tumours with depth of invasion <1 mm is virtually zero [III].[5] These tumours may therefore be treated by wide local excision alone.

LATERAL VULVAL TUMOURS

The management of regional lymph nodes can be modified for patients presenting with lateral vulval tumours. Although there is extensive lymphatic cross-over in the midline of the vulva, lateral tumours (i.e. those with the medial border at least 2 cm lateral to a line drawn between the clitoris and the anus) require only an ipsilateral inguinal node dissection. If the ipsilateral nodes are negative, the contralateral nodes are rarely involved [III].[6] However, should these nodes be positive, a contralateral node dissection should be undertaken. In a prospective trial, the outcome for 26 women who underwent ipsilateral lateral groin node dissection alone was similar when compared with historical controls [II].[7]

Inguinal node dissection

Surgical dissection of inguinal nodes is considered mandatory in early stage vulval cancer when depth of invasion is >1 mm. A randomized trial comparing inguinal node dissection with radiotherapy to the groin in women with clinically normal inguinal nodes found a survival advantage in favour of the surgical arm. However, this trial has been criticized because an inadequate dose of radiotherapy was given to the inguinal nodes.[8] A subsequent systematic review, of only three eligible studies, suggested that surgery is superior to radiotherapy [Ia].[9]

Attempts have been made to reduce the morbidity associated with this procedure. Unfortunately, superficial inguinal node dissection, which removes only the lymph nodes above

the cribriform fascia, is associated with a higher rate of inguinal recurrence compared with inguino-femoral node dissection, which removes tissue below the cribriform fascia and medial to the femoral vein. In a prospective clinical trial, 155 women underwent a superficial inguinal node dissection and although the overall survival rate was the same compared with a series of historical controls, the rate of inguinal node recurrence was significantly higher.[7] It is therefore recommended that a full dissection should still be performed in cases of early vulval cancer [II]. The routine removal of pelvic lymph nodes in early stage vulval cancer is not recommended. Recent data have suggested that by sparing the long saphenous vein, the short-term and long-term morbidity associated with lymphoedema may be reduced [III].

Another approach to reduce morbidity is the identification of the sentinel node at the time of node dissection. The idea depends on the sentinel node (i.e. the first node to drain the vulval tumour) being identified and, if histologically normal, the remainder of the inguinal lymph node dissection could be omitted. The most reliable technique is probably a hybrid of preoperative intra-lesional injection of radiolabelled technetium combined with intralesion injection of blue dye at the time of surgery and scanning of the nodal tissue for a radioactive signal. In the collected series to date, the sentinel node – the anatomical location of which is highly variable – has been identified in 100 per cent of cases and there have been no cases reported in which the sentinel node was normal but other nodes were positive for tumour. Larger clinical trials will be required to validate this promising technique fully [II].[10]

Advanced vulval cancer

Many patients with this condition will benefit from a multi-modality approach to their management. Neoadjuvant chemotherapy and radiotherapy can be used to shrink the tumour and so permit surgery, which may preserve urethral and anal sphincter function. Reconstructive surgery can potentially reduce physical morbidity by filling large tissue defects and may reduce psychological morbidity as well.

Surgery to the primary lesion

The size and location of the tumour will influence the surgical approach to the primary lesion. The surgical goal is to remove the tumour with at least a 1 cm disease-free margin. In the majority of cases a triple incision technique can be employed. Several clinical series have shown that the incidence of skin bridge recurrence between the primary lesion and the inguinal node dissection is low, even if there is evidence of lymphatic channel involvement [III].[11] However, if there is evidence of tumour within the skin bridge between the primary tumour and the inguinal nodes at the time of surgery, a radical vulvectomy with en-bloc inguinal node dissection should be considered. If extensive areas of vulval tissue need to be removed, reconstructive surgery with the use of skin grafts or myocutaneous flaps may be essential to achieve healing.

Management of inguinal nodes

In cases in which there is clinical suspicion of inguinal node involvement, an inguinal node dissection should be undertaken. As stated above, if there is concern about lymphatic permeation, an en-bloc dissection should be considered. In cases in which the nodes are fixed or ulcerated, biopsy of these or fine-needle aspiration should be considered, followed by radiotherapy to the inguinal and pelvic lymph nodes. Surgical removal of large inguinal or pelvic nodes should be attempted if feasible, since standard radiotherapy doses to the inguinal nodes may be inadequate to bring about a complete regression.

KEY POINTS

Surgical management of vulval cancer

- Vulval cancer should be managed in cancer centres.
- Vulval tumours should be excised with a minimum margin of 10 mm of normal epithelium. This will vary from a wide local excision to radical vulvectomy, depending on the size of the tumour and the nature of adjacent epithelium.
- Lymphadenectomy is required for all but superficially invasive squamous tumours.
- Routine lymphadenectomy is not required for basal-cell and verrucous carcinomas and melanomas.
- Lateral tumours initially require only ipsilateral lymphadenectomy.
- Formal inguino-femoral lymphadenectomy remains the procedure of choice.
- A triple incision technique will suffice unless there is evidence of skin bridge involvement at the outset, when an en-bloc approach should be used.
- Pelvic lymphadenectomy is not routinely used in the treatment of vulval cancer.
- Advanced disease requires a multi-modality approach.

THE MANAGEMENT OF OTHER VULVAL CANCERS

Basal-cell carcinomas and verrucous carcinomas of the vulva are usually only superficially invasive to a depth of 1 mm and are rarely associated with lymph node metastases. These tumours can be adequately managed by means of a wide local excision. Basal-cell carcinomas can be

treated with radiotherapy if surgery would compromise the sphincter function, but this is rarely necessary.

Melanomas of the vulva should be managed by wide local excision. Inguinal node dissection does not influence outcome in these cases, and management should be determined as for the criteria for other sites of cutaneous melanoma.

Cancer can develop within the Bartholin's gland and may be either squamous or adenocarcinoma. Its management is the same as for squamous vulval cancer.

Neoadjuvant therapy

Radiotherapy may be given preoperatively to the primary lesion to allow for tumour shrinkage. This is particularly useful if primary surgery would necessitate removal of the urethral or anal sphincters. A total maximum dose of 55 Gy may be given with concurrent 5-fluorouracil (5FU). Subsequent tumour shrinkage may then enable the preservation of sphincters.

Radical chemoradiotherapy with curative intent

Radical radiotherapy with chemotherapy may be used as an alternative to surgery in the management of advanced squamous vulval carcinomas. There are no published data comparing surgery with chemoradiotherapy in the primary treatment of vulval cancer. Radical radiotherapy alone in the UK has usually been confined to patients who decline surgery or in whom medical morbidity prevents surgery. The recommended dose of radiotherapy is 65 Gy with concurrent 5FU and cisplatin. In a study of 14 women who were not candidates for standard surgery (nine stage III and five stage IV), nine (64 per cent) had a complete response to radiation (50–65 Gy) in combination with cisplatin (50 mg/m^2) and 5FU (100 mg/m^2 per 24 $\times$ 96 hours).[12]

Adjuvant radiotherapy

Surgical margins

Postoperative radiotherapy should be considered in patients with close or positive surgical margins. There is no minimum disease-free margin at which radiotherapy should be considered. However, patients with <4.8 mm of disease-free margin have a 57 per cent chance of disease recurrence.[4] Where possible, consideration should be given to re-excision of the vulva to improve the disease-free margin rather than radiotherapy [IV].

Inguinal nodes

Postoperative radiotherapy should be considered in patients who have nodal involvement with metastatic disease. Several case series have found that prognosis is only affected when two or more nodes are involved [III]. The presence of extra-capsular spread in any lymph node is an adverse factor and warrants adjuvant treatment [III]. Adjuvant radiotherapy should be confined to the affected side and should include pelvic nodes as well. In a randomized trial comparing adjuvant pelvic radiotherapy with pelvic lymphadenectomy, in 114 women with positive inguinal nodes, there was a significant survival advantage (68 per cent vs 54 per cent at 2 years) in favour of radiotherapy [Ib].[13] A total dose of radiotherapy between 45 and 50 Gy without 5FU is recommended.

KEY POINTS

Non-surgical management of vulval cancer

- Vulval tumours can be treated by primary radical radiotherapy if surgery is declined or not possible.
- Adjuvant radiotherapy is recommended when surgical margins are inadequate (<8 mm) if re-excision might compromise function.
- Radiotherapy to the groin and pelvic node sites is recommended if more than one node is involved or there is evidence of any extracapsular spread.
- Radiotherapy may be used prior to surgery to attempt to reduce the morbidity and functional loss associated with surgery in large lesions.
- Radiotherapy with concurrent chemotherapy may improve outcome, but as yet there are no data in support of this approach.

Treatment-related morbidity

A more conservative approach to the management of vulval cancer and individualization of care have led to a reduction in the treatment-related morbidity. However, there still remains a significant rate of wound infection and wound breakdown. Lymphoedema of the legs is a major cause of long-term morbidity and there are also high levels of psychological and psychosexual morbidity associated with the disfiguring nature of the surgery employed.

Morbidity associated with recurrent disease

Recurrent disease affecting the vulva itself should be managed by further surgical excision and, if necessary, radiotherapy. Recurrence involving the inguinal nodes or pelvic nodes should be treated with radiotherapy. However, this can usually only be palliative, and most patients with groin recurrence die of disease.

Follow-up of treated patients

Patients should be followed up on a 3-monthly basis for the first 2 years following treatment, as this allows for the detection of early recurrence and the management of treatment-related morbidity. Once they have completed 2 years of follow-up, they may be seen 6 monthly for the following 3 years.

VAGINAL CANCER

Vaginal cancers are rare gynaecological tumours accounting for only 1–2 per cent of all gynaecological cancers. The majority of vaginal cancers are squamous in origin (about 85 per cent), but adenocarcinoma can also develop in young women between the ages of 17 and 21 and is associated with a higher incidence of metastatic disease to the lymph nodes and lungs. Melanoma and sarcomas are rare causes of vaginal cancer. Clear-cell adenocarcinomas of the vagina are linked to women with a history of in-utero exposure to diethylstilbestrol (DES). An increased incidence of this tumour was first reported in the mid-1970s, but there has been a steady decline in its incidence over recent years with the withdrawal of DES from clinical practice.

Aetiology

Little is known about the aetiology of vaginal cancer, but it is presumed to share similarities with vulval and cervical cancer. Vaginal intraepthelial neoplasia grade 3 (VaIN) is a recognized pre-cancerous condition affecting the vagina and it is frequently seen in combination with cervical intraepithelial neoplasia (CIN). It may occur in one of two ways: as a lateral extension of the CIN out onto the vaginal fornices at the time of treatment for CIN, or in women who have previously undergone hysterectomy for CIN, which was incompletely excised by this procedure. In these latter cases, the VaIN is often found within the surgical margin of the vaginal vault. The percentage of women who present with this condition and who subsequently develop vaginal cancer is unknown, but there is a significant risk of invasive disease. Factors that influence the outcome of vaginal cancer are the size of the tumour and the age of the patient.

Diagnosis

The diagnosis of vaginal cancer may be suspected at the time of colposcopic examination of the vagina. An adequate biopsy, which includes the entire thickness of vaginal epithelium, should be obtained for histological confirmation. This is important, as the depth of invasion of the tumour into the vaginal mucosa and muscle is significant in the staging of

Table 70.2   Staging of vaginal cancer

FIGO	Description	TNM
I	Tumour confined to vagina	$T_1N_0M_0$
II	Tumour invades paravaginal tissues but not to pelvic sidewall	$T_2N_0M_0$
III	Tumour extends to pelvic sidewall	$T_1N_1M_0$
		$T_2N_1M_0$
		$T_3N_0M_0$
		$T_3N_1M_0$
IVa	Tumour invades mucosa of bladder or rectum and/or extends beyond the true pelvis	T_4, any N, M_0
IVb	All cases with distant metastases	Any T, any N, M_1

FIGO, International Federation of Gynecology and Obstetrics classification; TNM, tumour, nodes, metastases, Union Internationale Contre le Cancer (UICC).

the disease (Table 70.2). A diagnosis of cancer of the vagina can only be made with certainty in the presence of a normal cervix or following hysterectomy, as described above.

Investigations

The cervix should be carefully examined if still in situ to exclude cervical involvement. An MRI of the pelvis will help to determine the extent of any spread from the vagina and also the status of the regional pelvic nodes.

Treatment

In planning definitive treatment, consideration should be given not only to the stage of disease at presentation, but also to the size and location of the tumour. Surgery in combination with pelvic radiotherapy, when appropriate, can be effective in the management of stage I and II disease, with survival rates of 68 per cent and 48 per cent respectively [III].[14]

Stage I vaginal cancer
TUMOUR <0.5 CM DEEP
Early vaginal cancer may be managed either by surgery or by intracavity radiotherapy. Surgery should include wide local excision or total vaginectomy with reconstruction of the vagina where possible. Intracavity treatment with 60–70 Gy to the tumour should be given and in cases where the tumour lies within the lower third of the vagina, external-beam radiotherapy to the pelvic and inguinal lymph nodes should be considered.

TUMOURS >0.5 CM DEEP
Surgery for this condition should include wide vaginectomy, pelvic lymphadenectomy and reconstruction of the vagina where possible. For lesions in the lower third of the vagina, inguinal lymphadenectomy should be performed as well. Radiotherapy for this condition should be a combination of brachytherapy to the tumour and external-beam

radiotherapy to the pelvic and inguinal nodes if the tumour is present in the lower third of the vagina.

Although surgery or radiotherapy can be used in the primary management of stage I disease, the usual practice in the UK has been to offer radiotherapy, which has the advantage of vaginal preservation.

Stage II vaginal cancer
Radical surgery can be considered for this condition and should include radical vaginectomy with lymph node dissection or possibly pelvic exenteration. Radiotherapy may also be used, with a combination of brachytherapy to the tumour and external-beam radiotherapy to the pelvic and inguinal lymph nodes.

Stage III and IV vaginal cancer
These cases should be managed by a combination of brachytherapy to the primary tumour and external-beam radiotherapy to the pelvis and inguinal lymph nodes.

Morbidity

The treatment-related morbidity can be significant. Sexual dysfunction due to vaginal atrophy and damage to the bladder and rectum are not infrequent. Recurrent vaginal cancer can be treated with radical pelvic radiotherapy if recurring after surgery. If disease recurs after radiotherapy, palliative surgery may be possible in selected cases.

Follow-up

Patients should be followed up on a 3-monthly basis for the first 2 years following treatment, as this allows for the detection of early recurrence and the management of treatment-related morbidity. Once they have completed 2 years of follow-up, they may be seen 6 monthly for the following 3 years.

KEY POINTS

Vaginal cancer

- There is limited published evidence concerning the treatment of vaginal cancers.
- Case series support the use of surgery in selected cases, with cure rates similar to those of primary radiotherapy.

SUMMARY

Vulval and vaginal cancers are rare and affect an older age range. Individualization of care has led to a reduction in morbidity without affecting cure rates. Multi-modality treatment is often required in advanced cases. All vulval and vaginal cancer should be managed at a cancer centre.

PUBLISHED GUIDELINES

Guidelines for the Management of Vulval Cancer. London: RCOG, 1999.

KEY REFERENCES

1. Rhodes CA, Cummins C, Shafi MI. The management of squamous cell vulval cancer: a population based retrospective study of 411 cases. *Br J Obstet Gynaecol* 1998; **105**:200–5.
2. Herod JJ, Shafi MI, Rollason TP, Jordan JA, Luesley DM. Vulvar intraepithelial neoplasia: long term follow up of treated and untreated women. *Br J Obstet Gynaecol* 1996; **103**:446–52.
3. Jones RW, Baranyai J, Stables S. Trends in squamous cell carcinoma of the vulva: the influence of vulvar intraepithelial neoplasia. *Obstet Gynecol* 1997; **90**:448–52.
4. Heaps JM, Yao SF, Montz FJ, Hacker NF, Berek JS. Surgical–pathological variables predictive of local recurrence in squamous cell carcinoma of the vulva. *Gynecol Oncol* 1990; **38**:309–14.
5. Sedlis A, Homesley H, Bundy BN et al. Positive groin lymph nodes in superficial squamous cell vulvar cancer: a Gynecologic Oncology Group study. *Am J Obstet Gynecol* 1987; **156**:1159–64.
6. Homesley HD, Bundy BN, Sedlis A et al. Assessment of current International Federation of Gynecology and Obstetrics staging of vulvar carcinoma relative to prognostic factors for survival (a Gynecologic Oncology Group study). *Am J Obstet Gynecol* 1991; **164**:997–1004.
7. Stehman FB, Bundy BN, Dvoretsky PM et al. Early stage I carcinoma of the vulva treated with ipsilateral superficial inguinal lymphadenectomy and modified radical hemivulvectomy: a prospective study of the Gynecologic Oncology Group. *Obstet Gynecol* 1992; **79**:490–7.
8. Stehman FB, Bundy BN, Thomas G. Groin dissection versus groin radiation in carcinoma of the vulva: a Gynecologic Oncology Group study. *Int J Rad Oncol Biol Phys* 1992; **24**:389–96.
9. van der Velden J, Ansink A. Primary groin irradiation vs primary surgery for early vulvar cancer (Cochrane Review). In: *The Cochrane Library*, Issue 3. Oxford: Update Software, 2001.
10. Makar APH, Scheistroen M, van der Weyngaert D, Trope CG. Surgical management of stage I and II vulvar cancer: the role of the sentinel node biopsy. Review of the literature. *Int J Gynecol Cancer* 2001; **11**:255–62.
11. Hacker NF, Leuchter RS, Berek JS, Castaldo TW, Lagasse LD. Radical vulvectomy and bilateral inguinal lymphadenectomy through separate groin incisions. *Obstet Gynecol* 1981; **58**:574–9.
12. Cunningham MJ, Goyer RP, Gibbons SK, Kredentser DC, Malfetano JH, Keys H. Primary radiation, cisplatin, and 5-fluorouracil for advanced aquamous carcinoma of the vulva. *Gynecol Oncol* 1997; **66**:258–61.
13. Homesley HD, Bundy BN, Sedlis A., Adcock L. Radiation therapy versus pelvic node resection for carcinoma of the vulva with positive groin nodes. *Obstet Gynecol* 1986; **68**:733–9.
14. Tjalma WAA, Monaghan JM, Lopes AB, Naik R, Nordin AJ, Weyler JJ. The role of surgery in invasive squamous carcinoma of the vagina. *Gynecol Oncol* 2001; **81**:360–5.

Chapter 71

Gestational Trophoblastic Disease

Barry W. Hancock

INTRODUCTION

Gestational trophoblastic disease (GTD) is an uncommon complication of pregnancy. An average consultant obstetrician may deal with only one new case every second year.

The term gestational trophoblastic disease describes a group of inter-related diseases, including complete and partial molar pregnancy, choriocarcinoma and placental site trophoblastic tumour, which vary in their propensity for local invasion and metastasis. Although persistent GTD most commonly follows a molar pregnancy, it may also be seen after any type of gestation, including term pregnancy, abortion and ectopic pregnancy. Gestational trophoblastic tumours produce human chorionic gonadotrophin (hCG), which is important in the diagnosis, management and follow-up of these patients, providing an example of an 'ideal' tumour marker. The first complete responses to methotrexate chemotherapy were described in the 1950s, and presently almost 100 per cent of patients are cured.

EPIDEMIOLOGY

The incidence of hydatidiform mole is difficult to assess accurately but appears to be gradually increasing. As GTD follows all kinds of pregnancies, the denominator for the incidence should ideally include all live births, stillbirths, abortions and ectopic pregnancies. However, the accepted convention has been to report incidence data according to the live-birth rate. Furthermore, reports from different countries often use different denominators, and figures for hospital-based populations are likely to overestimate the incidence compared with community-based figures, particularly in developing countries. Under-reporting may also occur, especially, but not uniquely, in communities where medical attention is sub-optimal.

Worldwide, the incidence of GTD reportedly varies between 0.5 and 8.3 cases per 1000 live births.[1] The UK figure is approximately 1.5 per 1000 births;[2] in contrast, the incidence is approximately twice as high in Japan and other Asian countries and also in native American Indians. There is also a significantly higher incidence in Asian women living in the UK.

Maternal age appears to be the most consistent risk factor associated with molar gestation. Age-specific incidence reports usually reveal a 'J curve', with extremes of reproductive life associated with an increased incidence. Pregnancies below the age of 15 years have a moderately increased risk, whereas those occurring over the age of 50 years are associated with a substantially increased risk. This increased incidence in the youngest and oldest age groups seems to be a consistent finding in all regions and races.

Women who have had a previous mole have an increased risk of further molar pregnancies. Following one mole, the risk is less than 2 per cent, but following two molar pregnancies it increases substantially up to 1 in 6; following three moles the risk may be as high as 1 in 2. Occasionally, family clusters have been seen, implicating an underlying genetic disorder in such cases.

Nutritional and socio-economic factors also appear to be important risk factors for molar pregnancy in some

Table 71.1 Risk factors for gestational trophoblastic disease (GTD)

Age	↑ <16 years, ↑↑↑ >45 years
Geographic	↑ Asia, ↑ Japan
Ethnicity	↑ American Indians, ↑ UK Asians
Previous GTD	↑ one episode, ↑↑↑ two or more episodes
Dietary	↑ carotene deficiency
Genetic	Rare family clusters and repetitive moles

Table 71.2 Pathological features of hydatidiform mole – a comparison between complete and partial mole

	Complete	Partial
Macroscopic	Often recognizable, with characteristic grape-like structures	Can resemble hydropic abortion; may have recognizable fetal tissues
Microscopic	Diffusely hydropic villi	Focal hydropic swelling of villi
	Atypical and hyperplastic trophoblast	Focal trophoblastic hyperplasia
	Usually diagnosable from uterine products	Often misdiagnosed as hydropic abortion or complete mole
Karyotype	Usually diploid (paternally derived)	Usually triploid (maternal contribution)

populations. In particular, low dietary intake of carotene and animal fat may be associated with an increased incidence of complete mole (Table 71.1).

In Europe and North America, choriocarcinoma following a complete hydatidiform mole (CHM) is of the order of 3 per cent. Hydatidiform mole is the most common antecedent to choriocarcinoma, with abortion or ectopic pregnancy being the next most common, followed by live births.[2] Although initially the risk of progression of choriocarcinoma from a partial mole was thought to be negligible, recent reports have shown a small but real risk of malignant transformation. Choriocarcinoma also occurs more frequently in women of older reproductive years.

PATHOLOGICAL FEATURES

Hydatidiform mole may be complete or partial and the histopathological features differ (Table 71.2).[3] Complete mole is recognized by the presence of characteristic grape-like structures, which represent swollen chorionic villi, and the absence of a viable fetus. The conceptus is entirely paternally derived and is a total allograft within the mother. The chorionic villi are diffusely hydropic and enveloped by hyperplasic and atypical trophoblast. Complete moles are usually diploid, the most common type being 46XX; in most cases a haploid sperm divides within an ovum without a nucleus. In contrast, partial moles usually have recognizable embryonic and fetal tissues, with focal hydropic swelling of the chorionic villi and focal trophoblastic hyperplasia. Partial moles are generally triploid, for example 69XXY; they result most often from dispermic fertilization of normal ova. When a fetus is present it often has the features of triploidy, including growth retardation and multiple congenital malformations.

In current-day practice, the earlier evacuation of suspected molar pregnancies has meant that there is more likelihood of misdiagnosis. Complete moles are now often characterized by subtle morphological abnormalities that may result in their misclassification as partial moles or non-molar abortions.

Triploidy is a commoner abnormality than androgenetic complete mole and, if most triploids are paternally derived, it would be expected that partial moles should be at least twice as common as complete moles. However, many studies have reported that complete mole is more common than partial mole, suggesting underdiagnosis of the latter. In a UK study, only a third of histologically confirmed moles registered were partial mole.[3] Expert review of referred cases suggested that up to one-half of partial moles are in fact either complete moles or hydropic abortions, which mirrors the experience of others.

The clinical entity of invasive mole occurs when a complete or, less commonly, a partial mole invades deeply into the myometrium.

Gestational choriocarcinoma is the malignant form of GTD and may originate from a previous hydatidiform mole or from a normal conception. The definitive histopathological diagnosis of choriocarcinoma requires the demonstration of a dimorphic population of both cytotrophoblast and syncytiotrophoblast without the presence of formed chorionic villi, plus evidence of myometrial invasion. However, because of the availability of a sensitive tumour marker, the majority of patients are treated without the benefit of a histological diagnosis. Gestational choriocarcinoma metastasizes widely, particularly to the lungs, pelvic organs and brain.

CLINICAL FEATURES

The majority of patients with CHM are diagnosed prior to 16 weeks of gestation, or often earlier nowadays. Abnormal vaginal bleeding during pregnancy is the usual means of presentation and this may be associated with anaemia. The clinical presentation of CHM has changed considerably over the past few decades. Excessive uterine size, anaemia hyperemesis, pre-eclampsia, theca lutein cysts, hyperthyroidism and metastatic disease are seen far less often, except in countries with less well-developed healthcare systems.

Invasive mole can produce heavy bleeding, lower abdominal pain or intraperitoneal haemorrhage. Occasionally, the bladder or rectum is infiltrated, producing haematuria or rectal bleeding. Invasive moles may regress spontaneously or they may embolize, particularly to the lungs, but they do not usually exhibit the progression of true malignancy.

Table 71.3 Clinical features of hydatidiform mole: a comparison between complete and partial mole

	Complete	Partial
Features	May be severe and/or accompanied by paraneoplastic sequelae	Often mild, resembling spontaneous miscarriage
Diagnosis	Usually suspected on clinical or ultrasound scan findings	Often unsuspected and retrospectively diagnosed after uterine evacuation
Persistent trophoblastic disease	In up to 20% of cases	In <0.5% of cases

The clinical features of partial mole are less severe than those of complete mole (Table 71.3) and this condition is frequently diagnosed on histological review of curettings from what appeared clinically to be a miscarriage. Even in earlier studies, increased uterine size, theca lutein cysts and pre-eclampsia were seen in only a small percentage of cases.[4]

DIAGNOSTIC INVESTIGATIONS

The increasing use of ultrasound in early pregnancy has probably led to earlier diagnosis of moles. However, while the ultrasound diagnosis of complete mole is usually reliable, that of partial mole is more difficult. In complete mole, a 'classic' pattern is seen, consisting of multiple small sonolucencies representing the numerous hydropic villi. The finding of multiple cystic spaces in the placenta and a ratio of above 1.5 in the transverse to antero-posterior dimension are suggestive of partial mole.[5] Fetal parts may be seen, but this also occurs in mole with co-existent normal fetus. In over half of cases the diagnosis of partial mole is not made by ultrasound. In locally invasive moles, increased areas of echogenicity are seen within the myometrium. Transvaginal ultrasound has allowed very early diagnosis in some cases.

Trophoblastic disease is virtually unique in that it produces a specific marker – hCG – which can be measured in urine and/or blood and correlates precisely with the amount of disease present. Human chorionic gonadotrophin is a large placental glycoprotein composed of two peptide subunits and is produced naturally during pregnancy. The alpha subunit is similar to those of other pituitary glycoprotein hormones, but the beta subunit is specific to hCG alone. Higher than normal levels of hCG (particularly when >200 000 IU/L) are suggestive of molar pregnancy, although levels with partial mole are only infrequently above the range for normal pregnancy. As a diagnostic marker for molar pregnancy, hCG measurement is therefore of limited value. It exists in a number of forms (e.g. nicked hCG, hCG missing the beta subunit C-terminal segment, hyperglycosylated hCG and free beta subunit) and when it is measured in trophoblastic disease it is important that the assay being used detects all main forms of hCG and its beta subunit fragments.[6]

EVACUATION OF MOLAR PREGNANCY

Suction curettage is the method of choice for evacuation of complete molar pregnancies;[7] because of the lack of fetal parts, a suction catheter of up to 12 mm is usually sufficient. Sharp curettage is now not generally recommended because of the possibility of uterine perforation and of increasing the risk of Asherman's syndrome (uterine synechiae). Medical termination of complete mole should be avoided where possible. There is theoretical concern about the routine use of potent oxytocic agents because of the possibility of forcing trophoblastic tissue into the venous spaces of the placental bed and disseminating disease to the lungs. It is recommended that, where possible, oxytocic therapy is only commenced once evacuation is complete. However, if there is significant haemorrhage prior to or during evacuation and some degree of control is needed, such agents may be used according to clinical judgement. It is also suggested that prostaglandin analogues should be reserved for cases for which oxytocic therapy is ineffective. Since evacuation of a large mole is a rare event, advice and help from an experienced colleague should be sought where appropriate. In partial molar pregnancies where the size of fetal parts deters the use of suction curettage, medical termination can be used. Data from the management of molar pregnancies with mifepristone are incomplete; evacuation of complete mole with this agent may be best avoided, as it increases the sensitivity of the uterus to prostaglandins.

The difficulty in making the diagnosis of partial mole before evacuation mandates the histological assessment of material obtained from incomplete miscarriages. Also, since persistent trophoblastic disease may develop after any pregnancy, all products of conception, obtained after repeat evacuation performed for persisting symptoms, should be histologically examined.

> Though there is much published on evacuation of molar pregnancy, the above text reflects mainly UK expert opinion and practice [IV].

REGISTRATION

In the UK, a trophoblastic registration scheme has been in operation since it was initiated by the Royal College of Obstetricians and Gynaecologists in 1973. Three supra-regional centres in London (Charing Cross Hospital), Sheffield (Weston Park Hospital) and Dundee (Ninewells Hospital) co-ordinate the registration and monitoring of all patients. However, only Charing Cross and Weston Park have the specialist facilities to offer appropriate chemotherapy.

Patients with the following should be registered:

- complete hydatidiform mole,
- partial hydatidiform mole,
- twin pregnancy with complete or partial hydatidiform mole,
- limited macroscopic or microscopic molar change judged to require follow-up.

Twin molar pregnancy

The incidence of twin pregnancy with mole (usually complete) and viable fetus appears to be lower (<1 in 200 molar pregnancies) than twin pregnancy with viable fetuses (about 1 in 100 normal pregnancies). A successful pregnancy outcome occurs in about one-third of cases. Persistent trophoblastic disease requiring chemotherapy may be more frequent, but treatment is invariably successful (as for single molar pregnancies). UK guidance is that 'if the twin pregnancy is associated with a partial mole then it should be allowed to proceed; in the case of association with complete mole then the pregnancy may proceed after appropriate counselling' [III].[7]

Ectopic molar pregnancy

As with normal pregnancy, hydatidiform mole may occur in ectopic sites, most often in the fallopian tube.[8] Tubal ectopic moles are rare and over-diagnosed, but strict follow-up of confirmed cases is essential, as these are more likely to require chemotherapy for persistent disease [IV].

Persistent trophoblastic disease

In a proportion (up to 20 per cent) of patients, trophoblastic disease persists, as evidenced by continuing clinical symptoms (particularly vaginal bleeding) and/or elevation of hCG levels. Excessive uterine size, markedly elevated hCG levels and prominent theca lutein cysts are the main factors predicting persistent trophoblastic disease.

The UK surveillance scheme involves periodic assays of urine and/or serum hCG being performed for up to 2 years, depending on the original histological diagnosis and rate of fall of hCG. This has ensured that the great majority of patients requiring chemotherapy for persistent disease are recognized early. We have been able to adopt a conservative approach using stringent criteria for the initiation of chemotherapy (Table 71.4). For example, whilst it is stressed that 'there is no clinical indication for the routine use of second uterine evacuation in the management of molar pregnancies', this may be recommended in selected cases with

Table 71.4 Defining persistent trophoblastic disease and the need for chemotherapy

High static or rising hCG levels after one or two uterine evacuations
Persistent uterine haemorrhage with raised hCG levels
Pulmonary metastases with static or rising hCG levels
Metastases in liver, brain or gastrointestinal tract
Histological diagnosis of choriocarcinoma or placental site trophoblastic tumour

hCG, human chorionic gonadotrophin.

persisting mild symptoms and lower levels of hCG. This will reduce by half the number of patients requiring chemotherapy [III]. We are also prepared to wait for up to 6 months before initiating treatment for patients whose hCG level continues to fall.

The indications for when to use chemotherapy vary internationally. The above guidance relies on retrospective, uncontrolled but substantial data from UK studies [III].

CHOICE OF CHEMOTHERAPY

Once the decision has been made to initiate chemotherapy, the most appropriate regimen is chosen by assessing the patient's prognostic risk.[9] This involves using a number of factors from the history, examination and investigations to allow the patient to be assigned to a risk group, which in turn facilitates the selection of the least toxic, most effective treatment for that individual (Table 71.5).

Although it is universally recognized that a single accurate and precise staging and classification system is needed, to date there is still a variety of staging and classification systems used by centres treating GTD, and this makes meaningful comparisons of treatment results difficult. In the UK we have used a variation of the World Health Organization (WHO) scoring system: 'low-risk' and 'high-risk' groups have been defined and the chemotherapy regimen dictated by risk (Table 71.6). Less than 10 per cent of all registered patients

Table 71.5 Risk factors in patients requiring chemotherapy

≥40 years old
Increasing time since evacuation/diagnosis
Increasing level of serum beta-human chorionic gonadotrophin
Postpartum (or unknown origin)
Increasing number of metastases
Increasing size of metastases
Metastases other than in the lungs
Previous chemotherapy

Table 71.6 Treatment of persistent gestational trophoblastic disease

Low risk	Methotrexate i.m. (low dose)
	Dactinomycin i.v. (cyclical)
High risk	Etoposide/methotrexate/dactinomycin-cyclophosphamide/ vincristine (EMA-CO) (i.v. cyclical, alternating)
	Methotrexate-etoposide/dactinomycin (M-EA) (i.v. cyclical, alternating)

in the UK require chemotherapy. The cure rate is above 95 per cent.

> There is considerable published evidence on the role of chemotherapy in persistent GTD, based mostly on non-randomized, controlled or non-controlled trials [II].

POSTPARTUM CHORIOCARCINOMA

This is a very rare and serious complication with a reported UK incidence of 1 in 50 000 live births. Most cases present with abnormal vaginal bleeding following delivery, and diagnosis may be delayed, many patients presenting with metastatic disease. Nevertheless, such patients are potentially curable with intensive chemotherapy.[10]

THE ROLE OF SURGERY

> **Indications for hysterectomy in the management of gestational trophoblastic disease**
>
> - Choice (older patient, localized disease, family complete).
> - Excessive uterine bleeding (before or during treatment).
> - Chemoresistant (localized) uterine tumour.
> - Placental site trophoblastic tumour.

Older patients who are fit and have completed their family can be offered a hysterectomy, which reduces the risk of persistent disease from 20 per cent to less than 10 per cent. Although hysterectomy eliminates the complications of local invasion, it does not prevent metastatic disease and therefore gonadotrophin follow-up is still required.

As GTD is highly chemosensitive, the need for surgical intervention once the diagnosis has been established is small. At present, there are essentially two further indications for hysterectomy, namely to control severe uterine

haemorrhage and to eliminate disease that is confined to the uterus and resistant to chemotherapy. In order to minimize the risk of causing trophoblastic emboli, the vessels draining the uterus should be ligated at an early stage and the uterine tissues should be handled as gently as possible. Conservative uterine surgery, whereby local excision of a bleeding invasive trophoblastic tumour is performed, may be reasonable in young women, as their disease may then be cured medically, thus preserving their fertility.

A rare problem is that of vaginal bleeding after completion of successful chemotherapy due to a post-molar arteriovenous malformation. Selective embolization or ligation may preserve fertility, but sometimes hysterectomy is necessary.

Surgery provides the cornerstone of management for the rare placental site trophoblastic tumours. These tumours have a slow growth rate and can present many years after term delivery, non-molar miscarriage or complete mole. The usual presentation is with local disease leading to vaginal bleeding or amenorrhoea, but they may also metastasize, particularly to the lung. Surgery alone is the treatment of choice for localized disease; chemotherapy is needed for metastatic tumour.

> There is some supporting evidence for the role of hysterectomy in GTD, but the above text relies mainly on retrospective, uncontrolled studies and expert opinion [III].

Surgery also has an important role, in selected patients, for the removal of chemotherapy-resistant metastases. Thoracotomy – for which the indications are previous multi-agent chemotherapy, a solitary lung lesion confined to one lung and no other sites of active disease – may achieve remission in over two-thirds of patients. Craniotomy is now recommended in the UK for the resection of accessible deposits before starting chemotherapy because of the risk of precipitating haemorrhage.

ROUTINE FOLLOW-UP

Patterns of clinical and hCG surveillance for further molar problems vary across the world, determined by local factors and also by knowledge of the difference in risk of sequelae between complete and partial moles. The clinical course of partial mole is almost invariably 'benign'. Persistent trophoblastic disease after partial mole is much less common than after complete mole and almost all cases are low risk. However, it has recently been confirmed that partial mole can transform into choriocarcinoma.[11] Therefore all patients with confirmed partial mole should undergo hCG follow-up.

The risk of molar problems is greatest in the first 12 months following diagnosis, although it is sometimes difficult to decide whether an increase in hCG levels during monitoring is recurrence of the original or occurrence of a second mole; genetic evaluation of the trophoblastic tissue from both episodes may help. It is convention to ask patients to avoid further pregnancy for 6–12 months following the molar pregnancy to enable efficient hCG follow-up. However, some patients either ignore this advice or accidentally become pregnant during this time; fortunately, in the vast majority of cases, the outcome is good. Current advice is therefore to avoid pregnancy for 6 months but, when it does occur, to allow the pregnancy to continue with careful clinical, ultrasound and hCG monitoring.

CONTRACEPTION

Early studies from London[12] suggested that patients who used oral contraceptives after evacuation of a molar pregnancy had a slower rate of hCG decrease and increased risk of developing persistent trophoblastic disease. In the UK we therefore still recommend avoiding oral contraception until the hCG level has returned to normal [IV]. However, numerous studies have noted no increased risk with oral contraceptive use and, on balance, North American clinicians consider the risks of early further pregnancy greater than the risks of using the oral contraceptive pill. However, there is agreement that intrauterine contraceptive devices should be avoided until hCG levels are normal, because of the risk of uterine perforation and bleeding.

KEY POINTS

These **RCOG recommendations**[7] are based on limited but robust evidence that relies on expert opinion and has the endorsement of respected authorities.

- Registration of any molar pregnancy is essential.
- Ultrasound has limited value in detecting partial molar pregnancies.
- In twin pregnancies with a viable fetus and a molar pregnancy, the pregnancy can be allowed to proceed.
- Surgical evacuation of molar pregnancies is advisable.
- Routine repeat evacuation after the diagnosis of a molar pregnancy is not warranted.
- The combined oral contraceptive pill and hormone replacement therapy are safe to use after hCG levels have reverted to normal.
- Women should be advised not to conceive until the hCG level has been normal for 6 months or follow-up has been completed (whichever is sooner).

PUBLISHED GUIDELINES

Royal College of Obstetricians and Gynaecologists. *The Management of Gestational Trophoblastic Disease.* Guideline No. 20. London: RCOG, 1999.

KEY REFERENCES

1. WHO. *World Health Organization Scientific Group on Gestational Trophobalstic Disease.* Technical Report Series 692. Geneva: WHO, 1983.
2. Bagshawe KD, Dent J, Webb J. Hydatidiform mole in England and Wales 1973–83. *Lancet* 1986; ii:673–7.
3. Paradinas FJ, Browne P, Dent J et al. Problems in the histological diagnosis of hydatidiform mole: a survey from the UK. *J Pathol* 1991; **163**:168A.
4. Berkowitz RS, Goldstein MR, Bernstein MR et al. Natural history of partial molar pregnancy. *Obstet Gynecol* 1983; **66**:677–82.
5. Fine C, Bundy AL, Berkowitz RS et al. Sonographic diagnosis of partial hydatidiform mole. *Obstet Gynecol* 1989; **73**:414–18.
6. Cole LA, Shahabi S, Butler SA et al. Utility of commonly used commercial human chorionic gondotrophin immunoassays in the diagnosis and management of trophoblastic disease. *Clin Chem* 2001; **47**:302–15.
7. Royal College of Obstetricians and Gynaecologists. *The Management of Gestational Trophoblastic Disease.* Guideline No. 20. London: RCOG, January 1999.
8. Burton JL, Lidbury EA, Gillespie AM et al. Over-diagnosis of hydatidiform mole in early tubal ectopic pregnancy. *Histopathology* 2001; **38**:409–17.
9. Fisher PM, Hancock BW. Gestational trophoblastic diseases and their treatment. *Cancer Treat Rev* 1997; **23**:1–16.
10. Dobson LS, Gillespie AM, Coleman RE, Hancock BW. The presentation and management of post-partum choriocarcinoma. *Br J Cancer* 1999; **79**:1531–3.
11. Seckl MJ, Fisher RA, Salerno G et al. Choriocarcinoma and partial hydatidiform moles. *Lancet* 2000; **356**:36–9.
12. Stone M, Dent J, Kardana A et al. Relationship of oral contraception to the development of trophoblastic tumour after evacuation of a hydatidiform mole. *Br J Obstet Gynaecol* 1976; **83**:913–16.

Index